GENERAL PATHOLOGY

GENERAL PATHOLOGY

EDITED BY

LORD FLOREY

Provost of The Queen's College
University of Oxford

Fourth Edition

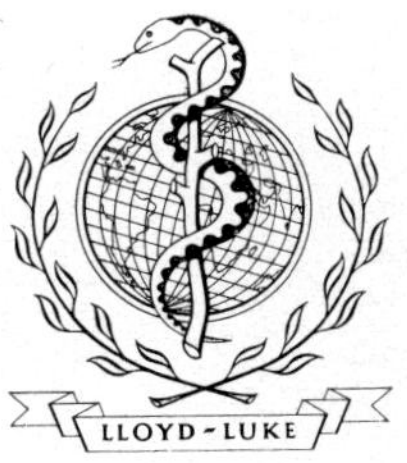

LLOYD-LUKE (MEDICAL BOOKS) LTD

49 NEWMAN STREET

LONDON

1970

FIRST EDITION 1954
SECOND EDITION . . . 1958
Reprinted 1959
THIRD EDITION 1962
Reprinted 1964
FOURTH EDITION . . . 1970

PRINTED AND BOUND IN ENGLAND BY
HAZELL WATSON AND VINEY LTD
AYLESBURY, BUCKS

SBN 85324 054 X

AUTHORS

E. P. ABRAHAM, M.A., D.Phil., F.R.S.
Fellow of Lincoln College, Oxford, and Professor of Chemical Pathology, Sir William Dunn School of Pathology, University of Oxford

I. BERENBLUM, M.D., M.Sc.
Head of the Department of Experimental Biology, The Weizmann Institute of Science, Rehovoth, Israel

R. J. BERRY, M.A., D.Phil., M.D.
Head of the Radiobiology Laboratory, Radiotherapy Department, Churchill Hospital, Oxford

G. V. R. BORN, M.A., D.Phil., M.B.
Vandervell Professor of Pharmacology, Royal College of Surgeons of England and University of London

M. L. FENWICK, M.A., Ph.D.
University Lecturer in Experimental Bacteriology, Sir William Dunn School of Pathology, University of Oxford

H. W. FLOREY, O.M., M.D., F.R.C.P., F.R.S.
Provost of The Queen's College, University of Oxford

C. E. FORD, D.Sc., F.R.S.
Head of Cytogenetics Section, Medical Research Council Radiobiological Research Unit, Harwell

J. E. FRENCH, D.M., D.Phil.
Fellow of St. Cross College, Oxford, and University Lecturer in Pathology, Sir William Dunn School of Pathology, University of Oxford

G. P. GLADSTONE, M.A., M.B., B.S.
Fellow of St. Cross College, Oxford, and Reader in Bacteriology, Sir William Dunn School of Pathology, University of Oxford

J. L. GOWANS, M.A., D.Phil., M.B., B.S., F.R.S.
Fellow of St. Catherine's College, Oxford, and Henry Dale Research Professor of the Royal Society, Sir William Dunn School of Pathology, University of Oxford

H. HARRIS, M.A., D. Phil., B.A., M.B., B.S., F.R.S.
Fellow of Lincoln College, Oxford, and Professor of Pathology, Sir William Dunn School of Pathology, University of Oxford

M. A. JENNINGS, D.M.
Fellow of Lady Margaret Hall, Oxford, and University Lecturer in Pathology, Sir William Dunn School of Pathology, University of Oxford

R. G. MACFARLANE, M.A., M.D., F.R.C.P., F.R.S.
Fellow of All Souls College, Oxford, and Professor of Clinical Pathology, Sir William Dunn School of Pathology, University of Oxford

G. W. PICKERING, M.D., F.R.C.P., F.R.S.
Master of Pembroke College, University of Oxford

J. C. F. POOLE, D.M.
Member of the Medical Research Council External Staff, Sir William Dunn School of Pathology, University of Oxford

A. C. RITCHIE, M.B., Ch.B., D.Phil.
Professor of Pathology, University of Toronto

A. H. T. ROBB-SMITH, M.A., M.D., F.R.C.P.
Director of Pathology, Radcliffe Infirmary, and Nuffield Reader in Pathology, University of Oxford

K. B. ROBERTS, M.A., D.Phil., M.B., B.S.
Professor of Physiology, Memorial University, Newfoundland

W. E. VAN HEYNINGEN, M.A., Sc.D.
Master of St. Cross College, Oxford, and Reader in Bacterial Chemistry, Sir William Dunn School of Pathology, University of Oxford

J. F. WATKINS, M.A., M.D.
Fellow of Wolfson College, Oxford, and University Lecturer in Bacteriology, Sir William Dunn School of Pathology, University of Oxford

PREFACE TO THE FOURTH EDITION

THIS edition of *General Pathology* was almost completed when Lord Florey died suddenly on 21st February, 1968. The chapters for which he was responsible are thus the last writings to issue from his pen. Some of his pupils had hoped to produce a Festschrift for his 70th birthday, but have been deprived of that pleasure. This book must serve instead. It remains a lasting memorial to Lord Florey's conception of the subject of Pathology, a conception which, by his instruction and by his example, he succeeded in diffusing throughout the world. The book has been extensively re-written, but its structure, style and scope remain the same. A new chapter on pathological consequences of chromosomal abnormality has been added.

June, 1969

PREFACE TO THE FIRST EDITION

PROGRESS in the medical sciences is now so rapid that even those who confine themselves to relatively narrow specialities find it increasingly difficult to master, or indeed to read, the great volume of literature that appears. Nevertheless, the student must try to grasp what is known of the general principles underlying the pathological changes that he will be called upon to diagnose and treat.

For many years it has been the custom at Oxford for every medical student to spend one year studying for an Honour School; in practice this is usually the Honour School of Physiology, which includes a good deal of biochemistry. The aim in the Honour School is not merely to teach facts, but to encourage students, both in the laboratory and by individual tuition, to think about the principles and problems of physiology and biochemistry, an appreciation of which is unquestionably required for the sound building of future clinical knowledge. Thus, it is hoped to give students early in their medical work some training in the deductive and inductive reasoning associated with experimental methods.

It is primarily for those who have read the Honour School of Physiology that a course in General Pathology and Bacteriology is given in Oxford. At present the course lasts for two terms of eight weeks each, and caters particularly for the better student. It is taken at the same time as the study of pharmacology, and immediately before clinical work begins. The lectures in this book are drawn from this course, but they may be of value to those more advanced in their medical work than the students for whom they were prepared; with increasing specialisation the more general aspects of pathology tend to become lost in the details of the subject.

It is to be emphasised that the lectures do not form a complete survey of General Pathology. For the most part they deal with subjects in which one or other of the authors has had a special interest. In particular they attempt to treat of some of the fundamental changes that take place in the body in response to injury, using this word in a broad sense, and to discuss some present-day views about the nature and causes of such changes.

It is hoped that some students will find sufficient stimulus from the lectures to carry an experimental outlook into clinical medicine and surgery, for these subjects have suffered, and continue to suffer in this country, from an approach that pays too little attention to experimental science. At the present day nearly all significant advances in the diagnosis, treatment and prevention of disease depend on the application of experimental methods.

H. W. FLOREY

December, 1953

ACKNOWLEDGEMENTS

IN the preparation of the previous editions of this book we received valuable assistance from a number of people: Dr. G. S. Dawes, Dr. A. Felix, Professor R. B. Fisher, Dr. Philip Geisler, Professor Peter Harris, Dr. J. Howard, Dr. Ruth Jordan (Mrs. Klemperer), Dr. C. I. Levene, Dr. G. B. Mackaness, Dr. V. T. Marchesi, Dr. R. H. Mole, Dr. William B. Ober, Dr. A. D. Osborne, Dr. M. Schachter, Dr. H. A. Sissons, Professor W. G. Spector, Dr. A. F. B. Standfast, Dr. G. M. Watson, Dr. D. W. Weiss, Professor R. E. O. Williams and Dr. J. A. H. Wylie. We were particularly indebted for photographs and other illustrative material to Lady Coghill, Dr. Don W. Fawcett, Dr. Hermes C. Grillo, Dr. R. W. Horne, Dr. Guido Majno, Professor A. A. Miles, Dr. William B. Ober, Dr. G. E. Palade, Professor A. Policard, Dr. Ashworth Underwood and Professor D. L. Wilhelm.

For the present edition we have also to thank Dr. E. P. Benditt, Dr. J. F. Burke, Professor E. S. Finckh, Dr. J. W. Grisham, Dr. M. J. Karnovsky, Dr. L. V. Leak, Dr. J. H. Luft, Professor G. V. J. Nossal, Dr. B. A. Warren and Dr. Dorothea Zucker-Franklin for providing illustrations.

We are indebted to Dr. P. W. Kent for advice on Chapter 6, Professor Peter Harris and Dr. Lawrence Youlten for advice on Chapter 12, and Dr. Nancy L. R. Bucher, Dr. J. J. Reynolds and Dr. T. P. S. Powell for advice on Chapter 17.

Chapter 10 is a revised version of the chapter originally written by Sir Roy Cameron (deceased). Chapter 31 originally written by Dr. F. Kingsley Sanders has now been rewritten by Dr. M. L. Fenwick.

We are again grateful to Miss Christine Court for half-tone and line drawings and copies of many graphs; and to Mrs. P. B. Loder for helpful criticism and proof reading of Chapters 14, 15, 25, 26, 32, 33, 27, 39 and 40.

The completion of this edition of the book, interrupted by Lord Florey's death, would not have been possible without the help rendered in many ways by Mrs. D. G. Finch-Mason and Miss D. Mackay.

The following acknowledgements are made in detail for each chapter:

Chapter 1.—FIGURES 1–4 by permission of the Bodleian Library; FIG. 5 from the original in the Hunterian Library in the University of Glasgow, with permission from the University Court; FIGS. 6, 7, 10–13, 15 by courtesy of the Wellcome Trustees; FIG. 8 from a print, supplied by the Ashmolean Museum, of an engraving in their possession; FIG. 9 from Holländer's *Die Medizin in der klassischen Malerei*, by courtesy of Ferdinand Enke.

We are indebted to Mr. McKenna, the University Librarian and Keeper of the Hunterian Books and MSS, and to Mr. Robert Cowper, one of the Glasgow University photographers, for their assistance in connection with FIG. 5.

Chapter 2.—FIGURES 1–3 from Lewis' *The Blood Vessels of the Human Skin*, by courtesy of Shaw & Sons, Ltd.; FIG. 8 by courtesy of the Editor *J. Physiol.* (*Lond.*); FIG. 9 by courtesy of the Editor *Brit. J. exp. Path.*

Chapter 3.—FIGURES 1, 44, 48, 49, 60, 69 by courtesy of the Editor *J. Path. Bact.*; FIGS. 3–7, 10, 20–23, 25, 26 by courtesy of the Editor *Brit. med. J.*; FIGS. 8, 11, 14, 45–47, 49–58, 61–68, 70, 76–79 by courtesy of the Editor *Quart. J. exp. Physiol.*; FIGS. 9, 15, 27–29, 31, 32 by courtesy of the Editor *Proc. roy. Soc. B.*; FIGS. 7, 16–18 by courtesy of the Editor *Fed. Proc.*;

FIGS. 13, 33, 84–87 by courtesy of the Editor *J. Cell. Biol.*; FIG. 19 by courtesy of the Editor *Amer. J. Anat.*; FIGS. 82, 83 and Table I by courtesy of the Editor *Brit. J. exp. Path.*

Chapter 4.—FIGURES 1, 2 from Adami's *Inflammation*, by courtesy of Macmillan & Co.; FIGS. 3–5 by courtesy of the Editor *J. Path. Bact.*; FIGS. 6, 7, 22 by courtesy of the Editor *Brit. J. exp. Path.*; FIG. 8 by courtesy of the Editor *C. R. Acad. Sci.* (*Paris*); FIGS. 11–14 by courtesy of the Editor *J. exp. Med.*; FIGS. 24, 25 by courtesy of the Editor *Quart. J. exp. Physiol.*; Plate A by courtesy of the Editor *J. Path. Bact.*; Table II from Topley and Wilson's *Principles of Bacteriology and Immunity*, by courtesy of Edward Arnold & Co.

Chapter 5.—FIGURE 2 by courtesy of the Editor *J. Physiol.* (*Lond.*); FIGS. 3–12 by courtesy of the Editor *Proc. roy. Soc. B.*

Chapter 6.—FIGURES 2–11 and Plates C and E by courtesy of the Editor *Quart. J. exp. Physiol.*; Plates B, D by courtesy of the Editor *Proc. roy. Soc. B.*; Plate F by courtesy of the Editor *J. Path. Bact.*

Chapter 7.—FIGURE 4 by courtesy of the Editor *Brit. med. Bull.*

Chapter 8.—FIGURE 5 by courtesy of the Editor *Nature* (*Lond.*); FIG. 8 by courtesy of the Editor *Brit. J. Haematol.*; FIG. 10 from a photograph by Dr. A. G. Sanders; Table I from Wintrobe's *Clinical Hematology*, by courtesy of Henry Kimpton.

Chapter 9.—FIGURES 4a, b, 14, 15a, 16, 17 by courtesy of the Editor *Brit. J. exp. Path.*; FIG. 5a by courtesy of the Royal College of Surgeons of England; FIG. 5b from *Modern Trends in Pathology 2*, ed. T. Crawford, by courtesy of Butterworth & Co.; FIG. 7 from *The Inflammatory Process*, eds. B. W. Zweifach, L. Grant and R. T. McClusky, by courtesy of Academic Press Inc.; FIG. 8 drawn by Miss Christine Court from a specimen in the museum of the Royal College of Surgeons of England by permission of the Curator; FIGS. 19, 20 by courtesy of Dr. J. C. F. Poole; FIG. 21 by courtesy of the Editor *J. Path. Bact.*

Chapter 10.—FIGURE 1 by courtesy of the Editor *The Lancet*; FIGS. 2, 3 by courtesy of the Editor *Ann. N.Y. Acad. Sci.*; Table II by courtesy of the Editor *Arch. Surg.*

Chapter 11.—FIGURE 1 by courtesy of the Editor *Fed. Proc.*; FIGS. 2, 3 by courtesy of the Editor *Amer. J. Physiol.*; FIG. 4 by courtesy of the Editor *Quart. J. Med.*; FIG. 5 by courtesy of the Editor *J. biol. Chem.*; FIG. 6 by courtesy of Academic Press Inc.; FIG. 7 by courtesy of the Editor *The Lancet*; Table I by courtesy of Dr. H. B. Stoner.

Chapter 12—FIGURES 1, 4, 5, 7 by courtesy of Dr. Samuel Oram; FIG. 2 from a photograph kindly lent by Sir Charles Lovatt Evans; FIG. 3 by courtesy of the Editor *Amer. J. Physiol.*; FIGS. 6, 9 by courtesy of Dr. Terence East; FIG. 8 by courtesy of Dr. H. M. Sinclair; Table I from Davson's *Textbook of General Physiology* (1951) by courtesy of J. and A. Churchill Ltd.

FIGURES 1, 4, 5–7, 9 are from the King's College Hospital Photographic Records.

Chapter 13.—FIGURES 1–3, 5 by courtesy of the Editor *Clin. Sci.*; FIG. 4 by courtesy of the Editor *Arch. intern. Med.;* FIG. 6 by courtesy of the Editor *Trans. Ass. Amer. Phycns.*

Chapter 14.—FIGURE 2, by courtesy of the Editor *J. exp. Med.*; FIG 3 by courtesy of the Editor *Fed. Proc.*; FIG. 8 by courtesy of the Editor *Proc. Nat. Acad. Sci.* (*Wash.*).

Chapter 15.—FIGURE 1 from Fulton's *Textbook of Physiology*, by courtesy of W. B. Saunders Co.; FIG. 2 by courtesy of Dr. A. D. Morgan and Professor N. F. Maclagan; FIG. 3 by courtesy of the Institute of Orthopaedics; the patient in FIG. 3 was under the care of the late Mr. V. H. Ellis at the Royal National Orthopaedic Hospital.

Chapter 16.—FIGURE 1 from Ham's *Histology*, by courtesy of J. B. Lippincott Co.; FIGS. 13, 14 by courtesy of the Editor *Anat. Rec.*; FIG. 15 by courtesy of the Josiah Macy, Jr. Foundation; FIG. 16 by courtesy of the Editor *Proc. Nat. Acad. Sci.*; FIG. 17 by courtesy of the Editor *Ann. N.Y. Acad. Sci.*; FIG. 19 from Eppinger's *Die Permeabilitätspathologie*, by courtesy of Springer-Verlag.

Chapter 17.—FIGURES 1, 2, 28–30 by courtesy of the Editor *Brit. J. exp. Path.*; FIGS. 5, 11, 13, 18 by courtesy of the Editor *Amer. J. Anat.*; FIG. 9 by courtesy of the Editor *Phil Trans. B.*; FIG. 12 by courtesy of the Editor *Anat. Rec.*; FIGS. 17, 24–27, 33, 34 by courtesy of the Editor *J. Path. Bact.*; FIGS. 21, 22 by courtesy of the Editor *Ann. Surg.*; FIG. 23 by courtesy of the Editor *J. Cell. Biol.*; FIGS. 35, 37 by courtesy of the Editor *Cancer Res.*; FIG. 32 by courtesy of the Editor *Arch. Path.*; FIGS. 40–46 by courtesy of Dr. A. H. T. Robb-Smith and Dr. William Holmes.

Prints for FIGS. 5, 11 were supplied by the Photographic Department of the Royal Society of Medicine.

Chapter 18.—FIGURES 4, 5 by courtesy of the Editor *J. Path. Bact.*; FIG. 6 by permission of the Bodleian Library; FIG. 7 by courtesy of the Editor *Proc. roy. Soc. B.*; FIG. 9 by courtesy of the Editor *Brit. med. J.*; FIG. 10 by courtesy of Academic Press Inc.; FIG. 11 by courtesy of

Mr. B. L. Shepperd; Fig. 12 by permission of the Editor, *Circulation*; Figs. 14, 15 by courtesy of Dr. J. C. F. Poole; Fig. 17 by courtesy of Mr. D. J. Tibbs; Fig. 18 by courtesy of Professor T. Crawford and Dr. N. Woolf; Tables I, II by courtesy of Professor J. N. Morris; Table III by courtesy of Professor J. C. F. Böttcher.

Chapter 19.—Figure 3 by courtesy of Dr. E. P. Evans; Figs. 4–6 by courtesy of Dr. Werner Schmid; Fig. 8 from Gaisford and Lightfoot's *Paediatrics for the Practitioner*, by courtesy of Butterworth & Co.; Figs. 9–12 by courtesy of Professor P. E. Polani.

Chapter 20.—Figures 1–5 by courtesy of the Editor *Biochem. J.*; Fig. 7 by courtesy of the Editor *Exp. Cell Res.*; Figs. 8, 9 by courtesy of the Editor *Brit. J. exp. Path.*;

Chapter 21.—The photomicrographs for Figs. 2–6 were supplied by Dr. William B. Ober.

Chapter 22.—The photomicrographs for Figs. 2, 3 were supplied by Dr. William B. Ober.

Chapter 25.—Figure 1 by courtesy of the Editor *Brit. med. Bull.*; Figs. 2, 3 by courtesy of the Editor *Parasitology*; Figs. 4, 9 and Table I from Lea's *Actions of Radiation on Living Cells*, by courtesy of the International Atomic Energy Agency; Fig. 6 by courtesy of the Editor *Brit. J. Radiol.*; Fig. 7 by courtesy of the *Radiologic Clinics of North America* and the W. B. Saunders Co.; Fig. 8 by courtesy of Dr. P. C. Koller; Fig. 10 by courtesy of the Editor *J. Genetics.*

Chapter 26.—Figure 1 by courtesy of the U.S. Armed Forces Institute of Pathology, Washington, D.C. from negative No. HP 144; Figs. 2, 3, 9 by courtesy of the Editor *J. Chimie Physique*; Fig. 4 reproduced from the Report of the Medical Research Council for 1962–63 with the permission of The Controller of H.M. Stationery Office; Fig. 5 reproduced with modification by courtesy of the late Dr. W. M. Court-Brown; Fig. 6 by courtesy of the Editor *Medicine* (*Baltimore*); Fig. 8 from *Symposium on Radiobiology*, ed. J. J. Nickson, reprinted with permission from John Wiley & Sons. Inc., and by courtesy of Drs. A. Lacassagne and R. Latarjet.

Chapter 27.—Figure 1 by permission of the Bodleian Library; Fig. 2 by courtesy of the Editor *Bull. Hist. Med.*

Chapter 28.—Figures 1, 2 from Jennison's "Atomizing of Mouth and Nose Secretions into the Air as revealed by Highspeed Photography", by courtesy of the Editor *Aerobiology*, A.A.A.S. Publn. No. 17; Table I by courtesy of the late Dr. D. W. Henderson.

Chapter 31.—Figures 1A–E, 2A–F by courtesy of Academic Press Inc.; Fig. 1F by courtesy of Dr. R. C. Valentine; Fig. 7 by courtesy of Mr. R. Burrows; Fig. 11 by courtesy of the Editor *The Lancet*; Fig. 12 by courtesy of the Rockefeller University Press.

Chapter 32.—Figure 1 from *The Nobel Prize Winners* by courtesy of the Central European Times Publishing Co. and the Wellcome Trustees; Fig. 3 from Boyd's *Fundamentals of Immunology*, 2nd edit. by courtesy of Interscience Publishers; Fig. 4 by courtesy of the Editor *J. Immunol.*; Fig. 5 from Schultze and Heremans' *Molecular Biology of Human Proteins*, by courtesy of Elsevier Publishing Co.; Fig. 6 by courtesy of the Editor *Proc. nat. Acad. Sci.* (*Wash.*).

Chapter 33.—Figure 1 from *The Enzymes*, by courtesy of the Editor, Dr. James B. Sumner, and the Academic Press Inc.; Figs. 3–6 by courtesy of the Editor *Endeavour*; Figs. 7–12 and Table I by courtesy of the Editor *J. Amer. chem. Soc.*
Prints for Figs. 7–12 were supplied by the Photographic Department of the Royal Society of Medicine.

Chapter 34.—Figures 1, 3 by courtesy of the American Association for the Advancement of Science (Copyright 1964); Fig. 2 by courtesy of the Editor *J. Immunol.*;

Chapter 35.—Figure 3 by courtesy of Blackwell Scientific Publications Ltd.; Fig. 7 by courtesy of the Editor *Antibiot. et Chemother.*

Chapter 36.—Figures 1, 3 by courtesy of the Wellcome Trustees; Fig. 2 by kind permission of Sir Patrick Coghill; Fig. 7 by courtesy of the Editor *Nature* (*Lond.*)

Chapter 37.—Figure 1 by courtesy of the British Postgraduate Medical Federation, University of London, and the Athlone Press; Fig. 2 by courtesy of the Editor *Austr. J. med. Sci.*; Fig. 3 by courtesy of the Editor *Virology*; Fig. 4 by courtesy of the Editor *The Lancet*.

Chapter 38.—Figure 1 by courtesy of the Wellcome Trustees; Fig. 3 by courtesy of the Editor *Amer. J. med. Sci.*; Fig. 5 by courtesy of the Editor *J. Pharmacol.*; Fig. 6 by courtesy of the Editor *Nature* (*Lond.*).

Chapter 39.—FIGURE 2 by courtesy of the Editor *J. Immunol.*; FIG. 3 from *Cellular and Humoral Aspects of the Hypersensitive State*, ed. H. S. Lawrence, by courtesy of Hoeber-Harper and Dr. Frank J. Dixon.

Chapter 41.—Plate G by courtesy of the Editor *Phil. Trans. B.*

Chapter 42.—FIGURES 1–3 by courtesy of the Wellcome Trustees; FIGS. 8, 13–16 by courtesy of the Editor *Brit. J. exp. Path.*; FIGS. 26, 27 by courtesy of the Editor *Amer. Rev. Tuberc.* Original prints were kindly supplied by Dr. Max B. Lurie (FIGS. 26 and 27.).

CONTENTS

Chapter 1

THE HISTORY AND SCOPE OF PATHOLOGY

By H. W. Florey

To-day we are perhaps more conscious than ever before of our debt to our predecessors, and not only to those of the immediate past but to those also of relatively remote times. The study of medical history is both interesting in itself, and may help to modify the view sometimes expressed that medical students and doctors are lacking in culture of any sort. Moreover some historical perspective is often advantageous when one is considering the multitude of advances that are now taking place in the theory and practice of medicine. I do not therefore consider it a waste of time to bring before you what seem to me to be some of the more important events in the development of pathology. Krumbhaar[1] when writing on the history of pathology remarked that "when we consider one of the broader definitions of Pathology—such as 'The study of the causes of and the effects (both structural and functional) produced by disease', we at once realise that a consideration of its history might properly be almost co-terminous with that of medicine."

Early Studies

The study of disease has no doubt been going on since the time that mankind emerged as a thinking animal, for many of its manifestations are easily seen and felt. There is evidence from mummies, bones, carvings and paintings of antiquity that pathological lesions similar to those of to-day existed, and certain ancient literary fragments contain recognisable descriptions of disease.[2] An Egyptian papyrus of about 2160 to 1788 B.C. notes diseases of women and cattle, and the Edwin Smith papyrus of 1600 B.C. describes fractures, dislocations, infections of wounds, tumours and a number of other conditions. The Ebers papyrus of about 1550 B.C. mentions "coryza, dysentery, mastoiditis, diseases of bones and joints, tumours, cysts, parasitic diseases, abscess, many diseases of the eye, gastro-intestinal tract and female genitalia". It is perhaps surprising that the Egyptians did not construct a firm foundation of anatomical knowledge, for their practice of embalming might be thought to have given them great opportunities for observation of the viscera. The internal organs were, however, apparently removed through small incisions and the Egyptians did not, in fact, contribute anything substantial to the knowledge of human anatomy. There are many references to disease in other ancient writings, for instance those of the Jews, the Assyrians, the Indians and the Chinese.

Though some cultures had well-developed pathological theories which to a certain extent controlled ancient medical practice, it was the Greeks who most profoundly influenced Western medicine. They invaded Greece and Asia Minor from the north, conquering the preceding Minoan civilisation, and not only came into contact with the medicine of their conquered subjects, but in

Asia Minor were influenced by doctrines coming from Mesopotamia and from Egypt. The nimble-witted Greeks absorbed other people's ideas and, as in all they did, added greatly to them by accurate observation and by a new philosophical outlook. They recorded the appearances of many disease conditions that can be recognised by careful clinical examination and such descriptions are still valid, but their studies of pathology were severely handicapped since, except for a short period in Alexandria, they made no systematic examinations of the body after death. The Alexandrian writings have apparently all been lost. With the lack of background founded on post-mortem observation there flourished physiological and pathological theories that had little foundation in ascertained fact. These theories, which may have originated with the Hindus before 2000 B.C., dominated physiological and pathological thought in Europe until the re-awakening of inquiry during the Renaissance began to make its effects felt in the fifteenth and sixteenth centuries.

The Greek views on pathology, based on "humours", to which "spirits" and other elaborations were later added, cannot detain us now, but as they dominated medical thought and paralysed rational progress in western medicine for at least 1500 years, they can rightly be deemed of great importance, perhaps historically the most important pathological theories yet propounded. Greek medicine came down to mediæval times partly through the works of the non-medical patrician Roman, Cornelius Celsus (about 30 B.C. to A.D. 38), who collated much of the knowledge of the time. But it was a Greek, Galen (A.D. 130–200) from Pergamum in Asia Minor, who, besides making many original observations, some of an experimental nature, put the pathological doctrines of the time into a form that was treated as authoritative until well after the Renaissance. It was not until the sixteenth century that a serious breach was made in the teachings of Galen, which had been erected into a dogma which no one challenged by further observation.

The ancient humoral theories still persist in some of the words that we commonly use, indeed much of medical terminology is of Greek origin. The humour, or fluid, that predominated was thought to govern, amongst other things, a man's temperament. Thus one was *sanguine* (from predominance of blood which was hot), another *phlegmatic* (phlegm was thought to be a product of the brain), another *jaundiced* (yellow bile from the liver) and a fourth *melancholic* (black bile from the spleen). Certain expressions such as "to vent one's spleen" come from the same era.

Though the theories that underlay the use of these words have gone, certain aspects of Greek medical thought survive to this day. In particular the oath of dedication that was taken by the followers of Hippocrates set a high standard of moral behaviour for the medical man towards his patients and their relatives. The fact that all medical practitioners to-day are expected, in addition to having professional skill, to adhere to a code of ethics in their practice is a continuance of the ideal that was first clearly formulated by Hippocrates. Though some of the original Hippocratic oath to which Greek medical men subscribed seems outmoded to-day, medical schools given to symbolistic rites still use it, and from time to time an attempt is made to formulate an "international oath" for medical practitioners that would bear a close resemblance to the oath of the Greeks.

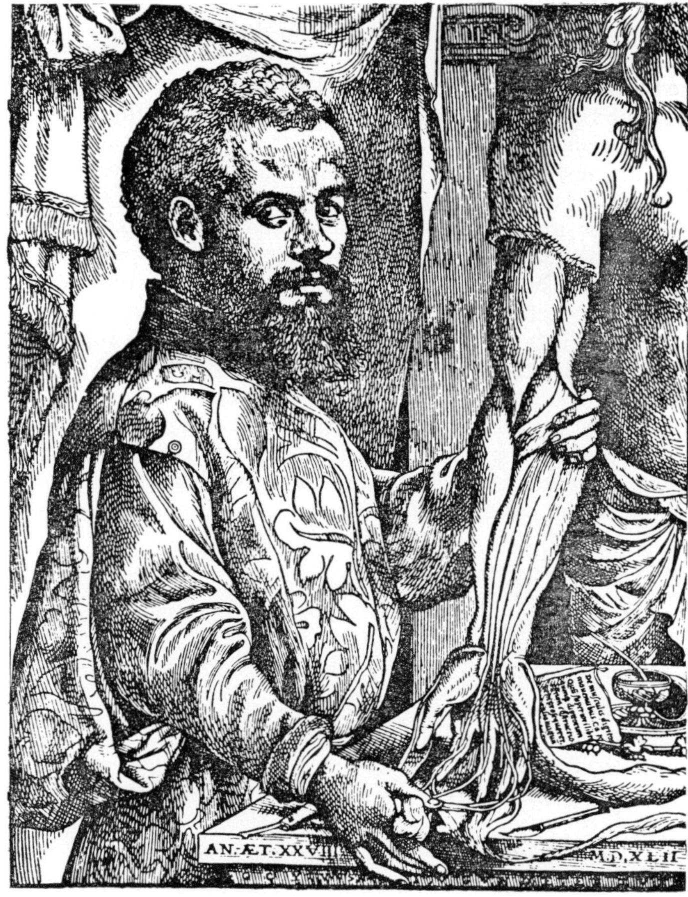

1/FIG. 1.—Vesalius (1514–64), from *De humani corporis fabrica*, 1543.

The Rise of Morbid Anatomy

With the Renaissance the scientific and medical atmosphere altered completely. The great sixteenth-century anatomists who worked for the most part in Italy, among whom the Belgian Vesalius stands supreme, founded the modern study of anatomy by their careful dissections and observations, their work often being illustrated by engravings of the greatest beauty (FIGS. 1–3). It was largely through their work that a beginning was made in challenging Galenic dogmatism.

It is worth recalling that Leonardo da Vinci (1452–1519) dissected some thirty corpses and made remarkable drawings of his observations. Unfortunately his great collection of drawings and notes, which he never published, passed into private hands at his death and was not seen for the next fifty years,

If his work had been known, there is little doubt that Leonardo would have been hailed as the originator of modern anatomical studies.

The word "anatomy"—literally a "cutting up"—first denoted the function at which the corpse was dissected. FIGURE 4 shows the somewhat feverish atmosphere to be found when Vesalius and others were examining a body, and one can perhaps glimpse the eagerness of the gathering of students before the revelations of the new method of exact dissection and the disregard of what the ancients had said. Just as hangings were public functions, so during the rise of interest in scientific matters anatomies attracted gatherings of laymen, often people of rank and education, for whom science in all its aspects was a fashionable hobby. The study of anatomy by dissection was fairly widespread in Europe by the end of the sixteenth century. FIGURE 5 shows an anatomy of the period in this country, and FIG. 6 one in Holland, a country which was to assume the lead in medicine during the seventeenth century. FIGURE 7 shows a dissection in eighteenth-century Holland, marked by the elegance of the participators—an elegance which might perhaps be copied by present-day anatomists and pathologists without harm. The illustration of an anatomy by Hogarth shows how by the eighteenth century the professor sat with a wand and somewhat disdainfully pointed out parts of the body laid bare by a bewigged attendant (FIG. 8).

As the dissection of bodies became more frequent, deviations from the usual were often noted, and in time substantial additions were made to pathological anatomy. Some information about disease conditions had been obtained by sporadic post-mortem examinations before the fifteenth century (FIG. 9), but it is in the writings of Antonio Benivieni (*ca.* 1440–1502), a Florentine surgeon, that we first encounter a description of some twenty post-mortem examinations "made specifically to determine the cause of death and explain symptoms".[1] Benivieni has been called the father of pathological anatomy and his book has been described as "the only book on pathology that owes nothing to anyone".

It was, however, Giovanni

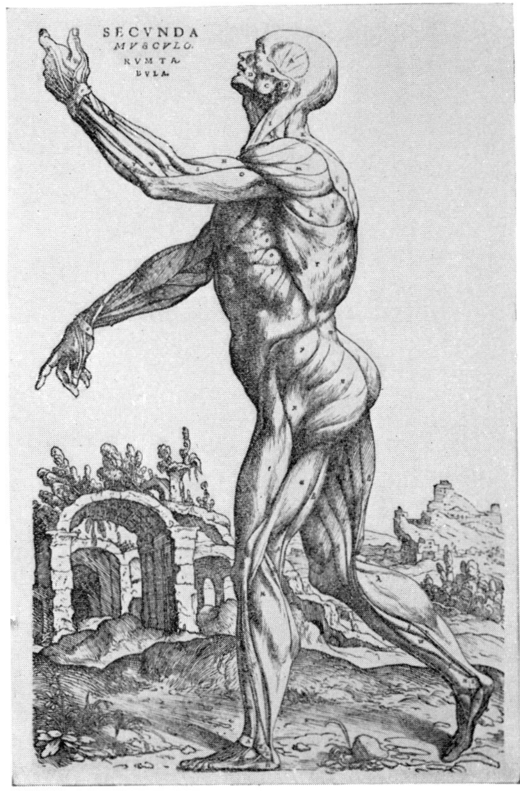

1/FIG. 2.—Second muscle tabula from the *Fabrica*.

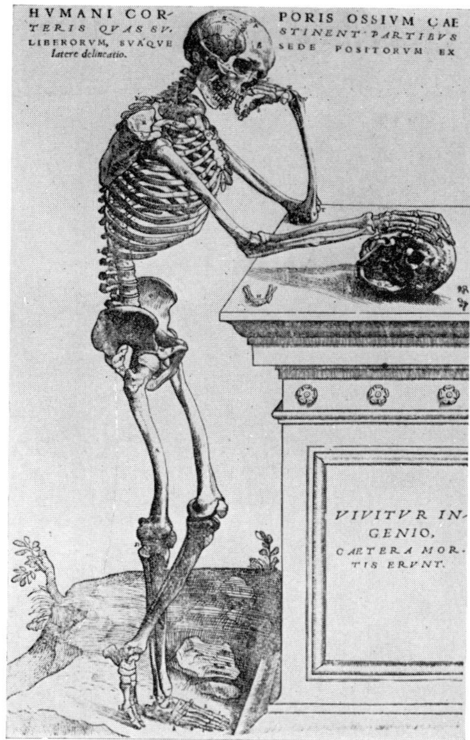

1/Fig. 3.—From the *Fabrica*. Note that the skeleton is depicted in a living position.

Battista Morgagni (1682–1771) (Fig. 10) who really put the scientific study of gross morbid anatomy on a firm foundation. He was a professor at Padua for no less than fifty-six years, during which time he made a vast number of morbid anatomical observations and added important facts to descriptive anatomy. His principal contribution was to correlate his post-mortem findings with the symptoms exhibited by the patient before death. His great book *De sedibus, et causis morborum per anatomem indagatis* was published in 1761. It takes the form of a series of letters to a friend, whose name is now unknown, and describes some 700 reports of patients and post-mortem examinations. "The life-history of the patient, the history of his disease, the events in connexion with his final illness and death, are all recounted with detail and care. The condition of the organs at the post-mortem examination is minutely described and an attempt is made to explain how the symptoms were the result of the lesions. Morgagni is justly said to have introduced the 'anatomical concept' into the practice of medicine. This concept is one of the main elements in modern diagnosis, and a modern physician, in reflecting on a case, considers first whether he is able to express the symptoms in terms of the lesion."[3]

In England John Hunter (1728–1793) (Fig. 11) and to a lesser extent his brother William (1718–1783) contributed greatly to pathology, as well as to normal and comparative anatomy. The great Hunterian Museum, with John Hunter's specimens, was almost completely destroyed in the second world war, but he made a lasting contribution to museum technique which still endures. A nephew and pupil of John Hunter—Matthew Baillie (1761–1823) (Fig. 12), a Balliol man—wrote the first systematic text on pathological anatomy in which the matter was arranged according to organs rather than by symptoms, which had been Morgagni's method.

Krumbhaar[1] has summed up the position as follows: ". . . By the end of the eighteenth century we find gross pathologic anatomy established as a firm basis for medical science; chiefly by the vast number of Morgagni's observations, on the whole well correlated with clinical records, and a beginning made with Baillie's text of systematic treatment of the subject as an independent discipline.

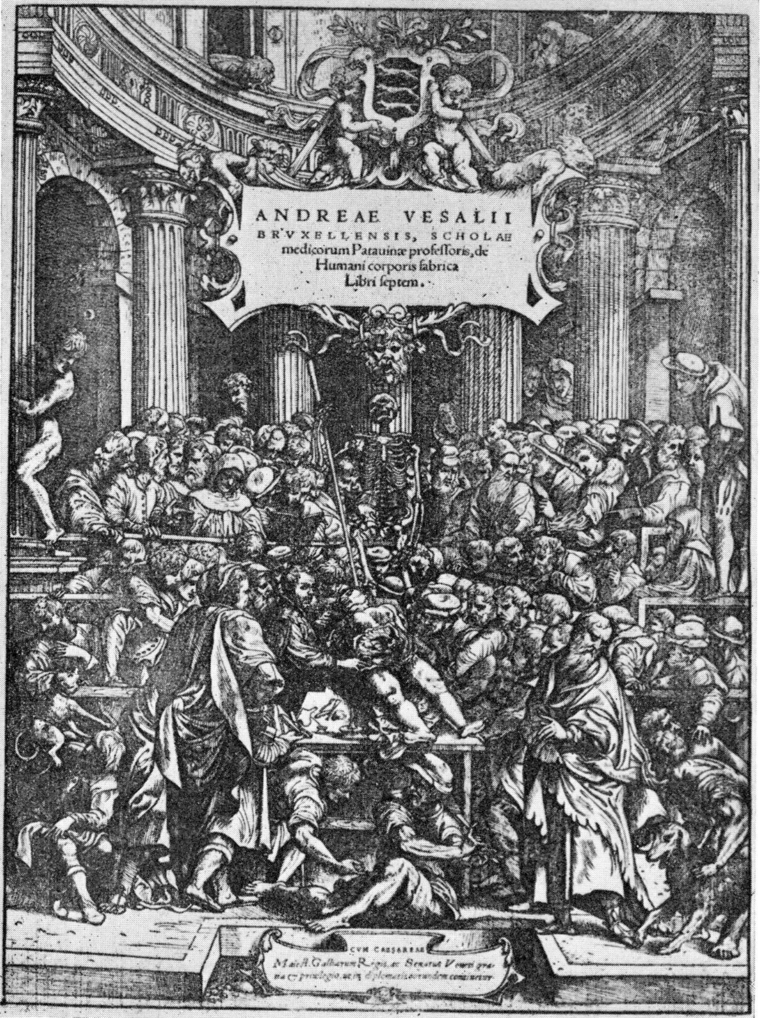

1/FIG. 4.—AN ANATOMY

The figure shows "a dissection scene at Padua. In the centre stands Vesalius dissecting a female body. At the head of the table stands an articulated skeleton. At its foot are dissecting instruments. Eager students throng around. In the foreground attendants are squabbling. On one side an attendant holds a monkey, one on the other a dog, for Vesalius had often to resort to animal in lieu of human anatomy. Shut off by a bar are members of the lay public. Gallants, grey-bearded scholars, monks and an enthusiastic bookworm may be discerned among them.

Other observers crowd in from every vantage point, even from the windows in the roof. The naked man to the left has been used by Vesalius to demonstrate the surface markings of the underlying organs. The whole scene is busy and vigorous in the extreme."[3]

Though, as we have seen, theoretic systems still held sway in academic pedagogy, the way for Bichat's study of the tissues, Rokitansky's gross descriptions, and Virchow's cellular pathology had been definitely opened."

The Pathology of Tissues and Cells

Bichat (1771–1802) died young of tuberculosis, but even in his short life he was able to become one of the founders of modern pathology. By dissection and by treating his material with "various chemical reagents as heat, air, water,

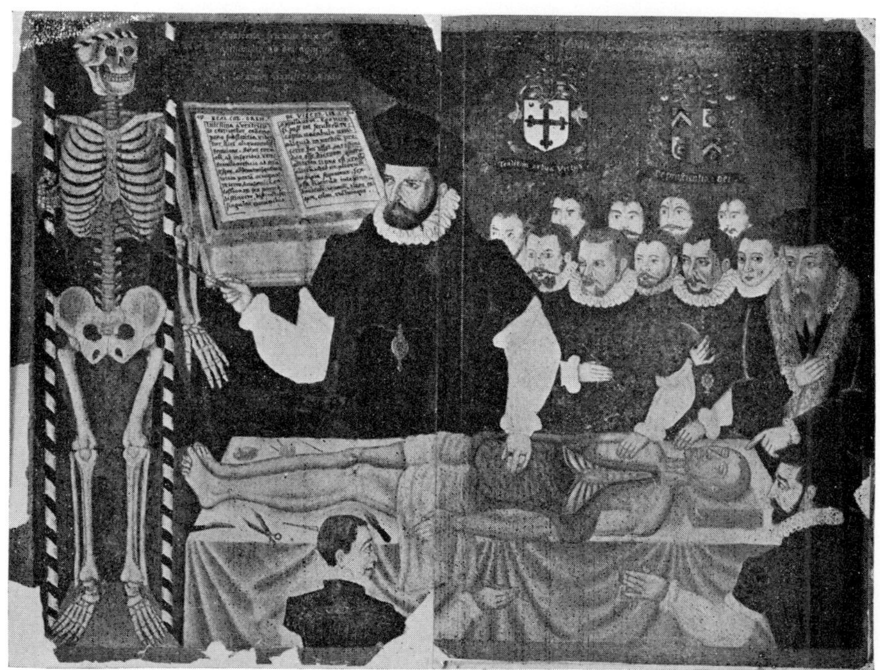

1/Fig. 5.—The London Guild of Barber-Surgeons began to pursue anatomical studies as early as 1462. This miniature-like oil painting was preserved because it was bound into a volume of Anatomical Tables of the Master of the Guild, John Banister. The scene shows John Banister (1533–1610) delivering the Visceral Lecture at the Barber-Surgeons' Hall, London, in 1581. A description of the picture was given by D'Arcy Power.[4]

acids, alkalies, salts, desiccation, maceration, putrefaction, boiling, etc." he arrived at the conception that organs were composed of tissues (from the French "tissu", a cloth) and that these were important units of the body. He distinguished twenty-one kinds of tissue which were combined to make up the organs. "He divided morbid anatomy into two parts: (1) the alterations common to each system wherever located (i.e. our general pathology) and (2) diseases peculiar to each region (i.e. our special pathology). Disease of a tissue is essentially the same, no matter in what organ the involved tissue may be".[1] The apogee of gross descriptive morbid anatomy was probably reached by the work of Carl Rokitansky (1804–1878) (Fig. 13) of Vienna, who is reported to have

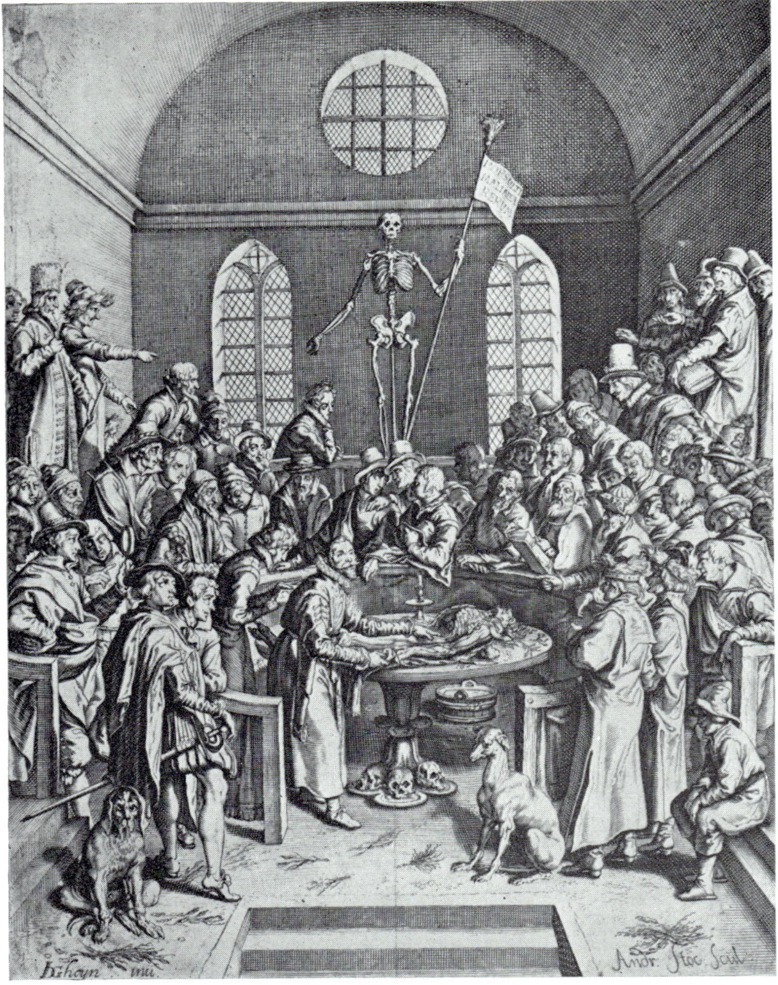

1/FIG. 6.—The scene in an anatomical theatre built in Holland in 1597 by Pieter Pavius. The grouping is similar to that in Vesalius' theatre (FIG. 4). The company consists of men of various ranks and ages; knights, learned men, country men and burghers, dressed in the appropriate clothes of the time. The skeleton that dominates the picture carries a flag bearing the inscription "*Mors ultima linea rerum*".

performed 30,000 autopsies himself and to have had access to material from 60,000.

Though additions to knowledge of gross morbid anatomy still continue to be made, it was the use of the microscope which paved the way for the revolution in thought on pathology with the introduction of the cell theory of the structure of the animal body. The origin of this theory was exhaustively considered by Cameron,[6] who pointed out that there were many predecessors who made contributions to the cell theory by way both of observation and deduction before those to whom the origination of the theory is usually attributed. The two scientists generally credited with establishing the cell theory are Schleiden (1804–1881), a botanist, and Schwann (1810–1882), a zoologist. Cameron considered that Schleiden's contributions had been over-emphasised and underlined the part played by Schwann, who recognised nucleated cells in animal tissues and promulgated the doctrine that animal and plant tissues were essentially similar in that they were made up of collections of cells.

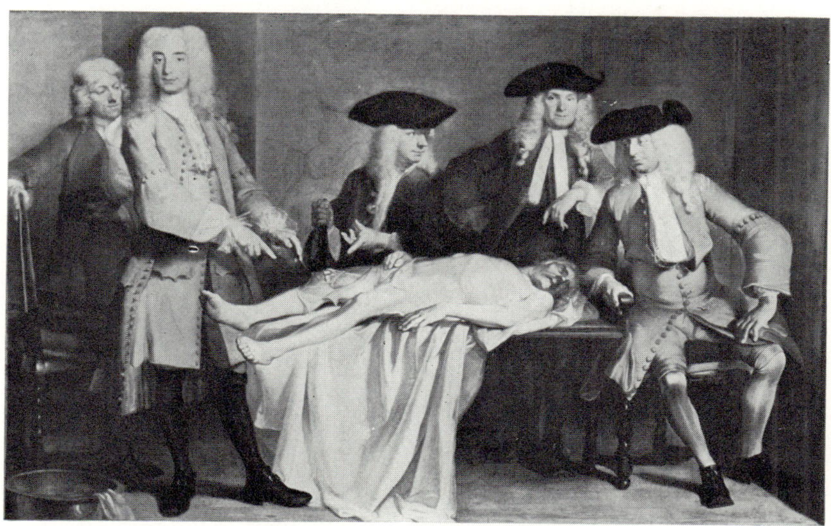

1/FIG. 7.—This picture of an anatomy painted by Cornelius Troost in 1728 has an artificial air of elegance perhaps associated with the fact that Professor Roëll, seen on the left conducting the anatomy, and his companions are described as surgeons and not primarily anatomists.

Though microscopical observations had been made on tissues by Malpighi (1628–1694) and by van Leeuwenhoek (1632–1723) with simple though powerful magnifying-glasses, and a number of subsequent biologists had made significant observations by the use of the microscope, it was not until the nineteenth century that improvements in the microscope—especially the development of achromatic lenses—enabled this instrument to be used to great advantage. Even so, Rokitansky, who worked in the nineteenth century, rarely used a microscope, and Bichat initiated the idea of tissues completely as a result of naked-eye observation. The studies by Virchow (1821–1905) (FIG. 14), a pupil of Johannes Müller, led through the use of the microscope to the initiation of the idea that the fundamental changes in disease can be traced to alterations in the cells of the body. His great book *Die Cellularpathologie in ihrer Begründung auf physiologische und pathologische Gewebelehre* appeared in 1858.[7] It was in substance a shorthand report of twenty lectures given to medical men, since Virchow was too busy to write out his lectures himself.

The nineteenth century saw the full efflorescence of morbid anatomy, both gross and microscopic. Great improvements were made in the compound micro-

THE REWARD OF CRUELTY.
Behold the Villain's dire disgrace!
Not Death itself can end.
He finds no peaceful Burial Place,
His breathless Corse, no friend.
Torn from the Root, that wicked Tongue,
Which daily swore and curst!
Those Eyeballs from their Sockets wrung,
That glow'd with lawless Lust!
His Heart expos'd to prying Eyes,
To Pity has no Claim;
But, dreadful! from his Bones shall rise,
His Monument of Shame.

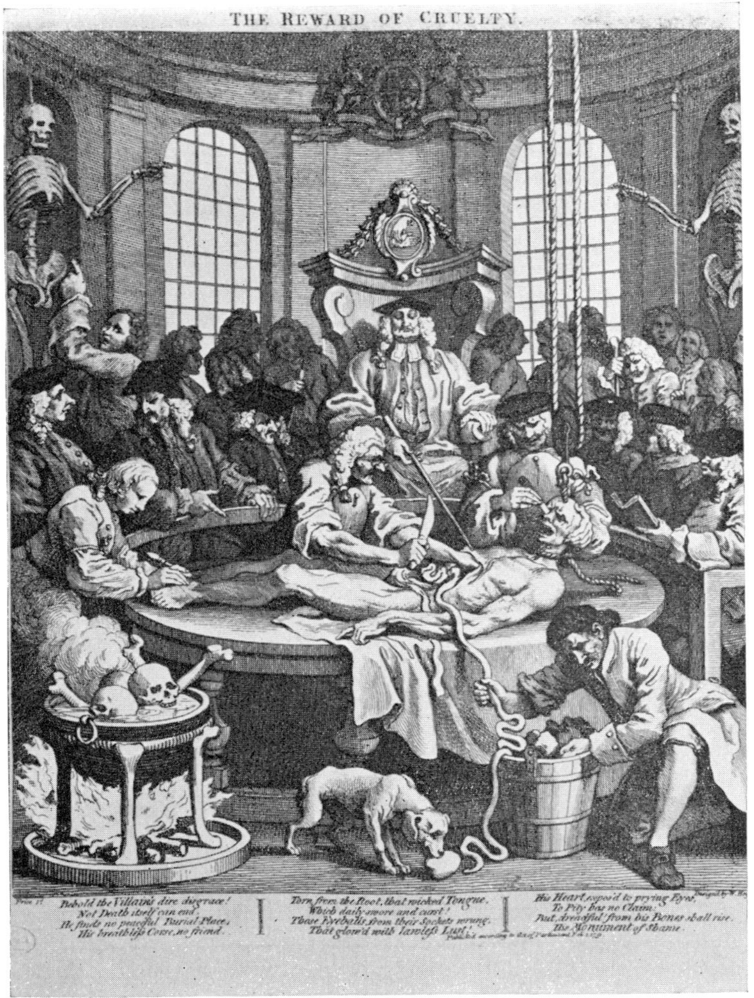

1/FIG. 8.—THE REWARD OF CRUELTY, the fourth of a series of four engravings entitled THE FOUR STAGES OF CRUELTY, by Hogarth.

The scene is the interior of a lecture-room in Surgeons' Hall. The corpse is that of Tom Nero, a former coachman, and the demonstrator is supposed to be John Freake (1688–1755), a famous surgeon and benefactor of St. Bartholomew's Hospital. The skeletons are those of James Field, an eminent pugilist, and Maclean, a romantic highwayman who had been hanged in the previous year.

An Act of 1752 provided that part of the death sentence should include a direction that the body after hanging should be delivered to Surgeons' Hall for dissection.

Though no doubt some of the features of the scene are exaggerated, it probably gives an insight into the conditions of an anatomy in the middle of the eighteenth century.

scope, and the embedding of tissues in such materials as soap, beeswax and paraffin wax was perfected so that thin sections could be cut, at first freehand and later by a microtome. The introduction of methods of staining the sections greatly extended the possibilities of microscopic study.

Thus much of the addition to knowledge of pathology since Virchow's day has consisted in exploring with ever-increasing refinements of microscopical and staining technique the intimate cellular changes associated with disease.

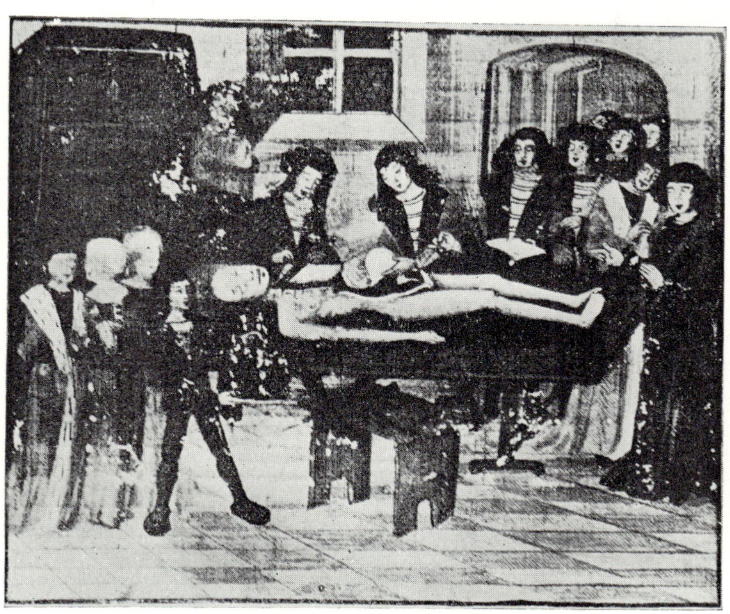

1/FIG. 9.—This figure is taken from Holländer's book[5] and reproduces a miniature, the earliest illustration of an autopsy that he was able to find. It appeared in a French translation published in 1363 of the Chirurgia Magna of Guy de Chauliac of Montpellier.

The miniature, now somewhat damaged, shows a female corpse in a hospital room. In the background is the bed of the dead woman, near which a nun prays for the departed soul. Two attendants are opening the corpse while the professor reads from a book. Students are entering through the door. In the foreground a nurse and some women are visible. From their clothing it is possible that these are women doctors.

As a result of this historicai process of growth, the morbid anatomical viewpoint has tended to dominate pathology and in many medical schools the teaching of pathology is still centred on the post-mortem room and the museum. No one should under-estimate the importance of the study of morbid anatomy both macroscopic and microscopic, any more than one should belittle the study of normal anatomy, but I have no hesitation in saying that it will be of only restricted value to the medical student and medical practitioner unless it is made the basis of an understanding of disordered function. From the point of view of the medical man his patients provide examples of disordered physiology or perhaps more often of disordered psychology, so that "pathology" must be conceived of in wide terms.

HIC EST VT PERHIBENT DOCTORVM CORDA VIRORVM PRIMVS IN HVMANI CORPORIS HISTORIA
JOANNES BAPTISTA MORGAGNVS
in Patavino Gymnasio e Primaria Sede
Anatomen adhuc docebat anno 1762.

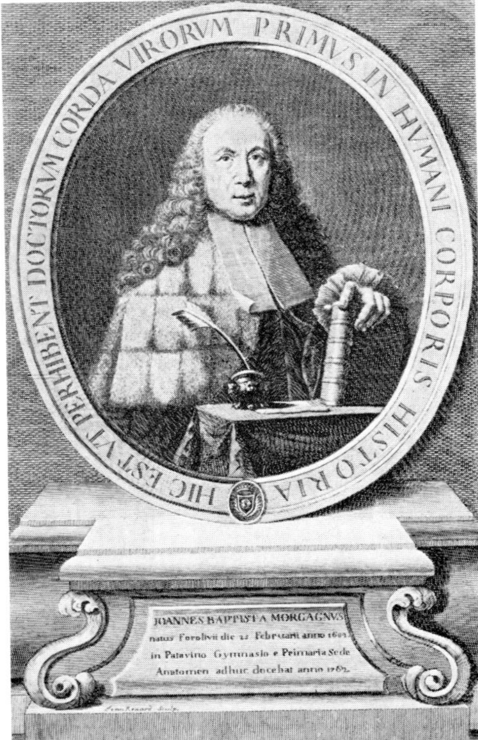

1/Fig. 10.—Giovanni Battista Morgagni.

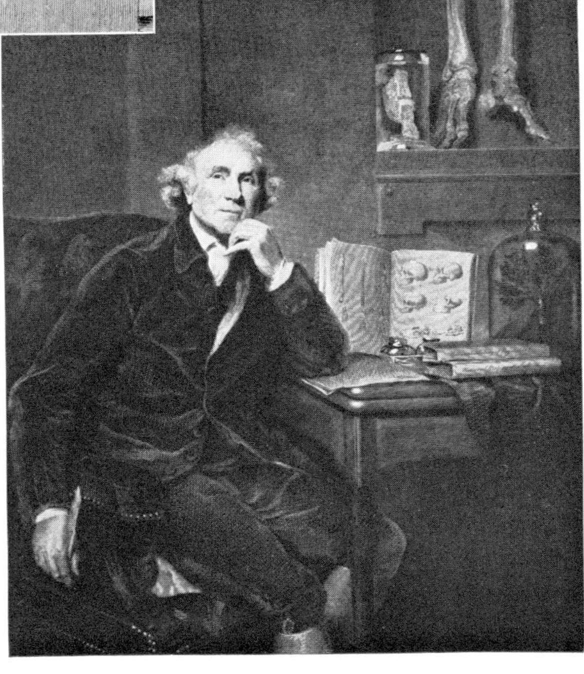

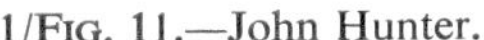

1/Fig. 11.—John Hunter.

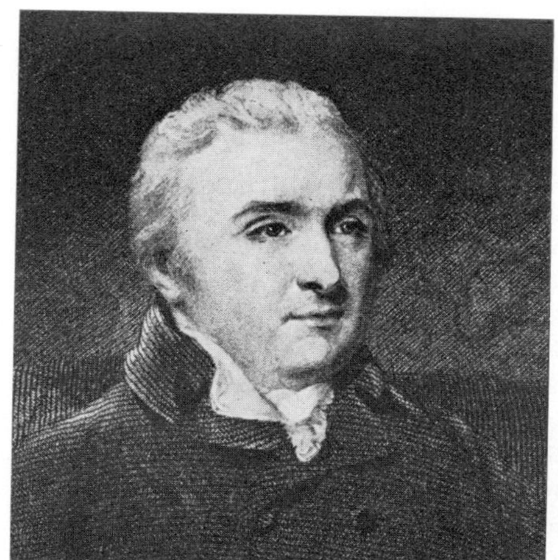

1/Fig. 12.—Matthew Baillie.

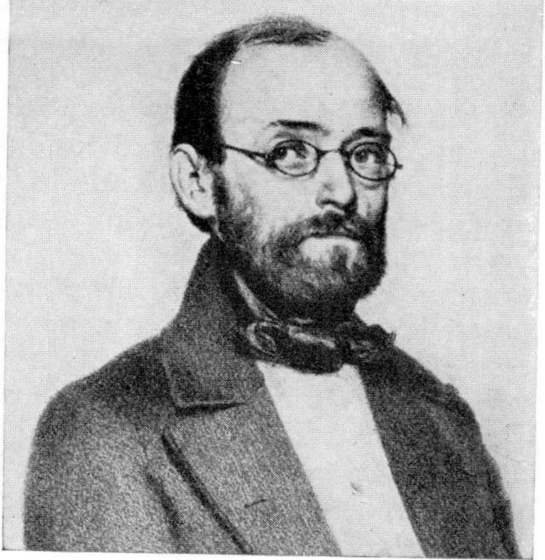

1/Fig. 13.—Carl Rokitansky.

Though some past morbid anatomists may have tended to emphasise the purely structural side of their observations one must not forget that it is largely due to the efforts of pathologists and physicians in correlating anatomical lesions with functional disturbances in patients that we have a fairly comprehensive knowledge of the march of pathological changes in diseased conditions. Nor should the difficulties of the morbid anatomists be under-estimated. At first they worked without the aid of the microscope, and even with this aid their task had difficulties that can be illustrated by a simple analogy. It is as if a full-length cinema film were taken, every two-hundredth frame extracted, the extracted frames jumbled together, and an observer was then asked to recon-

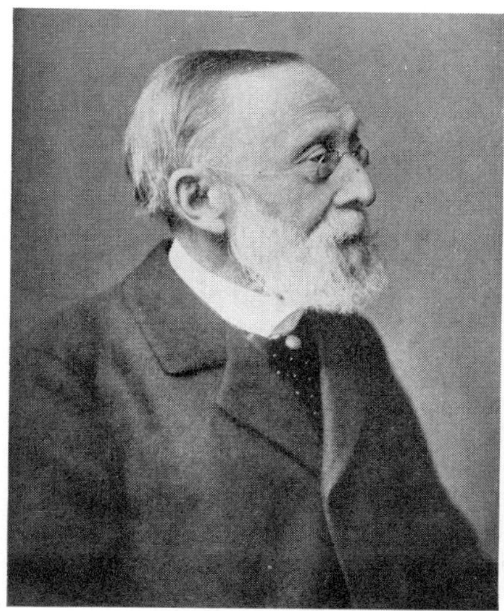

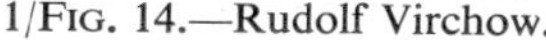

1/Fig. 14.—Rudolf Virchow.

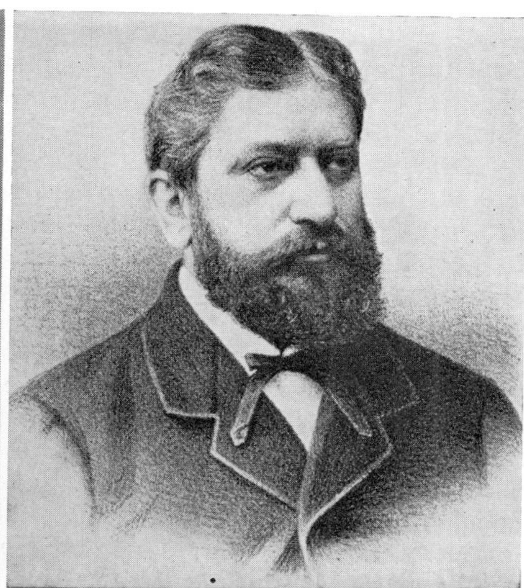

1/Fig. 15.—Julius Cohnheim.

struct the story of the film from them. Remember, then, that the great bulk of our knowledge of the origin and progression of most diseases has been slowly acquired by painstaking observations.

It seems unlikely that any more substantial additions will be made to morbid anatomy and histology by methods that have proved so fruitful in past centuries but a great impetus has recently been given to morphological studies by the introduction of the electron microscope. Knowledge of the detail of cell and tissue components has been immensely extended by observations made with it during the last fifteen years. The preparation of pathological tissues taken post-mortem from man for electron miscroscopy is usually unsatisfactory because destructive changes occur in cells very soon after death and these can be clearly seen by the electron microscope. Progress is however being made by the examination of tissue obtained fresh and fixed immediately at surgical operation or after the procedure for taking small pieces known as biopsy.

There is no doubt that much about the structure of normal and pathological tissues and cells will be learnt from electron micrographs in the future. Examples will be found showing what the new techniques are capable of in the chapters to follow.

Histochemistry, another branch of microscopical observation, is yielding much information, especially about the presence and sites of action of some enzymes, and sometimes spectacular results are obtained by the methods of autoradiography. This method depends on incorporating in cellular constituents radioactive substances, the emanation from which will affect silver salts in photographic emulsions. It is possible by this method to locate where certain cellular processes occur. Examples of the use of autoradiography also occur in the following chapters.

Experimental Pathology

Physiology and biochemistry are subjects that you have already studied extensively. From this work you will be familiar with the idea that information about the normal working of the animal body has largely been acquired by experiment, though to be sure the teaching of physiology in Oxford in the middle of the nineteenth century was by means of a Physiological Museum.

Though Galen and others in antiquity performed experiments, it was not until the scientific developments of the 16th and 17th centuries occurred that the firm foundations of modern physiology were laid by Harvey, who, arguing from anatomical knowledge, demonstrated by experiment that the blood circulates round the body. Pathologists were generally much behind physiologists in applying experimental methods to the elucidation of their particular problems. In the nineteenth century great progress in pathology began to be made by the experimental approach, and we shall have occasion later to refer particularly to work on inflammation. Though most of the great nineteenth-century German pathologists were morbid anatomists and histologists, many able experimentalists emerged towards the end of the century, of whom one of the greatest was Julius Cohnheim (1839–1884) (FIG. 15). He published a series of lectures on General Pathology in 1882 which were translated into English in 1889.[8] I strongly recommend you to read at least the introductory lecture, for much of its content has a very contemporary look and you may perhaps gather an added respect for your pathological forebears. To illustrate his point of view, here are a few quotations: "While in morbid anatomy we learn the modifications undergone by the morphological (or chemical) constitution of the individual organs in disease, morbid physiology teaches *how the functions of the affected organs are performed under abnormal circumstances*, i.e. subsequently to the action on the individual of conditions differing so considerably from those usually in operation as to derange the normal vital process." His outlook, which is that of many pathologists to-day, is well expressed as follows: "General pathology knows no other direction and no other classification than that which obtains in physiology. . . . Not merely the direction, . . . but above all, the method of investigation is the same in morbid as in normal physiology. You know what the most essential aid of physiology is, that one by which she has become an inductive natural science in the sense that chemistry and physics are such; it is experiment—and where purely physical and chemical experiments are inadequate—express physiological experiment. By experiment, as is well known, the single possible factors are tested as to their performances, and the conditions in which an organ works are varied in order to obtain information as to the significance of the individual factors. The results of physiological experiment are in the first place of service to pathology; then, however, we make use of pathological experiment, which was first practised in England by John Hunter, and in France by Magendie, yet was only raised to the rank it at present occupies as our most important fundamental aid by the researches of Traube and Virchow in the fifth decade of this century. One circumstance, as will be readily understood, makes experiment a still more pressing necessity in pathology than in physiology, namely, that we are in a very much higher degree dependent on chance for material for observation than is physiology. Normal men and animals are found at all times and in all places; it is by no means so with the diseases one desires to investigate. This dependence on contingency for material makes itself very intensely felt, even in the investigation of the anatomical side of the processes of disease. Every dead body is equally valuable so far as the anatomy of the normal lung is concerned, provided this organ has been healthy; it is otherwise with the inflamed lung. Here it is very different whether the individual has died on the second or third or as late as the eighth day; for inflammation of the lung is progressive, while anatomical examination can evidently only supply information as to the condition of the lung which prevailed at the moment of death. This gap is filled by pathological experiment."

It may reasonably be claimed that in many cases the difficulties of the experimental pathologist are greater than those of the physiologist, for he has often first to produce diseased or abnormal conditions before he can proceed to an experimental analysis of them. In most cases animals or their tissues have to be used for experiments, but with due precautions and allowance for species differences valid conclusions applicable to man can usually be drawn from them. Modern technical developments increasingly enable experiments and instrumental observations to be made safely on man. For example much has been learnt of cardiac function in man by direct catheterisation of the right side of the heart, isotopes can be used for studying metabolic conditions, and various tests of function of such organs as the kidney are successfully employed to analyse disease processes.

In many instances straight physiological experiments by one of the classical methods, namely the removal of an organ, has thrown great light not only on the physiological workings of the body but on many pathological conditions associated with malfunction of organs. This can most clearly be seen in investigations of the endocrine glands, and you are no doubt already familiar with some of the remarkable changes associated with removal of the pancreas and of the thyroid, parathyroid, adrenal and pituitary glands, and their correlation with conditions occurring naturally in man.

A good example of the influence on pathological conceptions of biochemical investigations is furnished by the glittering series of experiments by which the effects of vitamins on the functioning of the body have been elucidated. They have shown the profound pathological effects that the lack of these materials can produce.

A revolutionary influence was exerted on the experimental study of disease when Pasteur, Koch and others clearly showed, what some predecessors had already indicated, that many diseases were caused by the invasion of the body by micro-organisms. The science, and hence for you the study, of bacteriology is intimately related to what is often considered to be more strictly pathology. The techniques and conceptions of medical bacteriology, which are now being absorbed into the wider views of what is called microbiology, differ greatly from those of pathology, but the two subjects must be considered together in your studies and thought of as being complementary.

The discovery towards the end of the nineteenth century that many microbial diseases, comparable at least in some respects to those naturally occurring in man, could be produced in animals in the laboratory added vastly to our knowledge of infectious processes. We now have at our disposal, as a result of co-operation between chemists and pathologists using experimental methods, chemical substances which will control some of the worst plagues of mankind. In the following lectures you will be introduced to many of the extraordinarily interesting reactions that occur between the host and invading organisms, and from the study of these you should get some clear idea of how experiment, often combined with microscopic observation, has advanced our knowledge of pathology.

One other example of a subject in which experimental methods are widely used is in the study of the genesis of cancer, research that involves examination of the factors controlling normal and abnormal growth. It is particularly in this field that the examination of isolated tissues and cells growing *in vitro* has been used—yet another example of the diversity of techniques now available.

Such is now the interdependence of the experimental sciences that one can expect fundamental discoveries affecting our views on pathology to come from zoologists, anatomists, biochemists and physiologists, as well as from those more narrowly termed pathologists.

I have endeavoured to give you a brief glimpse of the way in which pathological knowledge has been acquired, and to put before you the idea that in this era of flourishing experimental science it is to experiment in the test-tube, in animals and, in favourable circumstances, in man that we must look for increase of the boundaries of our knowledge.

It is easy for a student, and hence a practitioner of medicine, to underestimate the difficulties of elucidating disease processes. Dubos[9] has well expressed this when referring to the work of Pasteur on silkworm diseases. He said, "The struggle against error, always imminent in these studies on silkworm diseases, is of peculiar interest because it provides a well-documented example of the workings of a scientific mind. As Pasteur himself said: 'It is not without utility to show to the man of the world, and to the practical man, at what cost the scientist conquers principles, even the simplest and the most modest in appearance.' Usually the public sees only the finished result of the scientific effort, but remains unaware of the atmosphere of confusion, tentative gropings, frustration and heart-breaking discouragement in which the scientist often labours while trying to extract, from the entrails of nature, the products and laws which appear so simple and orderly when they finally reach textbooks and newspapers." Perhaps in the following chapters you will from time to time see evidence of this groping. Our efforts as teachers will not have been in vain if we have managed to convey to you some of the difficulties presented in establishing even plausible pathological "doctrine".

The Analysis of Health and Disease

Although the extremes are easily recognised, it is difficult or impossible to draw a sharp line between health and disease. It is suggested from time to time that we do not know what "health" is and that criteria of health should be established. This is one of the objects of that somewhat nebulous subject "Social Medicine".

Many diseases are of gradual onset so that it is impossible to say exactly when they begin; in contrast, others occur suddenly, such for example as many diseases caused by bacteria or viruses. Diseases that persist for a long time are referred to as chronic diseases, and those that begin suddenly and run a short course are referred to as acute diseases. The latter are generally more severe in their immediate effects, though by no means the more damaging in the long run.

A disease condition may make a person feel ill in various ways—he has *symptoms*, for example he feels sick or giddy, he has pains in the limbs or a headache, or he itches. He may also present *signs*, that is, changes that can be discovered by an observer who, for example, may find the patient flushed, or that he has a rash, or a swelling, or a limp, or a derangement of the heart sounds or the respiratory sounds which may be heard on auscultation. The main reason why a patient consults his doctor is to be relieved of his symptoms. His medical attendant endeavours to do this by therapeutic procedures which may be directed to relieving the symptoms or, more rationally, to dealing with their underlying cause. Before rational therapeusis can be instituted it is necessary to decide what is the pathology of the condition—in other words, to make a *diagnosis*. To do this the physician brings to bear all that he can find out about the state of the patient's mind and body, and weighs up the evidence. Sometimes he can reach a conclusion with a high degree of certainty, but in many cases he cannot find out enough about what is happening in the body to base his diagnosis on anything more than probabilities. Increasingly it is possible to unravel the meaning of a disordered physiology by experimental physiological methods. No better example of this can be given than that of the elucidation of cardiac malfunction by the electrocardiograph, which measures and records the physical manifestations of muscle contraction and the propagation of impulses. This is just as much a pathological investigation as those that are based on morphology and chemistry.

Never be satisfied just because a name has been applied to a disease condition, for mental effort is apt to cease from that moment. Instead, a diagnosis should only be an aid to framing in your mind a clear picture of the alterations that have so far taken place in the body, and what further changes it is likely to undergo. The patient will want to know what is going to happen to him, in other words he will want a *prognosis*. Clearly, the giving of an intelligent prognosis demands an intimate knowledge of pathology.

For the intelligent student, who will later be the brilliant surgeon or the sage physician, the correct procedure in dealing with these complex matters is to approach each case in the way that those engaged in research approach their problems.

A research worker's aim is by his observations to clarify processes hitherto obscure and thus, as he hopes, to add something new to knowledge. Often he has to devise new biological situations from which deductions may be drawn. He amasses facts by observation and experiment, and his constant endeavour, by amplifying some points and by rejecting unworthy evidence, is to arrive at valid conclusions about the unknown. Clearly such work is not suited to everyone's liking or talent, but the practitioner of medicine can approach the diseases of his patients with the same attitude of mind. He uses known methods to collect the facts, after which he is called upon to synthesise these into some coherent story, much as a research worker endeavours to do. The acquisition of a knowledge of the current diagnostic methods will occupy a good deal of your time while studying clinical medicine and surgery.

Causes of Disease

In the course which you are now starting, one of our main occupations will be to consider in what ways cells react to the various forms of stimulus that can produce pathological changes. Let us briefly review what sort of stimuli these are.

All living things inherit the pattern of their structure from previously existing cells. In the case of highly developed animals inheritance passes through the sexual cells. It is not to be wondered at that in the very complicated processes of embryonic development the racial pattern is not always perfectly reproduced. Errors may be manifest in anatomical defects of such severity that independent life of the new individual is impossible or in relatively trivial lesions such as a hare lip or a cleft palate. Physiological defects may take the form of inborn metabolic errors such as are displayed in the condition of alcaptonuria, or in errors in the mechanism of blood coagulation such as occur in hæmophilia. It would seem possible that some diseases whose origin is at present obscure may be due to as yet undetected inborn metabolic errors.

Apart from inborn disease or the potentiality for disease, the body is constantly called upon to adjust its internal cellular and fluid environment to varying surrounding conditions. Claude Bernard expressed this long ago when he talked of the "milieu interne", and stated that "all vital mechanisms, however varied they may be, have but one object, that of preserving constant the conditions of life in the internal environment".

To help animals to survive, a number of physical protective mechanisms have appeared. The most spectacular, though evidently not the most effective, were those associated with the extinct reptiles. Even the delicate skin of man repels many physical assaults, including, particularly, those of bacteria. Bones of the chest and skull protect vital parts of our anatomy. Our internal structures are in some parts isolated from the outside world only by the thinnest of mucous membranes, sometimes not more than one cell thick, but these though not of much protection against mechanical injury, to which they are little exposed, are surprisingly well equipped to deal with other kinds of injury. We shall consider later the reactions which these structures can show to external noxious stimuli.

It is clear that mechanical insults of sufficient intensity can break down these physical barriers protecting us from the outside world, and can affect us in a number of ways. We will consider some of the consequences to the body in general when we come to consider traumatic shock. More subtle, and at first unnoticed, are the constant penetrations of bacteria through our external protections. We live in a world containing myriads of micro-organisms of very many different species. Fortunately only relatively few species have acquired the ability to live in the animal body and to cause disease, that is, to be pathogenic, but they are the cause of a high proportion of diseases. The study of what happens after these organisms gain entry into the animal body will occupy a considerable amount of our time.

Then there are numerous other external agents which can produce injury, such as heat, cold and radiations of many kinds. Of the last we are coming to be more and more conscious, and not without reason.

A great group of diseases is associated with disturbances of the endocrine glands, of the primary cause of which we are, in almost all cases, entirely ignorant. The biochemical changes associated with them are paralleled by the derangements associated with lack, or occasionally excess, of vitamins. Though these sometimes rather elusive nutritional changes are scientifically most interesting, we should not forget that simple under-nutrition from lack of the main food constituents leads to the development of pathological states which it is not always easy to relate to a particular deficiency. Many diseases are classed as "degenerations", in which cells change or die from causes that are largely unknown at present. A further great group of diseases is associated with the disordered growth of tissues.

From among this somewhat embarrassingly long list of the general causes of disease we will select for first discussion the phenomenon called inflammation.

The Study of Pathology

You are no doubt by now worried by the prospect of having to learn, digest, and select some of the vast accumulation of facts with which observation and experiment have furnished us. The course in general pathology which you pursue before going to work in hospital is designed to show you, as far as possible in a limited time, some of the fundamental reactions to disturbances which occur in the body. The changes discussed will be met with in one form or another in practically every pathological condition you encounter and many are common to most, if not all, mammals and even to other animals. There are still some who suppose that the study of pathology cannot be successfully or profitably begun until a student is actually working in a hospital. Cohnheim, with whom I heartily agree, said: "I do not presuppose that any one of you has already attended the clinics; on the contrary, I believe I can promise that it is precisely the pursuit of morbid physiology which forms the best preparation for, and introduction to, clinical study; you will thus be enabled to understand very much which would otherwise be simply retained by memory."[8]

You will acquire some morbid anatomical knowledge of a general nature, but it is not until you reach a hospital that you will be able to do what I have endeavoured to show was done by the great morbid anatomists and physicians of the past, that is to correlate the symptoms and signs in the living patient with the changes seen in the body after he or she is dead, and so to build up a knowledge of what is called special pathology.

Though no one person can see enough to build up a complete picture of the march of disease from his personal observations, generations of pathologists have clarified the morphological changes presented by many of the conditions you will meet with, and modern experimental science is making rapid strides in extending such knowledge. Such syntheses of knowledge are contained in many textbooks of pathology. You will not be able to learn about the many complicated methods for investigating the morbid physiology of the disease state in man until you are working among patients.

I should like to emphasise again that the study of pathology, conceived of in its widest sense, is of little value to one who is going to practise medicine unless it enables him to grasp clearly the functional changes that are produced by the anatomical changes so frequently caused by disease and seen post-mortem. For every sick person is essentially a functionally deranged organism. He may owe his symptoms to changes that are physically recognisable in his organs or to disorder in the workings of his mind or, if you prefer, of his central nervous system. A sick person is a person with morbid physiology or psychology, and the physician's business is to learn what the disorder—in its literal sense—is due to, and to apply this knowledge to remedy the defect—in other words, to "cure" the patient. The modern trend is to use pathological knowledge to prevent disease, if that is possible, rather than to cure it.

I cannot stress to you too much, therefore, the desirability of acquiring the point of view which will lead you to ask yourself in every case, "What do the observations, of whatever nature, that I make tell me about the *disease process* from which my patient is suffering?" Never be intellectually satisfied with a diagnosis or a label. But it must be recognised with sadness that such an exhortation will probably affect the conduct of only the most alert students and practitioners.

REFERENCES

1. Krumbhaar, E. B. (1937). *Pathology*. "Clio Medica" series, No. XIX. New York: Paul B. Hoeber, Inc.
   This short book covers the history of Pathology in an interesting way. It is recommended to the student.
2. Sigerist, H. E. (1951). *A History of Medicine*. Vol. I. "Primitive and Archaic Medicine." New York: Oxford University Press.
   A treatise on historical method and early medicine particularly in Egypt and Mesopotamia.

3. SINGER, C. (1928). *A Short History of Medicine*. Oxford: Clarendon Press.
This history of medicine should be read by all students.
4. POWER, D'A. (1913). *Proc. roy. Soc. Med.*, **6**, Sect. Hist. Med., 18.
A discussion of the anatomical studies of The London Guild of Barber Surgeons.
5. HOLLÄNDER, E. (1913). *Die Medizin in der klassischen Malerei*. Stuttgart: Ferdinand Enke.
For those who read German this book will give a most entertaining glimpse of medicine in classical painting. Good illustrations.
6. CAMERON, G. R. (1952). *Pathology of the Cell*. Edinburgh and London: Oliver & Boyd.
This book is an almost inexhaustible fount of information on many aspects of cellular pathology and physiology.
7. VIRCHOW, R. (1858). *Die Cellularpathologie in ihrer Begründung auf physiologische und pathologische Gewebelehre*. Berlin: A. Hirschwald.
8. COHNHEIM, J. (1882). *Lectures on General Pathology*. London: The New Sydenham Society, 1889, translation into English.
The introductory lecture is warmly recommended.
9. DUBOS, R. J. (1950). *Louis Pasteur, Free Lance of Science*. Boston: Little, Brown & Co.
An admirable biography and an exposition of biological experiment.

Chapter 2

INFLAMMATION

By H. W. Florey

The word "inflammation" is commonly used in medicine and by the lay public, but when its meaning is examined closely, difficulties of interpretation appear which in the past have given rise to much discussion. It is as well not to try to attach to it a narrow meaning, but rather to conceive of it as, in the words of Grawitz, "the reaction of irritated and damaged tissues which still retain vitality", or as in the definition of Burdon-Sanderson, who said, "The process of inflammation is the succession of changes which occurs in a living tissue when it is injured, provided that the injury is not of such a degree as at once to destroy its structure and vitality". Menkin has given a narrower definition which calls to mind the phenomena that we shall be principally interested in. Inflammation, he says, is "the complex vascular, lymphatic, and local tissue reaction elicited in higher animals by the presence of micro-organisms or of non-viable irritants". Ebert[1] objects to these definitions and proposes that "Inflammation is a process which begins following a sublethal injury to tissue and ends with complete healing".

The important idea to grasp at the outset is that inflammation is a process and not a state. The inflamed area undergoes continuous change. Fortunately it has proved possible to devise means by which the successive macroscopical and microscopical changes of inflammation can be watched in great detail in the living animal.

Historical Considerations

Inflammation has been studied from the earliest times. Pus is described in Egyptian papyri of the second millennium B.C. as being related to the demon of disease, and abscesses and ulcers were recognised. Hippocrates and his school made good observations on inflammation of the external parts, and their term "erysipelas"—literally a redness of the skin—has lasted to this day as a description of a certain infection of the skin characterised by a spreading red area, and "oidema"—swelling—is still used, though spelt œdema or edema. Fever and inflammation were conceived of as healing processes within certain limits, but as processes that might be harmful if these limits were exceeded. The doctrine of the four cardinal signs of inflammation, redness, swelling, heat and pain, was enunciated by Celsus (about B.C. 30 to A.D. 38), and to these Galen (A.D. 130–200), who was the first person to write extensively on inflammation, added a fifth sign, *Functio læsa*, and much later John Hunter (1728–1793) also called attention to the loss of function.

Boerhaave, who lived from 1668 to 1738 when Dutch medicine was supreme in Europe, laid much emphasis on the changed state of the blood vessels in inflammation. He believed that there was "an excess of blood in the inflamed part due to increased hydrostatic pressure and to the friction of the red arterial blood in the smallest canals".

With the rise of microscopy and its application to pathology more progress towards our present views was made. The work of Cowper, Haller and Spallanzani in the 17th and 18th centuries established that the redness of the inflamed part was due to the distension of the small blood vessels, and not, as at first believed, to the passage of blood into vessels not normally containing it or to the passage of blood into the tissues.

John Hunter, a surgeon and indefatigable collector of anatomical specimens, who had the outlook which to-day would be called that of an experimental biologist, reintroduced the important conception formerly adumbrated by Galen, that inflammation could be initiated by any injury, for instance an injury caused by pressure, friction, heat, cold or "air in wounds". He expressed his views in the following words: "But if inflammation develops, regardless of the cause, still it is an effect whose purpose it is to restore the parts to their natural functions."

A great step forward in understanding inflammation and in diffusing knowledge of it was taken by Cohnheim (1882) when he gave detailed and accurate descriptions of the events to be seen during inflammation of transparent tissue such as the web and tongue of the frog. In particular he called attention to the emigration of white corpuscles from the blood vessels. Though, as we shall see later, he was not the first to observe these phenomena, it was not until his descriptions appeared that due attention was paid to them and that they became an integral part of pathological doctrine. Cohnheim shared with Samuel, another pioneer in the investigation of inflammation, the view that the main feature of the reaction was an increased permeability of the vascular wall, a view which has subsequently been modified and extended.

The interpretation of the observations on inflammation gave rise to much controversy, especially after the promulgation by Metchnikoff of the theory that phagocytosis was the central phenomenon. Metchnikoff (1845–1916) was a Russian who worked in Odessa as a zoologist when a young man, though the bulk of his important work was done at the Pasteur Institute in Paris. He had no medical training, but his views, based on observations on many genera and species of animals, gained acceptance in spite of a sustained attack by German and English pathologists.

While Metchnikoff stoutly maintained that the cells which appeared during the inflammatory process were the chief protection of the animal body against microbial invasion, equally potent arguments for considering that the main protective function resided in the liquids of the blood—the so-called humoral view—were advanced by those who were founding the branch of medical science now known as immunology. We shall have occasion to follow these points in more detail later, when you will see that the different views have been synthesised into one generally accepted doctrine.

While Cohnheim, Samuel, Metchnikoff and many others were occupied in making observations on living tissues, many histologists and pathologists were examining fixed material from human inflammations and from experimental inflammations in animals. They furnished detailed descriptions of the histological appearances of inflamed tissues, and were able largely to deduce the march of the events in the inflammatory process.

At present the electron microscope with its great magnification and resolving power is being used to extend these observations, while at the same time much interest is being taken in the chemical and physical mechanisms involved in the many changes that occur. Thus the study of inflammation, which may justifiably be considered the backbone of pathology, continues to afford great interest to investigators. We are still far from being able to give a complete picture of what happens in the tissues or to explain how and why the sequence of events that follows tissue injury takes place.

MACROSCOPICAL OBSERVATIONS

In seeking the cause of the redness, heat, pain, swelling and loss of function known to the ancients, let us first consider those observations that can be made without the aid of the microscope.

Redness

Triple Reaction

We owe to Lewis and his colleagues an analysis of the phenomena that follow varying degrees of injury to the human skin.[2] He described what he called the "triple reaction", which consists at first of a central dull red area surrounded by a brighter red halo to be followed by swelling of the dull red area. This reaction can be elicited if a firm stroke is made with a corner of a ruler on the forearm or back. A red line appears in exactly the position where the ruler was applied. This dull red area is soon surrounded by a bright red halo stretching some 2 to 3 cm. around it (FIG. 1). Swelling or a weal then appears along the line of the stroke, which becomes paler (FIG. 2). This swelling increases and finally there is a pale weal surrounded by a wide red flare (FIG. 3).

You will notice that in these simple experiments two of the "cardinal signs" of inflammation, namely redness and swelling of the part injured, are very clear. A third "cardinal sign", heat, is also present, for the area of redness and swelling feels hot and if the temperature of the skin is measured during these changes it is found to rise. The suggestion first made by John Hunter, that many types of injury produce a similar inflammation, was confirmed by Lewis and his collaborators, for they showed that in addition to mechanical injury such diverse forms of stimulus as heat, cold, electric shock, ultra-violet and X-radiation and various chemical irritants, for example morphia and cantharides, all produced a similar "triple response".

Cause of the Triple Response

In view of the very diverse nature of the stimuli that produce inflammation, Ebbecke had proposed, shortly before Lewis's work, that injury might release a chemical substance which caused local vasodilatation. Lewis and his collaborators analysed the matter in detail and regarded the central dull red line following a ruler stimulus as being due to dilatation of small blood vessels—venules and capillaries—that are acted on directly by a chemical substance liberated in the injured tissue. In addition it stimulates sensory nerve-endings in the injured area, setting in motion an axon reflex through which arterioles outside the

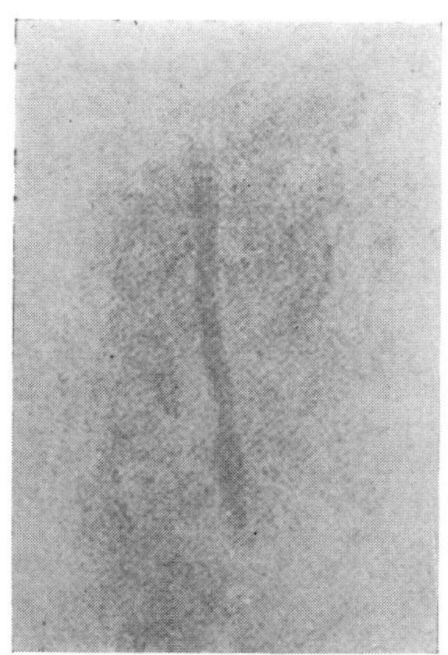

2/FIG. 1

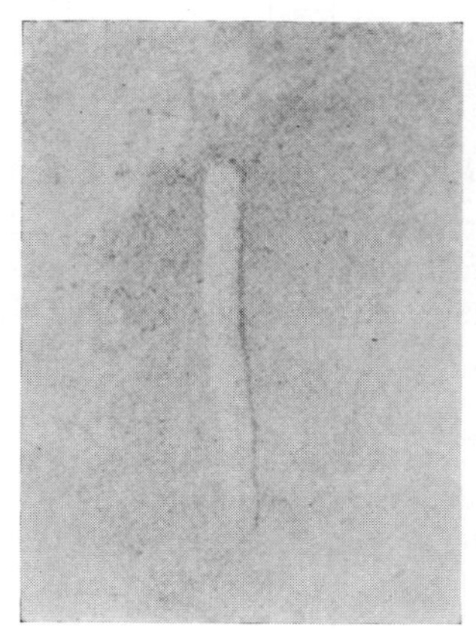

2/FIG. 2

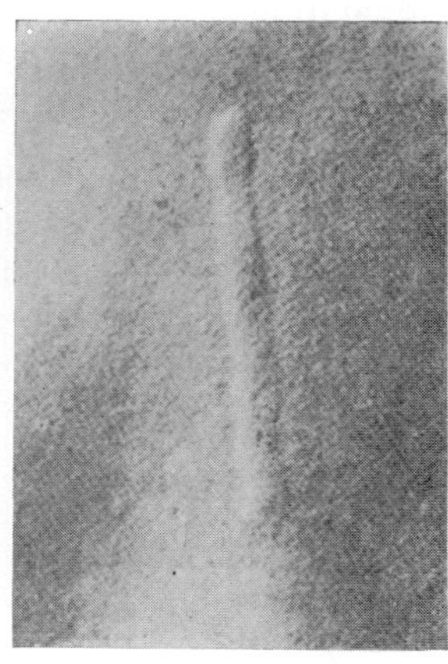

2/FIG. 3

DEVELOPMENT OF THE TRIPLE RESPONSE

The individual chosen for this experiment was subject to urticaria, that is to say these changes were produced easily and in an exaggerated form. But they are essentially the same in everyone.

2/FIG. 1.—*First stage.* 1½ minutes after stimulation. The thin dark line corresponds exactly with the ruler stroke. The injured area is surrounded by a diffuse flare which was actually bright red.

2/FIG. 2.—*Second stage.* The same skin at the end of 3½ minutes. The flare surrounding the stimulus is now more sharply defined and wealing has nearly reached its full height.

2/FIG. 3.—*Third stage.* The same skin at the end of 40 minutes. The lighting has been altered to display the weal more fully. The weal is pale, it has widened, and its edges are less sharply defined. (From Lewis.[2])

injured area are dilated. Thus the flare—the bright red halo round the site of injury—is produced.

Lewis thought that this substance which produced dilatation of the minute vessels was histamine or a histamine-like substance which he defined as "any substance (or substances) that is liberated by the tissue cells and exerts on the minute vessels and nerve endings an influence culminating in the triple response". There are now many substances of this nature to be considered. Often no clear-cut distinction is made between dilatation of the minute vessels in inflammation and an increase in their permeability, probably because most, if not all, of the substances that have to be considered can cause both reactions and it is easier to measure permeability changes than vascular dilatation in the intact animal. These substances will be discussed when we deal with the question of increased permeability.

H-ion Concentration

Dilatation of normal small blood vessels may be brought about by altering in their neighbourhood the H-ion concentration to beyond physiological limits.[3] Some observers (e.g. Schade[4]) maintain that tissue fluids become considerably more acid during the development of an inflammation and that the vascular dilatation is brought about, or at least maintained, by the increased H-ion concentration. Whether in fact this is an important mechanism for the production of vascular dilatation has never been proved.

The Role of the Axon Reflex in producing Arteriolar Dilatation

An axon reflex is illustrated in FIG. 4. A stimulus passes from a sensory nerve-ending up to the bifurcation of the axon, whence it travels antidromically towards the periphery again. Although travelling along a sensory nerve, this

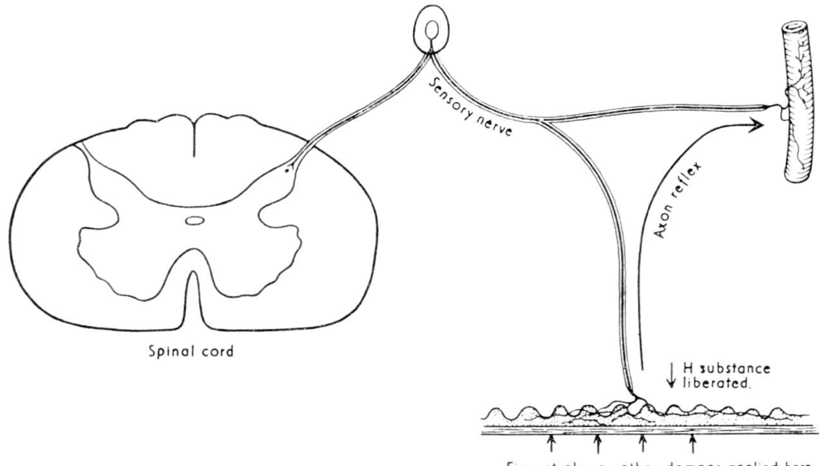

2/FIG. 4.—The mechanism of the axon reflex which dilates neighbouring arterioles when a stimulus is applied to the skin. The nerve impulse passes centrally along the axon to its place of division and then peripherally to the arteriole. This phenomenon occurs even after the division of the sensory nerve distal to the spinal root ganglion, provided that the peripheral nerve has not had time to degenerate.

antidromic impulse has the capacity to dilate the arterioles. One of the first workers to suggest that an axon reflex was involved in the vascular dilatation of inflammation was Bruce,[5] who, in studying the effects of mustard oil on the conjunctiva of the rabbit, found that vascular dilatation was much reduced by cocainisation and that if the nerves to the conjunctiva had been cut and given time to degenerate dilatation failed to occur. Bruce considered that these effects were due to the abolition of an axon reflex. Similarly, Krogh[6] noted that the strong capillary dilatation that followed the application of iodine to a frog's tongue was abolished if the sensory nerve endings had been paralysed by cocaine. From these and other experiments he also concluded that axon reflexes were involved in the inflammatory phenomena.

Lewis and Grant,[7] during their analysis of the "triple response", showed that a red central area surrounded by a brighter red flare appeared after the application of a test-tube containing hot water to normal skin, but that if the sensory nerves to the skin had been cut some days before the experiment, during which the nerve fibres had degenerated, only the central red area developed. If the experiment was done within six or seven days of cutting the sensory nerve and before the completion of nerve degeneration the peripheral flare could still be seen. These results were reasonably explained by the mechanism of the axon reflex. Thus the sensory impulses from the injured area seem to have a close connection with vascular dilatation in the surrounding parts.

The Role of the Vasomotor Nerves

Apart from this axon reflex, the question whether vasomotor or sensory nerves of blood vessels play a significant role in the reaction to injury and in inflammation has been the subject of enquiry for many years. Cohnheim held the view that the vasomotor nerves played no part in the development of inflammation, but their influence has been well shown by observations on the rabbit's ear which has a double innervation with both dilator and constrictor nerves. If the dilator nerves are cut, causing vasoconstriction, the inflammatory damage following a given insult is more severe than when the constrictor nerves are cut, which causes vasodilatation (see Adami, 1909). The possible influence of both the central and peripheral nervous system on inflammation is discussed in detail by Chapman and Goodell.[8]

However, while there are some observations showing that the nervous system can modify the manifestations of inflammation that follow injury, there is good experimental evidence that all the really essential phenomena of inflammation that we are going to study can take place in the absence of nervous connections, as was maintained by Cohnheim.

Heat

We have probably all experienced the sense of heat that an infection gives to a part. Even a small infection, say in the finger, makes that finger hotter than its neighbours. The explanation is that normally some parts, especially those more or less exposed to the air, are at a lower temperature than the interior of the body. When inflammation causes blood from the interior to pass more rapidly and in greater amount through the dilated vessels of some superficial part, the tissue becomes warmer than adjacent normal areas, in which the blood has more time to cool during its passage through the skin. The phenomenon of increased heat of an inflamed part is negligible under ordinary conditions except in lesions on the surface of the body. Further, since the skin alone has heat-sensitive nerves, other organs would fail to appreciate temperature differences that might occur.

It has been suggested that the rate of metabolic processes is increased in inflamed tissues, and it is true, as Gessler[9] showed, that such tissues consume much oxygen, but it has never been demonstrated that the increased metabolism is sufficient to play any significant part in the rise of temperature.

Pain

It cannot be stated with any finality what are the causes of pain associated with inflammation. It has been suggested that chemical substances are liberated that sensitise the nerve endings so that they react to slight stimuli by registering pain, but there is no proof of this. Certain substances, which will be considered in more detail when we discuss the increased permeability of inflamed blood vessels, have been shown to have very marked pain-producing properties. They have been tested by applying them in solution to the bared base of a blister raised on human skin by the application of cantharides or heat. Blister fluid, serum and 5-hydroxytryptamine cause pain when applied to such a bare surface. The 5-hydroxytryptamine was active at a dilution of 1 in 100,000,000 (10^{-8} g./ml.). It has been shown that pure bradykinin, a peptide, produces similar pain, described as burning, at a dilution of 10^{-7} to 10^{-6}. Both these substances occur widely in tissues and may take part in the inflammatory reaction[10], as will be discussed later.

Departures of body fluids from isotonicity may give rise to pain, for pain is caused by the injection of hypertonic and hypotonic solutions, and the osmotic pressure of tissues is altered during inflammation. The injection of isotonic solutions of potassium chloride is very painful, and as potassium is released from cells during acute inflammation there may be a disturbance of the sodium-calcium-potassium balance. The accumulation of hydrogen ions in inflamed areas may also contribute to the production of pain. What is certain is that inflammation occurring in tissues which become tense when relatively little fluid has collected in them, such as the tissues round the stem of the external auditory meatus and the alæ nasæ, and the subcutaneous tissue where skin is tightly stretched over bone, is much more painful than similar affections elsewhere. This suggests that pressure may be a factor in producing pain. It is very noticeable that when pus or fluid is evacuated from lesions in which it is under tension the pain and tenderness immediately lessen. This effect is almost certainly due to the relief of pressure, due to swelling, on the nerve endings.

SWELLING

Alteration of Capillary Permeability

Protein-containing fluid, known as an exudate, accumulates in the tissue, forming the weal following slight localised injury and the swelling in more serious types of inflammatory lesion. Analysis of fluid from weals and blisters shows its high protein content. Often inflammatory exudate contains enough fibrinogen to clot and form masses of fibrin, which can be readily seen when the exudate comes out on to a surface (FIG. 5). Fibrin can also be seen in appropriately stained histological preparations of many inflamed tissues (FIG. 6).

The rate of escape of fluid from an inflamed capillary has been estimated to be from 5 to 7 times greater than that from a normal vessel with similar levels of internal hydrostatic pressure and plasma protein. Thus inflamed small blood vessels are more permeable than normal, but in this context the word "permeability" has a somewhat restricted meaning.

The capillaries and the smallest venules are permeable freely at all times to water and to salts, amino-acids, glucose and other substances of small molecular size in the blood. They are not, however, freely permeable to proteins, though Drinker[11] stressed that small quantities can pass out of the capillaries of most tissues. Lymph issuing from the thoracic duct, coming in the quiescent animal mainly from the intestine and liver, will clot owing to its content of fibrinogen. Lymph from the liver may contain more than 4 per cent of blood proteins, while that obtained from the limbs of dogs by massage or after

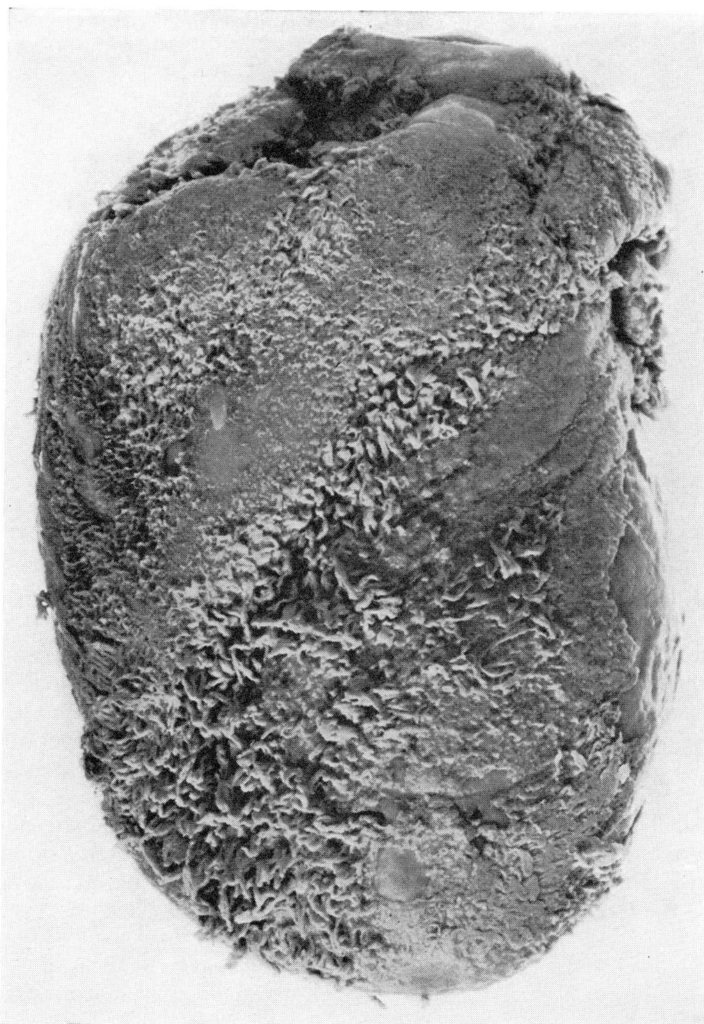

ACUTE FIBRINOUS PERICARDITIS

2/FIG. 5.—The pericardial surface has attached to it masses of fibrin, derived from the pericardial exudate caused by an acute inflammation.

muscle activity contains about 1·8 per cent. The protein content of lymph from various parts of the body of a number of animals has been tabulated by Yoffey and Courtice.[12]

It is to Starling[13] that we owe our present views on the balance of forces acting in the capillaries. He discovered that proteins in solution exert osmotic pressure, and he considered that the endothelial membrane of the small blood vessels let through water and salts freely but not proteins. The proteins of the blood therefore exerted an osmotic pressure across the capillary wall. In man

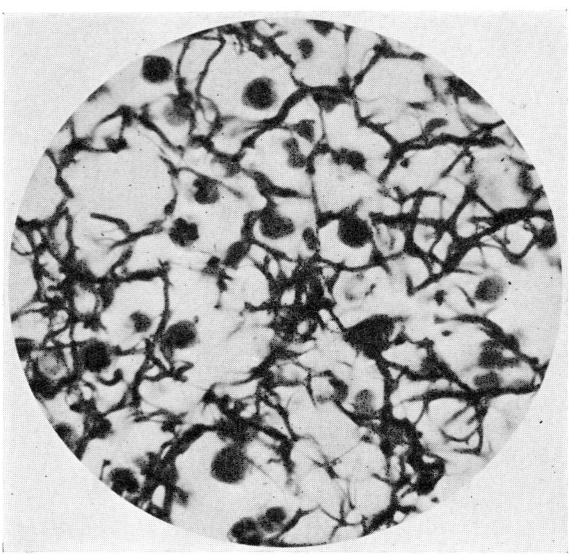

2/FIG. 6.—Shows fibrin strands that have formed in an inflammatory exudate.

this pressure is about 32 mm. Hg. Normally a rough balance of forces is struck between the hydrostatic pressure of the blood stream tending to press fluid out from the capillary and the osmotic pressure of the blood proteins tending to draw water into the capillary (FIG. 7). This matter is discussed further in Chapter 12.

If the capillary wall is altered so that proteins pass through it more freely than usual, the pressure relationships are altered too. Inflammation involves such a change. The capillaries become more permeable to protein; protein leaks into the tissue fluids; the osmotic balance being thus disturbed, more fluid is retained in the tissues outside the wall of the blood vessel. This effect is exagger-

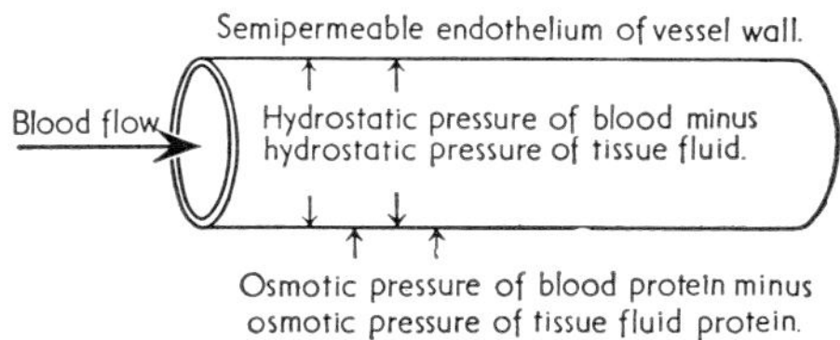

2/FIG. 7.—*Starling's hypothesis*. The hydrostatic pressure of the blood tends to filter fluid outwards through the vessel wall which is normally nearly impermeable to proteins. Fluid is attracted into the vessel from the tissue spaces by the osmotic effect of the proteins of the blood, which are in much greater concentration inside than outside the vessel. Normally these opposing osmotic and hydrostatic pressures are nearly balanced.

Inflammation. If the vessel wall becomes more permeable to proteins the concentration of proteins in the tissue spaces rises. The hydrostatic pressure then has less osmotic pressure to overcome, and more fluid passes out from the blood to the tissues.

ated by the fact that blood proteins and other proteins in the inflammatory tissue fluid may break down and so increase the number of molecules that can exert osmotic pressure, thus tending to reduce further the effective osmotic pressure of the proteins in the blood vessels. At the same time, as was shown experimentally by Landis[13a], the hydrostatic pressure in the smallest blood vessels is increased during inflammatory hyperæmia, and thus filtration pressure is increased.

Testing Increased Capillary and Venular Permeability

A reaction which indicates increased permeability is the rapid swelling of the paw or snout of the rat when "permeability factors" are given either locally or systemically. But the method most commonly used depends on the fact that certain dyes such as trypan blue, pontamine blue and T1824, known also as Evans' blue, do not pass readily through normal capillary walls after intravenous injection because they become associated with plasma proteins—albumin in particular. Provided that the concentration of dye in the blood is not too great, the colouring of any site or tissue is associated with the movement of protein molecules.

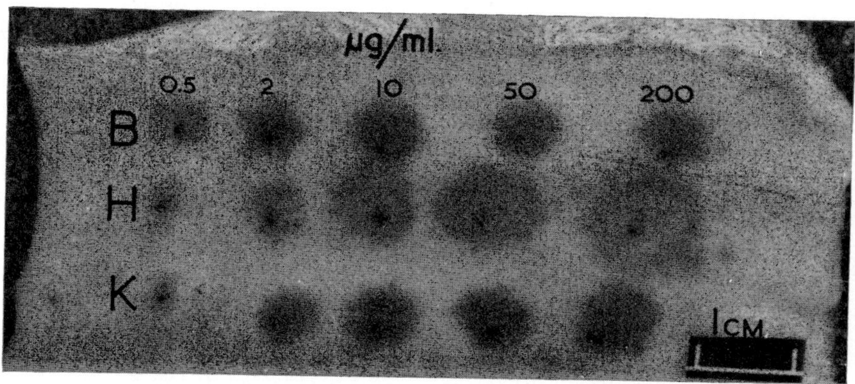

2/FIG. 8.—Blue staining of the skin of a guinea-pig in which pontamine blue was circulating. In the centre of the areas 0·1 ml. of solutions of B, bradykinin (not pure); H, histamine; K, serum kallikrein had been injected. (From Bhoola, Calle, and Schacter.[14])

The testing of permeability-increasing substances by the dye method is usually carried out by first injecting a solution of the dye intravenously into a rat, guinea-pig, or rabbit. The substance to be tested, dissolved in sodium chloride solution of suitable tonicity, is then injected intradermally into the shaved skin. Sometimes the abdominal skin is used, but some workers find that the dorsal skin gives more reproducible results. If the test substance increases the permeability of the small blood vessels with which it comes into contact the proteins and the dye associated with them leak out into the tissues, forming a coloured patch around the needle prick that is easily seen (see FIG. 8).[14] The diameter of the patch, and to some extent the intensity of the colour, gives an indication of the permeability-increasing power of the solution injected. One advantage of this method is that a number of injections can be made at one time into one animal, so that the activity of different solutions can be compared, and by using graded dilutions some sort of quantitative result can be obtained.

Miles and Miles[15] assayed the potency of permeability factors by plotting the log dose of permeability factor against the mean diameter of the area of exuded pontamine blue. Some workers have estimated the amount of exuded dye by extracting it in solvents from disintegrated tissue. Another refinement depends on attaching radioactive bromine, Br^{82}, to trypan blue and injecting this material intravenously. The Br^{82} does not accumulate in normal tissues but does so in injured areas. If a more firmly marked protein is required, either albumin or globulin can have radioactive iodine attached to it.

Some workers, for example Menkin and Spector, have made considerable use of inflammatory exudate collecting in a serous cavity of dogs or rats, generally in the pleura after the intrapleural injection of turpentine. An almost pure inflammatory exudate can be removed, measured and examined, and factors making for its production or suppression can be investigated.

Biphasic Nature of Response to Injury

The development of increased vascular permeability following relatively mild trauma is divided into two phases. The reaction of the skin of guinea-pigs to heating at 54° C. for 20 secs. shows this point well. The first phase of increased permeability is characterised by rapid onset and subsidence. The second occurs ½ to 1 hour after the decline of the initial reaction and the increased permeability of this phase is maximal for 3 to 4 hours, finally subsiding after 6 to 8 hours. Similar biphasic reactions have been found to occur in inflammation induced in other ways, the biphasic response to ultra-violet light being particularly clear cut (Logan and Wilhelm[16].) There are some differences in the responses of different species.

Chemical Mediators of Increased Permeability

Attention is now concentrated on the investigation of possible chemical "mediators" of the two phases of the permeability reaction. It can be said at once that little or nothing definite is known of the chemical mediator of the prolonged, later phase, and Wilhelm[17] after an exhaustive review of possible mediators pessimistically states—"Half a century of work on the identification of substances increasing vascular permeability and the other vascular events in the inflammatory process has resulted in little reliable information concerning relevant chemical mediators".

Nevertheless a number of more or less well characterised substances producing increased vascular permeability and other changes found in inflammation have now been investigated and some of them may possibly be involved in at least the first stage of the vascular alterations of inflammation.

Wilhelm divides those that have been "reasonably characterised" into:

(*a*) Proteases: such as plasmin, kallikrein and globulin permeability factor;
(*b*) Polypeptides: such as leukotaxine, bradykinin and kallidin;
(*c*) Amines: such as histamine and 5-hydroxytryptamine.

(a) Proteases

The importance of the proteases is probably not due to a direct effect on blood vessels but to the possibility that they may produce pharmacologically active polypeptides.

Plasmin is a protease which occurs in mammalian blood as an inactive precursor, plasminogen, which can be activated by dilution, by tissue extracts, by an activator in blood and tissue fluids, and by contact with glass. Tissues contain natural antagonists to plasmin.

Kallikrein occurs in saliva and urine and in an inactive form in pancreas and blood. It is a non-dialysable heat-labile protein. The inactive form kallikreinogen can be activated in a number of ways, the most important of which for present consideration is exposure to proteolytic enzymes. Serum kallikrein is also released by simple physical manipulation such as contact with glass or by dilution. Kallikrein can be sharply distinguished from plasmin, and is considered more likely to be involved as a permeability factor. Both these enzymes act on a variety of proteins.

Globulin permeability factor.—From several groups of investigators[18] evidence has come for considering that normal plasma contains a third permeability-increasing factor. It exists as an inert "pro-factor" until altered by certain procedures such as dilution of fresh serum in glass tubes, or exposure of undiluted serum to powdered glass, starch granules, cellulose or agar. The activated permeability factor is either an α- or a β-globulin according to the species of animal.

It is accompanied by an inhibitory globulin which is probably an α-globulin so that there is what is called a pro-PF/IPF system which is essentially the same in all species so far examined. There is good evidence that the globulin factor is an enzyme, but it does not appear to be a common type of protease and its substrate has not so far been identified. It can be sharply differentiated from plasmin but the distinction from kallikrein is not so sharp. It does not apparently owe its activity to the liberation of histamine or bradykinin.

(b) Polypeptides

The importance of the proteases lies in their products. Menkin[19] first called attention to the permeability-increasing properties of polypeptides by describing leukotaxine, which was an impure mixture.

Bradykinin and kallidin are two substances to which great attention has been recently paid. The kallikreins break down a kininogen, kallidinogen, an α_2-globulin found in plasma, to kallidin, one form of which is now known to be similar to bradykinin, a vasoactive polypeptide first discovered in the products of the reaction of a snake venom protease. Both substances have now been synthesised.

The structure of bradykinin is:

H. Arg. Pro. Pro. Gly. Phe. Ser. Pro. Phe. Arg.

Two kallidins have been found after the action of kallikrein from human urine on human plasma. One is identical with bradykinin and the other has an addition N-terminal lysine residue:

Kallidin-10

H.Lys.Arg.Pro.Pro.Gly.Phe.Ser.Pro.Phe.Arg.OH

Kallidin-9 or Bradykinin

Margolis and Bishop[20] believe that kininogen consists of two substrates one of which produces the decapeptide and the other the nonapeptide.

In the presence of Hageman factor (see Chapter 7 on Blood Coagulation) plasma kallikreinogen ("component A" of Margolis) is activated by foreign surfaces, organic solvents or acid. The resultant kallikrein then reacts with "component B", which is about one-third of the total kininogen, to produce nonapeptide. The remainder of the kininogen is the source of decapeptide which can be released by, amongst other things, glandular kallikrein.

Bradykinin is an extremely active substance in all species so far tested. At concentrations of 10^{-9} to 10^{-8} it increased permeability in the capillaries of guinea-pig and rat skin. This makes it on a molar basis about 15 times as active as histamine. It is also highly active in man.

Pharmacologically Active Amines

Histamine.—Lewis produced evidence that histamine or some substance with very similar properties was released on mild trauma to produce the "triple response".

Histamine is undoubtedly present in normal tissues, including the skin, for it is released by perfusing intact skin with organic compounds known as "histamine liberators", the most powerful of which is compound 48/80. Injected intradermally this substance produces a flare and weal. Erythema, œdema and pruritis occur after its intravenous or subcutaneous injection into laboratory animals or man.

Histamine is found in tissues particularly in relation to mast cells, which are capable of releasing it without degranulation. While stored histamine is presumably responsible for immediate reactions, it is possible that fresh production of histamine may play a part in slower or continued reactions. The histamine-forming enzyme, histidine decarboxylase, is present in many tissues and has been shown to increase in amount under a variety of experimental stimuli, for example in hypersensitivity and after burning.[21]

Although it is clear that histamine exists in tissues and that it can be released by a wide variety of procedures, it is not known for certain how it is held in the cell or how it is released. Whatever the mechanism, histamine is almost certainly released in the reactions of allergy which are considered in detail in Chapters 38–40. These reactions take place rapidly in certain tissues following the entry into the body of a foreign protein in a person whose cells have been "sensitised" by previous contact with the same protein. Allergic reactions have something in common with inflammatory reactions; for instance, one manifestation, common after the ingestion of a foodstuff to which the subject is sensitive, is urticaria, in which the skin shows swellings or weals, very much like the lesions produced by the firm stroke of the ruler. One of the reasons for believing that histamine is involved is that the administration of antihistamine drugs often reduces such reactions.

5-hydroxytryptamine (5 HT).—This amine, which used to be known as serotonin, is widely distributed in nature. It occurs in the stings of many animals and plants and is present in mammalian tissues in greatest concentration in the blood, intestine and brain. In the blood it occurs in the platelets, and in the gut in the argentaffin cells, but its precise location in the brain has not been determined. In the rat and mouse it is to be found in the mast cells, but in other species it is not so clearly connected with these cells. On present evidence it appears that 5 HT is stored in specific granules in the cell cytoplasm, e.g. in platelets, mast cells and the argentaffin cells of the intestine, from which it is readily liberated.

5 HT produces a flare on intradermal injection into man, but although it increases capillary permeability in the rat skin it does not have this effect in the skin of man. Its capacity as a pain-producer has been mentioned already.

Less is known about 5 HT than about histamine, but it is certainly a vaso-active amine which must be kept in mind as being possibly involved in acute inflammation.

Other Substances

Some other well defined substances are candidates for consideration as mediators.

Nucleosides and nucleotides.—Adenosine and adenylic acid are released from burnt tissues[22] and possibly are responsible for widespread changes following severe injury.[23] They appear to dilate arterioles rather than the more peripheral vessels. The capacity of nucleosides and nucleotides to increase capillary permeability has been investigated[24] in the rat and in man. In the rat the nucleosides inosine, adenosine, and guanosine, and the nucleotide inosinic acid were active. Inosine was inactive in man but xanthosine, which was inactive in rats, caused a response in some human subjects though not in others. The interesting possibility was raised by Spector and Willoughby[24] that the distinction between reactors and non-reactors to xanthosine might have a genetic basis.

Hyaluronidase.—A few minutes after the infliction of an injury to an area away from blood vessels it can be seen that the amorphous matrix of the connective tissue in that area changes from a gel to a fluid. This change could conceivably be due merely to the action of physical forces, but it is possible that the enzyme hyaluronidase, which depolymerises mucopolysaccharides of the connective tissues, may be involved.

Hyaluronidase is said to accumulate in inflamed tissues and it is actively produced by some bacteria, such as strains of staphylococcus, streptococcus and *Cl. welchii*, which invade tissues. Proteolytic enzymes could also be involved in this softening of the connective tissue.

Hyaluronidase has been stated both to increase capillary permeability and to have no effect on it. Probably it need not be seriously considered as a mediator of increased capillary permeability in inflammation.

Lactic Acid

Miles has suggested that the production of lactic acid by anærobic glycolysis during inflammation may be sufficient to increase the permeability of small blood vessels. He states that 50 μg of lactic acid suffices to increase the permeability in a gram of guinea-pig skin. Possibly the lactic acid could be produced by emigrated leucocytes.

Relationships of Permeability Substances to Inflammation

Wilhelm[17] has stated that proof that a substance is involved as a natural mediator can be obtained in three ways: (1) by isolating the permeability factor at the relevant period of the inflammatory process, (2) by suppressing the response with specific antagonistic drugs, or (3) by depleting the animal of the supposed permeability factor.

All the putative mediators so far mentioned have been extracted from inflammatory exudates such as can be produced in the pleural cavities of rats by injecting turpentine, but unfortunately this does not prove that they were there in an active form in which they could have initiated or maintained the inflamed state of the vessels. One of the prime difficulties in examining damaged tissues for likely substances is that such substances can readily be released from a combined or inactive form by procedures involved in extracting them.

The results following depletion of amines by drugs in rats has suggested that they may be involved in the first phase of inflammation, but somewhat more convincing evidence is provided by the use of antagonistic drugs.

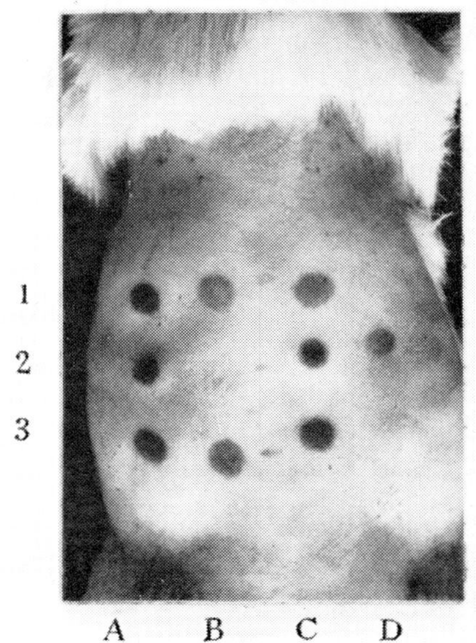

2/FIG. 9.—Suppression by an antihistamine drug of the immediate increase of capillary permeability after a burn.

Guinea-pig with pontamine blue in the circulation; a copper disc was applied to the shaved skin at 54° C. for 5 secs.; the antihistamine drug triprolidine was given intravenously.

The six burns making up lines A and C are controls and are strongly blue. The three other well-stained patches (B1, B3, D2) are burns made after a small dose of triprolidine (10 μg. per kg.). The three spaces with a faint reaction, hardly discernible in the photograph (B2, D1, D3), were burned after a larger dose of triprolidine had been given (making 100 μg, per kg. in all). (From Wilhelm and Mason.[30])

Unfortunately drugs such as the antihistamines are by no means specific. Nevertheless, the use of antagonistic drugs has provided the best evidence that histamine is involved in the first phase of inflammation due to injury by heat (see FIG. 9) and that 5-hydroxytryptamine is liberated in rats. This view has been strengthened by finding that the first phase of inflammation caused by ultraviolet light is similarly inhibited.[25] But no evidence has been produced that any of the substances so far considered are involved in the second, later and more prolonged phase of the inflammatory reaction.

If histamine is involved it would have to be continuously produced as it is rapidly inactivated in the tissues by diamine oxidases and by acetylating and other enzymes. Further the small blood vessels rapidly become immune to the effects of histamine; for example, the repeated pricking of histamine into the human skin produces diminishing results. From these considerations it is perhaps not surprising that the delayed response to burning is found to be unaffected by antihistamine drugs and that the amount of free histamine in the lesion at this stage is insufficient to maintain the observed effects. By experiments in man it has been shown that bradykinin, unlike histamine and 5 HT, does not produce a refractory state in the small vessels, so with this substance a more prolonged effect is possible.[25a]

A powerful argument against considering any of the "mediators" so far investigated as being involved in the late phase of inflammation is afforded by the fact that Cotran and Majno[26] and Miles[27] have both found that histamine, 5 HT, bradykinin, globulin permeability factor, plasma kininogenases and lactic acid all induce short-lived changes in the venules, while the second delayed phase of increased permeability is associated with capillary and not venular damage. This point will be dealt with again when the morphological changes occurring in vessels with increased permeability are discussed.

Other Suggestions about Increased Permeability

It is worth mentioning another possible mediator. It has been pointed out by Cotran and Majno[26] that the injection of a one per cent solution of lysolecithin over the cremaster muscle of the rat caused increased permeability in the capillaries as well as the venules, a phenomenon not seen with other mediators. Lysolecithin may be released in tissues through the action of complement.

The α-toxin of *Clostridium welchii* is a lecinthinase and it is one of the few substances that produce prolonged permeability changes. The lecinthinases are perhaps worth further study.

A different approach was used by Spector and Willoughby when they postulated that certain hormones might be released during inflammation and that these hormones in their active form might help to restore vascular permeability to normal. The arguments for this view stem from the observations that the substances dopa, dopamine, noradrenalin and adrenalin can suppress inflammation at least partially. If the enzymes in the tissues which inactivate these substances are suppressed then inflammatory swelling is reduced. Hence the enzymes monoamine oxidase, dopa decarboxylase and dopamine β-oxidase could be considered as mediators of the inflammatory response. These views, based on experiments with substances inhibiting enzyme reactions, need further elucidation before they can be accepted.

The great problem of finding a mediator for the delayed phase still remains to be solved. It remains to be seen whether one of the active globulin fractions which have been extracted from rabbit serum might meet the specifications.[31] Such globulins are active only in homologous species but they have a prolonged effect.

Those who wish to follow in detail the arguments about mediators that have occupied the attention of many workers during recent years may be referred to the reviews by Wilhelm,[17] by Spector and Willoughby[28] and by Miles.[27]

We perhaps should not forget that, as Hadfield and Garrod suggested,[29] the increase in the permeability of capillaries following injury may be due to a direct action of the noxious stimuli on endothelium as first suggested by Cohnheim, though even this could be caused by the upset of some chemical mechanism in the vessel wall. Some recent work on this point will be mentioned in Chapter 3.

Loss of Function

Diminution or lack of function of inflamed parts is usually caused by a reflex inhibition of muscle movements associated with pain, in addition to such mechanical disability as swelling may produce. In glandular organs it may be caused by interference with the activity of the specific cells, though how this is brought about is not clear—nor, indeed, has much work been done on this subject.

REFERENCES

1. Ebert, R. H. (1965). *The Inflammatory Process*, p.1. Eds. B. W. Zweifach, L. Grant and R. T. McCluskey. New York: Academic Press.
2. Lewis, T. (1927). *The Blood Vessels of the Human Skin and their Responses.* London: Shaw & Sons, Ltd.
3. Krogh, A. (1929). *The Anatomy and Physiology of Capillaries* (Silliman Memorial Lecture). New Haven: Yale University Press.
4. Schade, H. (1924). *Münch. med. Wschr.*, **71,** 1.
5. Bruce, A. N. (1910). *Arch. exp. Path. Pharmak.*, **63,** 424.
6. Krogh, A. (1920). *J. Physiol.* (*Lond.*), **53,** 399.
7. Lewis, T., and Grant, R. T. (1924). *Heart*, **11,** 209.
8. Chapman, L. F., and Goodell, H. (1964). *Ann. N.Y. Acad. Sci.*, **116**, 990.
9. Gessler, H. (1921). *Arch. exp. Path. Pharmak.*, **91,** 366.
10. Elliott, D. F., Horton, E. W., and Lewis, G. P. (1960). *J. Physiol.* (*Lond.*), **153,** 473.
11. Drinker, C. K., and Yoffey, J. M. (1941). *Lymphatics, Lymph, and Lymphoid Tissue.* Cambridge, Mass.: Harvard University Press.
    Gives a large bibliography of work on Lymphatics.
12. Yoffey, J. M., and Courtice, F. C. (1956). *Lymphatics, Lymph, and Lymphoid Tissue*, 2nd edit. London: Edward Arnold (Publishers) Ltd.
13. Starling, E. H. (1896). *J. Physiol.* (*Lond.*), **19,** 312.
13a. Landis, E. M. (1934). *Physiol. Rev.*, **14,** 404.
14. Bhoola, K. D., Calle, J. D., and Schachter, M. (1960). *J. Physiol.* (*Lond.*), **152,** 75.
15. Miles, A. A., and Miles, E. M. (1952). *J. Physiol.* (*Lond.*), **118,** 228.
16. Logan, G., and Wilhelm D. L. (1966). *Brit. J. exp. Path.*, **47,** 286.
17. Wilhelm, D. L. (1965). In *The Inflammatory Process*, p. 389. Eds. B. W. Zweifach, L. Grant and R. T. McCluskey. New York: Academic Press.
18. Miles, A. A. (1958–59). *Lectures on the Scientific Basis of Medicine*, **8,** 198.
19. Menkin, V. (1940). *Dynamics of Inflammation.* New York: The Macmillan Company.
    This gives a full bibliography on the subject.
20. Margolis, J., and Bishop, E. A. (1963). *Aust. J. exp. Biol. med. Sci.*, **41,** 293.
21. Schayer, R. W., and Ganley, O. H. (1959). *Amer. J. Physiol.*, **197,** 721.

22. WEDD, A. M., and DRURY, A. N. (1934). *J. Pharmacol. exp. Ther.*, **50,** 157.
23. GREEN, H. N., and STONER, H. B. (1950). *Biological Actions of the Adenine Nucleotides.* London: H. K. Lewis & Co.
24. SPECTOR, W. G., and WILLOUGHBY, D. A. (1957). *J. Path. Bact.*, **73,** 133.
25. LOGAN, G., and WILHELM, D. L. (1966). *Brit. J. exp. Path.*, **47,** 300.
25a. GREAVES, M., and SHUSTER, S. (1967). *J. Physiol. (Lond.)*, **193**, 255.
26. COTRAN, R. S., and MAJNO, G. (1964). *Ann. N.Y. Acad. Sci.*, **116,** Art. 3, 750.
27. MILES, A. A. (1964). *Ann. N.Y. Acad. Sci.*, **116,** Art. 3, 855.
28. SPECTOR, W. G., and WILLOUGHBY, D. A. (1965). In *The Inflammatory Process*, p. 427. Eds. B. W. ZWEIFACH, L. GRANT and R. T. MCCLUSKEY. New York: Academic Press.
29. HADFIELD, G., and GARROD, L. P. (1947). *Recent Advances in Pathology*, 5th edit. London: J. & A. Churchill.
30. WILHELM, D. L., and MASON, B. (1960). *Brit. J. exp. Path.*, **41,** 487.
31. MULLER, H. K., SALASOO, I., and WILHELM, D. L. (1968). *Aust. J. exp. Biol. med. Sci.*, **46,** 165.

There are many articles and books on various aspects of inflammation. The following may be consulted with profit:

METCHNIKOFF, E. (1893). *Lectures on the Comparative Pathology of Inflammation.* London: Kegan Paul, Trench, Trübner & Co.

ADAMI, J. G. (1909). *Inflammation.* London: Macmillan & Co.

LEWIS, T. (1927). *The Blood Vessels of the Human Skin and their Responses.* London: Shaw & Sons.

COHNHEIM, J. (1882). *Lectures on General Pathology.* London: The New Sydenham Society, 1889, tr. into English.

The Inflammatory Process, edited by B. W. ZWEIFACH, L. GRANT and R. T. MCCLUSKEY. (1965). New York: Academic Press.

The Acute Inflammatory Response. By a number of authors. Edited by Harold E. Whipple (1964). *Ann. N.Y. Acad. Sci.* **116,** Art. 3, 747–1084.

Chapter 3

INFLAMMATION

BY H. W. FLOREY

MICROSCOPICAL OBSERVATIONS

Structure of Small Blood Vessels

THE lining of all blood vessels consists of flattened endothelial cells which, when viewed in cross section with the light microscope, are so thin as to present little evidence of cellular structure other than the nucleus (FIG. 2). When appropriately stained by silver nitrate or some other methods and viewed *en face*, endothelial cells are seen to be large nucleated plates apparently joined together at their periphery by a darkly stained substance which has been called "cement". A "typical" cell is about 3 microns thick in the neighbourhood of the nucleus but it thins out to 0·2 micron or less at the periphery. FIGURE 1 illustrates these points, but it should be noted that the flat endothelial cells of other species do not have precisely the same shape as those of the rabbit.

Electron microscopy has during recent years considerably extended our knowledge of the structure of endothelial cells. They have the usual cell constituents such as a nucleus, mitochondria, endoplasmic reticulum with attached ribosomes, a Golgi complex, and centrosomes. They also contain multivesicular bodies, "dense" bodies, and elongated structures which were first described by

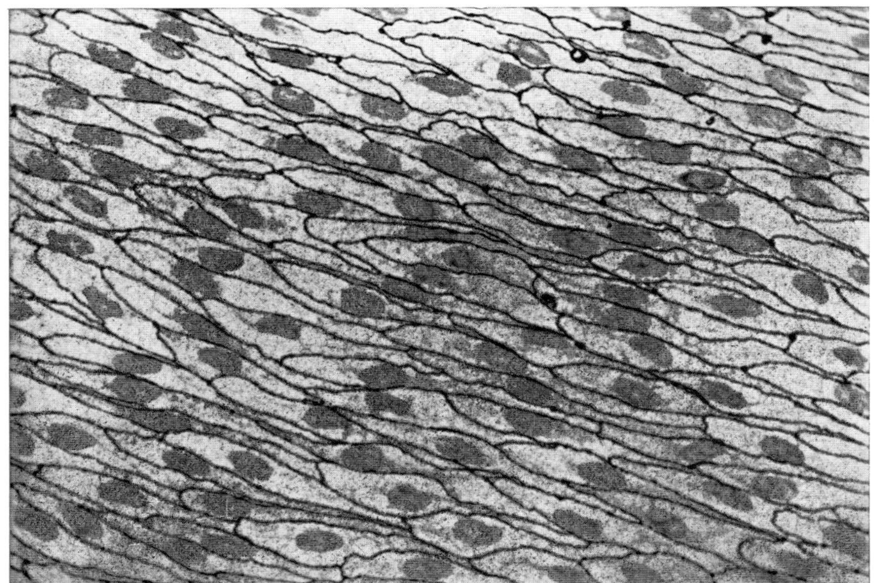

3/FIG. 1.—Endothelium from the aorta of a rabbit viewed *en face*. The flat nucleated cells are outlined by treatment with silver nitrate. (× 360.) (From Poole, Sanders and Florey.[10d])

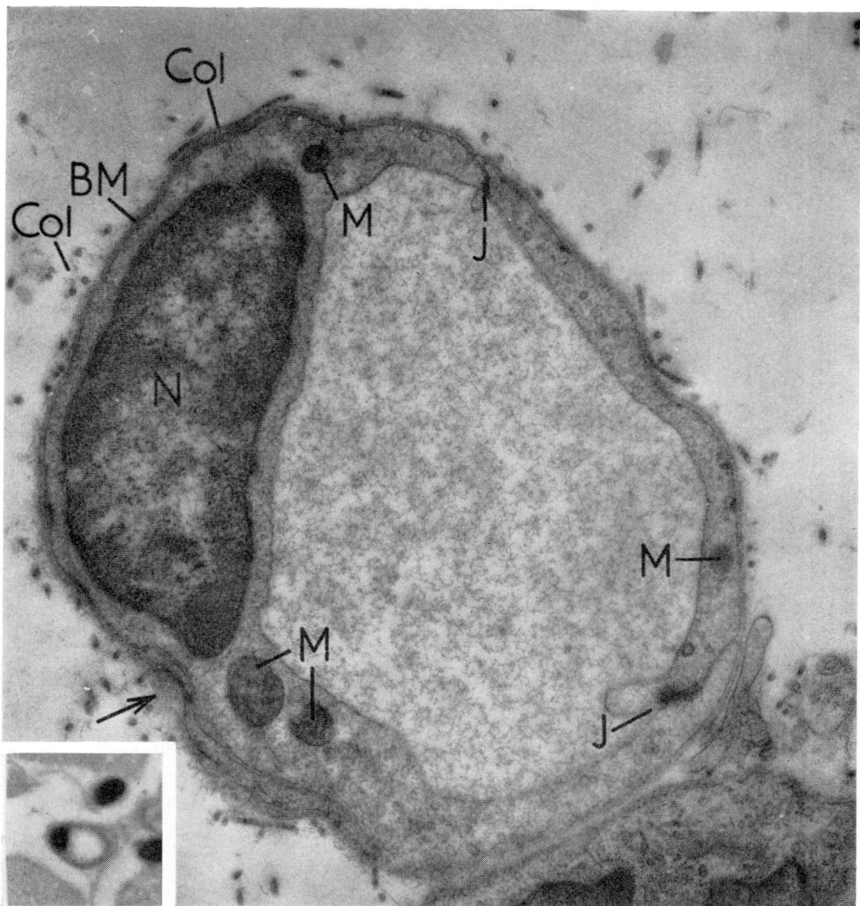

3/FIG. 2.—Electron micrograph of a cross section of a capillary from the subcutaneous tissue of a guinea-pig. This shows a nucleus (N), mitochondria (M), and cell junctions (J) with electron-dense zones near the lumen which have been called attachment belts, adhesion plates or desmosomes. The cytoplasm contains very numerous vesicles, as first described by Palade.[12] A basement membrane (B)M surrounds the vessel. The basement membrane appears fibrillary in certain parts, e.g. at (↑). Collagen fibres (Col) cut longitudinally and transversely can be seen external to the basement membrane. Some fine fibres in relation to the collagen fibres are also seen. (× 17,500.)

For comparison, in the bottom left-hand corner is a cross section of a capillary of a rabbit's tongue viewed in a light microscope with a 2 mm. oil immersion lens. (× 1300.)

Weibel and Palade[1] (FIGS. 2, 3, 4, 5 and 6). Sometimes fine fibres are seen within the cytoplasm.

The wall of a capillary may be formed of a single cell bent round to enclose a lumen so that in a cross section only one cell junction appears, or in one cross section there may be two or more junctions, indicating that at that point more than one cell contributes to the circumference.

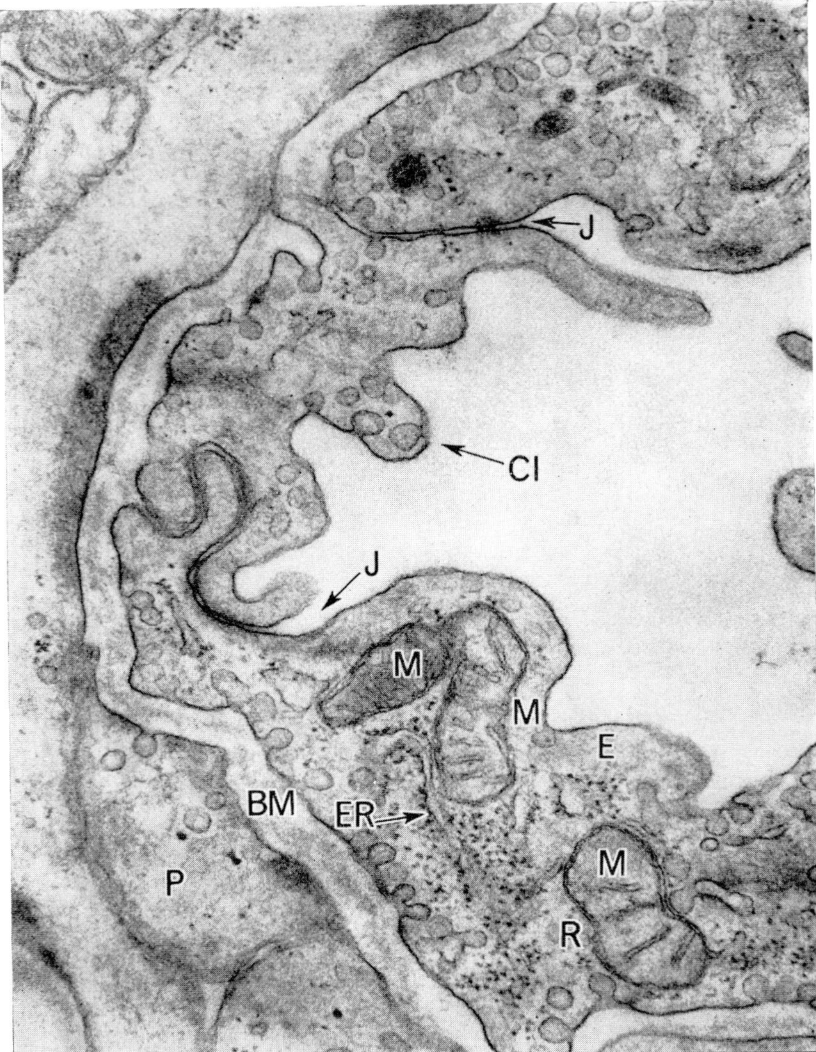

3/FIG. 3.—This picture shows parts of three endothelial cells (E) and two junctions (J). The space between the cells varies in width and at the constricted portions the cytoplasm is darker. These areas are sometimes referred to as "tight junctions." Mitochondria (M), ribosomes (R) and endoplasmic reticulum (ER) are present. Caveolæ intracellulares (CI) are present on both surfaces of the cells. The basement membrane (BM) is between the endothelial cells and one surface of a pericyte (P) which also contains caveolæ. (× 50,000.) (From Florey.[10c])

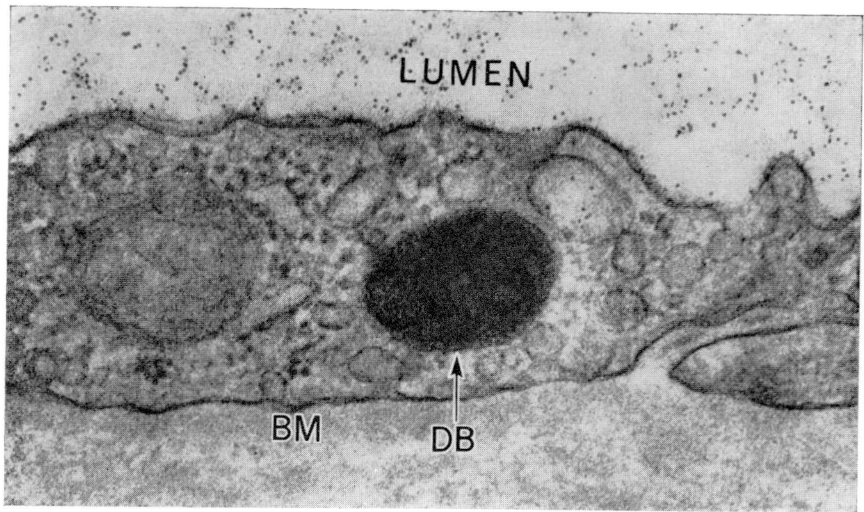

3/Fig. 4.—A "dense" body (DB) in the endothelium of a pancreatic capillary. The fine particles in the lumen are molecules of ferritin which have been injected intravenously. The basement membrane is marked BM. (× 86,000.) (From Florey,[10c])

Two structures which are of particular interest in a consideration of the changes in acute inflammation are a vesicular system and the intercellular junction.

The surface membrane of endothelial cells is infolded into the substance of the cell so that in their simplest form flask-shaped structures which have been called caveolæ intracellulares are formed (Fig. 7). Like the outer plasma

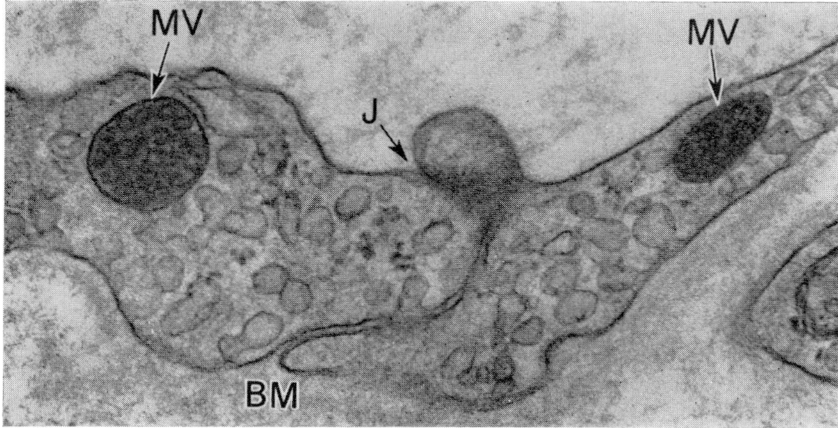

3/Fig. 5.—Two multivesicular bodies (MV) in two endothelial cells of the pancreas. These bodies are globular and are bounded by a unit membrane. Within this membrane numerous small vesicles are enclosed. Caveolæ intracellulares can be seen. The junction (J) between the two cells is shown and the basement membrane (BM). (× 63,000.) (From Florey.[10c])

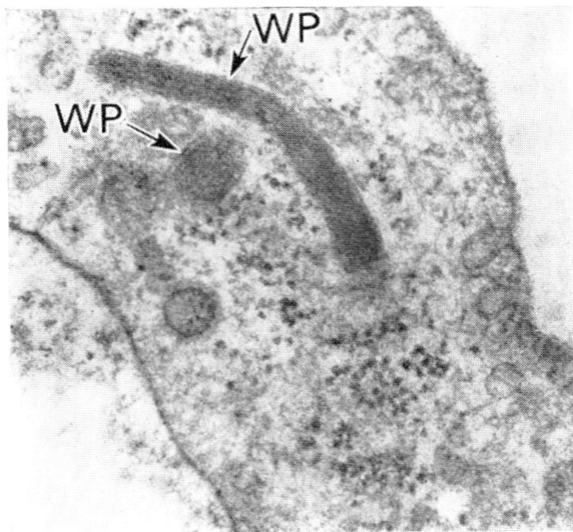

3/FIG. 6.—Bodies (WP) first described by Weibel and Palade are present in this endothelial cell from the aorta of a rat. One body is cut longitudinally and the other transversely. Their function is unknown. (× 73,000.) (From Florey.[10c])

membrane of the cell the caveolæ are bounded by a "unit membrane" which is composed of two darkly staining leaflets with a less electron dense layer between them (FIG. 8). There are frequently more caveolæ on the external surface than on the luminal surface. Though usually having a simple flask-shaped appearance they are sometimes multiple, a number of caveolæ opening into one another and to the surface by a common orifice (FIG. 9). Apparently isolated vesicles are encountered within the body of the cell. The caveolæ and vesicles are some 500–700Å in diameter.

Another type of vesicle—a "coated" vesicle or an acanthosome—is occasionally met with. Such vesicles appear to be quite distinct from the smooth vesicles just described (FIGS. 10 and 11).

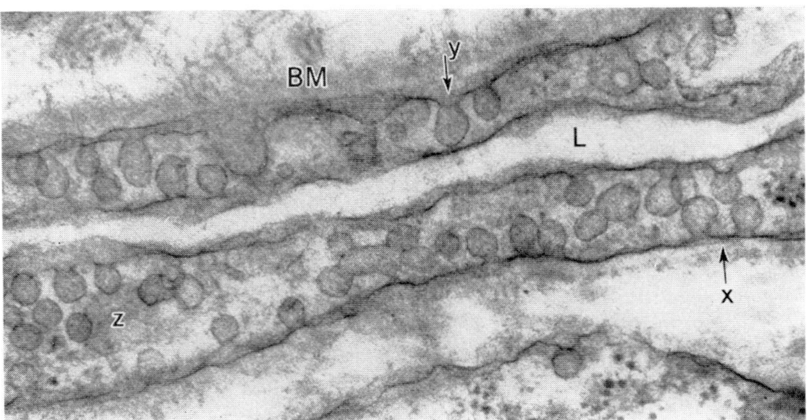

3/FIG. 7.—Endothelium of a cardiac capillary to show caveolæ intracellulares. They appear to be infoldings of the plasma membrane of the cell. They are on both the luminal (L) and external surfaces of the cell. In some places they appear to touch one another—for example at X—and some appear almost to span the full width of the cell (Y). At Z there may be some vesicles which are isolated in the cell but this appearance may be due to the angle at which the section is cut. (× 70,000.) (From Florey.[10c])

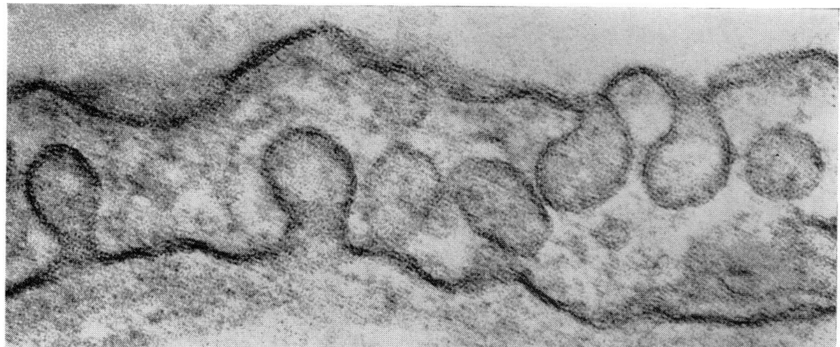

3/FIG. 8.—Caveolæ intracellulares in an endothelial cell of a cardiac capillary of a mouse. The walls of the caveolæ are continuous with the unit membrane enclosing the cell. A basement membrane can be seen at the lower part of the picture. (× 160,000.) (From Florey.[10a])

Much attention has been paid to the area in which endothelial cells meet—the cell junctions. Ideas on their precise structure have undergone an evolution but even now finality has not been reached. Based on the picture furnished by staining with silver nitrate and examination in the light microscope it was supposed that the cells were held together by cement much as is a brick wall (FIG. 1). Chambers and Zeifach,[2, 3] on the basis of observations on the living frog,

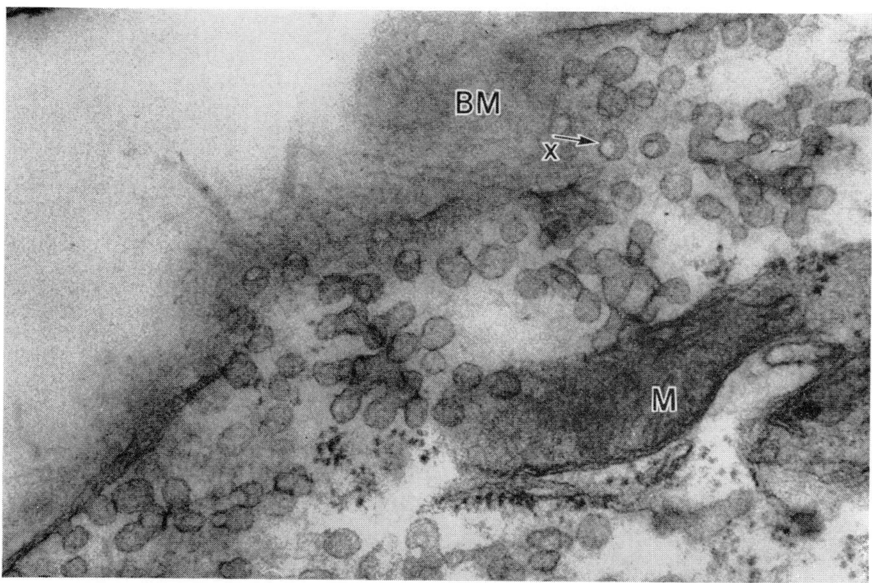

3/FIG. 9.—An endothelial cell cut obliquely is shown. It can be seen that caveolæ intracellulares are not always simple invaginations but that they may join one another to form clusters. The pale areas seen in some vesicles—for example at X—are the mouths of caveolæ sectioned parallel to the cell surface. M is a mitochondrion and BM the basement membrane. (× 75,000.) (From Jennings and Florey.[10])

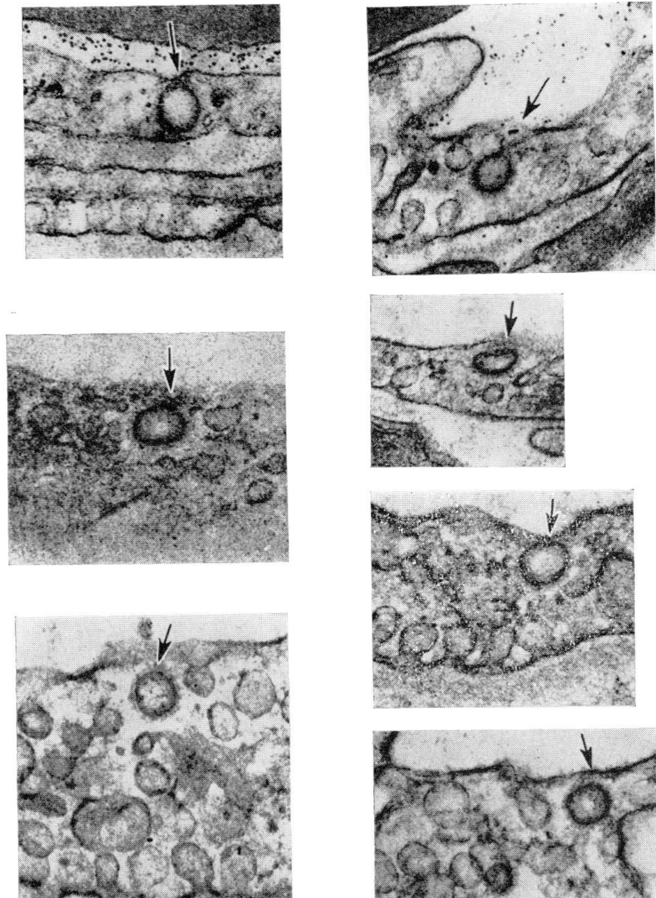

3/FIG. 10.—A collection of "coated vesicles" and corresponding caveolæ from endothelial cells of a number of organs. These coated vesicles (arrows) are more prominent and larger than the usual caveolæ intracellulares and associated vesicles. They have a coat of fine "bristles" and appear to have a dense lining. They are sometimes called acanthosomes. (× 70,000.) (From Florey.[10c])

propounded the view that the cement was secreted by the endothelial cells and that it was a calcium proteinate. With the advent of the electron microscope it was discovered that the space between endothelial cells was very narrow, being only some 150 to 200 Å wide and it was concluded that there could be no substantial amount of cement, as had been suggested by silvered preparations. The profiles of the junctions are often sinuous showing that the free edges of the cells are interdigitated.

It was found that there were areas in the profiles of the junctions seen in electron microscopic sections in which the cell membranes and the adjacent cytoplasm were denser than those of the rest of the cell in the immediate neigh-

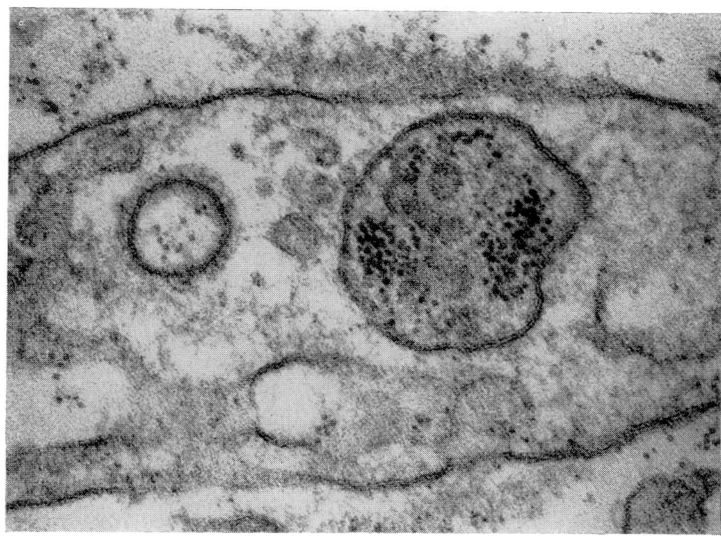

3/FIG. 11.—A multivesicular body containing ferritin is shown together with an acanthosome which also contains molecules of ferritin. The ferritin had been injected intravenously. The function of acanthosomes is not known but they are capable, like the multivesicular bodies, of segregating fine particles or large molecules. (× 120,000.) (From Florey.[10a])

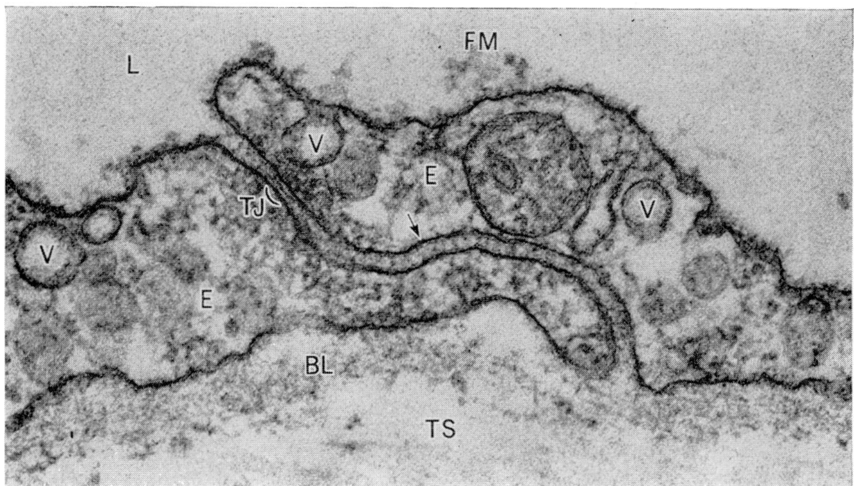

3/FIG. 12.—Junction between two endothelial cells (E) in capillary wall separating vessel lumen (L) from tissue space (TS). The unit membranes of the endothelial cells are visible intermittently (indicated at arrow) with dense cytoplasmic layer and paler outer layer. Flocculent material (FM) appears to attach to the luminal surface of the endothelial cells (outer leaflet of unit membrane). The tight junction (TJ) characteristically displays the central dark element (fused outer layers of units) separated symmetrically by two light zones (central, lipid layers of units) from two dark lines which are the cytoplasmic layers of the unit membranes of each endothelial cell. Vesicles (V) also show unit membrane. Basement lamina (BL) is granular and discontinuous. Mouse diaphragm. (× 100,000.) (From Luft.[7])

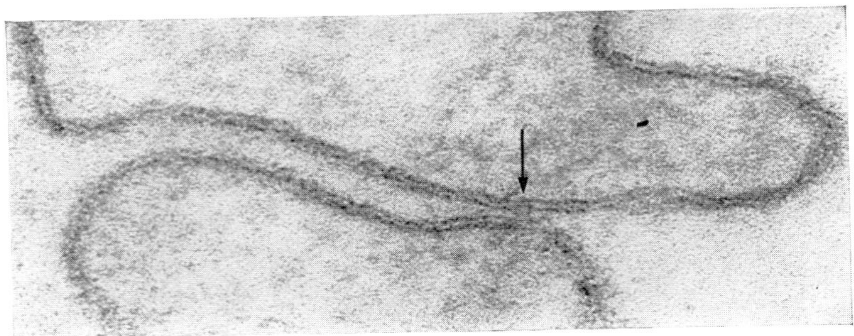

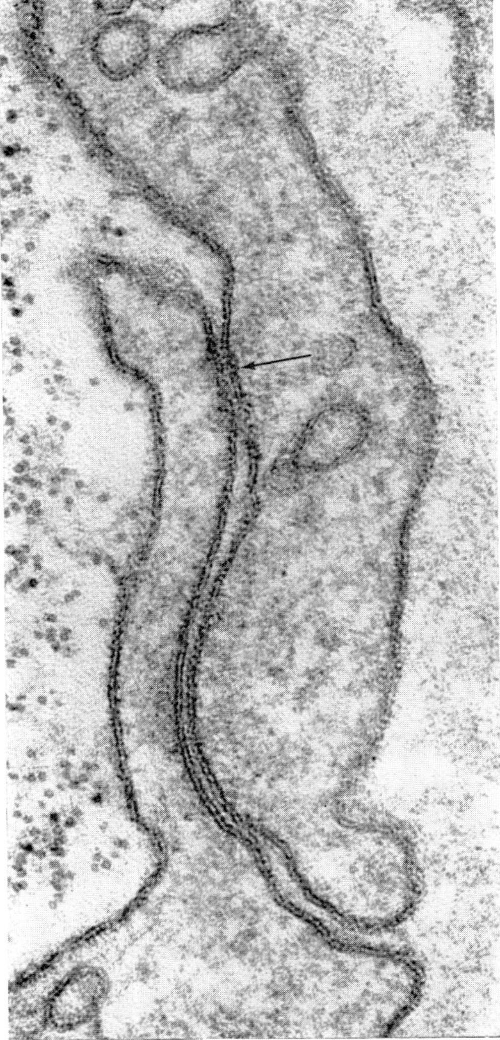

3/Fig. 13 (*above*).—An intercellular junction in a cardiac capillary of a mouse. The junction at the level of the arrow has a gap of about 40 Å between the adjacent unit membranes of the plasmalemmata. This gap contains amorphous electron opaque material. The lumen of the capillary is to the right. (× 250,000.) (From Karnovsky.[6])

3/Fig. 14 (*left*).—Junction between endothelial cells in a small vessel of the adrenal cortex of a mouse. The external leaflets of the plasma membranes are touching at the arrow but do not appear to be completely fused. Ferritin was injected intravenously 25 min. before the specimen was taken. None of the ferritin, the molecules of which can be seen in the lumen at the left of the picture, has passed into the junction. (× 170,000.) (From Florey.[10a])

bourhood (FIGS. 2 and 3). Such areas have been given different names at different times. The terms adhesion plate and attachment belt convey the idea that it is believed that in this area the cells are attached firmly to one another. The area has sometimes been called a desmosome on the assumption that it is similar to the desmosomes found between epithelial cells.

Improved technique has revealed further detail in this special area of the junctions. Muir and Peters[4] published pictures in which a dark line was shown extending over a considerable distance along the apparent gap between the plasma membranes at the attachment belt. This line they interpreted as being due to the fusion of the outer leaflets of the adjacent "unit membranes" which bound the endothelial cells. This type of structure can be seen in FIG. 12. It is not without interest that their most striking pictures were obtained from the brain, the small vessels of which have now been demonstrated visually to be less permeable to large molecules than vessels elsewhere[4a]. Farquhar and Palade[5] demonstrated very clearly the fusion of the outer leaflets of unit membranes at junctions between epithelia but similarly beautiful illustrations of fusion at endothelial junction have been hard to find. Nevertheless the conception of what became known as the "tight junction" has been launched and taken firm hold. But the idea that the outer leaflets of the plasma membranes of endothelial cells are fused over a considerable distance has been challenged by Karnovsky[6], who has succeeded in resolving the unit membranes of the cells contiguous to a junction over their whole length. Pictures have been secured showing that although the outer leaflets touch at certain points they may not necessarily be fused. Indeed in contiguous sections one section may show touching or fusion at some point while the corresponding area in the next section does not show it. These pictures have been obtained after prolonged staining with uranyl acetate, a procedure which may extract some cell constituent and so enable a clearer view of the membranes to be secured than after other methods of dealing with the tissue (FIGS. 13 and 14).

The space between endothelial cells can sometimes look "empty" but even after simple fixation with osmium tetroxide and staining with uranyl acetate it is possible to see that some electron dense material is present in the junctions (FIG. 15). Luft[7] has published some striking pictures obtained after staining with ruthenium red which is used by botanists for staining pectin. With this stain a dense material is present in spaces between collagen bundles in the connective tissue, in the basement membrane surrounding capillaries, and in the space between endothelial cells, although here it is mainly seen in the area between the external surface and the "tight junction", a distribution which Luft is inclined to attribute to his technical procedures. In addition to the places mentioned dense material is present in caveolæ intracellulares and on the luminal surface of endothelial cells (FIGS. 16, 17 and 18).

Luft suggests that the caveolæ intracellulares may be the area from which the dark staining material is secreted after being manufactured in the endothelial cell. He is inclined to believe that the material is an acid mucopolysaccharide which his technique retains in the tissues better than other methods, as well as staining it. We are thus back at the conception that there is an extremely thin layer of "cement" of a mucopolysaccharide nature between endothelial cells and that there is a thin layer of the same material covering the surface of

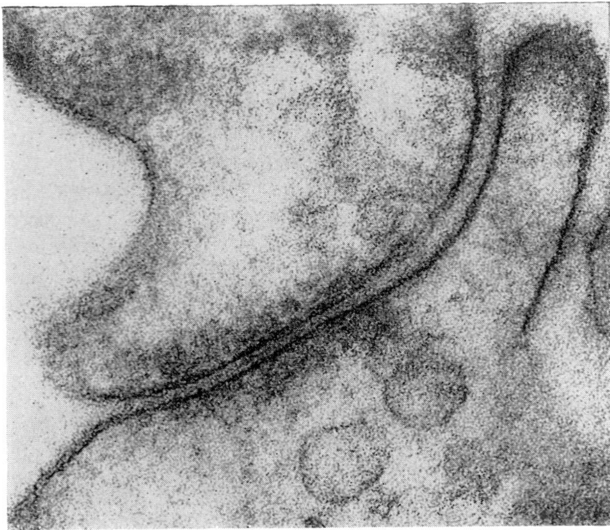

3/FIG. 15.—A junction between two endothelial cells. The space between the cells is filled with some dense material. The dense area in the surrounding cytoplasm associated with the narrowest part of the junction can be seen. (× 150,000.) (From Jennings and Florey.[10])

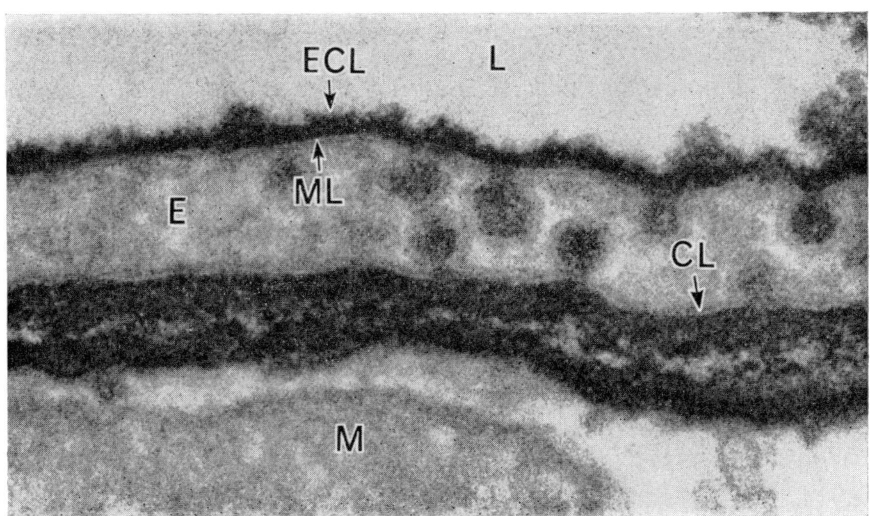

3/FIG. 16.—Portion of capillary wall. Endothelial cell (E) separates lumen (L) from muscle cell (M). Two layers of the unit membrane are visible; the cytoplasmic leaflet (CL) (pale since no uranyl/lead staining was used), and the lighter middle layer (ML). The density of the ruthenium red-labelled endocapillary layer (ECL) begins at the outer leaflet of the unit and extends several hundred Ångstroms into the lumen to end in an irregular, fluffy, indeterminate boundary. (× 140,000.) (From Luft.[7])

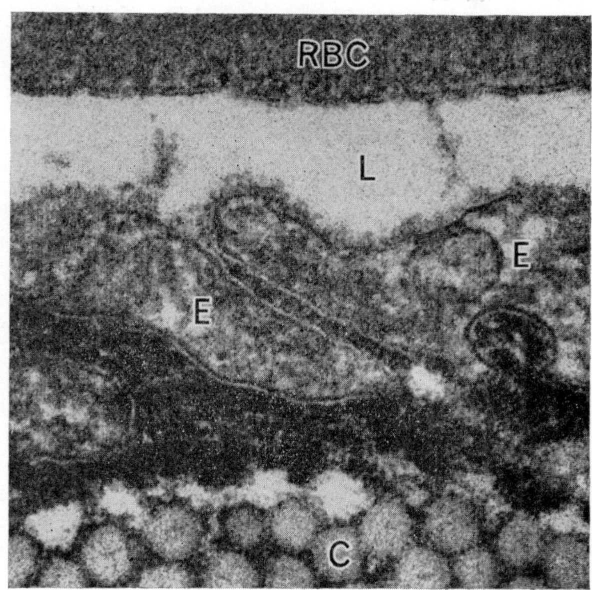

3/FIG. 17.—Junction from capillary, with erythrocyte (RBC) in lumen (L). Collagen fibrils (C) in the tissue space are outlined by material reactive to ruthenium red. A tongue of density extends from the tissue space along the junction toward the lumen but is stopped at the "tight" segment. Unit membrane is visible. (× 140,000.) (From Luft.[7])

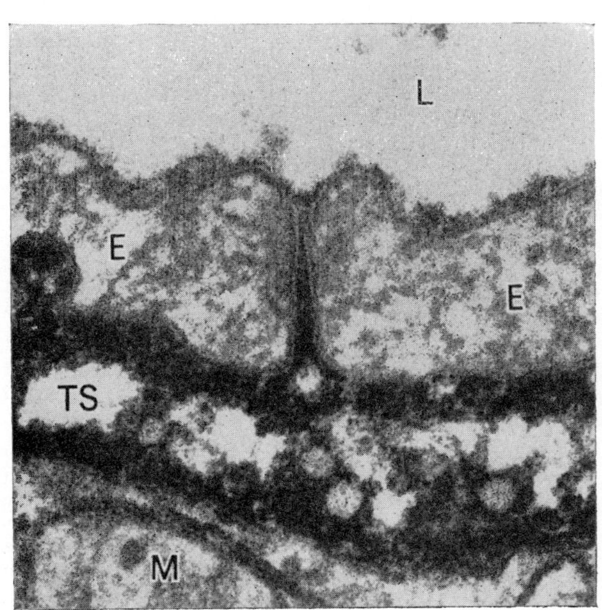

3/FIG. 18.—Junction from capillary, showing possible penetration of ruthenium red density from the tissue space (TS) through the tight segment and into the lumen (L). The tight junction is slightly widened (distance from centre-to-centre of the light, lipid layers is about 75Å.) (× 140,000.) (From Luft.[7])

endothelial cells which corresponds to the endocapillary layer of a protein nature proposed by Chambers and Zweifach[2, 3] on theoretical grounds.

While the discussion of the nature of the gap between endothelial cells has engaged attention the nature and function of the darkened cytoplasm seen in relation to "tight junctions" seems to have passed out of sight. Perhaps it is involved in the passage of large molecules between neighbouring cells (for it has been shown that such transfers do in fact occur between some types of cell), and it may have some function in communication between cells.

In addition to the suggestion that the caveolæ of endothelial cells may secrete mucopolysaccharide and their possible role in the transport of material across the vessel wall, it has been shown by Marchesi and Barrnett[8] that the caveolæ in the capillaries of skeletal muscle contain phosphatases (possibly adenosine triphosphatase) as judged by histochemical reactions. It has not been demonstrated what function this serves.

Endothelial cells secrete an activator of fibrinolysin[9] (FIG. 19) but whether the caveolæ are involved is not known. Finally it has been suggested[10] that the caveolæ are a means of increasing the surface area of cells so that diffusion of small molecules across the cell membrane can take place more readily.

In the region of the cellular junctions, and sometimes elsewhere, profiles of "flaps" are not infrequently seen on the internal surfaces of endothelial cells which may have some function in the intake of larger particles, but this is not certain (FIG. 20).

A basement membrane surrounds small blood vessels such as capillaries and small venules. It consists of two zones the outer of which is electron dense and in some preparations appears to be composed of very fine fibres, though it is possible that the fibrillary appearance is artifactual. The inner zone is electron transparent. Together the two zones are about 500 Å thick and they are stated to increase in thickness with age. The basement membrane is closely applied to the endothelial cells and follows the shape of the vessels (FIG. 21). Perhaps it is an elastic structure and some have supposed that it is important in maintaining the integrity of the small blood vessels. The chemical composition of the basement membrane is still disputed although some evidence has been produced that it is of a collagenous nature. As we have seen, Luft considers that it contains a mucopolysaccharide similar to that occurring in the intercellular junctions.

3/FIG. 19.—Endothelial cells removed after freezing from the inferior vena cava of a dog. The cells were covered by a 1 per cent bovine fibrin clot and the preparation was then incubated for 45 min. The endothelial cells (E) are surrounded by an area in which the fibrin has been dissolved, the edge of the lysis being marked by arrows. The fibrin film is intact over a group of subendothelial cells (SEC). (× 60.) (From Warren.[9])

3/FIG. 20.—"Flaps" on the internal surface of endothelial cells. They occur particularly near junctions between endothelial cells, but they are to be found elsewhere. They may be associated with the ingestion of large particles, but their function is unknown. (× 60,000.) (From Florey.[10c])

3/FIG. 21.—Endothelial cell of a cardiac capillary. This shows the double nature of the basement membrane (BM), which is composed of a lighter part adjoining the external membrane of the cell and a parallel darker part. It is sometimes said that the basement membrane is fibrillary. While this appears to be so, the appearance may be a fixation artifact, as the coagulated plasma in the lumen and on the surface of the endothelial cell does not look strikingly different from the basement membrane. L, lumen. (× 75,000.) (From Florey.[10c])

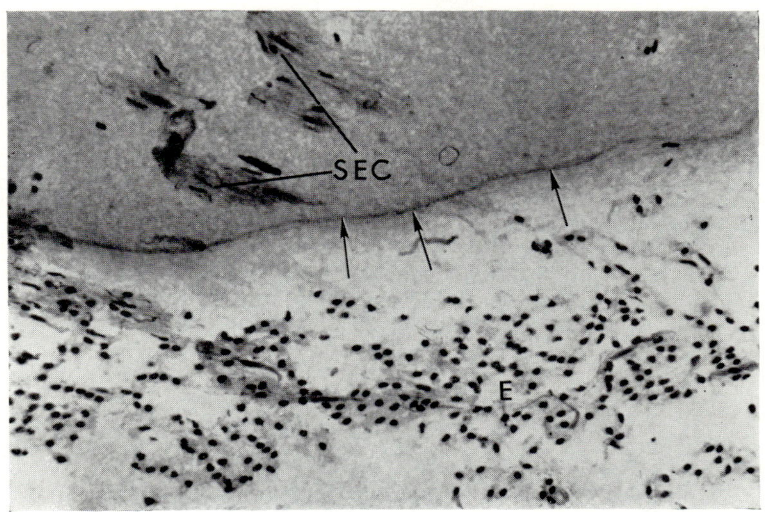

3/Fig. 19

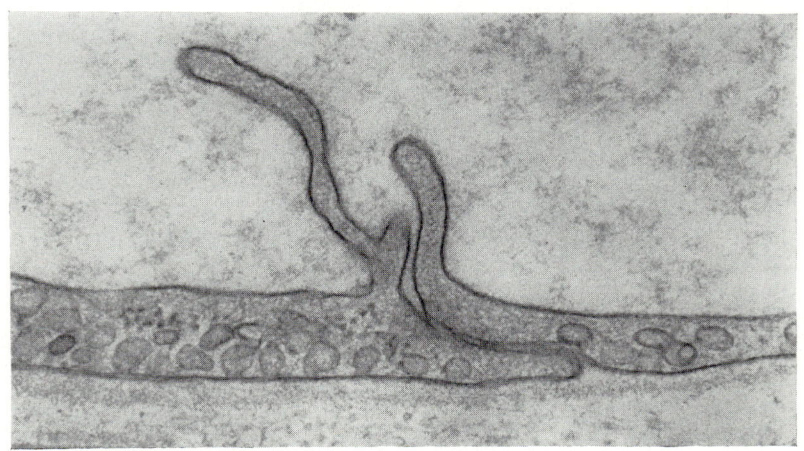

3/Fig. 20

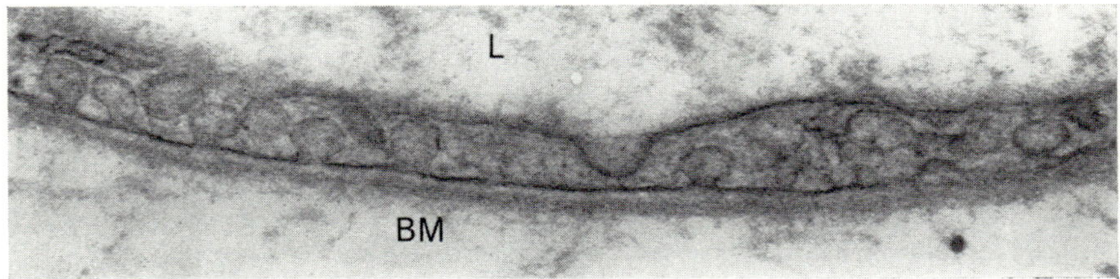

3/Fig. 21

The basement membrane often appears to be closely associated with surrounding collagen fibres (FIG. 22) and other finer fibrils the precise nature of which is not known. This association may have some relation to that other basement membrane which has long been described as the result of light microscopic examination and which can be coloured with polysaccharide stains such as periodic acid-Schiff. It is impossible with the light microscope to see the narrow and apparently well-defined basement membrane of electron microscopy and the exact relationship between the two structures remains to be determined.

It seems probable that the vascular basement membrane is elaborated by the endothelial cells, though in the large arteries of some animals no distinct basement membrane exists round the endothelium.

Closely connected with capillaries and venules are flat cells with many

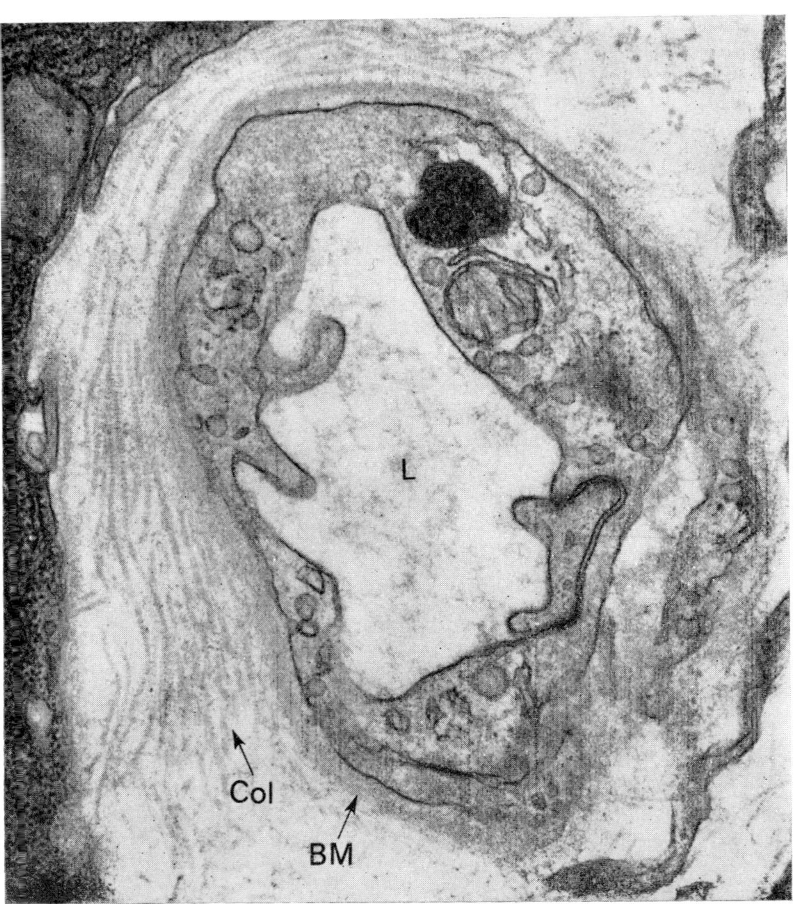

3/FIG. 22.—Capillary in pancreas. The vessel is surrounded by a basement membrane (BM) which is intimately associated with collagen (Col) fibres, which are oriented concentrically to the capillary. L, lumen. (× 42,000.) (From Florey.[10c])

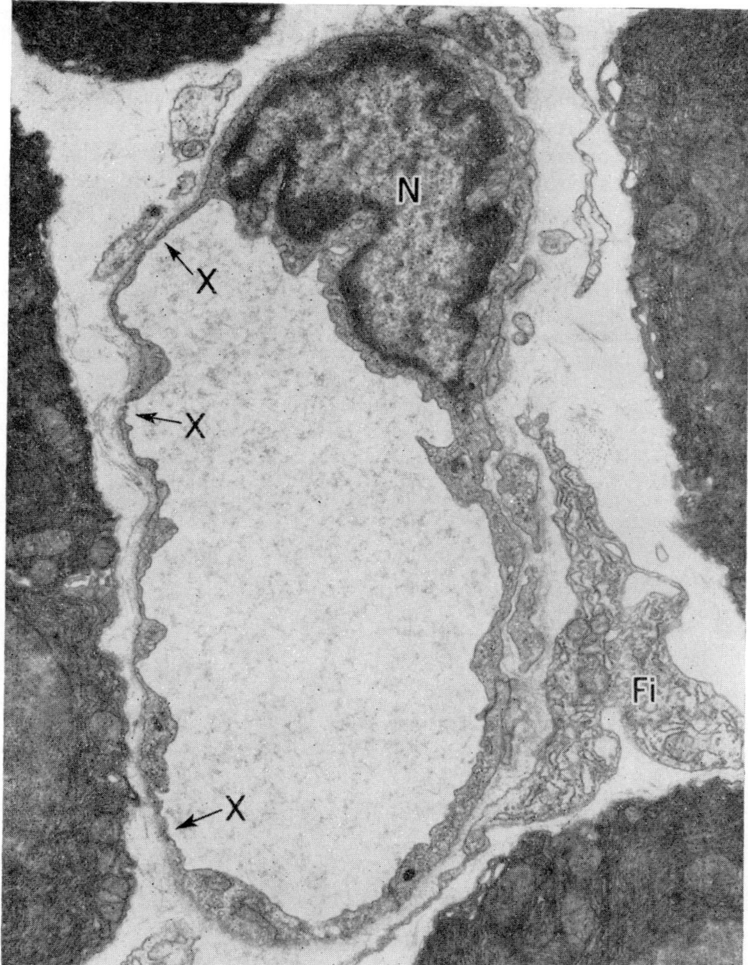

3/FIG. 23.—A capillary from the pancreas. The endothelial cells are of varying thickness and at certain points (X) are very tenuous. A fibroblast (Fi) is in the space between the capillary and the surrounding acinar cells. N is a nucleus. (× 9,000.) (From Florey.[10c])

elongated processes which are commonly called pericytes or adventitial cells. A nucleus is only rarely encountered by electron microscopy but cross sections of their fine processes which are enclosed in the basement membrane are common. The pericytes contain organelles similar to those of endothelium, and caveolæ intracellulares, which are often more common on the external than on the internal surface, are present. Some workers consider that transitional forms between pericytes and smooth muscle cells exist.

The above description of endothelium, particularly that of capillaries and venules, applies to vessels in cardiac and skeletal muscle and subcutaneous tissue and it is on vessels of this type that most of the observations on acute inflammation have been made. Nevertheless the electron microscope has demonstrated that the endothelial cells of all fine vessels do not have the same structure. Those in the glomeruli of the kidney, and in the pancreas, intestine, pituitary gland, adrenal and thyroid glands, and in some other tissues (see review by Majno) have "pores" or areas of extreme thinness which are in certain cases closed by a single plasma membrane or even possibly by the outer leaflet only of the unit membrane.[11] Elsewhere such fenestrated endothelial cells have areas in which cytoplasm contains caveolæ and other structures of the usual appearance (FIGS. 23 and 24).

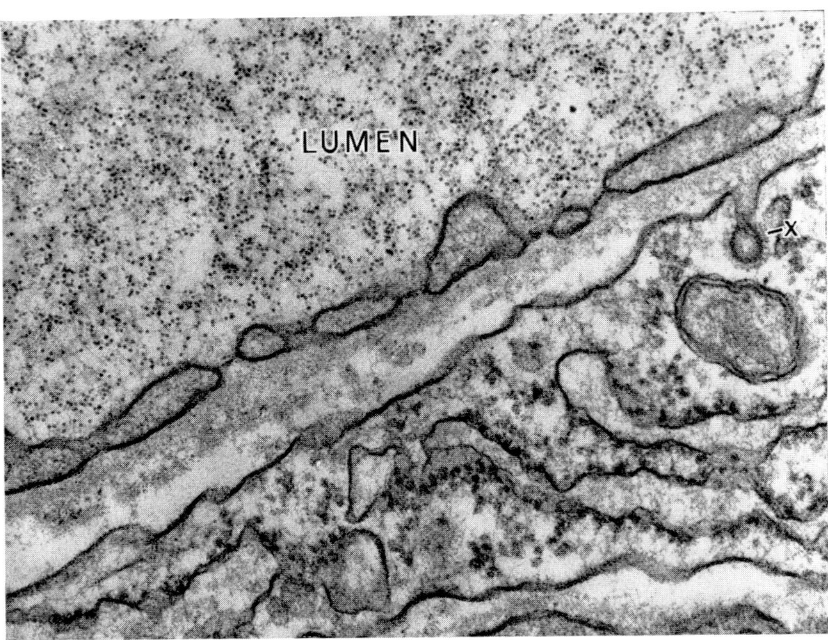

3/FIG. 24.—Portion of an endothelial cell from the pancreas of a mouse to show the "pores' across which a thin membrane stretches. Ferritin which had been injected intravenously is present in high concentration in the lumen but very little has escaped extravascularly—the "pores" not being very porous. At x there is an acanthosome in an epithelial cell of the pancreas. (× 68,000.)

The endothelial cells of the lungs have extensive tenuous areas of cytoplasm contained between two plasma membranes as well as thicker areas with the usual caveolæ (FIG. 25). In most species the sinusoids of the liver and bone marrow are commonly described as being lined by endothelium between the cells of which are substantial gaps through which the plasma in the lumen of the vessel can pass freely to the extravascular spaces. Nevertheless it is not uncommon to find well marked junctions between very tenuous endothelial cells (FIG. 26). The endothelium of the cerebral capillaries is closely invested by neuroglia, and is remarkable in that it contains very few of the caveolæ intracellulares which are so prominent in the capillaries of cardiac and skeletal muscle.

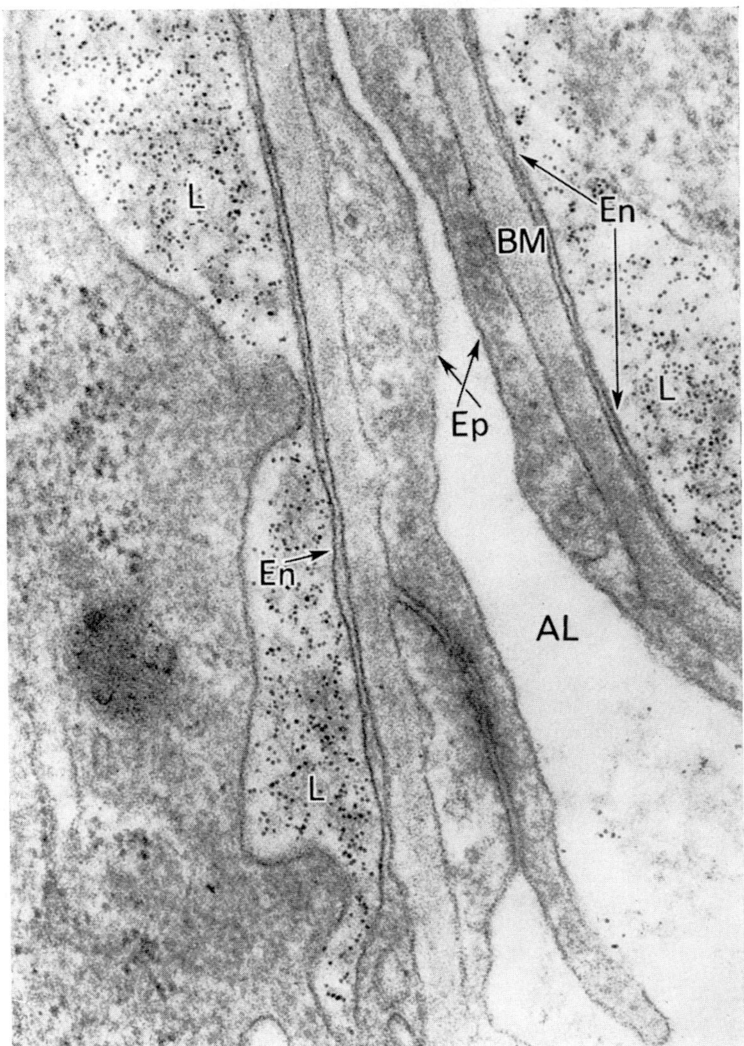

3/FIG. 25.—Capillaries bordering an alveolus of lung. The very tenuous nature of the endothelium (En) can be seen. It consists of a thin layer of cytoplasm sandwiched between two unit membranes. The thick basement membrane (BM) is shared with the epithelial cells (Ep) lining the alveolus (AL). The endothelium of the capillaries also contains thicker areas with caveolæ. A small portion of such an area is at the extreme bottom of the picture. Ferritin is within the lumens (L) of the capillaries. (× 90,000.) (From Florey.[10c])

Thus the electron microscope has shown clearly that the wall of a small blood vessel is not simply a nucleated membrane, the structure and properties of which could be likened to a semi-permeable membrane made of cellophane.

Transport across the Capillary Wall

As we saw in Chapter 2 one of the striking features of acute inflammation is the increase in the permeability of small blood vessels, so that they allow the passage even of large concentrations of plasma proteins into the surrounding

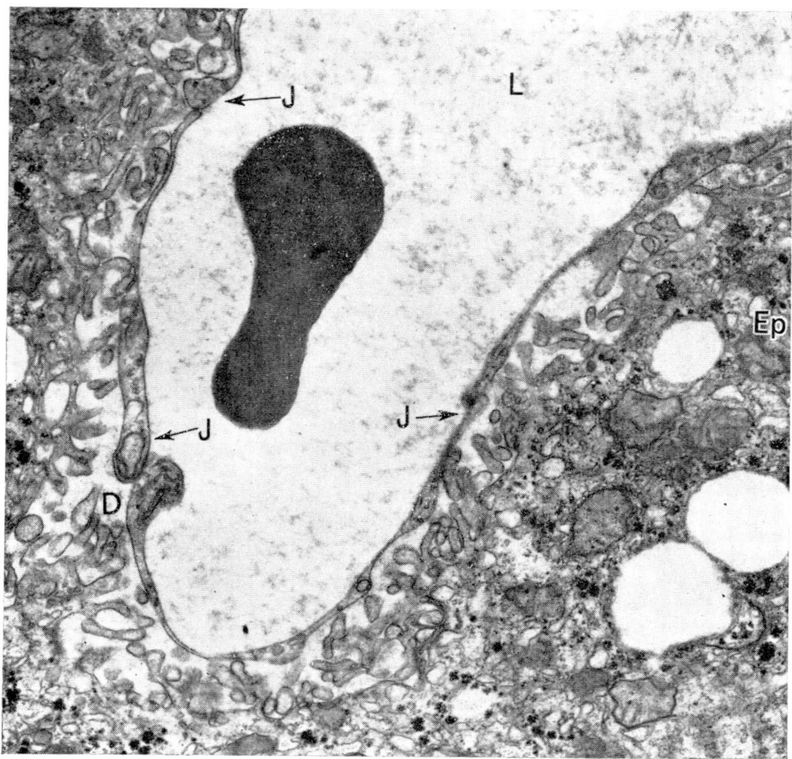

3/Fig. 26.—Endothelial cells lining a liver sinusoid and connected by junctions (J). The very tenuous cytoplasm rests on the villi of the underlying epithelial cells (Ep) in the space of Disse (D). L, lumen. (× 18,500.) (From Florey.[10c])

tissue. Can morphological changes be seen in the capillaries and venules which explain the increased permeability? Before discussing this it will be necessary to look briefly at the theories that have been put forward to explain the physiological transfer of water and dissolved substances across the walls of small blood vessels.

No morphological basis emerged from the older observations for the idea that fluids and large molecules leaving a normal capillary traversed the cell cytoplasm, but certain mathematical and experimental considerations led to the conclusion that the endothelial cells of capillaries might have pores in them which theoretically might be cylinders of a radius of from 30–45 Å and which existed at a density of 1–2 × 10^9 per sq. cm. of endothelial surface. Through these pores water and lipid-insoluble molecules of various sizes could pass. There is no reason to suppose that the pores need actually be cylindrical. Even the large protein molecules of plasma could penetrate through such pores, but the restriction to the passage of protein molecules would be sufficient to allow of a considerable degree of molecular sieving at normal rates of filtration. Not all capillaries are equally permeable, those of the glomeruli, for example, being estimated to be 100 times more permeable than those of muscle. From most normal capillaries relatively few large molecules do in fact escape.

It should be possible to see pores of the postulated size with the electron microscopes now in use, but although technical procedures would appear to be adequate to demonstrate them none has been found.

It has been suggested by their discoverer Palade[12] that the caveolæ intracellulares and associated vesicles play a part in transporting fluid and dissolved substances across the endothelial cells. He proposed that the plasma membrane of the luminal surface of the endothelial cell enfolds and engulfs plasma from the lumen by a process which has been called micropinocytosis. The caveolæ intracellulares thus formed and containing plasma are pinched off after reaching a certain size and pass as vesicles across the cytoplasm to the outer surface of the cell, where the reverse process takes place and the quanta of plasma are discharged on to the basement membrane. This idea led to the postulate that the basement membrane and not the endothelial cell itself is the area in which the semi-permeable qualities of capillaries and venules really reside. If this were so we might expect to see some changes in the basement membrane in vessels made more permeable by inflammation.

Palade tested his hypothesis by using tracer particles visible in the electron microscope. Subsequently others have used similar methods but unfortunately without being able to reach conclusions which are free from reservations. It is certain that after intravenous injection molecules of ferritin, which have a diameter of about 100 Å, and particles of colloidal gold and saccharated iron oxide, some of which may be as small as 50 Å, can find their way in small numbers into caveolæ on the luminal side of the endothelium and that a few particles penetrate to the exterior of the vessel, though the mode of their passage in the external part of the cell is difficult to determine.

Occasionally it is possible to find intravenously injected saccharated iron oxide in caveolæ on both surfaces of endothelial cells and in vesicles apparently in the endothelial cytoplasm (FIG. 27) and Bruns and Palade have made similar observations with ferritin.[12a] Although the number of particles found in caveolæ at any one time is very small, especially on the outer side of the cell, such observations may indicate a possible route of transport of large molecules from blood to tissues.

Observations have been made on the behaviour of ferritin and saccharated iron oxide using the perfused heart of the rat. Rat hearts perfused with appropriate saline solutions can be kept beating for hours and it is possible to add marker particles at considerable concentration to the perfusion fluids. In such circumstances ferritin can be made to enter caveolæ intracellulares and vesicles at

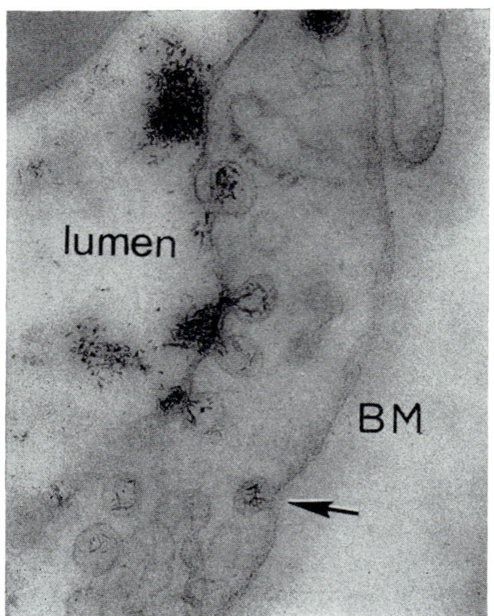

3/Fig. 27.—Saccharated iron oxide was injected intravenously into a mouse. Particles of saccharated iron oxide are entering caveolæ intracellulares from the lumen of a cardiac capillary. They are seen in apparently detached vesicles and in one caveola (arrow) abutting on the basement membrane (BM). (× 85,000.) (From Jennings and Florey.[10])

a concentration that differs little from that in the lumen of the vessel (Fig. 28). Particles are also found in the basement membrane and surrounding tissue spaces. Saccharated iron oxide behaves similarly (Fig. 29). The results of these experiments can be interpreted to show that marker particles enter vesicles and are ferried across the endothelial cell to be discharged beneath the basement membrane. But ferritin does not enter vesicles readily in the rat heart-lung pre-

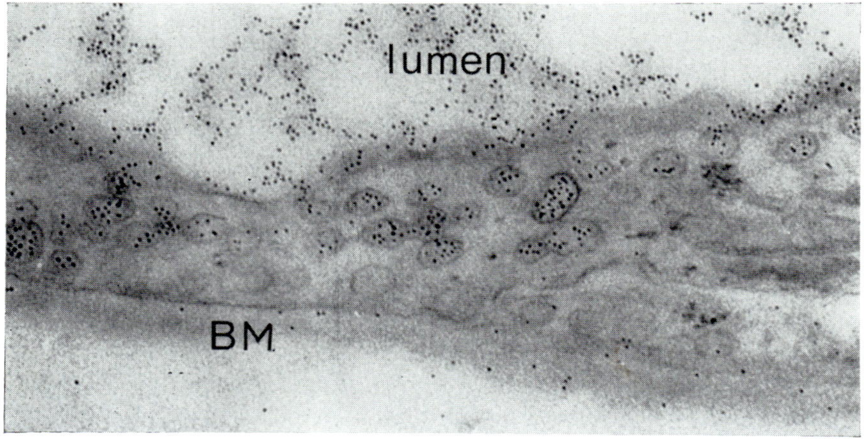

3/Fig. 28.—Ferritin molecules contained in fluid perfusing an isolated rat heart have entered the caveolæ and vesicles, the concentration being greater in those nearest the lumen. Some ferritin is found in the basement membrane (BM). (× 63,000.) (From Jennings and Florey.[10])

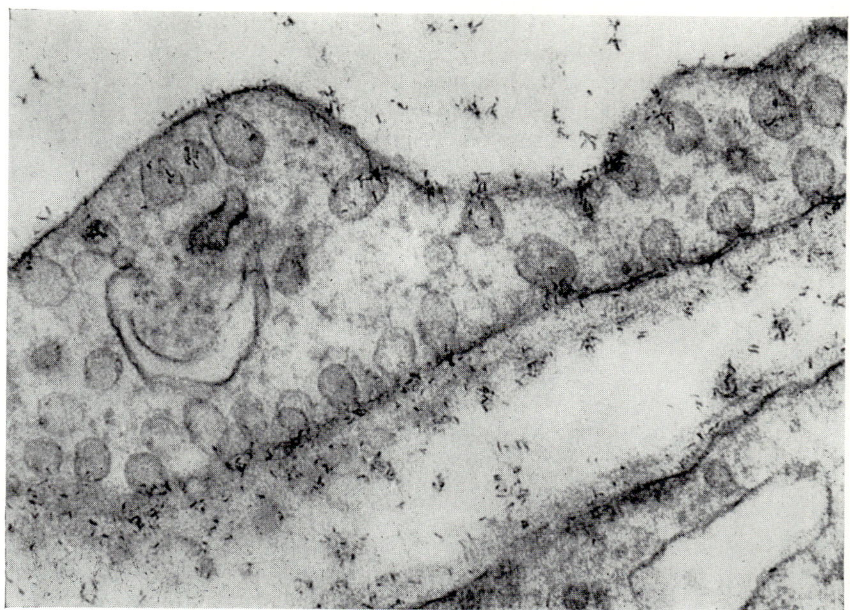

3/FIG. 29.—A capillary from a rat's heart perfused for 15 min. with McEwen's solution containing particles of saccharated iron oxide. The picture shows particles of the saccharated iron oxide in both the luminal caveolæ and those abutting on the basement membrane. Numerous particles are seen in the basement membrane as well as in the pericapillary space. (× 70,000.) (From Jennings *et al.* [10b])

paration devised by Simpson-Morgan. In this blood is pumped by the heart to be aerated in the lungs and thence back to the heart, all other organs being excluded. Ferritin in sustained high concentration can be made to flow in the blood for hours in such a preparation and the endothelium preserves its structure. Even after two hours little ferritin is found in the caveolæ and only a few particles can be seen outside the small vessels.

The presence of plasma proteins in the fluid in the blood vessels in the Simpson-Morgan preparation and their absence from the fluid used to perfuse the isolated heart may be responsible for this difference in behaviour. This might be attributed to the ferritin molecule adsorbing plasma proteins and so being substantially larger than appears in electron micrographs, but Marrack[13] was unable to show any such adsorption to ferritin. Possibly the presence of mucopolysaccharide on the cell surface, as described by Luft, may explain the different behaviour, for in perfused hearts polysaccharide might be washed away and so give free entry to the luminal caveolæ.

These discrepant observations have led to attempts to see whether any procedures could be devised to interfere with the vesicles since they have been assumed not to be static but to be in process of constant formation and movement. Nothing so far tried has been found to inhibit their formation or to destroy them[10] and one explanation of this might be that the vesicles are in fact either semi-permanent structures or are formed very slowly and are resistant to change.

This type of investigation has been taken further by Karnovsky[6] who injected intravenously the protein peroxidase prepared from horse-radish, which has a molecular weight of 40,000, and a diameter of about 40 Å. It was detected by the use of a histochemical test the product of which is opaque to electrons. One minute after intravenous injection the peroxidase was found in the vesicles of the endothelium in the cardiac capillaries. After three minutes the peroxidase was also found in the basement membrane and in the caveolæ on the external surface of the endothelium (FIG. 30).

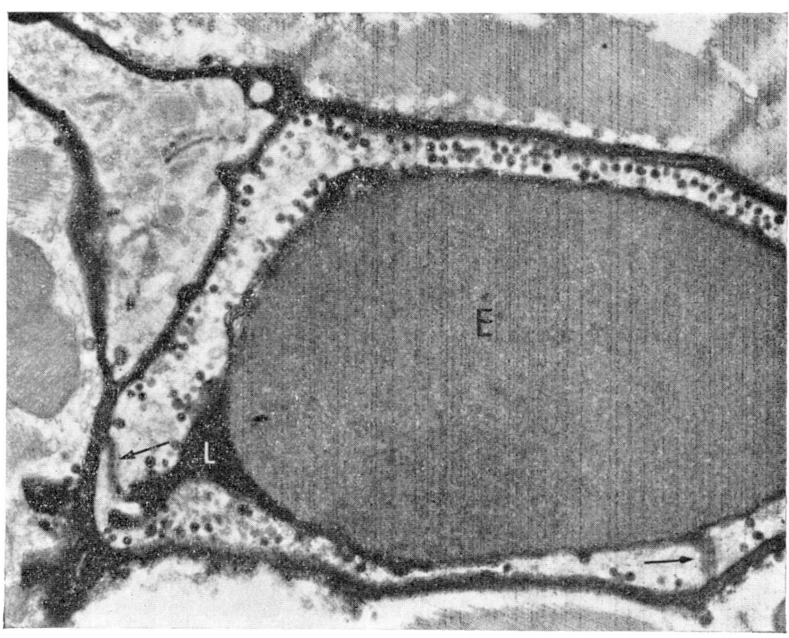

3/FIG. 30.—A cardiac capillary from a mouse killed 12 min. after the intravenous injection of horse radish peroxidase. The presence of peroxidase is indicated by the black reaction product. Peroxidase is present in the lumen (L) around the erythrocyte (E). Peroxidase is also present throughout the two intercellular clefts (arrows) and extends into the basal lamina and the extracellular spaces. The cleft on the right is cut tangentially. The micropinocytic vesicles and caveolae also contain peroxidase. (× 17,000.) (From Karnovsky.[14])

Palade's suggestion about the possible role of the caveolæ and vesicles in transport was most stimulating, but attention has turned increasingly to the junction between cells as a possible route, particularly for water and the smaller solutes and it has been suggested that it is in the region of the "tight" junction that the pores postulated by physiologists may exist[6, 11]. Particles of saccharated iron oxide are found in the intercellular junctions of perfused hearts but they do not penetrate completely as they are held up at least for a time at the narrow part or "tight" junction (FIG. 31). It is possible that small proteins do in fact pass relatively easily down junctions in the living animal, for Karnovsky[6] found peroxidase throughout the junctions as well as in the caveolæ intracellulares

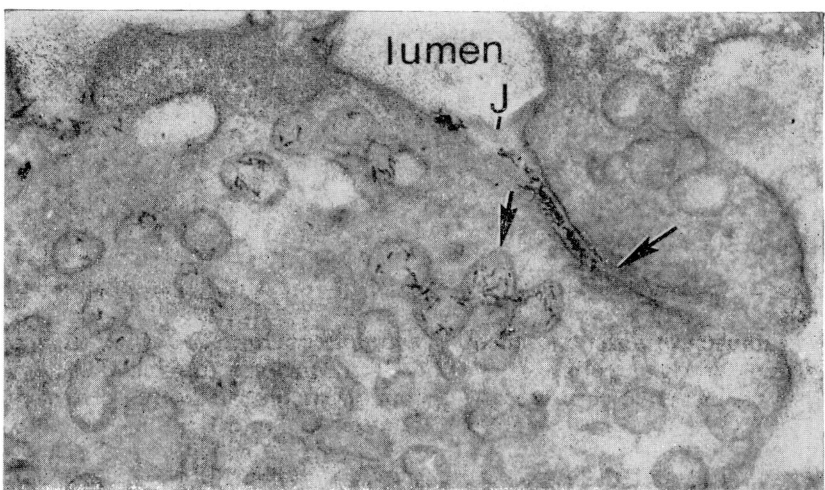

3/FIG. 31.—Capillary from a rat's heart perfused with McEwen's solution containing saccharated iron oxide for 15 min. Particles have entered caveolæ (arrow) and a junction where they are held up at the narrow portion (arrow). (× 99,000.) (From Jennings and Florey.[10])

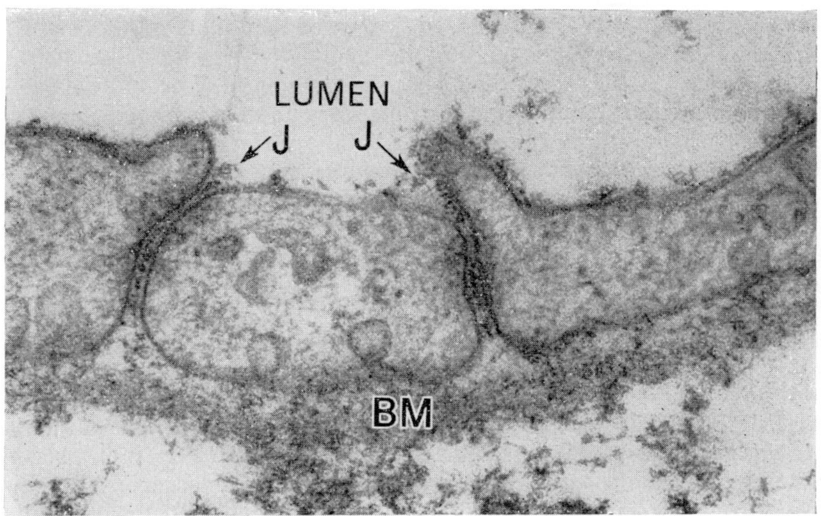

3/Fig. 32.—Capillary from a rat's heart perfused with a solution containing dinitrophenol for 35 min. Saccharated iron oxide was present in the perfusate for the last 15 min. The junctions (J) have a usual appearance and particles are passing through them in a central layer, though none are present in the narrow areas. The flow, as judged by the accumulation of particles outside the vessel, is considerable. BM, basement membrane. (× 99,000.) (From Jennings and Florey.[10])

(FIG. 30). Its presence in the external caveolæ might largely be explained by entry into them from the basement membrane.

That the area of the tight junction may possibly be labile is shown by the fact that the intercellular junctions may "relax" slightly so that particles readily pass right through. Thus after adding substances of various kinds to the fluid perfusing a heart the junctions retain their general shape but they are not tight (FIG. 32). Except in a few special situations, such as the renal glomerulus and the liver, no actual gaps or very permeable pores have been found, though there is growing evidence of the specialisation of capillaries in various organs.

In the relatively simple capillaries of muscle and connective tissue, on which most of the physiological work has been done, it now seems that the junctions may transmit water and solutes and small proteins, their "tight" areas being the site of the postulated "molecular sieving". Larger molecules may go slowly through the cells, possibly in the vesicles. However, there is still no absolute agreement as to how, under physiological conditions, substances pass the endothelial barrier.

The Small Blood Vessels in Inflammation

The increased permeability that has been shown to occur in inflammation and under the influence of certain vasoactive substances such as histamine might be due to an intensification of the physiological mechanism of fluid transport or it might be due to some quite different process.

Majno and Palade[16] and Majno, Palade and Schoefl[17] have examined the changes in blood vessels when they become more permeable under the influence of vasoactive substances. Using the cremaster muscle of the rat, which is a thin sheet of tissue about 250μ in thickness, they showed that dilute solutions of 5 HT and histamine act on the venous ends of the small blood vessels to alter their permeability. Other vasoactive agents such as bradykinin and serum permeability factor behave similarly. Majno and his colleagues injected a suspension of very fine carbon particles intravenously, and a solution of histamine or serotonin locally into the scrotum. After 1 hour the cremaster muscle was fixed, spread out, and examined by a low magnification of the microscope. FIGURES 33 and 34 show that in these conditions carbon is trapped in the venous ends of the small vessels.

The appearance presented by these preparations under low magnification suggests that the vessels have carbon attached to their walls or even that they are blocked, but examination with the electron microscope of similar preparations in which mercuric sulphide particles of a diameter of about 100 to 150 Å were injected instead of carbon has given a more accurate view. The authors found it quite striking that the small vessels such as would allow the passage of only one red blood corpuscle at a time as a rule appeared to be quite normal. In larger vessels (venules) there were dense accumulations of HgS particles between the endothelium and the basement membrane and there were scarcely any particles within or adhering to the endothelial cells. It was found that there were occasional gaps in the endothelium from 0·1 to 0·4μ in diameter but that the basement membrane was intact at these points. The sequence of events leading to the escape of the particles would seem to be as follows: gaps open in the wall of the venule, plasma passes through, but as the basement membrane remains intact the HgS particles are filtered off while probably water and plasma protein

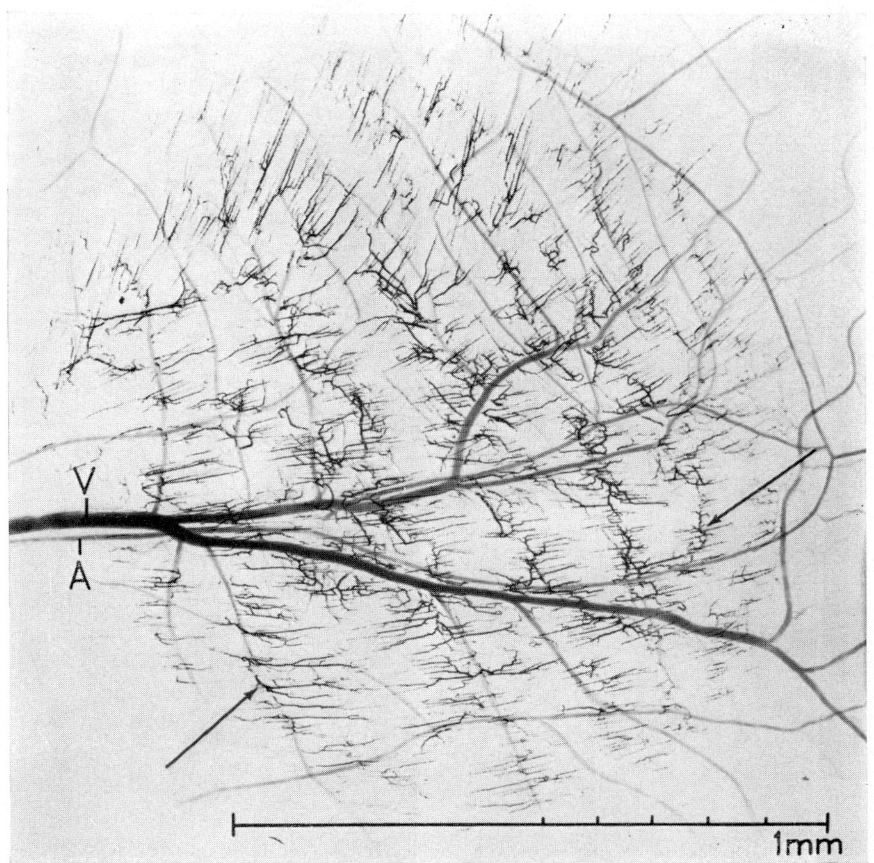

3/FIG. 33.—From a rat with colloidal carbon particles circulating in the blood and serum permeability factor injected locally in the scrotum. One hour later the thin cremaster muscle was removed and spread out whole, fixed and cleared. Blood vessels which had become more permeable show up black, as carbon had passed through their walls and accumulated between the endothelium and periendothelial sheath.

The branching disposition of these more permeable vessels (two of which are indicated by arrows), with other evidence, clearly indicates that they are venules and not the true capillaries. (From Majno *et al.*[17])

pass on into the tissue spaces. The particles accumulate and spread out in the subendothelial layer. With the light microscope the particles look as though they are on the luminal surface or in the endothelium, but they are in reality outside it. Not only are the electron-dense particles seen to have escaped, but blood platelets, chylomicra and fragments of red corpuscles can be observed. Escaped plasma may clot, for fibrin can also be recognised. The gaps can be shown to be places where two contiguous endothelial cells have separated. FIGURE 35 shows some of these points.

That these gaps are really along the intercellular junctions was shown in

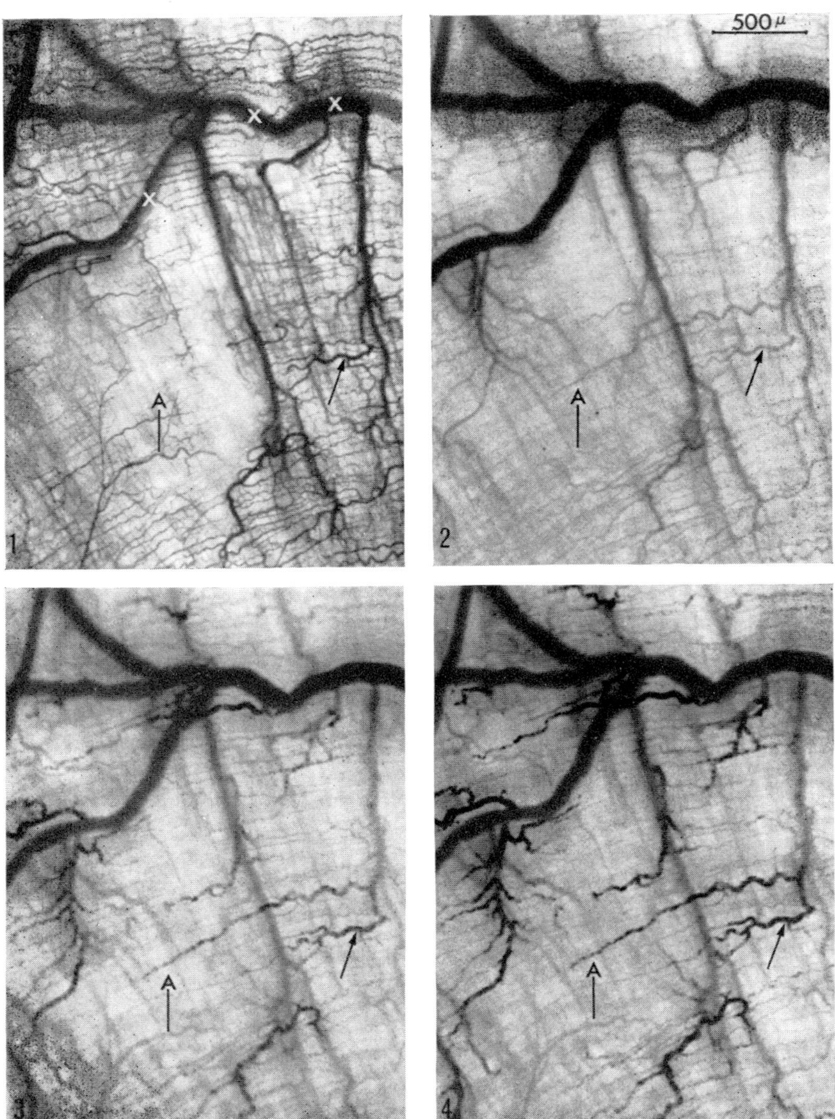

3/Fig. 34.—This series of pictures illustrates the topography, and the speed, of vascular leakage as induced by mediators of the histamine type. This sequence shows a thin striated muscle (rat cremaster) viewed in the living state, under the microscope. (1) Four seconds after an injection of carbon black through the jugular vein. The carbon emphasizes the arteriole (A) and flows into the venous tree. Note evidence of laminar flow at XXX. (2) Two minutes later the carbon black is evenly distributed in the blood stream; the arteriole A has become almost invisible; no vessel has retained any carbon. Immediately after this picture was taken, bradykinin (0·01 mg./ml.) was dripped onto the muscle. (3) 1′ 40″ later the arteriole A is dilated; leaking venules (arrow) have started to "label" with carbon. (4) 2′ 40″ after bradykinin: the carbon labelling is intense. Note that only the first 3–4 orders of venular branches are affected. The larger vein has not constricted throughout the sequence—venous constriction is not a necessary part of the phenomenon. (From Majno *et al.*[20a])

the following way. A rat was injected intravenously with a carbon suspension, and histamine was injected locally into the cremaster. After 1 hour carbon had collected in the venules. The rat was killed, the plasma washed out of the vessels with a solution of glucose and the intercellular "cement lines" stained by silver nitrate. In such a preparation it was easy to demonstrate that the deposits of carbon were aligned along the brown "cement lines".

As Majno and Palade pointed out, these findings do not introduce a new idea, for the possibility of the existence of gaps in vessel walls in inflammation was widely discussed in Cohnheim's day. The present observations illustrate very clearly that the main, if not the exclusive, lesion following the application of several of the vasoactive substances which are possibly involved in inflammation is in the venules, and that the gaps lead to the subendothelial space, where particles are trapped. Thus in the circumstances attending the increased permeability following the injection of vasoactive substances fluids and substances in solution as well as larger objects such as red blood cells, seem to be going between rather than through the cytoplasm of cells.

FIGURE 36 shows that in the inflammation produced by mechanical trauma in the mesentery of the rat carbon particles escape from the vessel and accumulate in the subendothelial space in a way similar to that occurring after the action of vasoactive substances.

Investigations by "labelling" methods similar to those of Majno and Palade have shown that in the prolonged or secondary phase of inflammation due, for example to mild burning, the capillaries proper may be extensively affected[18]. Hurley and his colleagues concluded that the pattern of damage depended on the anatomical distribution of capillaries and venules in the particular tissue burnt[18a], and they argued that their results were best explained if the leakage in the secondary phase of inflammation were due to direct damage to the vessel walls. Alterations in the endothelial cells as well as gaps in the wall were seen by the electron microscope[18b, 18c]. There is thus a difference between the primary and secondary responses in the main site of the lesion in the vascular tree, as well as the differences in their relation to permeability increasing substances which were described in Chapter 2.

Nevertheless the essential change leading to increased permeability in the capillaries as in the venules is a separation of endothelial cells at their junctions.

The material such as carbon which is temporarily held up by the basement membrane eventually finds its way into the tissue around the small vessels by passage at discrete spots, often where the basement membrane splits to envelop a portion of a pericyte, or where it has become thin or disappeared over a collection of carbon[19]. No other morphological change in the basement membrane during inflammation has been recorded.

Majno and Leventhal[20] have demonstrated that the nuclei of endothelial cells in venules treated by vasoactive substances become very folded and tend to bulge into the lumen of the vessel (FIG. 35). This appearance, they believe, indicates a contraction of the endothelial cell, and they have suggested that this contraction is sufficiently violent to tear the endothelial cells apart at the junctions.

No observations have supported the view that during the inflammatory process or after the action of vasoactive drugs the system of caveolæ and vesicles becomes more active; indeed, it seems that it is not involved at all in the increase

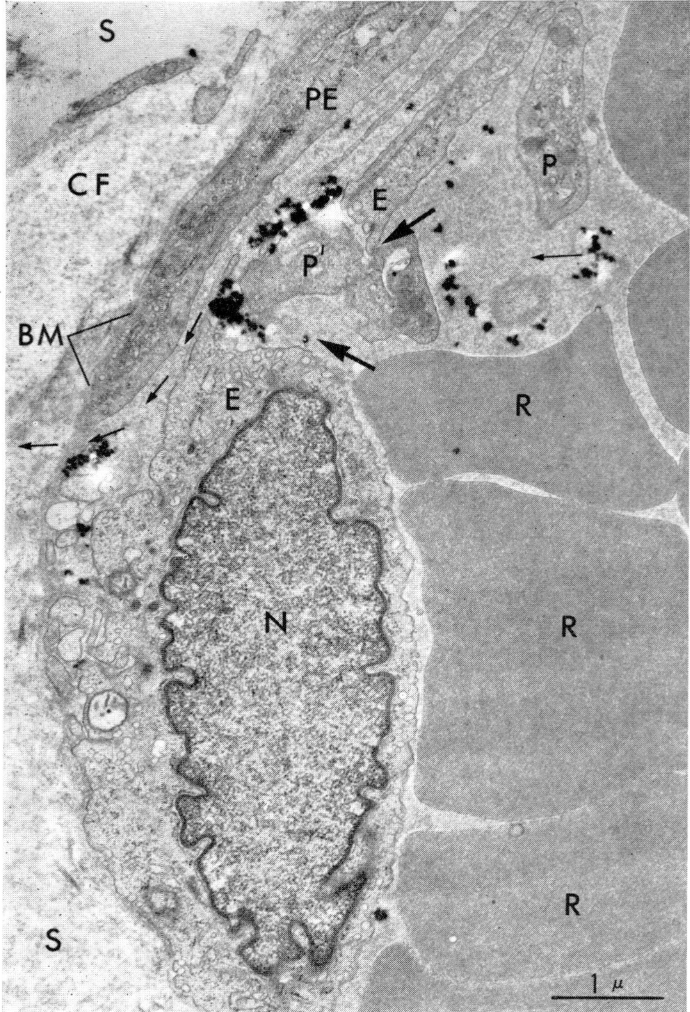

3/FIG. 35.—Wall of venule, three minutes after local injection of bradykinin (0·01 mg./ml.). The two endothelial cells E have become separated, leaving a gap (between the large arrows) which is partially filled by a platelet P[1] (another platelet P is in the lumen just above). The very dark particles are colloidal carbon black which was injected intravenously. Plasma is escaping through the gap, carrying carbon particles with it: the "escape route" is marked by small arrows. As the plasma reaches the basement membrane BM, the latter acts as a filter, retaining the carbon black. In the nucleus (N) of the endothelial cell note the many small folds and indentations: this is possibly the effect of contraction of the endothelial cell caused by bradykinin. The lumen of the venule (right) contains red blood cells (R), tightly packed because stasis has occurred through loss of plasma. CF = cross section of a collagen fibre, S = extracellular space. (Rat striated muscle: × 15,000.) (From Majno *et al.*[20a])

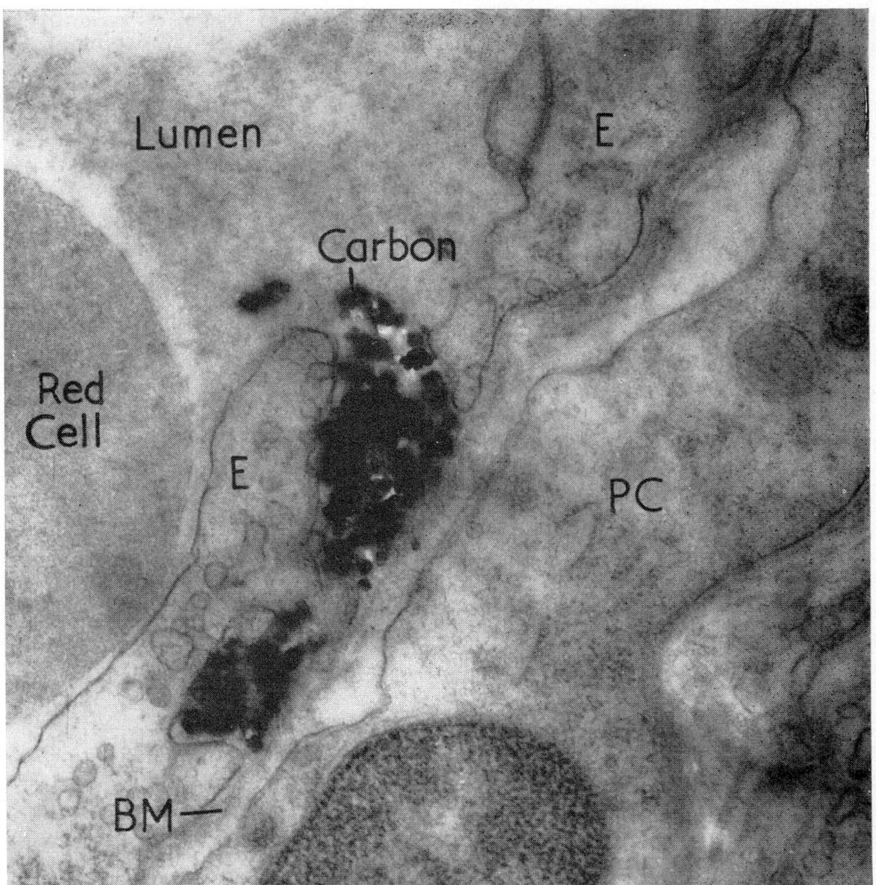

3/FIG. 36—Inflamed venule in the mesentery of a rat. A carbon suspension was injected intravenously 1 min. after injuring the mesentery mechanically and the tissue was fixed 3 min. later. Carbon particles are present in a space in the wall of the venule. This space may well be at the junction of two endothelial cells. (× 41,000.) (Preparation by V. Marchesi.)

of vascular permeability. It is possible that the wide gaps between endothelial cells in inflammation may be an exaggeration of the small changes that may occur in the tight junctions under physiological conditions, but on the other hand it is possible that the loosening of the junctions may be a truly pathological effect.

It is interesting to note that descriptions of the events in acute inflammation rest almost exclusively on observations on one type of blood vessel—namely those with structures such as are met with in subcutaneous tissue and skeletal muscle.

Behaviour of Leucocytes and Earliest Changes in the Vessels

We will now consider what changes in inflammation can be seen by the use of the light microscope. We owe a great deal of our knowledge of acute inflammation to observations carried out on living animals by using transparent portions of their anatomy.

For this purpose amphibia, such as the frog, have been found to be convenient. The frog has three useful transparent parts—the tongue, the web of the foot, and the mesentery. Cold-blooded animals also have a great advantage over mammals in that the tissues do not have to be kept warm. Waller,[21] about 1846, was apparently the first to use the frog's tongue to study the fine circulation in the living animal. FIGURE 37, which is taken from his article, shows how the tongue was pulled out over a hole in a piece of cork until it was so thin as to be transparent. The tongue is in some ways better than the web, in particular because it contains no pigment cells.

Cohnheim,[22] who contributed so much to our understanding of inflammation, also used the frog's tongue. In more recent times this organ has been used by Krogh and his collaborators,[23] and the tadpole's tail by the Clarks.[24]

The description of events following injury given in practically all textbooks of pathology is a paraphrase of that given by Cohnheim in Chapter 5 of his *Lectures on General Pathology* (1882).[25] I recommend the student to read it. Cohnheim, however, was not the first to describe some of the fundamental changes of inflammation that can be seen with the aid of the microscope.

According to Grant, Dutrochet was the first to describe the sticking of leucocytes to the walls of small vessels and their emigration. His observations and those of William Addison (1843)[26] have largely been forgotten. Indeed, I had to cut the pages of the latter's article on inflammation in a journal which had been in the possession of the Bodleian Library for over a century.

Addison described very clearly the adherence of "lymph globules", i.e. white blood cells, to the walls of the vessels of the frog's web, which he examined with magnifications of 250 and even 500 times. He recognised that adherence of white cells to the vessel walls became conspicuous in inflammation; it was "very much increased in vessels that have been irritated or excited, when the lymph globules became so numerous as to line the whole interior of some vessels, while the current of red corpuscles passes over them" (FIG. 38).

Addison described other changes in the circulation, including oscillating flow. He noted that the white corpuscles passed from the blood vessels into the tissues. Unfortunately he had no clear idea of how the vessel wall was constituted, and did not observe the actual emigration of the white cells. He stated that "the colourless corpuscles appear to form pus corpuscles".

Waller (1846)[27] published observations of a similar kind and stated that the "spherules" (white blood cells) adherent to the inner surface of the blood vessels could be aptly compared to "so many pebbles or marbles over which a stream runs without disturbing them". This is a description which with all our present knowledge it is hard to improve upon, as will be seen later.

He went on to make the observation that white cells emigrated from the blood vessels into the surrounding tissues and, like Addison, deduced that so-called pus corpuscles were emigrated white blood cells.

According to Cohnheim, Thoma (1878)[28] was the first clearly to demonstrate that the phenomena of inflammation which had been described in amphibia occurred in mammals. In general, mammals have no external part as suitable as the web or tongue of the frog, and observation of the mesentery is technically

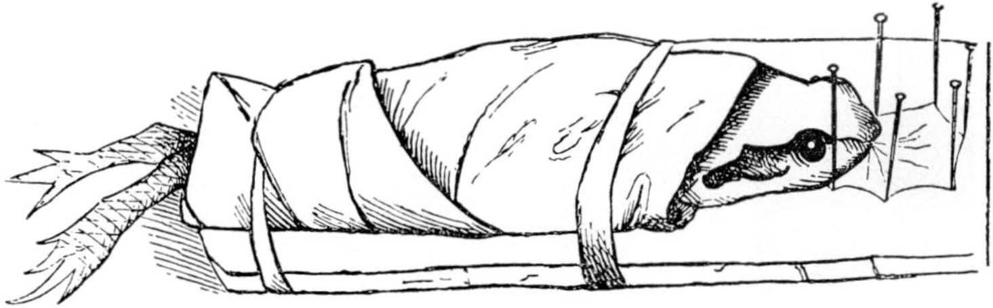

3/FIG. 37.—An illustration from Waller's paper[27] showing the way in which he pinned out the frog's tongue so that it became thin enough for him to observe the vessels with a microscope.

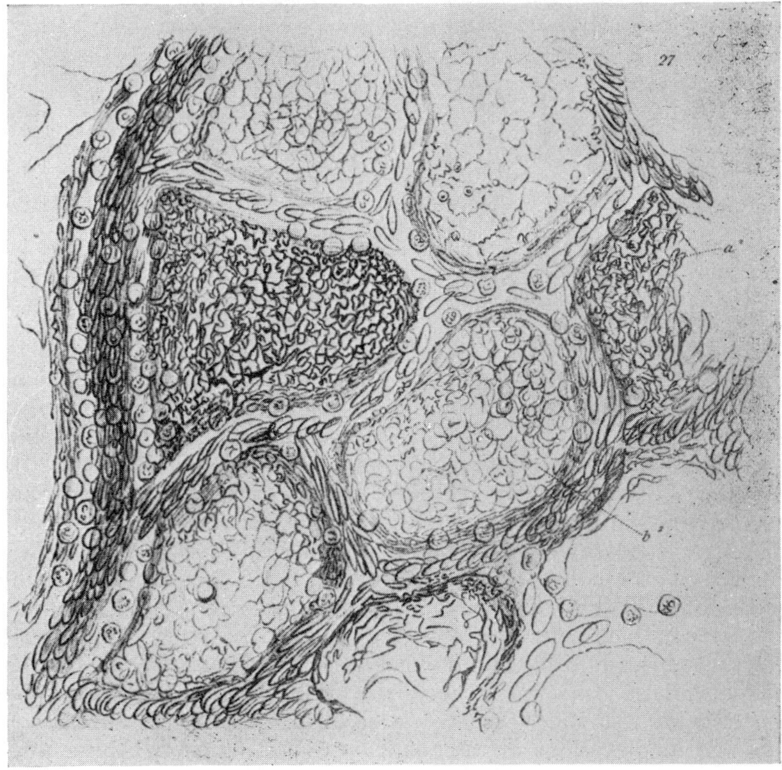

3/FIG. 38.—"Inflamed vessels in the web of a frog's foot; showing the accumulation of the lymph globules, and the peculiarity of their situation; apparently lying among the fibres forming the wall of the vessels, and exterior to their boundary." (From Addison.[26])

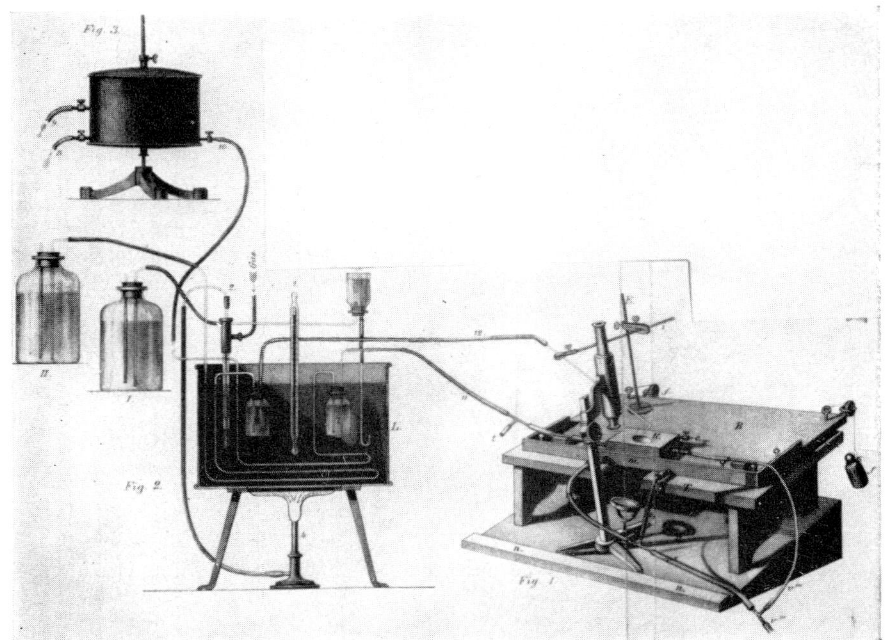

3/FIG. 39.—The apparatus used by Thoma for the observation of the circulation in mammalian mesentery with the aid of what to our eyes seems a primitive microscope. The apparatus to the left is designed to secure a warm fluid to bathe the mesentery continuously. (From Thoma.[28])

more difficult in mammals as it must be maintained at body heat. Thoma surmounted the difficulties, but only by the construction of a most elaborate apparatus (FIG. 39). This apparatus and its successors were made obsolete, as far as the observation of many vascular and cellular changes are concerned, by an invention of Sandison, later elaborated by the Clarks and a number of collaborators. This preparation is based on the old observation of Ziegler that if two coverslips are fixed slightly apart and planted in the peritoneal cavity of an animal, vessels and connective tissue will grow between them. Applying this to a more accessible part, they punched a hole in a rabbit's ear, fixed a transparent plate on each side, and observed the new tissue elements and blood vessels growing out into the blood clot that at first filled the gap. The distance between the plates determines the thickness of the new tissue and thus the amount of detail that can be seen with the microscope. There have been many variants and modifications of the Sandison-Clark chamber. FIGURE 40 shows the sort of picture one sees at low magnification in tissue that is some 30μ thick. The phenomena of inflammation may be seen clearly, and even the $\frac{1}{12}$-in. oil immersion lens can be used successfully, giving magnifications of 1,000 times or more. Observations on these elegant preparations have actually not added a great deal to what was known about inflammation by Cohnheim and some of his predecessors.

The accumulated evidence from observations on living tissue and from histological preparations can be synthesised to give the following picture of the march of events when an injury is inflicted on a vascular tissue in mammalia, including man—events that are closely akin to those occurring in other animals such as amphibia.

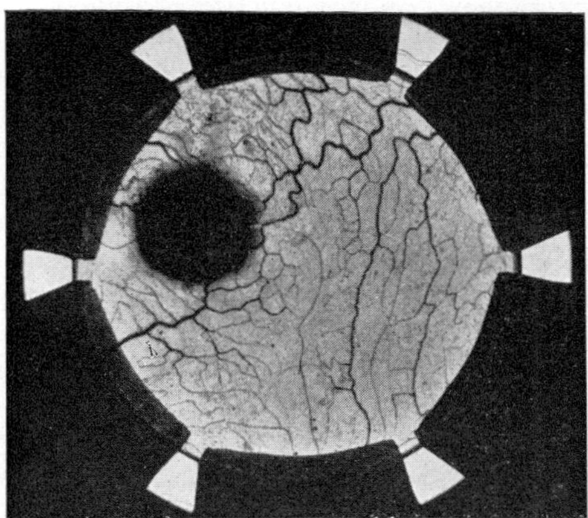

3/FIG. 40.—The appearance under low magnification of the table of an ear chamber. The covering of new tissue about 30μ thick is complete. The 6 projections are the buffers raised above the level of the table, upon which the cover-slip rests. Their height determines the depth of the chamber and hence the thickness of the newly formed tissue. The round black shadow with a diffuse edge is made by the silver pin in the bottom of the chamber, which can be removed if it is desired to infect the tissue by inserting, for example, tubercle bacilli.

Immediately after the infliction of an injury there may be a fleeting contraction of the arterioles. Allison, Smith and Wood[29] have shown that a burn of the tissue in a transparent chamber causes arteriolar contraction around it which may last for as long as 5 minutes. This is gradually relaxed and arteriolar dilatation appears within 30 minutes of the injury. The diameters of the smallest vessels also become enlarged and some that were previously carrying little or no blood now carry a rapid stream. This increased rate of blood flow may continue for a long time—a time measured sometimes in hours, its duration depending on the degree of initial injury. At the beginning of this rapid flow it is possible to see in the venules (but not in the capillaries in the mammal) that the flowing contents are divided into different zones. There is a peripheral plasmatic zone in contact with the endothelium which is free from both red and white corpuscles, these being concentrated in an axial corpuscular stream. With the passage of time the rate of blood flow begins to diminish, though the blood vessels are still widely dilated, and with this slowing leucocytes appear in the marginal stream in the venules and tend to stick to the vessel walls. At first the leucocytes stick momentarily and are then displaced to be washed away by the blood stream. As they begin to adhere more closely some are pushed slowly along by the blood stream, becoming flattened and elongated in the direction of the flow so that they have the appearance of blobs of jelly being pushed along over a sticky surface. Gradually some of the cells adhere more firmly until even a relatively swift stream of plasma and red corpuscles cannot dislodge them.

Allison *et al.*[29] have shown that under certain conditions leucocytes adhere only to the side of a vessel nearest to an injury. They consider that this supports the idea that the apparently increased stickiness of the vessel wall is caused by products diffusing from the site of injury.

There are conflicting views on why leucocytes appear in the periphery of the blood stream during the development of inflammation. It was at one time taught that white corpuscles had a lower specific gravity than red corpuscles and so tended to be thrown to the periphery of the stream. Fåhraeus[30] pointed out that most of the observations had been made on frogs, in which the erythrocytes are nucleated and are considerably larger than the leucocytes. Fåhraeus and his pupil Vejlens showed that the relative positions of leucocytes and erythrocytes in streaming blood depended partly on the relative sizes of the two, the larger cells tending to travel in the central fast portion. In mammals when the blood stream is slow the erythrocytes tend to aggregate and so to form masses larger than individual leucocytes. These masses take the centre of the stream and force the leucocytes to the periphery. The tendency for the red cells to clump intravascularly is increased in diseases associated with infection, such as pneumonia, where the suspension stability of the red cells is greatly reduced (see Chapter 8). If a similar reduction is artificially brought about by adding gelatine solution the leucocytes tend to accumulate at the periphery of blood flowing in capillary tubes. Though no doubt these forces may be of great importance, one has the impression, after watching the circulation in a chamber in the rabbit's ear, that a good deal of the phenomenon of "pavementing", as it is called, depends on the chance impinging of leucocytes on an altered vessel wall, though what the alterations are is not known.

With an adequate injury some of the leucocytes sticking to the wall begin

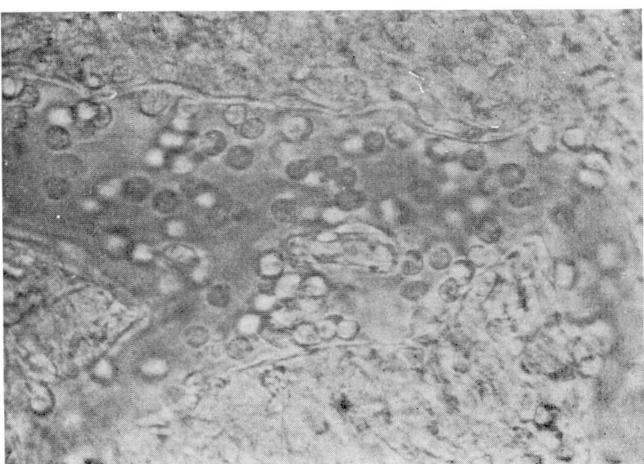

3/FIG. 41.—Leucocytes adhering to the wall of a venule. Owing to movement the red cells are not visible as such but appear as a grey background. From a transparent chamber in a rabbit's ear. (× 560.)

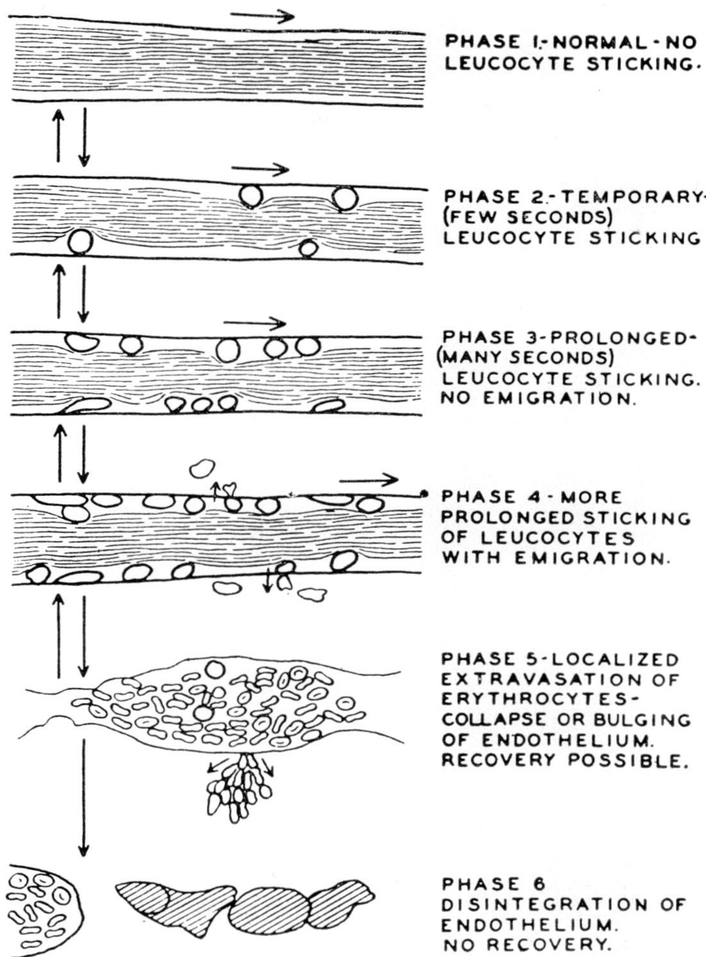

3/FIG. 42.—Successive stages of inflammatory change showing the sticking and emigration of leucocytes, extravasation of erythrocytes and disintegration of endothelium. The arrows on the left indicate the reversibility or otherwise of the changes in the endothelium. (From Clark and Clark.[24])

to make their way through it by active movements. By this active migration, the nature of which will be considered later, the leucocytes pass out of the vessels into the surrounding tissue in which they continue their movements. Their passage through the vessel wall is known as emigration. Probably all forms of white blood cell can stick to the vessel wall, but the lymphocyte does not appear to adhere readily. Sometimes it is possible, when the circulation is slow and there are few red corpuscles present, to observe the leucocytes that are adherent to the vessel wall moving about actively upon the inside of the vessel by amœboid motion (FIG. 41). It seems likely that the same process takes them out

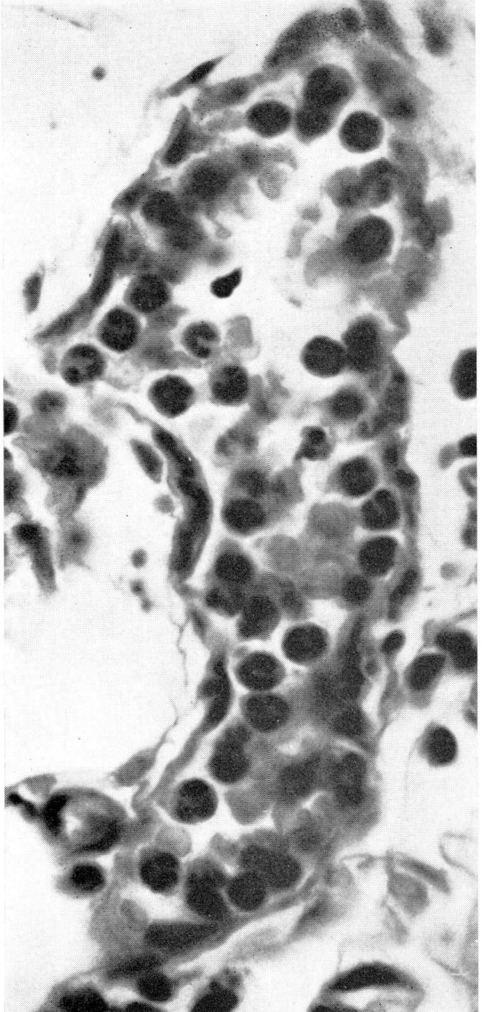

3/FIG. 43.—A venule in a spread of rat mesentery fixed and stained with hæmatoxylin and viewed by the light microscope. The tissue had been inflamed by mechanical trauma and the specimen shows large numbers of leucocytes along the margins of the vessel. During life they adhered to the vessel wall, but on fixation they rounded up, so that they now appear slightly separated from the endothelial cells, which are plainly seen. Most of the leucocytes are polymorphs. It was from such preparations that the electron micrographs showing leucocyte emigration in the rat were obtained. (× 1120.)

through the vessel wall when the necessary conditions are present. In acute inflammation granulocytes migrate in far greater numbers than monocytes and lymphocytes. Granulocytes take from about 2 to 12 minutes to penetrate the vessel wall and thereafter they may move through a clear space in the tissue at as much as 20μ in 1 minute.

Allison *et al.*[29] noted that a defect seemed to exist in the vessel wall for a short time after the passage of a leucocyte, for one or more additional cells would follow the same route to the perivascular space. This phenomenon can be well seen in a film prepared by Ciba.[31]

It has been considered that emigration requires a certain level of blood pressure, for Cohnheim and recently Miles noted that it stopped when the

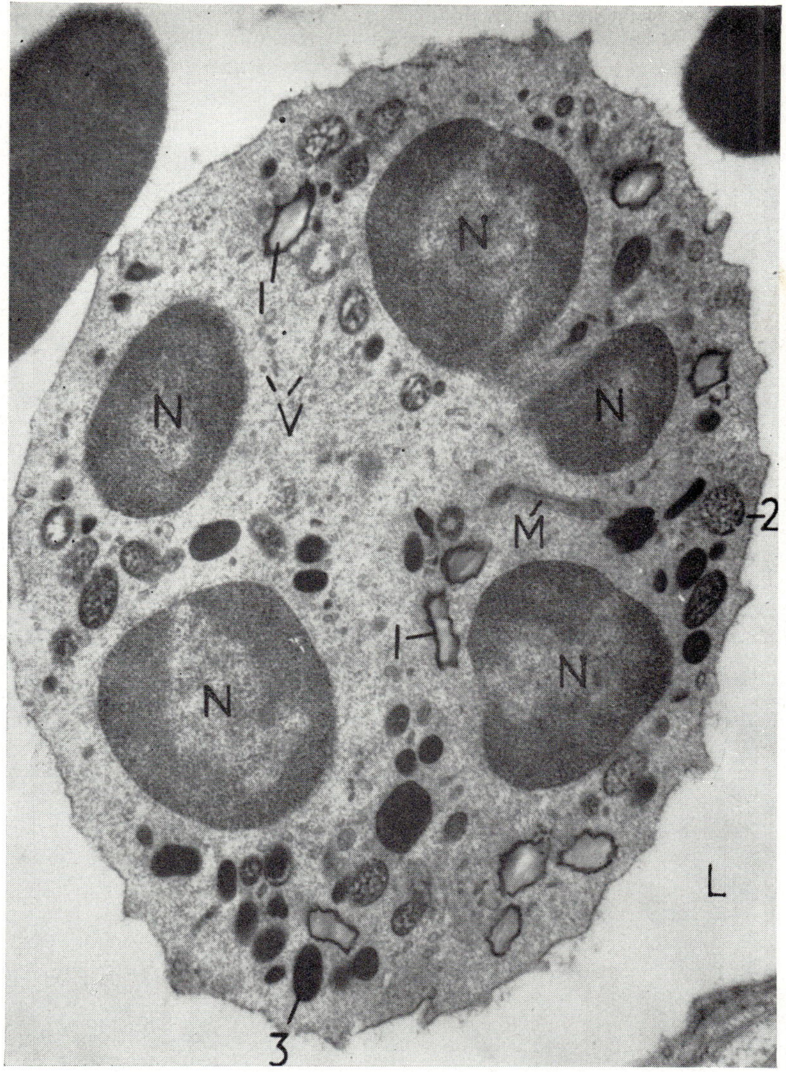

3/Fig. 44.—Polymorphonuclear leucocyte floating free in the lumen of a venule. 1, 2 and 3 indicate three kinds of granule easily distinguishable. N marks a part of the nucleus and M a mitochondrion. A few small vesicles (V) are scattered in the cytoplasm. (× 17,500.) (From Florey and Grant.[33])

vessels reached a condition of stasis, but this is now denied by Allison *et al.* and by Zweifach.[32]

In addition to the white cells some red cells emerge, as was described by Cohnheim and others, and in general it can be said that the greater the intensity of the inflammatory reaction the greater the number of red cells that escape.

They are passive in the matter, being pushed out by the blood pressure through tiny breaches in the vessel walls, possibly sometimes through holes by which leucocytes have previously escaped. The process is known as diapedesis of the red cells. A recapitulation of what we have been describing is given in FIG. 42.

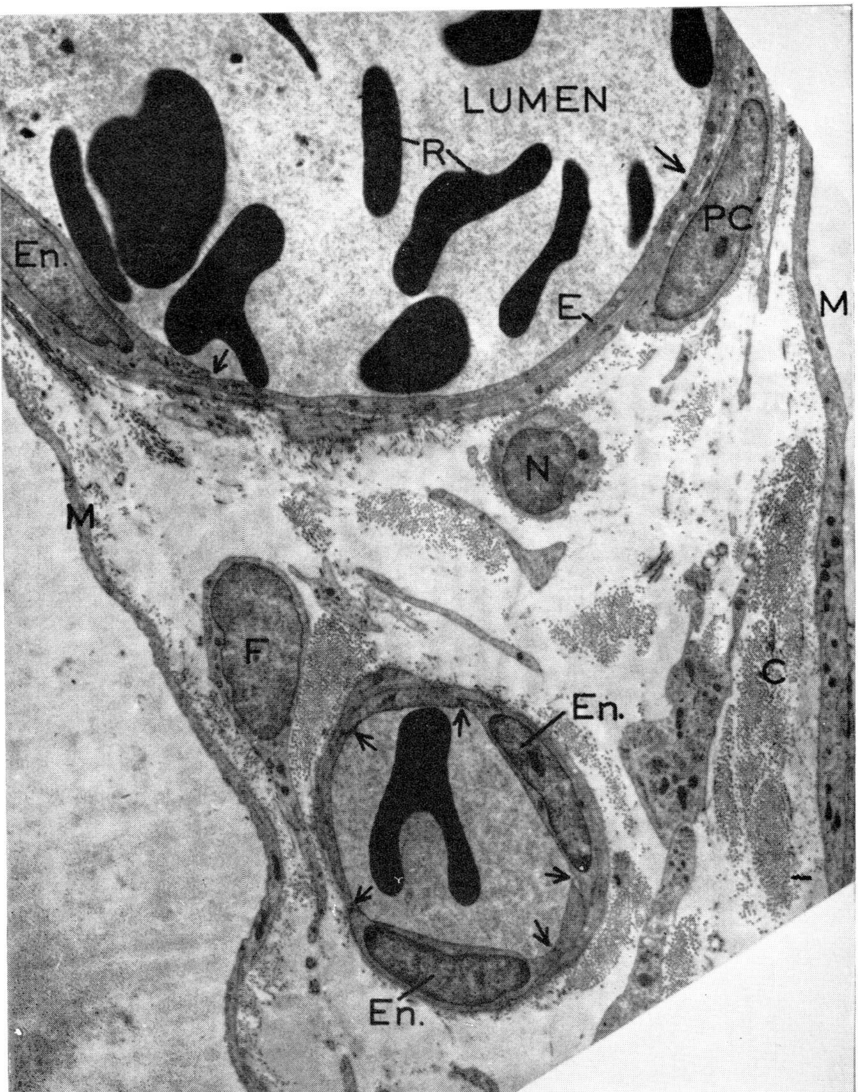

3/FIG. 45.—Electron micrograph cross section of normal mesenteric venule and capillary. The vessels are contained in connective tissue bounded by a covering of mesothelium (M). E = endothelial cell. En = nucleus of endothelial cell. R = red cell. PC = periendothelial cell. F= fibroblast. N = nucleus of a connective tissue cell. Arrows mark intercellular junctions. (× 4,500.) (From Marchesi and Florey.[34])

Observations with the Electron Microscope

The process of emigration has now been investigated with the electron microscope which has revealed in more detail how the leucocytes penetrate the walls of the small blood vessels in inflammation. The observations have mostly been made on venules in the inflamed mesentery of the rat and in inflamed rabbit-ear chambers. Most, if not all, of the emigration in these tissues under the conditions observed takes place through the venules.

FIGURE 43 shows the appearance at a high power of the light microscope of an inflamed vessel in a rat's mesentery. It was from vessels in this condition that electron micrographs were obtained. Polymorphonuclear leucocytes are easily recognised in electron micrographs because of their rich and varied content of granules. FIGURE 44 shows a rabbit polymorph in a capillary. These cells contain at least three distinct kinds of granule. Light grey, round or elongated profiles are mitochondria. In the cytoplasm near the nucleus some small vesicles can usually be recognised. The hyaloplasm in pseudopodia is finely granular and free from the larger granules.

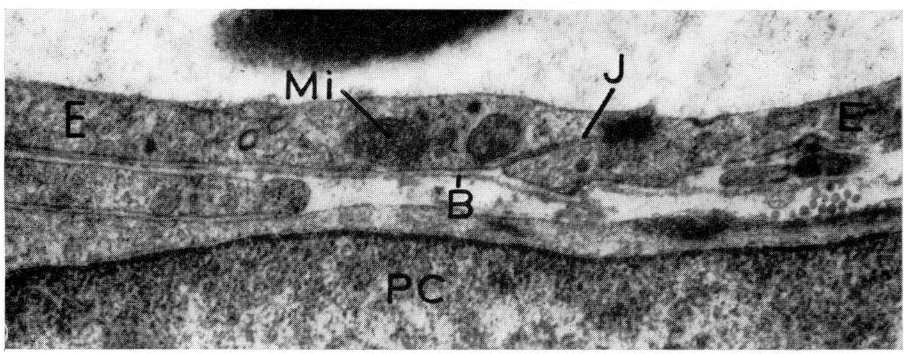

3/FIG. 46.—A junction (J) between two endothelial cells. An electron dense "tight" area is seen at the end of the junction nearest the lumen of the vessel. The basement membrane (B) spans the junction. Mi = Mitochondrion. E = endothelial cell. PC = periendothelial cell. (× 31,500.) (From Marchesi and Florey.[34])

FIGURES 45 to 70 should be consulted in conjunction with the following description.

The electron micrographs of vessels in which "sticking" is taking place show that the leucocytes come into intimate contact with the inflamed endothelium, and that there is no electron-dense material on the endothelial surface, or any other evidence that a "cement" is secreted to which the leucocyte adheres. Indeed, no alteration of the surface of the endothelium of such venules in rat mesentery has so far been detected. Occasionally in the rabbit-ear chamber inflamed by ultraviolet light some electron-dense material can be seen on the surface of the endothelium, but this is not particularly associated with the adhering leucocytes. (FIG. 48).

Once in contact with the endothelium, and in some unknown way tending to adhere to and move about on it, the leucocyte puts out pseudopods. If one is put out near a cell junction it will force its way down the junction, and our present information is that passages of leucocytes through the wall are made through or at least very close to a junction. Precisely how the pseudopod breaks the junction apart is not apparent. It may be by the physical force of the leucocyte's movements or it may be associated with some enzyme action.

While it is certain that leucocytes can force apart an intercellular junction, it is not quite clear whether or not the endothelium itself is sometimes penetrated.

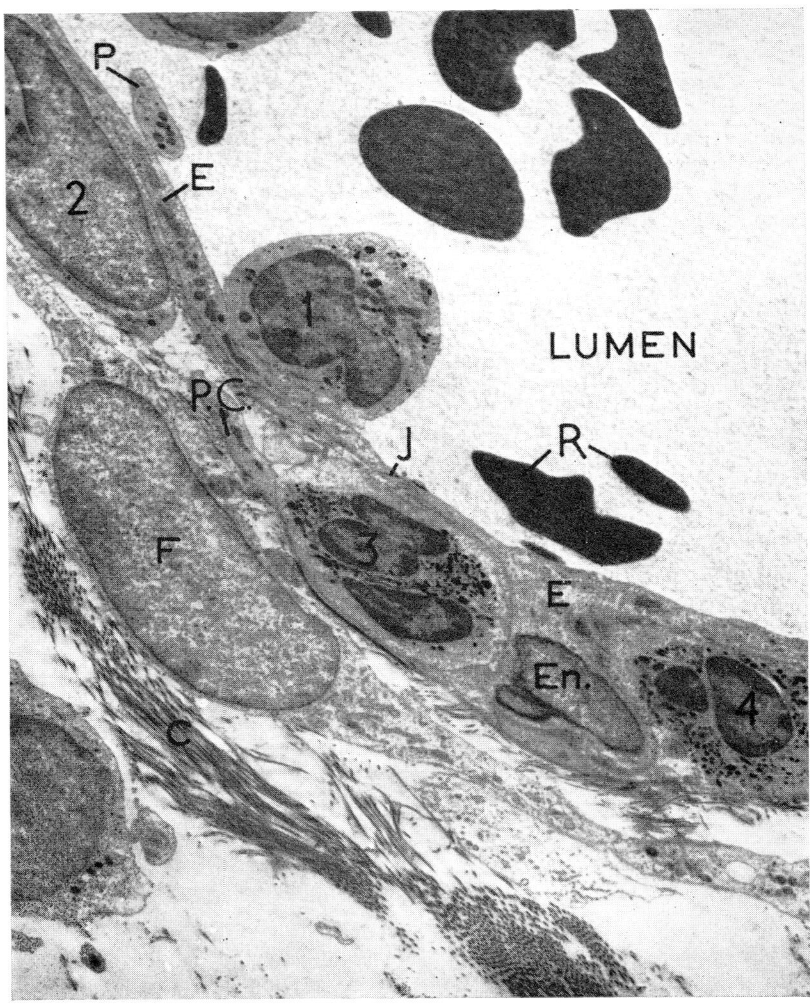

3/Fig. 47.—Inflamed venule of a rat. Cell 1 is a polymorphonuclear leucocyte in contact with and apparently adherent to the endothelium. Cells 2, 3 and 4 are polymorphs which have already passed through the endothelium (E). En = endothelial cell nucleus. PC = periendothelial cell. **P** = blood platelet. R = red cell. F = fibroblast. C = collagen. (× 6000.) (From Marchesi and Florey.[34])

In many photographs the leucocyte is apparently penetrating to one side of an intercellular junction, and though serial sections of some of these cells have shown another point at which they are within the junction, it is at least possible that the junctions are traumatised and neighbouring cytoplasm torn by the vigorous motions of the leucocyte. That the force of the movement of a leucocyte's pseudopod can deform cells can be appreciated by observing its effect on periendothelial cells (FIG. 64).

The leucocyte may push its way straight through the junction, the basement membrane, the perivascular sheath, and perivascular collagen fibres, to emerge

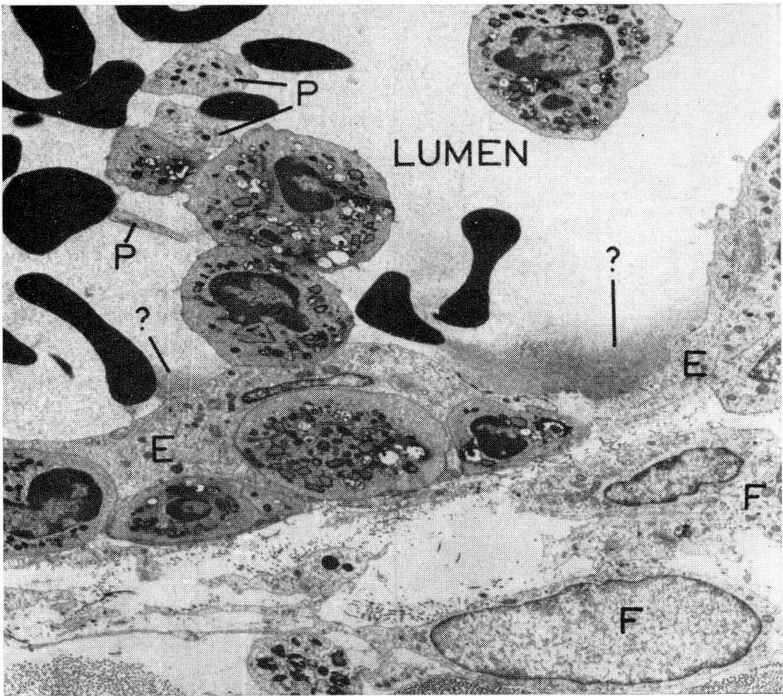

3/FIG. 48.—Inflamed venule in rabbit ear chamber. Polymorphonuclear leucocytes are adhering to one another and to the endothelium (E). Some have passed through the endothelium and are in the subendothelial space. At the ? is some electron dense material which might be due to an alteration of the surface of the endothelium. PP are platelets and FF fibroblasts. (× 5250.) (From Florey and Grant.[33])

into the connective tissue around the venule. Frequently, however, the advancing pseudopod seems to be held up mechanically for a time and diverted to pass parallel to the endothelium. It may peel off the basement membrane from the endothelial cells, or it may pass between the basement membrane and the periendothelial cells and fibres. The pseudopod finding its way between these structures is sometimes long and relatively tenuous. A number of leucocytes that have partially migrated may be held up in the periendothelial space, forming a ring outside the endothelium. After the leucocyte has travelled parallel to

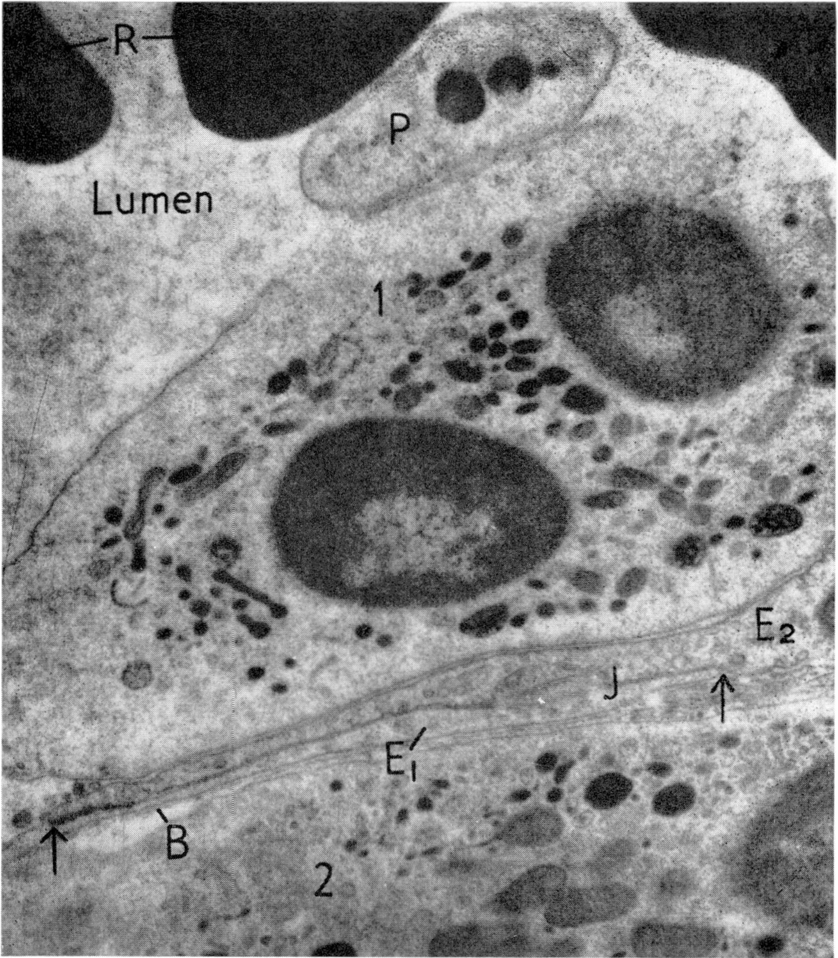

3/FIG. 49.—Cell 1 is a polymorph adherent to the endothelium of an inflamed venule of a rat. Cell 2 is a polymorph outside the endothelium and its basement membrane (B). At this point the endothelium is made up of two cells (E1 and E2) joined by a long overlapping intercellular junction (J). The ends of the junction are marked by arrows. A small part of the nucleus of E2 appears on the right. (× 20,000.) (From Marchesi.[35])

3/FIG. 51 (*see opposite*).—Higher magnification of part of FIG. 50. The body in the junction (arrow) has a discrete membrane and is separating the plasma membranes of the endothelial cells (E1 and E2) which were contiguous in FIG. 49. The intercellular junction appears to be intact on both sides of the body. (× 39,000.) (From Marchesi.[35])

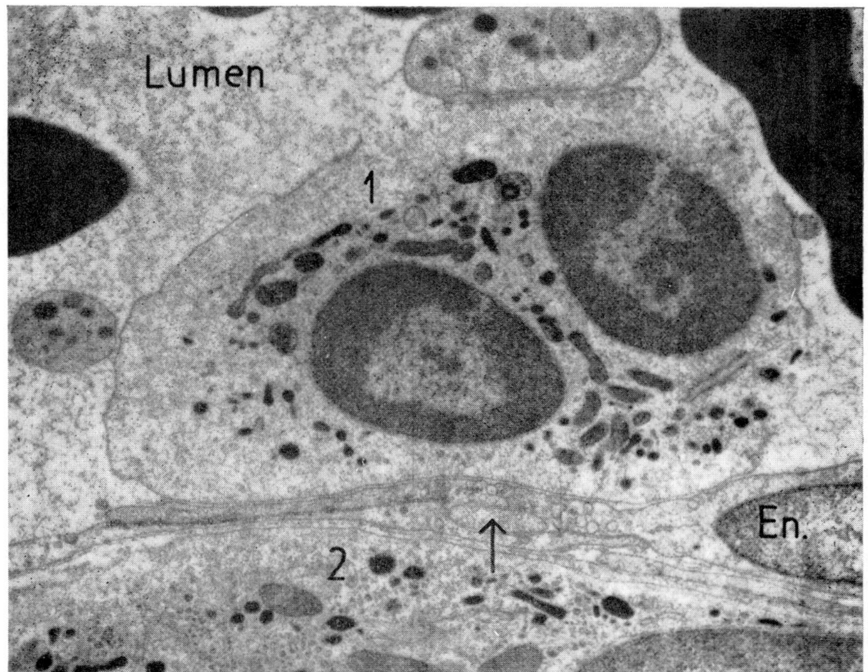

3/FIG. 50.—A section of the same cell as in FIG. 49 from a little farther into the block. In this plane a body (arrow) is apparent within the intercellular junction. This is seen at higher magnification in FIG. 51. (× 19,000.) (From Marchesi.[35])

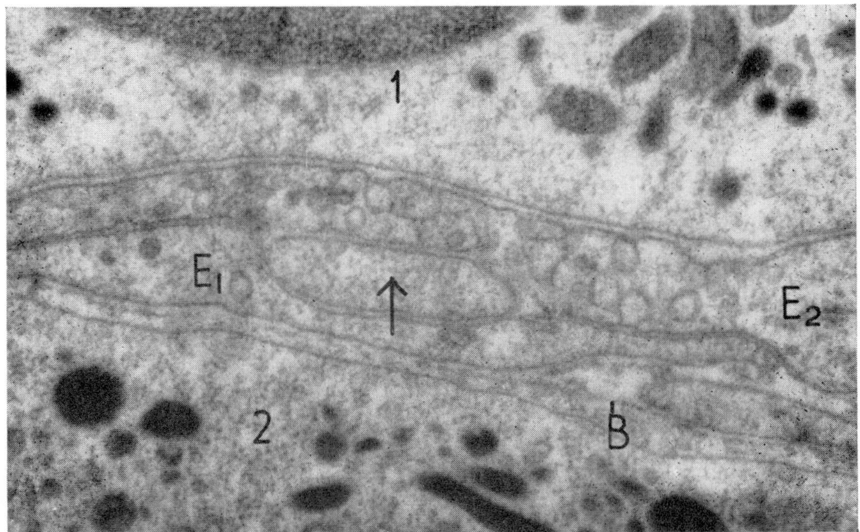

3/FIG. 51.

3/FIG. 52 (*see opposite*).—A section still farther into the block than FIG. 50. Cell 1 is now seen to have a pseudopod (Ps) extending into the endothelium. It is apparent that the body seen within the intercellular junction in FIGS. 50 and 51 was an extension of this pseudopod. (× 19,000.) (From Marchesi.[35])

3/FIG. 53 (*see opposite*).—Higher magnification of part of FIG. 52. The pseudopod is apparently opening up the intercellular junction, but ahead of it the junction looks morphologically intact (arrow). (× 39,000.)

the vessel wall for a certain distance a pseudopod eventually finds its way into the surrounding connective tissue, to be followed by the rest of the leucocyte, which eventually becomes quite free from the vessel wall.

It is noteworthy that holes do not appear to be left in the endothelium after the passage of a leucocyte. The edges of the endothelium which are pushed apart keep in close contact with the emigrating cell and come together again after its passage without being altered in any perceptible way. The intercellular junctions must be quite tough, for they may be observed to be intact when they occur in endothelium which is stretched thinly over leucocytes caught in the periendothelial space.

Eosinophil leucocytes and monocytes penetrate the wall of the venule in a comparable way, and possibly the same may be true of the rare basophil. So far no lymphocyte has been seen penetrating the wall of an acutely inflamed vessel. Occasionally a red cell is found in the periendothelial space. It apparently reaches there by passing through a hole in the endothelium, possibly following a leucocyte though this is by no means certain. Descriptions have been given of the rapid "explosive" emergence of red cells from venules. They are certainly not actively motile like the leucocytes and are presumably forced through openings in the vessel wall by the pressure within the vessel. Occasionally intracellular objects which look like platelets can be seen in inflamed endothelium.

Although electron micrographs have clarified some details of leucocyte emigration, it is interesting to reflect that Arnold[36] showed that leucocytes left venules by going through the areas stained by silver nitrate, that is, through the intercellular junctions (FIG. 71), and that Zweifach[37] from observations on living vessels described the pause in the progress of leucocyte emigration that occurs after the cells have passed the endothelium proper and are held up by the periendothelial structures.

Changes in the Blood Flow and in the Vessel Walls

While emigration is taking place the blood stream usually becomes slower and slower until, after oscillating to and fro, it finally stops. Stasis has occurred. Stasis may come on very rapidly before any of the phenomena of leucocyte emigration have had time to occur. It can be particularly well seen in preparations of mammalian mesentery, in which the slightest roughness in handling makes the blood flow stop completely, the vessel being filled with a yellowish translucent glassy mass in which individual red corpuscles are not recognisable in the living preparation. In fixed and stained preparations the packed corpuscles inside a vessel in stasis have a hyaline ("glassy") look quite distinct from the appearance of a merely congested vessel on the one hand and of a thrombosed

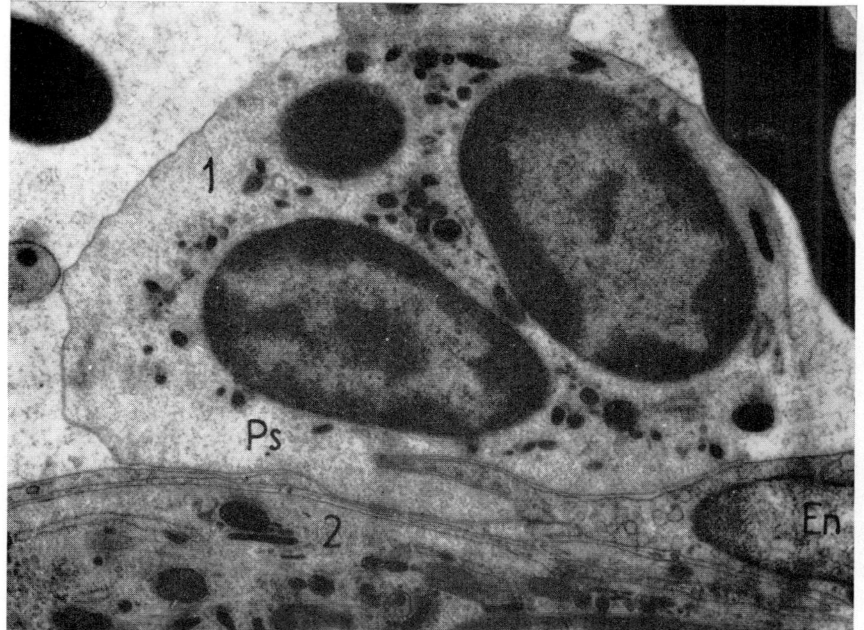

3/Fig. 52.

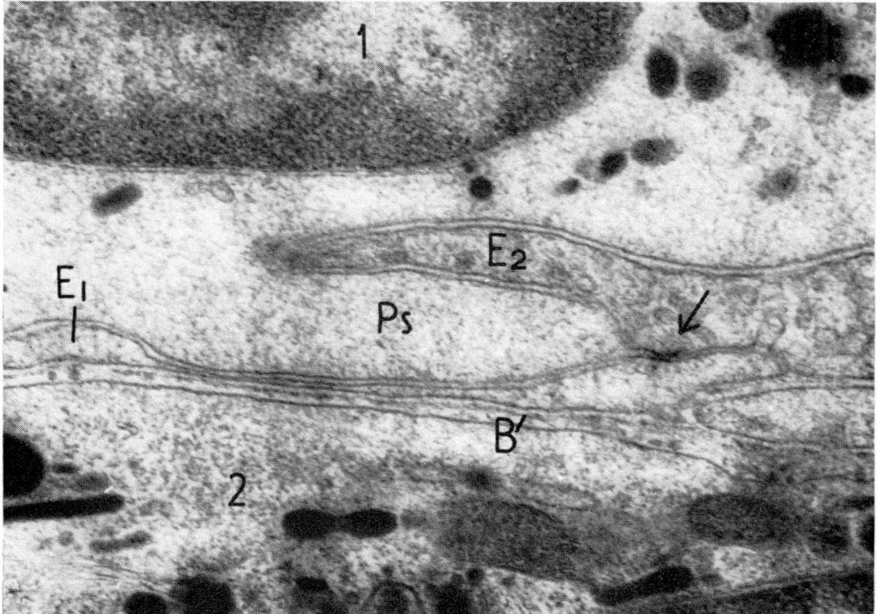

3/Fig. 53.

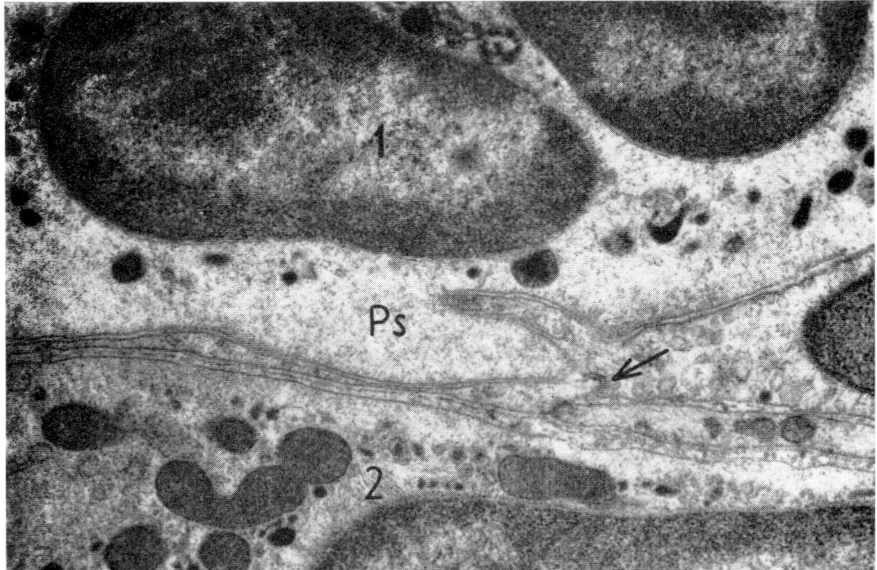

3/FIG. 54.—A section still farther into the block than FIG. 52. In this plane of section the pseudopod (Ps) extends farther into the junction, but there is still a small area of contact between the two endothelial cells (arrow). (× 24,000.) (From Marchesi.[35])

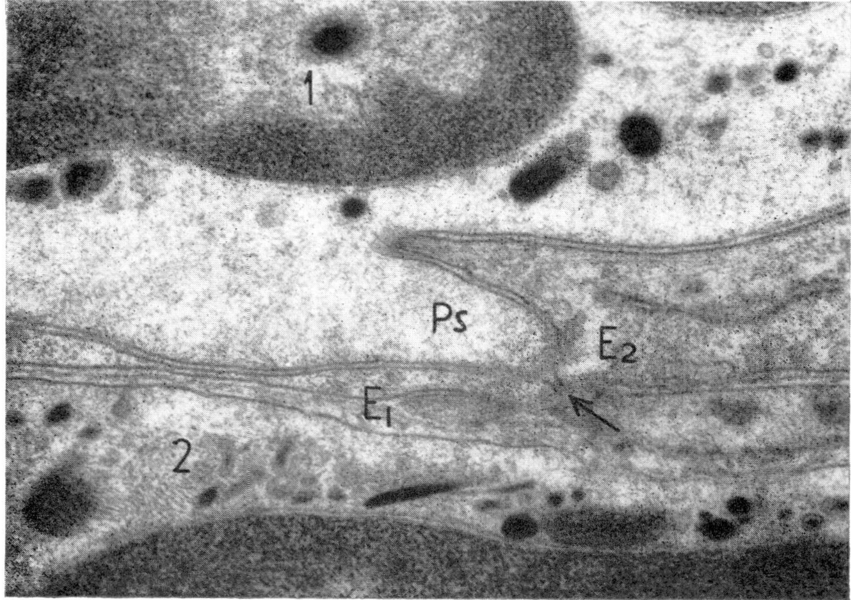

3/FIG. 55.—A section still farther into the block than FIG. 54. The remaining area of contact between cells E1 and E2 is beginning to separate (arrow) in front of the advancing pseudopod. (× 31,000.) (From Marchesi.[35])

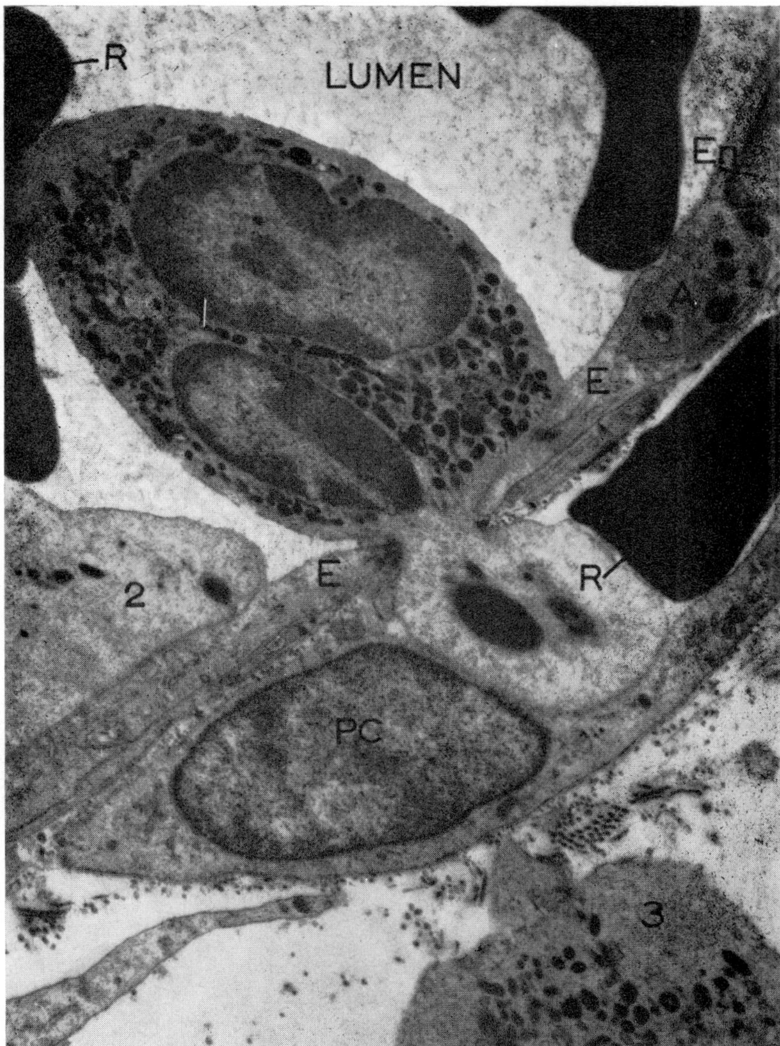

3/FIG. 56.—Inflamed venule of rat. Cell 1 is a polymorph passing through the endothelium and coming into contact with a periendothelial cell (PC). The hyaloplasm of the advancing pseudopod is almost free of granules. A red cell (R) is seen in the periendothelial space. An intracellular object (A) is enclosed by endothelial cytoplasm; this might be a platelet or the tip of a polymorph (see also FIG. 63). Cell 2 is a polymorph adherent to the endothelium and cell 3 has passed into the connective tissue. (× 13,500.) (From Marchesi and Florey.[34])

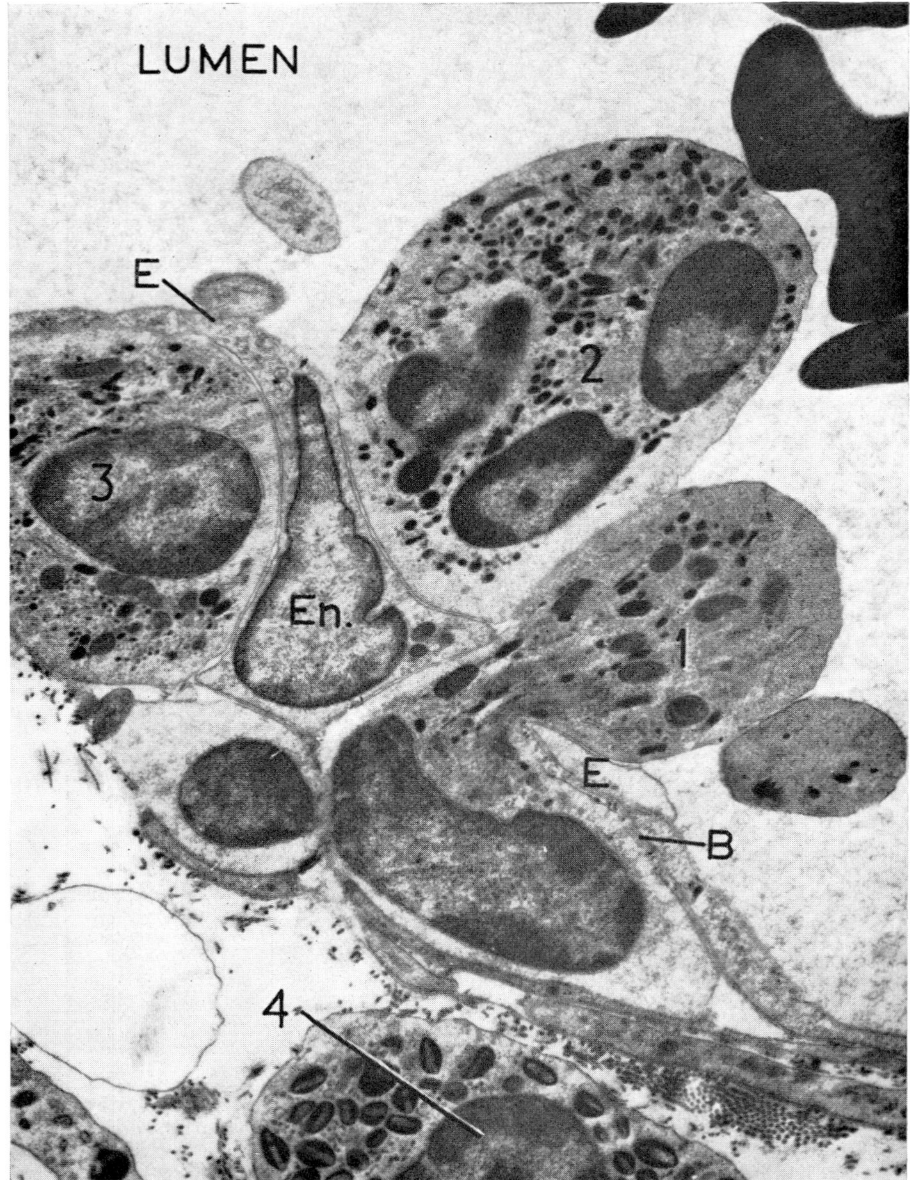

3/Fig. 57.—Inflamed venule of a rat. Cell 1 is a polymorph passing through the endothelium and, in combination with cell 3, severely distorting it. Cell 2 is adherent to the endothelium and to cell 1. Cell 3 is in the subendothelial space. Cell 4 is an eosinophil in the connective tissue. Portions of endothelium are indicated by EE, and En is an endothelial nucleus. (× 11,500.) (From Marchesi and Florey.[34])

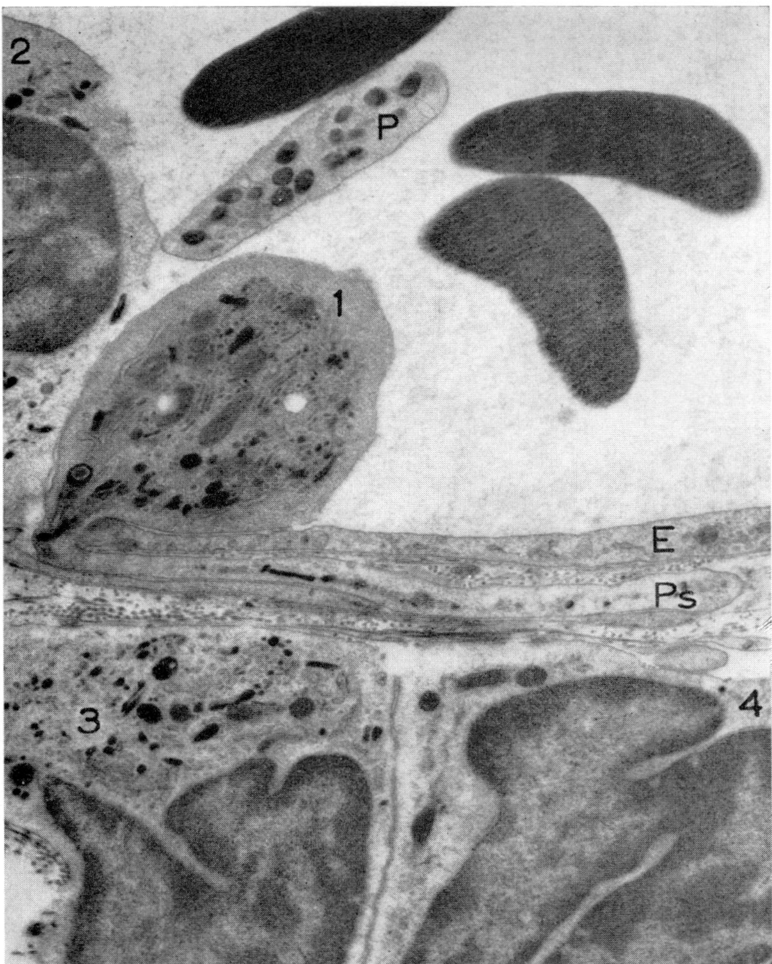

3/FIG. 58.—Inflamed venule of a rat. A polymorph (1) has penetrated the endothelium (E) and has sent out a particularly long pseudopod parallel to the endothelium. 2, 3 and 4 are also polymorphs. P is a platelet. (× 15,500.) (From Marchesi.[34])

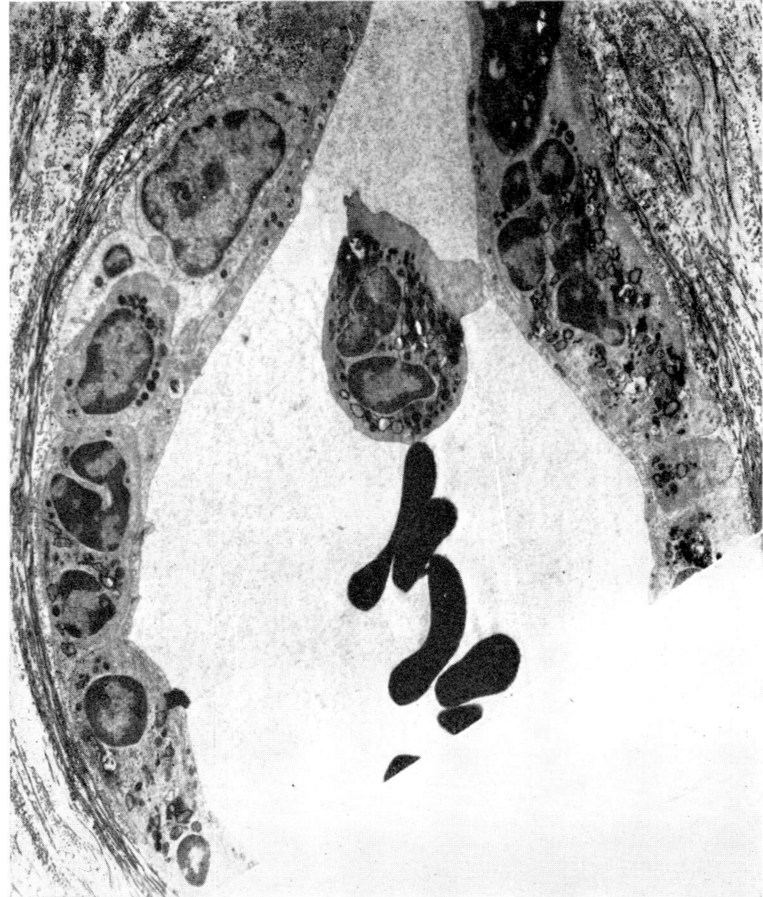

3/FIG. 59.—Rabbit ear chamber. Several leucocytes have passed through the endothelium of a venule and are, for the time being, arrested as an almost continuous layer between the endothelium and its surrounding sheath of connective tissue. There is one polymorph leucocyte in the lumen. (× 4500.) (From Florey and Grant.[33])

vessel on the other. In spite of their appearance the corpuscles remain intact and the condition can be reversed,[38] and a good circulation can be re-established in the vessel previously in stasis. It is now generally agreed that stasis is brought about by the alteration of capillary permeability which, while allowing fluid to escape, retains the red blood corpuscles. It is to be supposed that re-establishment of the flow is made possible by concurrent recovery of the capillary wall towards its normal state.

It will be remembered that the blood flow, after being accelerated at the beginning of inflammation, gradually became slower, although the fine vessels remained widely dilated, a phenomenon at first sight difficult to explain. A number of circumstances conspire to make it more difficult for the blood to flow

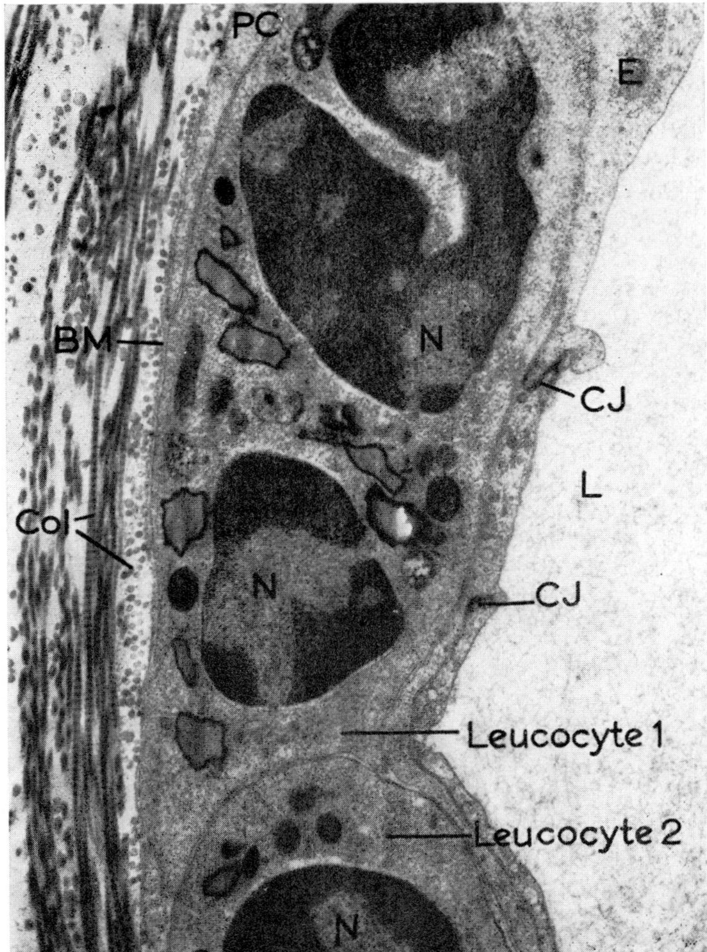

3/FIG. 60.—Two leucocytes in a subendothelial position. There are two intact cell junctions (CJ) in the endothelium (E) and the basement membrane (BM) of the endothelial cells is well shown, stripped away from them by the leucocytes. Bundles of collagen fibres (Col) in the periendothelial sheath run at right angles to one another, those near the basement membrane being cut transversely and those farther away longitudinally. PC = periendothelial cell. (× 17,500.) (From Florey and Grant.[33])

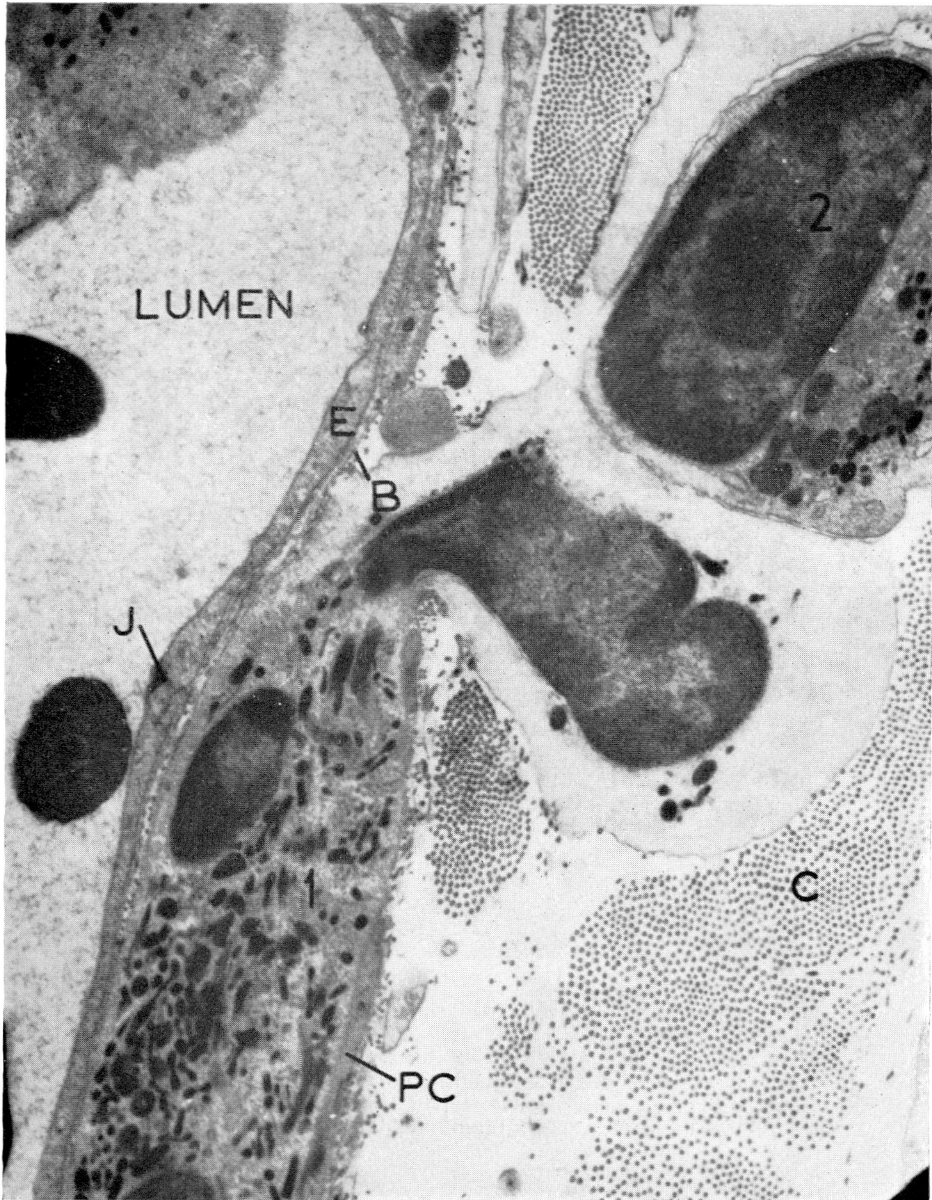

3/FIG. 61.—Inflamed venule of a rat. Cell 1 is a polymorph which has been flattened between the basement membrane and a periendothelial cell and is now turning to send a pseudopod of clear hyaloplasm among the collagen fibres of the connective tissue. Note the orientation of granules in the apparent direction of movement. Cell 2 is a polymorph in the connective tissue. (× 14,000.) (From Marchesi and Florey.[34])

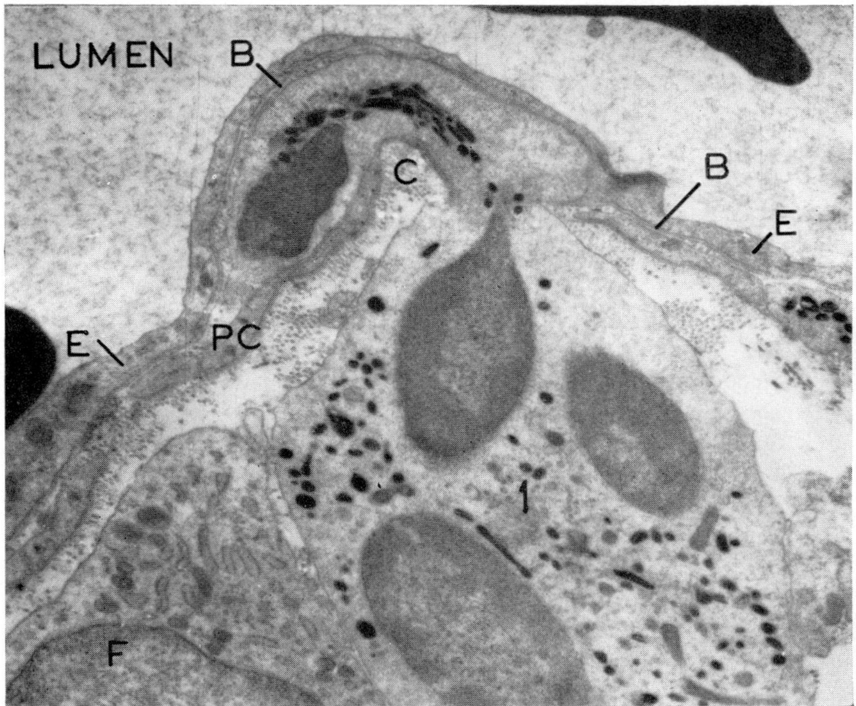

3/Fig. 62.—Inflamed venule of a rat. A polymorph (1) is spreading out into the connective tissue. F = fibroblast. E = endothelium. B = basement membrane. PC = periendothelial cell. C = Collagen. (× 13,500.) (From Marchesi and Florey.[34])

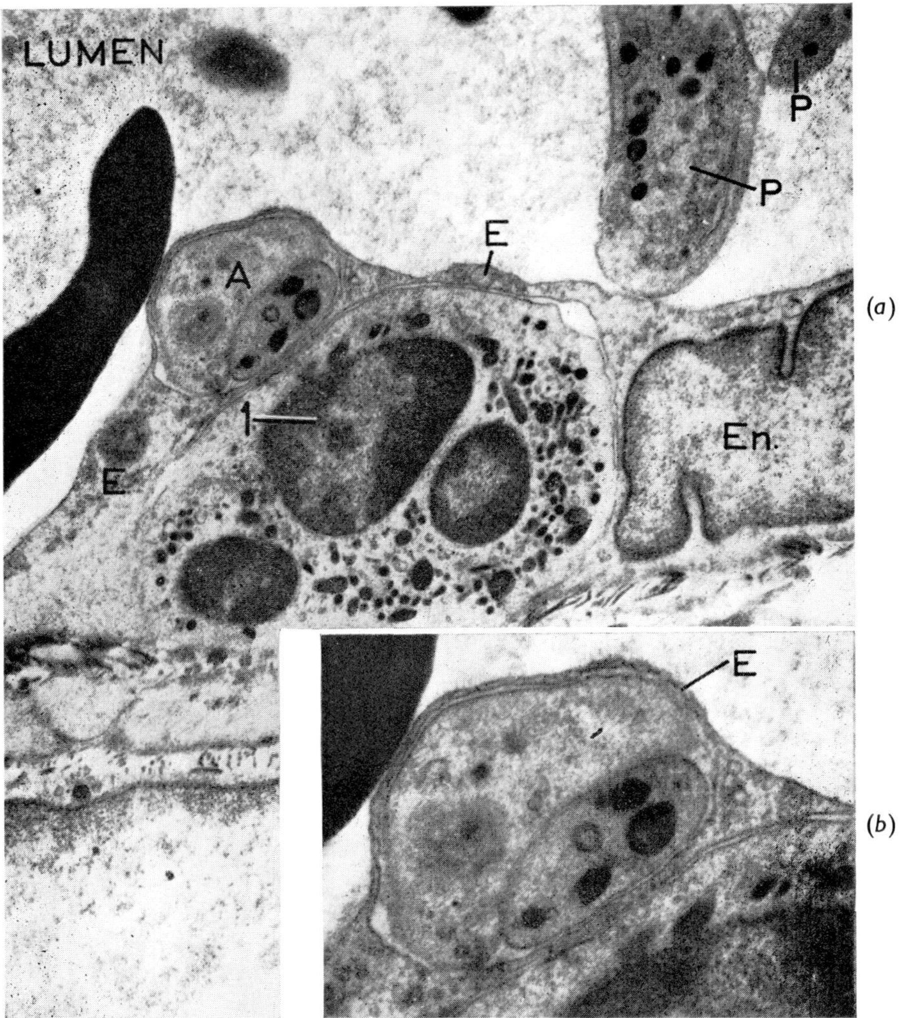

3/Fig. 63.—Inflamed venule of a rat. (*a*) Cell 1 is a polymorph in the subendothelial space. At A is an intracellular object which is seen enlarged in (*b*). The object seems to be entirely surrounded by endothelial cytoplasm, without a cell junction. It is composed of two portions, the smaller of which might be a platelet. The other portion might be the clear hyaloplasm of a leucocyte. The endothelium over these structures is tenuous and looks like a string of irregular-sized beads, but it seems to be intact. (× 22,000.) (From Marchesi and Florey.[34])

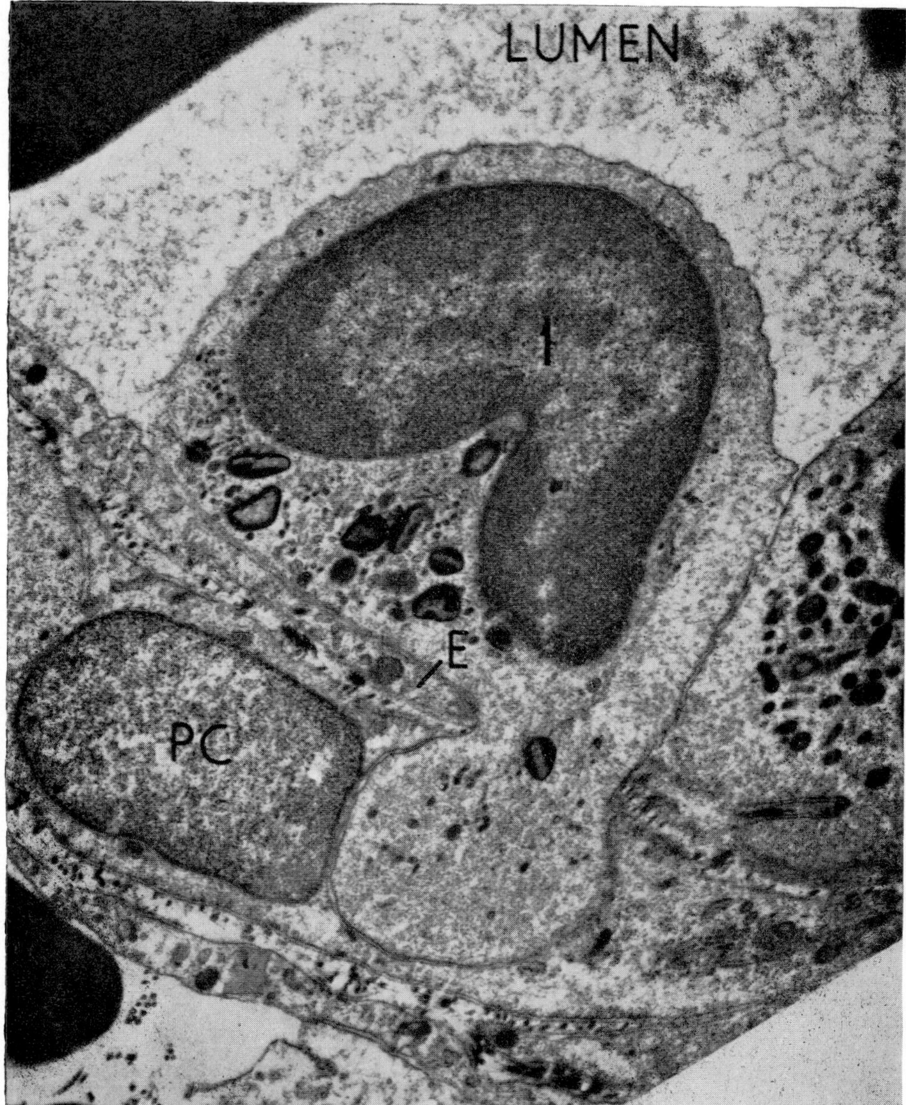

3/FIG. 64.—Inflamed venule of a rat. Cell 1, containing the characteristic granules of an eosinophil, is passing through the endothelium (E). It has penetrated deeply into a periendothelial cell (PC). (× 18,000.) (From Marchesi and Florey.[34])

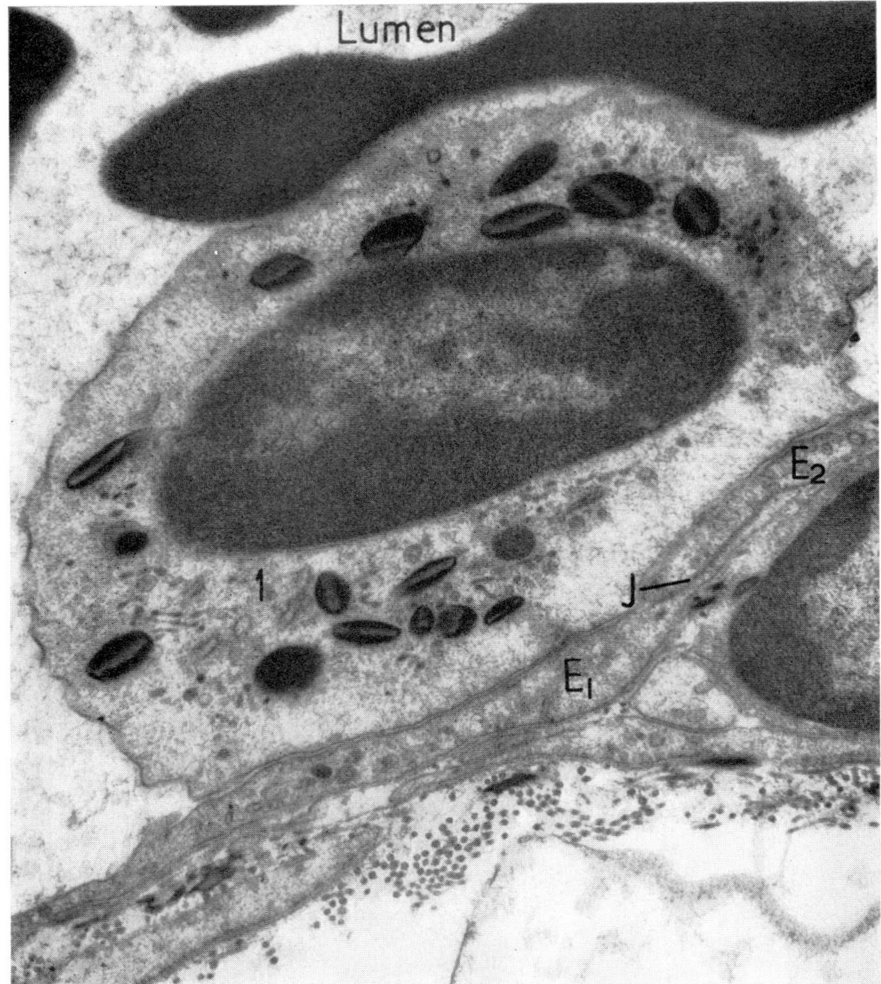

3/Fig. 65.—Inflamed venule of a rat. Cell 1 is an eosinophil flattened against a venule wall. An apparently intact intercellular junction (J) joins the endothelial cells E1 and E2. (× 24,000.) (From Marchesi.[35])

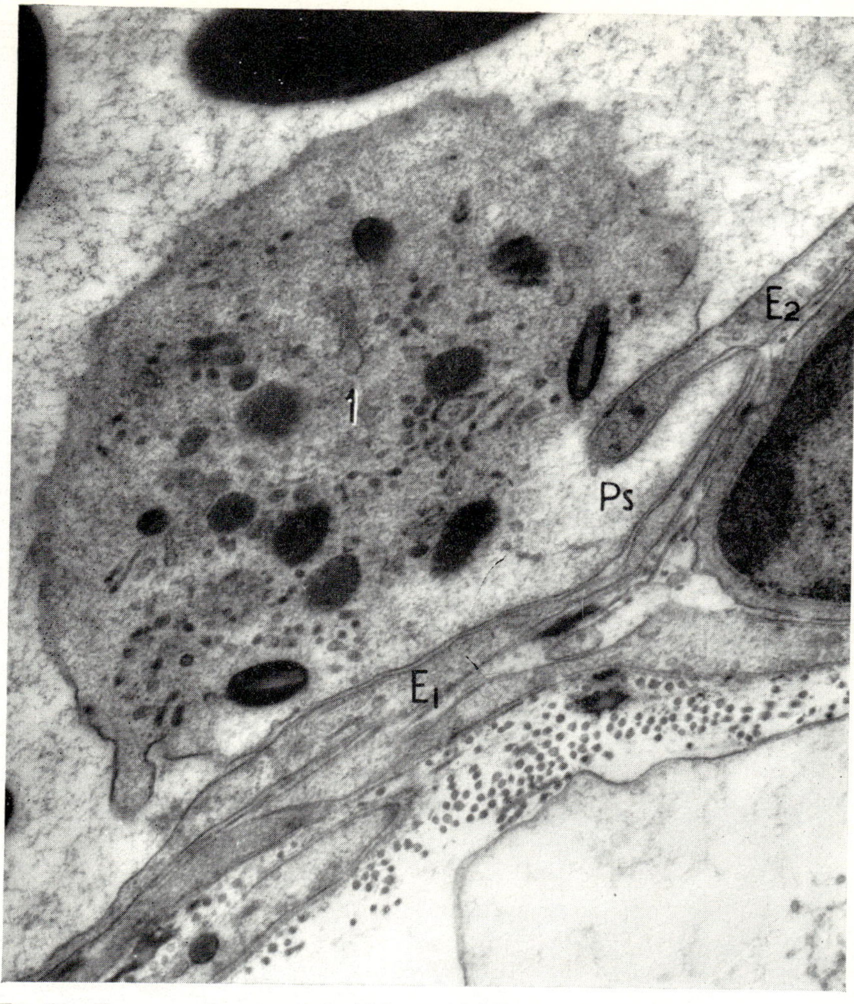

3/FIG. 66.—From a section near that which provided FIG. 65. In this plane the eosinophil has a pseudopod (Ps) extending into the intercellular junction between E1 and E2. (× 24,000.) (From Marchesi.[35])

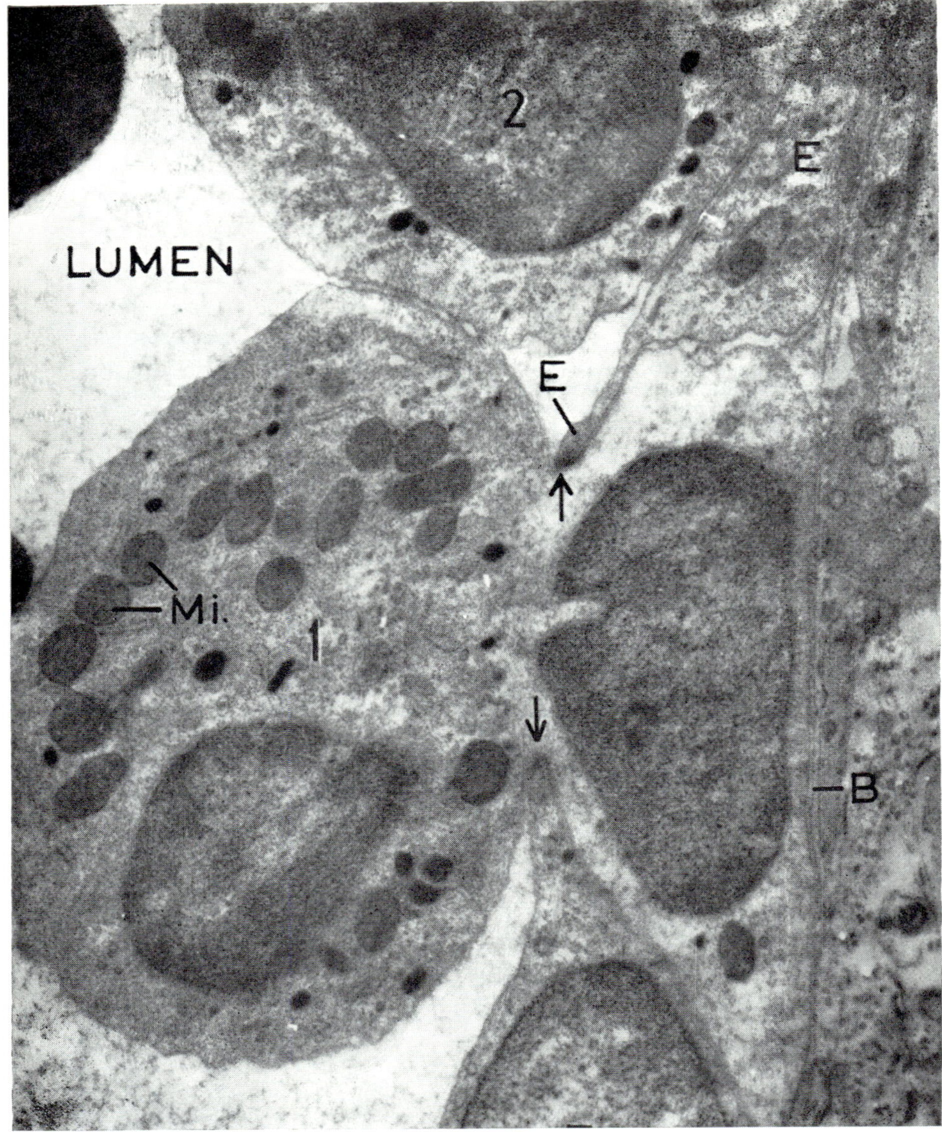

3/Fig. 67.—Inflamed venule of a rat. Cell 1 is passing through the endothelium (E) and is flattened against the basement membrane (B). The number and shape of the mitochondria and the few granules make it almost certain that this is a monocyte. The electron-dense material at the arrows may be parts of an adhesion plate (tight area of a junction). Cell 2 is a leucocyte adherent to the vessel wall. (× 28,500.) (From Marchesi and Florey.[34])

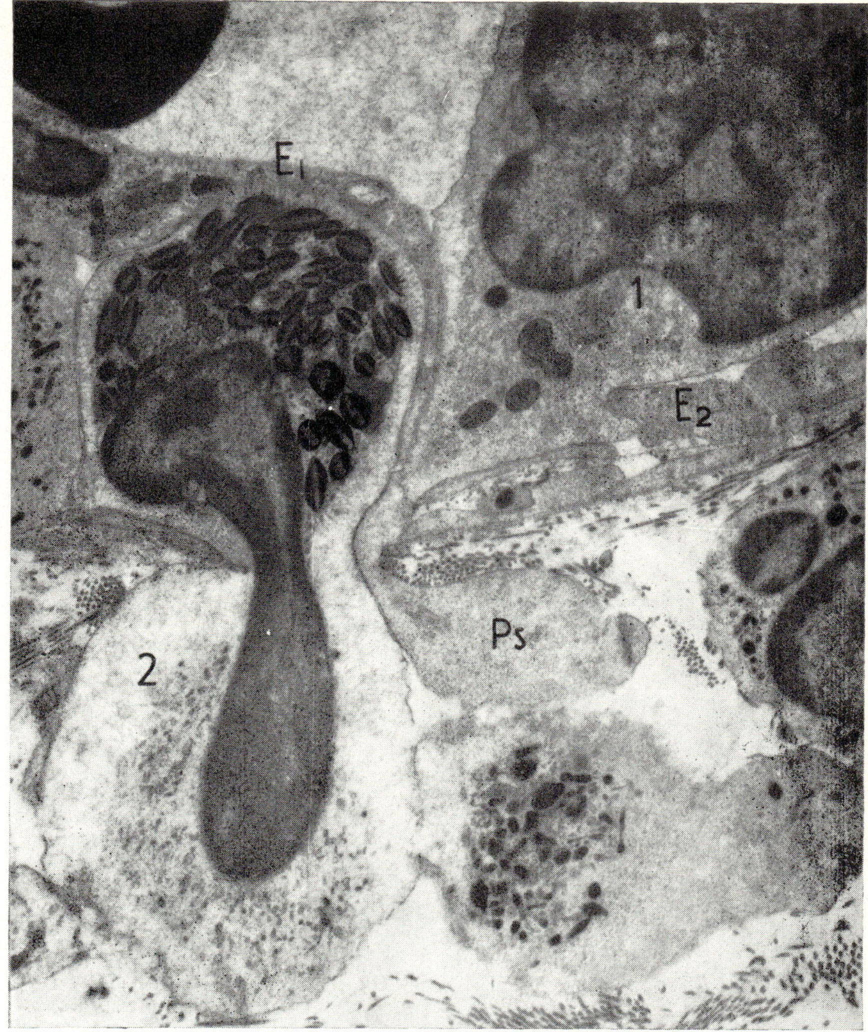

3/Fig. 68.—An eosinophil (2) and a monocyte (1) penetrating the wall of a venule together. The eosinophil is already on the outside of the endothelium and is beginning to emerge into the surrounding tissue, while the monocyte is just beginning to penetrate it. The eosinophil's granules are well shown bunched up in the hind portion of the cell. The advancing pseudopod contains only fine granules. The monocyte is almost free from granules, the grey objects being mitochondria. Ps = pseudopod of monocyte. (× 12,000.) (From Marchesi.[35])

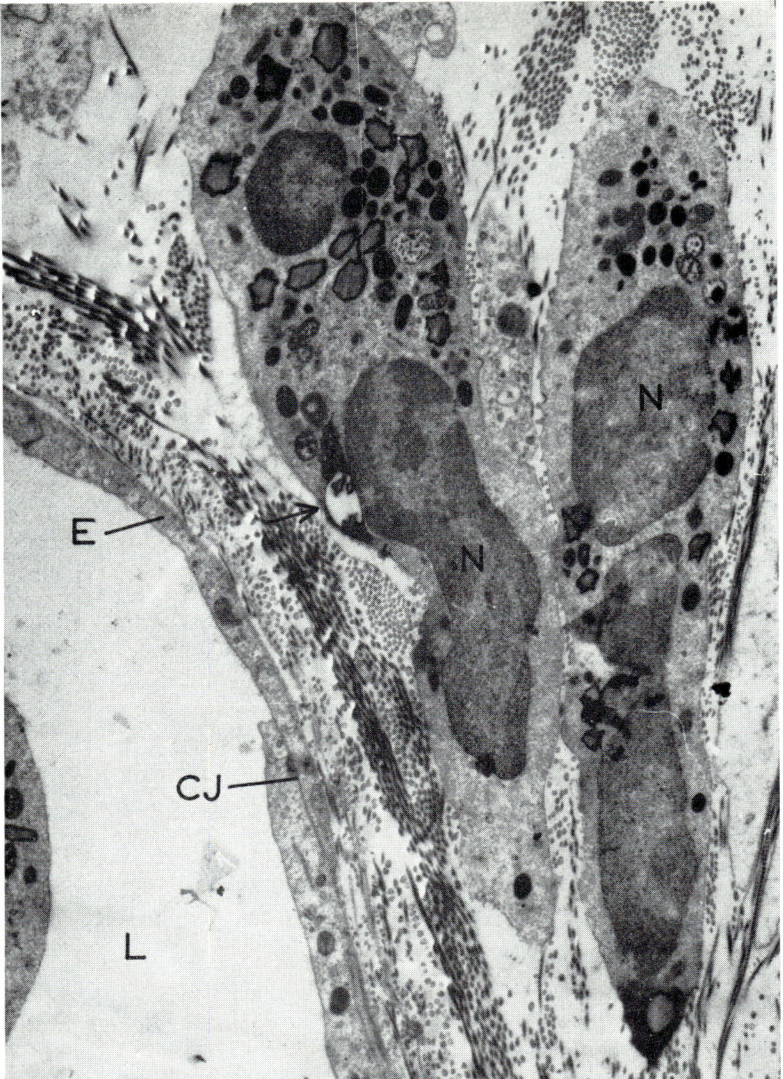

3/Fig. 69.—Ear chamber of rabbit. Two polymorph leucocytes are free in the connective tissue surrounding a venule. The endothelium of the venule (E) has a cell junction (CJ). A portion of a polymorph is seen in the lumen of the vessel. The granules of the migrated leucocytes had the same appearance as those of the leucocytes in the vessel lumen. The arrow indicates what appears to be a partly empty granule. L = lumen. (× 10,500.) (From Florey and Grant.[33])

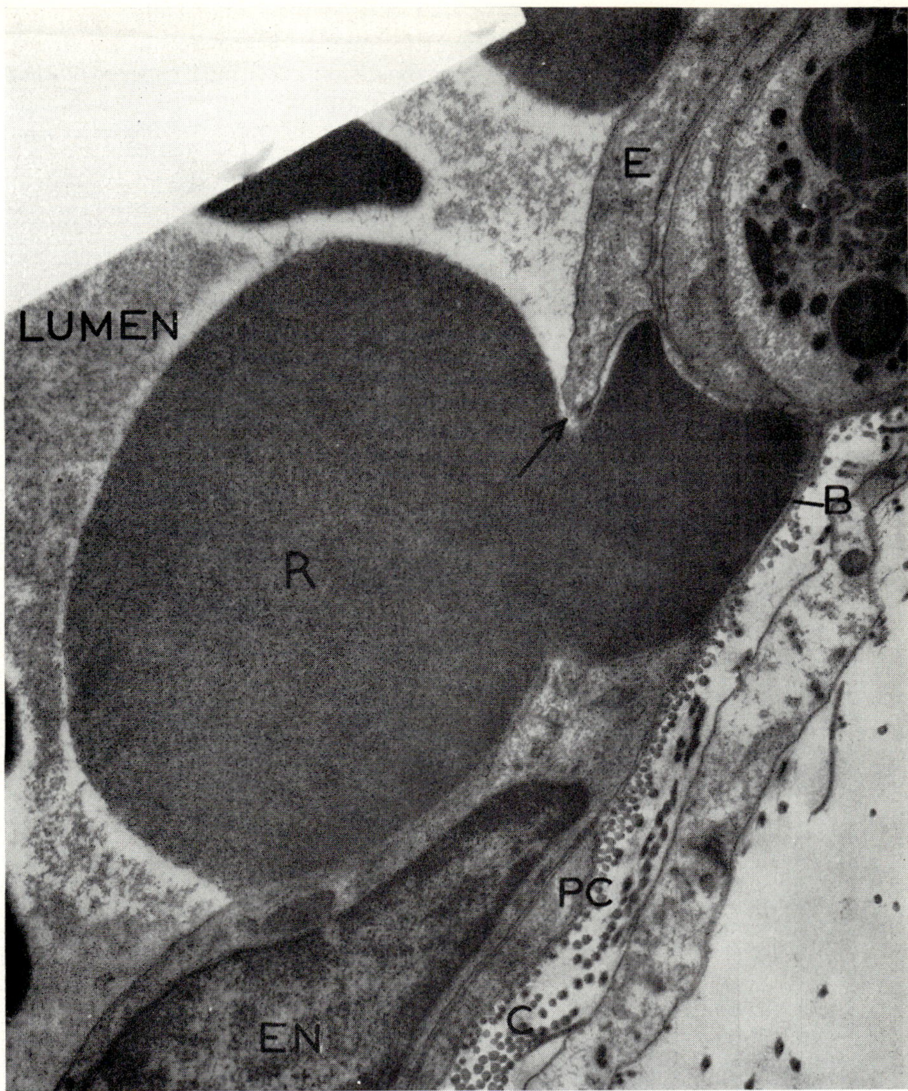

3/Fig. 70.—Inflamed venule of rat. Red cell (R) passing through the endothelium (E). There is possibly an adhesion plate at the arrow. En = nucleus of endothelial cell. PC = periendothelial cell. C = collagen. B = basement membrane. (× 21,000.) (From Marchesi and Florey.[34])

through the fine vessels. Even if loss of fluid through the capillary walls does not go so far as to produce stasis the corpuscles may be suspended in a reduced amount of plasma with the result, which has been confirmed experimentally, that the blood becomes more viscous. Landis attributed the rise in capillary pressure that takes place during the development of stasis to the increased difficulty of forcing viscous blood through the fine vessels. With increasing escape of fluid outside the vessels it is possible also that the venules are somewhat compressed mechanically and so pressure is put up in the vessels feeding them.

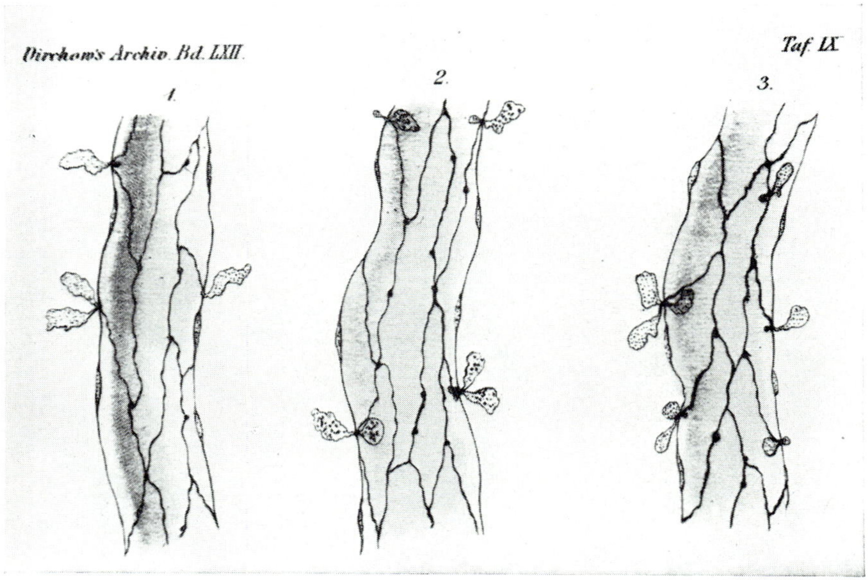

3/FIG. 71.—*1.* A small inflamed vessel, called a capillary by the author, from the tongue of a frog. The intercellular borders have been stained with silver. Leucocytes are penetrating the walls at points on the intercellular junctions.
2. A similar preparation from a frog mesentery.
3. A similar preparation from a frog bladder. (From Arnold, 1875.[36])

The cause of the adhesion of the leucocytes to the walls of inflamed vessels awaits elucidation. It might of course be due to changes in the leucocytes themselves, but although they do sometimes adhere to one another in inflamed areas it has been observed in chambers in the rabbit's ear that a leucocyte can bowl along in the peripheral stream till it comes to a localised area of inflammation, then adhere to the wall, and again be carried along normally when the inflamed area is passed. Red cells and platelets can also occasionally be seen to adhere to the walls of inflamed vessels. It is disappointing that so far the electron microscope has not given any clear evidence of the existence of a change in the endothelial surface although it is always possible that technical advances may disclose something more than can be seen at present.

Evidence of some change in the endothelium is provided by visible roughness in the form of "spikes". The red cells can be seen to catch on these spikes and be bent double round them by the force of the blood stream (FIG. 72). The Clarks described how compression of an inflamed capillary could result, on release, in the formation of delicate threads of endothelial substance stretching across the lumen from side to side. Red cells were often temporarily suspended on the threads. There was very firm sticking of leucocytes to the vessel walls at the time this was observed. Further consideration is given in the next chapter to the sticking of leucocytes to vessel walls and their subsequent migration.

The fact that many types of stimuli call forth the same inflammatory response has already been mentioned. Probably the most frequent cause of inflammation is invasion of the body by pathogenic bacteria, and although the general phenomena are the same in all acute inflammations there may be great differences in the relative proportions of fluid and cells that pass out from the inflamed vessels.

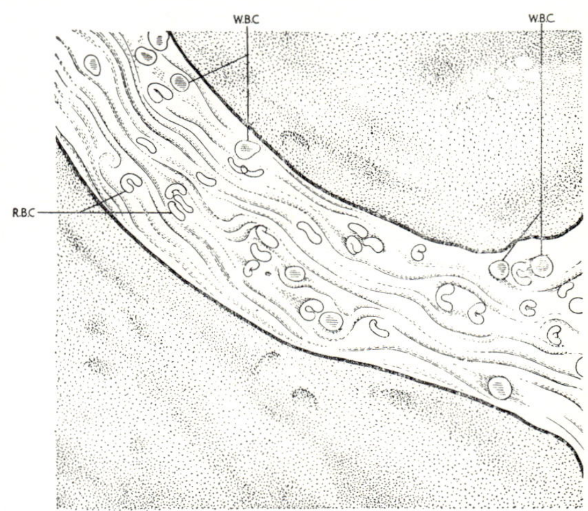

3/FIG. 72.—"Spikes" on endothelial surface of a venule. Red corpuscles are caught and bent double on these "spikes", the exact nature of which is unknown. The freely flowing red cells are represented by stream lines.

(A drawing from a photograph of the phenomenon as seen in a transparent chamber in a rabbit's ear.)

When a tissue is fixed and prepared for microscopic examination in the usual way the granulocytes round up and appear as in FIG. 73. These round cells were moving about actively in the tissues by the projection of their pseudopods until they were killed by noxious agents present in inflamed tissues or by a fixative used to preserve the tissues, or they may have died many hours or days after death of the body as a whole.

THE LYMPHATIC SYSTEM

Blood vessels can be relatively easily studied because they contain a red fluid that makes them conspicuous, but lymphatics, which are very numerous in nearly all the tissues of the body, contain colourless fluid and in normal circumstances any changes that they may undergo are not appreciated. For experimental purposes they can be injected with coloured or opaque fluids of one sort or another. The older anatomists studied them in great detail and some of the beautiful preparations made during the nineteenth century have never been surpassed. FIGURE 75 from Sappey's anatomical work[40] shows the great profusion of lymphatic capillaries and collecting trunks in the breast. Nearly all parts of the body are as richly supplied with such vessels.

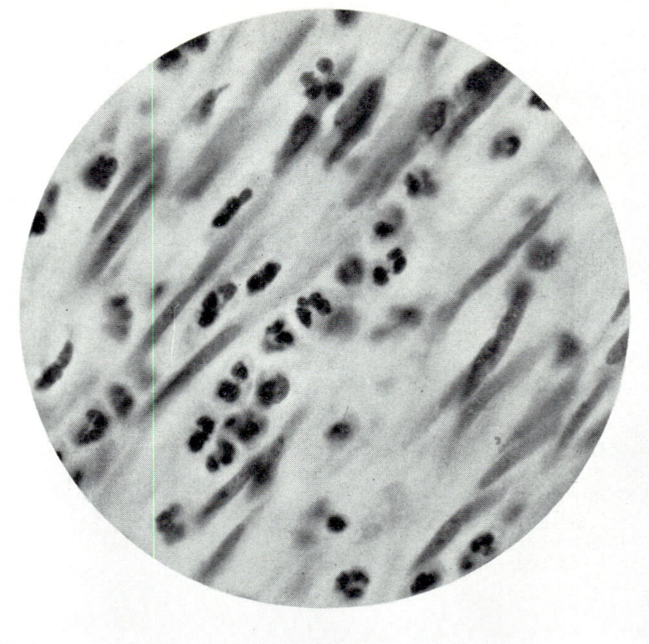

3/Fig. 73.—Shows the separation of smooth muscle fibres in the wall of the appendix by inflammatory œdema fluid and by granulocytes, which have become rounded up during fixation.

It is possible to see lymphatics in the living human skin when they are injected with such dyes as Patent blue V or pontamine blue, as was shown by Hudack and McMaster[39] (Fig. 74). A fine needle is inserted into the skin and the injection made through it without attempting to enter any individual lymphatic vessel. Fluid thus injected enters and shows up the lymphatic capillaries. The richness of the plexus of vessels is well shown in the figures, and it is clear that intradermal injection, quite a common clinical procedure, must in all probability be associated with injection into the lymphatics.

Recent technical improvements have made easier the investigation of the lymphatic system. Non-toxic radiopaque dyes have been developed and they can be used even for injection into man, a circumstance which has been taken advantage of, particularly in surgery. The invention of small calibre polyethylene tubing has greatly facilitated the cannulation of small lymphatics for lymph does not clot readily in it. Indeed experiments lasting many days can be performed on animals and long observations made on man. It could be maintained that much of the spectacular advance in our knowledge of lymphocytes (see Chapter 5) owes its origin to the polyethylene tube. The cannulation of lymphatics such as are present in a digital cleft of man enables the anatomy of the lymphatic system to be shewn up so that it is possible to follow and examine its condition in disease. In particular it has been shewn that the lesions in what are called idiopathic primary œdemas are aplastic, hypoplastic, varicose and dilated lymphatics. The condition is not due to blockage of lymphatics as was at one time believed.

Structure of Lymphatics

The lymphatics possess some of the physiological properties of small blood vessels, but they are generally credited with being normally more readily permeable to large protein molecules and particles such as chylomicra. If this were so it might be expected that with the electron microscope some morphological

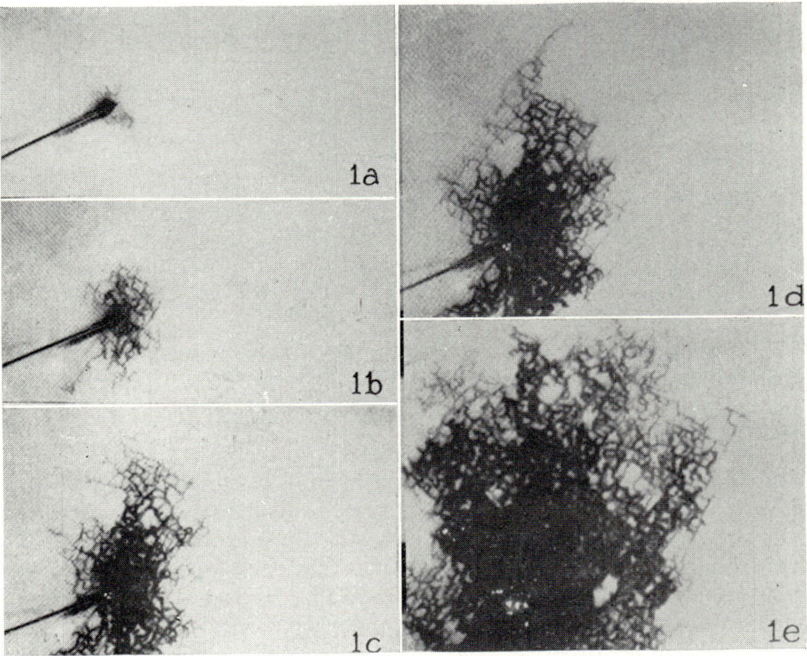

3/FIG. 74.—The lymphatic network shown up by the injection of an 11 per cent solution of Patent blue V into the skin of man. The successive pictures were taken from a cinematograph film. (From Hudack and McMaster.[39])

differences between the two types of vessel might be demonstrable. It is true that the structure of lymphatic endothelium from some areas, for example the wall of the intestine, bears a close resemblance to that of blood vessels (FIGS. 76, 77, 79), but there are certain differences. In the absence of comprehensive investigation on the lymphatics it is impossible to say whether differences in morphology exist between lymphatic endothelial cells from different organs of the striking character met with in blood vessels, e.g. those between the blood vessels of the adrenal and the cardiac muscle. However, at least in some places such as the diaphragm, the intestine and the ears of guinea-pigs and mice the basement membrane is absent or only present in patches. But the distinction is not absolute for

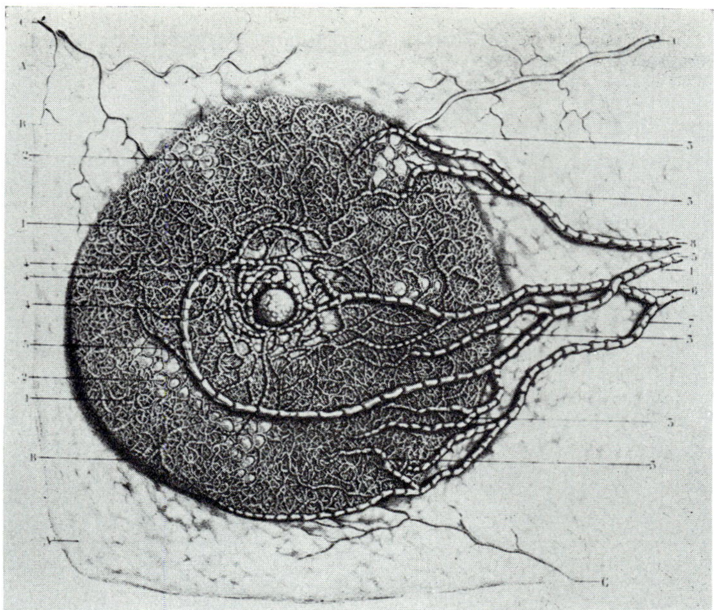

3/FIG. 75.—Shows the very complex network of lymphatics in the breast. The vessels unite to form trunks which have a beaded appearance due to the presence of valves. (From Sappey.[40])

it is possible to find lymphatic endothelium with a well-marked basement membrane (Casley-Smith and Florey[41]; Kato[42]) (FIG. 76).

Although the lymphatic endothelial cells may in general be very like those of blood vessels from the skin or heart, in certain areas, e.g. the guinea-pig ear, they project numerous processes both into the lumen and into the connective tissue surrounding the vessels. There are also very deep indentations in the wall which give the vessels a most irregular appearance (see e.g. Leak and Burke[43]). At small areas of the junctions between endothelial cells electron densities are found corresponding to those seen in blood vessels, but some junctions are without such areas. As yet the minute examination such as is at present being made of endothelial junctions in blood vessels has not been accorded to lymphatic endothelium, nevertheless observers are now agreed that completely open junctions can be observed in the lymphatics of normal diaphragm, intestine, mouse and guinea-pig ear, and rabbit thoracic duct (Kato[42]). For example, open junctions containing carbon particles have been found in diaphragmatic lymphatic capillaries after the intraperitoneal injection of carbon (FIG. 78), and fat particles have been found in open junctions of lacteals of the villi during the absorption of fat from the intestine.

These open junctions cannot be looked on as conferring a very porous structure on lymphatics for lymphatics can be injected with colloidal carbon without any obvious leaks being demonstrated under the small magnification of the light microscope (FIG. 80), but their existence is probably of importance not only under physiological conditions but during inflammation. It is possible

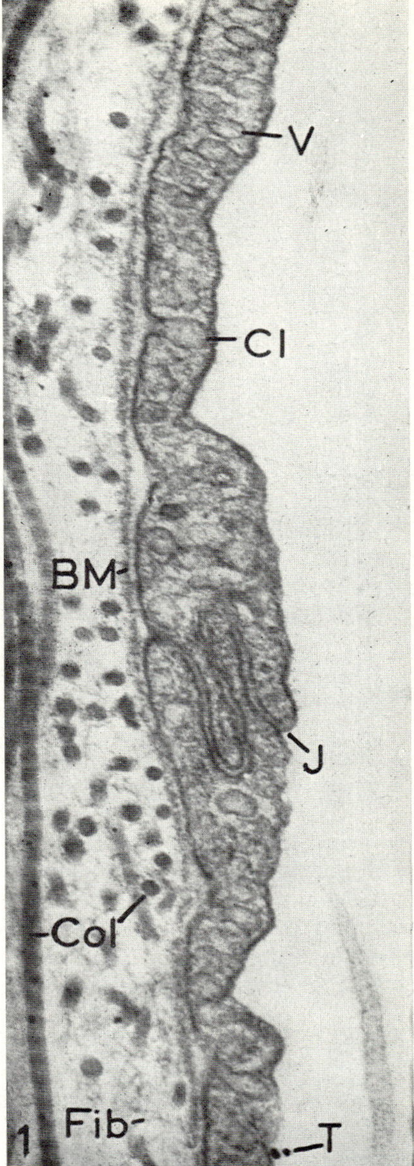

3/Fig. 76.—Endothelial cells from a lymphatic of a mouse's ear. The picture shows a junction (J) between two endothelial cells, numerous intracellular vesicles (V) and deep caveolæ intracellulares (CI), a prominent basement membrane (BM) and collagen fibres (Col) in transverse and longitudinal section. Between the collagen fibres there are numerous fine, irregular fibrils (Fib). At T two particles of thorium dioxide are seen in the lumen. (× 70,000) (From Casley-Smith and Florey.[41])

that lymph may escape in small amounts from normal lymphatics, even from those constituting main trunks.

Lymph Flow in Inflammation

Under physiological conditions fluid from the tissue spaces passes into the lymph capillaries and thence via the collecting trunks and lymph nodes back to

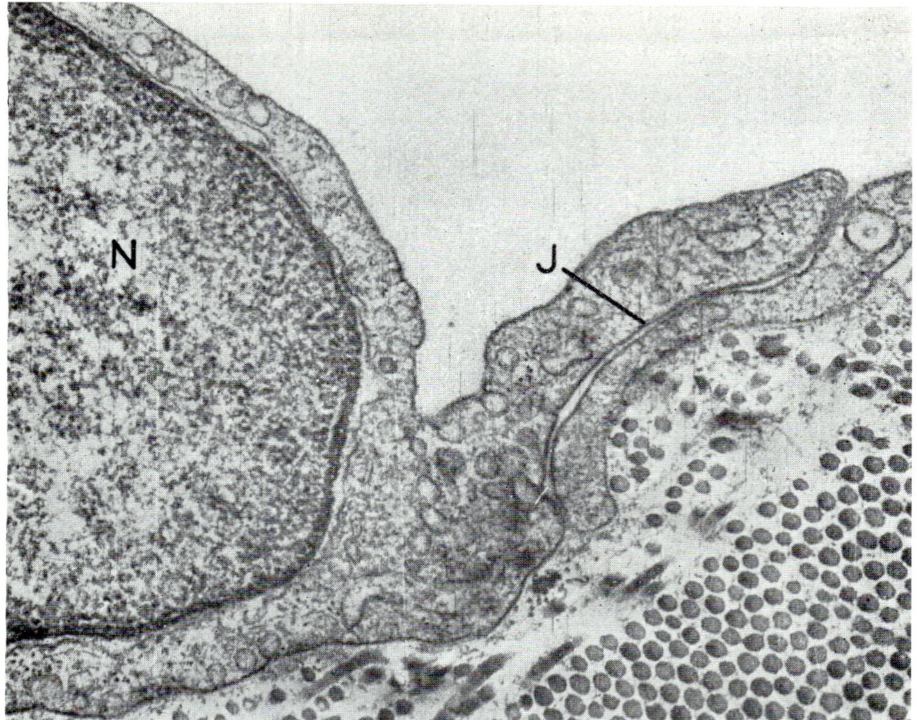

3/FIG. 77.—Endothelial cells of a lymphatic from a rat's colon. The picture shows a junction between two cells (J), many intracellular vesicles and a nucleus (N). (× 50,000) (From Casley-Smith and Florey.[41])

the veins. Large-sized molecules and particles such as chylomicra are removed from the tissue spaces in this fluid, and under pathological conditions foreign particles such as bacteria and even red blood cells and leucocytes may find their way into lymphatics and be transported to the nearest lymph node. Under physiological conditions there may be a flow of lymph only during considerable activity of the part, for instance when the muscles of a limb are contracting

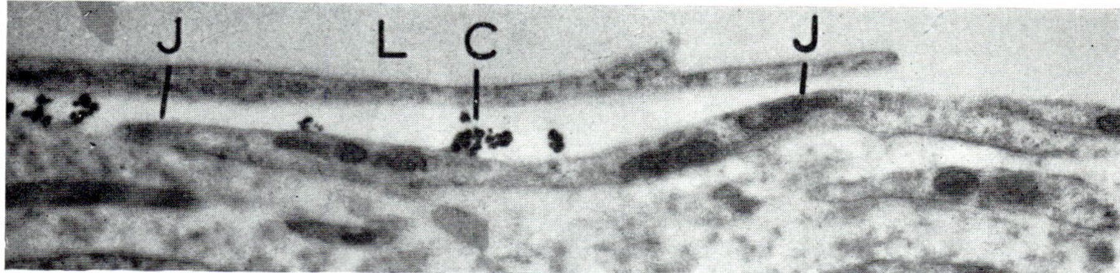

3/FIG. 78.—An open junction (J) between two endothelial cells in a lymphatic of the mouse's diaphragm. Carbon was injected into the peritoneal cavity and has found its way into the open junction. It can be seen at C. L is the lumen of the lymphatic vessel. (× 20,000) (From Casley-Smith and Florey.[41])

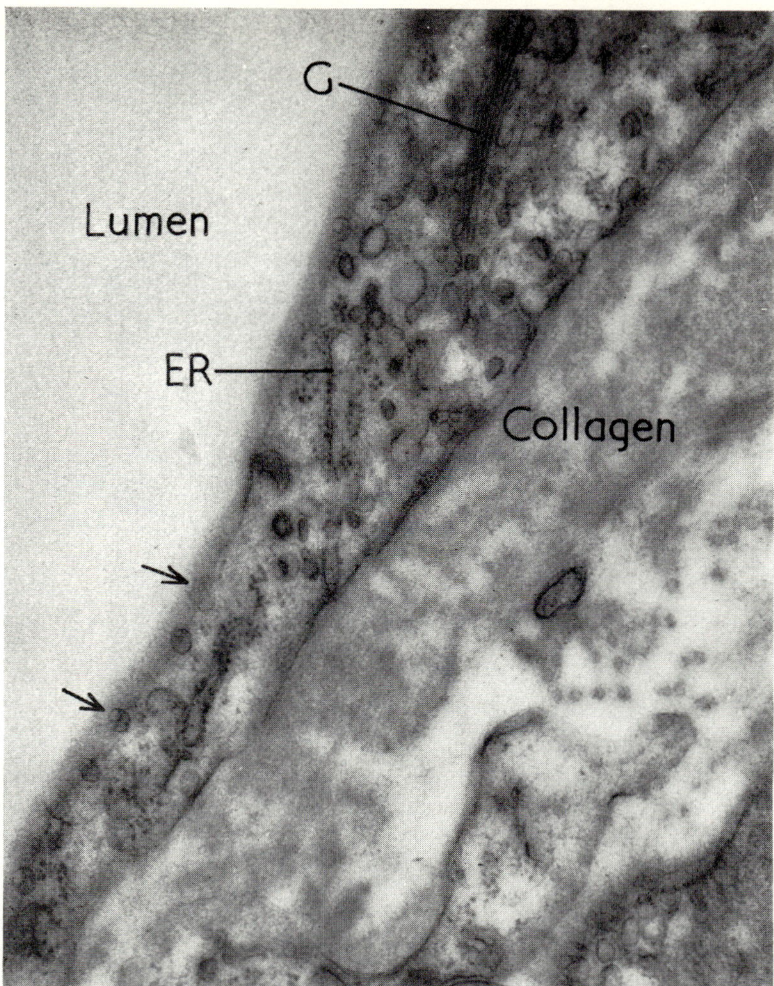

3/FIG. 79.—Rat colon. This picture illustrates some of the organelles of lymphatic endothelium. A Golgi complex is shown (G), also many tubular endoplasmic reticular elements, often lined with RNA particles (ER). There are some free RNA particles, many vesicles, and caveolæ intracellulares. The luminal plasma membrane is sectioned obliquely. Cross sections of openings of caveolæ intracellulares in this membrane can be seen at the arrows. (× 61,000) (From Casley-Smith and Florey.[41])

vigorously. If, however, the limb be inflamed, then the flow of lymph rich in protein is considerable and it may easily clot, as was first pointed out by Cohnheim.

Starling in 1894[44] stated that if the foot of a dog was kept in water at 60° C. for 5 minutes the lymph flow was increased and the lymph became richer in protein—an observation similar to that of Samuel, who showed that from 7 to 8 times as much lymph may drain away from an inflamed as from an uninflamed region. Such observations have been confirmed many times.

Drinker and his colleagues investigated lymph production in detail and under many conditions. They found that changes in flow, pressure and protein concentration occurred when the part producing the lymph was subjected to external temperatures of between 50° and 60° C., and that the lymph flow was

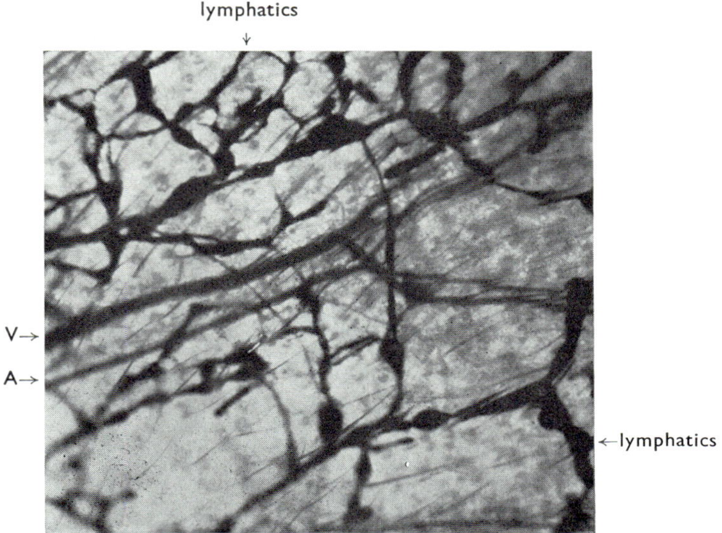

3/FIG. 80.—The lymphatics in the ear of a living mouse have been injected with carbon. The closed network of lymphatic vessels of very irregular calibre is shown. The smooth walled artery and vein are indicated by A and V.

enormously increased in the presence of sterile inflammation. There was no measurable normal lymph pressure in the leg of an anæsthetised dog, but pressure rose to 120 cm. of lymph during inflammation. It is thus clear that the increased blood flow associated with inflammation has a parallel in increased flow of lymph.

Attempts have been made by other means to investigate what happens to the permeability of lymphatics following mild injury. Thus McMaster and Hudack[45] applied in the mouse the same elegant injection method that they used in man. They spread the mouse's ear over a white background and injected a solution of a poorly diffusible dye such as pontamine blue into the skin at the edge of the ear through a very fine glass needle. The dye soon entered neighbouring lymphatics which were clearly shown up. A fine suspension of carbon can be injected in a similar way, though in this case the needle has to be inserted into a lymphatic, a procedure which can easily be accomplished by trial and error. McMaster and Hudack found that a slight scratch, which did not obviously damage the skin, made the lymphatics beneath the line of scratch permeable to pontamine blue, which escaped into the surrounding tissues (FIG. 81). Fine carbon particles did not escape, but hæmoglobin readily passed through the injured walls. Heating the ear to 43° C., the application of xylol, and even scratching at the ear by the mouse itself increased the permeability.

It can be objected that, especially in inflammatory conditions, the passage of fluid is from the tissues into the lymphatics and not vice versa, as occurs in the experiments just quoted. This may be true but the experiments certainly demonstrate that normal lymphatics are not sieves and that mild trauma may injure their walls. The possible ways in which large molecules or particles pass from the outside to the inside of lymphatics have been investigated with the electron microscope in ways parallel to those employed on endothelium of blood vessels. As a result of this it is well established that following injury many more open

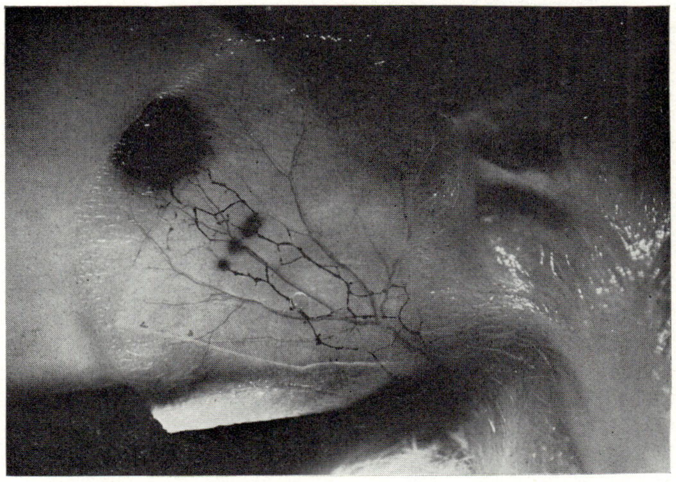

3/Fig. 81.—Ear of a living anæsthetised mouse photographed by reflected light 6 minutes after the entry of standard pontamine blue solution into the lymphatic capillaries. Ten minutes previously the ear was stroked transversely across the middle with a blunt wire. Immediately before taking the photograph a fragment of coverslip was placed upon the ear, which had been coated with paraffin oil to increase visibility.

Sharply localised ecchymoses of dye appeared along the line of "tache", although this latter was so weak as not to elicit any reaction of the blood vessels. Under normal conditions no such escape occurs in ½ hour. (From McMaster and Hudack.[45])

junctions between endothelial cells occur than in normal tissue and it may well be that the absence or poor development of anchoring devices, such as "adhesion plates" or "tight junctions" are supposed to be, may facilitate the solution of continuity under relatively mild stress. The caveolar system is also supposed to be involved in fluid transport because particles can be found in vesicles after injection into the tissues, but following the results of investigations on blood vessels it would be wise to reserve judgment on the role they play, which in any case would seem to be small. The view that particles or large molecules such as protein pass directly through the cytoplasm of lymphatic endothelium needs much greater proof than has been so far supplied.

At the present time it seems most probable that just as fluid escapes from

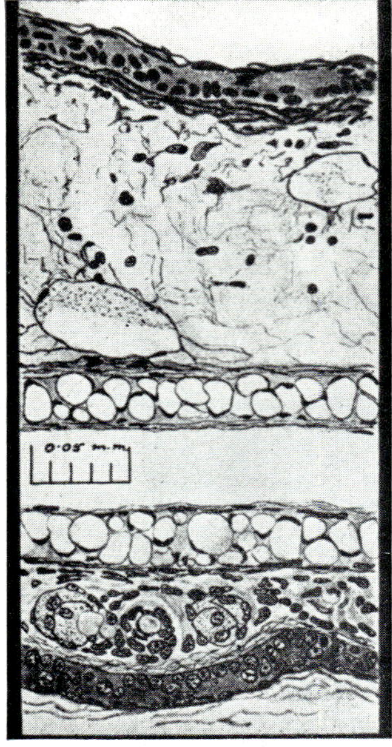

3/FIG. 82.—The upper picture is from a mouse's ear in which œdema was produced by the application of heat. Cross-sections of dilated lymphatics containing a fine coagulum can be seen. Fine fibres are attached to the walls of the lymphatics. For comparison a section of a normal ear is shown below. No lymphatic channels are visible. (From Pullinger and Florey.[46])

inflamed blood vessels through open endothelial cell junctions so it gains access to lymphatic vessels by a similar process. The intimate chemical mechanism involved is no clearer than is that operating on blood vessels.

The increased flow of lymph during inflammation is due to the increased exudation of fluid from the blood vessels. It is well established that the plasma protein molecules which escape from the blood vessels under either physiological or pathological conditions do not re-enter blood vessels but are drained back into the blood via lymphatics—in other words lymphatics can be conceived of as an elaborate drainage system for the tissues. Although it is certain that the fluid in the lymphatics originates from the blood and that the lymphatic capillaries are more permeable during acute inflammation it is not yet certain what conditions in the tissues ensure the passage of fluid from the tissue spaces into the lymphatics.

It might be argued that increased pressure in the tissue spaces associated with the out-pouring of fluid from the blood vessels would have the effect of compressing the lymph capillaries, for the pressure in them is presumably somewhat less than in the extravascular spaces. Indeed, Adami[47] stated that the lymphatics were collapsed in inflamed tissues. It is not very difficult to show, however, that the lymphatics are in fact dilated by the swelling of the tissues. Dilated lymphatic capillaries in œdematous tissues of tadpoles and chicks have been described by Clark and Clark,[48] and the upper part of FIG. 82 shows dilated lymphatics in the ear of a mouse made œdematous by the application of heat. In the lower, unheated ear, lymphatics cannot be recognised. This observation of the dilatation of lymphatics during inflammatory swelling continues to be confirmed.

It will be remembered that in such tissues as the skin an axon reflex dilates the arterioles in the neighbourhood of an injured area. But another factor is involved, for the finer blood vessels become paralysed by the inflammatory processes or, at least, they do not respond to stimuli which produce contraction in normal vessels. Thus Meltzer and Meltzer found that they did not contract to adrenalin, and Jacobj[49] showed that there was paralysis of their contractile elements, since they did not react to stimulation of the sympathetic nerves. When there is loss of tone the vessels are widely dilated by the hydrostatic pressure of the blood inside them.

This state of things cannot apply to the lymphatics, which have the lowest pressure in the gradient blood: tissue: lymph. A clue to the mechanism by which lymphatics are dilated was given by Gaskell[50] many years ago. He showed that the lymphatics of the larynx had fine fibres attached to their walls and he suggested that when fluid distended the tissue spaces the fibres were separated and a force applied to them which tended to stretch them. This pull on the fibres opened the lymphatics. Heimberger[51] showed that similar fibres were attached to the lymphatic capillaries at the base of the nail.

In some experiments by Pullinger and Florey[46, 52] the lymphatics of the mouse's ear were injected with carbon in fine suspension so that they could be identified with certainty, and swelling of the tissue was then induced. Sections of such ears, when appropriately stained, showed a multitude of fibres attached to the walls of the dilated lymphatics (FIG. 83). Thus it was not unreasonable to

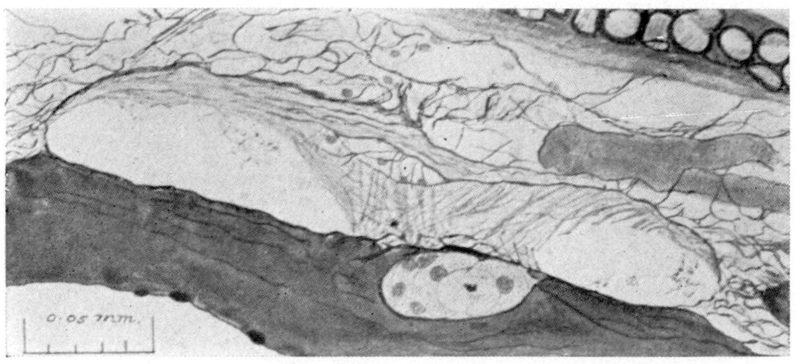

3/FIG. 83.—Tangential section of a lymphatic of a mouse's ear to show a network of fibres in the wall. These fibres are continuous with those in the surrounding connective tissue. The dark layer at the bottom of the picture is epithelium. (From Pullinger and Florey.[46])

postulate that the fluid accumulating in the tissues during the swelling associated with inflammation or during the formation of œdema from other causes (see Chapter 12) stretches the fibres attached to the outside of the endothelial walls of lymphatics and so a pull is exerted on the walls which will hold them open against an interstitial pressure greater than that within the lymphatics.

Following examination of œdematous tissues with the electron microscope this view was challenged by Viragh *et al.*[53], who maintained that the collagenous fibres attached to lymphatics break down during œdema caused by dextran injection and that the lymphatics therefore cannot be held open by them. They postulated that the lymphatics are held open by the increased amount of fluid entering them "due partly to pinocytosis". The latter statement should be received with considerable reserve. They described many patent intercellular junctions in dextran œdema and suggested that fluid is forced through them and so keeps them open.

But Leak and Burke[43, 54, 67] have demonstrated the existence of fine fibres 4 mμ in diameter between the lymphatic endothelium and the adjacent collagen fibres (see FIGS. 84–87). Many of these fine fibres are attached to the plasmalemma of the endothelial cells at areas of increased electron density. It is suggested that

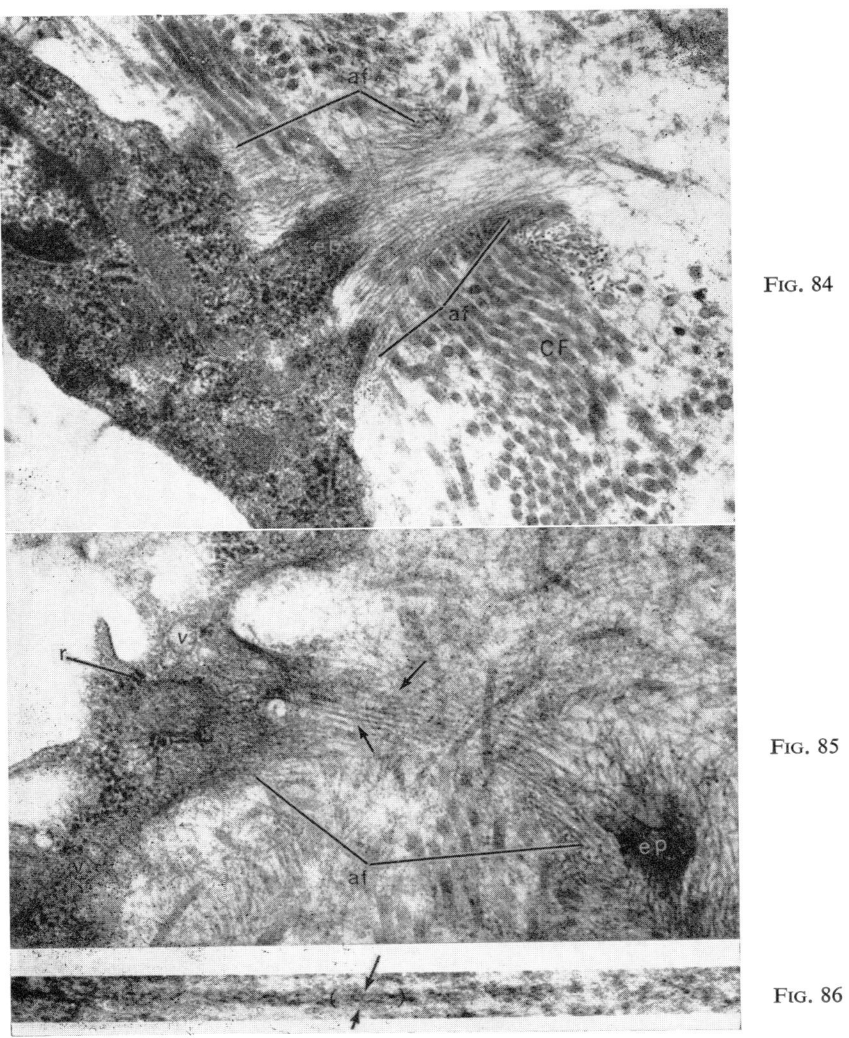

3/FIG. 84.—Anchoring filaments (af) emanate from the lymphatic endothelial processes (ep) and continue for varying distances among collagen bundles (CF). The lumen of the lymphatic is seen at lower left. (× 25,000.) (From Leak and Burke.[67])

3/FIG. 85.—Cytoplasmic bleb (ep) represents a portion of endothelial cell projection which is surrounded by the anchoring filaments (af) that extend from the main part of lymphatic wall. Some of the filaments exhibit a beaded pattern (arrows) along their long axis. This grazing section across the endothelial surface illustrates the insertion of anchoring filaments on the outer leaflet of the unit membrane, or within the surface layer which resides exterior to the outer leaflet of the trilaminar unit membrane. Ribosomes (r) and vesicles (v) are observed in the cytoplasm. The lumen of the vessel is at upper left. (× 36,000.) (From Leak and Burke.[67])

3/FIG. 86.—Enlarged magnification of anchoring filaments from Fig. 85 which demonstrates the beaded pattern that is present in these filaments (arrows). (× 170,000.) (From Leak and Burke.[67])

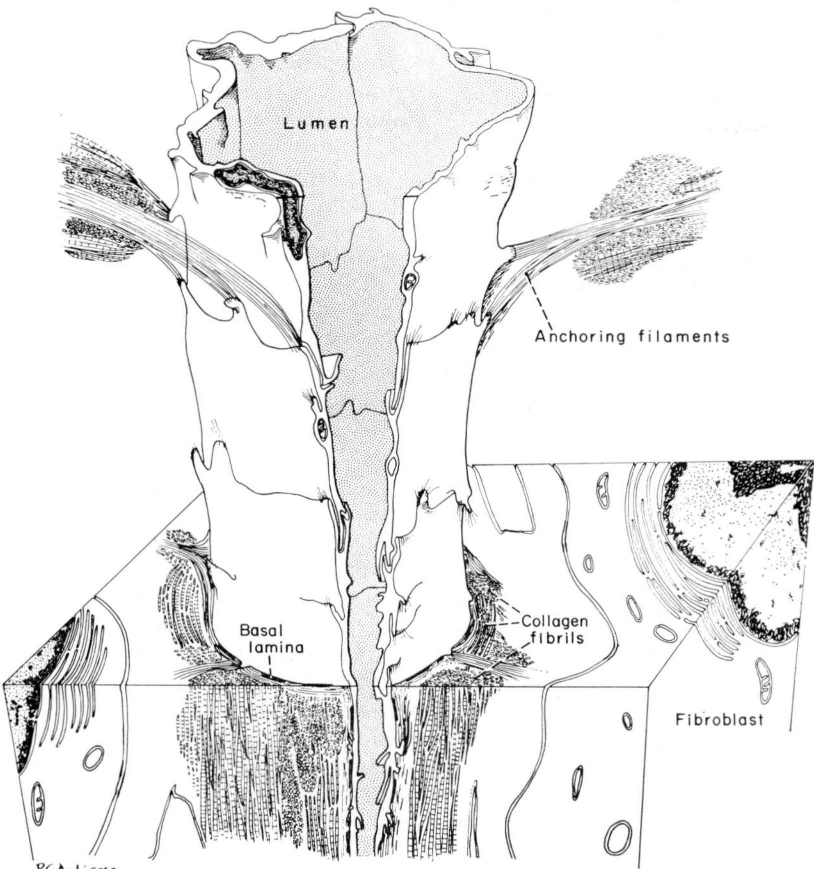

3/Fig. 87.—A three-dimensional, interpretative diagram of a lymphatic capillary that was reconstructed from collated electron micrographs. The three-dimensional relation of the lymphatic capillary to the surrounding connective tissue area is illustrated. The lymphatic anchoring filaments appear to originate from the endothelial cells, and extend among collagen bundles, elastic fibres, and cells of the adjoining tissue area, thus providing a firm connection between the lymphatic capillary wall and the surrounding connective tissue. Irregular basal lamina and collagen fibres are as marked. (From Leak and Burke.[67])

these filaments stabilise the lymphatic capillary especially when the intercellular junctions are partially or completely open. They found that the inner overlapping segments of intercellular junctions were not stabilised by the fine filaments and they envisage that this area might act as a "swinging flap". Casley-Smith[55] agreed that these fine fibres exist and are attached both to endothelium and collagen fibres. He found lymphatics open in dextran œdema and suggested that the endothelial projections into the surrounding connective tissue might be due to the pull exerted on portions of the cell by the fibres.

For the present it would seem that the concept that lymphatics are dilated in inflammation by fibres pulling on the external surface of the endothelium can be allowed to stand.

As a result of the examination of histological and electron microscopical sections it is common to conceive of connective tissue, such as exists subcutaneously, as composed of fibres of collagen and elastin embedded in some continuous hydrophilic "ground substance". Day[56] has given reasons arrived at by experiment for believing that connective tissue is composed of membranes and that this membranous structure is elastic, so that when excess fluid is introduced pressure is exerted which tends to force it into lymphatics in the neighbourhood. It may well be that the elasticity of such a membranous structure, which is thought not to be freely permeable to large molecules, could supply some of the force which moves inflammatory fluid from the connective tissues into the lymphatics.

Once in the lymphatics the lymph finds its way first to the regional lymph nodes and then into the veins by the thoracic and right lymphatic ducts. It is usually considered that the passage of lymph along the lymphatic trunks is passive, being effected by the pressure on them of the parts of the body concerned or assisted by the movements of the thorax. However, a number of animals have been shown to have rhythmically contractile lymphatic trunks. Recently unanæsthetised and freely running sheep have been investigated by Hall, Morris and Woolley[57] who have shown that the lymph from many parts of the body is propelled by the rhythmic intrinsic contractions of lymphatic trunks. No observations on the effect of inflammatory or other œdema on such pulsations have been recorded but it is possible that when there is extensive œdema the rhythmic contractions would be increased in size and frequency. The contractility of human lymphatics has not been thoroughly investigated.

Thus, to summarise, just as the finer blood vessels dilate and become more permeable to large molecules during inflammation, so the lymphatic vessels undergo parallel changes, which facilititate the removel of the excess fluid and large molecules poured into the tissues from the blood vessels. Though no doubt this is the commoner process, there is also the possibility that in a limited lesion, such as a weal, lymph may escape from the lymphatic vessels which have become more permeable and add to the fluid collected in the extravascular spaces.

Removal of Particles by the Lymph

Particulate matter such as colloidal carbon as well as dyes have been used to trace lymphatics and to observe their behaviour. In a few parts of the body quite large objects such as red cells readily enter lymphatics under physiological conditions. This is particularly true of the rich lymphatic plexus which occurs in the underside of the diaphragm. In this situation it has been shown by many workers that particles injected into the peritoneal cavity pass successively through the junctions between the mesothelial cells of the peritoneum, through a connective tissue membrane, and through the junctions between the endothelial cells of the underlying lymphatic lacunes. So free is the passage of red cells from blood injected intraperitoneally that it is possible to transfuse fœtuses or small children by this route.

Physiologically, fat particles in the form of chylomicra enter undamaged lymph capillaries of the intestine during fat absorption. When there are many chylomicra in the blood some can escape from normal small blood vessels and appear in the lymph of the cervical lymphatics. In conditions of mild inflammation blood corpuscles can penetrate lymphatics which otherwise are relatively impermeable. This can be seen, for instance, if the mesentery of a guinea-pig or rat is brought through an incision in the abdominal wall and, with suitable precautions to keep it warm and moist, examined microscopically. At first there are no red cells in the lymph, but soon the inflammation set up by handling the tissues damages capillaries and lymphatics enough to allow red blood cells to leave the one and enter the other. Red corpuscles, often in large numbers, can then be seen floating in the lymph, which in these two species is moved forward by contractions of the lymphatic trunks.

In the same way bacteria can enter lymphatics. They may lodge in and inflame the walls, causing lymphangitis, and pass also to the regional lymph nodes, where they may be filtered off and remain. In acute bacterial inflammation there is an increase in lymph flow which helps to remove the inflammatory exudate that comes from small blood vessels. This flow of fluid may have a useful function in diluting and removing toxins produced by bacteria in the tissues.

Lymph Nodes as Filters

It has long been known that lymph nodes can arrest small particles reaching them by the lymph stream. According to Drinker and Yoffey it was Virchow in 1860 who first clearly formulated the "barrier theory" of the function of lymph nodes.

The structure of the lymph nodes is such that it is not difficult to conceive that they act as "filters". The afferent lymphatics enter the node through a number of channels "which pierce the capsule obliquely and open into the marginal or cortical sinus. This sinus is a large vessel, bounded on the outside by the capsule of the node and on the inside by the lymphocytic parenchyma. The sinus is traversed by fibrous trabeculæ and blood vessels and, like all the sinuses, is crossed and recrossed by a fine mesh of reticulum, an important structure for the filtering function of the node. From the cortical sinus irregular but numerous cleft-like channels, the intermediary sinuses, pass between the masses of lymphoid tissue towards the hilus of the gland where they rejoin the cortical sinus to form the efferent lymph vessel."[58]

The reticulum mesh crossing the sinuses may form a kind of mechanical filter for the lymph passing through the node, but the efficiency of this mechanism is greatly increased by the fact that attached to the trabeculæ and to the surrounding sinus walls are many phagocytic cells (FIG. 88).

The structure of lymph nodes has been investigated by electron microscopy[59] and it has been shown that the fibres in the trabeculæ which stain as reticulin and which permeate a node have a core of collagen with sometimes some elastic tissue. The trabeculæ are everywhere clothed in cells which are considered to be reticulum cells and which have properties distinct from those of fibroblasts, smooth muscle cells and other common cellular constituents of connective tissue. The sinuses are lined by distinctive litoral cells which may themselves be phagocytic, although specific observations on this point are scanty. There are gaps between the litoral cells into which cells having the appearance of macro-

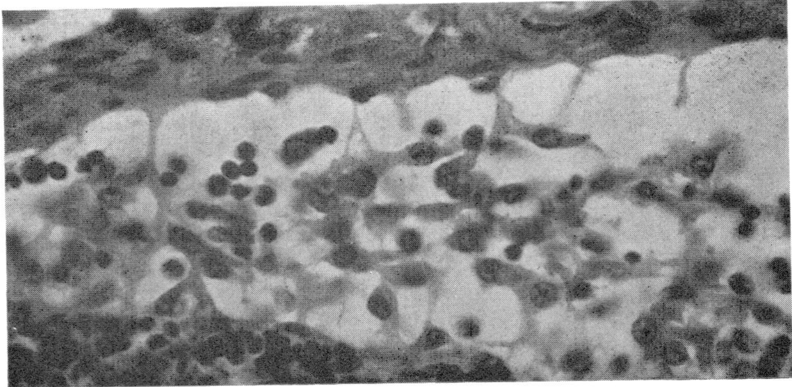

3/FIG. 88.—A sinus in a lymph node in which there has been a considerable hyperplasia of sinus-lining cells. These stretch across the sinus and it is easy to comprehend how they would act as a mechanical filter quite apart from their phagocytic powers.

phages protrude. These no doubt are phagocytic. The peculiarities of the post-capillary venules are considered in Chapter 5.

In view of the greatly increased interest in the activities of the lymph node and it cellular contents a closer examination of the properties of the cells lining the sinuses might be of interest. The node is also probably a kind of "settling" chamber, for on reaching it the contents of the afferent lymphatics suddenly enter a large space so the rate of flow of the lymph must be retarded, and it has been shown experimentally that the slower the rate of flow the more efficient is the filtration of particles.

The character of the particle passing through the node plays a part in deciding whether it is arrested; thus red cells, which are easily deformed, pass more readily through a node than anthrax bacilli, which usually occur in chains and are relatively rigid. The work of Widdicombe, Hughes and May showed that the character of bacteria could affect their arrest.[60] Table I shows this point.

3/TABLE I

Injection into inflowing lymph of	*No. of expts.*	*Dose*	*Lymph flow ml./hr.*	*Percentage recovery in outflowing lymph*
B. subtilis spores . .	9	339–339,000	0·8–2·8	21·4 (±14·7)
B. subtilis vegetative cells .	4	150–565,000	1·6–3·7	19·0 (±12·3)
B. anthracis spores . .	4	910– 12,250	1·4–1·6	9·2 (± 2·0)
B. anthracis vegetative cells .	4	1550–159,000	0·5–2·4	0·03 (± 0·05)

The ranges of dose and lymph flow are given. The figures for recovery are means with the standard deviations.

(*From Widdicombe* et al.[60])

Allowing for the correlation between rates of lymph flow and recovery of cells there was no significant difference between the percentage recoveries of spores and vegetative forms of *B. subtilis* and of *B. anthracis* spores, but the recovery of vegetative forms of *B. anthracis* was significantly lower than that of the other three bacterial forms.

The measurements made by Drinker and his colleagues[61] led them to the conclusion that the nodes were very efficient in filtering out red cells and bacteria such as streptococci, both of which were almost completely removed by the dog's popliteal node (FIGS. 89, 90 and 91). Widdicombe and his colleagues did not find rabbit nodes as efficient as this in removing erythrocytes. When large numbers of cells were used as many as 26 per cent passed through.

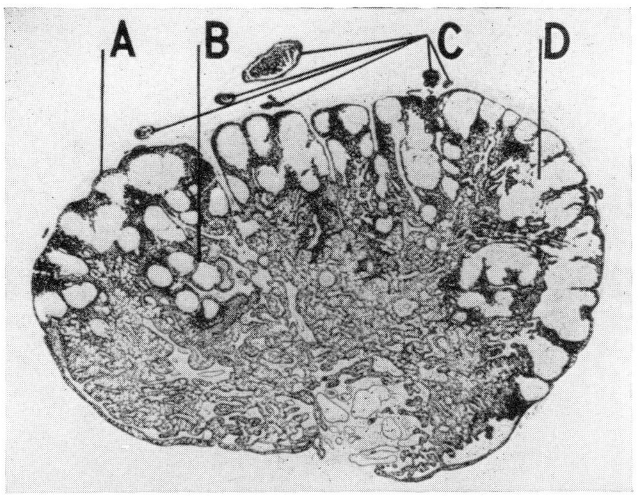

3/FIG. 89.—A popliteal lymph node of a dog injected through the afferent lymphatics with a dilute suspension of carbon. The outline and course of the sinuses appear dark, running between uncoloured areas of tissue. A. cortical sinus; B. intermediate sinus; C. afferent lymphatics in the capsule; D. lymphocyte collections. (From Drinker, Field and Ward.[61])

Drinker and his colleagues pointed out that the capacity of nodes as filters was reduced if they were massaged. A deduction that impinges on practical medicine is made from these experimental observations. Bacteria are much less likely to enter lymphatics from inflamed areas, and to be forced out of lymph nodes, if the limb or the part that is inflamed is motionless. This principle is applied in the treatment of wounds by immobilisation in plaster. The immobilisation helps to prevent spread of the infection.

The efficacy of a lymph node as a filter of bacteria is greatly increased by the occurrence of an inflammatory reaction in it.[62] Smith and Wood[63] showed that after the injection of pneumococci into the foot pad of rats the organisms reached the node where they caused a substantial emigration of polymorphs into the intermediary sinuses. These polymorphs phagocytosed the bacteria, even though the latter were encapsulated and little susceptible to phagocytosis in the

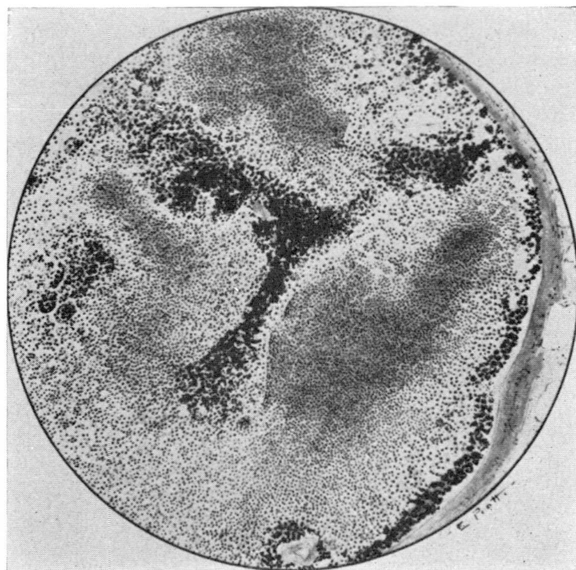

3/FIG. 90.—Section of a popliteal node of the dog. A suspension of streptococci had been perfused through it. The black material in the sinuses consists of streptococci both free and attached to cells. The cortical sinus is at the right of the picture. (From Drinker, Field and Ward.[61])

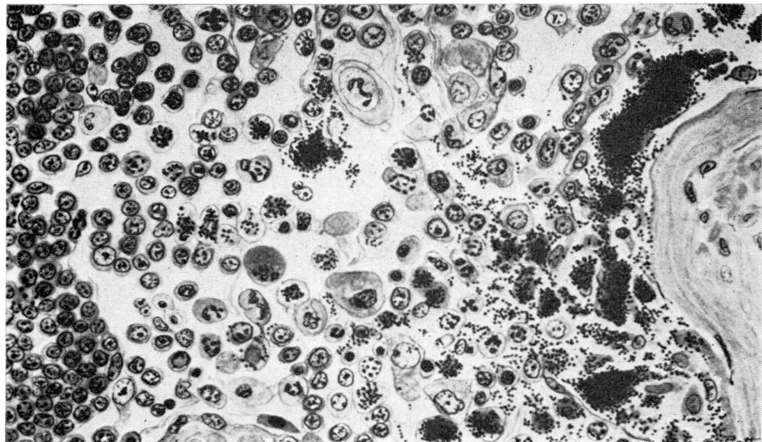

3/FIG. 91.—Higher magnification of a sinus in a lymph node perfused with a suspension of streptococci. The organisms have not penetrated into the mass of lymphocytes on the left. Some but not all of the cocci are intracellular. (From Drinker, Field and Ward.[61])

absence of antibody, and by their action and that of other phagocytic cells the pneumococci disappeared within 18 hours. During the course of the inflammatory reaction not only were the sinuses dilated at an early stage, but the exit into the efferent lymphatics was partially blocked "simulating a log-jam at the narrow outlet of the node".

Some of the polymorphs present in inflamed nodes arise at the initial site of infection, where they find their way into lymphatics and are transported to the nearest node. Polymorphs that have ingested bacteria may subsequently die and their remains be ingested by the sinusoidal cells together with their bacterial content. The inflammatory reaction is associated with painful swelling of the nodes. It is, for example, not an uncommon experience to suffer from swollen, tender, painful nodes in the neck as an accompaniment of sore throat. If a pyogenic organism of sufficient virulence is concerned, the inflammation there may go on to abscess formation. For instance, suppuration of the axillary nodes in connection with a neglected septic lesion on the hand is not uncommon.

Although Widdicombe and his colleagues, from their own work and that of others, had to conclude that under certain conditions the lymph node was not a very efficient filter, that is to say it did not stop all bacteria or particles from entering the efferent lymph, Yoffey and Courtice[64] point out that lymph nodes in natural disease are rarely confronted with as many organisms as are presented to them during experiments.

Beside bacteria other infecting agents, for instance the spirochæte of syphilis, may be arrested at least temporarily in regional lymph nodes. Among cells that may be arrested in the same way cancer cells are of particular importance, since once lodged there they may multiply and form secondary growths (metastases). Lymph nodes are the commonest of all sites for cancer metastases.

Some viruses at least are not effectively arrested by the lymph nodes. For instance, vaccinia virus which had been instilled intranasally into rabbits was not held up by the draining nodes but, on the contrary, entered the blood in a constant stream by way of cells travelling in the cervical lymph ducts.[65] On the other hand ectromelia virus enters the macrophages of lymph nodes and can multiply in and destroy them. Probably the relationship between virus and the cells of the node in their phagocytic and immunological capacities is complex and differs from one virus to another.[66]

REFERENCES

1. Weibel, E. R., and Palade, G. E. (1964). *J. Cell Biol.*, **23,** 101.
2. Chambers, R., and Zweifach, B. W. (1940). *J. cell. comp. Physiol.*, **15,** 255.
3. Chambers, R., and Zweifach, B. W. (1947). *Physiol. Rev.*, **27,** 436.
4. Muir, A. R., and Peters, A. (1962). *J. Cell Biol.*, **12,** 443.

4a. Reese, T. S., and Karnovsky, M. J. (1967). *J. Cell. Biol.*, **34,** 207.

5. Farquhar, M. G., and Palade, G. (1963). *J. Cell Biol.*, **17,** 375.
6. Karnovsky, M. J. (1967). *J. Cell Biol.*, **35,** 213.
7. Luft, J. H. (1966). *Fed. Proc.*, **25,** 1773.
8. Marchesi, V. T., and Barrnett, R. J. (1963). *J. Cell Biol.*, **17,** 547.
9. Warren, B. A. (1964). *Brit. med. Bull.*, **20,** 213.
10. Jennings, M. A., and Florey, Lord (1967). *Proc. roy. Soc. B.*, **167,** 39.

10a. Florey, Lord (1968). *Quart. J. exp. Physiol.*, **53,** 1.

10b. JENNINGS, M. A., MARCHESI, V. T., and FLOREY, H. (1962). *Proc. roy. Soc. B.*, **156,** 14.
10c. FLOREY, Lord (1966). *Brit. med. J.*, **2,** 487.
10d. POOLE, J. C. F., SANDERS, A. G., and FLOREY, H. W. (1958). *J. Path. Bact.*, **75,** 133.
11. LUFT, J. H. (1965). "The Ultrastructural Basis of Capillary Permeability" Chapter 3 in *The Inflammatory Process*. New York: Academic Press.
12. PALADE, G. E. (1953), *J. appl. Physics*, **24,** 142. (1960). *Anat. Rec.*, **136,** 254.
12a. BRUNS, R. R., and PALADE, G. E. (1968). *J. Cell Biol.*, **37,** 244 and 277.
13. MARRACK, J. R. (1966). Personal communication.
14. KARNOVSKY, M. J. (1967). Personal communication.
15. FAWCETT, D. W. (1959). In *The Microcirculation*, p. 1. Eds. REYNOLDS, S. R. M., and ZWEIFACH, B. W. Urbana: Univ. Illinois Press.
16. MAJNO, G., and PALADE, G. E. (1961). *J. biophys. biochem. Cytol.*, **11,** 571.
17. MAJNO, G., PALADE, G. E., and SCHOEFL, G. (1961). *J. biophys. biochem. Cytol.*, **11,** 607.
18. COTRAN, R. S., and MAJNO, G. (1964*a*). *Amer. J. Path.*, **45,** 261.
18a. HURLEY, J. V., HAM, K. N., and RYAN, G. B. (1967). *J. Path. Bact.*, **94,** 1.
18b. HAM, K. N., and HURLY, J. V. (1968). *J. Path. Bact.*, **95,** 175.
18c. COTRAN, R. S. (1967). *Exp. molec. Path.*, **6,** 143.
19. COTRAN, R. S., and MAJNO, G. (1964*b*). *Ann. N.Y. Acad. Sci.*, **116,** Art. 3, 750.
20. MAJNO, G., and LEVENTHAL, M. (1967). *Lancet*, **2,** 99.
20a. MAJNO, G., GILMORE, V., and LEVENTHAL, M. (1967). Personal communication.
21. WALLER, A. (1846). *Phil. Mag.*, **29,** 271.
22. COHNHEIM, J. (1872). *Untersuchungen ueber die Embolischen Processe*. Berlin: A. Hirschwald.
23. KROGH, A. (1929). *Anatomy and Physiology of the Capillaries* (Silliman Memorial Lectures). New Haven: Yale Univ. Press.
24. CLARK, E. R., and CLARK, E. L. (1935). *Amer. J. Anat.*, **57,** 385.
In the list at the end of this paper a number of references are given to work on the tadpole's tail.
25. COHNHEIM, J. (1882). *Lectures on General Pathology*. London: The New Sydenham Society, tr. into English 1889.
26. ADDISON, WILLIAM (1843). *Trans. provinc. med. surg. Ass.*, **11,** 233.
27. WALLER, A. (1846). *Phil. Mag.*, **29,** 397.
28. THOMA, R. (1878). *Virchows Arch. path. Anat.*, **74,** 360.
29. ALLISON, F., Jr., SMITH, M. R., and WOOD, W. Barry, Jr. (1955). *J. exp. Med.*, **102,** 655.
30. FÅHRAEUS, R. (1929). *Physiol. Rev.*, **9,** 241.
31. CIBA FOUNDATION. Film entitled "Analysis of the Effect of Vasoactive Substances on the Blood Vessels of the Mesorchium of the Rat".
32. ZWEIFACH, B. W. (1954). *Trans. Fifth Connective Tissue Conference*, p. 38. New York: Josiah Macy, Jr. Foundation.
33. FLOREY, H. W., and GRANT, L. H. (1961). *J. Path. Bact.*, **82,** 13.
34. MARCHESI, V. T., and FLOREY, H. W. (1960). *Quart. J. exp. Physiol.*, **45,** 343.
35. MARCHESI, V. T. (1961). *Quart. J. exp. Physiol.*, **46,** 115.
36. ARNOLD, J. (1875). *Virchows Arch. path. Anat.*, **62,** 487.
37. ZWEIFACH, B. W. (1955). *Ann. N.Y. Acad. Sci.*, **61,** 670.
38. FLOREY, H. (1926). *Proc. roy Soc. B*, **100,** 269.
39. HUDACK, S., and MCMASTER, P. D. (1933). *J. exp. Med.*, **57,** 751.
40. SAPPEY, M. P. C. (1885). *Description et iconographie des vaisseaux lymphatiques considérés chez l'homme et les vertébrés*. Paris: Delahaye et Lecrosnier.
41. CASLEY-SMITH, J. R., and FLOREY, H. W. (1961). *Quart. J. exp. Physiol.*, **46,** 101.
42. KATO, F. (1966). *Nagoya med. J.*, **12,** 221.

43. LEAK, L. V., and BURKE, J. F. (1967). *Anat. Rec.*, **157,** 276.
44. STARLING, E. H. (1894). *J. Physiol.* (*Lond.*), **16,** 224.
45. MCMASTER, P. D., and HUDACK, S. (1932). *J. exp. Med.*, **56,** 239.
46. PULLINGER, B. D., and FLOREY, H. W. (1935). *Brit. J. exp. Path.*, **16,** 49.
47. ADAMI, J. G., and NICHOLLS, A. G. (1911). *Principles of Pathology*, Vol. 2. London: Oxford Univ. Press.
48. CLARK, E. L., and CLARK, E. R. (1921). *Anat. Rec.*, **21,** 127.
49. JACOBJ, W. (1923). *Arch. exp. Path. Pharmak.*, **98,** 55.
50. GASKELL, W. H. (1876). *Arb. physiol. Anstalt, Leipzig*, **11,** 143.
51. HEIMBERGER, H. (1926). *Z. ges. exp. Med.*, **51,** 112; (1927). *ibid.*, **55,** 17.
52. PULLINGER, B. D., and FLOREY, H. W. (1937). *J. Path. Bact.*, **45,** 157.
53. VIRÁGH, SZ., PAPP, M., TÖRÖ, I., and RUSZNYÁK, I. (1966). *Brit. J. exp. Path.*, **47,** 563.
54. LEAK, L. V., and BURKE, J. F. (1966). *Amer. J. Anat.*, **118,** 785.
55. CASLEY-SMITH, J. R. (1967). *Brit. J. exp. Path.*, **48,** 680.
56. DAY, T. D. (1959). *Quart. J. exp. Physiol.*, **44,** 182.
57. HALL, J. G., MORRIS, B., and WOOLLEY, G. (1965). *J. Physiol.* (*Lond.*), **180,** 336.
58. DRINKER, C. K., and YOFFEY, J. M. (1941). *Lymphatics, Lymph and Lymphoid Tissue*. Cambridge, Mass.: Harvard Univ. Press.
59. CLARK, S. L. (1962). *Amer. J. Anat.*, **110,** 217.
60. WIDDICOMBE, J. G., HUGHES, R., and MAY, A. J. (1955). *Brit. J. exp. Path.*, **36,** 473.
61. DRINKER, C. K., FIELD, M. E., and WARD, H. K. (1934). *J. exp. Med.*, **59,** 393.
62. OPIE, E. L. (1910). *Arch. intern. Med.*, **5,** 541.
63. SMITH, R. O., and WOOD, W. B. Jr. (1949). *J. exp. Med.*, **90,** 555 and 567.
64. YOFFEY, J. M., and COURTICE, F. C. (1956). *Lymphatics, Lymph and Lymphoid Tissue*, 2nd edit. London: Edward Arnold (Publishers) Ltd.
65. YOFFEY, J. M., and SULLIVAN, E. R. (1939). *J. exp. Med.*, **69,** 133.
66. MIMS, C. A. (1964). *Bact. Rev.*, **28,** 30.
67. LEAK, L. V., and BURKE, J. F. (1968). *J. Cell Biol.*, **36,** 129.

Reference may be made to the following excellent reviews:

The Acute Inflammatory Response (1964). By numerous authors. Ed. HAROLD E. WHIPPLE. *Ann. N.Y. Acad. Sci.*, **116,** Art. 3, 747.

The Inflammatory Process (1965). By numerous authors. Eds. ZWEIFACH, B. W. GRANT, L., and MCCLUSKEY, R. T. New York: Academic Press.

MANJO, G. (1965). "Ultrastructure of the Vascular Membrane", in *Handbook of Physiology*, Section 2. *Circulation*, **3,** 2293. Washington, D.C.: Amer. Physiol. Soc.

ALLEN, LANE (1967). "Lymphatic and Lymphoid Tissues," in *Ann. Rev. Physiol.*, **29,** 197.

MAYERSON, H. S. (1963). "The Physiologic Importance of Lymph", in *Handbook of Physiology*, Section 2. *Circulation*, **2,** 1035. Washington, D.C.: Amer. Physiol. Soc.

Chapter 4

CHEMOTAXIS, PHAGOCYTOSIS AND THE FORMATION OF ABSCESSES. THE RETICULO-ENDOTHELIAL SYSTEM

By H. W. Florey and M. A. Jennings

The observations considered in Chapter 3 show that there is now a comprehensive picture of the morphological changes occurring during the emigration of leucocytes from the blood vessels. However, there is a considerable gap in knowledge concerning the intimate mechanism by which the leucocytes stick to the walls of the small vessels and what forces are involved in the migration.

EMIGRATION FROM THE VESSELS

Adhesion of Leucocytes

It has to be admitted that it is not known why leucocytes adhere to the walls of small vessels following types of injury caused by stimuli as diverse as mechanical injury or bacterial products. The leucocytes appear *in vivo* as though adhering to a sticky surface and it would be simplest to suppose that the endothelial surface was stimulated or damaged by noxious stimuli to release some material to which leucocytes adhered. This explanation has in fact been offered many times but unfortunately no unequivocal evidence for the existence of sticky material has been produced. The demonstration by Luft that a substance possibly of a mucopolysaccharide nature exists on the surface of normal endothelium makes it possible to consider that this may increase during inflammation. Even if this were so there is no reason to suppose that it would form a surface to which leucocytes would cling for it is present in normal vessels to which leucocytes do not adhere. It does not seem likely that a fibrin deposit on endothelium can account for the phenomenon because heparin has no effect on the adhesion. It is however possible by the appropriate administration of the calcium chelating agent trisodium ethylenediamine tetra-acetic acid (EDTA) to reverse the sticking of leucocytes caused by injury as observed in rabbit ear chambers or rat mesentery[1]. As a result of their experiments Thompson and his colleagues concluded that calcium is intimately concerned in the phenomenon of leucocytic adhesion but precisely how is unknown. It has been proposed by Bangham[2] that calcium forms a binding cationic bridge between cells and that their mutual repulsion is overcome when a covalent bond is formed between calcium and the negatively charged carboxyl groups on the cell surfaces, but the distance between leucocytes and endothelium during sticking is probably too great to allow of this happening.

The possibility exists that the endothelial surface is not altered but that the leucocytes are altered to become adhesive. For this there is no evidence though to be sure leucocytes can be seen to adhere to one another in vessels in an inflamed ear chamber.

Emigration of Leucocytes

We have seen that the mechanism by which leucocytes adhere to inflamed endothelium is obscure, and the situation is little better with regard to reasons for their emigration from blood vessels.

Before examining emigration further it will be necessary to consider chemotaxis which has been defined as "a reaction in which the direction of locomotion in the cell or organism is determined by a substance in its environment"[3] The phenomenon is widely encountered in unicellular organisms, in cells such as spermatozoids of plants and in animals of increasing complexity, as Metchnikoff and others showed in their studies of comparative pathology.[4, 5] (Figs. 1 and 2). What is of particular interest in inflammation is whether the motile cells present in the blood are attracted to inflamed spots and if so what chemical substances produce the effect.

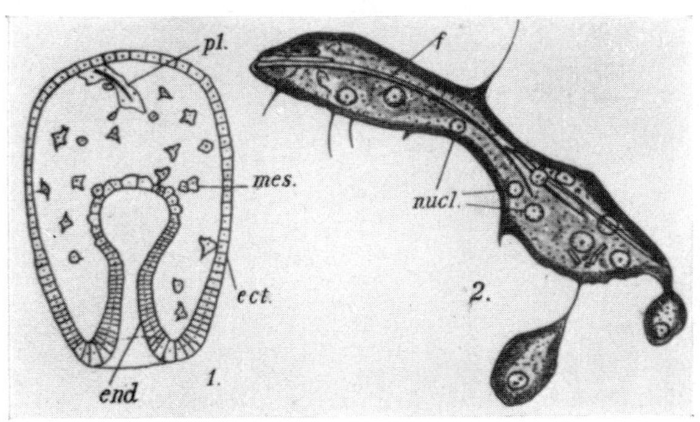

4/Fig. 1.—Response to Injury in Metazoa

(1) Transverse section of body cavity of larva of *Astropecten*: *ect.*, ectoderm; *end.*, endoderm; *mes.*, mesodermal wandering cells; *pl.*, "plasmodium" composed of mesodermal cells fused together round a foreign body that has punctured the ectoderm.

(2) Higher magnification of the "plasmodium": *f.*, foreign spicules; *nucl.*, nuclei of fused mesodermal cells. (From Adami.[4] Redrawn from illustrations of Metchnikoff.)

Five readily distinguishable types of blood cell are recognised as being involved in inflammation in mammals such as man, viz.:

1. Cells known under a variety of names to all of which some objection can be raised. *Neutrophil* is the name that Hirsch[6] favours though the names granulocyte or polymorphonuclear leucocyte are frequently encountered in the literature.

The characteristics of this cell have been briefly considered in Chapter 3. In the living state these cells, which range from 10 to 15 microns in diameter, are motile and their movement can conveniently be watched on glass slides by light microscopy. They constantly change their shape and if they are moving forward a pseudopod consisting of hyaloplasm devoid of granules or organelles is thrust out in the direction of movement. The trailing portion may be constricted into a tail-like structure. Large numbers of granules which are about 0·2 microns in diameter are a prominent feature in the cytoplasm. They are for the most part

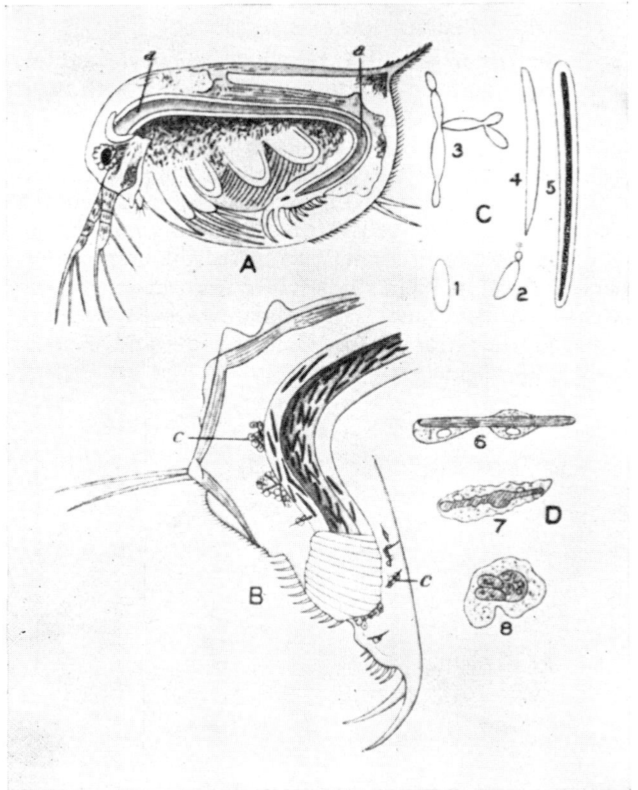

4/Fig. 2.—Response to Invasion in Metazoa

Daphnia or water flea invaded by a yeast. The organisms are indicated by deep shading below the intestinal canal (*a*) in A, and by dark lines in the high-power view of the hind end of the gut, B, where those that have penetrated the intestinal wall are seen being engulfed by leucocytes in the body cavity (*c*). C, stages of development of the parasite—5 represents a spore form. D, stages in the ingestion and destruction of a spore by two leucocytes. (From Adami.[4] Redrawn from illustrations of Metchnikoff.)

near the nucleus and in a moving portion of the cell may be in Brownian motion. No verbal description can convey the fascination of the movements of these cells and every student of pathology should be given an opportunity to see them. Many excellent cine films have been made but none more beautiful than that of Comandon[7] produced nearly 40 years ago. Fixed preparations of some blood cells in movement can be seen in Chapter 3.

In the living state the many-lobed nucleus is difficult to see but it must be very elastic for neutrophils can pass through extremely narrow channels and strikingly elongated nuclei are sometimes seen, for example between the epithelial cells of the intestine when neutrophils are passing into the intestinal lumen. The significance of the granular content will be considered under phagocytosis

2. *Eosinophil*.—This cell has many features in common with the neutrophil

though its nucleus does not become so multilobed and in some species such as the rat is annular. The eosinophil is distinctive by reason of its cytoplasmic content of granules which stain intensely with acid dyes such as eosin. These granules vary in size from about 1·0 micron in the horse to 0·2 micron in the rat. Under the electron microscope these granules are seen to consist of membrane bounded structures containing a dense matrix, part of which may be of a crystalline nature (see 3/Fig. 65). In the living state on a glass slide the eosinophils are motile, moving much in the same way as neutrophils though they have usually been considered to be more sluggish. But Greenwood[8] has found that eosinophils of the sheep, man and pig can move as fast as or faster than neutrophils, though they may be slower to start moving (see 3/Fig. 68).

3. *Basophil.*—Very little is known about the activities and properties of the basophils of the blood, which constitute normally 0·05 per cent or less of the circulating leucocytes. They seem to be formed in the bone marrow, along with other granulocytes, but they have resemblances to the mast cells of the tissues, which have similar basophil granules with metachromatic staining properties. It is thought that like those of the mast cells their granules contain histamine and heparin; it has been calculated that in man about half of the total blood histamine is located in the basophils[9, 10].

The granules of blood basophils and tissue mast cells do not stain with the common histological stains, so that these cells do not stand out in ordinary sections, and not much is known about their behaviour in, for example, acute inflammation. When antigen is applied to sensitised animal tissues, with the production of anaphylaxis, mast cells are disrupted and histamine released[11]. If such release occurs in anaphylactic states in man it is possible that blood basophils as well as mast cells participate in the reaction.

The basophils are thought to be motile and to stick to inflamed endothelium.

4. *Monocyte.*—These cells are the largest mononuclear cells in the blood measuring some 12 to 15 microns when spread in a blood smear. They differ from the cells previously mentioned in being devoid of large granules but relatively rich in cytoplasmic organelles such as mitochondria, Golgi apparatus, and vacuoles which probably represent endoplasmic reticulum. They possess a large nucleus which is kidney shaped or at least indented. In the living state on a glass slide they are found to be slowly motile thrusting out broad pseudopods. They move more quickly when not in contact with glass but with fibrin in a plasma clot.

5. *Lymphocyte.*—These cells have been much studied both alive and in fixed specimens. When lymphocytes from the blood are observed alive [12, 13] in, for example, an appropriate medium in a warm chamber they are seen to be motile. Similarly when fragments of spleen or lymph node in tissue culture are watched, lymphocytes are seen emigrating into the surrounding fluid. They can be seen moving in the natural tissue juice in chambers in the rabbit's ear. In freshly shed blood they exhibit no movement for some time, but within about 8 hours are moving vigorously. Both in tissues and *in vitro* their movement is generally characteristic, as their relatively large compact nucleus goes in advance, trailing a small tail of cytoplasm behind. On occasion, however, they may apparently move with a leading peudopod, and they may put out blunt pseudopods when not actually moving. The knowledge of the lymphocyte has increased greatly of recent years and this cell is considered in detail in Chapter 5.

Thus there are five types of motile cell that occur in the blood and which are known to appear in inflamed tissues.

Are these motile cells subject to chemotactic influences?

CHEMOTAXIS

Granulocytes

Large numbers of experiments have been performed on the chemotaxis of leucocytes both *in vitro* and *in vivo*, particularly in amphibian and mammalian tissues. Many of the methods used have been criticised adversely by Harris[14] who devised a procedure by which the movements of isolated leucocytes could be continuously photographed at a magnification of about 250 times. He showed clearly that certain bacteria and starch grains are chemotactic for neutrophils (FIGS. 3, 4 and 5). It is clear that when the leucocytes come within some 100 microns of bacteria their random locomotion changes and they proceed towards the bacteria in a reasonably straight line. Why this should occur is not known. It is usually supposed that a substance exists around the attracting object in a diminishing concentration gradient and that the cells have some mechanism which directs them to the more concentrated areas, but what this mechanism is is unknown.

From watching leucocytes that have emigrated from injured blood vessels into tissues that are free of infection there would appear to be no evidence to suggest that once external to the vessels they move in any particular direction. But there is no doubt that many kinds of bacteria can attract neutrophils, which will move freely towards them. This will happen even if the bacteria kill the leucocytes when they get close. For example products of *Ps. pyocyanea* and of some strains of *C. diphtheriae* are chemotactic but leucocytes are destroyed by these organisms. Although tissue breakdown products have been generally believed to be chemotactic, Harris was unable to show by his method that dead fragments of tissue, autolysing tissue, or tryptic or peptic digests had any attractive power under the same conditions as those in which bacteria were found to be chemotactic.

Boyden[15] devised another excellent technique and amongst other things was able to demonstrate that antigen-antibody complexes were strongly chemotactic. This action proved to be due to the release from the serum of a complex comprising certain components of complement. Under appropriate experimental conditions the same complex can inhibit chemotaxis.[16] If this clue is followed up perhaps some better understanding of the chemical nature of chemotaxis may be obtained.

There are some reports that claim to show that certain substances, e.g. aluminium silicate, repel leucocytes. Other work has, however, not confirmed the existence of this example of "negative" chemotaxis.[17] Of more immediate interest to pathology, it has been maintained that certain bacteria can repel polymorphs. Such statements need to be treated with reserve and even if true it has yet to be clearly demonstrated that negative chemotaxis plays any role in the development of inflammatory responses.

McCutcheon[18] considered that it had yet to be proved that chemotaxis to particles was due to the production of a chemical substance that produced a field of diminishing concentration around the particle. He suggested that the

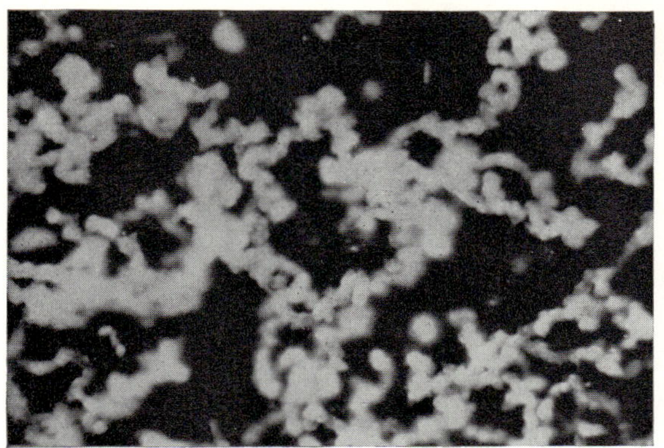

4/FIGS. 3 to 5.—A plasma clot about 20μ thick was placed between a microscope slide and a coverslip to which living granulocytes were adhering. The substance or solution to be tested for chemotaxis was inserted in one part of the clot and the preparation incubated at 37° C. and observed microscopically with dark ground illumination at a magnification of about 250 times.

Photomicrographs were taken with a slow high-contrast film which was constantly exposed for from 5 to 15 minutes. Figure 3 shows the pattern traced out by the granulocytes when moving at random. (From Harris.[14])

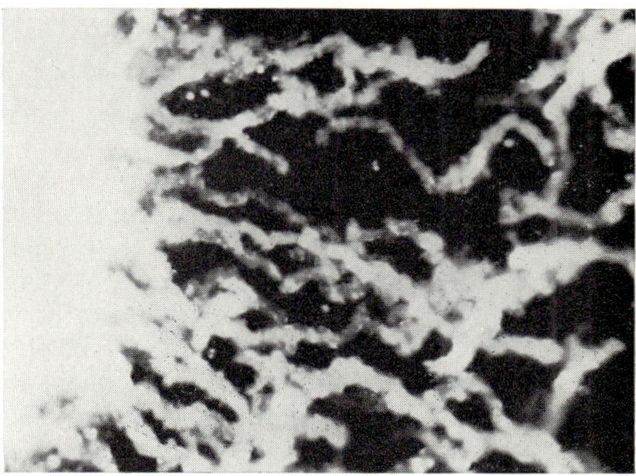

4/FIG. 4.—The pattern traced out by the granulocytes in the presence of a clump of *Staphylococcus albus*, which is on the left. It will be seen that, within a certain range of the clump, all the traces converge directly upon it. (Exposure 15 minutes. ×250.) (From Harris.[14])

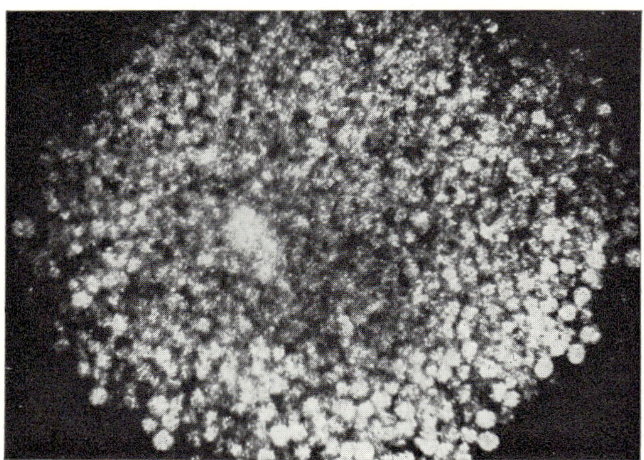

4/FIG. 5.—Later stage in the phagocytosis of *Staph. albus*. The clump of bacteria has been almost entirely replaced by an aggregate of granulocytes, engaged in phagocytosing the organisms. (From Harris.[14])

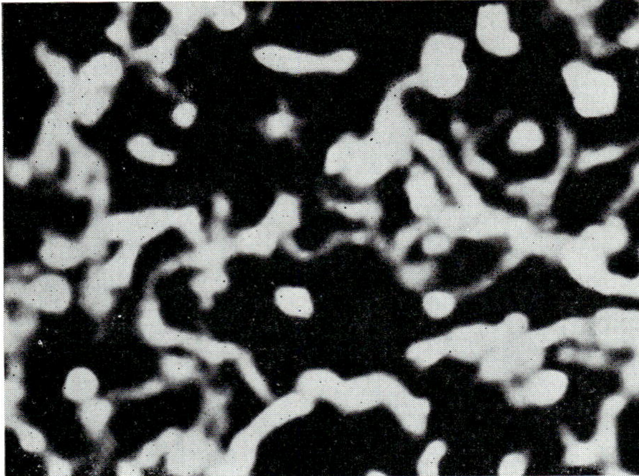

4/FIG. 6.—The pattern traced out by monocytes when moving at random. (Exposure 1 hour. ×250.) (From Harris.[14])

hypothesis is worth exploring that particles adsorb substances from the surrounding plasma and in this way set up a concentration gradient in their neighbourhood.

Eosinophils seem to respond chemotactically to the same stimuli as affect neutrophils.

Monocytes

It was at one time believed that the monocyte was not responsive to chemotactic influences *in vitro*, and the idea was held that if this cell was subject to chemotaxis at all, it was certainly less so than the granulocyte, but when a photomicrographic trace method was adapted for the study of monocytes positive results were obtained. When monocytes collected from the peritoneal cavity of a rabbit or other animal are placed in contact with glass they adhere closely to it for many hours, and sometimes for two or three days. During this period they do not move about spontaneously or react to chemotactic stimuli, but later they

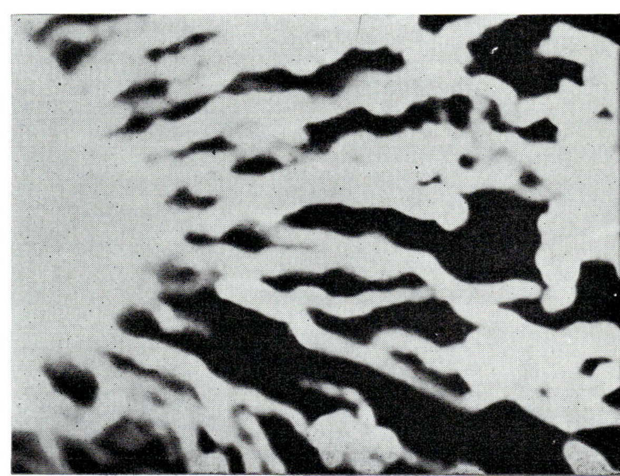

4/FIG. 7.—The pattern traced out by monocytes in the presence of a clump of *Mycobacterium tuberculosis* (H37Ra), which is on the left. Within a certain range of the clump all the traces converge directly upon it. (Exposure 1 hour. ×250.) (From Harris.[14])

become actively motile and then chemotaxis may be clearly demonstrated (FIGS. 6 and 7). Starch grains and certain bacteria were found to be chemotactic for the monocyte, just as for the granulocyte. With monocytes, too, crushed and autolysed tissues were not chemotactic. The evidence so far obtained shows that the monocyte reacts *in vitro* chemotactically in the same way and to much the same extent as the neutrophil and. apparently, to the same sorts of stimuli.

Lymphocytes

So far nothing has been found to attract lymphocytes *in vitro* using methods similar to those used for neutrophils.

FACTORS AFFECTING CHEMOTAXIS

Chemotaxis exerted by *Staph. albus* on polymorphonuclear leucocytes can occur in the absence of serum, complement or glucose and in solutions that have had chelating agents added to remove as much calcium and magnesium as possible. The tonicity of solutions in which chemotactic experiments are carried out can be varied widely without affecting chemotaxis.

The cells remain motile in solutions containing up to 0·011 M sodium cyanide or 0·005 M sodium azide and it therefore appears that they may be active at least for a time in the absence of oxygen, moreover they can survive and remain motile in solutions that do not contain a source of energy. Chemotaxis cannot be inhibited without impairing the motility of the cell.[17] It is thus clear that chemotaxis can occur in tissues even under what would at first sight appear to be extremely adverse conditions.

Sequence of Cells appearing in Inflamed Tissues

It has already been mentioned that polymorphs and monocytes adhere to the walls of inflamed vessels and migrate into the surrounding tissues, but the predominant cell in acute inflammatory exudates is the first named. With the passage of time, in certain circumstances the granulocyte ceases to be the commonest cell in an exudate, and is replaced by the monocyte or macrophage. The sequence in which the predominant cells appear in peritoneal exudates has been studied in great detail [19, 20, 21, 22]. Borrel[19], Opie[23] and Vorwald[24] found that for the first twenty-four hours even tubercle and typhoid bacilli caused a polymorph reaction like that to *Staph. aureus*, but later the cell type changed until the macrophage was predominant.

The mechanism underlying such a sequence has been the subject of considerable discussion. Menkin[25] considered that increasing acidity of the exudate kills off the sensitive polymorph. His views have not been generally accepted and it is fair to say that at present no conclusive evidence is to hand to explain why at the beginning of an inflammation the wandering cells are chiefly polymorphs while later they are of the mononuclear type. As there is no striking difference in the chemotactic response *in vitro* of monocytes and polymorphs the development of different stimuli at different stages of inflammation seems unlikely to be a cause. This was borne out by a careful reinvestigation of the numbers of the two cells leaving the small vessels under different conditions, which led Paz and Spector[26] to suggest that there was no specific differential emigration. They found that both types always emigrated together, but that polymorphs tended to wander away or to die *in situ*, leaving the long-lived monocytes conspicuously on the field. If the inflammation was relatively mild the few polymorphs soon disappeared, while if it was severe with much emigration, as in a pyogenic infection, the polymorphs remained obvious at the site of injury, especially if bacteria continued to be present and to promote the exodus of new cells from the vessels.

It seems that the factors which best account for the sequence of cells in inflamed tissues may prove to be in the nature and properties of the cells themselves.

Mechanism of Emigration

We may now consider some possible mechanisms by which leucocytes emerge from blood vessels during inflammation.

It has sometimes been supposed that the actual emigration of leucocytes from the blood vessels of an inflamed area is due to the chemotactic action of substances liberated in the tissues. Such a suggestion is at present only speculation. Even if chemical changes following, for instance, bacterial or thermal damage alter the vessel walls so that leucocytes are induced to emigrate, it does not follow that there is any chemotactic action. As we have seen, there is no clue as to how leucocytes adhere to inflamed endothelium, but after adhesion their intrinsic movements may be the main cause of their passing through the vessel wall.

In some of their experiments Hurley and Spector[27] probed further into the possibility that substances which cause emigration from the blood vessels are liberated in damaged tissues. By the use of a standardised histological technique they determined whether injected substances caused leucocyte emigration or not. Emigration was promoted by a substance or substances in extracts of burnt skin and of polymorphonuclear leucocytes, and in serum incubated with a number of tissues. The system causing emigration was thought to consist of a precursor present in serum, an activator present in certain tissues, and the activated principle. This last could be distinguished from permeability-increasing substances and was thought to be a protein. There was no evidence that it was chemotactic *in vitro*.

Histamine, which may be involved in increasing capillary permeability, is generally held not to cause leucocyte emigration and this has been confirmed[28]. Adenosine, adenylic acid and guanosine, substances shown by Bennet and Drury[29] to be liberated in damaged tissue, attracted leucocytes into the conjunctival sac of rabbits when dropped into the sac in solution, but this effect has not been further investigated.

It seems likely that peptides and permeability globulin have at the most a weak action in promoting emigration. Bradykinin, kallidin, serotonin and constituents of polymorph granules have all been found not to cause leucocyte accumulations in skin.[28]

PHAGOCYTOSIS

We have already noted that Metchnikoff and others studied the activities of living cells in inflammation. Among the phenomena that they noted was the ingestion of small particles by certain cells—the process of phagocytosis. As this is one of the most important phenomena exhibited by some types of inflammatory cell it has been extensively investigated, especially as many of the cells concerned can be handled *in vitro* without much difficulty. The cells of mammalia, especially man, naturally occupy most of our attention, but phagocytosis is a property of cells present even in the simplest animals[4].

In man the important wandering phagocytic cells are the neutrophil polymorphs and the monocytes, both of which emigrate into the tissues from the blood, though in the early stages of acute inflammation the former appear in vastly greater numbers than the latter. There are also large numbers of "fixed" phagocytic cells in various organs of which the liver, spleen and lymph nodes are the most important, but these will be considered when the reticulo-endothelial or macrophage system is dealt with. For the present we will confine our attention to the cells that emigrate from the blood into the tissue spaces.

The process of phagocytosis consists of the intake into the cell of material from the surrounding medium. The term *phagocytosis* has usually been limited to the intake of solid particles such as bacteria and fragments of cells or of material from outside the cell, while the term *pinocytosis* has been used for the intake of fluid. There is now some doubt whether any distinction need be drawn between the two processes and in this discussion the term phagocytosis will generally be used. Both result in the formation of an intracytoplasmic vacuole containing foreign material and bounded by a portion of cell membrane which has been invaginated. Both processes, and especially pinocytosis, have been studied extensively in unicellular oranisms such as *Amoeba*, which depend for their nutrition on this form of ingestion. The activities of phagocytic cells in higher animals have been investigated in numerous ways. They can be traced *in vivo*, for example, by injecting visible particles such as carbon or bacteria living or dead by routes which will bring them into contact with phagocytic cells. The consequent uptake can be studied in fixed tissues or in living preparations as in the rabbit ear chamber. Much information about the process of phagocytosis has been obtained from isolated cells in suspension or in tissue culture. Sources from which living macrophages have been harvested for investigations *in vitro* are described later in this chapter in connection with the reticulo-endothelial system. Generally they can be detached from suitable internal surfaces such as the serous membranes in useful numbers simply by washing the surfaces with physiological saline, but to obtain polymorphonuclear phagocytes it is necessary to introduce a mildly irritating substance such as an 0·1 per cent solution of glycogen in saline. Such a solution injected into the peritoneal cavity of a rabbit will yield a cell suspension comprising 99 per cent of polymorphs when the cavity is washed out 4 hours later.[30]

As seen by the light microscope it has been found that if the particle to be phagocytosed is small, such as a single bacterium, it apparently sinks into the cytoplasm immediately after contact with the leucocyte, but if the particle is relatively large, for instance a clump of bacteria, clear protoplasm in the form of pseudopodia flows along and around the object until it is surrounded and thus becomes incorporated in the interior of the cell.

Though visual methods for studying phagocytosis give a very clear idea of the process, other methods which avoid the possibility of chemotaxis are sometimes used. Briefly, they involve the rotation of tubes containing suspensions of particles and leucocytes, so that the number of contacts between cell and particle is governed by chance. Fenn[31], who employed this method extensively, was able to show that under these conditions the number of particles ingested was proportional to the expected number of collisions and the size of the particles.

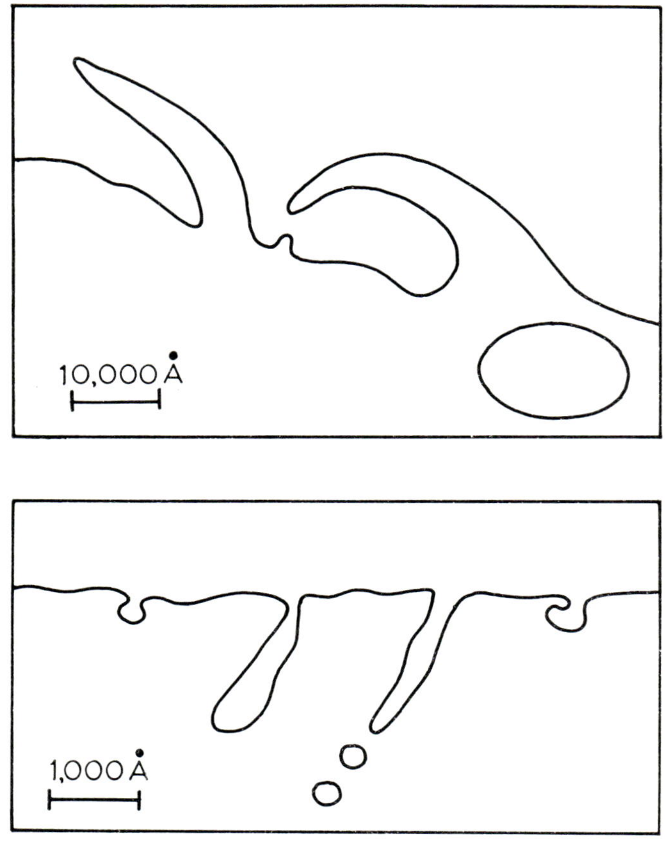

4/Fig. 8.—Pinocytosis and Micropinocytosis

The upper picture shows pinocytosis, which can be watched by the light microscope. Membranes waving on the surface of the cell enclose a drop of fluid which becomes isolated and enters the cell cytoplasm.

Below is shown micropinocytosis which has been deduced from electron micrographs. Invaginations of the cell membrane are thought to become nipped off at the opening so that a droplet of fluid enters the cell. Note difference in scale of the two drawings. (From Policard and Bessis.[121])

Lewis[32] observed with the light microscope the process, which he called pinocytosis, by which monocytes and macrophages in tissue culture incorporated substantial droplets of liquid medium into their cytoplasm (Fig. 8). Macrophages have on their surfaces membranous pseudopodia which undulate and wave about in a remarkable fashion. Sometimes these membranes enfold a droplet of fluid from the surrounding medium so that it is pushed into the cytoplasm, where it proceeds towards the centre of the cell. The droplets, which initially may be of various sizes, decrease in volume and finally may leave only a small refractive granule. In active cells the incorporation of droplets may be rapid and the small droplets may fuse to form larger ones. The amount of fluid which can be taken up by this process has been estimated to be as much as one-third of the volume of the cell in an hour. No doubt the cell must also lose fluid but there is no evidence that this is done by extrusion or "reverse pinocytosis". The undulating membranes can sometimes be observed under favourable conditions on macrophages in living tissue in the rabbit ear chamber. Not all cells have the undulating membranes observed on macrophages, but the latter may only be exhibiting a special form of the pseudopod-like activity which enables polymorphs to engulf bacteria.

Pinocytosis and phagocytosis follow respectively the adhesion of protein to the cell surface and the contact of a particle with it. They were formerly thought of as in some sense automatic or purely "physical" reactions following on these events, but the application of metabolic inhibitors or the lowering of temperature have been found to inhibit phagocytosis, and it is now generally believed that they are energy consuming processes requiring both glycolysis and oxidative phosphorylation[33, 34, 35]. Probably different cells or cells in different situations have different requirements; for example, it was found that phagocytosis by lung macrophages was more depressed by lack of oxygen than was phagocytosis by polymorphonuclear leucocytes[36, 37].

Conditions Affecting Phagocytosis

Many factors affecting phagocytosis have been investigated.

A wide variety of anions and certain nucleosides and nucleotides stimulate pinocytosis by macrophages[38]. Phagocytosis can be promoted by reducing the charge on bacteria by means of cations which unite with the ionised groups on the surface. Aluminium, chromium and iron ions do the same. The influence of calcium ions in increasing phagocytosis is striking, especially in accelerating it. Mudd and Mudd[39] considered that such effects were principally due to alterations in the adsorption of serum components on the surface of test particles or bacteria. Possibly this effect is produced because proteins normally repelled by electronegative bacteria will fix themselves to the bacterium when the charge on it is reduced. The effect of hydrogen ions is less definite. Most observers think that phagocytosis occurs best at about neutrality, but Loos stated that maximal phagocytosis occurred at a pH of 6·6.

Fever often occurs in infectious disease and might possibly influence phagocytosis. The data on this matter are not very satisfactory. It is stated that human leucocytes phagocytose the greatest number of organisms at 37° C., and that the normal body temperature seems best also in other species, for example 41° C. in the chicken and pigeon. Other data, however, suggest that within limits the efficiency of leucocytes in taking up particles increases with rise of temperature.

Leucocytes appear to be rather resistant to changes in osmotic pressure. Those of the horse, for instance, ceased to phagocytose in serum only after it had been considerably diluted and recovered phagocytic power as soon as they were restored to something approaching the usual surroundings. Phagocytosis appears to be maximal in isotonic or somewhat hypotonic solutions (0·5 per cent

NaCl). The effect of hypertonic solutions is apparently inhibitory, and this may be of some interest in view of the suggestion that pus is hypertonic.

The effect of surface tension is no doubt of great importance, and it has been proposed that the act of phagocytosis depends on the relationship of the interfacial tensions between phagocyte, particle and surrounding medium. Many important data bearing on this have been discussed by Mudd *et al.* in *Physiological Reviews*[40], but what exactly these mean in terms of the properties of cell membranes is still obscure[41].

Associated with surface properties is the question of the viscosity of leucocytes. During locomotion these cells undergo local changes of viscosity, but it is not known whether "softening" occurs when the cell is in contact with a foreign body, thus affecting phagocytosis. It has been suggested that the greater viscosity of mononuclear cells, compared to polymorphs, may account for their slower rate of phagocytosis.

Opsonins

A most important influence on the ability of polymorphs to phagocytose bacteria, and possibly other particles, is exerted by components of blood plasma known collectively as opsonins. The question of opsonins is bedevilled by a somewhat confused terminology, but the position now seems to have been reached of recognising that the important point about opsonins, which are proteins, is that they coat the surface of bacteria. It is conceivable that polymorphs find it difficult to get hold of the surface of uncoated and of capsulated bacteria. Possibly the polysaccharide or polypeptide on the surfaces of capsulated bacteria make them slippery, certainly colonies of such organisms are "mucoid". In opsonisation the important process is the anchoring of a sufficient amount of protein sufficiently firmly to change the surface properties of the bacteria. It does not seem to matter much what protein is involved in this process, for many proteins have been described as opsonins.

The surest way to fix protein to a bacterial surface is by forming a specific union of antibody with the polysaccharide, or in the case of the anthrax bacillus polypeptide, antigen on the bacterial surface. For this reason the best opsonins are antibodies. Antibodies and antigens, the substances giving rise to them, are considered extensively in Chapters 32 and 33.

The opsonising antibodies which are specific for each bacterium, and thermostable, are capable of fixing themselves in large amount to the bacterial surface and for this reason they are effective even with capsulated organisms. Although these specific antibodies occur in large amount after specific immunisation, small amounts of them exist in "normal" serum as the result of an unrecognised stimulus—perhaps due to unappreciated infection by the bacterium concerned, or to the stimulus of antigens in food, or to stimulus by other bacteria with an immunological relationship to the specific bacterium. These antibodies do not differ from the antibodies deliberately produced by specific immunisation but they are present in too small amounts to act as opsonins alone. The antigen-antibody complex which they form on the surface of the bacterial cell will, however, fix complement, a complex globulin component of normal serum, and the globulin of the antibody together with that of complement is sufficient to act as an opsonin. As complement is thermolabile the opsonising mixture of globulins will appear to be thermolabile; hence the idea that there are thermolabile opsonins. The reason for the thermolability given above receives support from the observation that thermolabile opsonin can be produced by diluting immune antibody, which is thermostable, until its opsonic capacity just disappears and then restoring opsonic capacity by adding complement.

Besides the specific fixation of protein to the bacterial cell, protein can be made to stick by unspecific means. A bacterial cell is strongly electro-negative because at physiological pH values there is an excess of ionised acid over basic groups on its surface. The surface will therefore adsorb basic proteins. The basic proteins protamine, globin and lysozyme have, in fact, been shown to be opsonins, but only lysozyme is known for certain to be present in tissues under physiological or pathological conditions.

Tullis and Surgenor[42] described two proteins, one a β globulin and the other an α_1 globulin, which are opsonic without the aid of complement and which are not basic proteins. They called these substances P.P.F. (phagocytosis-promoting factors). Most of their experiments were done using starch grains, although it was claimed that the same results were obtained with staphylococci.

Surface Phagocytosis

It has been demonstrated[43] that, although in the usual type of experiment phagocytes will not ingest encapsulated pneumococci in the absence of immune serum, they can be made to do so by altering the experimental conditions. If instead of a simple fluid in a smooth-walled vessel the preparations were furnished with strands of fibrin or of desoxyribonucleic acid or pieces of filter paper or even of lung and bronchi, phagocytosis took place. The effect was apparently mechanical. It looked as though, if the bacteria became trapped on the surfaces provided by fibrin, alveolar wall and so on, or even between two leucocytes, the phagocytes could manage to ingest them. This attractive idea of "surface phagocytosis" was questioned by Lerner,[44] but Smith and Wood[45] produced further evidence in its favour, and their hypothesis found more support when Cohn[46] showed that staphylococci were ingested more quickly in the peritoneal cavities of mice than under comparable conditions of opsonization *in vitro*. The most likely reason for this was thought to be that phagocytosis was enhanced by the presence of tissue structures. It now seems quite likely that the mechanical assistance given to phagocytes by tissue surfaces can play an important part in resistance to some bacterial infections.

In summary it may be said that certain serum proteins promote phagocytosis through their adsorption on the surfaces of particles such as bacteria. Some bacteria can be phagocytosed in the absence of serum, others must be brought into contact with proteins, including complement, in normal serum, while still others which are virulent—especially if encapsulated—can only be ingested in the presence of specifically immune serum.[40] There is a possibility that even these last can be ingested without immune serum if the mechanical conditions are suitable.

Electron Microscopic Observations

When phagocytosis is observed in electron micrographs it becomes clear that even particles as small as single bacteria do not simply sink through the surface of the cell as they seem to do under the light microscope. Instead the area of contact between particle and cell increases until the particle is enveloped by cell membrane. Pseudopod formation is not so marked as with larger particles, but the end result is the same and for that matter is the same as after the ingestion of fluid. That is to say, foreign material comes to be contained in an invagination of the cell membrane which through the meeting of cell surfaces soon becomes pinched off and forms a free vacuole in the cytoplasm bounded by a unit membrane, known as a phagocytosis vacuole or phagosome (FIGS. 9 and 10). The foreign material may be considered for a time as still external to the cell though entirely within it, much as material in the bronchial and gastro-intestinal tracts may be considered as external to the body.

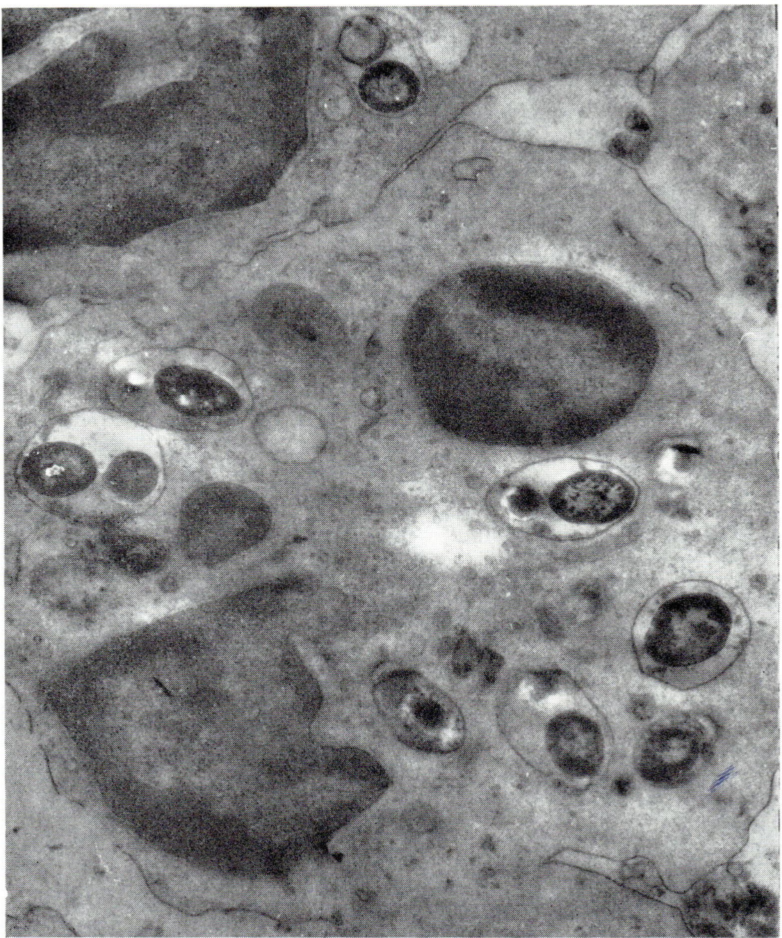

4/FIG. 9.—Rat polymorphs which have ingested pneumococci. The pneumococci are contained in "phagocytosis vacuoles". The vacuoles are clearly bounded by a discrete membrane. (× 13,500)

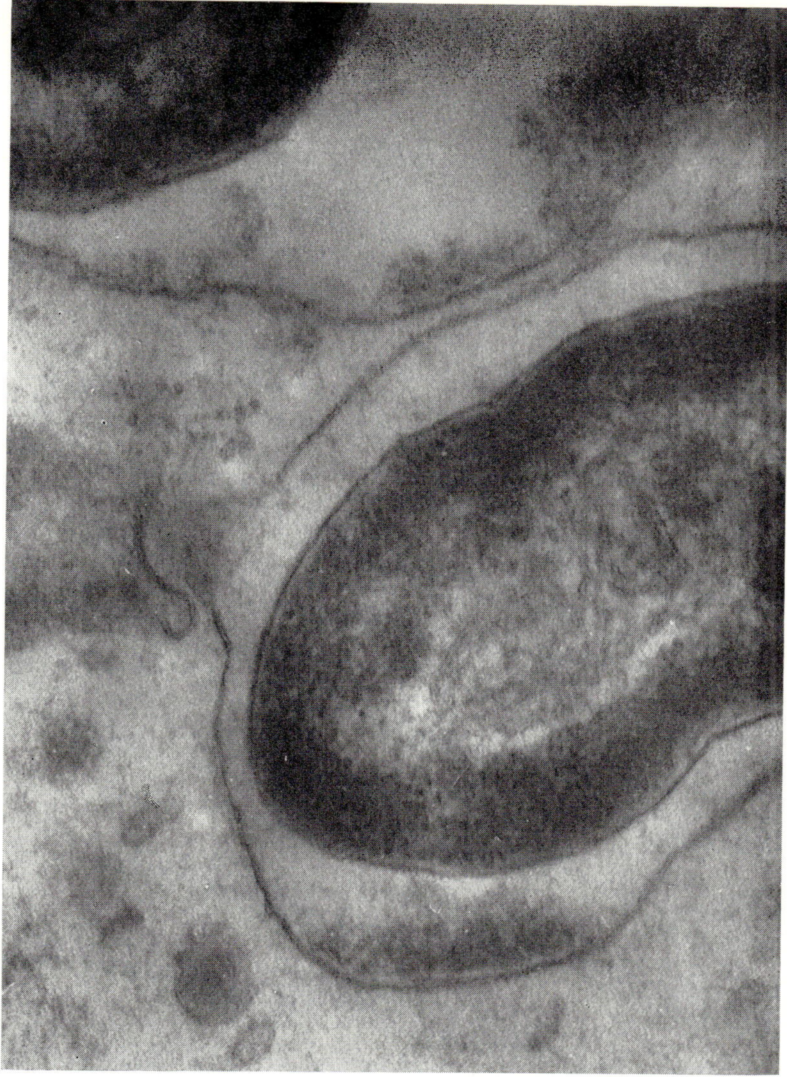

4/FIG. 10.—Rat polymorph. Parts of two phagocytosis vacuoles containing pneumococci. A double or "unit" membrane can be seen to surround the vacuole. Some internal structure can also be recognised in the bacterium which morphologically has not undergone any apparent change at this stage. (× 87,500)

Similar intake of particles into membrane bounded vesicles may be seen in many other types of cell beside the phagocytes. It has been studied, for example, in fibroblasts in tissue culture.[47] But it should be noted that virus particles may be found free in the cytoplasm soon after entry into tissue cells, as might be expected from the intimate relationship between the metabolism of the virus and that of its host cell. It is stated, however, that phagocytes have a capacity which is not found in other cells to restrain the growth of viruses in their cytoplasm.[48]

When we come to consider smaller materials, for example particles of ferritin or other large protein molecules, the precise mode of entry into cells is harder to ascertain. Do such materials enter the cell by permeating the cell membrane, or does their entry, too, depend on membrane activity of the kind already described, that is, the infolding and inversion of part of the membrane itself? It seems very possible that both modes of entry may occur; it seems clear from the use of labelled materials that the second certainly does. Electron microscopy has shown that small indentations or infoldings of the plasma membrane are quite common in a variety of cells, including phagocytes, and it seems to be well established that labelled material such as particles of colloidal gold or bacterial antigenic material, can enter macrophages by this route.[49, 50] Because of its small scale, electron microscopists have referred to this process as micropinocytosis (FIG. 8). As they travel into the cell the vesicles seem to fuse with each other and with larger ones to form substantial phagocytic vacuoles packed with the foreign material. This process has been illustrated by Cohn and his colleagues[49] for macrophages in tissue culture and is shown in FIGS. 11 and 12 from the work of Nossal and his colleagues[50] in living animals. Thus materials of molecular size may come to be retained in membrane bounded structures in the cell cytoplasm. Information of this sort which is coming to hand bearing on the uptake of foreign proteins into body cells may be of great

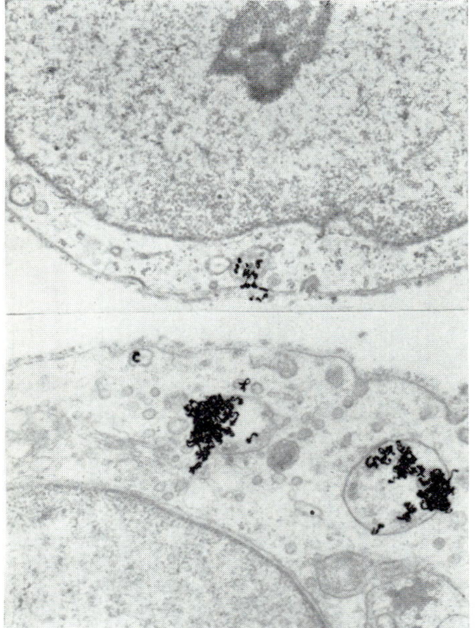

4/FIG. 11.—Electron microscopic autoradiographs of parts of two macrophages (litoral cells) in the medullary sinus of a rat's popliteal lymph node, 30 min. after the injection of *Salmonella* flagella antigenic material labelled with ^{125}I into the related foot pad. The upper cell shows labelled antigen on the cell membrane and in a vesicle close to the surface. The lower cell shows antigen in two small vesicles, one of which is still close to the surface, and in two larger vesicles. (× 15,600.) (From Nossal, Abbott and Mitchell.[50])

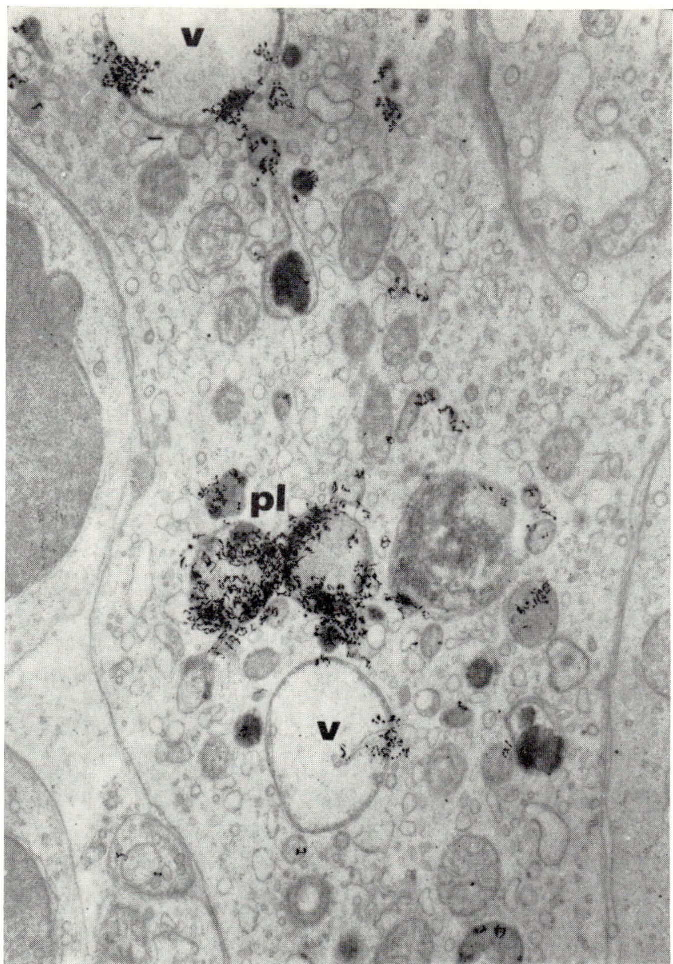

4/FIG. 12.—From a similar lymph node to that shown in Fig. 11, one day after the injection of labelled flagella antigenic material. The broad macrophage process contains membrane bounded vesicles of various sizes, and much of the labelled antigen seems to be in the vesicles v = large vacuole. pl = a region where several vesicles of different sizes may be fusing together. × 15,000.) (From Nossal, Abbott and Mitchell.[50])

interest in connection with our attempts to understand the mechanisms of antibody formation, though it is possible that this is only one of various ways in which such proteins may be dealt with by phagocytic cells.

What happens to Ingested Particles?

Particles such as carbon may remain in macrophages for a very considerable time. Polymorphs have a much shorter life, so that inert and indigestible material which they have taken up is quite soon, by their death, deposited in the tissues where it may remain or be taken up by macrophages. If, however, the materials are digestible, both polymorphs and macrophages can completely demolish the particles.

It used to be disputed whether leucocytes could take up and kill living organisms or whether they could only ingest those that had been killed already. Metchnikoff's views on the importance of phagocytosis in protecting the body against invasion by pathogenic organisms had to meet severe criticism from those who maintained that organisms were killed by various agencies in the blood and tissue fluids, the phagocytes merely disposing of the bodies. Metchnikoff himself provided some evidence that live organisms were ingested. He injected a suspension of *Vibrio metchnikovi* into the anterior chamber of the eye of an immunised animal. The organisms were taken up by phagocytes. When one of these leucocytes was isolated and put in a hanging drop of broth, the broth killed the leucocyte and the ingested organisms grew out of the killed cell.

Similar experiments have been described by Wood and his collaborators. Smith and Wood[51] found that Friedländer's bacilli which had been phagocytosed alive by rat granulocytes were killed in about 30 minutes, though they were not digested for several hours. Rogers and Tompsett[52] showed that both virulent and avirulent staphylococci may be ingested by granulocytes. The former are not killed, but multiply vigorously in the cytoplasm of the leucocytes and it is the cells that die, liberating living cocci into the surrounding fluids. The avirulent organisms, though they survive in the granulocytes for a short time, are killed and digested in the space of some four hours.

The question of the fate of staphylococci after ingestion was later investigated by a different method.[53, 54] Selected polymorphonuclear leucocytes were disrupted by an electric shock at different intervals after the ingestion of bacteria, the process being watched continuously by phase contrast microscopy. The ingested cocci were released into the surrounding medium. When released 20 minutes after ingestion coagulase negative organisms did not grow, but 60 per cent of coagulase positive organisms subsequently underwent division. The authors concluded that virulent staphylococci could live for some time inside the leucocyte and even undergo division while still in the cell.

These experiments leave little room for doubt that, at least under some conditions, leucocytes do ingest living bacteria and that sometimes this leads to death of the cell through continued multiplication of the organisms. In other cases the cell is in the ascendancy, though precisely how it kills the organisms after ingestion is not yet entirely clear. Macrophages as well as polymorphs can kill staphylococci with considerable efficiency. Neutrophil polymorphs can ingest but are unable to kill tubercle bacilli and *Brucella* and *Listeria* organisms. If taken up by polymorphs these bacteria are released when the cells die and may then be ingested by macrophages. The presence of multiplying tubercle bacilli within a macrophage may kill the cell, but on the other hand if they come from immunised animals the macrophages may be able to restrain the growth of or even kill the tubercle bacilli. Their ability to do this seems to be related to the state of immunity of the animal as a whole, but the mechanism of this so-called cellular immunity is still obscure. The matter will be found discussed in Chapters 37 and 42.

The Role of the Granules

The old observation that polymorphs lose their granules soon after ingesting bacteria has been illustrated with great elegance by light microscopy.[55] The degree of degranulation is directly related to the quantity of material engulfed. The meaning of such observations has been made clearer through the great magnification and resolving power achieved with the electron microscope. The

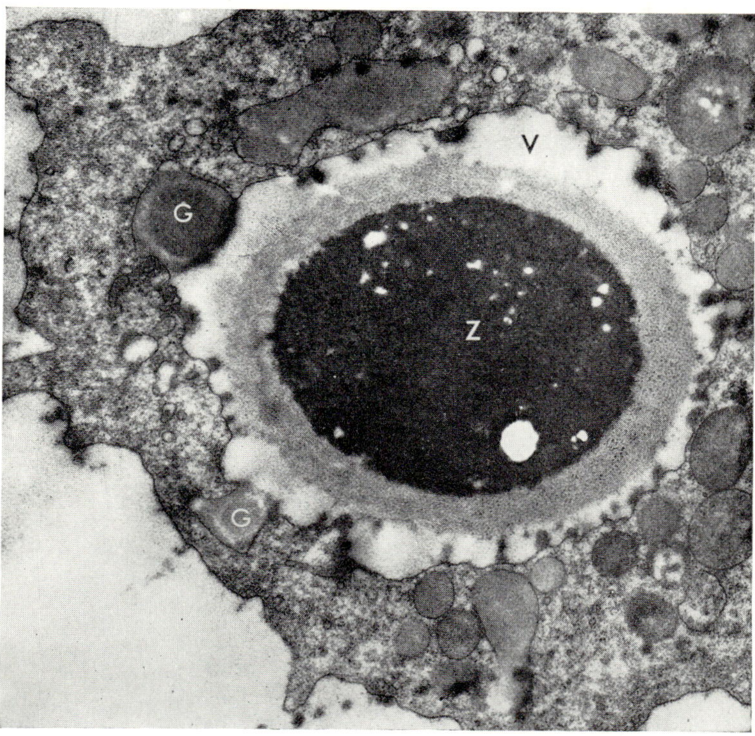

4/FIG. 13.—Part of a neutrophil polymorph which was fixed after $1\frac{1}{2}$ min. of incubation with the particulate material zymosan. It contains an ingested particle of zymosan (Z) which has an electron dense core and stippled periphery. The membranes of two cytoplasmic granules (G) seem to have fused with the membrane of the phagocytic vacuole (V). (× 23,000.) (From Zucker-Franklin and Hirsch.[56])

granules are found to be membrane bounded structures and they have been shown to contain a variety of hydrolytic enzymes. They are in other words the lysosomes of the phagocytic cells, large and prominent in polymorphs, smaller and less conspicuous but apparently with a similar constitution in macrophages. Through some means not understood the granules impinge on the phagocytic vacuoles with breaking down of the contiguous membranes between the two structures, and their reconstitution in continuity between granule and vacuole. Thus the contents of the phagocytic vacuole become exposed to whatever substances the granule may contain (FIGS. 13 and 14). Eosinophils that have ingested

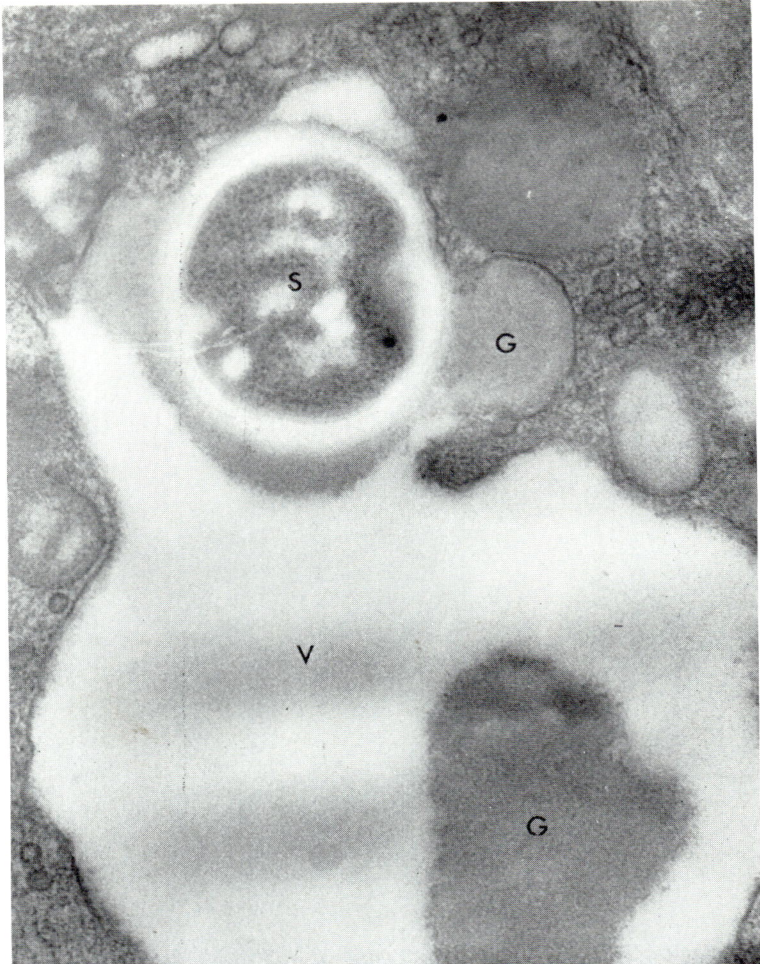

4/FIG. 14.—Part of a neutrophil polymorph which was fixed after 2 min. of incubation with staphyloccoci. It has engulfed a staphylococcus (S) which has a core of varied density and a pale peripheral zone. The contents (G) of the cytoplasmic granule on the right, whose membrane has fused with that of the phagocytic vacuole (V), seem to be emerging into the vacuole and surrounding the staphylococcus. Other material in the vacuole may also be granule contents. (× 63,000.) (From Zucker-Franklin and Hirsch.[56])

bacteria apparently form phagocytic vacuoles in the same way as polymorphs, but, at least under some conditions, the electron-dense crystalline structures of the granules remain discrete for a time even after the vacuoles have been formed[57].

We have already seen that living bacteria ingested by phagocytes can sometimes be killed and digested by them. By what means is this brought about? Antibacterial substances which have been found in polymorphs, and which may be mainly in the granules, include proteolytic enzymes, lysosyme, whose substrate is a complex polysaccharide, hydrogen peroxide, lactic acid, and a group of cationic proteins.

Antibacterial Constituents. 1. Enzymes

The enzymes in the granules of polymorphs are said to include acid and alkaline phosphomonoesterase, acid ribonuclease, acid deoxyribonuclease, cathepsin, β-glucuronidase, lysozyme, a nucleotidase, peroxidase, lipase, and a diphosphopyridine nucleotide oxidase[58]. Macrophages also contain enzymes associated with the granules, but less was known about their constitution until it was discovered that the injection of rabbits with BCG greatly increased the yield of cells obtainable by washing out the lungs. Qualitatively the enzymes in the granules seem to be the same in "stimulated" macrophages as in those obtained from natural animals. Enzymes found include acid phosphatase, acid ribonuclease, cathepsin, β-glucuronidase, lysozyme and lipase.

On the basis of electron microscopic work with macrophages developing in culture, acid phosphatase seems to pass from the Golgi saccules, which are regarded as lysozomes in this context, to the dense bodies which appear to be a late stage of the phagocytosis vacuoles[49]. In both polymorphs and macrophages enzymes pass from the granule fraction to the soluble fraction of the cells soon after the ingestion of dead bacteria. This finding is not easy to explain because the granules seem to discharge into the membrane bounded phagocytic vacuoles, but degradation products of the bacteria soon leave the vacuoles and possibly enzymes follow the same course.

Proteolytic ferments such as trypsin do not kill organisms, and there is not much reason to think that others can do so. Indeed, there is evidence that living bacteria can thrive in the presence of many proteolytic enzymes[59]. But the digestive capacity which proteases confer on polymorphs and monocytes is of particular importance for helping in the clearance of dead bacteria and other debris. Also liberated enzymes are active in the tissue fluids after the death and dissolution of the phagocytes.

One enzyme found in phagocytes, lysozyme, is known to have a direct effect on living bacteria. Lysozyme, by acting on certain amino-polysaccharides present in the cell walls of some Gram-positive cocci (not those that are pathogenic), rapidly lyses the organisms. Its range of action may be more extensive than this, for many other organisms, particularly the coagluase negative staphylococci, are killed by exposure to lysozyme at an acid pH or in the presence of complement or antibody. Thus lysozyme may be more important to the killing of intracellular bacteria than was previously supposed. It is said that organisms whose walls contain the substrate for lysozyme are more quickly degraded intracellularly than those without this substrate.

2. Hydrogen Peroxide. Acids

Hydrogen peroxide is said to be present in bactericidal concentrations in polymorphs.

Macrophages and polymorphs have glycolytic activity and produce lactic acid under both aerobic and anærobic conditions. The contents of a phagocytic vacuole are said to have a pH near 4, and it is possible that this is associated with the production of organic acids. Some of these have antibacterial properties, but there is no proof at present that the lethal capacity of phagocytes resides in their ability to form acids.

3. Basic Proteins

Leucocytes were said many years ago to contain strongly bactericidal substances, named "endolysins" or "leukins"[60, 61]. Cohn and Hirsch[62] separated a material, phagocytin, which was associated with the granules of polymorphs, was strongly bactericidal, and did not appear to be an enzyme. The lysosome fraction of rabbit polymorphs has now been shown to contain a group of basic proteins with antibacterial and bactericidal action against a variety of pathogenic organisms including staphylococci[63]. The proteins of this group differ in amino-acid composition but share certain distinctive properties such as a high arginine-lysine ratio and a high concentration of cystine. When more is known of these substances the way in which bacteria are killed by cells may become clearer, as they appear to have quite potent antibacterial properties.

Disposal of Intercellular Bacteria

Examination of the fate of radioactively labelled bacteria after ingestion by polymorphs[64] shows that in the first two hours of intracellular residence *in vitro* very considerable breakdown occurs of nucleic acids, fats and proteins. Ribonucleic acid is more readily degraded than deoxyribonucleic acid. Although digestion of the organisms seems to occur, at least at first, inside the phagocytic vacuole the acid soluble breakdown products rapidly leave the cell and do not accumulate inside it.

When living instead of dead bacteria have been ingested degradation takes place more slowly but follows the same course, and if the organism has been treated with immune serum before ingestion degradation is also slowed, presumably because globulin complexes have to be attacked. Phagocytes from animals that have been immunized against a bacterium do not have any enhanced ability to digest that organism, which suggests that the cellular immunity of macrophages against tubercle bacilli is not specifically due to improvements in their enzyme action[65].

From experiments of this kind it is clear that the digestive processes of phagocytes can sometimes deal effectively with living organisms as well as with dead ones, killing the organisms by chemical action and degrading their components. Opsonized organisms, as we have seen, may be hard for the cell to ingest, but once inside the cell they can be dealt with similarly, the globulin complex on the cell wall being broken down successfully in the phagocytic vacuole.

Dispersion of Organisms

As already noted, the organism may not be killed after ingestion, but may multiply intracellularly and eventually kill the leucocyte. In this case the leucocyte, wandering in the tissues and perhaps into the lymphatics before it dies, may aid in disseminating virulent bacteria. This very likely takes place in tuberculosis, for a macrophage may live for some time and migrate about while carrying living tubercle bacilli. In leprosy and kala-azar macrophages seem to be the natural habitat for the disease-producing organisms. Sometimes an organism may actually be protected by its intracellular position from bactericidal substances present in the blood and tissues.[66, 67]

Evidence that Polymorphonuclear Leucocytes help to protect the Body

At the present time there is no dispute about the fact that phagocytosis is a very important protective mechanism against bacterial invasion. One of the best demonstrations of this fact, by Rich and McKee,[68] is based on the observation of Camp and Baumgartner[69] that if acute inflammation occurs when there are less than about 1,000 leucocytes per cu. mm. of blood an insignificant exudation of leucocytes takes place, though other features remain the same. Rich and McKee largely deprived rabbits of their polymorphs by administering benzol, which damages the bone marrow, and compared the course of pneumococcal infection in these and healthy animals, using both rabbits immunised against pneumococci, and non-immune animals. In the non-immune few pneumococci were phagocytosed in any case, so that the presence or absence of leucocytes did not make much difference to the course of the infection. The animals died of fatal septicæmia in a few days, and the slightly longer survival of those with leucocytes was attributed not to phagocytosis, but to the release of antibacterial substances from dead leucocytes.

It was only in animals actively or passively immunised that the effect of leucocytes showed clearly. The specific antibodies both made the bacteria susceptible to phagocytosis (as discussed earlier) and made them adhere together as they multiplied instead of drifting off singly and in pairs through the tissues. Even in the absence of leucocytes death was delayed in immunised animals by the clumping together of bacteria at the site of infection, though eventually spread of the bacteria by the blood stream (septicæmia) took place. But in immune rabbits that had a normal complement of leucocytes, the bacteria were removed by phagocytosis while they were still kept localised by clumping, and of the four groups this was the only one in which the animals survived.

The conditions in these experiments were such as to show that, where infecting bacteria are susceptible to phagocytosis, phagocytes may have a life-saving action. It is likely that some chemotherapeutic agents depend for their complete effectiveness on the action of phagocytes, as did immune bodies in the above experiments.

There are some conditions in man in which there is a great lack of leucocytes in the circulating blood (leucopenia), or even complete suppression of the formation of granulocytes (agranulocytosis). The latter state can be caused by drugs of a variety of chemical constitutions. In such conditions pathogenic bacteria entering the tissues may grow freely and cause serious or fatal illness where in a healthy person the infection would soon be overcome. A more subtle defect of the leucocytes has also been described. There is a rare, genetically determined disease in which the polymorphs, though present in normal or raised numbers, seem unable to deal with staphylococci although they can ingest them. The patients have recurrent staphylococcal infections which antibiotics do little to control. It has been suggested that the polymorphs of these patients may lack some important bactericidal constituent[70].

It has been shown that the vascular dilatation of inflammation is necessary for the collection of leucocytes in the tissues. Thus if adrenalin is injected into an area two hours after the inoculation of *Staph. aureus* and the injection is repeated at 2-hour intervals, the vascular changes are prevented and at the end of 6 hours there is no emigration of leucocytes, though in control areas not injected with adrenalin many polymorphs are present. Because of this effect on the leucocytes, adrenalin injections greatly reduce the numbers of organisms such as *Cl. septicum* and streptococci necessary to establish infection.

The Fate of Polymorphs in Tissue

A large number of polymorphs may migrate from damaged vessels into the tissues following an aseptic injury. What happens to these cells? The Clarks have watched them in transparent chambers. At first they move briskly about at random near the blood vessels, passing freely over the surfaces of macrophages lying in the tissues. After a time they become sluggish and their numbers diminish until in a few days none can be seen. It will be remembered that these cells do not divide. Probably most of them, as they age, break up and are phagocytosed by macrophages, but some may first pass through a stage of degeneration in which the nucleus swells into a rounded form, so that they are difficult to distinguish from lymphocytes (known to pathologists as "small round cells") in fixed specimens. The Clarks[71] watched *in vivo* such a change occurring in some polymorphs segregated in a blind end of a lymphatic. A similar change to a mononuclear form was noted in tissue cultures[72] and in blood removed from the axillary vein and incubated, though here it apparently occurred much more quickly.[73]

There is other evidence that polymorphs have a relatively short life, for example it has been reported that granulocytes disappeared from the rabbit in 3 to 4 days after the production of new cells was prevented by poisoning the bone marrow with benzol. A life span of less than 4 days was indicated in a human patient in whom polymorphs completely disappeared 4 days after the onset of the disease known as agranulocytosis, in which the bone marrow ceases to produce these cells.[74] Kline,[75, 76] using radioactive phosphorus, found a life span of 13 days. In whole blood *in vitro* a life span of about 3 days was indicated.[77] It is stated that after death polymorphs may continue their phagocytic activities in the body for as long as 11 days,[78] and that they may live for 7 days in undiluted homologous blood serum.[79]

The Fate of the Monocytes

These phagocytic cells of the blood when they emigrate into the tissues have a much longer life than the polymorphs. Under favourable conditions they can phagocytose tissue debris and grow in size until they are 30μ or more in diameter, and are indistinguishable from macrophages arising in the tissue (histiocytes). They may also form multinucleated giant cells. These changes can be conveniently watched in transparent chambers in the rabbit's ear and are described in detail in Chapter 17.

The behaviour of cells around a spot composed of minute carbon particles of indian ink was clearly seen in an ear chamber. The mica lid of a chamber with fully grown tissue was removed and replaced by one on which a small spot of indian ink mixed with serum had been dried. FIGURE 15*a* shows the blob of carbon after a few hours. Very soon many polymorphs were seen in the neigh-

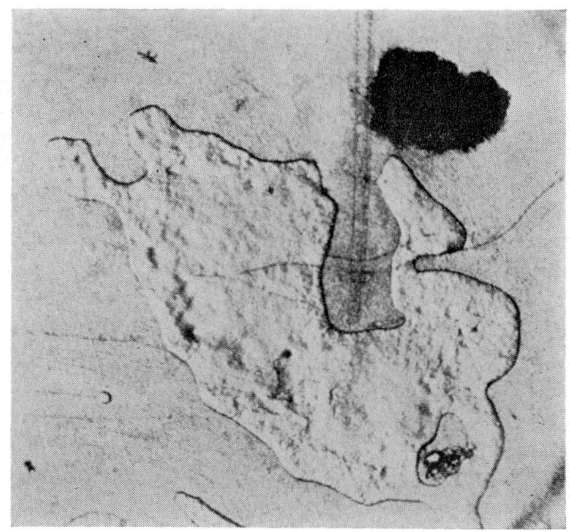

4/FIG. 15.—(*a*) Chamber in rabbit ear with fully healed tissue over the central table, most of which is shown in the picture. The mica lid has been removed and replaced by one carrying a small spot of indian ink, which appears at the right-hand upper corner. Below it is a bubble of air that was included during the replacement of the lid, but this was soon absorbed.

bourhood of the carbon, some of which they ingested. These polymorphs disappeared within a day or two, and macrophages appeared and gradually invaded the spot of carbon, phagocytosed the material and began slowly to disperse over the surface and into the substance of the tissue (FIG. 15*b*, *c*, *d* and *e*). The carbon-containing macrophages were watched for 75 days, when they still appeared to be intact living cells scattered through the tissue of the chamber.

Macrophages probably persist in tissues for much longer than this. Tattooing lasts for years, and much of the pigment is held within macrophages, at any rate for a long time. Loaded macrophages may, however, slowly leave the tissue, and it is probably partly through their movement into the lymphatics that the regional lymph nodes come to contain foreign material.

In some instances when macrophages gather round foreign objects they appear to fuse with one another to produce what are known as "foreign body giant cells". What precisely is the stimulus to the formation of multinucleated

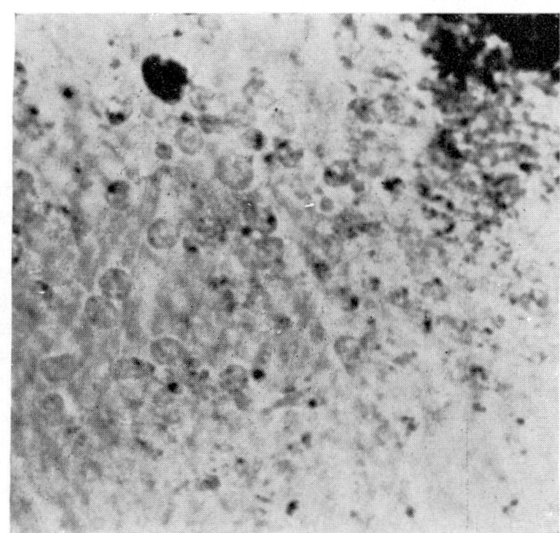

4/FIG. 15.—(*b*) Later the same day. Numbers of polymorphs are to be seen near the mass of ink (just seen at right upper corner). Some already contain carbon.

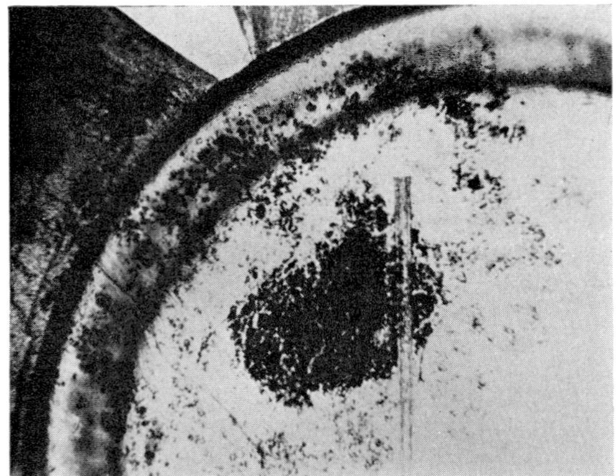

4/FIG. 15.—(*c*) Twenty-four days later. The carbon has been extensively invaded and ingested by macrophages, and is being dispersed by their migration.

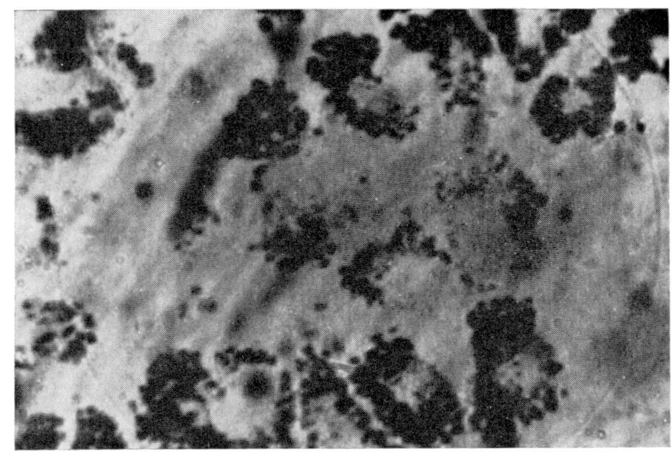

4/FIG. 15.—(*d*) High-power view taken on same day as last figure. The cells crammed with carbon granules are typical macrophages. The clear area in each cell is occupied by the nucleus.

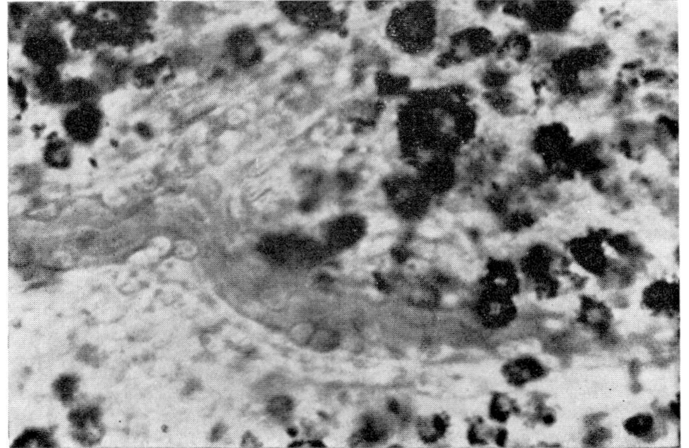

4/FIG. 15.—(*e*) This shows the size to which loaded macrophages can grow. Some are hardly bigger than the polymorphs clinging to the vessel wall, while others have up to three times their diameter.

cells is not clear, but they are found almost invariably around such foreign material as silk or cat-gut sutures. FIGURE 16 shows them forming around a piece of boiled liver that had been inserted into the peritoneal cavity of a guinea-pig.

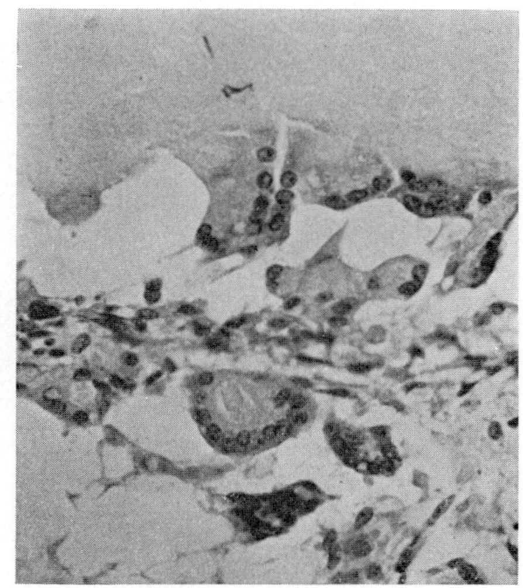

4/FIG. 16.—Macrophages and giant cells around a piece of boiled liver that had been inserted into the peritoneal cavity of a guinea-pig two weeks earlier. Above four giant cells are pressed against the foreign body, their cytoplasm filled with its substance and almost indistinguishable from the main mass of liver. Below are macrophages and several more giant cells.

FORMATION OF ABSCESSES

We have followed the vascular reactions accompanying injury, especially those caused by bacteria, and we have examined the migratory cells which appear in the tissues when the conditions are appropriate. We will now go on to examine in some detail the events that follow the implantation in the tissues of pus-forming or pyogenic organisms, as they are generally called.

The results of the implantation of a not very virulent *Staphylococcus aureus* can be observed in human skin, where pimples and boils due to such an organism are frequent. The sequence of events can be followed in a laboratory animal, for instance a rabbit, by taking material for section from one or a series of animals at different times after the inoculation of staphylococci just under the skin. Within an hour or two after inoculation the blood vessels contain marginated leucocytes, and a few polymorphs have already emigrated into the tissues. The bacteria soon begin to divide, and as they increase in number a considerable amount of toxin of various kinds is liberated by them. Probably the α-hæmolysin and the δ-hæmolysin are the principal toxins which damage the tissue cells in the neighbourhood, causing them to swell and show other signs of degeneration. When the concentration of toxins becomes sufficiently great, together with some impairment of the circulation from stasis in the blood vessels, the cells at the centre of the lesion die. By about ten hours after inoculation many bacteria can be seen free in the tissues, though many others have been ingested by the neutrophil leucocytes which by this time are present in large numbers. In course of time many of these die also, from either the action of bacterial toxins, the growth of bacteria within them, or the termination of their natural span of life.

By about 20 hours there is a great collection of cells and cocci, and the fibrils of the connective tissue are widely separated by œdema fluid. After 48 hours there is a well-developed abscess (FIG. 17).

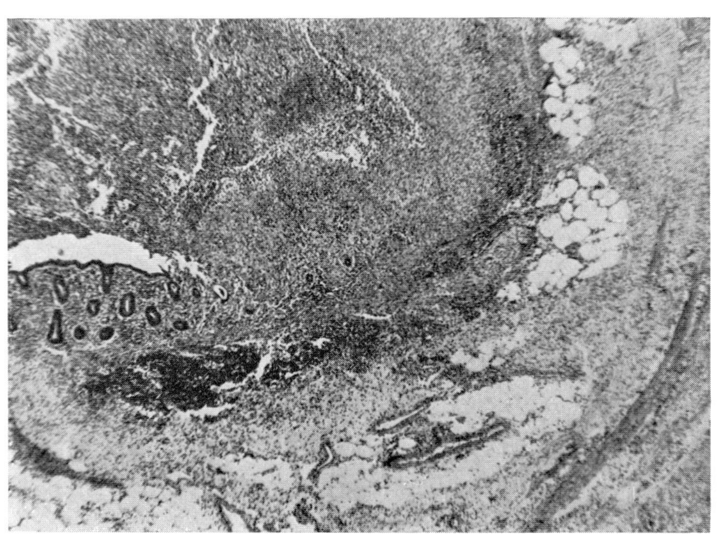

4/FIG. 17.—AN ABSCESS IN THE APPENDIX OF MAN

Part of the circular muscle can be seen on the right, and part of the mucosa on the left. The rest of the mucosa has broken down. Pus fills the lumen and is seen in the left upper part of the picture.

Pus

The essential feature of an abscess, differentiating it from inflammation caused by, say, moderate mechanical trauma or a non-pyogenic organism, is that there is substantial death of tissue, including any leucocytes that may be in the dying area, with subsequent liquefaction. In the case we are considering the tissue is killed by toxins of the *Staphylococcus*. Where the bacteria reach their maximal development these toxic substances kill tissue cells and emigrated leucocytes. The dead cells, particularly the polymorphs, liberate enzymes—proteases, peptidases and lipases—which proceed to digest the dead cells, fibrin, and other structures. The digested liquid product is pus—the yellow or greenish fluid in the centre of an abscess (FIG. 18).

Pus can be made to form in the absence of bacteria by the injection of certain chemicals. Thus bacterial proteins derived even from non-pathogenic organisms, certain vegetable proteins, turpentine, mercury, croton oil and 5 to 10 per cent. silver nitrate solution all produce abscesses on injection. They all cause an accumulation of leucocytes and necrosis of tissue with subsequent liquefaction of the cells and tissue constituents.

If pus is examined, by making and appropriately staining a smear, it is seen to consist of amorphous debris among which cells—the "pus corpuscles" of the older pathologists—can be recognised as polymorphs in various stages of disintegration. If due to an organism such as the staphylococcus, bacteria are often present in large numbers lying in the fluid and sometimes intracellularly as well. Pus is highly infective from its content of bacteria, many of which are alive.

As pus is formed chiefly by the action of enzymes liberated from dead polymorphs and other cells, and possibly to some extent by enzymes from bacteria, it may reasonably be expected to contain all types of breakdown products arising from proteins and other cellular contents as well as constituents of exuded blood plasma.

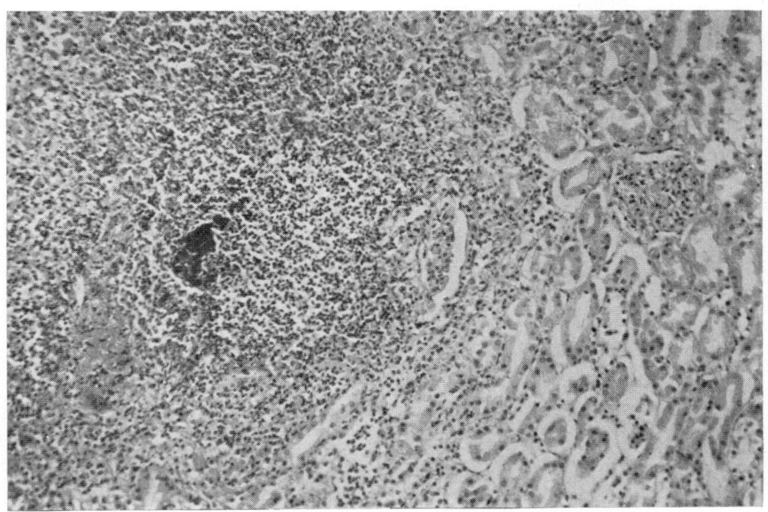

4/Fig. 18.—An Abscess in the Kidney

Kidney tubules and a glomerulus can be recognised at the right of the picture. The pus, consisting of vast numbers of polymorphs in an area from which the kidney tissue has disappeared, is at the left. The dark mass in the pus is a colony of infecting bacteria.

In the fluid part of pus—the so-called pus serum—cholesterol, lecithin, fats, soaps and a number of other components of tissue breakdown are present. Perhaps of most interest are desoxyribonucleoprotein and desoxyribonucleic acid, which arise mainly from the nuclei of the polymorphs. These substances can be present in such amounts that the pus is very viscous and difficult to evacuate from a cavity like the pleura. "Enzymic surgery" has even been used in an endeavour to render such pus more fluid, so that it could be washed away. For this purpose two enzymes known as streptodornase and streptokinase have been used in combination, the first breaking down desoxyribonucleoprotein and DNA with the formation of nucleotides, nucleosides, purine and pyrimidine compounds, and the second, streptokinase, activating plasminogen to plasmin, a proteolytic enzyme.

Amino-acids are present in pus but apparently not in such quantities as one might suppose, probably because they are among the products most readily absorbed into the blood stream. It has been suggested that this may partly explain why large amounts of urea are excreted by persons with extensive suppuration. Many other breakdown products are recorded as occurring in pus so that it is a pathological product containing a very extensive range of different substances.

Outside the liquefied area phagocytes continue to accumulate, and these, with strands of fibrin, can sometimes form so substantial an investment that the old name for it was a "pyogenic membrane". It is unlikely that the organisms will spread through such a zone of leucocytes, and if the pus drains away, either by natural rupture through a surface or by surgical intervention, healing occurs rapidly. But for rapid healing to occur the pus must escape. The body only

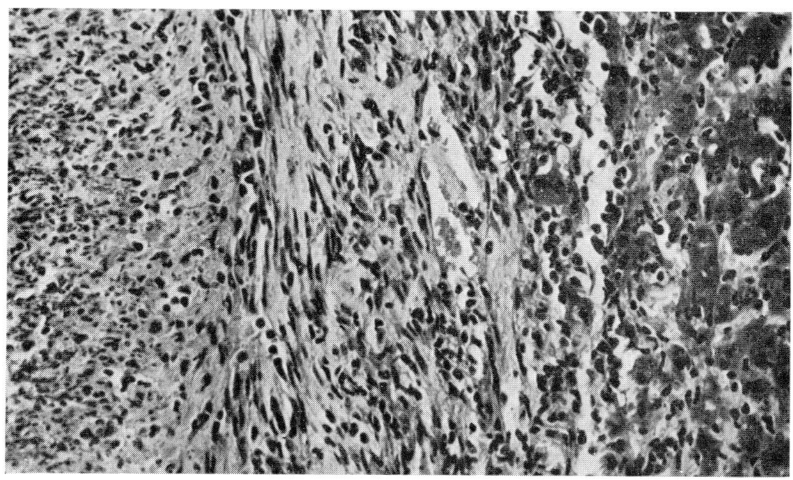

4/FIG. 19.—Part of the wall of an abscess caused by staphylococci in the liver of a mouse. The pus, which is at the left of the picture, is surrounded by granulation tissue.

slowly absorbs and removes dead material, and, in the absence of drainage even though few live bacteria are present, swelling and mild inflammation may go on for a long time, merging eventually into the process known as chronic inflammation, in which the predominant cell is the macrophage and fibrous tissue is laid down concurrently with continuing inflammation (FIG. 19). If this state of things continues for a long time very large amounts of fibrous tissue may be formed, eventually encapsulating the necrotic material.

THE RETICULO-ENDOTHELIAL OR MACROPHAGE SYSTEM

We have so far concentrated our attention on phagocytic cells that circulate in the blood and emerge from it to move about in the tissues. It was recognised, however, during the last century that there were also phagocytic cells normally existing in the tissues. They did not appear to be derived from the blood and were given a multitude of confusing names. Some order began to appear when it was discovered by Ribbert in 1904 that lithium carmine injected in solution into the circulation was taken up in considerable amounts by certain cells, which were thereby "vitally stained". Soon after, it was found that solutions of the electro-negative dyes, pyrrhol blue, isamine blue and trypan blue (to which others have since been added) would vitally stain cells. We owe the earliest systematic observations made with such dyes to Goldmann, who examined many tissues.

The name "reticulo-endothelial system" was coined by Aschoff and Landau to designate the group of cells whose striking property was the ability to abstract highly diluted dye from the circulating blood, and to concentrate it to such an extent that it formed deeply coloured granules or vacuoles in the cytoplasm.

The dyes taken up in this way have large molecules, made larger by conjunction with albumin of the plasma and tissue fluids. Such dye-albumin complexes escape slowly from normal blood vessels, trypan blue and vital new red leaving the vessels the most readily. On the basis of their similar reaction to vital staining it was suggested that the cells of the reticulo-endothelial system had important common functions to perform, although the cells were widely separated in the body.

The cells of the reticulo-endothelial (or R.E.) system are also voracious phagocytes of particulate material such as bacteria, which they take up as readily as a dye that is in solution. When there is an increased call for their activities the reticulo-endothelial cells of an organ can rapidly increase in number, partly by local mitosis, but also by immigration from elsewhere.

It is no longer profitable to follow Aschoff in including in the system cells such as fibroblasts that can take up some dye but have not the same capacity to concentrate it as the endothelial cells. What is useful is to recognise, as he did, that in a number of organs there are cells lining the blood or lymph channels which probably subserve common functions. Cells with similar properties, known as macrophages or histiocytes, occur in connective tissues. Monocytes which circulate in the blood can be considered to be part of the system, for they can transform into macrophages on leaving the circulation. The microglia of the central nervous sytem can become local phagocytes.

The main groups of cells in the system are set out in Table I.

Macrophages of Connective Tissues and Body Spaces

The phagocytic cells scattered through the *connective tissues* used sometimes to be referred to as "resting wandering cells", but are now usually called histiocytes. They apparently have two main sources of origin, arising from unidentified precursors in the connective tissue itself or from the monocytes of the blood. The connective tissue histiocytes are certainly phagocytic, but it is by no means clear that they wander much. No directional movements have been observed *in vivo*.

In Chapter 17 it is described how blood monocytes can be labelled and traced through slightly damaged vessel walls into healing tissues, where they enlarge and become indistinguishable from the resident histiocytes. There is good evidence that many of the macrophages in inflammatory lesions may have been circulating monocytes which originated in the bone marrow[80, 81].

The *peritoneal* and *pleural spaces* contain resident populations of macrophages. For experimental purposes the peritoneal space of small animals is often injected with oil or some other foreign substance, a procedure which increases

4/TABLE I

Macrophage or reticulo-endothelial system

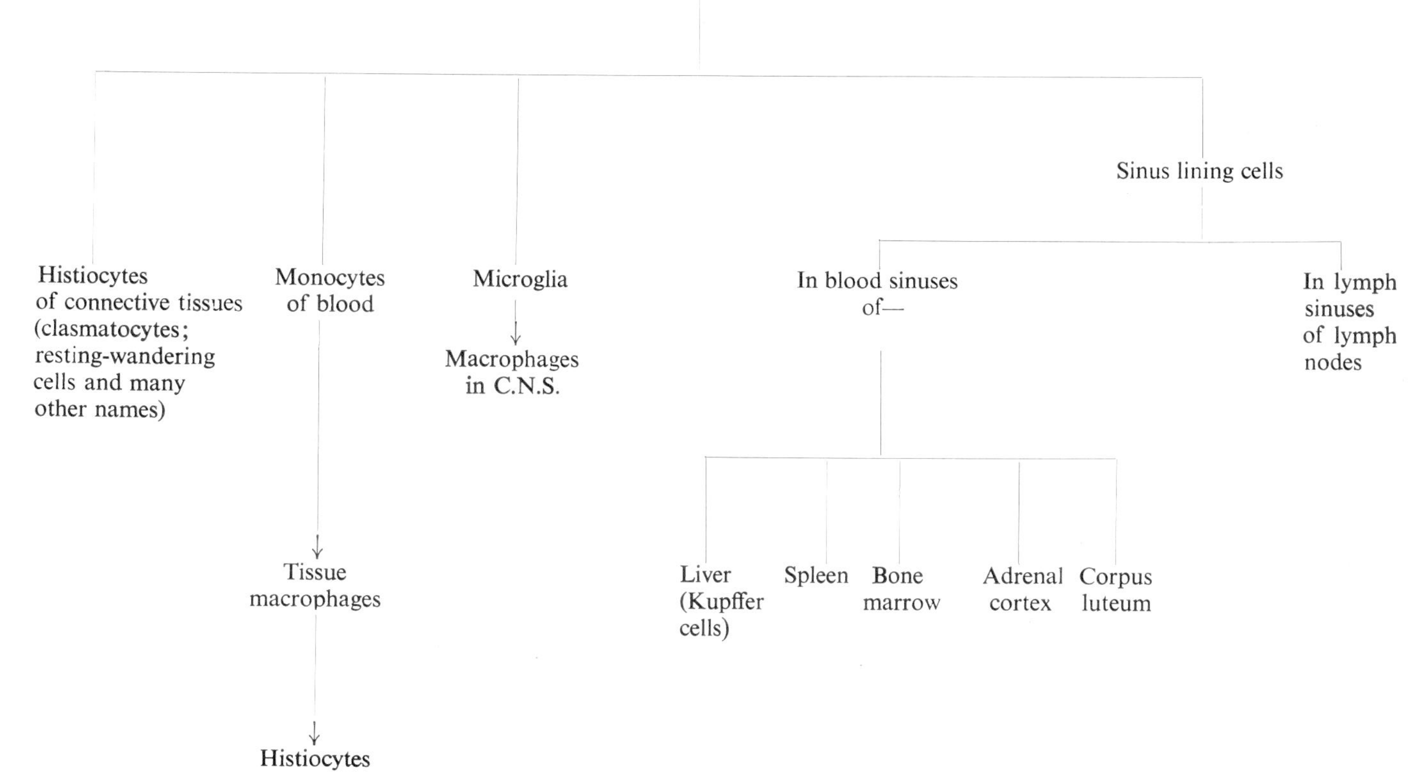

the number of cells obtainable when the cavity is washed out. However, simple washing of the cavity with a suitable saline solution produces a suspension of cells which includes many macrophages[82]. While some of these were probably free in the cavity it is likely that others were situated at or near the surface of the serous membrane and were washed off in the course of the manipulations, for macrophages form part of the surface over the milk spots, though not, it seems, elsewhere in the peritoneum[83]. These cells can readily be visualised by injecting carbon into the serous cavity when, since they are avidly phagocytic, they can be seen blackened, particularly along the course of the vessels and aggregated in the milk spots. The omentum is very rich in such cells. They are clearly able to take up foreign material from the serous cavities of the living animal without difficulty.

Mitoses are sometimes seen in the macrophages of milk spots and of peritoneal washings, and peritoneal macrophages can divide in culture[84] but, as in other situations, under local stimulation many macrophages may be added from the blood having been formed in the bone marrow.[85] There is also evidence that under intense antigenic stimulation peritoneal macrophages can develop from small lymphocytes.[86]

The *lung* is particularly rich in phagocytes, for there is a constant demand for their activity to keep the alveoli clear of dust particles or any other solid material. They emerge into the alveolar spaces and are seen there as large round cells often containing particles such as carbon (from the air), hæmosiderin (from extravasated red blood cells), and so on. Many of these cells probably pass up the bronchial tree and are expectorated or swallowed. There is some uncertainty as to whether they also enter the interstitial tissues of the lung and carry their load to the lymphatics. Certainly, as may be seen in the lungs of any town dweller, much particulate matter can enter the lymphatics and reach the hilar glands, but some may be carried there in tissue fluids and lymph rather than within cells.

The exact origin of these pulmonary cells is not entirely clear. They evidently come from the walls of the alveoli, where they might have migrated from the blood vessels or have been local histiocytes. It has been shown that two thirds or more of cells washed out of the lungs of mice through the airways originated in the bone marrow.[87] Cells loaded with particles that had been injected intravenously, and presumed to come from the liver, have also been found in the alveoli,[88, 89] but whether this represents a usual source of lung macrophages is not known.

Phagocytic cells of local importance are found in the *central nervous system* where they are derived from the local connective tissue cells, the microglia. They are not stained on the intravenous injection of such dyes as trypan blue, which do not pass out of the cerebral blood vessels, but they can be shown up by injecting dyes or carbon into the brain. They become conspicuous when engaged in cleaning up the debris after damage to the brain and spinal cord, and in such conditions often become loaded with lipid material from the breakdown of myelin and present a foamy appearance in paraffin sections.

Phagocytes lining Sinusoids

It is to be noted that only certain vessels contain highly phagocytic cells. The vessels concerned are all sinusoidal, that is to say they are thin-walled vessels in

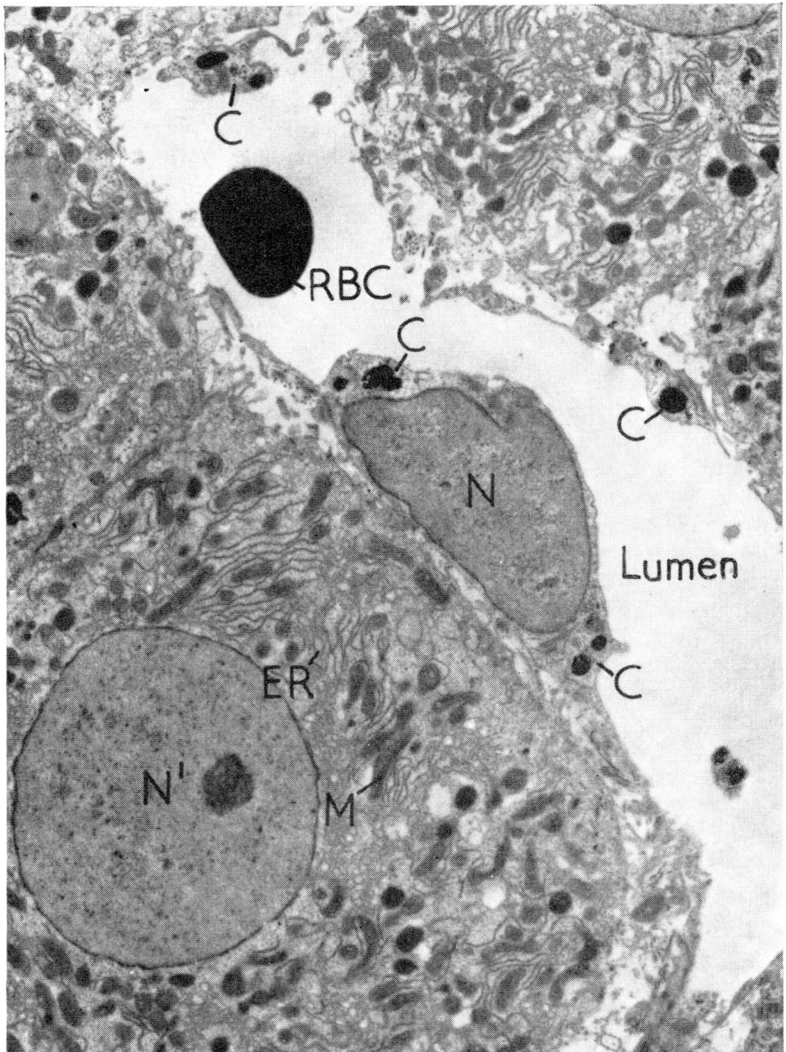

4/Fig. 20.—Kupffer cells lining a sinusoid in the liver. Carbon has been ingested by the endothelial cells and is indicated by C. N is the nucleus of a Kupffer cell and N¹ of an epithelial cell. Large numbers of mitochondria (M) are seen in the epithelial cell. Endoplasmic reticulum (ER) appears as prominent black fibres. (× 6000)

the wide channels of which the flow slackens. The phagocytic cells are flattish "squames" which rest on the wall, but they thicken and become prominent after taking up foreign material.

Some of these sinusoids are on the blood circulation and some on the lymph circulation. The liver contains more phagocytes than any other organ. In this situation they are known as Kupffer cells. Spleen, bone marrow and adrenal gland

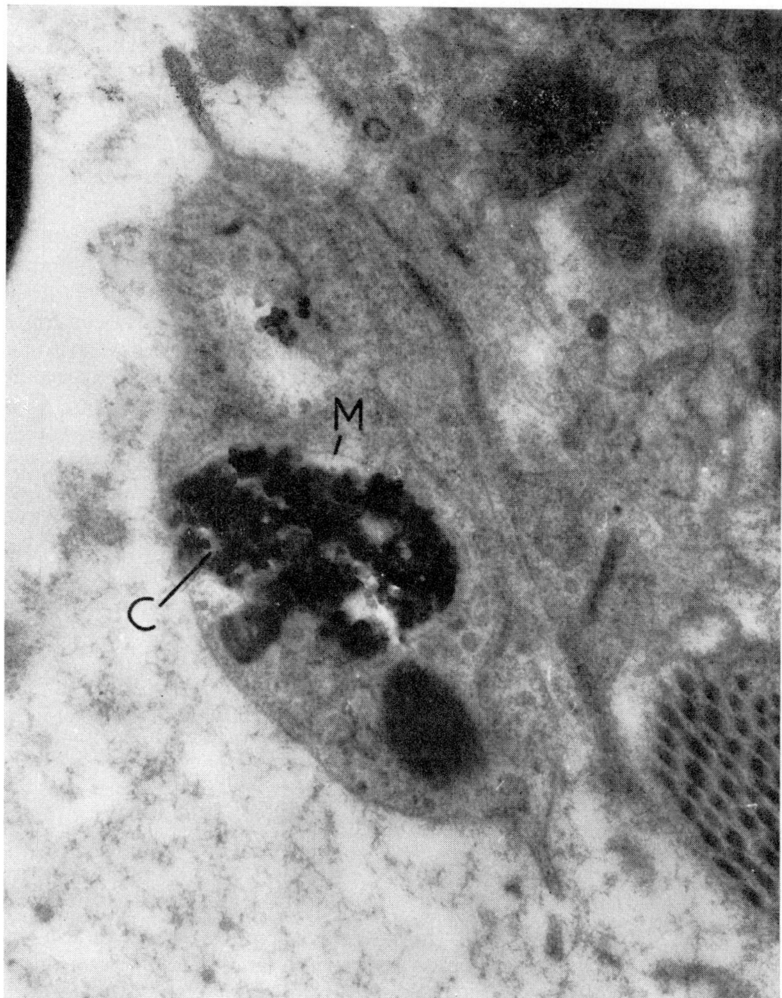

4/FIG. 21.—Kupffer cell showing ingested carbon (C) inside a vacuole, the limiting membrane (M) of which can be seen in places (× 33,000)

contain cells with similar activities. It was at one time thought that sinuses in the parathyroid gland and in the islets of Langerhans were similar to those of the adrenal and thymus, but the cells lining them do not take up colloidal thorium dioxide and are evidently of a different nature.[109] The sinuses of the corpus luteum at certain phases of its growth contain phagocytic cells. The pituitary gland also contains some sinusoidal phagocytes on the blood stream. Sinuses carrying lymph and lined by similar cells form a network in the substance of all lymph nodes.

The sinusoids of the *liver* have an apparently discontinuous lining of endothelial cells, many of which are flat or have flat portions of cytoplasm. It appears that these cells can in general be phagocytic, but a certain number of plump, more actively phagocytic cells are seen (FIGS. 20 and 21), and if through disease or experimental intervention there is an unusual call for the phagocytosis of material from the blood many cells may become prominent from their content of ingested material. Such phagocytic cells projecting into the sinusoids are the classical Kupffer cells, and are easily demonstrated by light microscopy, for instance after the intravenous injection of carbon, but it has not yet been shown whether or not all the lining cells have this potentiality.

The number of actively phagocytic cells in the liver can increase both in natural disease and, for example, in the condition known to experimentalists as reticulo-endothelial blockade (see below) and in strong graft versus host reactions. The local Kupffer cells can certainly proliferate, but it has been found that both bone marrow cells and small lymphocytes can provide new Kupffer cells under intense immunological stimulation such as can be applied experimentally. Under these conditions one or the other precursor may preponderate according to the particular stimulus used. It is considered that under relatively normal conditions the bone marrow cells are probably more important than lymphocytes as an external source of new Kupffer cells.[90] These cell transformations are discussed in Chapter 5.

The vascular system of the *spleen* is more complex than that of the liver, and the related phagocytic cells include both reticulo-endothelial cells, arranged round the fibrillary reticulum, and free macrophages[91]. Under intense immunological stimulation most of the dividing phagocytes in the spleen were found to have originated in the bone marrow.[92]

Compared to those of the liver and spleen the phagocytic cells resident in the *bone marrow* have received little attention, but it has been suggested that the sinus lining cells, which are discontinuous, are also the active reticulo-endothelial phagocytes[93].

The disposition and function of macrophages in the *lymph nodes* are discussed in Chapter 3.

FUNCTIONING OF THE RETICULO-ENDOTHELIAL SYSTEM

This short survey of some of the more conspicuous parts of the reticulo-endothelial system gives evidence of its variety, and brings forward some of the ideas that are developing at this time about the cell transformations that may give rise to phagocytes. These evidently have a bearing on its ability to meet major fluctuations in the demands made upon it. Little is yet understood about general factors, such as the levels of circulating hormones, which may alter its activity, or the changes that may take place in the cells under stimulation.

Differences between Macrophages

While the constituent cells of the reticulo-endothelial system seem to have, in the main, common functions, the means by, or extent to which these are performed seem not to be identical in all parts of the system. For example, if lung alveolar macrophages are compared *in vitro* with peritoneal macrophages it is found that the former depend for their energy more on oxidative phosphorylation and the latter more on anærobic glycolysis; lung macrophages also have a greater concentration of lysosomal enzymes. In some experimental situations liver and spleen macrophages can be shown to discriminate between red blood cells treated with stronger or weaker antibodies, and Kupffer cells can destroy or neutralise antigen more effectively than spleen cells[92]; such specialisations may have a place under natural conditions in, for example, the disposal of aged red blood cells.

On the basis of their morphology and staining, their mitotic rate in culture, and their speed of spreading and attachment to glass, Bennett[94] placed the macrophages that he examined in three groups that behaved somewhat differently, firstly those of bone marrow, spleen and liver, secondly those of peripheral blood and peritoneal cavity, and thirdly those of the lung alveoli.

Phagocytic Activities

The experimental trick known as "reticulo-endothelial blockade" stemmed from the well-established physiological method of investigating the function of an organ by removing it and studying the consequences. Although the reticulo-endothelial system was too much scattered to be excised, it was hoped that its effects could largely be eliminated by loading the cells with ingested particles. This was done by the intravenous injection of such particulate materials as thorium dioxide (Thorotrast) or finely divided carbon (Hydrokollag or indian ink). Easton[88] showed that when Thorotrast is repeatedly injected in mice over a few days the main uptake is in the liver, spleen and bone marrow, and that, surprisingly, particles accumulate in the lungs. This seemed to be because the loaded and proliferating cells in the liver sinusoids tended to move towards the central veins of the lobules and some left the liver in the hepatic vein and were caught in the lung capillaries. Many of these eventually passed into the alveoli and so into the airways.

Although the remarkable capacity of the system to hypertrophy in response to demand stood in the way of the clarification of function that was hoped for, these experiments have led to a better understanding of the reaction between macrophage and circulating particle. For example, it has been found that while an initial dose may block the uptake of another dose of the same material it may not block uptake of material of a different type, and that the kind of stabilising agent used in suspending the particles may affect the result.[95] The amount of uptake may be related more to the concentration of particles left in the circulation than to the quantity already ingested.[96] This suggests that properties of the surface of the cell and particle may be more important in determining uptake than the amount already ingested. Electron micrographs of the spleen during the height of blockade induced with thorium dioxide supported this view by showing that the bulk of the particles were packed round the surfaces of the macrophages rather than being inside them[91] and the same was found when the blockade produced by large doses of steroids was examined.[97] Such experiments have a bearing on the function of macrophages in disposing of bacteria, the ingestion of which varies enormously with the properties of the organism and its state of opsonization, which profoundly affects its surface. It is of interest that the kinetics of particle uptake in the frog, fowl and chick embryo seem to be similar to those in small mammals.[98]

Phagocytosis in Infection

Owing largely to the work of Metchnikoff the cells of the reticulo-endothelial system have for long been considered to take part in the protection of the body against invasion by infecting micro-organisms. It was noted earlier that the monocyte emerges from the blood and is capable of being attracted by bacteria. In the tissues it can ingest, in many cases kill, and finally digest the organisms. Much work has been done to show that the macrophages which collect in inflammation do in fact play a prominent part in ridding the tissues of bacteria, and it is possible that they may be more effective in dealing with them than the more easily and quickly mobilised polymorphs. (Some of this work has been summarised by Gay.[99])

The macrophages lining the sinusoids are also a defence against infection. Thus is was discovered by Wyssokowitsch as long ago as 1886 that bacteria injected intravenously are to a great extent removed by the liver and spleen. This observation has been repeated many times, and it is interesting to follow by serial blood culture the dramatic removal of very many organisms within a few hours (Table II).

4/TABLE II

Living pneumococci per ml. of circulating blood at stated times after the intravenous injection of 3 strains of pneumococcus of differing virulence into normal rabbits

Time after injection	*Avirulent*	*Slightly Virulent*	*Highly Virulent*
Immediately	8,900,000	1,030,000	1,070,000
2 hours	206	20,800	137,000
5 hours	20	340	25,000
24 hours	0	1,300	1,510,000
48 hours	—	134	animal dead
96 hours	—	0	—

(*From Topley and Wilson.*[100])

As the table shows, even a virulent organism is removed from the circulation at first, but then, following growth inside the phagocytic cells and their death and rupture, it reappears to produce a septicæmia which leads to death. If the organism is not so virulent it is destroyed by the phagocytes after ingestion. The cells of the reticulo-endothelial system are called upon, no doubt, to remove from time to time the bacteria that invade the blood stream of most people in small numbers, particularly from the oral cavity and the intestine. Many people have some dental sepsis and it is, at first, a startling thought that even biting hard sweets may force bacteria from an unhealthy tooth into the circulation. The extraction of septic teeth or removal of septic tonsils causes a bacteriæmia (circulation of bacteria in the blood) that is demonstrable by culture in a substantial proportion of cases. But the efficiency of the cells we have been discussing is very great, and after a quite short time—perhaps only a few minutes—the organisms are completely removed from the blood, which is thereby sterilised. Cells in the lymph nodes behave in a similar way (see Chapter 3).

Not only are the sinusoidal reticulo-endothelial cells involved in defence against bacteria, but they may play an important part in abstracting protozoal and fungal invaders from the blood stream. Free malarial parasites may be taken up as well as those contained in red cells that they have invaded and damaged. In disease caused by *Histoplasma capsulatum* the parasitic fungus is found in large numbers in the phagocytic cells. The cells may ingest parasites without being able to kill them. In spite of much phagocytosis of *Histoplasma capsulatum* the death rate from the disease is high. Similarly the macrophages by no means always kill tubercle bacilli that they have ingested.

Many viruses are taken up by reticulo-endothelial cells, opsonins being of importance in their ingestion as they are with the ingestion of bacteria. Macrophages may contain useful amounts of interferon when infected with virus, and were found to be exceptional among the various types of cell tested in containing some even before infection.[101, 102] The macrophages may be able to destroy the virus or they may become the site of viral multiplication. In young mice the resistance of the Kupffer cells was shown to increase in parallel with the resistance of the whole animal to a viral hepatitis infection.[103] In some experimental infections it appears that liver cells are only infected by virus that has been through a cycle of multiplication in Kupffer cells first. Other experiments have shown a parallel in different strains of a virus between virulence and ability to multiply in macrophages.[104]

Beside ingesting and killing invading organisms macrophages play a part in the production of antibodies, that is they contribute to the humoral defence mechanisms (Chapter 35). They seem to be the main site of the acquired immunity which resides in cells rather than in the body fluids, as discussed above. There is no doubt that in some diseases, for example in tuberculosis, cellular immunity plays a part in the resistance of the infected individual.[65]

Activities in Tissue Injury

When tested *in vitro* macrophages have much the same ability as polymorphs to ingest foreign material such as bacteria or inert particles, though their phagocytic power seems to be less dependent on the presence of serum factors. Bacteria if not virulent are generally digestible and so are disposed of by the cell that has ingested them, but inert material, or resistant organisms such as the tubercle bacillus, survive beyond the life of any polymorph and so may be re-ingested by macrophages. Macrophages are also able to recognise and ingest old ("effete") cells of the same individual, a capacity lacking in polymorphs.[105] After hæmorrhage or tissue injury macrophages containing red blood cells, cell fragments, and lipid or pigment granules derived from digested cell components, may be present in quantity in the area.

Hæmoglobin and red cells are dealt with in the tissues as they are physiologically in the circulation. The red corpuscles are ingested locally by macrophages or histiocytes and in a very short time all recognisable structure of the erythrocyte is lost (Fig. 22). Whether the red cell or hæmoglobin is the starting material, the phagocytic cells produce hæmosiderin and bilirubin, the latter being now recognised as the same as the pathologist's hæmatoidin that is seen microscopically in old scars or dead areas in the form of yellow crystals (Plate A). The transformation of pigments is responsible for the alterations that take place in the colour of a bruise as it ages.

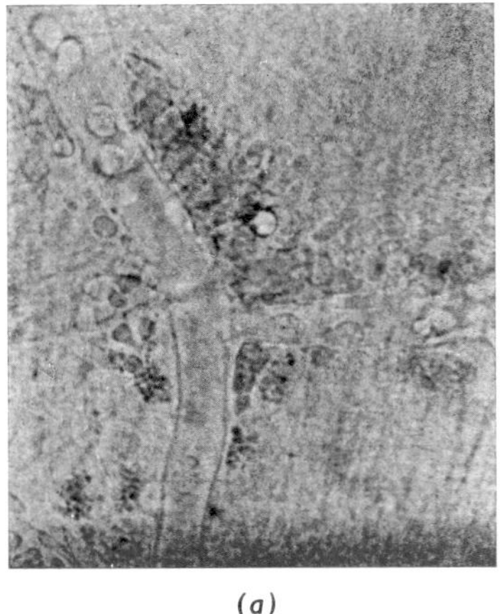

(a)

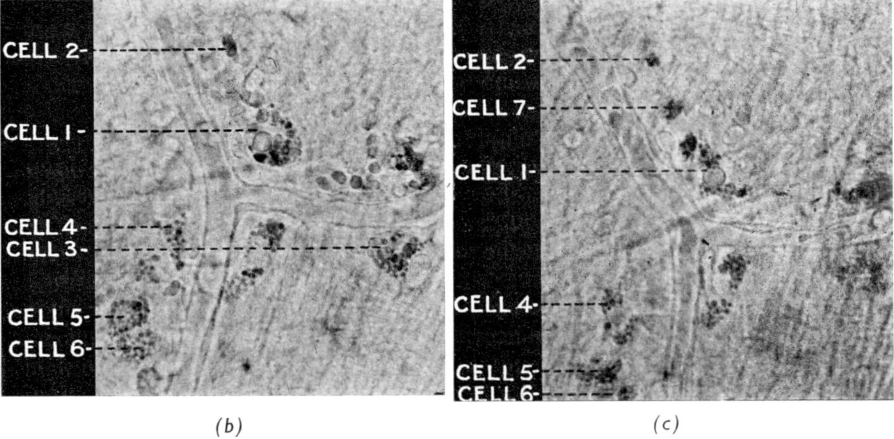

(b) (c)

4/FIG. 22.—THE REACTION OF HISTIOCYTES TO A SMALL HÆMORRHAGE, AS SEEN IN A TRANSPARENT CHAMBER IN THE RABBIT'S EAR

(*a*) 3 hours after injury. Around the vessel and its branch is a small hæmorrhage. The vessels are dilated. The finer dark granules are aggregates of an injected dye within tissue macrophages.

(*b*) 20 hours after injury. A large part of the hæmorrhage has been cleared away. Histiocyte (1) has been most active and is packed with ingested red cells. Histiocyte (3) also contains several red cells in various stages of digestion. Histiocyte (2) appears to contain only one large dye vacuole. Histiocyte (4) has moved closer to cells (5) and (6).

(*c*) 68 hours after injury. The hæmorrhage has been cleared away and the tissue is practically normal again. Intact red cells can no longer be recognised within the histiocytes. A new histiocyte (7) has moved into the field and now lies next to histiocyte (1). It did not move until most of the hæmorrhage had been cleared away, however, and took no active part in phagocytosing the extravasated red cells. (From Ebert and Florey.[110])

PLATE A

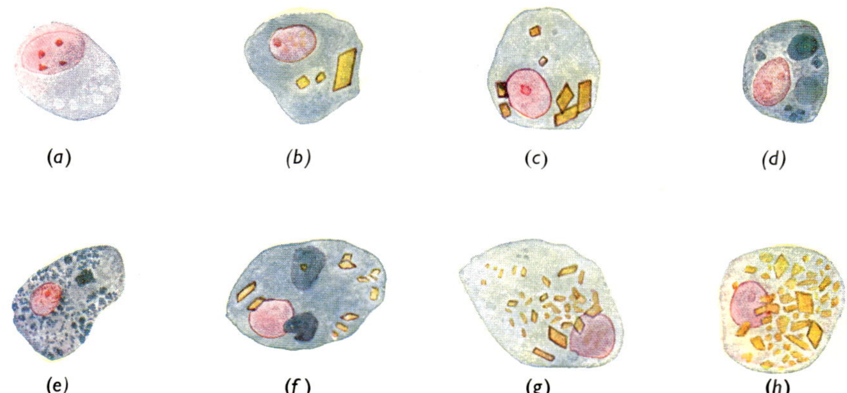

(*a–c*) MACROPHAGES OF MOUSE AFTER SUBCUTANEOUS INJECTION OF HÆMOGLOBIN

(*a*) 2 days, showing diffuse Prussian blue reaction for iron, due to hæmosiderin.
(*b*) 12 days, showing early formation of crystals of hæmatoidin.
(*c*) 16 days, later stage with diminution of hæmosiderin.

(*d–h*) MACROPHAGES AFTER INJECTION OF ERYTHROCYTES

(*d*) and (*e*) Cells containing abundant hæmosiderin several days after injection.
(*f–h*) Hæmatoidin formation in isolated cells, 10, 15 and 29 days respectively after injection (From Muir and Niven.[111])

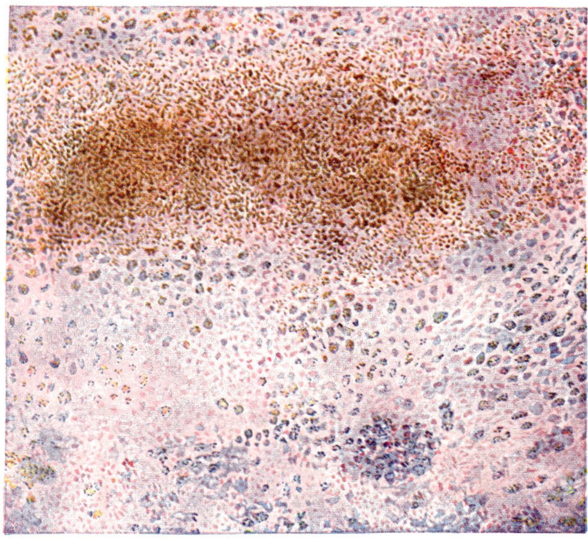

(*i*) Spread preparation of subcutaneous tissue of mouse 12 days after injection of mouse erythrocytes. The brown area is a large collection of iron-free phagocytes containing crystalline hæmatoidin and represents its formation on a massive scale. This area is surrounded by collections of hæmosiderin-containing phagocytes free from hæmatoidin. At the junction of the two areas phagocytes containing both kinds of pigment are seen. (From Muir and Niven.[111])

Physiological Activities

Red Blood Cells and Iron Metabolism

Physiologically the cells of the reticulo-endothelial system play an important part in dealing with red blood cells that are "effete" or "worn out", which in some way they are able to recognise. It is now generally considered that the human red cell survives for some 120 days in the circulation. Macrophages *in vitro* can distinguish old from young red blood cells in the sense that they ingest the former much more often than the latter. In perfused livers old red blood cells were taken up by the Kupffer cells, but young cells were not.[106] There is, however, some doubt as to whether the red cells are dealt with entirely intracellularly, evidence having been produced that phagocytosis of red cells by the cells of the spleen is rather a rare event. It may be that some red cells are lysed in the blood and the products are then taken up and dealt with. In either case the hæmoglobin becomes intracellular and undergoes a series of changes mediated by enzymes. The chief effects are the splitting off of an iron-free pigment, bilirubin, which escapes from the cell, becomes associated with plasma proteins and is carried to the liver to be excreted in the bile; and the formation of iron-containing pigment, probably a mixture of substances, though still often known to pathologists as hæmosiderin.

Iron is tenaciously retained by the body, where it enters into combination with a protein—apoferritin—with which it forms ferritin, containing some 23 per cent of iron. The exact relationship between hæmosiderin and ferritin is not clear, but electron micrographs of cells containing the light microscopist's hæmosiderin often show much ferritin to be present. It is thought that ferritin forms the main iron store of the body, which is called upon normally, as well as after hæmorrhage, to furnish iron for new corpuscles. It is stored in organs rich in reticulo-endothelial cells such as the liver and spleen and in the bone marrow where it is seen in macrophages and in intercellular spaces in close association with the erythroblasts.[107] It also occurs in the intestine where it may be manufactured from absorbed iron. It thus appears that physiologically the reticulo-endothelial system is intimately concerned with iron metabolism.

Fat Metabolism

Macrophages containing fat are often found in the tissues after inflammation or injury, when the fat is thought to be derived from cell debris that they have taken up and digested. But it is apparent that the reticulo-endothelial cells can also take up fat from the blood, for if fat emulsions are injected intravenously, or cholesterol is added to the food, the phagocytic cells in the liver and elsewhere may contain fat that is easily demonstrable. In the intimal lesions of atheroma fat-containing cells, some of them probably macrophages, are common, and in cholesterol-fed rabbits such cells are plentiful in the aortic intima and have been found in passage through the endothelium overlying lesions (see Chapter 18).

Findings of this kind have led to the question whether the reticulo-endothelial system may play some part in the normal metabolism of ingested fat, or in the disposal of excessive fat loads in the blood. No satisfactory answer to this question has yet emerged. The experimental findings are difficult to interpret and tend to be contradictory. For example, from the account already given it will be clear that experiments depending on "blockade" of the reticulo-endothelial system by some other particle may not be very informative about the capacity of the system to deal with fat. However, a good deal has been learnt, mainly by experiments *in vitro* with isolated macrophages, about the capacity of these cells to degrade and to synthesise fats of various kinds. This and other relevant information has been brought together in a review by Day.[108]

Phagocytosis by other Cells

The cells of the R.E. system that we have been considering are very conspicuously phagocytic. The ordinary endothelium lining blood vessels and lymphatics does not possess this property to anything like the same extent. The appearances in the light microscope that have been interpreted as showing considerable amounts of carbon accumulated in the endothelium of small blood vessels under inflammatory conditions (e.g. Gözsy and Kátó[122]) are probably to be explained by the carbon leaving the blood stream to enter the space between the endothelium and the periendothelial sheath of the small blood vessels (see Chapter 3). But Cotran[112] has shown that when colloidal carbon is repeatedly injected into the blood stream so that large amounts continue to circulate a good deal can be taken into large vesicles in the endothelium, and it is now clear that the endothelial cells of small blood vessels and of arteries such as the aorta can take up particles even when there is no prolonged overloading of the circulation.[112a, 113] They are found to a small extent in the small caveolæ and vesicles

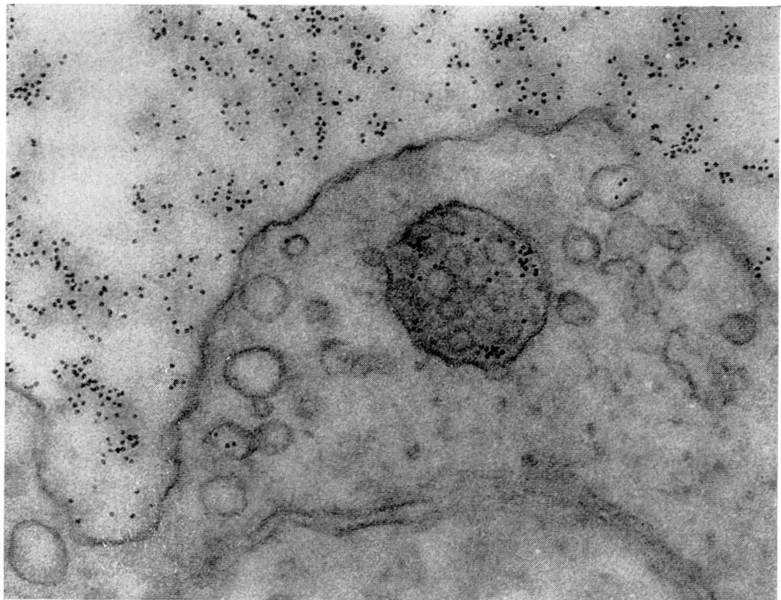

4/FIG. 23.—Part of an endothelial cell in a pulmonary capillary 15 min. after the introduction of ferritin into the circulation. Ferritin is present in the lumen of the vessel, in a caveola and a vesicle of the endothelium, and is already accumulating in a multivesicular body. Within the body it is mostly free in the main compartment, not inside the small vesicles. (× 99,000.)

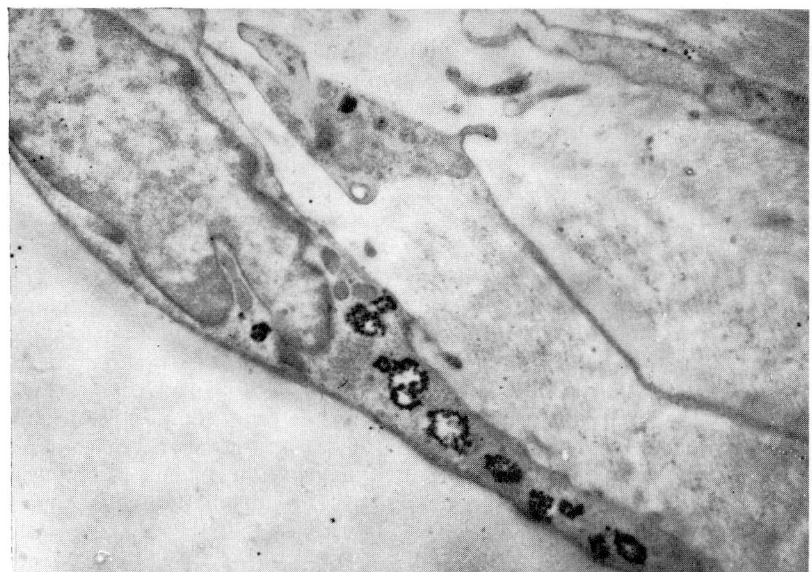

4/FIG. 24.—Iron oxide has been taken up by an endothelial cell of a lymphatic vessel in the diaphragm. The dark-appearing iron oxide is segregated in vacuoles. (× 11,000) (From French, Florey and Morris.[123])

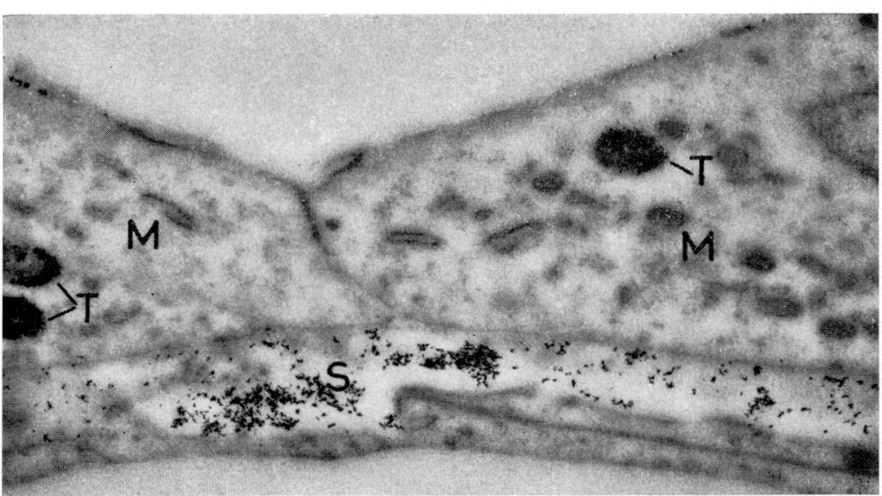

4/FIG. 25.—A suspension of thorium dioxide was injected into the peritoneal cavity of a rabbit. The particles are penetrating the diaphragm to gain entry into the lymphatics. Some particles can be seen free on the peritoneal surface (at the top of the picture), some particles (T) are in vacuoles in the cytoplasm of mesothelial cells (M), and some are free in the space (S) between the mesothelial cells and the endothelium of the lymphatic, which is at the bottom of the picture. (× 20,000) (From French *et al.*[123])

(see Chapter 3) but are sometimes concentrated in larger rounded bodies, some of which are of the type known as multivesicular bodies, that is, large vesicles bounded by a unit membrane and containing smaller vesicles also bounded by unit membranes. Within a few minutes of the introduction of thorium dioxide, ferritin, or colloidal ferric hydroxide into the circulation collections may be found in these bodies, and quite soon some may contain a marked concentration of particles (FIG. 23 and see 3/FIG. 11). It is not certain how materials reach this destination. Sometimes it seems to be through the fusion of small vesicles with each other and with larger vesicles, but it is possible that particles can sometimes cross the cytoplasm or arrive in other ways.

The lymphatic endothelium in the diaphragm and probably in other sites can take up particles such as colloidal thorium dioxide and colloidal ferric oxide and can segregate them in vacuoles (FIG. 24). Particles can also be taken up in certain circumstances by the mesothelial cells lining the peritoneal cavity (FIG. 25). Possibly in these situations uptake is by means of pinocytic vesicles which join to form large vacuoles. There is no reason for supposing that the particles are in transport through the cell. What role this phagocytic property of endothelium and mesothelium plays in physiological activity or under pathological conditions is not at present known.

Phagocytosis by the Blood Platelets

It is somewhat extraordinary that in the discussions that occur on the various mechanisms by which particulate matter can be removed from the blood stream little or no mention is made of the properties of the platelets. As can be observed in the minute circulation in a rabbit's ear, individual platelets quickly disappear from the circulation after the injection of carbon suspensions such as are commonly used for determining the phagocytic powers of the reticulo-endothelium. The platelets adhere to the carbon and agglutinate round it.[114] Much work has been done on this phenomenon, work which seems usually to have been omitted from discussions on the functioning of the reticulo-endothelial system. It has been shown by the examination of histological sections that such clumps of platelets and particles are trapped at least temporarily in small vessels in the lung and elsewhere[115]. The platelets appear to be very important in defence against circulating organisms, for Govaerts[116] demonstrated that platelets agglutinate about bacteria as well as about carbon particles and foreign erythrocytes. It has been suggested that in certain experiments all bacteria injected intravenously were cleared by the platelets within the first 5 to 10 minutes.[117, 118]

Observations with the electron microscope have shown that platelets have the ability to take up a number of different particles including bacteria by a process which resembles the phagocytosis of particles by leucocytes (see Chapter 8). It remains uncertain whether platelets play any important part in the breakdown or elimination of materials which they take up in this way, but it may be significant that platelets with ingested particles are apparently themselves more susceptible to uptake by cells of the reticulo-endothelial system[119]. It seems that the platelets may play a more important part than has hitherto been generally recognised in helping to clear the blood of foreign materials.

THE OMENTUM

If a suspension of carbon which is not agglutinated in the presence of body fluids is injected intraperitoneally much of it is abstracted by the omentum, which becomes jet black, while the rest of the peritoneal surface and the mesentery appear of normal colour. If the layers of the omentum be separated and spread out it can be seen that the blood vessels are outlined by masses of black material that cannot be removed by gentle rubbing (FIG. 26). Smaller materials such as vital dyes may be taken up in a similar way (FIG. 27).

Microscopical examination shows that these black masses are not extracellular, but are made up of histiocytes crammed with carbon. The performance of the phagocytes is even more remarkable than might appear at first sight, for as we have seen, the macrophages along the vessels are shielded from the peritoneal cavity, in which the carbon suspension is placed, by a layer of flat mesothelial cells on either side, and the carbon particles must pass through or between these cells to reach them.

What functions this rich complement of phagocytic cells normally serves is not known, but they may evidently be involved in clearing up bacteria and debris if perforation of the abdominal or intestinal wall causes leakage of foreign material into the peritoneal cavity.

We might take this opportunity to have a further look at the lowly omentum, which usually has scant attention paid to it by physiologists and pathologists, though in bygone days it was used to ornament the carcases of sheep hanging in butchers' shops. Physiologically it acts as a fat depot, and the omentum of a well-fed cat or sheep is reminiscent of a Victorian lace curtain from the pattern formed by the abundant fat along the blood vessels. It is also remarkable in that it contains many mast cells, easily demonstrated by their intense metachromatic staining with toluidine blue. The metachromasia is considered to be due to heparin, which the granules contain as well as histamine and 5-hydroxytryptamine. The function of these cells normally or in disease is not clear, but they degranulate in some experimental injuries and anaphylactic reactions.

The omentum is of particular interest because of its ability to help in sealing off damaged or inflamed areas. Thus in human disease it may be found adherent to an acutely inflamed or perforated appendix, or to an area in which a peptic ulcer is about to perforate the wall of the stomach or duodenum. Through its action in these cases it may prevent the escape of gastric or intestinal contents, or may localise them and prevent general peritonitis. Substantial foreign bodies, such as a bullet, or a cotton swab accidently left in the peritoneal cavity at operation, may become enwrapped in omentum. This capacity of the omentum once caused a surgeon to call it "the abdominal policeman". "It travels around the abdomen with considerable activity, and is attracted by some sort of information to neighbourhoods in which mischief is brewing." The fact is that it has no intrinsic powers of movement, but is constantly moved relatively to other abdominal structures by the peristalsis of the gut and the movements of the diaphragm during breathing.[120] Thus it soon comes into contact with any part of the peritoneum that is inflamed or damaged. Its tendency to stick to the roughened surface is helped by the fact that exudate seems to come particularly readily from its vessels. Dense fibrinous adhesions soon form, which may

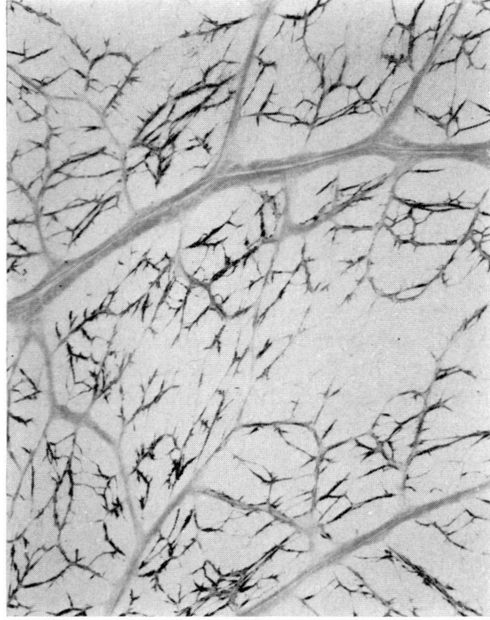

4/Fig. 26.—The omentum of a cat into whose peritoneal cavity a suspension of carbon (Hydrokollag) had been injected. The histiocytes lying along the blood vessels have taken up the carbon, thus outlining the finer vessels with black.

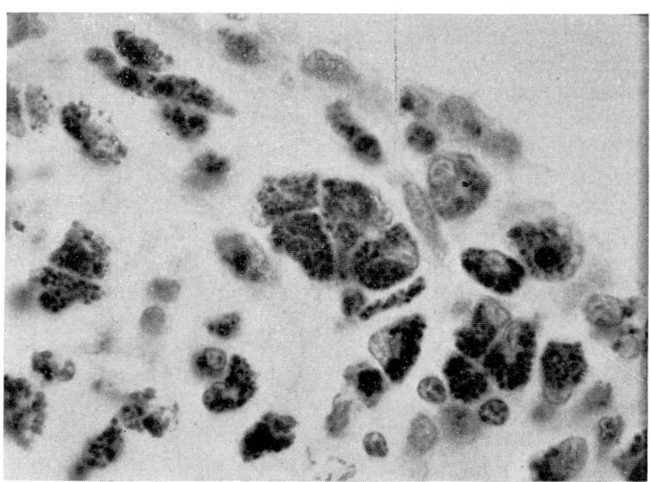

4/Fig. 27.—Histiocytes in the omentum of a mouse which had received 12 intraperitoneal injections of trypan blue. The granules in the cells are collections of blue dye that has been taken up.

later either largely disappear or become organised, in which case after a sufficient time the damaged structures may become firmly united or encapsulated by mature fibrous tissue formed in the way discussed in Chapter 17.

At the end of an abdominal operation on the gastro-intestinal tract the surgeon sometimes tucks the omentum round the suture lines and may even insert a stitch to keep it in place, in the hope that it will help to prevent leakage. Where the blood supply of the heart has been reduced by disease of the coronary vessels, attempts have been made to improve the circulation by bringing part of the omentum through the diaphragm and sewing it to the myocardium. Experiments on dogs gave some grounds for supposing that a collateral circulation could be set up in this way.

Altogether, one may say that this organ that looks like a lace curtain is not entirely without interest, for it functions as a protection against injury and many people have been preserved from death by its action.

REFERENCES

1. Thompson, P. L., Papadimitriou, J. M., and Walters, M. N.-I. (1967). *J. Path. Bact.*, **94,** 389.
2. Bangham, A. D. (1964). *Ann. N.Y. Acad. Sci.*, **116,** Art. 3, 945.
3. McCutcheon, M. (1942). *Arch. Path.*, **34,** 167.
4. Adami, J. G. (1909). *Inflammation.* London: Macmillan & Co.
5. Leber, T. (1888). *Fortschr. Med.*, **6,** 460.
6. Hirsch, J. G. (1965). *The Inflammatory Process*, p. 245. Eds. Zweifach, B. W., Grant, L., and McCluskey, R. T. New York: Academic Press.
7. Comandon, J. A film prepared at the Pasteur Institute. This is an admirable demonstration of many of the phenomena of chemotaxis and phagocytosis.
8. Greenwood, B. (1968). *J. Physiol.* (*Lond.*), **196,** 108P.
9. Graham, H. T., Lowry, O. H., Wheelwright, F., Lenz, M. A., and Parish, H. H., Jr. (1955). *Blood*, **10,** 467.
10. Fredricks, R. E., and Moloney, W. C. (1959). *Blood*, **14,** 571.
11. Mota, I., and Ishii, T. (1960). *Brit. J. Pharmacol.*, **15,** 82.
12. McCutcheon, M. (1924). *Amer. J. Physiol.*, **69,** 279.
13. Ebert, R. H., Sanders, A. G., and Florey, H. W. (1940). *Brit. J. exp. Path.*, **21,** 212.
14. Harris, H. (1953). *J. Path. Bact.*, **66,** 135; *Brit. J. exp. Path.*, **34,** 276.
15. Boyden, S. (1962). *J. exp. Med.*, **115,** 453.
16. Ward, P. A., and Becker, E. L. (1968). *J. exp. Med.*, **127,** 693.
17. Lotz, M., and Harris, H. (1956). *Brit. J. exp. Path.*, **37,** 477.
18. McCutcheon, M. (1955). *Ann. N.Y. Acad. Sci.*, **59,** 941.
19. Borrel, A. (1893). *Ann. Inst. Pasteur*, **7,** 593.
20. Durham, H. E. (1897). *J. Path. Bact.*, **4,** 338.
21. Beattie, J. M. (1903). *J. Path. Bact.*, **8,** 129.
22. Cappell, D. F. (1929). *J. Path. Bact.*, **32,** 595.
23. Opie, E. L. (1910). *Arch. intern. Med.*, **5,** 541.
24. Vorwald, A. J. (1932). *Amer. Rev. Tuberc.*, **25,** 74.
25. Menkin, V. (1956). *Biochemical Mechanisms in Inflammation.* Springfield, Ill.: Charles C. Thomas.
26. Paz, R. A., and Spector, W. G. (1962). *J. Path. Bact.*, **84,** 85.
27. Hurley, J. V., and Spector, W. G. (1961). *J. Path. Bact.*, **82,** 403 and 421.

28. WARD, P. A., COCHRANE, C. G., and MÜLLER-EBERHARD, H. J. (1965). *J. exp. Med.*, **122**, 327.
29. BENNET, D. W., and DRURY, A. N. (1931). *J. Physiol. (Lond.)*, **72**, 288.
30. COHN, Z. A., and MORSE, S. I. (1959). *J. exp. Med.*, **110**, 419.
31. FENN, W. O. (1921). *J. gen. Physiol.*, **3**, 439, 465, 575.
32. LEWIS, W. H. (1931). *Bull. Johns Hopk. Hosp.*, **49**, 17.
33. CHAPMAN-ANDRESEN, C., and HOLTER, H. (1964). *C.R. Lab. Carlsberg*, **34**, 211.
34. BRUMFITT, W., GLYNN, A. A., and PERCIVAL, A. (1965). *Brit. J. exp. Path.*, **46**, 215.
35. COHN, Z. A. (1966). *J. exp. Med.*, **124**, 557.
36. OREN, R., FARNHAM, A. E., SAITO, K., MILOFSKY, E., and KARNOVSKY, M. L. (1963). *J. Cell Biol.*, **17**, 487.
37. OUCHI, E., SELVARAJ, R. J., and SBARRA, A. J. (1965). *Exp. Cell Res.*, **40**, 456.
38. COHN, Z. A., and PARKS, E. (1967). *J. exp. Med.*, **125**, 213 and 457.
39. MUDD, E. B. H., and MUDD, S. (1933). *J. gen. Physiol.*, **16**, 625.
40. MUDD, S., MCCUTCHEON, M., and LUCKÉ, B. (1934). *Physiol. Rev.*, **14**, 210. This article has a very full list of references.
41. DINGLE, J. T. (1968). *Brit. med. Bull.*, **24**, 141.
42. TULLIS, J. L., and SURGENOR, D. M. (1956). *Ann. N.Y. Acad. Sci.*, **66**, 386.
43. WOOD, W. B., SMITH, M. R., and WATSON, B. (1946). *J. exp. Med.*, **84**, 387.
44. LERNER, E. M., 2nd (1956). *J. exp. Med.*, **104**, 233.
45. SMITH, M. R., and WOOD, W. B., Jr. (1958). *J. exp. Med.*, **107**, 1.
46. COHN, Z. A. (1962). *Yale J. Biol. Med.*, **35**, 12.
47. GORDON, G. B., MILLER, L. R. and BENSCH, K. G. (1965). *J. Cell Biol.*, **25**, No. 2, part 2, 41.
48. KANTOCH, M. (1961). Quoted by Mackaness (1964). *Microbial Behaviour in vivo and in vitro*, p. 213. Eds. SMITH, H., and TAYLOR, J. 14th Symposium, Society for General Microbiology. London: Cambridge Univ. Press.
49. COHN, Z. A., FEDORKO, M. E., and HIRSCH, J. G. (1966). *J. exp. Med.*, **123**, 757.
50. NOSSAL, G. J. V., ABBOT, A., and MITCHELL, J. (1968). *J. exp. Med.*, **127**, 263.
51. SMITH, M. R., and WOOD W. B. (1947). *J. exp. Med.* **86**, 257.
52. ROGERS, D. E., and TOMPSETT, R. (1952). *J. exp. Med.*, **95**, 209.
53. ROGERS, D. E., and MELLY, M. A. (1960). *J. exp. Med.*, **111**, 533.
54. MELLY, M. A., THOMISON, M. B., and ROGERS, D. E. (1960). *J. exp. Med.*, **112**, 1121.
55. HIRSCH, J. G., and COHN, Z. A. (1960). *J. exp. Med.*, **112**, 1005.
56. ZUCKER-FRANKLIN, D., and HIRSCH, J. G. (1964). *J. exp. Med.*, **120**, 569.
57. ZUCKER-FRANKLIN, D., DAVIDSON, M., and THOMAS, L. (1966). *J. exp. Med.*, **124**, 521.
58. COHN, Z. A., HIRSCH, J. G., and WIENER, E. (1963). *Lysosomes*, p. 126. Eds. DE REUCK, A. V. S., and CAMERON, M. P. Ciba Foundation Symposium. London: J. & A. Churchill.
59. SALTON, M. J. R. (1953). *J. gen. Microbiol.*, **9**, 512.
60. KLING, C. A. (1910). *Z. Immun.-Forsch.*, **7**, 1. (Review).
61. PETTERSSON, A. (1905). *Zbl. Bakt.*, **39**, 423.
62. COHN, Z. A., and HIRSCH, J. G. (1960). *J. exp. Med.*, **112**, 983.
63. ZEYA, H. I., and SPITZNAGEL, J. K. (1968). *J. exp. Med.*, **127**, 927.
64. COHN, Z. A. (1963). *J. exp. Med.*, **117**, 27 and 43.
65. LURIE, M. B., and DANNENBERG, A. M. (1965). *Bact. Rev.*, **29**, 466.
66. ROUS, P., and JONES, F. S. (1916). *J. exp. Med.*, **23**, 601.
67. MAGOFFIN, R. L., and SPINK, W. W. (1950). *J. Lab. clin. Med.*, **36**, 959.
68. RICH, A. R., and MCKEE, C. M. (1934). *Bull. Johns Hopk. Hosp.*, **54**, 277.
69. CAMP, W. E., and BAUMGARTNER, E. A. (1915). *J. exp. Med.*, **22**, 174.
70. HOLMES, B., QUIE, P. G., WINDHORST, D. B., and GOOD, R. A. (1966). *Lancet*, **1**, 1225.

71. CLARK, E. R., CLARK, E. L., and REX, R. O. (1936). *Amer. J. Anat.*, **59,** 123.
72. LEWIS, W. H., and RUBIN, M. I. (1932). *Anat. Rec.*, **53,** 249.
73. RICHTER, K. M. (1942). *J. Morph.*, **71,** 53.
74. ROBERTS, and KRAIKE (1930). Quoted from E. V. Cowdry. *A Textbook of Histology* (1938). London: Henry Kimpton.
75. KLINE, D. L., and CLIFTON, E. E. (1952). *Science*, **115,** 9.
76. KLINE, D. L., and CLIFTON, E. E. (1952). *J. appl. Physiol.*, **5,** 79.
77. JEANNERET, H., and FISCHER, R. (1941). *Schweiz. med. Wschr.*, **71,** 204.
78. CROSS, H. B. (1921). *Bull. Johns Hopk. Hosp.*, **32,** 238.
79. DE HAAN, J. (1922). *Pflügers Arch. ges. Physiol.*, **194,** 448.
80. SPECTOR, W. G., and LYKKE, A. W. J. (1966). *J. Path. Bact.*, **92,** 163.
81. VOLKMAN, A., and GOWANS, J. L. (1965). *Brit. J. exp. Path.*, **46,** 50 and 62.
82. MIMS, C. A. (1964*a*). *Brit. J. exp. Path.*, **45,** 37.
83. FELIX, M. D. (1961). *J. nat. Cancer Inst.*, **27,** 713.
84. ARONSON, M., and SHAHAR, A. (1965). *Exp. Cell Res.*, **38,** 133.
85. VOLKMAN, A. (1966). *J. exp. Med.*, **124,** 241.
86. MACKANESS, G. B. (1964). *Microbial Behaviour in vivo and in vitro*, p. 213. Eds. SMITH, H., and TAYLOR, J. 14th Symposium, Society for General Microbiology. London: Cambridge Univ. Press.
87. PINKETT, M. O., COWDREY, C. R., and NOWELL, P. C. (1966). *Amer. J. Path.*, **48,** 859.
88. EASTON, T. W. (1952). *Amer. J. Anat.*, **90,** 1.
89. CORDINGLEY, J. L., and NICOL, T. (1967). *J. Physiol. (Lond.)*, **190,** 7P.
90. BOAK, J. L., CHRISTIE, G. H., FORD, W. L., and HOWARD, J. G. (1968). *Proc. roy. Soc. B*, **169,** 307.
91. WEISS, L. (1964). *Bull. Johns Hopk. Hosp.*, **115,** 99.
92. HOWARD, J. G., BOAK, J. L., and CHRISTIE, G. H. (1966). *The Lymphocyte in Immunology and Hæmopoiesis*, p. 216. Symposium held at Bristol, 1966. London: Edward Arnold.
93. WEISS, L. (1961). *Bull. Johns Hopk. Hosp.*, **108,** 171.
94. BENNETT, B. (1966). *Amer. J. Path.*, **48,** 165.
95. MURRAY, I. M. (1963). *J. exp. Med.*, **117,** 139.
96. DRUTZ, D. J., KOENIG, M. G., and ROGERS, D. E. (1967). *J. exp. Med.*, **126,** 1087.
97. WIENER, J., COTTRELL, T. S., MARGARETTEN, W., and SPIRO, D. (1967). *Amer. J. Path.*, **50,** 187.
98. KENT, R., (1966). *J. reticuloendoth. Soc.*, **3,** 271.
99. GAY, F. P. (1930–31). *Harvey Lect.*, **26,** 162.
100. TOPLEY and WILSON's *Principles of Bacteriology and Immunity* (1946). 3rd edit., revised by G. S. Wilson and A. A. Miles. London: Edward Arnold.
101. ACTON, J. D., and MYRVIK, Q. N. (1966). *J. Bact.*, **91,** 2300.
102. SMITH, T. J., and WAGNER, R. R. (1967). *J. exp. Med.*, **125,** 559.
103. GALLILY, R., WARWICK, A., and BANG, F. B. (1967). *J. exp. Med.*, **125,** 537.
104. MIMS, C. A. (1964*b*). *Bact. Rev.*, **28,** 30.
105. VAUGHAN, R. B. (1965). *Brit. J. exp. Path.*, **46,** 82.
106. JENKIN, C. R., and KARTHIGASU, K. (1962). *C.R. Soc. Biol. (Paris)*, **156,** 1006.
107. SORENSON, G. D. (1962). *Amer. J. Path.*, **40,** 297.
108. DAY, A. J. (1964). *J. Atheroscler. Res.*, **4,** 117.
109. BAILLIF, R. N. (1960). *Ann. N.Y. Acad. Sci.*, **88,** 3.
110. EBERT, R. H., and FLOREY, H. W. (1939). *Brit. J. exp. Path.*, **20,** 342.
111. MUIR, R., and NIVEN, J. S. F. (1935). *J. Path. Bact.*, **41,** 183.
112. COTRAN, R. S. (1965). *Exp. molec. Path.*, **4,** 217.
112a. STILL, W. J. S., and PROSSER, P. R. (1964). *J. Atheroscler. Res.*, **4,** 517.
113. FLOREY, Lord (1967). *Proc. roy. Soc. B*, **166,** 375.

114. Stehbens, W. E., and Florey, H. W. (1960). *Quart. J. exp. Physiol.*, **45,** 252.
115. Dudgeon, L. S., and Goadby, H. K. (1931). *J. Hyg.* (*Lond.*), **31,** 247.
116. Govaerts, P. (1921). *Arch. int. Physiol.*, **16,** 1.
117. Tocantins, L. M. (1938). *Medicine* (*Baltimore*), **17,** 155.
118. Tait, J. (1918). *Quart. J. exp. Physiol.*, **12,** 1.
119. French, J. E. (1967). *Brit. J. Hæmat.*, **13,** 595.
120. Florey, H. W., and Carleton, H. M. (1926). *J. Path. Bact.*, **29,** 97.
121. Policard, A., and Bessis, M. (1958). *C.R. Acad. Sci.* (*Paris*), **246,** 3194.
122. Gözsy, B., and Kátó, L. (1960). *Ann. N.Y. Acad. Sci.*, **88,** 43.
123. French, J. E., Florey, H. W., and Morris, B. (1960). *Quart. J. exp. Physiol.*, **45,** 88.

REVIEWS

Chemotaxis

Reviews by H. Harris in *Physiol. Rev.* (1954). **34,** 529 and *Bact. Rev.* (1960). **24,** 3, are exhaustive considerations of this subject and can be recommended to anyone seeking further information.

Phagocytosis

L. J. Berry and T. D. Spies, *Medicine* (*Baltimore*), (1949). **28,** 239. A review of this subject with a large number of references.

De Reuck, A. V. S., and Cameron, M.P., Eds. (1963). *Lysosomes* (Ciba Foundation Symposium). London: Edward Arnold. Certain articles deal with intracellular events in phagocytes.

Wolstenholme, G. E. W., and O'Connor, M., Eds. (1961). *Biological Activity of the Leucocyte* (Ciba Foundation Study Group). London: J. & A. Churchill.

Reticulo-endothelium

R. H. Jaffé (1938). Article on the reticulo-endothelial system in *Handbook of Hæmatology*, Vol. 2. Ed. Downey, H. London: Hamish Hamilton Medical Books.

D. E. Rogers. Host mechanisms which act to remove bacteria from the blood stream. *Bact. Rev.* (1960), **24,** 50.

Cellular Immunity

G. B. Mackaness and R. V. Blanden. *Progr. Allergy* (1967), **11,** 89.

Chapter 5

LYMPHOCYTES

By J. L. Gowans

In Chapter 3 we described how lymph is filtered as it percolates through the sinuses of lymph nodes so that it is freed of bacteria and other foreign material by the phagocytic activity of the lining macrophages. The lymph, besides being filtered, emerges from the nodes richer in cells. These lymph-borne cells or "lymphocytes" are swept along the lymphatic vessels and finally enter the blood by way of the thoracic duct and other major lymphatic trunks in the neck.

When cells from a main lymph duct of a normal animal are examined in smears 90 per cent. or more can be seen to vary little in size and staining properties; they have cell diameters in the range of 6–8μ, deeply staining nuclei and a narrow rim of cytoplasm. These are "small" lymphocytes. The remainder of the cells are larger and vary considerably in size; the chromatin of their nuclei is less condensed and some possess strongly basophilic cytoplasm. Lymphocytes are conventionally classified on grounds of size into "small", "medium" and "large" but this is quite arbitrary because a frequency distribution of lymphocyte diameters does not show three distinct peaks. However, in practice, limits can be set and a satisfactory distinction made between the minority of larger cells and the great majority which are small and possess relatively uniform morphological features. To this morphological distinction can be added an important functional difference: when lymphocytes are studied in short term cultures *in vitro* it is only the medium and large cells which synthesize DNA and which divide; the small lymphocyte under these conditions is a non-dividing cell. In special circumstances small lymphocytes can be provoked to divide but when freshly isolated from blood or lymph they are never in the stage of DNA synthesis.

An examination of cells in the living state shows that all the lymphocytes in lymph, irrespective of size, share a number of properties. All have the same characteristic mode of locomotion, they are not phagocytic, they do not adhere to glass or plastic surfaces and they do not respond chemotactically to any materials which have so far been tested.[1]

Large Lymphocytes

There is good evidence that the large and medium lymphocytes in lymph originate by cell division in the lymph nodes although precisely where in the nodes has not been established. Thus, it is not known whether the large and medium lymphocytes described in the germinal centres of lymph nodes are identical with those found in the blood and in the lymph. The fate of these large cells after entry into the blood stream has been traced in autoradiographic experiments by first labelling their DNA with tritiated thymidine. A few divide to form small lymphocytes but in the rat, at least, this process only occurs on a very small scale. Many of the remainder have been shown to leave the circulation rapidly, enter the tissues, particularly the submucosa of the intestine, and develop into cells identified by conventional microscopy as plasma cells.[2] In the electron microscope some of the large cells in normal rat lymph show a moderate amount of endoplasmic reticulum but nothing comparable to that seen in plasma cells.[3] The implication here is that the large lymphocytes complete their development into plasma cells in the tissues.

The efferent lymph from an antigenically stimulated node contains greatly increased numbers of large and medium lymphocytes but again, although a proportion can be shown to be making antibody,[4] none have the ultrastructural features of mature plasma cells.[5] Recently it has been shown that when lymph from the efferent lymphatic of such a stimulated node is drained away through a cannula the animal does not develop the usual systemic immunity.[5] It is thought that when antigen is localized to a single regional site the immune response can be disseminated throughout the animal by cells, presumably large and medium lymphocytes, which enter the blood in the lymph and then colonize other nodes by migrating into them from the blood.

Small Lymphocytes

We have described the small lymphocyte as a small motile cell which enters the blood by way of the major lymph ducts. It possesses no arresting morphological features: the electron microscope shows little besides a few oval mitochondria in a scanty cytoplasm and a nucleus containing one or two nucleoli (Fig. 1). The small lymphocyte is anomalous in that it is a non-dividing cell yet it is very easily killed by X-irradiation. Other radio-sensitive cells, for example in the bone marrow, the intestinal epithelium and the testis, show a high mitotic activity.

The small lymphocyte, defined by the criteria of size and morphology, has a wide distribution in the body. In addition to making up about 20–30 per cent of the blood leucocytes in man it is the major cell type in the lymph nodes, spleen, Peyer's patches and in the lymphoid tissue embedded in the root of the lungs. Cells of identical morphology are distributed diffusely throughout the submucosa of the intestine and in the bone marrow; and in pathological material they are also particularly associated with areas of chronic inflammation, with the stroma of tumours, and with certain lesions which are the result of an immunological reaction in the tissues, for example the homograft reaction (see Chapter 41). The identification of these "small round cells" in normal and pathological tissues and in exudates is not easy. They may be identical with the small lymphocyte present in blood, lymph and lymphoid tissue but recent work has emphasized that such a conclusion may not always be warranted. For example, we shall see that the "small lymphocytes" in bone marrow have very different properties from those in the lymph nodes and the lymph. Even among the small lymphocytes in lymph two classes of cells with widely differing life spans have been identified. The lesson to be learned from much of the recent work on lymphocytes is that apparent identity of morphology may conceal important differences in function.

Origin and Life Span of Lymphocytes

At one time it was thought that small lymphocytes possessed a life span of, at the most, a few days. This was partly because lymphocytes died rapidly when

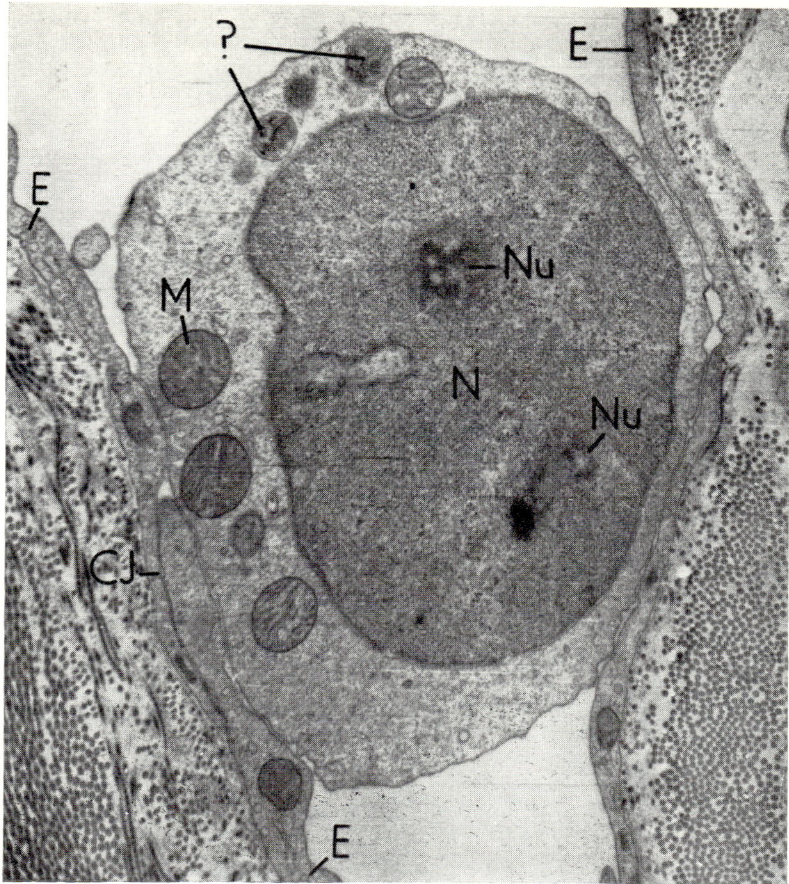

5/Fig. 1.—Small lymphocyte in lymphatic of normal colon of a rat. The picture shows a nucleus with two nucleoli (Nu), four mitochondria (M) and two bodies of doubtful nature (?). The wall of the lymphatic (E) is surrounded by collagen fibres. A junction between two endothelial cells is shown at CJ. (× 19,000)

attempts were made to cultivate them *in vitro* and partly because of the rapid rate of cell turnover in the blood which we will discuss later. Ideas on this point have now changed radically as a result of studies on the incorporation and persistence of radioactivity in the DNA of lymphocytes after the administration to the animal of DNA precursors. Otteson[6] was the first to suggest that some lymphocytes might have a long life span. He deduced the existence of two populations of cells by giving ^{32}P to human subjects and observing the rate of decay of radioactivity in DNA isolated from peripheral blood lymphocytes; about 80 per cent of the cells were estimated to have a mean life span of 100–200 days. The early autoradiographic studies with tritiated thymidine also pointed to a long life span because very few small lymphocytes became labelled either in the blood or the lymph after short courses of administration to man and a variety of experimental animals. Thus, after a 12-hour infusion of tritiated thymidine into a rat all the large and medium lymphocytes in the thoracic duct are labelled, but only about 1 per cent of the small (FIG. 2). Detailed studies have now been made on the life span of lymphocytes in rats by giving either a continuous infusion or repeated injections of tritiated thymidine. The aim was to ensure that the radioactive precursor of DNA was available continuously and

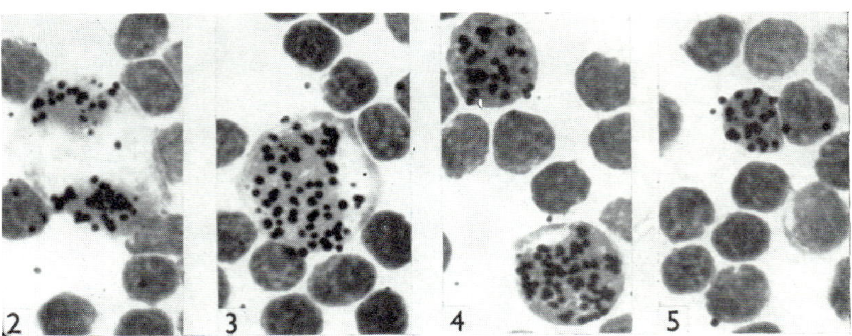

5/FIG. 2.—Autoradiographs of radioactively-labelled thoracic duct lymphocytes from a rat given tritium-labelled thymidine. From left to right: large lymphocyte dividing; large lymphocyte; two medium lymphocytes; small lymphocyte. Administration of ^{3}H-thymidine for short periods labels a high proportion of the larger lymphocytes, but very few of the small. (× 1500) (From Gowans.[23])

that consequently all newly formed cells which enter the blood or the lymph would be labelled. In experiments of this kind it has been found that it takes over 200 days of continuous infusion to label 90 per cent of the small lymphocytes in the peripheral blood.[7] The important point here is that even after this period 10 per cent of small lymphocytes remained unlabelled; that is, they must have been formed before the start of the infusion some seven months previously. Studies on the rate of decrease in the proportion of labelled small lymphocytes in the blood and the lymph after stopping the administration of tritiated thymidine suggest that there are two populations of small lymphocytes in the rat, one with a circulating life of less than 14 days and another which circulates for many weeks.[7, 8] It has been calculated that about 90 per cent of the small lymphocytes in thoracic duct lymph of rats are of the long-lived variety, while the corresponding values for blood, lymph nodes and spleen are 66, 75, and 25 per cent.[9]

Evidence of a different kind has recently substantiated the idea that at least some lymphocytes in man have an exceptionally long life.[10] The evidence is based on the fact, which we will consider later, that small lymphocytes will enlarge and divide when incubated *in vitro* with a bean extract, phytohæmagglutinin. This provides a convenient method for obtaining a population of cells in mitosis and thus for examining the pattern of their chromosomes. When blood lymphocytes from patients who had received therapeutic X-irradiation some years previously were incubated with phytohæmagglutinin, chromosome abnormalities of such severity were found that it could be inferred that the cells must have been entering their first division since irradiation. It was concluded from this study that small lymphocytes in these patients had a mean life of about five years while some had survived without dividing for up to ten years.

The origin of long-lived small lymphocytes is not certain although the thymus probably makes some contribution in the growing animal. An observation consistent with this view is that removal of the thymus from rats at one month of age eventually causes a reduction in the output of lymphocytes from the thoracic duct, although the effect takes some weeks to develop.[11] The origin of short-lived small lymphocytes is not known but thymus and bone marrow have been suggested as possibilities.

The idea that the thymus exports lymphocytes is a plausible one because it is normally the seat of vigorous cell division. Cells have been shown to leave experimental thymus grafts and enter the lymph nodes[12] and one suggestion is that the thymus exerts its influence on the development of lymphoid tissue by populating it with cells in this way (see Chapter 41). The difficulty has been to obtain convincing evidence that cells are continuously leaving the normal, intact thymus of the animal. One approach has been to infuse tritiated thymidine directly into the thymus and then to study the appearance of labelled cells elsewhere in the animal. When suitable controls are employed to insure that the isotope has not leaked from the thymus into the general circulation such experiments have shown that the lymph nodes, particularly of young animals, do derive cells from the thymus.[13] These experiments have not yet told us whether such thymus-derived cells are of the long- or the short-lived variety nor the number of cells which are contributed by the thymus to the peripheral lymphoid tissue.

Whatever the contribution of the thymus it is clear that small lymphocytes can also be formed in lymph nodes. Thus, labelled small lymphocytes can be detected in the efferent lymph of a single lymph node when tritiated thymidine is carefully infused into its afferent lymphatic.[14]

Output of Lymphocytes from the Lymph Ducts

Large numbers of lymphocytes continually escape from the nodes into the lymph, eventually to enter the blood via the major lymph ducts. No good evidence has yet been produced that lymphocytes enter the blood directly from the nodes, that is by migrating across the walls of blood vessels within them. On the other hand, in the spleen which filters blood rather than lymph, lymphocytes enter and leave the lymphoid nodules by traversing blood vessels directly.[15]

The number of lymphocytes entering the blood each day has been estimated by collecting lymph from the thoracic, cervical, subclavian and right lymph ducts, measuring its total volume and determining the concentration of cells in samples of it. In the rabbit the output of cells is sufficient to replace all the lymphocytes in the blood about 11 times a day.[16] Similar calculations based on the output from the thoracic duct alone have shown that the blood lymphocytes are also replaced several times daily in man and in the calf, sheep, dog, cat, guinea-pig, rat and mouse, the rate of replacement being more rapid in the smaller animals.[17] The pig is a curious exception in that its thoracic duct lymph contains very few lymphocytes; this interesting anomaly has not yet been explained.[18]

If large numbers of lymphocytes are continually entering the blood from the lymphatic ducts, an equal number must be continually disappearing from the blood. The magnitude of the turnover can be illustrated by measurements on the rat in which about 10^9 lymphocytes enter the blood each day from the thoracic duct alone; this is greater than the number of cells contained in the largest lymph node in the rat, the mesenteric node, and would replace the blood lymphocytes about 10 times daily. We have already discussed the fate of the large and medium lymphocytes which make up less than 10 per cent of the cells in lymph. We must now consider the ideas which have been put forward to explain the large-scale disappearance of small lymphocytes from the blood. Until recently this problem had been the centre of some controversy and it had always been hoped that its solution would give a clue to the function of small lymphocytes.

The Fate of Lymphocytes

Recirculation

Sjovall,[19] in 1936, was the first to suggest the hypothesis which in broad outline is now thought to account for the rapid turnover of the blood lymphocytes. He proposed that the lymphocytes which enter the blood from the lymphatic ducts leave the blood again in the tissues, pass into the lymphatic vessels, and are returned once more into the blood. On this hypothesis the rapid turnover of the blood lymphocytes would be more apparent than real since the same cells would be continually disappearing from the blood and reappearing in it. It was originally suggested that lymphocytes continually enter the tissue spaces and return to the blood by way of the peripheral lymphatics. A small-scale recirculation of lymphocytes probably does take place through most of the tissue spaces of the body because samples of peripheral lymph obtained from the limbs and from the intestine contain some lymphocytes.[20] However, the number of cells returning to the blood in this way can account for only a small fraction of the normal lymphocyte output from the main lymph ducts.

The idea of a rapid turnover of the blood lymphocytes was originally based on acute experiments in which measurements on cell output were made on samples of lymph collected during the day of lymphatic cannulation. Mann and Higgins[21] showed that if the drainage of thoracic duct lymph from unanæsthetised rats was continued for more than one day a considerable fall in lymphocyte output occurred, although the daily volume of lymph draining away remained unchanged. It was later found that this fall in lymphocyte output could be prevented if the lymph and living lymphocytes collected from the thoracic duct were continuously returned into the blood of the rat, as they would have been in the intact animal.[22] This suggested that the continuous entry of living lymphocytes into the blood was in some way essential for maintaining the normal output of cells from the thoracic duct.

The problem was further investigated by slowly transfusing into the blood of one rat lymphocytes obtained from the thoracic duct of other rats of the same inbred strain. The use of an inbred strain insured that the transfused cells were not destroyed in the recipient animal by a homograft reaction. Such transfusions resulted in a substantial increase in the output of lymphocytes from the thoracic duct of the recipient animal.[23] A possible explanation was that the transfused cells were passing in large numbers from the blood into the thoracic duct lymph, but to prove the point it was necessary to show that the transfused cells and the extra cells issuing from the thoracic duct were identical. This was established by transfusing radioactively-labelled lymphocytes. The transfusion of lymphocytes

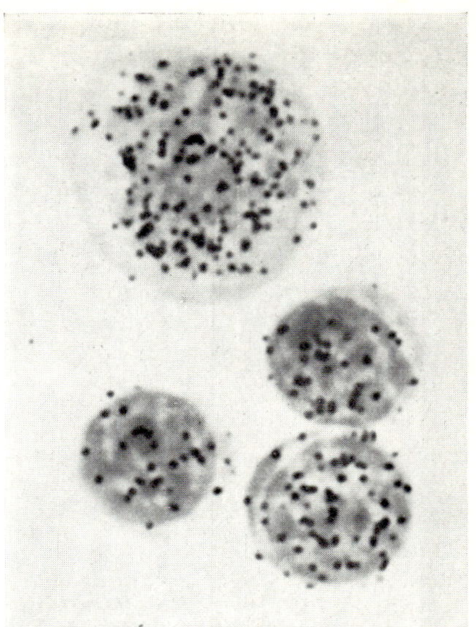

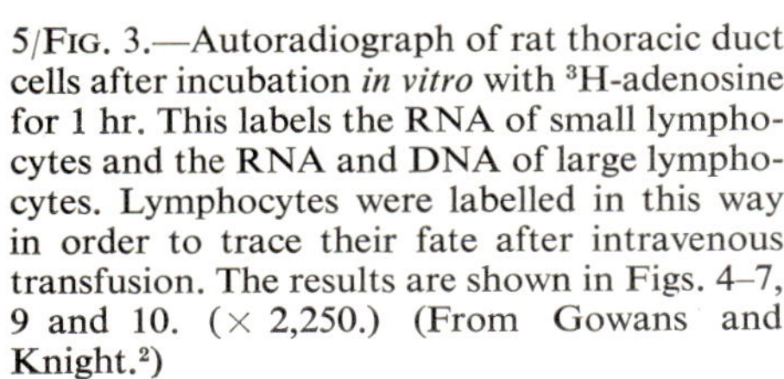

5/FIG. 3.—Autoradiograph of rat thoracic duct cells after incubation *in vitro* with ^{3}H-adenosine for 1 hr. This labels the RNA of small lymphocytes and the RNA and DNA of large lymphocytes. Lymphocytes were labelled in this way in order to trace their fate after intravenous transfusion. The results are shown in Figs. 4–7, 9 and 10. (× 2,250.) (From Gowans and Knight.[2])

labelled with either ^{32}P or with ^{51}Cr resulted in the appearance of radioactive lymphocytes in the thoracic duct lymph, in numbers which indicated that a large fraction of the transfused cells was being recovered.[23, 24] When the RNA of the transfused small lymphocytes was labelled by first incubating the cells *in vitro* with tritiated adenosine (FIG. 3), individual labelled cells which had migrated from the blood could be identified and counted in the thoracic duct lymph by the technique of autoradiography[2] (FIG. 7).

It has been possible to trace in detail the route taken by tritium-labelled small lymphocytes after their transfusion into the blood.[2] Lymphocytes were shown to leave the blood stream by passing through the walls of the so-called "post-

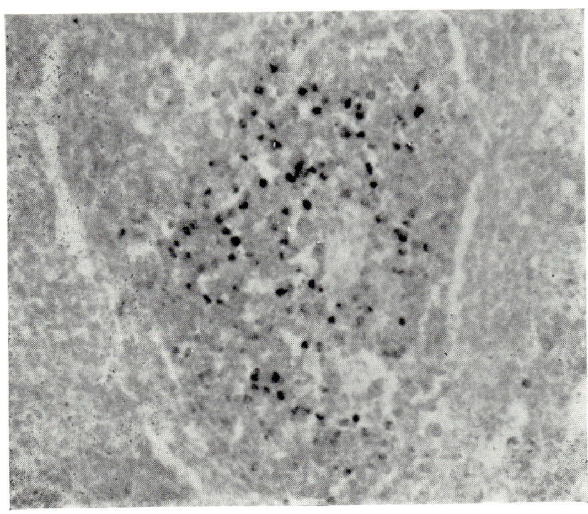

5/FIG. 4.—Autoradiograph of the spleen 24 hr. after a transfusion of labelled lymphocytes. The white pulp around the central arteriole contains many labelled small lymphocytes. In FIGS. 4 and 5 the individual labelled cells appear as black dots. Prolonged exposure of these autoradiographs has led to a confluence of the silver grains over each cell thus allowing photography at low power. (× 125.) (From Gowans and Knight.[2])

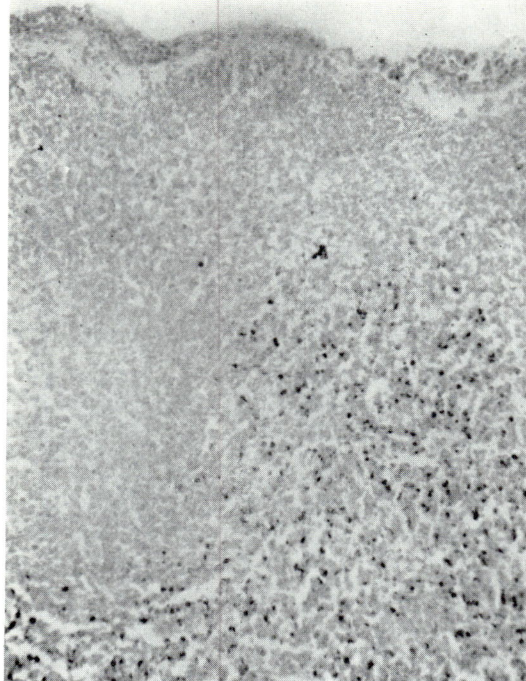

5/Fig. 5.—Autoradiograph of brachial lymph node 24 hr. after a transfusion of labelled lymphocytes. The deeper part of the cortex contains many labelled small lymphocytes but they have not entered the germinal centre (left) nor the cortical zone immediately under the marginal sinus. (× 80.) (From Gowans and Knight.[2])

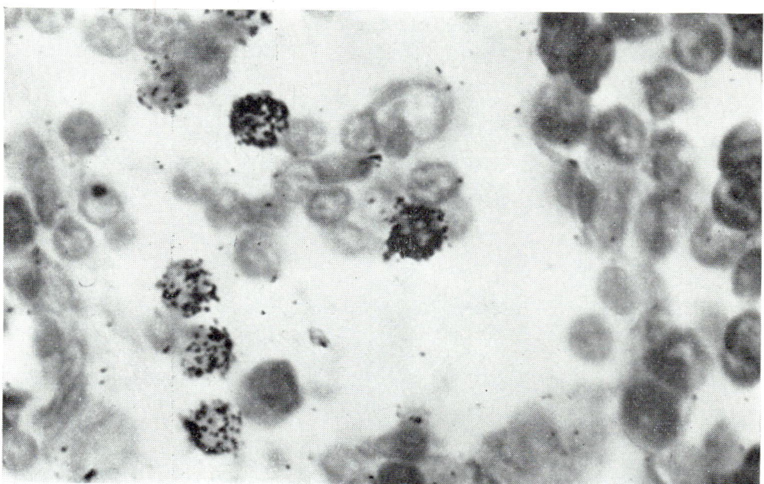

5/Fig. 6.—Autoradiograph of medullary lymph sinus of a cervical lymph node 24 hr. after a transfusion of labelled lymphocytes. The lymph channel contains labelled small lymphocytes which had originally been infused into the blood. (× 800.) (From Gowans and Knight.[2])

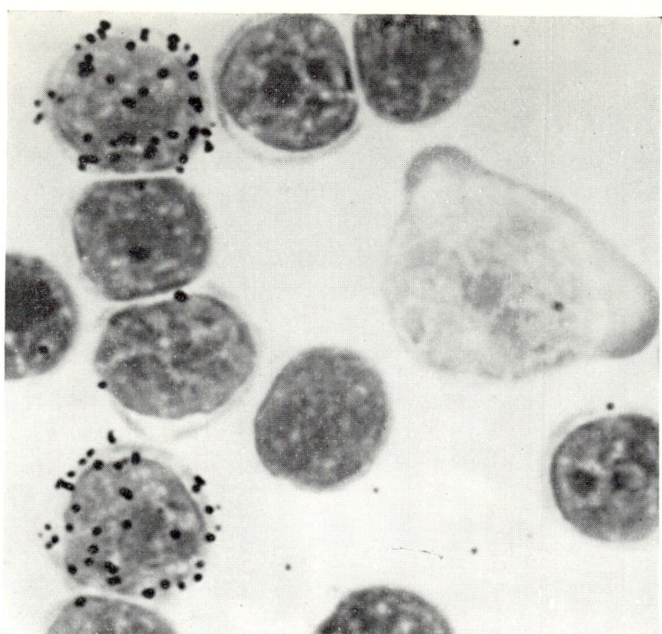

5/FIG. 7.—Labelled small lymphocytes in the lymph from a rat whose thoracic duct was cannulated one day after an intravenous transfusion of labelled lymphocytes. The labelled cells have circulated from the blood into the lymph. (× 2,250.) (From Gowans and Knight.[2])

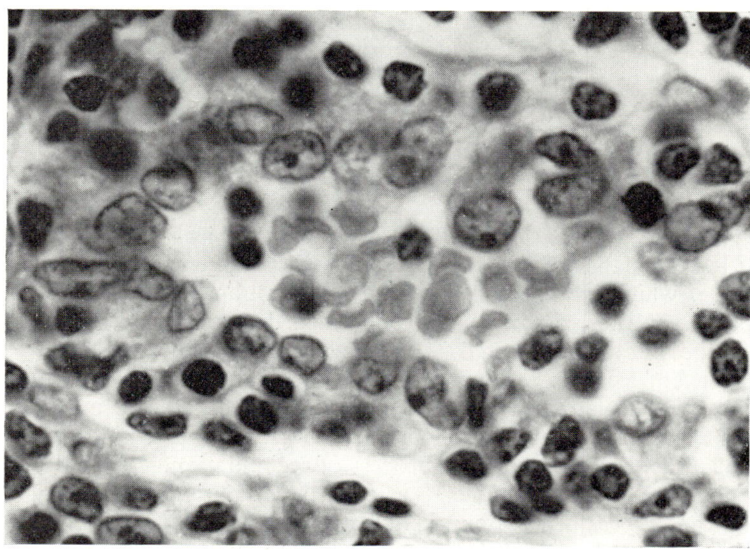

5/FIG. 8.—Post-capillary venule in a cervical lymph node from a normal rat. The lumen contains erythrocytes and leucocytes and is lined by an endothelium with large pale nuclei. Many small lymphocytes lie under the endothelium between layers of connective tissue. (× 1,080.) (From Gowans and Knight.[2])

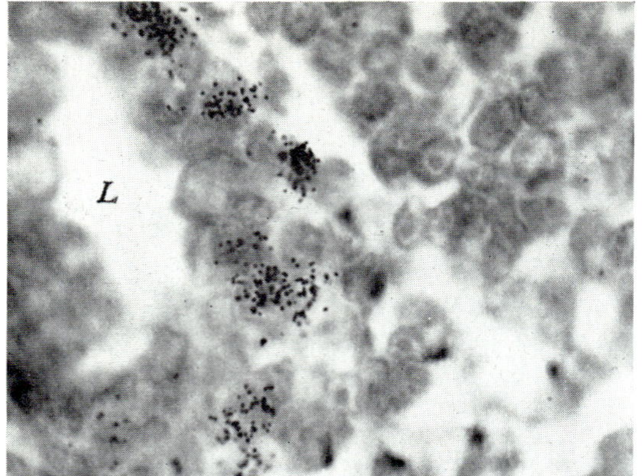

5/Fig. 9.—Autoradiograph of post-capillary venule in a mesenteric lymph node 15 min. after the start of a transfusion. Labelled cells have penetrated the endothelium from the lumen of the vessel (L) but they have not yet migrated into the node. (× 1,250.) (From Gowans and Knight.[2])

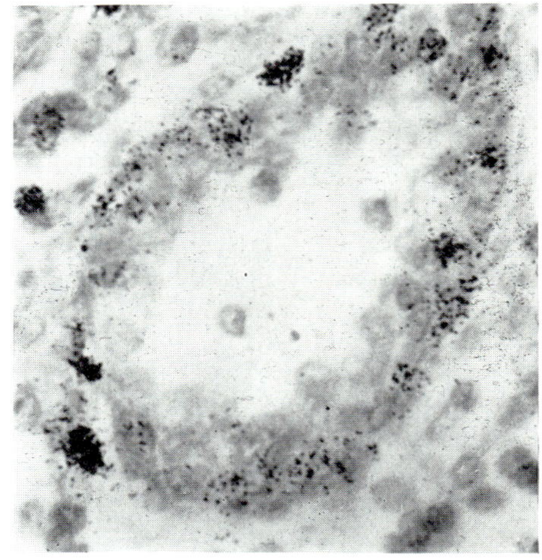

5/Fig. 10.—Autoradiograph of post-capillary venule in a cervical lymph node 30 min. after the end of a continuous 8 hr. transfusion. Many labelled cells have accumulated under the endothelium of the vessel and large numbers have entered the cortex of the node. (× 800.) (From Gowans and Knight.[2])

capillary venules" in the cortex of lymph nodes and in Peyer's patches (Figs. 8, 9 and 10). The labelled cells then accumulated in large numbers in those areas of the nodes which are normally rich in small lymphocytes (Fig. 5). Later they were detected in the lymph sinuses from which they were carried in the lymph back into the blood (Figs. 6 and 7). Labelled small lymphocytes were also found in high concentration in the white pulp of the spleen (Fig. 4) but only trivial numbers were detected in the thymus. Thus, the transfused cells made their way into those areas where small lymphocytes are normally located in the animal but the thymus was excluded from the process of recirculation.

At this stage it is reasonable to ask if a recirculation of lymphocytes is a normal physiological process or whether it is an abnormal phenomenon which occurs only when lymphocytes are transfused into an experimental animal. One compelling reason for believing it to be a normal process is that it is the only explanation which reconciles a high output of lymphocytes from the lymph ducts with the fact that more than 80 per cent of the emerging cells have a long life

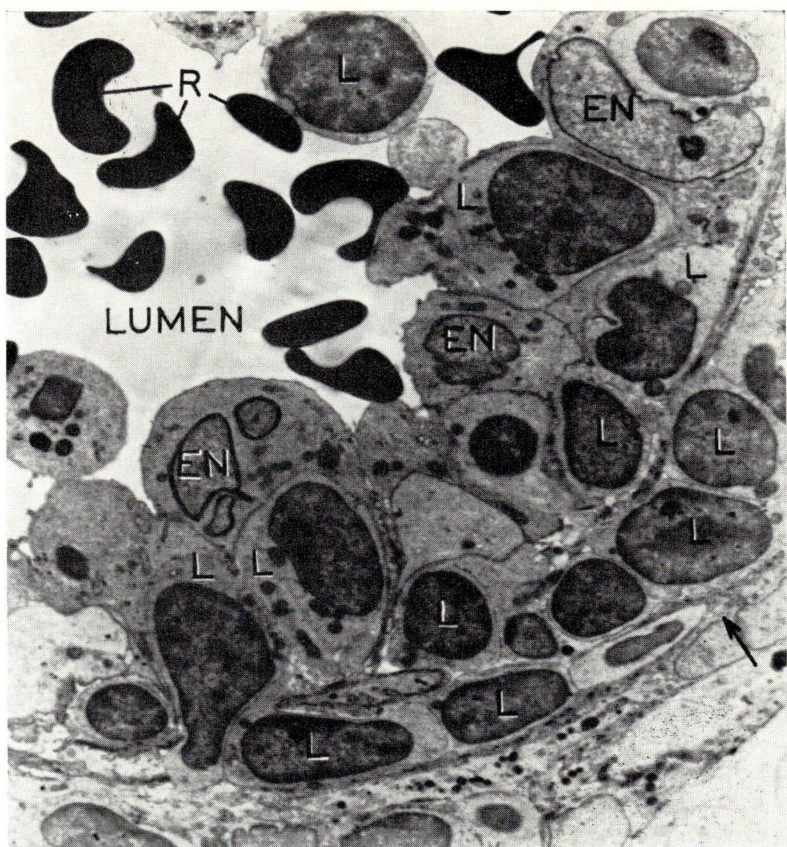

5/FIG. 11.—Electron micrograph of a post-capillary venule in the cortex of a normal rat lymph node. The lumen of the vessel contains a small lymphocyte (L) and some erythrocytes (R). The endothelial cells and their nuclei (EN) are distorted by numerous lymphocytes (L) apparently passing through the vessel wall. The presence of many lymphocytes between the endothelium and the periendothelial sheath (arrow) suggests that the sheath as well as the endothelium may form a barrier to their passage. In the bottom left of the picture one lymphocyte is penetrating the sheath. (× 3500.) (From Marchesi and Gowans.[3])

span. Another reason comes from examining the morphology of lymph nodes from normal animals. This supports the idea that the post-capillary venules are normally the site of a large-scale migration of lymphocytes. These vessels have an unusual endothelium and under the electron microscope many intact small lymphocytes can be seen apparently penetrating it and accumulating in groups between it and the periendothelial connective tissue (FIG. 11). A morphological study cannot decide the direction in which the cells are moving or whether they are moving at all. But the morphological evidence combined with the experimental demonstration that lymphocytes can pass from the blood into the nodes strongly argues that an active migration in this direction is a normal process. A study of serial sections in the electron microscope revealed an unexpected feature

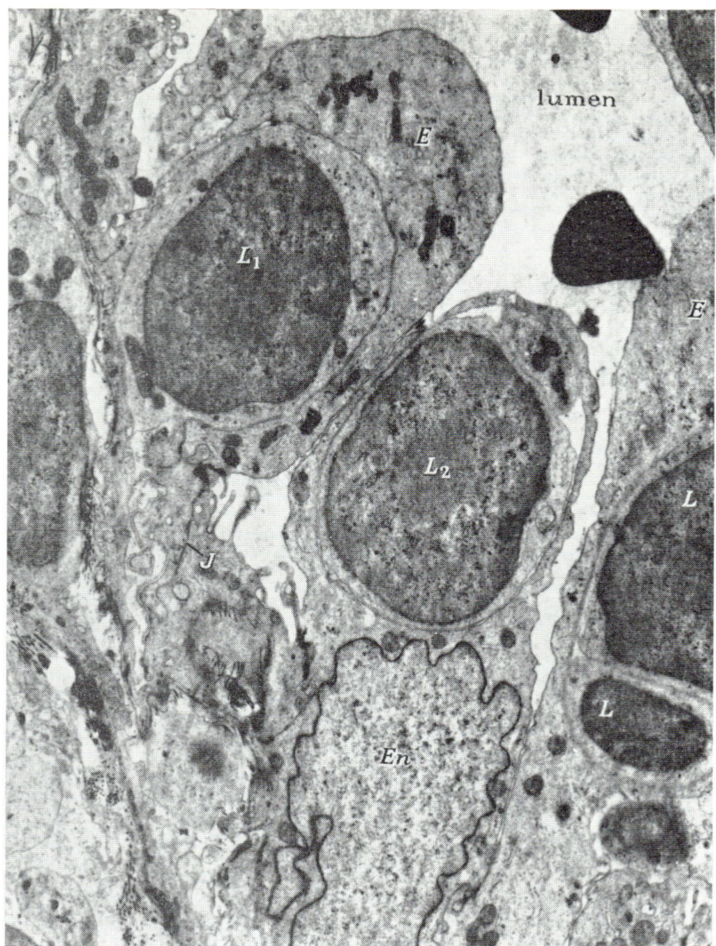

5/FIG. 12.—Electron micrograph of part of a post-capillary venule from a normal rat lymph node. L_1 and L_2 are small lymphocytes in the endothelium (E) of the vessel. L_2 appears to be completely enclosed by the cytoplasm of the endothelial cell whose nucleus is marked En. An intact intercellular junction is seen at J. (× 4,500.) (From Marchesi and Gowans.[3])

of the migration of lymphocytes through the walls of post-capillary venules[3]. Lymphocytes do not pass through intercellular junctions but actually enter the cytoplasm of endothelial cells and traverse it (FIG. 12). On the other hand, when the nodes are inflamed, polymorphs and monocytes pass through cell junctions of the venules as they do in inflamed vessels elsewhere (see Chapter 3). The nature of the special affinity which small lymphocytes possess for the endothelium of post-capillary venules and which is presumably the basis of the accurate "homing" of small lymphocytes into lymph nodes is not known. Some recent evidence suggests that sugar groupings on the surface of lymphocytes may be involved.[25]

The experiments in rats have shown that a large pool of long-lived small lymphocytes recirculates from blood to lymph through the lymph nodes; in the adult rat this pool amounts to at least 10^9 cells. It is not known what fraction of all the small lymphocytes in the animal recirculates. Certainly some remain "fixed" in the nodes and it is not clear in what way these differ from the remainder. The extent to which the short-lived small lymphocytes recirculate is also uncertain.

Evidence for recirculation is available for other species than the rat. A particularly clear cut demonstration comes from experiments, to which reference has already been made, where tritiated thymidine was infused into the afferent lymphatics of single lymph nodes in sheep.[14] The low proportion of labelled cells emerging in the efferent lymphatic showed that the great majority of cells leaving the node were not formed within it nor were they contributed by the afferent lymph; they must have been derived from the blood. Equally striking are studies on unanæsthetized calves showing that a profound lymphopenia and a sharp reduction in the output of lymphocytes from the thoracic duct is brought about when lymphocytes are killed by irradiating blood with γ-rays as it passes through an extracorporeal circuit.[26]

Although the process of recirculation explains the rapid turnover of the blood lymphocytes it unfortunately does nothing to clarify the problem of their ultimate fate and function. Independent evidence from immunological studies has recently led to suggestions about the functional significance of lymphocyte recirculation which will be considered later.

Function of Lymphocytes

Marrow Lymphocytes

It has been suggested that small lymphocytes migrate from the blood into the bone marrow where they provide stem cells from which erythrocytes and granulocytes develop. This migration, it was argued, occurred on a scale large enough to account for the rapid turnover of the blood lymphocytes. There is no doubt that marrow contains many small lymphocytes but recent work has shown that they label rapidly with tritiated thymidine (they are "short-lived") and that they are most probably produced within the marrow and not derived from cells which migrate into the marrow from the blood.[27] The evidence now suggests that the marrow "small lymphocytes" and those in the lymph nodes and the lymph are quite distinct populations of cells.

There is thought to be a cell-type in the marrow which can give rise to granulocytes and erythrocytes, and which can also populate lymphoid tissue and thus give rise to lymphocytes.[28] The problem is to identify this pluripotent stem cell morphologically and to this end the rival claims of marrow small lymphocytes, "transitional" lymphocytes[29] and "monocytoid" cells[30] are still being debated. There is no evidence that small lymphocytes from lymphoid tissue or lymph can act as hæmopoietic stem cells. For example, whereas injections of small numbers of marrow cells will rescue mice from a lethal dose of irradiation by repopulating their bone marrow, large numbers of lymphocytes from the thoracic duct have no effect on survival or on marrow regeneration.[31]

Lymphocyte Depletion

The classical method of revealing the function of an organ or tissue is to remove it and to observe the effect. It is impossible to remove all the lymphoid tissue from an animal because much of it is diffuse and embedded in other organs. Nevertheless it has been possible to remove by surgery the spleen, thymus, all the lymph nodes and some of the Peyer's patches from adult rats. These severe operations did not result in the obvious abnormalities.[32] It was notable, for example, that the activity of the hæmopoietic tissue was unimpaired.

A number of experimental procedures which cause a severe wasting disease in animals appear to have as their basis a gross reduction in the quantity of lymphoid tissue. Fatal wasting diseases can result from neonatal thymectomy where the lymphoid tissue fails to develop, from graft-versus-host reactions where the lymphoid tissue is destroyed immunologically, or in heavily irradiated animals treated with small doses of syngeneic bone marrow which restores their bone marrow but not their lymphoid tissue (see Chapter 41). In each of these examples it is reasonable to suppose that the deficiency of lymphoid tissue causes the wasting disease, and the simplest explanation is that the animal succumbs from chronic infections of either bacterial or viral ætiology which the absence of lymphoid tissue makes it unable to combat. This interpretation is favoured by the observation that while conventional mice waste after neonatal thymectomy, germ-free mice do not.[33] Unfortunately, the infectious processes held to be responsible for the wasting diseases have not been identified with any certainty. Another much more speculative hypothesis states that small lymphocytes normally exert a trophic or nutritional activity towards the tissues of the body and that it is the withdrawal of this influence which results in the wasting.[34] The difficulty in evaluating this idea is the vagueness with which it is formulated and, consequently, the difficulty of putting it to any kind of experimental test.

Animals thymectomized at birth may show in later life severe defects in immunological responsiveness affecting particularly their ability to reject homografts (see Chapter 41). It has been suggested that these defects can be attributed to a lack of small lymphocytes in lymphoid tissue.[35] Interestingly enough, the areas in the spleen and lymph nodes in which small lymphocytes are lacking (the so-called "thymus-dependent" areas), are precisely those through which small lymphocytes have been shown to recirculate, namely the periarteriolar lymphoid sheath of the spleen and the deeper part of the cortex of lymph nodes where the post-capillary venules are located.[35] These experiments suggest, in an imprecise way, that small lymphocytes are an essential component of an animals' immunological apparatus, but the argument becomes more persuasive with the demonstration that injections of thoracic duct lymphocytes will restore immunological competence to neonatally thymectomized mice.

A more specific depletion of small lymphocytes can be produced in rats by cannulating the thoracic duct and draining cells from the fistula for several days.[37] This procedure causes an acute depletion of small lymphocytes in the "thymus-dependent" areas of the nodes and the spleen and a marked lymphopenia. It does not shorten life but it causes an impairment of primary immunological responsiveness which recovers slowly after the fistula is closed. Drainage of cells for five days abolishes the primary antibody response to sheep erythrocytes and to tetanus toxoid, and it abolishes the response to first set homografts of skin provided that only weak antigenic differences separate the donor from the recipient.[38] The immunological deficiency of the depleted animal can be corrected by injecting pure suspensions of small lymphocytes so, again, the experiments show that small lymphocytes play some undefined part in immunological responses. It could be objected that the deficiencies brought about by this method of lymphocyte depletion are not very profound but in reply it can be pointed out that many small lymphocytes remain in lymphoid tissue despite prolonged drainage from the fistula. Chronic drainage from a thoracic duct fistula has been employed as an immunosuppressive procedure during kidney grafting in man but although it is a relatively safe manœuvre, its therapeutic success has only been marginal.

Immunological Functions

The experiments which deplete animals of lymphocytes indicate that small lymphocytes play an important part in immunological responses. The analysis of the precise nature of their role can best be understood against the background of a more comprehensive account of the cellular aspects of immunity which is given in Chapters 35 and 41. Here we will merely outline the main conclusions and the kinds of experiments upon which they are based.

The most direct evidence for the involvement of small lymphocytes in immunological processes comes from experiments employing suspensions of small lymphocytes prepared from either thoracic duct lymph or blood. By suitable manipulations it is possible to obtain suspensions of cells from thoracic duct lymph which contain more than 99·9 per cent small lymphocytes. Such purified suspensions have been shown to possess powerful immunological activity. The most important single observation is that an intravenous injection of rat[39] or mouse[40] small lymphocytes into a genetically appropriate member of the same species will cause a lethal graft-versual-host reaction (see Chapter 41). The importance of this observation is that there is only one possible interpretation of it: that small lymphocytes interact with foreign antigens in the tissues of the host and initiate the immunological response which finally kills it. This, and other evidence considered in Chapter 41, point to the small lymphocyte as the cell which initiates homotransplantation reactions, for example the reaction against skin or kidney homografts.[41]

The interaction of lymphocytes with transplantation antigens is only the first step of the immunological response. How does this interaction finally lead to the destruction of the foreign tissue? It is now known that some small lymphocytes react to transplantation antigens by enlarging and then dividing to produce more lymphocytes.[39, 42] One idea is that these new lymphocytes are the effectors of the response. These are the cells, it is argued, which migrate from lymphoid tissue, pass into the blood, enter the graft and, by some unknown means, destroy it. Although this is a plausible scheme it is still speculative. There is good evidence that the agents which destroy solid tissue grafts are lymphocytes (see Chapter 41), but it has not been shown that the new lymphocytes which are produced in the way we have just described possess specific destructive properties.

Unfortunately, the claim that small lymphocytes initiate homograft reactions does not solve the problem of their function for the simple reason that grafting is not a normal biological hazard. It has been suggested that animals need a mechanism for recognizing and destroying antigenic variants which may arise in their tissues. If such aberrant cells were also potentially neoplastic then a mechanism for rapidly eliminating them would clearly be of great importance. The evidence for this intriguing idea is rather slender. A less satisfying possibility is that homograft reactions are completely artificial; they merely illustrate the workings of a system whose real function is to protect the animal against invading bacteria and viruses.

The use of purified suspensions of cells has shown that small lymphocytes certainly play a part in responses which lead to the production of circulating antibody. A simple experiment showed that an injection of small lymphocytes from normal but not from immunologically tolerant donors would restore the primary antibody response to sheep erythrocytes in heavily X-irradiated rats.[43] Equally striking is the ability of small lymphocytes from immunized donors to confer secondary reactivity on irradiated recipients. For example, irradiated rats will give brisk secondary responses to an injection of tetanus toxoid when they have received lymphocytes from donors immunized some months previously with the same antigen.[44] Here the lymphocytes were not making antibody at the time of transfer but were carrying a property sometimes referred to as "immunological memory". Thus, small lymphocytes from non-immunized donors will confer primary immune responsiveness while those from immunized donors confer secondary responsiveness. The reactions which can be transferred by small lymphocytes mirror the immunological status of the donor animal.

The simplest explanation of the two experiments outlined in the previous paragraph is that the small lymphocytes interact with antigen, or with antigen which has been processed by macrophages, and that they then enlarge, divide and give rise to antibody-synthesizing cells in the host. This has, in fact, been shown to be the case: the donor small lymphocytes evolved into cells secreting hæmolysin against sheep erythrocytes in the first experiment, and into plasma cells making anti-tetanus toxoid in the second.[59] This does not mean that all antibody responses are initiated by small lymphocytes nor that their only role in antibody formation is to provide the precursors of antibody-producing cells. These matters are considered further in Chapter 35.

There are suggestions that transplantation reactions and reactions involving the synthesis of antibody may be initiated by two different populations of cells. This notion comes from studying the effect of removing particular lymphoid organs on the development of immunological reactivity in birds.[45] Removal of the thymus leads to a severe impairment of transplantation immunity but leaves the ability to form antibody relatively unaffected. Removal of the bursa of Fabricius, a lympho-epithelial structure associated with the distal end of the gut, affects predominantly the ability to make antibody. In mammals there is no convincing evidence that the immunological apparatus is composed of two functionally distinct systems of cells although it has been suggested that some of the lymphoid tissue embedded in the gut of mammals may be the homologue of the avian bursa. By the same token it is not known whether the ability of thoracic duct cells to engage in both types of response reflects the existence in mammalian lymph of two separate populations of small lymphocytes with different intrinsic properties.

The picture which emerges from the immunological studies suggests that small lymphocytes may play a dual role in immunological responses. There appear to be "uncommitted" lymphocytes which initiate primary responses and "committed" lymphocytes which mediate the destruction of homografts or carry immunological memory; and one may be produced from the other by antigen-induced cell division. Unfortunately, the experiments have given us no information about the properties of individual cells, only about populations of cells. Changes in the reactivity of a population of lymphocytes could theoretically be brought about simply by altering the relative proportions of cells with different, fixed reactivities. Thus, one influential view holds that committed and uncommitted lymphocytes do not exist: all small lymphocytes possess full reactivity and immunization merely generates more cells of a specific class by inducing division in the members of it.[46] This assumes that individual lymphocytes are pre-adapted to react to particular antigens, a view embodied in "elective" as opposed to "instructive" theories of immunity. These are highly speculative matters and they are considered at greater length in Chapter 34.

If the small lymphocytes of an animal are heterogeneous with respect to immunological reactivity, either for genetic reasons or as a consequence of immunization, then a possible function can be seen for the process of lymphocyte recirculation. Theoretically this could make available to a regionally stimulated lymph node all the lymphocytes in the animal which are potentially reactive to a particular antigen. There is, as yet, no evidence that a selective process of this kind operates in lymphoid tissue during either primary or secondary responses. However, it has recently been shown that the size of the antibody response which can be induced in the spleen is related to the concentration of lymphocytes in the blood perfusing it at the time of antigenic stimulation.[15] It seems that a traffic of lymphocytes through a lymphoid organ may have an important influence on the efficiency of the inductive events in antibody formation. The nature of this influence remains to be determined.

Transformation of Lymphocytes

Small lymphocytes have been regarded by many workers as primitive cells capable under suitable conditions of development into other cell types. It has been alleged, for example, that small lymphocytes can transform into fibroblasts, erythrocytes, granulocytes and macrophages. In the past, evidence for such transformations has come from the examination of fixed and stained specimens from which a sequence of development has been constructed from a series of static events. The weakness of evidence of this kind explains the controversy which has surrounded the subject for so long. Controversy is now no longer necessary since techniques exist for performing decisive experiments.

Small lymphocytes have now been shown to undergo morphological transformations both *in vivo* and *in vitro*. We have already described how small lymphocytes under certain conditions will develop into antibody-forming cells *in vivo*. The differentiation into large, basophilic cells which occurs under the impact of transplantation antigens *in vivo* has also been mentioned. These large cells are non-phagocytic and they give rise by successive divisions to lymphocytes of progressively decreasing size, ending with small lymphocytes. The experiments which uncovered this phenomenon made use of radioactive and chromosomal markers in order to establish with certainty that the new dividing cells had originated from small lymphocytes. [39, 42] Studies on a graft-versus-host reaction have also provided a third example of lymphocyte transformation *in vivo*, the new cells in this instance, being macrophages. The background to this second study is worth considering in a little detail.

The claim that lymphocytes can transform into macrophages, which is embedded in much of the older hæmatological literature, has recently been reinvestigated by modern techniques. Autoradiographic experiments with tritiated thymidine have shown that blood monocytes and the macrophages which emigrate from blood vessels into areas of sterile inflammation are derived from rapidly dividing precursors in the bone marrow.[47] No evidence of an origin from either small or large lymphocytes was obtained.[48, 49] More recently the Kupffer cells formed during regeneration of the liver after partial hepatectomy in mice have also been shown to originate from the bone marrow.[50] However, new Kupffer cells are also produced in the liver when a graft-versus-host reaction is induced in F_1 hybrid mice by an injection of parental-strain thoracic duct lymphocytes. Here, surprisingly, the use of a chromosome marker showed unequivocally that the dividing phagocytic cells were derived from the injected lymphocytes, and most probably from small lymphocytes.[50] It seems that under intense antigenic stimulation mononuclear phagocytes may develop from certain small lymphocytes although usually they are derived from a precursor in the bone marrow.

The phenomenon of lymphocyte transformation *in vitro* has a relatively recent history. It stems from the observation, made in 1960, that mitoses can be induced in human blood leucocytes by incubating them *in vitro* with a bean extract, phytohæmagglutinin.[51] This material agglutinates red blood cells and was used in a procedure for separating leucocytes from blood. The mitogenic effect was discovered by chance and was soon exploited to facilitate studies on human karyotypes. Experiments with tritiated thymidine strongly suggested that the cell in human blood which responds to phytohæmagglutinin is a small lymphocyte.[52] The crucial evidence comes from observations on single living small lymphocytes photographed at all stages of their enlargement and subsequent division.[53]

Prior to their division under the influence of phytohæmagglutinin small lymphocytes enlarge into cells with prominent nucleoli and with a strongly basophilic cytoplasm which is often vacuolated. The large cells are motile but not phagocytic and in the electron microscope their cytoplasm contains scanty endoplasmic reticulum and abundant free ribosomes.[54, 55] These morphological characteristics do not relate them with certainty to any other normal or abnormal human leucocyte although there are similarities to the large cells which arise from small lymphocytes during transplantation reactions in rodents, including the formation from them of more small lymphocytes.

The biological significance of lymphocyte transformation by plant extracts is not known. Somewhat more illuminating is the observation that transformation *in vitro* can also be brought about by a number of antigenic materials when the lymphocytes come from specifically immunized donors. Thus tuberculin, tetanus and diphtheria toxoids, and TAB vaccine will stimulate lymphocytes only from subjects who have been previously immunized.[56] The obvious interpretation of this specific stimulation is that the lymphocytes are carrying immunological memory and that the changes *in vitro* mirror in some way secondary immune responses. There is as yet no convincing evidence that the responses *in vitro* are accompanied by specific antibody production; indeed, there is still a dispute as to whether immunoglobulin of any kind is synthesized.

A further example of lymphocyte transformation *in vitro* is that which occurs when lymphocytes from two unrelated individuals are cultured together.[57] This is thought to be the result of a primary immune response to the mutually foreign histocompatibility antigens. Attempts have been made to relate the degree of transformation and cell division to the strength of the antigenic differences which would determine the fate of homografts exchanged between the two individuals *in vivo*, the aim being to develop a technique for selecting donors in human tissue transplantation. It seems unlikely that this method will gain general acceptance as a routine test in the face of the mounting success of serological methods of tissue typing (see Chapter 41).

A final example of lymphocyte transformation is that brought about in rabbit lymphocytes by specific anti-allotypic sera, that is, by antisera directed against genetically determined antigenic components of their immunoglobulins (see Chapter 32). These experiments are of great theoretical interest since they show that small lymphocytes, even from new-born animals, contain immunoglobulin or at least its genetically controlled antigenic determinants. It is an intriguing possibility that the induction of primary immune responses *in vivo* may involve the combination of antigen with receptors of the kind revealed by these experiments.

REFERENCES

1. Harris, H. (1953). *Brit. J. exp. Path.*, **34,** 599.
2. Gowans, J. L., and Knight, E. J. (1964). *Proc. roy Soc. B*, **159,** 257.
3. Marchesi, V. T., and Gowans, J. L. (1964). *Proc. roy. Soc. B*, **159,** 283.
4. Cunningham, A. J., Smith, J. B., and Mercer, E. H. (1966). *J. exp. Med.*, **124,** 701.
5. Hall, J. G., Morris, B., Moreno, G. H., and Bessis, M. C. (1967). *J. exp. Med.*, **125,** 91.
6. Ottesen, J. (1954). *Acta physiol. scand.*, **32,** 75.
7. Robinson, S. H., Brecher, G., Lourie, I. S., and Haley, J. E. (1965). *Blood*, **26,** 281.
8. Caffrey, R. W., Rieke, W. O., and Everett, N. B. (1962). *Acta hæmat.* (*Basel*), **28,** 145.
9. Everett, N. C., Caffrey, R. W., and Rieke, W. O. (1964). *Ann. N.Y. Acad. Sci.*, **113,** 887.
10. Buckton, K. E., Court Brown, W. M., and Smith, P. G. (1967). *Nature* (*Lond.*), **214,** 470.
11. Schooley, J. C., and Kelly, L. S. (1964). In *The Thymus in Immunobiology*, p. 236. New York: Hoeber Harper.
12. Harris, J. E., and Ford, C. E. (1964). *Nature* (*Lond.*), **201,** 884.
13. Weissman, I. L. (1967). *J. exp. Med.*, **126,** 291.
14. Hall, J. G., and Morris, B. (1965). *J. exp. Med.*, **121,** 901.
15. Ford, W. L., and Gowans, J. L. (1967). *Proc. roy. Soc. B*, **168** 244.
16. Hughes, R., May, A. J., and Widdicombe, J. G. (1956). *J. Physiol.* (*Lond.*), **132,** 384.
17. Gowans, J. L. (1966). *Int. Rev. exp. Path.*, **5** 1.

18. Binns, R. M., and Hall, J. G. (1966). *Brit. J. exp. Path.*, **47** 275.
19. Sjövall, H. (1936). *Acta path. microbiol. scand.*, Suppl. 27.
20. Yoffey, J. M., and Drinker, C. K. (1939). *Anat. Rec.*, **73** 417.
21. Mann, J. D., and Higgins, G. M. (1950). *Blood*, **5**, 177.
22. Gowans, J. L. (1957). *Brit. J. exp. Path.*, **38**, 67.
23. Gowans, J. L. (1959). *J. Physiol. (Lond.)*, **146**, 54.
24. Shorter, R. G., and Bollman, J. L. (1960). *Amer. J. Physiol.*, **198**, 1014.
25. Gesner, B. M., and Ginsburg, V. (1964). *Proc. nat. Acad. Sci. (Wash.)*, **52**, 750.
26. Cronkite, E. P., Jansen, C. R., Cottier, H., Rai, K., and Sipe, C. R. (1964). *Ann. N.Y. Acad. Sci.*, **113**, 566.
27. Osmond, D. G., and Everett, N. B. (1964). *Blood*, **23**, 1.
28. Barnes, D. W. H., and Loutit, J. F. (1967). *Lancet*, **2**, 1138.
29. Moffatt, D. J., Rosse, C., and Yoffey, J. M. (1967). *Lancet*, **2**, 547.
30. Caffrey Tyler, R. W., and Everett, N. B. (1966). *Blood*, **28**, 873.
31. Gesner, B. M., and Gowans, J. L. (1962). *Brit. J. exp. Path.*, **43**, 431.
32. Sanders, A. G., and Florey, H. W. (1940). *Brit. J. exp. Path.*, **21**, 275.
33. McIntire, K. R., Sell, S., and Miller, J. F. A. P. (1964). *Nature (Lond.)*, **204**, 151.
34. Loutit, J. F. (1962). *Lancet*, **2**, 1106.
35. Miller, J. F. A. P., Mitchell, G. F., and Weiss, N. S. (1967). *Nature (Lond.)*, **216**, 992.
36. Parrott, D. M. V., de Sousa, M. A. B., and East, J. (1966). *J. exp. Med.*, **123**, 191.
37. McGregor, D. D., and Gowans, J. L. (1963). *J. exp. Med.*, **117**, 303.
38. McGregor, D. D., and Gowans, J. L. (1964). *Lancet*, **1**, 629.
39. Gowans, J. L. (1962). *Ann. N.Y. Acad. Sci.*, **99**, 432.
40. Hildemann, W. H., Linscott, W. D., and Morlino, M. J. (1962). In *Ciba Symposium on Transplantation*, p. 236. London: J. & A. Churchill.
41. Gowans, J. L. (1965). *Brit. med. Bull.*, **21**, 106.
42. Ford, W. L., Gowans, J. L., and McCullagh, P. J. (1966). In *Ciba Symposium on The Thymus*, p. 58. London: J. & A. Churchill.
43. McGregor, D. D., McCullagh, P. J., and Gowans, J. L. (1967). *Proc. roy. Soc. B*, **168**, 229.
44. Ellis, S. T., Gowans, J. L., and Howard, J. C. (1967). *Cold Spr. Harb. Symp. quant. Biol.*, **32**, 395.
45. Warner, N. L., and Szenberg, A. (1964). *Ann. Rev. Microbiol.*, **18**, 253.
46. Brent, L., and Medawar, P. B. (1966). *Proc. roy. Soc. B*, **165**, 281.
47. Volkman, A., and Gowans J. L. (1965). *Brit. J. exp. Path.*, **46**, 62.
48. Volkman, A., and Gowans J. L. (1965). *Brit. J. exp. Path.*, **46**, 50.
49. Spector, W. G., Walters, M. N. I, and Willoughby, D. A., (1965). *J. Path. Bact.*, **90**, 181.
50. Boak, J. L., Christie, G. H., Ford, W. L., and Howard, J. G. (1968). *Proc. roy. Soc. B.* In Press.
51. Nowell, P. C. (1960). *Cancer Res.*, **20**, 462.
52. MacKinney, A. A., Stohlman, F., and Brecher, G. (1962). *Blood*, **19**, 349.
53. Marshall W. H., and Roberts, K. B. (1965). *Quart. J. exp. Physiol.*, **50**, 361.
54. Marshall, W. H., and Roberts, K. B. (1963). *Quart. J. exp. Physiol.*, **48**, 146.
55. Tanaka, Y., Epstein L. B. Brecher, G., and Stohlman, F. (1963). *Blood*, **22**, 614.
56. Robbins, J. H. (1964). *Science*, **146**, 1648.
57. Bain, B., Lowenstein, L., and MacLean, L. D. (1965). In *Histocompatibility Testing*, p. 121. Washington, D.C.: Nat. Acad. Sci.
58. Sell, S., and Gell, P. G. H. (1965). *J. exp. Med.*, **122**, 923.
59. Ellis, S. T., Gowans, J. L., and Howard, J. C. (1969). *Antibiot. et Chemother. (Basel)*, **15**, 40.

Chapter 6

THE SECRETION OF MUCUS AND INFLAMMATION OF MUCOUS MEMBRANES

By H. W. Florey

We have now given fairly extensive consideration to some of the reactions occurring in tissues following various kinds of trauma, the most important, from the point of view of future practitioners of medicine, being those caused by the presence of pathogenic bacteria. Pathogenic bacteria do not induce changes until they have passed certain barriers which are a first line of defence against their invasion. Thus the skin of animals is, in general, impervious to micro-organisms, so that solution of its continuity is necessary for infection to occur.

While it is difficult for bacteria and viruses to pass the barrier of the skin, the much more delicate mucous membranes which line the respiratory, alimentary and genito-urinary tracts are more easily penetrated. Inflammation of mucous membranes is characterised by phenomena common to all tissues—namely, vascular dilatation, increased permeability of blood vessels with the formation of an exudate from the plasma, and emigration of leucocytes, which may penetrate to the surface as well as into the subepithelial layers of the mucous membrane. In addition two features are to be noted that do not occur in other tissues, namely the secretion of mucus by some mucous membranes and the desquamation or shedding of the epithelial cells by all. In this chapter we will consider some of the properties of mucous membranes and some of the phenomena that occur when they are inflamed.

Since it is one of the characteristics of certain inflamed mucosæ to produce "mucus" or "mucin", it is as well to give some thought to what we mean by these terms. They are both used for the secretions coming from certain mucous membranes, and they are sometimes also used loosely for the characteristic viscosity-raising substances in these fluids. From personal experience we all know that the inflammatory secretion that comes from the nose soon after the beginning of a common cold, or that is coughed up from an inflamed trachea, is sticky viscid material. This stickiness, which imparts character to secretions of normal as well as inflamed mucous membranes, is due to the presence of "muco-substances". It has been known for many years that when mucins are hydrolysed with dilute acids reducing sugars and hexosamines are formed, and that they sometimes yield sulphate and/or phosphate, and sometimes also uronic acids. But until the last few years very little was known of their structure. However, the composition of the various mucous secretions and the chemical structure of their constituent biopolymers are now receiving vigorous attention, though the findings are outside the scope of this book. In general it may be said that the mucous secretions frequently contain at least one viscosity-raising agent or "muco-substance", usually a glycoprotein, together with serum proteins and enzymes. In mucins from epithelial tissues with high rates of cellular renewal nucleoproteins may also be present. The composition and structure of the constituents of a particular mucous secretion may be highly characteristic of the organ or tissue in which it is produced.

According to current information glycoproteins are complex molecules of high molecular weight (10^5–10^6) in which a number of oligosaccharides or polysaccharides are attached to a protein. The viscous glycoproteins in mucins have a large number of side chains (e.g. 600 to 700 in sheep submaxillary gland mucin) each of which terminates in a sialic acid residue, so that the whole assembly has a strongly ionic character. Glycoproteins of a non-viscous nature, such as those found in serum (α_1-acid glycoprotein, immunoglobulin, fetuin) or in bone, have a small number (1 to 10) of oligosaccharide side chains which, however, may be of considerable complexity.

Epithelial mucins are produced by special cells. These differ in morphology according to the situation in which they are found, and their histochemical and other staining reactions show that their products differ from organ to organ and from cell type to cell type. There is also evidence that there are differences between the mucins produced by the same organ in different species. The common and striking property of all these secretions is the remarkably high viscosity imparted to them by small amounts of their constituent muco-substances, for example the viscous juice from the duodenum of the pig or rabbit, which has the consistency of egg white, may contain only 0·15 per cent of viscosity-raising material.

Mucus contains not only its particular muco-substances but ions such as bicarbonate, chloride, sodium and calcium. In some situations it is probable that the alkaline properties due to bicarbonate are of importance.

Pathological Mucous Secretions

Mucinous fluids are secreted for physiological purposes, the most obvious example of this kind being saliva. In pathological states of the mucous membranes, particularly in inflammation, mucus, secreted in greater amounts than normal, is added to the exudate that seeps out through the epithelium. For example, sputum, which comes from the trachea and airways of the lungs in a variety of diseases, is always sticky, though the adjectives used to describe it range from "watery" to "viscid" or "tenacious". It usually contains leucocytes, disintegrating epithelial cells and bacteria. Enzymes are liberated from the disintegrating cells. These produce protein and other degradation products. Where bacterial infection is intense the exudate may be yellow, when it is known as muco-pus, the opaque yellow appearance being due to the presence of polymorphs. As the condition clears up, one of the signs of amelioration is that the exudate becomes less and less yellow and opaque, until only a practically clear mucous jelly is secreted. Some exudates, however, such as pus accumulating in a closed space, are viscous because of their content of desoxyribonucleic acid and desoxyribonucleoprotein, derived largely from the nuclei of dead polymorphs.

Mucin Production by Epithelial Cells

When still within the cell the material is known to histologists as "mucigen". It is very difficult to preserve intracellular mucigen satisfactorily for histological examination. The cells that elaborate it tend to change soon after death so that human post-mortem material is seldom satisfactory, although the introduction of apparatus for the removal of small portions of mucosa from the gastro-intestinal tract and bronchial tree of man has made it possible to obtain fresh human specimens. But as in many other instances, we are to a large extent dependent on experiments and observations on animal tissues to provide more exact information than can be obtained from man.

Mucigen in cells takes the form of granules or small droplets. Not only do the cells tend to undergo changes soon after death, but most fixatives disrupt the granules. Their form in life is not preserved and the intracellular mucin appears as an amorphous mass or even as a network outlining the exploded granules. By special means, depending somewhat on the organ, it is possible to preserve the granules for cytological study, but in most ordinary specimens the mucigen granules have been transformed by the fixative into a rather formless meshwork.

GASTRO-INTESTINAL TRACT

The Stomach

In many animals, including man, the stomach is completely lined by a columnar epithelium, composed in some species of particularly tall cells. The cytoplasm at the free end of each cell contains a collection of very small mucigen granules (Plate B, Fig. *e*). Similar cells line the foveolæ leading to the glands and show a regular decrease in size towards the base of each pit. Others of a different form exist in the neck of each peptic gland and may sometimes be found scattered even as far as the bases of the glands. These latter cells are known by a number of names, but we will follow Babkin and call them "mucous cells of the neck". They are rounded or wedge-shaped cells, generally stuffed with mucigen and with the nucleus compressed at the base of the cell or into the thin end of the wedge where it passes down between the oxyntic cells (Plate B, Fig. *f*). In the cat and some other species the mucin they contain stains differently with certain stains from that of the surface cells. In the pyloric antrum of the stomach the glands are composed entirely of mucous cells, not unlike the mucous cells of the neck (Plate B, Fig. *a*), and at the cardiac end there is a collection of similar mucus-producing glands known as the cardiac glands. In the pig the cardiac area is of considerable extent, but in most species it is small.

The stomach is thus provided with a very substantial number of cells that on histological and histochemical grounds are considered to contain mucigen. The various types of gastric mucous cell do not, however, have identical staining reactions, and from this, and also from the fact that only some of them seem to be able to incorporate sulphate labelled by ^{35}S, it seems likely that they do not all produce the same kinds of muco-substance (Plate C, Figs. *a*, *b*, *f*, *g*, *h*).

Secretion of Gastric Mucus

Fundal gastric juice, which is secreted in response to stimuli arriving *via* the vagi and to a hormone, gastrin, elaborated in the pyloric mucosa, contains hydrochloric acid and the enzymes pepsin and rennin. It contains in addition "dissolved" mucin and shreds of floating mucin, both coming from the mucous cells that have just been described.

There is relatively little firm information about the control of the production of the mucus constituent. This is partly because some of the cells seem to be continuously active, producing a certain amount of mucus in the absence of any stimuli related to digestion, and partly because the mucous cells have a remarkable capacity to replenish their contents as fast as it is discharged, so that very vigorous artificial stimulation is needed before any histological sign of emptying can be seen. Indeed, if the surface epithelial cells are exposed to a strong irritant they generally fall off their basement membrane more or less intact, rather than discharge their mucous content. Neighbouring cells spread out to make good these defects, and there is in the pits an area of vigorous mitosis from which losses are replaced.

In fasting, the surface of the stomach is covered by a clinging layer of mucus, which may perhaps come from the surface cells and pits, though there is no direct evidence for this. During fasting, also, the pyloric region of cats and dogs, and probably of man, slowly produces a thick egg white-like secretion which is alkaline, and when collected with exposure to air can have a pH as high as 8·4; presumably this comes in the main from the pyloric glands. The "dissolved mucus" in the freely flowing gastric juice secreted during digestion may partly be the response of the mucous neck cells of the fundus to feeding. In animals the flow of mucus from the pyloric part of the stomach usually increases during digestion, so this may also contribute to the digestive juice.

A mucous secretion can be produced from both fundus and pylorus by vagal or vago-mimetic stimulation, although some of the experimental findings are of a contradictory nature.[2a] The infusion of large quantities of acetylcholine through the blood vessels of the fundus and other parts of the stomach of dogs produced large quantities of alkaline juice which was described as often forming a jelly.[3] Apparently in these experiments, in which the stimulation was no doubt very great, pepsin and acid were not secreted for reasons that are obscure. The mucous neck cells were emptied of their mucigen granules, and the surface epithelium, though not exhausted, was partly emptied. In other experiments electrical stimulation of the vagus in the decapitate cat, which produced large quantities of acid gastric juice, sometimes reduced the mucigen content of the mucous neck cells but often did not do so although the peptic cells were completely emptied. Similarly the pyloric glands were sometimes though not always exhausted by vagal stimulation (PLATE B, FIGS. *a* and *b*). The appearance of the surface epithelial cells was never altered by this stimulus, and it has been suggested that in so far as these cells discharge their contents the effect is a mechanical one due to movements of the mucosa. It is not yet known whether gastrin has any effect on mucous cells, but possibly some of the inconsistencies found in experiments by vagal stimulation may be accounted for by the complex interactions which are known to exist between gastrin and the vagus.[3a]

In addition to these vagal effects, the secretion of alkaline mucus has been found to follow the electrical stimulation of freshly cut sympathetic nerves to the stomach, and a similar juice may appear as a "paralytic" secretion some few days after the cutting of the splanchnic nerves in cats.

Thus the present position is that mucus is normally secreted by the stomach, and that probably the mucous neck cells and the pyloric glands are under the control of the vagus nerve, and that there may also be other influences.

Apart from the question of remote control it is certain that the layer of mucus that normally covers the stomach epithelium can be increased by local stimulation, either mechanical or chemical. Thus rubbing the surface with a glass rod has been seen to produce mucus in a Pavlov pouch in the dog, and in the stomach of man.[4] The local application of a variety of chemical substances produces a considerable flow of mucus, and, if the substances are sufficiently concentrated, the shedding of epithelial cells.[5] There is some evidence that at least some of this mucus comes from the glands rather than from the surface cells.

Perhaps those who swallow strong alcoholic liquors on to an empty stomach—a current social habit—may be more interested to know that alcohol also appears to stimulate the production of mucus. One of the symptoms presented by chronic alcoholics is vomiting in the morning of a fluid rich in mucus. In experiments in the cat it has been shown that the application of 50 or 60 per cent ethyl alcohol for five minutes to the gastric mucosa, or of 1 per cent acetic acid for 30 minutes, produces a thick layer of mucus in which there is much shed epithelium. Shedding of epithelium is caused by even 20 to 30 per cent alcohol. It may interest the reader to recall that sherry contains from 16 to 22 per cent and neat gin from 51 to 59 per cent of alcohol (PLATE B, FIG. *g*).

One can envisage a gradation from the normal small amount of mucus produced physiologically on the surface to a greatly increased secretion caused by the strong mechanical and chemical stimuli to which the stomach of man is sometimes subjected.

The secretion of mucus is characteristic of acute gastritis and is often found also in "chronic gastritis" (the name covers a variety of long-lasting conditions, not all of them inflammatory). Biopsy specimens of the stomach in acute gastritis following an excess of alcohol show damage to the superficial epithelium, but there are generally signs that the losses are being repaired from the pits. After acute gastritis induced experimentally the epithelium is readily repaired. Similar shedding and restoration of the surface epithelial cells has been seen as a result of contact of food substances.[6]

In chronic gastritis the glands may show various abnormalities and sometimes come to consist entirely of mucous cells. From such stomachs no acid or pepsin is secreted. The surface epithelium may be surprisingly normal, or may be hypertrophied or flattened. Not infrequently in this condition areas of the stomach undergo metaplasia to an intestinal type of mucosa.

Function of Gastric Mucus

The gastric mucus presents itself firstly as a layer of thick material clinging to the mucosa and secondly as "dissolved mucus" in the gastric juice. It has for long been considered that, at least in the first form, it protects the mucosa from the acid and pepsin of the gastric juice as well as from mechanical damage, but the exact way in which it does this is not altogether clear.

It used to be thought that muco-substances were buffers and that this helped to protect the mucosa from acid gastric juice. It is now known that these substances are practically devoid of buffering power but that in the pylorus and duodenum they are secreted with a considerable amount of bicarbonate. We do not know what cells the bicarbonate comes from, but it is possible that even in the fundus the mucous cells are secreting an alkaline product.

PLATE B (*opposite*)

(*a*) Pyloric mucosa of a cat. Surface and gland cells both contain plenty of mucin which in both situations stains by the periodic acid-Schiff method. Harris's hæmatoxylin, periodic acid-Schiff and tartrazine. (× 75.)

(*b*) Pyloric mucosa from the same cat as FIG. *a* after electrical stimulation of the vagi for 6 hr. The mucin of the gland cells has been largely voided, but the superficial cells contain as much as at the beginning of the experiment. Staining as for FIG. *a*. (× 75.)

(*c*) Brunner's glands of a rabbit. The cells are full of mucin granules and the nuclei are compressed to the bases. Harris's hæmatoxylin, mucicarmine and metanil yellow. (× 225.)

(*d*) Brunner's glands from the same rabbit as FIG. *c* after the passage of N/20 HCl for 6 hr. 20 min. Most of the mucin has been evacuated from the cells and the nuclei are now clearly seen in a rounded condition. Note the red-staining granules of mucigen above the nuclei as well as the undischarged residue at the free borders of the cells. Staining as for FIG. *c*. (× 225.)

(*e*) Cat stomach. Superficial epithelium lining a gastric pit. Every cell contains a column of fine mucin granules. Harris's hæmatoxylin, mucicarmine and tartrazine. (× 900.)

(*f*) Cat stomach. Mucoid neck cells in a fundal gland. They contain red-staining mucin granules and are interspersed between round, pale oxyntic cells. Staining as for FIG. *e*. (× 900.)

(*g*) Fundal mucosa of cat stomach. The stomach had been filled with 20 per cent. alcohol for 5 hr. 40 min. Mucin which stains red is being discharged from the superficial cells, and mucin staining black is being discharged up the ducts and on to the surface from the mucoid neck cells. Indulin, mucicarmine and metanil yellow. (× 75.)

(From Florey.[1])

From the days of Claude Bernard, who envisaged the gastric mucosa as "enclosing the gastric juice within a container as impermeable as one of porcelain", the mucus has often been stated to impede the diffusion of pepsin or hydrochloric acid. In most of the experiments claiming to show this no direct comparison has been made with the speed of diffusion through water. This is admittedly not easy to arrange, but when such an experiment is done it appears that the mucus in the concentration in which it lines the stomach offers little hindrance to the diffusion of these substances—a result not surprising, perhaps, when the very low concentration of glycoprotein is considered.

Further reflection will show that an ability to slow down the rate of diffusion of a solute need not be postulated to explain the protective effect of the coat of mucus. Within this sheet separating the mucosa from the more or less fluid contents of the lumen mixing will not occur, and provided that the mucosa forms some alkali there will be a pH gradient across the thickness of the sheet; however acid the contents of the stomach, for example, the mucosa and a thin layer of the mucus coating it will always be alkaline. Similarly with pepsin, as this diffuses from the stomach contents through the mucus towards the mucosa, it will be met by alkali diffusing from the mucosa, so that even if it reached the mucosa without being irreversibly inactivated the milieu would be too alkaline to permit of peptic digestion.[7] Even if the mucus itself were gradually broken down by the digestive action of the gastric juice, as has been suggested, it could still form an effective barrier as long as its constant slow secretion kept pace with such degradation.[7a]

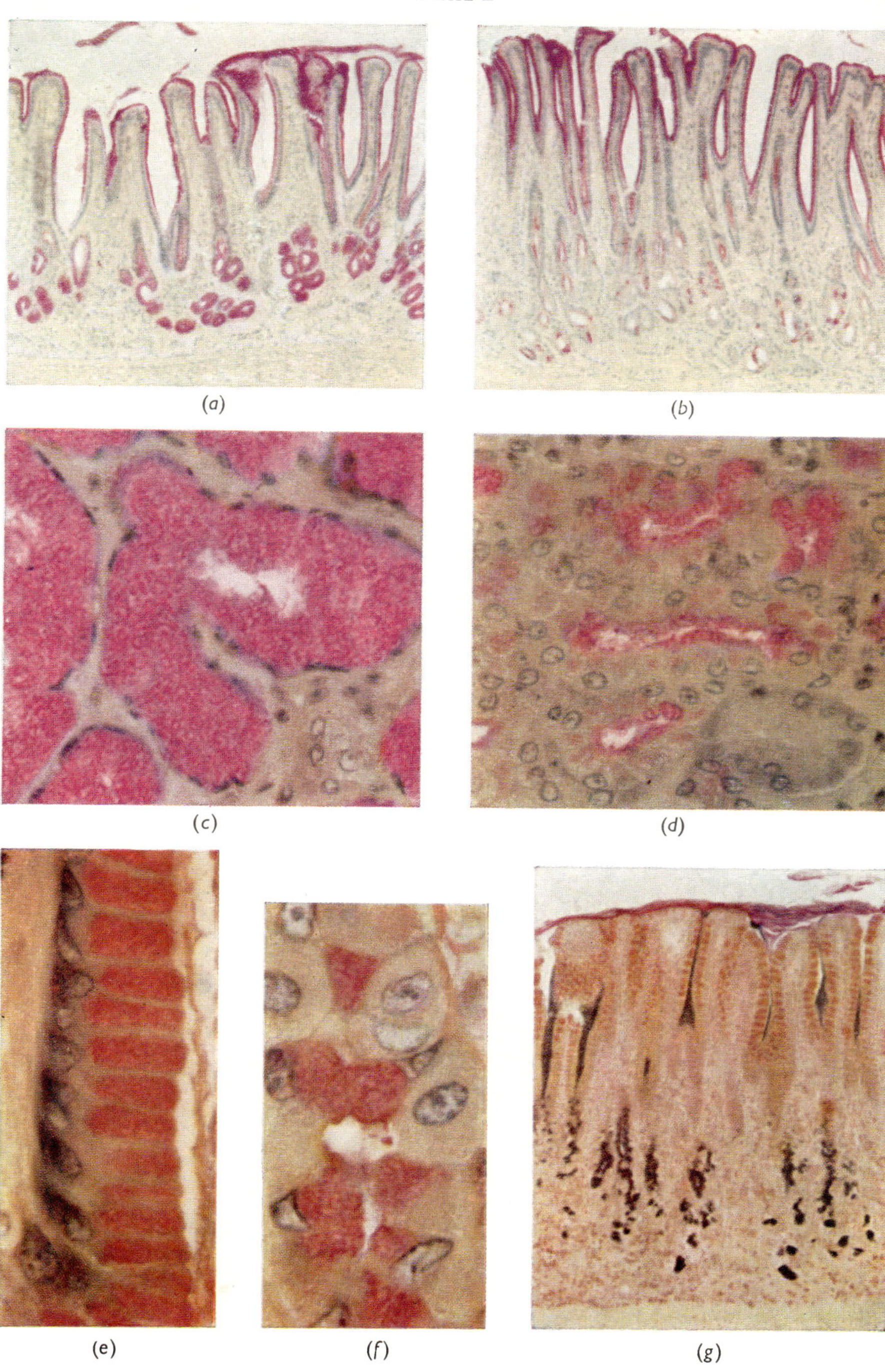

(a) (b)

(c) (d)

(e) (f) (g)

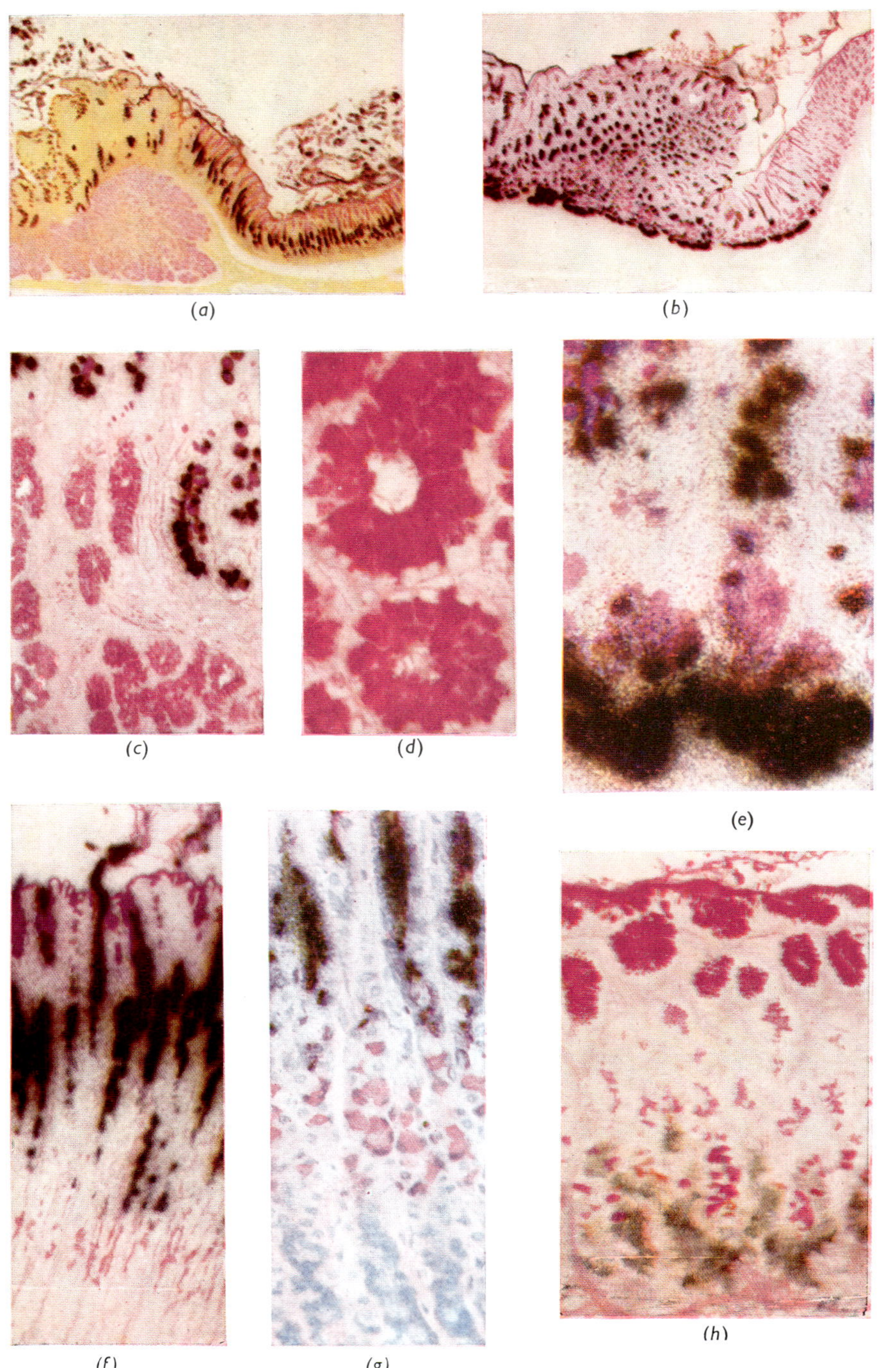
(a)
(b)
(c)
(d)
(e)
(f)
(g)
(h)

PLATE C (*opposite*)

Animals were injected intravenously with $Na_2{}^{35}SO_4$ and were killed at various intervals afterwards. The figures show histological sections of their tissues with overlying autoradiographs. Photographic emulsion was placed over the sections and exposed for from 2 to 10 weeks. When the emulsion was developed sites where radioactivity had affected the film were shown by black granules of silver. Except in FIG. *h* the concentration of radioactivity is in the mucus, i.e. it shows which cells are forming sulphated glycoproteins.

The granules are focused sharply so the mucin, stained red by the periodic acid-Schiff method, is slightly out of focus. No nuclear stain was used except for FIG. *g*.

(*a*) Pylorus and duodenum of rat killed 2 hr. 10 min. after injection. There is radioactivity in the pyloric gland and duct cells (R) and in the goblet cells of the duodenal crypts (L). The surface and upper parts of the ducts in the pylorus and the Brunner's glands in the duodenum (lower L) are inactive. (× 20.)

(*b*) Pylorus and duodenum of guinea-pig killed 2 hr. after injection. Here the duodenal goblet cells and Brunner's glands (L) are radioactive but in the pylorus (R) only a few gland acini next to the duodenum show any radioactivity. (× 20.)

(*c*) Duodenum of cat killed 6 hr. after injection. Goblet cells in the crypts (upper part of picture) are radioactive but Brunner's glands (below) show no activity. (× 120.)

(*d*) Higher magnification of Brunner's glands from the same cat as FIG. *c*. No radioactivity. (× 480.)

(*e*) Duodenum of guinea-pig killed 6 hr. after injection. Goblet cells in the crypts (upper part of picture) and Brunner's glands (below) are radioactive. (× 300.)

(*f*) Fundus of stomach of rat killed 3 hr. after injection. At the bottom of the picture are mucoid neck cells and at the top surface cells, both without radioactivity. In between, the cells of the gastric pits are producing strongly radioactive mucin which is passing to the surface. (× 120.)

(*g*) Fundus of stomach of rat killed 1 hr. 10 min. after injection. As in FIG. *f*, cells in the pits are radioactive and the mucoid neck cells are inactive. Peptic cells, stained blue at the bottom of the picture, are inactive. (× 280.)

(*h*) Fundus of stomach of cat killed 6 hr. after injection. No radioactivity in surface, pit or mucoid neck cells, but some radioactivity in the (unstained) peptic cells. Presumably a sulphated compound is associated with pepsinogen in the cat. (× 120.)

(From Jennings and Florey.[2])

This dynamic protective mechanism would enable a small quantity of alkaline mucus to protect the mucosa from a harmful change of pH, even though the alkali present could neutralise only a small proportion of the acid. The same considerations apply to the beginning of the duodenum.

The fundus would clearly share in such a mechanism of protection from the gastric juice, but it has its own problem in that the acid and pepsin of the juice are emerging from the fundal glands themselves. Though there is some uncertainty about the exact form in which the oxyntic and peptic cells secrete their products, it seems likely that an active acid-pepsin mixture is passing up the ducts. Perhaps it is because the other cells lining the ducts are all mucus-secreting cells that no damage is caused to the mucosa during its passage.

There has been considerable discussion of the origin and composition of the "dissolved mucus". It is obvious that a small volume of mucigen liberated from the cells swells to give rise to a large volume of "visible mucus", and it seems reasonable that the slow hydration might proceed further to give "dissolved mucus". Certainly if "dissolved mucus" is concentrated by, for example, filtration, its physical properties come to resemble those of "visible mucus". If the solution or attrition of the mucus on the luminal surface of the "visible mucus" coat is dynamically balanced by secretion of mucigen granules by the mucosa, it will follow that the actual concentration of mucus—and hence its mechanical strength—will be greatest where it is emerging from the ducts and mucous cells of the mucosa, which would explain why it is extremely difficult to remove the mucous coat from the surface; perhaps the fact that mucus is more sticky above than below pH 7 contributes to this firm bonding.

The Duodenum

All mammalia possess, just distal to the pylorus, deep glands that extend for a greater or less distance down the duodenum, though rarely past the entry of the pancreatic duct. These glands were first described with precision by Brunner in 1686. Brunner's glands, which in many species appear to be anatomically continuous with the pyloric glands, are composed of acini having the histological structure of mucous glands. The acini for the most part lie beneath the muscularis mucosæ, and empty by ducts into the overlying crypts of Lieberkühn.

Fistulæ made from the first part of the duodenum in a number of species produce a slightly opalescent alkaline viscous juice somewhat of the consistency of egg white. As fistulæ from other parts of the small intestine do not spontaneously produce any flow of juice (when they are mechanically stimulated, a watery fluid appears) it has been concluded that the mucinous juice which spontaneously flows from the duodenum comes from Brunner's glands. It has been shown in the cat, dog and pig that this secretion occurs more when the animal is fed than when it is starved. It can be produced by stimulating the vagus electrically, or by causing a dilute solution of hydrochloric acid to flow over the mucous membrane (Plate B, Figs. *c* and *d*). Furthermore if the duodenum is completely transplanted beneath the skin, so that all its original nerves are severed and it derives a new blood supply from the subcutaneous tissues, mucous secretion still follows the administration of food. Clearly in this case some hormone carried by the blood stimulates secretion. It was demonstrated over 30 years ago that the impure secretin then available acted as such a hormone, but conclusive proof that the action was not due to an impurity had to wait until pure natural and synthetic secretin were produced. Following this it was clearly shown that secretin stimulates Brunner's glands in the dog as effectively as does feeding.[8] There is some reason to treat with reserve at present[8a] the claim that has been made that cholecystokinin is also a hormone for Brunner's glands.[8b]

Thus the part of the intestine immediately adjoining the stomach has a highly organised apparatus for the production of a very viscid alkaline fluid following the ingestion of food. The juice apparently contains no enzymes of importance except a weak amylase and enterokinase. Lysozyme is present in the pig. The juice from fistulæ in a number of different species contained little organic matter—about 0·5 per cent—but, as was stated above, very small amounts of mucin can impart a striking degree of viscosity to an aqueous solution. Neutralising power differed considerably from species to species. In the goat 1 ml. of juice neutralised only 0·04 ml. of N/10 HCl, but in the rabbit the figure was 0·8 ml., while the values for the cat, dog and pig were about 0·25 to 0·5 ml. The neutralising power of these juices is due to their bicarbonate content. With so much bicarbonate present the pH of the juice as collected is high, between 8 and 9, these high values being due to the loss of CO_2 during collection. The muco-substances which give the juice its viscosity are not the same in all species (PLATE C, FIGS. *c*, *d*, *e*) and ultrastructural differences between the glands of different species give further evidence that the products are not always the same[9].

Function of Duodenal Juice

Just where acid gastric content is ejected from the stomach we find an alkaline viscous secretion produced. As has been discussed above, it is reasonable to consider that this juice may play a part in protecting the delicate villi of the duodenum from the possible deleterious effects of the acid chyme. Experiments have shown that the passage of N/10 HCl over the first part of the duodenum activates the secretion of mucus containing bicarbonate and that no damage is suffered by the villi, while the same strength of acid perfused at the same rate over those parts of the small intestine not furnished with Brunner's glands damages the villi severely. It is thus possible that during emptying of the stomach the duodenal villi have a continuous stream of mucous secretion ejected over them from the numerous ducts of Brunner's glands. One can envisage the presence of a constantly replaced alkaline film of mucus which impedes the access of gastric contents to the epithelial cells. Thus with the further strong neutralising power of the pancreatic juice and bile, the cells of the surface of the villi adjacent to the stomach are never subjected to an acidity which they cannot easily bear.

Some experiments on pigs lend support to this idea. It was possible by various types of operation on the stomach and intestine to compare the reactions of the duodenum and ileum to gastric contents, or to undiluted gastric juice. These experiments all led to the conclusion that the duodenum had much more capacity than the ileum to resist the destructive properties of gastric juice.

In the rabbit and possibly other animals the viscous juice may play a further role by suspending and separating food particles, thus allowing better access for the pancreatic enzymes. The fluid part of the secretion is no doubt absorbed in the lower part of the intestine and much of the mucin is incorporated in the fæces.

Peptic Ulceration

A very common lesion in civilised man is the condition called peptic ulceration. The ulcers occur for the most part towards the pyloric end of the stomach and in the duodenum just distal to the pylorus. More rarely they occur in the fundus. An important characteristic of these ulcers is their tendency not to heal but to become fibrosed and "chronic".

Many theories have been propounded to explain this kind of ulceration, and much thought and experimental work has been devoted to understanding why the acid gastric juice does not digest the normal stomach. Not only is intact mucosa not damaged by the gastric juice, but surgical incisions and areas deprived of mucosa usually heal rapidly. Curiously, no one seems to have worried very much about why the pancreatic juice does not digest the small intestine.

In some patients, particularly those with duodenal ulcer, a readily detectable excess of fundal juice is secreted and there is hypermotility of the gastric musculature. It is not unreasonable to suppose that these effects, possibly due to excessive vagal activity, might expose the duodenum unduly to ejections of unbuffered juice from the stomach. But excess secretion is not always found, and there is a strong case for believing that in peptic ulceration there is likely to be some element of lowered resistance locally in the mucosa, perhaps due to a vascular condition such as spasm or unusual distribution of the blood vessels. It has increasingly been realised, however, that the chemical phase of gastric secretion is likewise a very powerful mechanism, and the possibility must be considered that a prolonged output of gastrin, such as might be caused, for example, by the retention of food residues in the stomach, might be a cause of ulceration through the stimulating effect on fundal secretion. These questions are still being argued[10], and they are of importance to the patient as well as the scientist, since the surgeon is likely to base his decision whether to operate, and his choice of operation, in part at least on the particular views he holds about causation.

The Small and Large Intestines

Another cell producing mucus, commonly called a goblet cell from its supposed resemblance to a wine glass, is found throughout the intestine and reaches its maximum numbers in the colon and rectum. Though this cell can generally with some justice be likened to a goblet when it occurs in the small intestine, it may vary much in appearance. In the small intestine its fundamental characteristic in its "full" condition is that the cytoplasm towards the free border of the cell is greatly bellied out by its content of mucigen droplets. In some cases the basal part of the cell containing the nucleus is joined to the mass of mucigen droplets by a narrow stem (Plate D, Figs. *a* and *b*). Sometimes in the small intestine and always in the colon the cells have a shorter, more squat form (Plate D, Figs. *c* and *e*). Goblet cells occur also among the ciliated epithelial cells of the nose, trachea and bronchi in many mammals, including man. Much study has been made of the goblet cells of amphibia and many lowly species of animal, but here attention will be confined to those occurring in mammals.

In the intestine there is a constant shedding or desquamation of epithelial cells from the tips of the villi in the small intestine and from the surface of the mucosa in the large. These are replaced by cells newly formed throughout the crypts, in which region mitoses are common. Mitoses are never seen at the site of loss.

As new cells are formed in the crypts those above slide towards the surface, moving (in the jejunum of the young rat) at the rate of between 1 and 1·5 cell diameters an hour, so that gaps caused by the shedding of cells from the exposed surface are continually made good. The journey from the crypts of the small intestine to the tips of the villi is said to take 2 to 3 days in the rat and mouse and about 6 days in man. Studies in the small intestine of the rat show that mitoses take place in all parts of the crypt except a narrow band at the external end. While most of the new cells toward the base of the crypt go on to further divisions most of those toward the external end must differentiate to form the specialised covering of the villi, and some changes in the cell enzymes have been identified in this area which may perhaps be correlated with the initiation of differentiation. If cell loss is for any reason increased, as it may be during variations in feeding and in hormone balance or under the influence of a diurnal rhythm, as well as after pathological damage, there cannot be much acceleration of the already short cell cycle; compensation is more likely to be by way of a temporary outward movement of the level at which differentiation starts.[11] Some of the factors affecting cell renewal and the abnormalities which may take place in disease have been reviewed by Creamer.[11a]

There has been much discussion as to whether goblet cells are of a different kind from the ordinary epithelial cells. At any rate there is evidence that once a cell starts to make mucin it probably retains this capacity, though even this cannot be stated with absolute certainty.

Discharge and synthesis in goblet cells.—The granules or droplets of mucigen issue from the goblet cell into the lumen of a crypt or of the intestine, where they dissolve into a homogeneous mass (PLATE D, FIGS. *b* and *e*). The apparently "full" goblet, the type that predominates in a normal intestine, is not in the static state that its appearance suggests but is continuously synthesising and discharging mucin. By injecting labelled sulphate it can be shown that ^{35}S is incorporated near the cell nucleus into the mucigen of even "full" goblets and moves steadily forward with the mucigen within the cell until it is discharged at the surface within about 24 hours. There is no marked change in the total amount of mucin in the cell during this time (PLATE E, FIGS. *a–j*). Electron microscopic autoradiography has confirmed that sulphation of the mucopolysaccharides takes place in the Golgi region, and has further shown that the incorporation of glucose into complex carbohydrates takes place there. When glucose-6-H^3 had been injected into young rats the interval from the appearance of radioactive material in the Golgi region of colonic goblet cells to its discharge in mucigen droplets at the cell surface was about 4 hours, and it was calculated that a fresh Golgi saccule, enclosing a new droplet, was released from each stack of Golgi membranes every 2 to 4 minutes.[12] Thus it seems that the mucin molecule is finally put together, and the carbohydrate component probably synthesized, by the Golgi apparatus and that this goes on continuously and is balanced by continuous discharge.

Sometimes cells are found in which a residue only of mucin is present at the free border, while a few discrete granules of mucigen occupy the Golgi body area just above the nucleus. It is difficult to resist the view that these cells represent goblets in which discharge has been faster than synthesis, and this is confirmed by the fact that if an irritant is applied at the surface of the mucosa so as to induce an excessive flow of mucin many or all of the goblets are found in this partially discharged state within quite a short time (PLATE D, FIGS. *g–k*). Such cells begin immediately to replenish their contents, and there is evidence of heightened synthetic activity during this time. If the irritant is removed, full goblet cells are found again within a few hours.

The Effects of Local Irritation on the Colon

One effect of an irritant, whether chemical or mechanical, seems to be to speed up discharge of the goblet cells—compare FIGS. *h* and *o* of PLATE E. When the colon of an animal is stimulated by mustard oil much mucus is seen to be formed. As the goblet cells discharge their mucigen it dissolves in the alkaline watery fluid that is also produced, so that mucus of an egg white-like consistency pours into the gut lumen. This mucus contains desquamated cells and emigrated leucocytes, and perhaps fluid that has exuded from the blood vessels, for under a powerful irritant the discharge of mucin is not always adequate to protect the tissue from the injurious substance. The superficial cells die and desquamate into the lumen of the intestine. Œdema develops in the stroma supporting the epithelial cells and in the submucosa, and there is dilatation of the lymphatics draining the mucosa. Polymorphs appear in the stroma, and some make their way into the lumen to join the desquamated epithelial cells. In other words, inflammation takes place. The increased rate of loss of epithelial cells leads to spreading of neighbouring cells to help cover the defect and to an increase of mitoses in the usual position, the lower part of the crypts. No doubt this is what occurs in inflammation of the human gut such as is caused by infection with dysentery bacilli, when one of the signs of infection is the passage of liquid fæces containing much mucus.

A strong irritant is not essential for producing changes in goblet cells. Even the simple manœuvre of washing out solid fæces with saline or perfusion with normal saline or water will produce histologically recognisable discharge of the goblet cells.

Recovery from Inflammatory Changes

The process of recovery of an inflamed mucosa has been followed histologically in animals, mainly rats and cats, after the application of dilute mustard oil.

If the stimulus is sufficiently violent no granules of mucigen recognisable by histological means may remain, but in an hour or two granules appear again in the Golgi body area and build up a column which reaches to the surface. Such a stage had been reached in rats 6 hours after removal of the irritant, and by 24 hours the mucosa had a full complement of goblets of normal size and shape. During this process the uptake of ^{35}S from injected $Na_2{}^{35}SO_4$ is greatly increased (PLATE E, FIGS. *h* and *o*), showing that there is an increased rate of synthesis of sulphated glycoproteins. Methionine labelled with ^{35}S is concentrated in the epithelium, but the radioactivity does not enter the mucin (PLATE E, FIG. *p*.)

If surface epithelium has been lost there is immediate temporary "patching" of the gaps by spreading out of neighbouring cells, so that though groups of detached epithelial cells may be seen lying free in the lumen it is not apparent where they have come from. Within a few hours increased mitosis in the crypts begins to produce new cells which slide upwards and form a more effective covering. The inflammation in the interstitial tissue subsides as inflammation does elsewhere.

Only if damage has been very severe, with considerable necrosis of the mucosa, are more serious results seen. In such cases damage seems to progress even after the irritant has been removed; 3 days later the wall of the colon

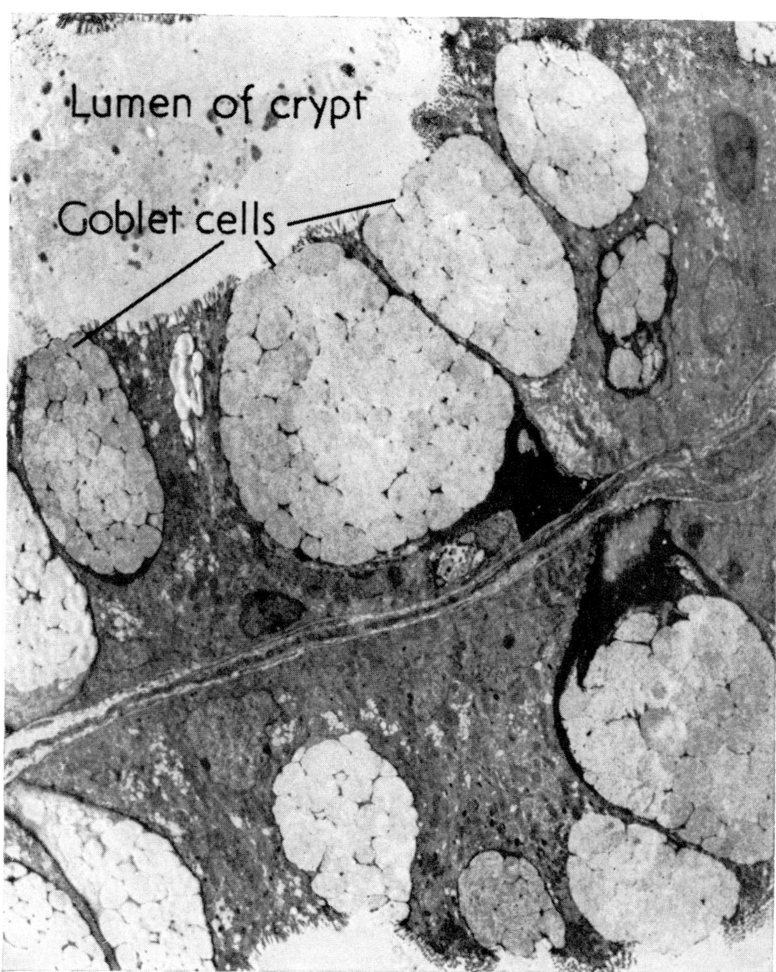

6/FIG. 1.—The bases of two crypts of the colon of a mouse. Numerous goblet cells crammed with mucigen droplets can be seen between the ordinary epithelial cells, the "brush borders" (microvilli) of which can be recognised. The cytoplasm and nuclei are much denser in the goblet cells than in the other cells. The cells of one crypt are separated from those of the other by a thin layer of fibres. (× 2800.)

is still thickened by œdema, and it may be almost impossible to find an intact epithelial cell. In these cases healing would include some fibrosis, but eventual complete covering by epithelium and re-formation of glands (though these might be irregular) could be expected.

This picture of recovery seen in animals is no doubt applicable to man recovering from inflammation and ulceration in the colon such as occurs in bacillary or amœbic dysentery. It has some application also to a disease known as "ulcerative colitis", in which there may be severe chronic inflammation in the

PLATE D (*opposite*)

(*a*) Full goblet cell from small intestine of the pig to show the stem of the goblet and the granular structure of the mucigen which distends the cup. Harris's hæmatoxylin, mucicarmine and metanil yellow. (× 900.)

(*b*) Goblet cell from small intestine of the pig to show the discharge of mucin from the free border of the cell. Mucigen granules can be seen above the nucleus in the stem of the cell. Staining as for FIG. *a* (× 900.)

(*c*) Goblet cell from small intestine of the pig to show a shorter form. Note granular contents, the absence of a stem and compression of the nucleus at the base of the cell. Staining as for FIG. *a* (× 900.)

(*d*) Goblet cell from the growing edge of an artificial ulcer in the colon of the cat. Note the granules just above the nucleus in the Golgi body area and the collection of granules towards the free end of the cell. Harris's hæmatoxylin, periodic acid-Schiff and tartrazine. (× 900.)

(*e*) Colon of cat to show goblet cells emptying their content into the lumen of a crypt. The granules are undergoing solution to form homogeneous mucus. Staining as for FIG. *d*. (× 900.)

(*f*) Partially emptied goblet cell from the colon of a cat. Staining as for FIG. *d*. (× 900.)

(*g*) Goblet cell from the duodenum of a rabbit through which N/15 HC1 had been perfused for 4 hr. The cell has voided some of its mucin. Granules are present above the nucleus and some pink mucus is still within the theca. Staining as for FIG. *d*. (× 900.)

(*h*) From the same specimen as FIG. *g* to show more complete emptying of a goblet cell. Here again granules are well seen in the supranuclear region. (× 900.)

(*i*) Rat colon stimulated by mustard oil. The goblet cells of the crypt have largely discharged their mucin and are now similar in shape to the ordinary cylindrical epithelial cells. Staining as for FIG. *d*. (× 900.)

(*j*) Transverse section across the crypts of normal colon of the rat. The goblet cells are full of mucin. Harris's hæmatoxylin, mucicarmine and metanil yellow. (× 900.)

(*k*) From the same rat as FIG. *j*. Transverse section of the crypts in a loop of colon which had been filled with dilute mustard oil for 6 hr. In response to the irritation the goblet cells have almost completely discharged their mucin. Staining as for FIG. *j*. (× 225.)

(From Florey.[1])

interstitial tissues, and breakdown of the epithelium. The cause of these changes is not known, though some hypersensitivity reaction has been suggested; bacterial infection does not seem to be responsible. The fæces may contain mucus and blood, and the crypts often show an excessive number of goblet cells. As damage proceeds the epithelium makes vigorous attempts at regeneration, with mitotic activity in the crypts and spreading of young cells over bared surfaces.

Observations with the Electron Microscope

Investigation of the fine structure of the goblet cells of the colon of the rat and mouse has added some details to our knowledge of the process of the elaboration of mucigen, and its discharge on stimulation by mustard oil.

FIGURE 1 gives a general picture of the appearance of full goblet cells in a crypt of the colon of a mouse. Goblet cells from an unstimulated colon contain

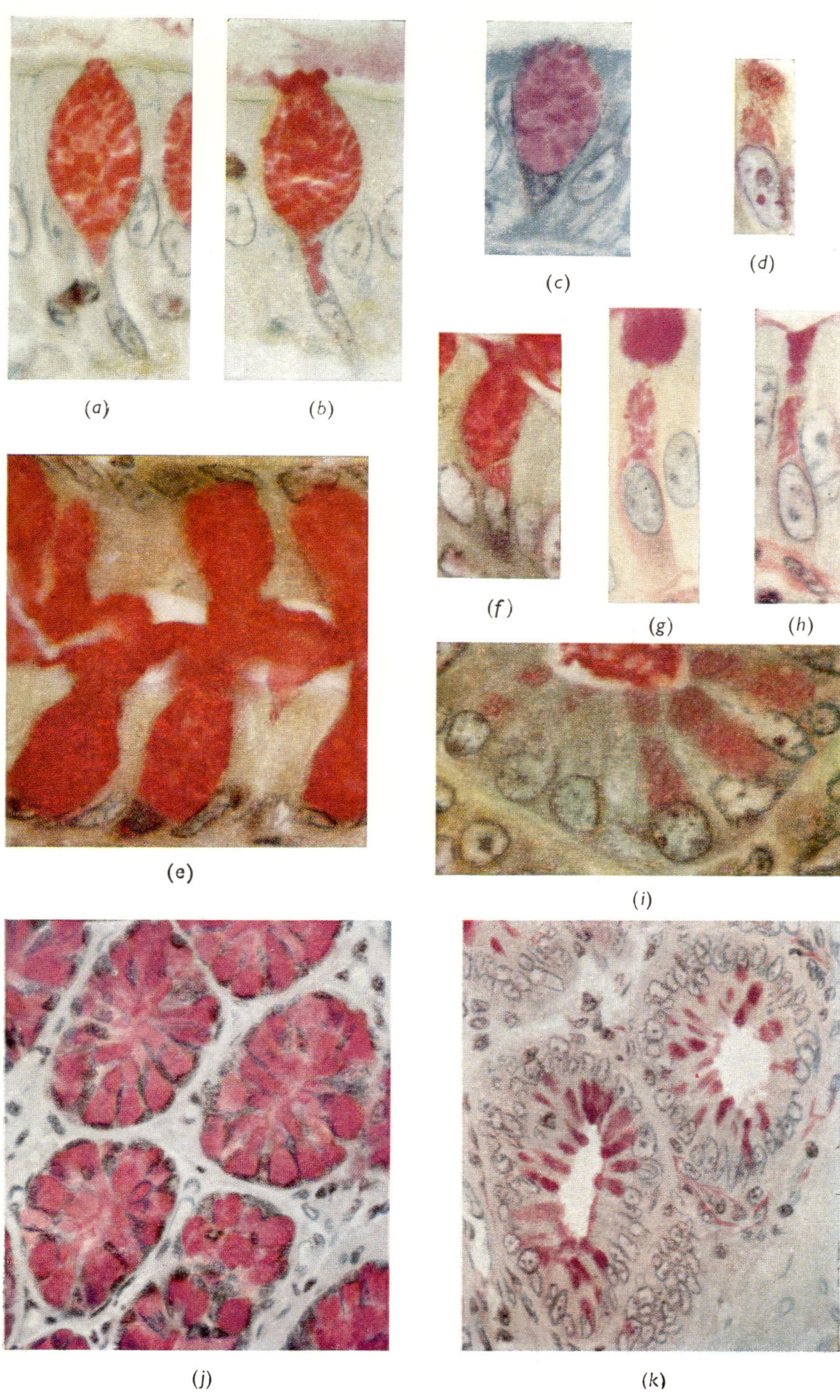

(a)
(b)
(c)
(d)
(e)
(f)
(g)
(h)
(i)
(j)
(k)

PLATE E

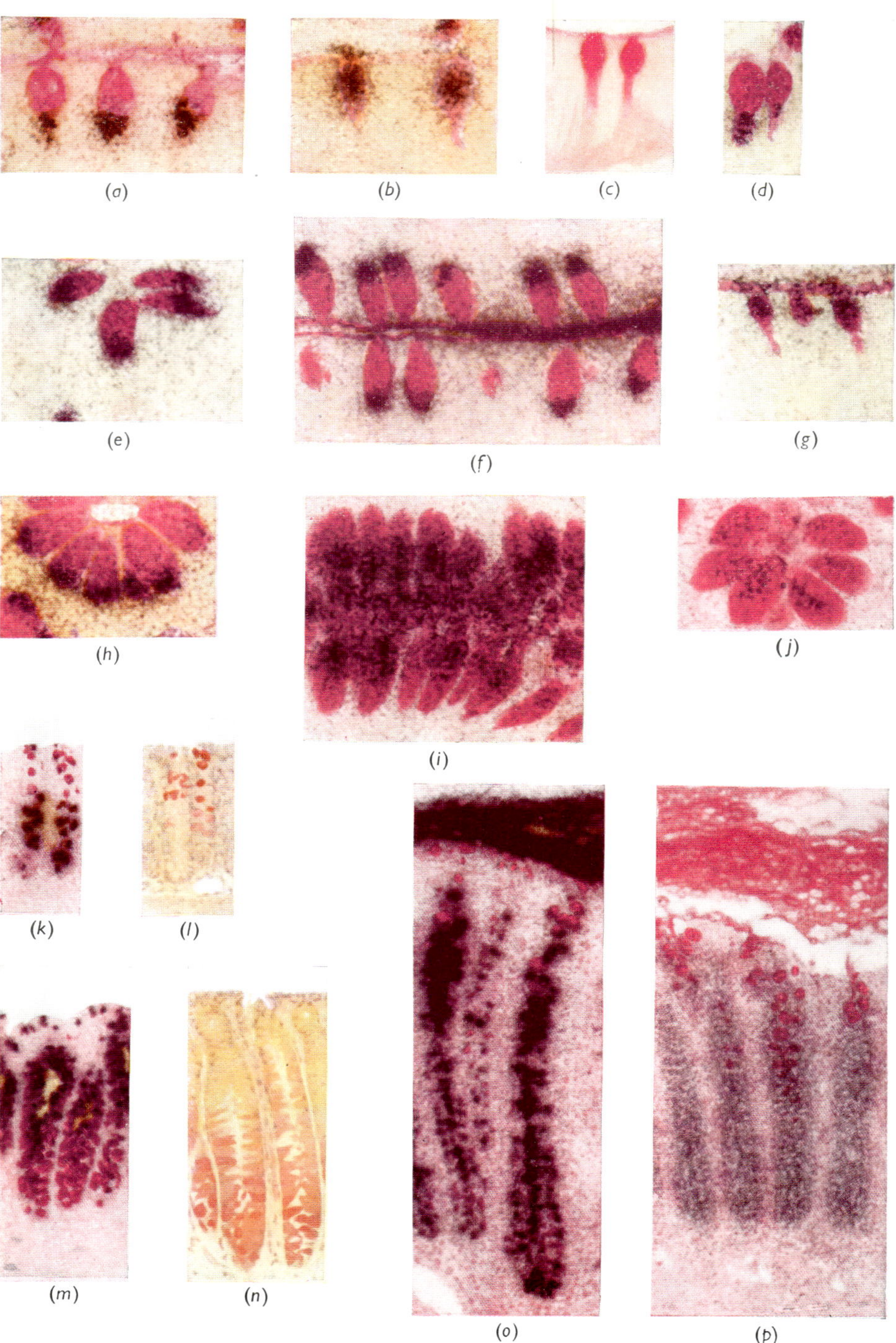

PLATE E (*opposite*)

Autoradiographs of intestine prepared in the same way as those in PLATE C. All the animals were injected with $Na_2{}^{35}SO_4$ except that shown in FIG. *p*.

(*a, b* and *c*) Ileum of mice killed 3¼, 6 and 12 hr. after injection respectively. In all the pictures the lumen of a crypt is at the top. The nuclei of the goblet cells are not stained, but are just below the mucus mass in each cell. At 3¼ hr. radioactivity is present in the mucus in the supranuclear region; at 6 hr. radioactivity is general in the goblet and some radioactive mucus has been secreted on to the surface; at 12 hr. all the radioactive mucus has left the cell. (× 480.)

(*d* and *e*) Ileum of rats killed 1 hr. 10 min. and 3 hr. after injection. In FIG. *d* the lumen of a crypt is at the top, in FIG. *e* four goblet cells are grouped round a crypt lumen which is faintly seen in the upper part of the picture. Radioactivity is concentrated in the mucus in the supranuclear region. (× 480.)

(*f*) Ileum of cat killed 2¼ hr. after injection. A crypt runs across the centre of the picture. Radioactivity is concentrated in the mucus of the supranuclear region and there is already some radioactive mucus in the lumen. (× 480.)

(*g*) Ileum of guinea-pig killed 6½ hr. after injection. The mucus mass in the goblets is radioactive and radioactive mucus has been secreted into the crypt lumen. (× 480.)

(*h, i* and *j*) Colons of mice killed 3¼, 12 and 24 hr. after injection respectively. At 3¼ hr. radioactivity is localised in the mucus in the supranuclear region, at 12 hr. it is general in the mucin mass and radioactive mucin has been secreted into the lumen of the crypt. At 24 hr. only a trace of activity is left. (× 480.)

(*k, l, m* and *n*) Colons of guinea-pig (*k, l*) and rabbit (*m, n*) killed 6½ and 6¼ hr. after injection respectively. FIGURES *k* and *m* are autoradiographs and FIGS. *l* and *n* are ordinary sections from the same blocks stained by the periodic acid-Schiff method and tartrazine.

FIGURES *k* and *m* show that in these species some colonic goblet cells take up ^{35}S more vigorously than others, and that the position in the crypts of the cells showing the most radioactivity is different in the two species. FIGURES *l* and *n* show that the intensity of ^{35}S incorporation is inversely proportional to the strength of the P.A.S. reaction. (× 120.)

(*o*) Colon of mouse killed 2½ hr. after injection. The goblet cells had discharged most of their mucus in response to the irritant dilute mustard oil, which was applied to the mucosa for 4 hr. before the injection was made. The general radioactivity of the mucus in the goblet cells, in the crypt lumens and on the surface shows how greatly synthesis and discharge were speeded up in response to irritation. Compare with FIG. *h*. (× 175.)

(*p*) Colon of mouse killed 2½ hr. after injection of ^{35}S-methionine. Similar stimulus to that described for FIG. *o*. Radioactivity is present generally in the epithelium, but there is none in the mucus. Compare with FIG. *o*. (× 175.)

(From Jennings and Florey.[2])

profiles corresponding to the droplets seen by the light microscope. These droplets are contained within a thin rim of cytoplasm, known as the theca, and are separated by apparently discontinuous bands of cytoplasm. They discharge, under physiological conditions, by breaking through the thin cytoplasmic surface of the cell (FIG. 2). Between the "goblet" and the nucleus can be seen an abundant collection of smooth membranes which is the Golgi complex. Between these membranes oval or round expansions occur which vary in size from just perceptible separation of the membranes to large profiles which look much like mature mucigen droplets (FIG. 3).

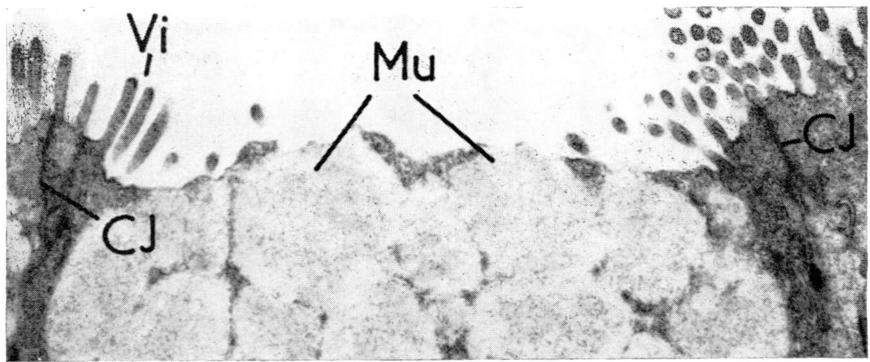

6/FIG. 2.—The free surface of a goblet cell in a rat's colon. The globules of mucin (Mu) are penetrating the thin cytoplasmic covering of the cell. The boundary of the goblet cell is shown by the cell junction (CJ). Microvilli are visible on the goblet cell as well as on the ordinary epithelial cells. (× 21,000.) (From Florey.[13])

In the rest of the cell there is an abundance of rough membranes, that is, the endoplasmic reticulum which is studded with ribonucleoprotein granules (ribosomes). These membranes are often arranged more or less parallel to the nuclear membrane (FIG. 3). No droplets can be seen between them. Mitochondria are sometimes found at the periphery of the theca but never between the mature droplets.

Goblet cells, both nuclei and cytoplasm, are strongly osmiophilic and they stand out in contrast to the principal epithelial cells. It is thus easy to see, especially when the goblets have been discharged, that there are very intricate interdigitations between the two types of cell (FIGS. 4 and 10). The goblet cells are joined to neighbouring cells by well-defined desmosomes (FIG. 5). The part of the theca abutting on the lumen possesses microvilli similar to those covering the principal cells (FIGS. 2, 5, 8 and 9).

When mustard oil is applied to the colon there is apparently a massive discharge of the mucin content of the goblet cells (FIG. 6). As with the light microscope, exhausted goblet cells always display some droplets of mucigen scattered through the cytoplasm (FIG. 7), usually with sharply defined bounding membranes (FIGS. 8 and 9) in contrast to the somewhat ill-defined cytoplasmic investment of mature droplets in full cells. An extensive Golgi complex, displaying a wide range of droplet size between the membranes, can always be recognised in discharged cells (FIG. 10), endoplasmic reticulum is plentiful, and there are many mitochondria (FIG. 11).

These observations extend those made with the light microscope on many kinds of mucus-producing cells which showed that mucigen droplets appear

6/FIG. 3 (*see opposite*).—Part of a goblet cell from the normal colon of a rat. Two stacks of Golgi saccules are clearly seen (one marked GC). Externally the saccules are flattened and have no visible lumen, but they become progressively more dilated towards the interior of the cell and their contents increasingly resemble the fully formed mucigen droplets to the left of the picture (Mu). No recognisable mucigen droplets can be seen in the endoplasmic reticulum studded with ribosomes (ER). The constituents of the goblet cell are dense compared with those of the neighbouring epithelial cells. The plasma membrane (Me) of neighbouring cells can be seen about the dark prolongations of the goblet cell. (× 31,000.) (From Florey.[13])

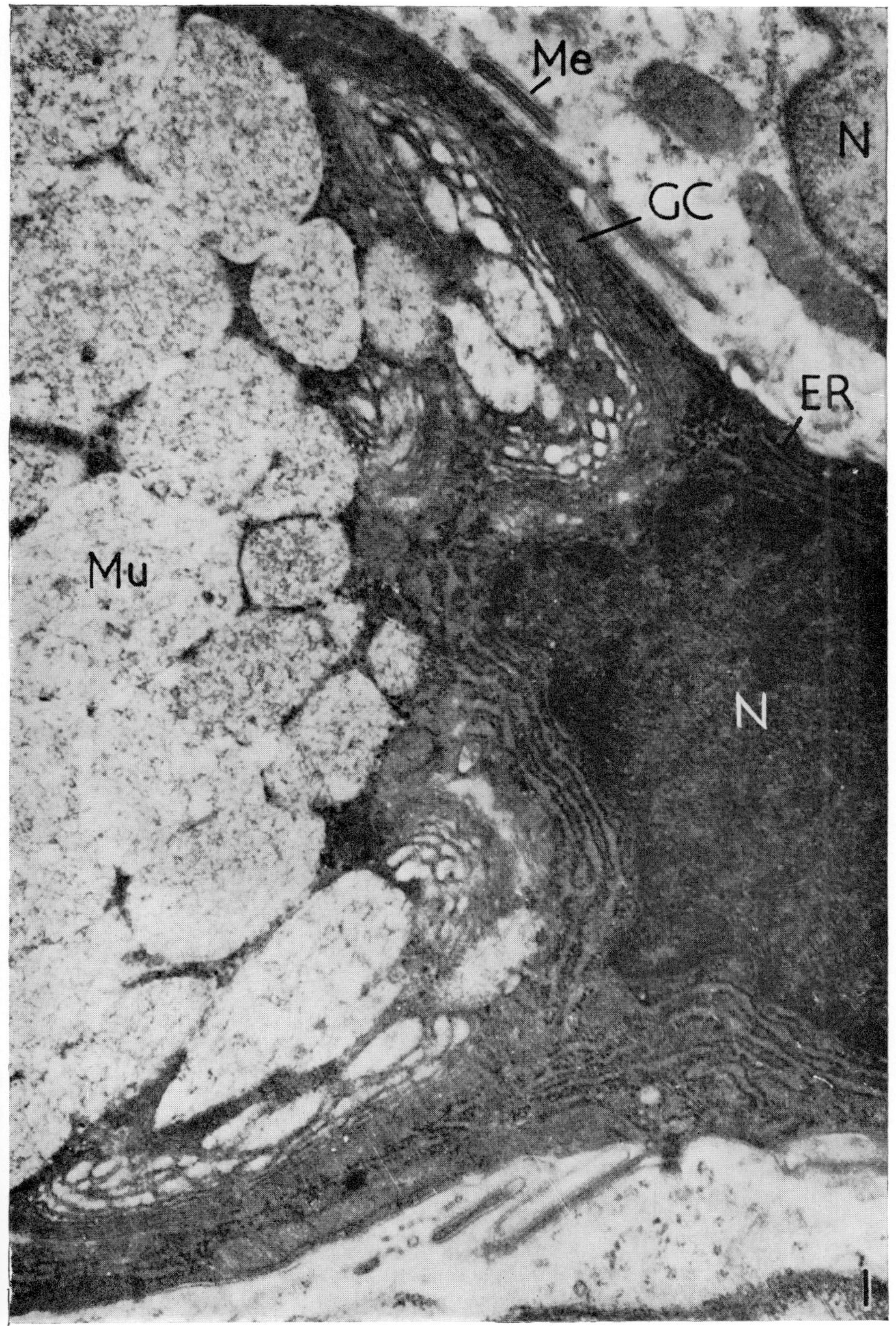

6/FIG. 3.

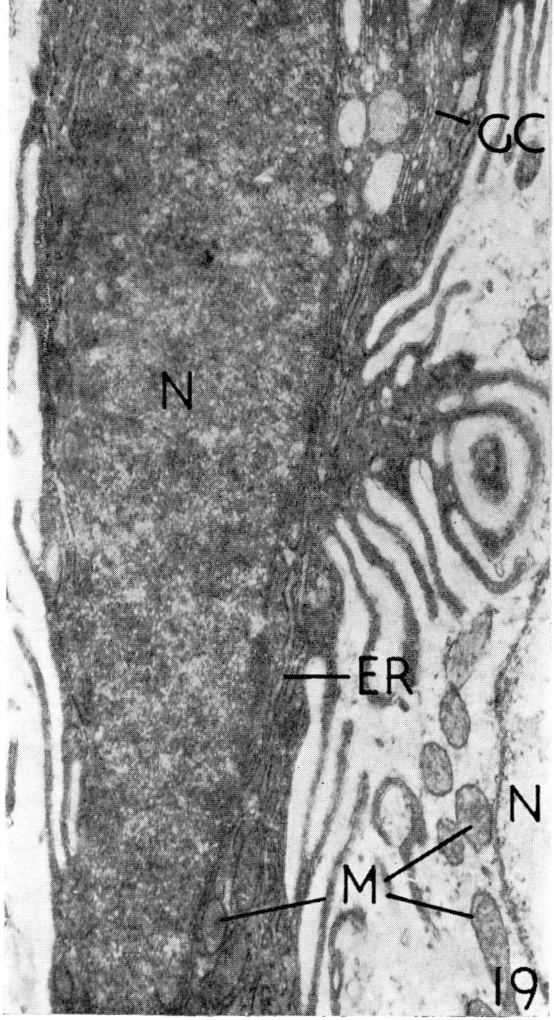

6/Fig. 4.—A longitudinal section of an exhausted goblet cell. The smooth Golgi membranes (GC) and the rough membranes (ER) are both seen, as are the complex interdigitations between the goblet cell and the less dense neighbouring epithelial cells. Both kinds of cell contain mitochondria (M). The nucleus (N) as well as the cytoplasm is denser in the goblet cell. (× 17,000.) (From Florey.[13])

first in the supranuclear region—the region of the Golgi complex. It now appears that recognisable collections of mucigen can first be seen between the lamellæ of the smooth membranes which make up the Golgi complex. No doubt the rough membranes are engaged in the synthesis of material which contributes to the glycoproteins but, as described above, there is reason to think that glucose and sulphur may be attached in the Golgi region. The collections of mucigen increase in size until they leave the Golgi area as membrane-bounded droplets. These pass towards the free pole of the cell, accumulating there in such amounts as to bulge out the cell walls. Finally the globules of mucigen are discharged through the surface layer of the theca, which breaks down (Fig. 2) but can

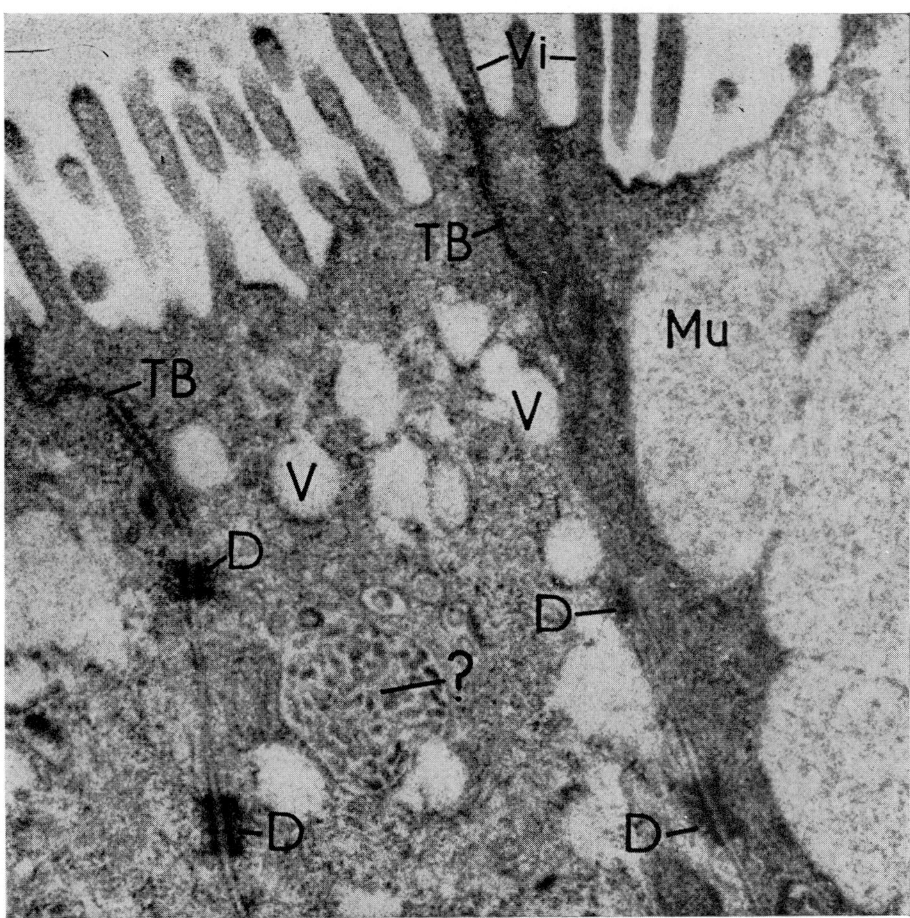

6/FIG. 5.—The apposed surfaces of a goblet cell containing mucigen (Mu) and an ordinary epithelial cell. The apposed membranes or junctions bounding the cells show a number of dense structures, the desmosomes (D) possibly representing regions of cell-to-cell communication. Close to the free surface the cell membranes are denser than elsewhere and are called terminal bars (TB). Microvilli (Vi) are present on both epithelial and goblet cells. The epithelial cell contains vesicles (V) and an unidentified structure (?). (× 41,000.) (From Florey.[13])

apparently be reconstituted. Mucin is continuously elaborated to replace that lost at the cell surface so that usually the cell remains full. When under conditions of irritation the cells discharge their globules quickly the same process of continuous replacement goes on in the Golgi complex, and is apparently accelerated to make good the loss.

Exactly how water and salts are added to the mucigen globules to form the thick mucin which appears at the surface is not clear, for no morphological evidence of the passage of water through the goblet cells or their neighbours has been obtained.

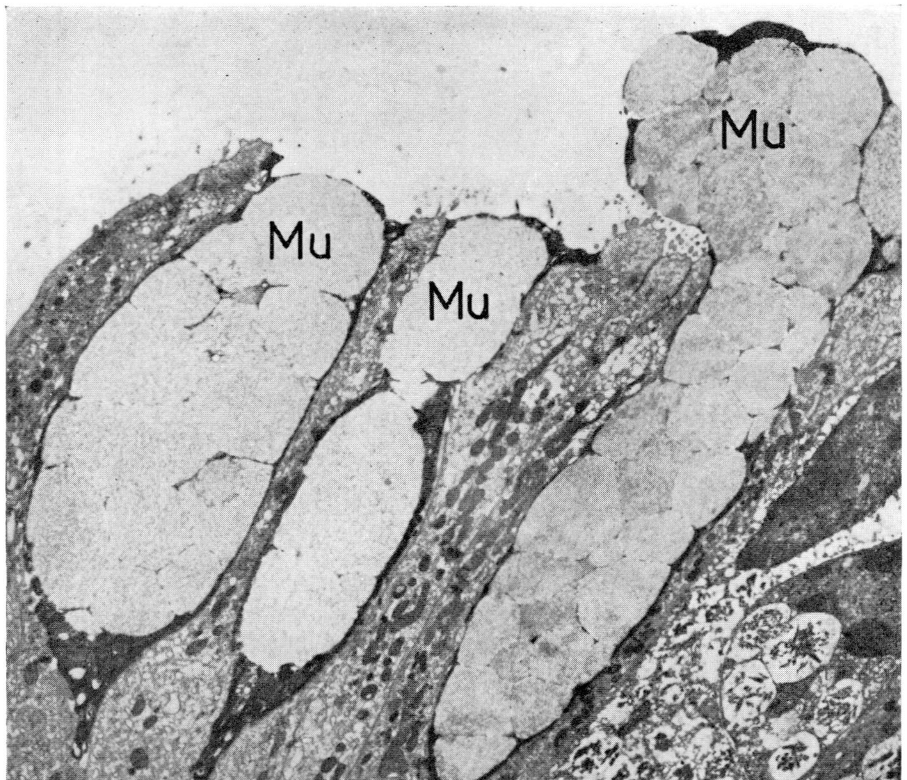

6/Fig. 6.—Goblet cells in the colon of a rat. They are discharging their mucigen (Mu) in response to irritation by dilute mustard oil. (× 7,000.) (From Florey.[13])

Mechanisms of Discharge and Synthesis of Mucus in the Colon

Our knowledge of the mechanisms by which the changes described above are brought about is very small. The emptying of goblet cells is probably an active secretory process, for if the vessels of the colon are perfused by plasma containing cyanide, thus paralysing cell mechanisms dependent on oxygen, no secretion takes place in response to mustard oil.

It has long been known that pilocarpine will cause violent movements of the smooth muscle of the intestine, and that fæces coated with mucus and eventually a mucous fluid are expelled from the rectum in cats and dogs given large doses. Histological investigation shows that this drug to a large extent empties the colonic goblet cells.

In the decerebrate cat faradic stimulation of the peripheral ends of the cut nervi erigentes—the nerves supplying the colon—caused that organ to secrete considerable amounts of fluid of variable viscosity. In some experiments it was so viscid that it clung together and fell from a test-tube in a single drop of 10 ml., while in other cases it was as fluid as water. Histological examination showed

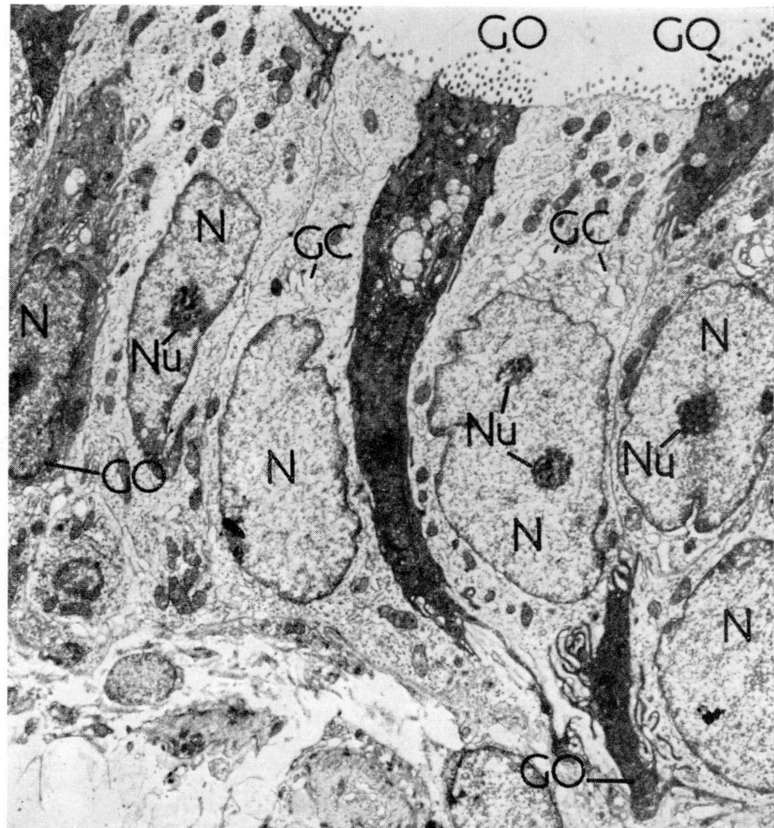

6/Fig. 7.—Goblet cells (GO) from which most of the mucin content has been exhausted by stimulation with mustard oil, though there are still some mucigen droplets in the discharged cells. The goblet cells are much darker than the ordinary epithelial cells, and the bizarre prolongations and interdigitations of the goblets with neighbouring cells can be seen. Nuclei (N) containing nucleoli (Nu) can be recognised in the epithelial cells which also display a Golgi complex with vacuoles (GC) above the nucleus. (× 5000.) (From Florey.[13])

that in many experiments the goblet cells had been evacuated. The fact that under appropriate conditions stimulation of nerves provokes a considerable colonic secretion may have some bearing on the disease condition known as "mucous colitis", in which large amounts of mucus are passed, though there is no demonstrable inflammatory lesion in the colon—in fact no "-itis".

In spite of this well-defined action of the nerves we do not know what part, if any, the nerves play in the reaction to inflammation in the colon of an intact animal. The inflammatory production of mucus by the goblet cells proceeds in response to local irritation if the nerves are divided. Mucus is secreted in a piece of colon isolated from all its intraperitoneal connections, and hence from its nerve supply, by being transplanted into the belly wall of the dog. Cocainisation of the mucosa does not inhibit the secretion caused by local irritation.

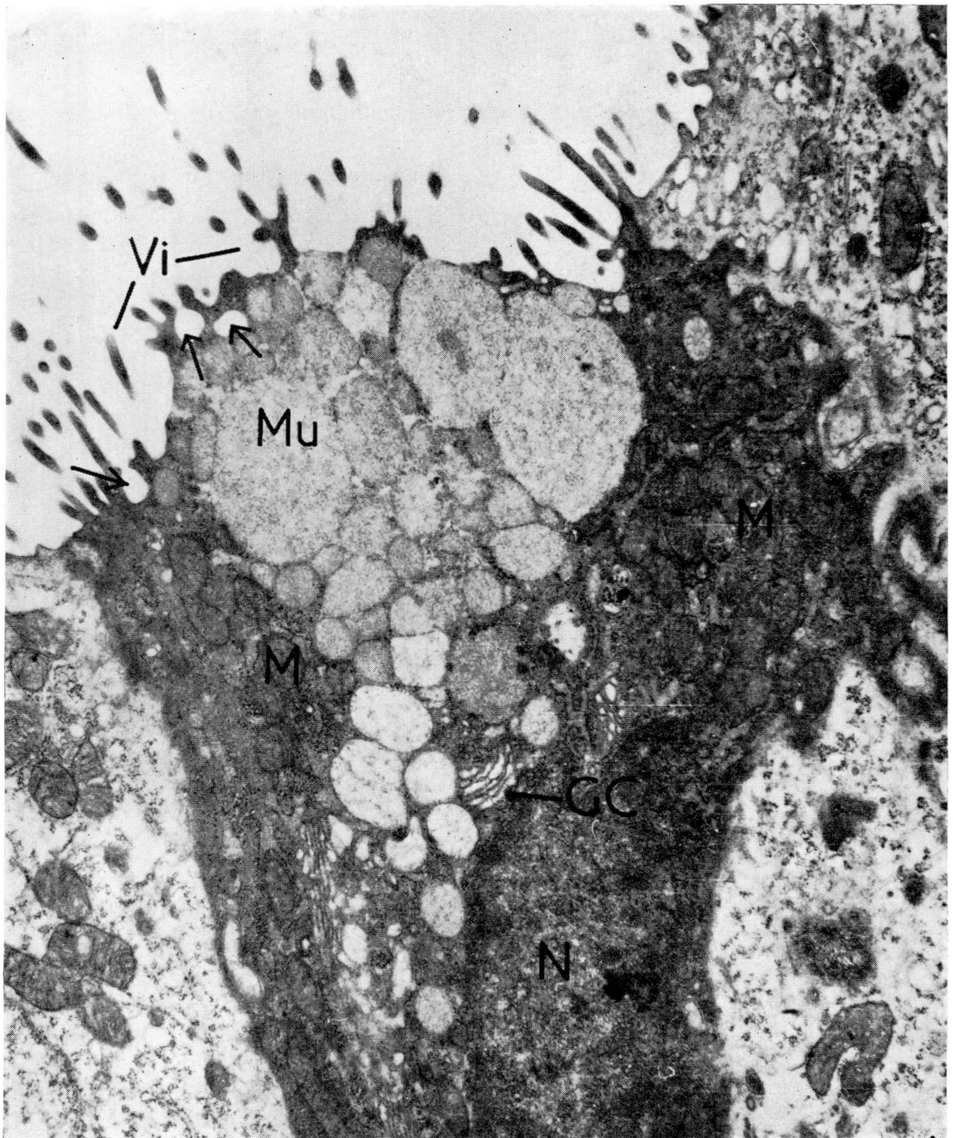

6/FIG. 8.—A goblet cell in the colon of a rat discharging in response to the application of dilute mustard oil. Much of the mucin (Mu) has already left the cell. Circular profiles of droplets of mucigen, clearly defined by a membrane, are present in the region of the Golgi complex (GC) which shows well the dilated saccules in the inner parts of the stacks. Many mitochondria (M) can be recognised. Microvilli (Vi) are reforming on the surface of the cell. The arrows are pointing to spaces from which mucigen droplets may have been discharged. (× 16,000.) (From Florey.[13])

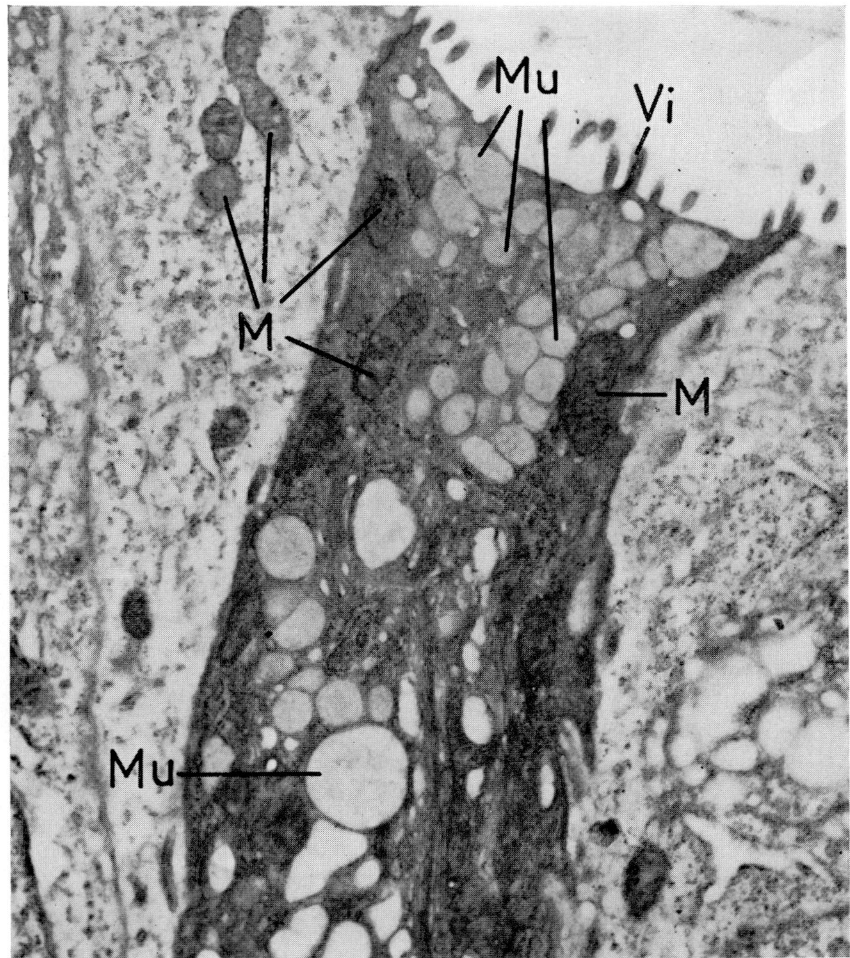

6/FIG. 9.—A goblet cell in the colon of the rat discharging following the application of dilute mustard oil. This picture shows mucigen droplets (Mu) bounded by well-defined surface membranes. Droplets near the free border of the cell are smaller than some in the depths. The surface of the cell is completely reformed and shows microvilli (Vi). Numerous mitochondria (M) can be seen both in the goblet cell and the neighbouring epithelial cells. (× 16,000.) (From Florey.[13])

It seemed possible that histamine, which may be responsible for some of the changes that develop in inflamed connective tissues, might play a part in mucous secretion following irritation. But the application of histamine locally to the mucosa of the colon did not cause any discharge of the goblet cells. The effects of other postulated mediators of inflammatory responses have not so far been ascertained.

Cortisone, which in large doses interferes with the synthesis of mesenchymal muco-substances, had no effect on the rate at which colonic epithelial mucin was replaced after a period of inflammation.

The Small Intestine

The small intestine seems to respond to local irritation in much the same manner as the colon, though there has been less experimental work on it. The goblet cells can be evacuated by applying irritants locally. It has not been possible to demonstrate any nervous control of their activity and it is at present uncertain whether the extrinsic nerves play any part in their emptying in response to a stimulus causing inflammation.

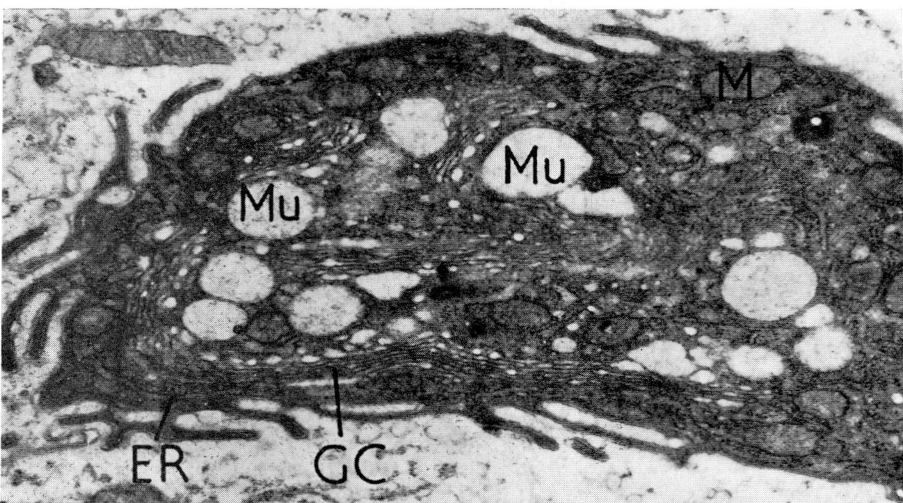

6/Fig. 10.—A cross section of an exhausted goblet cell in the supranuclear region. Small droplets of mucigen can be seen in dilated saccules of the numerous Golgi stacks (GC). Some larger droplets (Mu) are also seen. The endoplasmic reticulum (ER) lined with ribosomes does not contain droplets. Mitochondria (M) are plentiful. The interdigitations with neighbouring cells are well shown. (× 19,000.) (From Florey.[13])

Functions of Mucus produced by Intestinal Goblet Cells

As mucus produced by goblet cells is a slimy substance it has naturally been suggested that its physiological function is to lubricate the passage of fæces. While this may well be its most important normal function in those places where the fæces are semi-solid or even hard, namely in the colon and rectum of man and of those animals producing dry fæces, it seems unlikely that it performs this function in the small intestine where the contents are fluid.

Some observations show that particles which might impinge on and perhaps damage the villi are caught up and held in the mucus on the surface. If the small intestine of the cat be opened and spread out for observation under suitable conditions, particles of a suspension of graphite can be seen caught on strands of mucus, which when defined in this way have a lace-like appearance. The villi protrude and retreat through this covering, and in so doing bring

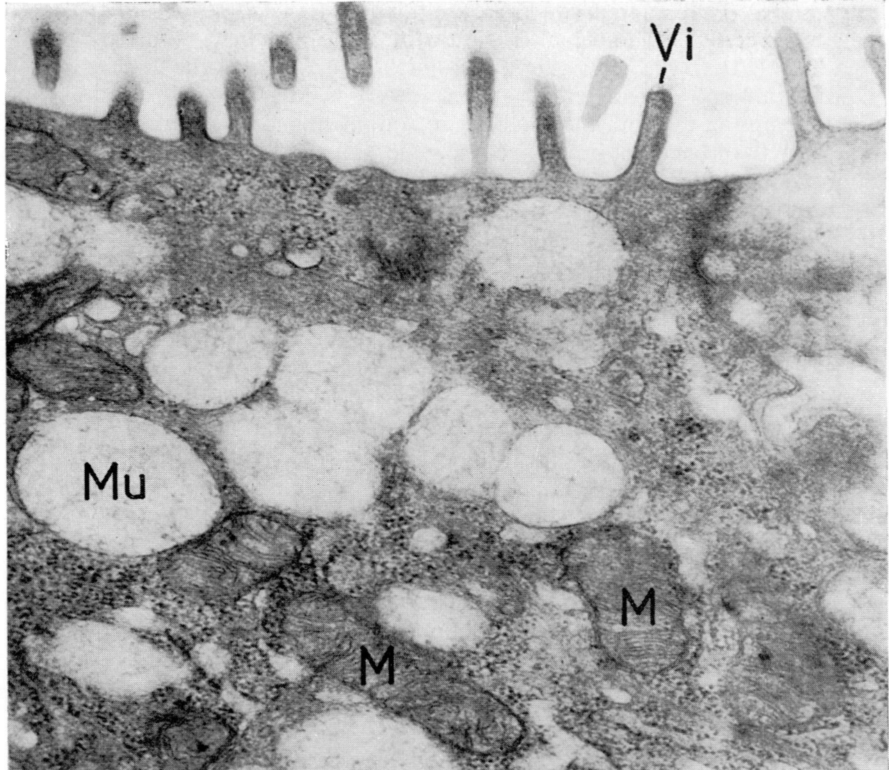

6/FIG. 11.—The surface of an exhausted goblet cell which shows reformed microvilli (Vi). Numerous droplets of mucigen (Mu), some of which show a clearly defined bounding membrane, are present. Several mitochondria (M) can also be recognised. (× 38,000.) (From Florey.[13])

any graphite particles which may have adhered to them into contact with the mucus. The particles are trapped in the mucous layer, and the villi are thus cleaned.

When a starved cat is given a suspension of graphite by stomach tube the carbon passes into the intestine, and in some places may come into intimate contact with the free borders of the epithelial cells. From this situation it may be caught in mucin exuding from goblets and by the movements just described the carbon may be rolled up into little balls 1 mm. or so in diameter, which gradually fuse until by the time the colon is reached all the carbon is collected into a black desiccated mass that is held together by mucin.

No doubt indigestible food particles and the bacteria that grow in the intestine are compacted together in a similar way by normal mucous secretion and thus mechanically kept from damaging the epithelial cells. This mechanism is not by any means perfect, for it was found that bacteria inserted into the intestine of the guinea-pig came into direct contact with the epithelial cells and even lay apparently in the brush border, oriented in line with the microvilli (PLATE F,

FIGS. *a* and *c*). That bacteria can grow comfortably in the crypts of the cat's colon seems to be certain, the normal slow flow of mucus not being sufficient to dislodge them (PLATE F, FIG. *d*), though a quicker discharge of the goblets caused by an inflammatory agent removes them (PLATE F, FIG. *b*).

It is tempting to think that mucous secretions might themselves be inimical to the growth of bacteria, but so far lysozyme, the only antibacterial constituent demonstrated, has not been shown to protect the body from bacterial invasion. Any protection that the intestinal mucous secretions afford must be largely attributed to their physical properties. We can look on the vigorous secretory response of the goblet cells of the colon and small intestine to an irritant, either artificial or in the form of pathogenic bacteria and their products, as an attempt to dilute the irritant, to push it away from the epithelial cells by a viscous fluid, to help to evacuate it, and, if it is solid, to "wrap it up".

MUCOUS SECRETION IN THE RESPIRATORY PASSAGES

It is regrettable that only too often most of us have viral infections of the nasal passages and of the trachea which are unpleasant in themselves and prepare the way for bacterial invaders. The nose, trachea and bronchi are furnished with a double set of cells producing mucus. Some are deeply placed in the mucosa and gathered together into gland acini; their secretion is collected by ducts that empty on to the surface of the mucosa (FIG. 12). The cells of the acini appear non-granular and distended or granular, and this difference in appearance

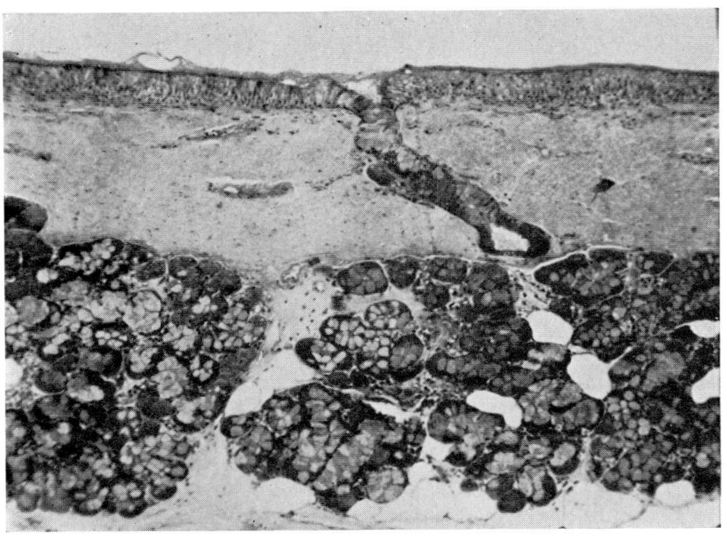

6/FIG. 12.—TRACHEA OF THE PIG

Mucicarmine stain. Glands consisting of "serous" cells (pale) and "mucous" cells are seen in the depths of the mucosa. A duct leading from the acini can be seen emerging on to the surface, which is covered by a thin layer of mucus. To the material from the glands mucus from the superficial goblet cells is added.

PLATE F

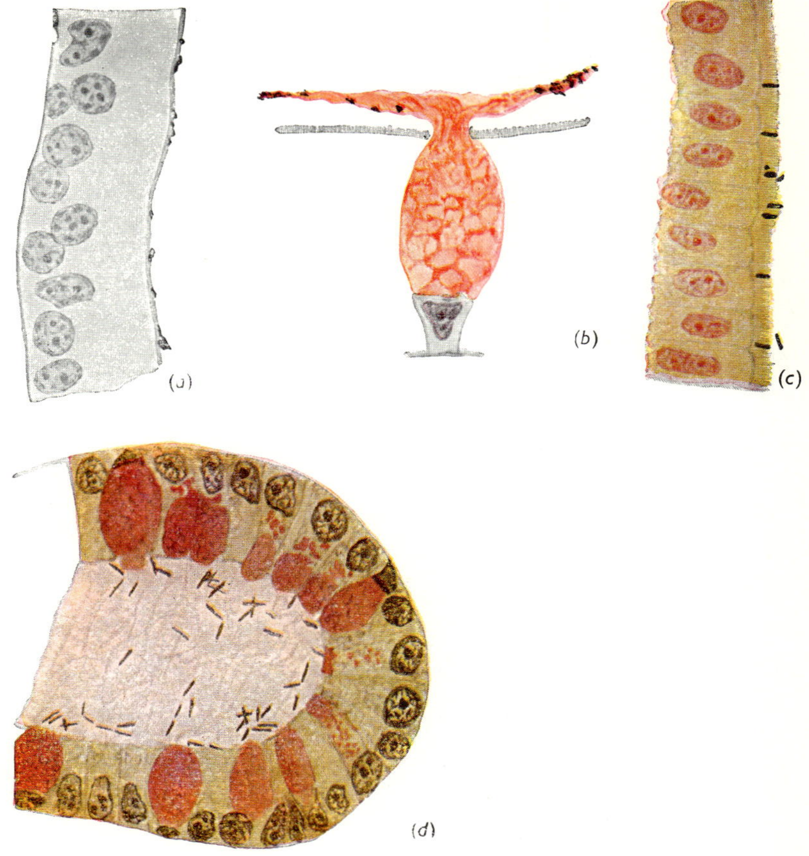

(*a*) Cat. Hydrokollag by stomach tube. Minute particles of carbon in direct contact with epithelial cells of small intestine.

(*b*) Cat. Discharging goblet cell "picking up" particles of carbon which adhere to the mucus.

(*c*) Cat. Non-pathogenic bacilli inserted into the striated borders of epithelial cells of small intestine.

(*d*) Cat. Colon. Bacteria growing in mucus at bottom of crypt.

All drawings made with Zeiss 2 mm. apochromatic lens and Watson 7× holoscopic eyepiece. (From Florey.[14])

is linked with differences in histochemical staining for glycoproteins.[15] The combined use of staining techniques and autoradiography has suggested that numerous different acidic compounds are produced in the glands.[16] At all events the secretion emerging from the ducts is a viscid, mucous fluid. In addition to these glands, goblet cells of a form somewhat similar to those of the intestine are scattered among the ciliated epithelium that lines the respiratory passages. The appearance and renewal of the surface cells have been the subject of some study.[20] Sometimes narrow, partially discharged goblets can be seen. In the finer airways near the part of the lung in which gas exchange occurs no mucus is produced. The deep glands are generally coterminous with the cartilage in the bronchi, though the cartilage may sometimes extend farther.[17]

It has been calculated that the volume of the deep glands in man is about 40 times that of the goblet cells, so they presumably produce the bulk of the mucous secretion in the bronchi and trachea. In the cat and rabbit about 2 ml. of secretion per kg. of body weight is produced in 24 hours.[18] On the basis of these figures a man might secrete from 100 to 150 ml. daily.

Stimulation of the vagus nerve in the cat excites secretion from the glands of the trachea, but the goblet cells do not appear to be in any way affected by the nerves or by the administration of pilocarpine to a point that exhausts the deep glands. Although these two facts are perfectly clear it is not so obvious what happens when the tracheal mucosa is irritated, for it seems that the deep glands secrete under local stimulation even in a heavily atropinised animal and that the goblet cells are very easily caused to desquamate. It would seem reasonable to suppose that the deep glands are set in action reflexly, though of this there is no proof.

Possible Protective Actions

We have at present no clear evidence exactly how infectious agents penetrate the layer of mucus over the epithelial cells and subsequently invade the respiratory mucosa. We have all had experience of a virus infection in the common cold. It often begins with a feeling of discomfort in the nostrils which may be accompanied by sneezing. This is soon followed by the production of a clear watery fluid which may be in sufficient quantity to drip steadily from the nostrils if allowed to do so. From its consistency it would appear to have little mucin in it. In the course of two or three days this watery secretion stops, to be followed by an obviously mucous secretion which gradually increases in viscosity. If the mucosa is invaded by pathogenic bacteria such as pneumococci or staphylococci the secretion becomes yellow from the accumulation of polymorphs and cellular debris—so-called muco-pus—before healing finally occurs in about two weeks.

One would like to believe that the mucous fluids produced by these mucosæ participate in protecting them from bacterial and viral invasion. There is some evidence of a mechanical protective function, for by appropriate microscopical examination the cilia of the nasal passages and of the trachea can be seen to keep constantly moving a thin coat of mucus, which finds its way to the back of the throat and is swallowed. This moving coat is composed of two layers, a relatively fluid layer in which the cilia beat and a viscous one on top. The correct functioning of the cilia appears to depend on the maintenance of these two layers.

In the trachea the streams of mucus move in a spiral, and in the normal nose there are also well-defined streams. These streams of mucous fluid often move rapidly, at a rate of some 3 cm. a minute for example. If during an experiment some carbon is dropped on to the surface it adheres to the sticky strands of mucus, and these are rolled up into larger and larger balls. No doubt this mechanism is highly effective in removing dust particles, for otherwise it is difficult to see why our air passages should not rapidly become gummed up in dirty atmospheres, such as those of hot, dusty climates and the smoke and vapour laden air of modern industrial cities. It can be deduced that many bacteria also are removed in this way, for the bronchi are usually sterile. The nose, however, contains bacteria, some of which may be pathogens. Perhaps one of the most dangerous organisms harboured by the nose in these days is penicillin-resistant *Staphylococcus aureus*. Nasal carriers are not infrequently responsible for the spread of antibiotic-resistant and other organisms in hospital.

There is another possible protective action. Some viruses can become adsorbed to certain mammalian cells. For experimental purposes it is usual to use erythrocytes as the test cell, and adsorption of virus to them leads to their agglutination (hæmagglutination). After being adsorbed for a few hours the virus liberates itself by enzymically splitting off from the glycoprotein of the red cell surface a sialic acid (N-acetylneuraminic acid from human erythrocytes) which is believed to be the point of attachment of the virus. Certain glycoproteins or mucins can inhibit the hæmagglutination, though they are rendered inactive in this respect if their sialic acid is split off first. It is possible that a similar adsorption, perhaps to the epithelial cells, may take place when viruses invade the respiratory tract, and it seems plausible to suggest that in that case the mucins produced there might play some part in inhibiting attachment of the virus. More work needs to be done to substantiate such a view, but those interested in the somewhat complicated experiments which have led to these interesting possibilities may like to consult an article by Burnet.[19]

Chronic Inflammation

We have seen how stimuli that produce inflammation cause the production of mucous secretions. If a relatively mild irritation is continued for some time we find that the common columnar or ciliated epithelial cells become replaced by goblet cells. A good example of this was seen in a "patch" of small intestine which was opened and grafted, mucosal side outwards, into the belly wall of a dog. In specimens examined histologically two years later the villi were much deformed, and the cells covering them and lining the crypts of Lieberkühn were found to be almost entirely goblet cells (FIG. 13).

It is now recognised that the disease called chronic bronchitis causes many thousands of deaths annually besides being responsible for much chronic disability, especially during the winter months. It is particularly prevalent in Great Britain and has been called the "English disease". The prime characteristic of chronic bronchitis is the production of excessive amounts of mucus which is coughed up in the form of sputum.

Histological changes are seen only in bronchitics with at least a ten years' history of disease. The most severe changes occur in patients with over twenty years' history.[21] The trachea, bronchi and bronchioles may be lined with an almost complete layer of goblet cells, i.e. these cells are greatly increased in number and extend more peripherally than in the normal mucosa. The thickness of the layer of acini of the deep glands may be double or treble that in the normal mucosa, i.e. the acini are greatly increased in volume. The so-called serous glands and the demilunes of serous cells found in some mucous glands disappear completely.

These changes do not seem always to be due to infection for they may be present in the absence of cells typical of either acute or chronic inflammation, though of course bacteria often colonise the diseased respiratory tract.

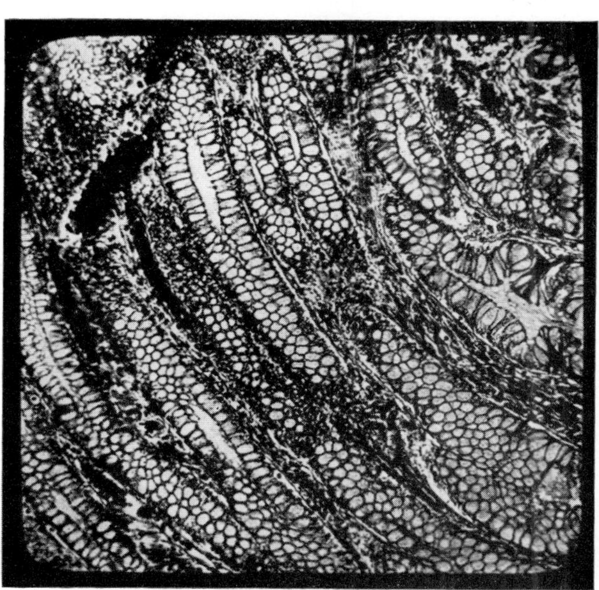

EFFECT OF CHRONIC IRRITATION

6/FIG. 13.—A "patch" of small intestine was inserted into the abdominal wall of a dog 2 years before this section of it was prepared. The epithelial cells of the crypts of Lieberkühn have largely been replaced by goblet cells.

It is suggested that the initial lesion is not an infection but rather a hypertrophy of the mucus-producing apparatus.[17] As has been mentioned above, long-continued mild irritation can cause an increased production of goblet cells in the small intestine. The same seems to be true of the trachea and bronchi and to apply to gland as well as goblet cells. Precisely what agents could produce such an effect in the human respiratory tract awaits discovery. Sulphur dioxide (at a concentration much higher than that encountered in the air of towns) produced gland and goblet cell hypertrophy in rats,[17a] and Reid[17] concluded that a variety of irritants, of which infection was only one, contributed to the increase of mucous-secreting cells in chronic bronchitis. Cigarette smoking and residence in a city have been shown to be correlated in man with hypertrophy of the bronchial glands[22], and with chronic bronchitis.[23]

Once the disease is established it seems likely that the excessive amount of mucus is not moved quickly out of the bronchi and trachea and that bacteria can readily colonise the relatively stagnant secretion. These bacteria may irritate the surface of the bronchi and bronchioles further, and may invade their walls and sometimes those of the alveoli nearest to them. Glynn[21] points out that in asthma, in which there is increased bronchial secretion, there may be a great increase in the number of goblet cells, though the deep glands are not hypertrophied.

Metaplasia in Mucous Membranes

Metaplasia can occur in mucus-secreting epithelia. Sometimes it is clearly due to prolonged irritation or infection but sometimes, particularly in the stomach, the cause is not known. In the trachea and bronchi the ciliated epithelium and goblet cells may be replaced by stratified and sometimes keratinising epithelium. In the stomach the mucous cells of the surface may be replaced by principal and goblet cells of intestinal type, and gastric glands may give place to intestinal crypts which, though irregular, may be complete with Paneth cells. Conversely, in the upper part of the intestine goblet cell epithelium may be replaced by epithelium of the gastric surface type.

REFERENCES

1. Florey, H. W. (1955). *Proc. roy. Soc., B*, **143,** 147.
2. Jennings, M. A., and Florey, H. W. (1956). *Quart. J. exp. Physiol.*, **41,** 131.

2a. Menguy, R., and Thompson, A. E. (1966–67). *Ann. N.Y. Acad. Sci.*, **140,** Art. 2, 797.

3. Morton, G. M., and Stavraky, G. W. (1949). *Gastroenterology*, **12,** 808.

3a. Gregory, R. A. (1968). *Proc. roy. Soc., B*, **170,** 81.

4. Wolf, S., and Wolff, H. G. (1947). *Human Gastric Function.* 2nd edit. London and New York: Oxford University Press.
5. Sober, H. A., Hollander, F., and Sonnenblick, B. P. (1950). *Amer. J. Physiol.*, **162,** 120.
6. Grant, R. (1945). *Anat. Rec.*, **91,** 175.
7. Heatley, N. G. (1959). *Gastroenterology*, **37,** 313.

7a. Skoryna, S. C., and Waldron-Edward, D. (1966–67), *Ann. N.Y. Acad. Sci.*, **140,** Art. 2, 835.

8. Love, J. W., Walder, A. I., and Bingham, C. (1968). *Nature (Lond.)*, **219,** 731.

8a. Love, J. W. (1969). *Personal communication.*

8b. Stening, G. F., and Grossman, M. I. (1968). *Lancet*, **1,** 1435.

9. Friend, D. S. (1965). *J. Cell Biol.*, **25,** 563.
10. Dragstedt, L. R., Woodward, E. R., Linares, C. A., and de la Rosa, C. (1964). *Ann. Surg.*, **160,** 497 (and Discussion).
11. Cairnie, A. B., Lamerton, L. F., and Steel, G. C. (1965). *Exp. Cell Res.*, **39,** 528 and 539.

11a. Creamer, B. (1967). *Brit. med. Bull.*, **23,** 226.

12. Neutra, M., and Leblond. C. P. (1966). *J. Cell Biol.*, **30,** 119; (1969). *Scientif. Amer.*, **220,** 100.
13. Florey, H. W. (1960). *Quart. J. exp. Physiol.*, **45,** 329.
14. Florey, H. W. (1933). *J. Path. Bact.*, **37,** 283.
15. McCarthy C., and Reid, L. (1964). *Quart. J. exp. Physiol.*, **49,** 81 and 85.
16. Lamb, D. (1966). *Proc. Path. Soc. Gt. Brit. & Irel.*, July.
17. Reid, L. (1958–59). "Chronic Bronchitis and Hypersecretion of Mucus." *Lectures on the Scientific Basis of Medicine*, **8,** 235. University of London: The Athlone Press.

17a. Lamb, D., and Reid, L. (1968). *J. Path. Bact.*, **96,** 97.

18. Perry, W. F., and Boyd, E. M. (1941). *J. Pharmacol. exp. Ther.*, **73,** 65.
19. Burnet, F. M. (1951). *Physiol. Rev.*, **31,** 131.

20. Blenkinsopp, W. K. (1967). *Exp. Cell Res.*, **46,** 144.
21. Glynn, A. A. (1961). *Brit. med. J.*, **1,** 127.
22. Field, W. E. H., Davey, E. N., Reid, L., and Roe, F. J. C. (1966). *Brit. J. Dis. Chest.*, **60,** 66.
23. Holland, W. W., and Reid, D. D. (1965). *Lancet*, **1,** 445.

General References

Descriptions of a number of the experiments mentioned in this chapter will be found in the following books and papers in addition to the above references:

Babkin, B. P. (1950). *Secretory Mechanism of the Digestive Glands,* 2nd edit. New York: Paul B. Hoeber, Inc.
This contains a review of work done on the secretion of mucus by the stomach.
Florey, H. (1930). *Brit. J. exp. Path.*, **11,** 348.
Florey, H. (1932). *ibid.*, **13,** 349.
Florey, H. W., and Harding, H. E. (1935). *Proc. roy. Soc., B,* **117,** 68.
Florey, H. W., and Harding, H. E. (1935). *Quart. J. exp. Physiol.*, **25,** 329.
Wright, R. D., and Florey, H. W. (1938). (Section A). *ibid.*, **28,** 207.
Jennings, M. A. (Section B). *ibid.*, **28,** 221.

Various aspects of the biology of mucous secretions are discussed in the following symposia:

"Mucous Secretions" (1963). *Ann. N.Y. Acad. Sci.*, **106,** Art. 2, 157.
"The Role of the Mucous Barrier in Defense vs. Peptic Ulceration". Part II of a Symposium (1966–67). *Ann. N.Y. Acad. Sci.*, **140,** Art. 2, 762.

Chemistry of Mucins

Information about the chemistry of the glycoproteins may be found in the following:

Zilliken, F., and Whitehouse, M. W. (1958). *Advanc. Carbohyd. Chem.*, **13,** 237.
Blix, G. (1959). *Proc. 4th Int. Congr. Biochem., Vienna,* 1958, **1,** 94. Oxford: Pergamon Press.
Gottschalk, A. (1960). *The Chemistry and Biology of Sialic Acids and Related Substances.* London: Cambridge Univ. Press.
Spiro, R. G. (1963). *New Engl. J. Med.*, **269,** 566.
Grant, P. T., and Simkin, J. L. (1965). *Ann. Rep. Progr. Chem.* (1964), **61,** 491. London: The Chemical Society.
Gottschalk, A., Ed. (1966). *Glycoproteins.* Amsterdam: Elsevier Publishing Co.
Spiro, R. G. (1966). *Methods in Enzymology,* **8,** 26. New York: Academic Press.
Balazs, E. A., and Jeanloz, R. W. (1966). *The Amino Sugars,* Vol. 2B. New York: Academic Press.
Kent, P. W. (1967). *Essays in Biochemistry,* **3,** 105. New York: Academic Press.

Chapter 7

THE REACTIONS OF THE BLOOD TO INJURY

1. The Reactions of the Plasma

By R. G. Macfarlane

Normal blood in healthy tissues flows through even the smallest vessels with ease. There is no tendency for the red cells, leucocytes, or platelets to adhere to each other, or to the vascular walls, and the plasma in which they are suspended slips along the endothelium with relatively little frictional drag. But any physical or chemical damage to the tissues is liable to produce a marked change in this flow pattern. In vessels so damaged, but not actually disrupted, the resulting changes form part of the complex inflammatory reaction. Leucocytes adhere to the endothelium and, though the vessels may dilate, the blood flow may become slower, or even stop. Plasma fluid escapes through the vessel wall, causing œdema and a rise of extravascular pressure, and the blood remaining in the vessels becomes increasingly viscous, until the red cells are packed into adherent masses. These changes, and the later leucocyte emigration, are discussed in Chapter 3.

In the case of vessels disrupted by trauma the pattern of events is different. The first effect is, of course, the escape of blood externally or into surrounding tissues. In normal individuals this bleeding is quite rapidly stopped by a series of reactions comprising vascular constriction, and the platelet aggregation and fibrin formation which form the so-called "hæmostatic plug". Other, less obvious hæmostatic factors include the opening up of vascular shunts which by-pass the injured area, the increasing local blood viscosity and red cell packing due to plasma loss through the vascular walls or through incompletely formed hæmostatic plugs, and the rising pressure of œdema fluid or blood in the extravascular tissue spaces.

These reactions, which are familiar to every observer of the microcirculation, have underlying mechanisms shown by recent research to be of considerable complexity. They involve the interaction of the products of tissue breakdown with the blood cells and platelets and with a series of plasma factors. In this chapter it is proposed to consider mainly these latter reactions in the blood plasma to local injury. They include blood coagulation and clot retraction, the formation of kinins, and fibrinolytic activity. Changes in the red cells, leucocytes and platelets will be described in Chapter 8.

BLOOD COAGULATION

The circulating blood *in vivo* normally has no demonstrable tendency to coagulate. It has been suggested that a sort of microscopic fibrin formation may occur continuously on vascular and blood cell surfaces at a rate normally balanced by an opposing rate of fibrinolysis. This idea has some attractive features but not much factual support, and it is more likely that the clotting process is a specific reaction to injury. The triggers which fire this reaction have proved difficult to identify, but considerable clarification of a previously confused picture of events has been achieved during the past few years. The basic observations are apparently simple. Though blood in contact with normal vascular endothelium remains fluid, contact with almost any other sort of surface causes clotting within a few minutes; also the addition of damaged tissue or tissue extracts to the blood will cause clotting within a few seconds even without contact with a "foreign" surface. Ionised calcium is required for these reactions, and citrates, oxalates, and chelating agents such as ethelene diamine tetra acetic acid (EDTA) which remove ionised calcium prevent the clotting effect of either foreign surfaces or tissue extracts, while the addition of more calcium to such decalcified blood restores clotting activity. Microscopic examination of a blood clot shows that its solidity is due to an interlacing network of fine strands (fibrin) and salt fractionation of normal plasma allows the separation of a specific protein (fibrinogen) which is the precursor substance from which these strands are derived. The change from soluble fibrinogen to solid fibrin is brought about by the action of thrombin, which can be extracted from the serum of freshly clotted blood. But thrombin does not exist as such in normal circulating blood, it is present as an inert protein precursor, prothrombin, which also can be separated by fractionation.

These observations were the basis of a theory formulated by Morawitz in 1905,[1] which is still the backbone of the more complex picture generally accepted today. Often referred to as the "classical theory", it can be set out as follows:

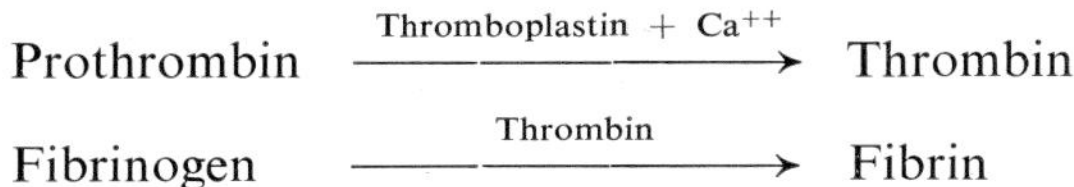

$$\text{Prothrombin} \xrightarrow{\text{Thromboplastin} + Ca^{++}} \text{Thrombin}$$

$$\text{Fibrinogen} \xrightarrow{\text{Thrombin}} \text{Fibrin}$$

Thus four factors are postulated: thromboplastin, calcium, prothrombin, and fibrinogen, and two products, thrombin and fibrin. Of these, thromboplastin was rather ill-defined. It was supposed to be the active principle responsible for the activity of extracts of certain tissues, particularly brain and lung which can cause clotting in 15 or 20 seconds, and the clotting of blood in wounds was supposed to be due to the release of a similar agent from any damaged tissue. However as Lister had demonstrated in 1863,[2] blood taken by careful venepuncture without admixture with tissue juice still clots, though at a later time, on contact with surfaces such as glass. It was then supposed that surface contact damaged blood cells and platelets to release some thromboplastin which caused clotting in a few minutes. Thromboplastin remains a controversial factor and, while attempts to define it have not been successful, they have led to discoveries which have clarified other parts of the clotting mechanism.[3]

The Thrombin-Fibrinogen Reaction

As regard the other factors and their interaction, there has been a steady growth of knowledge firmly established on a biochemical basis. The experiments of Lorand,[4] and Bailey and Bettelheim,[5] showed that thrombin is a proteolytic enzyme capable of splitting the fibrinogen molecule. Fibrinogen is a protein of high molecular weight, and with an elongated molecule, and it owes its stability in solution to negatively charged terminal groups including glutamic acid. The action of thrombin is to split off the glutamic acid-containing portion, which makes its appearance as an acidic peptide ("fibrinopeptide"); the larger remaining portions of the original fibrinogen molecule, now referred to as fibrin monomer, having lost negative charges, polymerise by end-to-end and side-to-side bonding to produce visible fibres. At this stage, however, fibrin formation is not complete and the newly polymerised fibrin is soluble in urea. During a later stage in physiological clotting secondary, probably amide, linkages are formed between the fibrin molecules, the final product being urea-insoluble. These secondary linkages depend on a factor (fibrin-stabilising factor, or Factor XIII) which is present in plasma or serum, but absent from purified preparations of fibrinogen and thrombin.[6] These reactions may be summarised as follows:

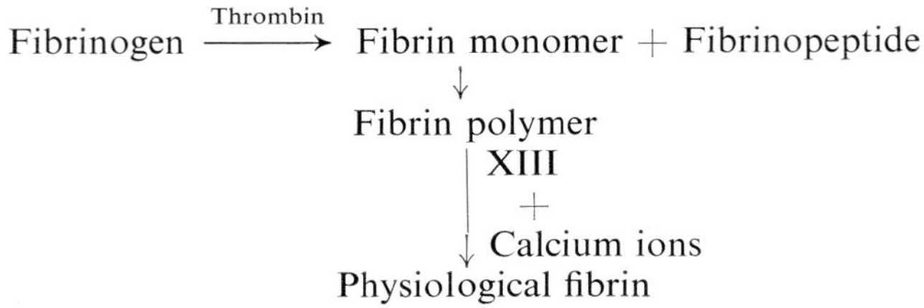

The reaction between thrombin and fibrinogen and the polymerisation of fibrin can take place within 3 or 4 seconds of adding a potent preparation of thrombin. A "unit" of thrombin is usually defined as that amount which will cause the clotting of 1 ml. of a specified solution of fibrinogen in 15 seconds at 37° C. During physiological coagulation a great excess of thrombin is formed since 1 ml. of human plasma generates about 200 units.

The Formation of Thrombin

The work of Seegers[7] and his collaborators over the past 25 years has added greatly to our knowledge of prothrombin and thrombin generation and has stimulated much research in other centres. The convincing demonstration that purified prothrombin can be converted quantitatively into thrombin under certain conditions (such as in 25 per cent citrate solution) without the addition of other blood or tissue products shows that prothrombin can be the sole precursor substance of thrombin. Prothrombin is an α_2 globulin which is present in normal plasma in concentrations of 10–15 mg. %. It has a molecular weight of about 68,000 whereas thrombin has a molecular weight of about 30,000 and since prothrombin can be activated by certain proteolytic enzymes, such as trypsin, it seems likely that activation involves splitting of the prothrombin molecule.

The physiological activation of prothrombin has been a major subject for blood coagulation research since Quick[8] introduced his test for prothrombin deficiency in 1935. This test was based on the classical theory, and relied on the assumption that tissue "thromboplastin" activates prothrombin directly. Thus in a system containing adequate fibrinogen and calcium, the clotting time on the addition of an excess of thromboplastin (brain extract) should be a measure of the prothrombin concentration. This test became widely used and was invaluable in revealing the prothrombin deficiency associated with obstructive jaundice and in the control of the therapeutic use of the dicoumarol drugs.[9] These block the synthesis of prothrombin in the liver and are used in the prevention and treatment of thrombosis.

But anomalies soon appeared. When the results of this test were compared with other methods for estimating prothrombin and it became clear that other plasma factors must be concerned with the activation of prothrombin which also affect the clotting time. Owren,[10] who did pioneer work in this field, named the first additional factor to be recognised Factor V, being the fifth clotting factor. Other new factors soon followed, often discovered more or less simultaneously in different laboratories and given different names. Confusion was finally ended by the establishment of an International Nomenclature Committee, which ruled that clotting factors with a good claim to real existence

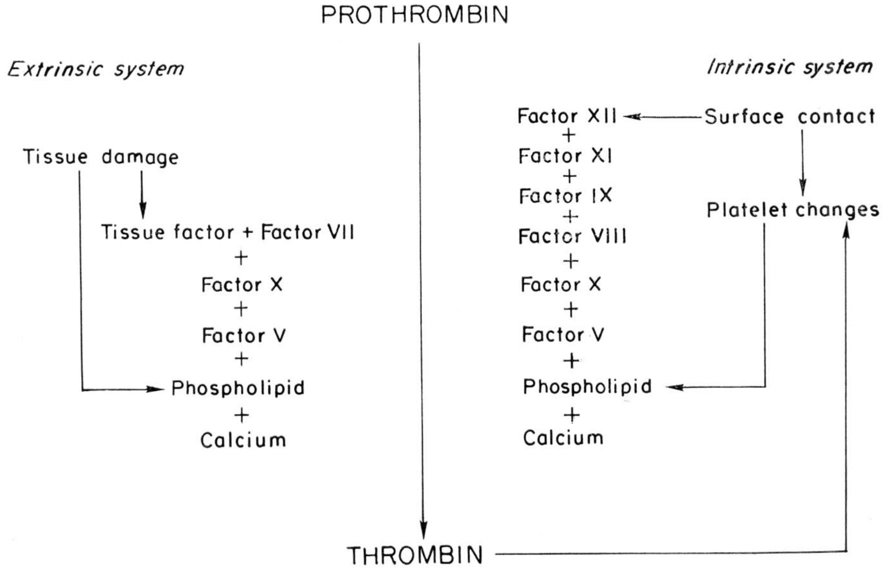

PROTHROMBIN

Extrinsic system

Tissue damage

Tissue factor + Factor VII
+
Factor X
+
Factor V
+
Phospholipid
+
Calcium

Intrinsic system

Factor XII ← Surface contact
+
Factor XI
+
Factor IX
+
Factor VIII
+
Factor X
+
Factor V
+
Phospholipid
+
Calcium

Platelet changes

THROMBIN

7/FIG. 1.—The Factors concerned with the activation of prothrombin following tissue damage (extrinsic system), or surface contact (intrinsic system).

should be known by Roman numerals. This ruling, which is accepted by most workers, not only resolved the multiple terminology which had reached chaotic proportions, but it disposed of a host of supposed "factors" which were derived products or transitory phenomena or simply artefacts. The result of this sorting out was the recognition of three plasma factors which are required for the activation of prothrombin by tissue thromboplastin, which, as shown on the left-hand side of FIG. 1, are Factors V, VII, and X.

Despite these advances, the nature of tissue "thromboplastin" remained in doubt. It has a phospholipid component, and it was believed that some specific phospholipid, such as phosphatidyl ethanolamine, is the active principle. But no pure phospholipid preparation has a specific activity comparable to the crude tissue extract. In recent studies the immensely powerful coagulant action of the venom of Russell's Viper has provided a clue.[11] This venom requires the presence of phospholipid for its action, but, though ethanolamine phosphatide is highly effective, other phosphatides will also serve, and their action seems to depend on their physical properties and electric charge rather than on a specific chemical constitution. Russell's Viper venom requires Factors V, and X and calcium for its activation of prothrombin and, by using a specific antiserum which neutralises the venom when required, it is possible to analyse the order of the reactions which take place in a mixture of venom, Factors V, and X, phospholipid and prothrombin. It was shown that the venom reacts with Factor X to form a new product which subsequently activates prothrombin in the presence of Factor V and phospholipid. Esnouf and Williams[12] then showed that the coagulant factor in the venom is an esterase which splits the Factor X molecule to produce an active derivative. This is itself an esterase, which has been called activated Factor X or "Xa". The reaction can therefore be written as follows:

$$\text{Factor X} \xrightarrow{\text{R.V.V.}} \text{Xa}$$

$$\text{Prothrombin} \xrightarrow{\text{Xa + V + phl}} \text{Thrombin}$$

It appears from recent work that, while Factor V and phospholipid are potent accelerators of the reaction of Xa with prothrombin, the latter reaction can proceed slowly in their absence. Very similar observations have been made with tissue thromboplastin, which also causes the activation of Factor X. But it requires Factor VII (as well as Factor V) to achieve this, whereas the venom does not, and tissue extracts cause rapid prothrombin conversion without the addition of the phospholipid which is needed for venom action. The simplest hypothesis explaining these facts is illustrated in FIG. 2. This supposes that tissue extracts contain a mixture of two components, an active agent (tissue factor) which is a labile protein or lipoprotein, and a stable phospholipid, which acts as a co-factor. Tissue factor activates Factor X, in the presence of Factor VII and the phospholipid functions in the later reaction between Xa, Factor V and prothrombin.

The Intrinsic System

Tissue factor is one of the two triggers which can operate the clotting mechanism, and it seems to be less important physiologically than the other, which is the stimulus provided by surface contact. This operates through a chain of factors which have only become recognised during the past 10 years. For nearly a century, the main interest of coagulation workers was in the tissue activated (or extrinsic) system, and the supposition that the clotting of blood following surface contact was due to the release of minute amounts of "thromboplastin" from cells and platelets offered no explanation of the failure of the blood to clot on contact with glass in such conditions as hæmophilia. In these conditions the blood clots normally on the addition of normal (or hæmophilic) tissue extract, and no fault can be found in the cells or platelets. Thus the hæmostatic defect occurs despite the apparently normal functioning of the tissue-activated system. The demonstration, in Oxford, that, following contact activation the blood generates its own "thromboplastin" (prothrombin activator) which is as powerful as any tissue extract, gave an incentive to explore the mechanism in detail.[13] The introduction of the "thromboplastin generation test" by Biggs and Douglas[14] provided the means to analyse both clinical cases and experimental data which has been widely used.

At least six factors are involved in the activation of prothrombin following contact, these being Factors XII, XI, IX, VIII, X and V. Phospholipid is also required and is normally provided by the platelets (see FIG. 1). The factor sensitive to surface contact is Factor XII (Hageman Factor), which then reacts with Factor XI, as shown by Ratnoff and his colleagues,[15] which in turn reacts with Factors IX and VIII to cause the activation of Factor X. There is evidence that Xa is produced during this reaction[16] as it is by Russell's Viper venom or by tissue extracts and Factor VII. Thus the intrinsic and the extrinsic systems have a common meeting point at Factor X.

The Nature of the Clotting Factors

A few of the clotting factors have been isolated in forms sufficiently pure to allow their properties to be defined.

Fibrinogen is a protein with a molecular weight of about 340,000. Electron microscopy and physical data suggest that its molecule is about 450 Å long with one central and two terminal knobs about 50 Å in diameter.[17] The amino acid sequences of peptides split off from the fibrinogen molecule have been determinated. Fibrinogen is the plasma protein most easily precipitated by salt (25 per cent saturation with $(NH_4)_2SO_4$) or by heat (47° C.), and is normally present in concentrations of 200–600 mg. per 100 ml. of plasma.

Prothrombin is a protein classified electrophoretically as an α_2 globulin. It has a molecular weight of about 68,000 and a rod-shaped molecule. It is relatively stable, and is readily absorbed by inorganic gels such as aluminium hydroxide or barium sulphate, a property utilised in its isolation. Its concentration in normal plasma is about 10–15 mg. per 100 ml., and it is not present in normal serum. One milligramme of purified prothrombin will produce about 2000 units of thrombin, and normal plasma can generate about 200 times as much thrombin as is needed to cause clotting in 15 seconds.

Factor V, classed as α globulin, is estimated to have a molecular weight of about 290,000. It is labile, losing activity on heating to 50° C., and on storage at 4° C. for more than a few days. It is not absorbed by inorganic gels.

Factor VII, classed as a β globulin has an estimated molecular weight of about 60,000. It is relatively stable, and is adsorbed by inorganic gels.

Factor X, has a molecular weight of 86,000. It is relatively stable, and is absorbed by inorganic gels. It is present in normal plasma in concentrations of about 1–2 mg. per 100 ml.

Factor VIII, is extremely labile, and is difficult to separate from fibrinogen. Various estimates of its molecular weight have been made, and they lie within the range of 300,000 to 400,000. Factor VIII is not readily absorbed by inorganic gels, but is destroyed or removed by almost any process which precipitates or alters the fibrinogen with which it is usually associated. From estimates of specific activity it can be calculated that the concentration of Factor VIII in normal plasma is probably less than 100 μg. per 100 ml.[18]

The other clotting factors have not yet been purified sufficiently to allow their physical and chemical properties to be determined.

Little is known about *Factor IX*, apart from the fact that it migrates electrophoretically with the α globulins, is relatively stable and is absorbed by inorganic gels. Observations, suggest that it is present in even smaller concentrations than Factor VIII in normal plasma. Little is also known about *Factors XI and XII.* Factor XII is said to be a sialoglycoprotein.[19]

From this brief summary of some of the known properties of these factors, it will be seen that they can be divided into two main groups. In the first are fibrinogen, Factor V and Factor VIII which are all labile substances with high molecular weights, not absorbed by inorganic gels and readily destroyed by proteolytic agents such as thrombin and plasmin. Their synthesis in the body is not dependent on vitamin K. The second group consists of prothrombin, and Factors VII, IX and X. These are all relatively stable and are readily absorbed by inorganic gels. Their molecular weights where known, are in the range of 60–100,000 and their most striking similarity is their dependence on vitamin K for their synthesis by the liver in vivo. Their production is therefore depressed (but not always simultaneously or to the same extent) by dicourmarol drugs. These similarities have led to the suggestion that Factors VII, IX, and X may be molecular variants of prothrombin, and Seegers[7] goes further in maintaining that they are actually derivatives of prothrombin produced during its conversion to thrombin.

The Function of the Clotting Factors

For many years the mode of action of clotting factors was unknown. An idea that enzymatic action is involved is illustrated by such names as "kinase", "fibrin ferment" and "thrombase" in use 50 years ago. But it was not until 1950 that it was demonstrated that fibrin formation is dependent on the proteolysis of fibrinogen by thrombin shown to be an enzyme with esterase action on synthetic substrates. Prothrombin is thus a proenzyme, and its activation may also be brought about by enzyme action. For example, trypsin and certain snake venoms can activate prothrombin, but the physiological activator seems to be the derivative of Factor X (Xa) which has esterase activity. Factor X, as already mentioned, appears to be activated by both the intrinsic and the extrinsic clotting systems, and also by certain extraneous enzymes, such as that contained in Russell's Viper venom. Thus, the activation of Factor X seems to be analogous to prothrombin activation, Factor X being a proenzyme activated by specific proteolysis. Milstone's plasma "thrombokinase" which he showed has esterase activity[20] very probably corresponds with Xa. The activation products of Factors XII and XI are said to have esterase activity, one activating the other. It seems likely that Factor IX is activated by activated Factor XI, and that subsequently Factor VIII is activated. The result of these reactions is the production of an activator of Factor X.

As a hypothetical generalisation, therefore, the clotting sequence from surface contact to prothrombin activation might be set out as shown in FIG. 2, the letter "a" designating the active (enzyme) form of the factor concerned.[21] Calcium is required for most of the reactions, and phospholipid may be required at stages other than that shown, for example it appears to accelerate the activation of Factor VIII. Factor V seems to act as a co-factor, and it is probable that phospholipid is a surface-active catalyst absorbing and orienting Factor V, Xa and prothrombin in such a way as to promote the rapid conversion of the latter.

Factor X is also activated by tissue factor and Factor VII, this being an alternative pathway linking tissue injury with the final result of fibrin formation.

In this view the clotting mechanism is a cascade of proenzyme transformations. Since each molecule of enzyme is capable of reacting with many molecules of substrate and since each substrate yields a new enzyme, there is likely to be a gain in activity from one stage to the next. Such a cascade would function as a biochemical amplifier, and the multiplicity of factors might represent the evolutionary development of a highly efficient mechanism designed to convert a minute

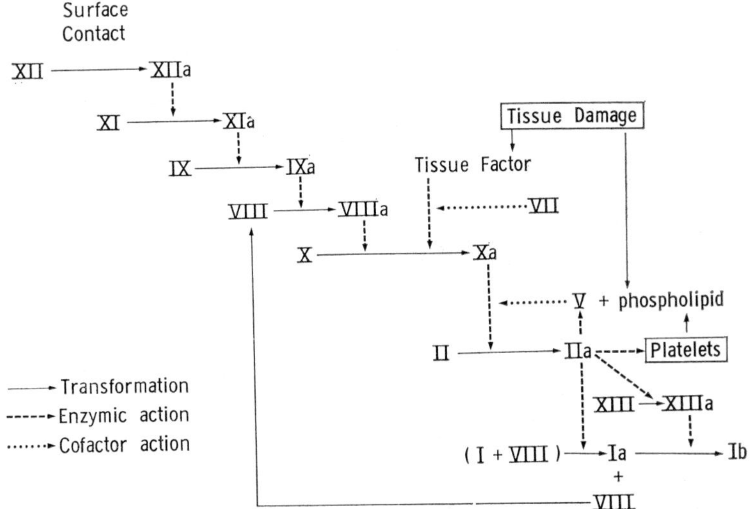

7/FIG. 2.—A scheme for the interaction of the clotting Factors using the Roman numerical nomenclature system. The letter "a" designates the activated form or derivative. (Common synonyms: XII = Hageman Factor, XI = PTA, IX = Christmas Factor, VIII = Anti-hæmophilic factor, X = Stuart-Prower factor, II = prothrombin, IIa = thrombin, I = fibrinogen, Ia = fibrin, Ib = stabilised fibrin, XIII = fibrin stabilising factor).

stimulus into the sudden and large effect of fibrin formation. It is possible that the extrinsic (tissue activated) pathway represents the simpler clotting mechanism which seems to predominate in some lower animals. The intrinsic system, on which the efficiency of mammalian clotting depends, involves more stages and might therefore be expected to provide greater amplification. It is interesting that this part of the mechanism is also involved in two other reactions to injury, such as the formation of kinins and the activation of the proteolytic enzyme plasmin. It is possible, therefore, that a pre-existing system of enzyme activators may have become "plugged in" to the more primitive clotting mechanism by adaptation and the natural selection of its greater efficiency.

Physiological Coagulation

There is little doubt that in physiological clotting the initial stimulus is contact of the blood with a particular type of surface. It seems unlikely that admixture with tissue juice is the predominant factor in promoting clotting in traumatised areas, since the tissue activated system seems to function normally in hæmophilic patients. The precise quality of surfaces which cause activation of the clotting system is not yet defined. It was for many years supposed that it depended upon the "wettability" of the surface. For instance, the skin, the cotton fabrics used to dress wounds, and the originary glass, metal or rubber apparatus used in the laboratory are all wettable and promote clotting, whereas certain oils, resins waxes, silicones, and some plastics are non-wettable and do not promote clotting. These latter substances, particularly silicone, are used to coat laboratory apparatus so that blood may remain fluid for a longer time without the addition of an anticoagulant. However, "wettability" is not the simple determining factor. Collodion is wettable but is relatively inert in promoting clotting, whereas nylon is non-wettable and is highly active in this respect, and it is unlikely that the blood does not wet the vascular endothelium in life. The electric charge of the surface in contact with blood is considered to be a factor in determining clotting, and it has been shown that the endothelial surfaces normally carry a negative charge as do the platelets and other formed elements of the blood. Experimental reversal of this charge *in vivo* by electrical means promotes rapid thrombosis of the vessel concerned.[22] It has been shown that certain long-chain saturated fatty acids can accelerate clotting *in vitro* and cause thrombosis when injected *in vivo*.[23] This effect is apparently related to activation of Factor XII, and its investigation may help to clarify the mechanism of contact activation and may also have a bearing on the problem of thrombosis. There is some evidence that the endothelial surface and the surfaces of sulphated compounds may have a local anticoagulant action similar to that of heparin,[24] which is a negatively charged sulphated mucopolysaccharide. Thus in the normal vascular and lymphatic spaces of the body the absence of activating contact and the presence of inhibitors may be responsible for the fluidity of the blood and lymph.

Physical changes of the endothelial surface which occur following trauma, inflammation or disease, or contact of the blood with extravascular surfaces may initiate the cascade effect, a rising wave of activity propogated down the chain until it culminates in the most explosive generation of thrombin and rapid fibrin formation. Certain autocatalytic processes increase the rate of activation, as shown in Fig. 2. These mainly concern thrombin which seems to have at least three effects other than its action on fibrinogen. Firstly, it seems to potentiate the interaction of Factors VIII and IX, possibly by "mobilizing" Factor VIII from an association with fibrinogen in a highly reactive but unstable form.[25] Secondly, it acts on the platelets, causing their aggregation and the release of platelet phospholipid which acts as an accelerator of the activation of prothrombin by Xa and Factor V. Thrombin also activates Factor XIII. From the point of view of hæmostatic efficiency, it seems that the rate of fibrin formation, once started, is important. In hæmophilia, the normal amount of fibrin is ultimately formed, but the process is slow and hæmostatically ineffective.

During the propagation of the normal wave of activation, the stimulus passes from one stage to the next before the factors concerned are fully activated. This is illustrated by the fact that, following contact activation, fibrin formation is usually complete when less than half of the available thrombin and less than

10 per cent of the available Xa have appeared. The analogy of a wave can be carried further, because activity at each stage rises to a maximum and then falls. This fall is due to the natural destruction or inactivation of any activated clotting factor which takes place in normal plasma or serum. Thrombin, for example is rapidly inactivated by normal serum and it has been calculated that the mean survival of a thrombin molecule is only about 24 seconds.[7] Activated Factor VIII disappears even more rapidly, and it seems likely that its very short survival brings the natural activation process to a halt soon after thrombin appears, and before all the available Factor X has been activated. The activation of Factor IX also ceases before it is complete, and in consequence normal serum contains the unconsumed residue of Factors IX and X, and also Factor VII.

The Inhibition of Clotting

The disappearance of clotting activity within a few minutes of fibrin formation is probably of the greatest importance in preventing thrombosis by the propagation of activation into the circulation. But very little is known about the factors involved. Various "antithrombins" have been described and numbered from 1 to 6, some of which inhibit polymerisation of fibrin monomer. The disappearance of thrombin itself is ascribed to a factor known as antithrombin III, which has been studied particularly by Seegers[7] and his colleagues. The antithrombin activity seems to be associated with a lipoprotein present in the α_2 globulin fraction of normal serum. It is destroyed by heating to 56° for 10 minutes, by solvents such as alcohol, ether or chloroform. Its action is potentiated by heparin, and it may be that the main antithrombin effect of heparin is due to this potentiation. Other enzyme inhibitors in normal serum, such as antitrypsin and antiplasmin have also been studied in relation to antithrombin but it is not yet clear if their effects are due to a single substance or to specific enzyme inhibitors. Nor is it known how these factors operate; they may form competitive inhibitors or substrates, or they may destroy the enzymes enzymatically.

Much less is known about the destruction of Xa, and practically nothing about the disappearance of other activated factors. There is evidence that activated Factor VIII is destroyed by thrombin itself.[25] If this is so it is an example of an automatically self-limiting process. The electronic analogy would be a feed back of the output of an amplifier so that when it reaches a certain level an earlier stage is switched off.

Practical use is made of the anticoagulant action of certain substances for laboratory and clinical purposes. Citrates, oxalates and EDTA, and certain ion exchange resins remove or depress ionised calcium and thus inhibit several stages of the clotting process which require calcium ions. Citrate is widely used as a relatively non-toxic anticoagulant in blood transfusion. Heparin not only inhibits thrombin, but also the formation of prothrombin activator. It is used as an anticoagulant in the laboratory, and also *in vivo* for surgery involving an extracorporeal circulation, and in renal dialysis. Other sulphated macro-molecules, such as dextran sulphate have an action similar to that of heparin. Clotting can also be delayed by preventing contact of the blood with activating surfaces. Blood taken by means of apparatus coated with silicone or certain plastics will remain fluid from 30 minutes to an hour or more, if the technique of avoiding contact is efficient.

The Assessment of Clotting Efficiency

In practice, it is important to detect faults in the clotting mechanism, but its inherent complexity may make this a difficult or fallacious process. The "clotting time" of the whole blood was usually regarded as a good general index, but is now known to be dangerously misleading in some cases. The clotting time measures the time occupied by all the stages of coagulation from surface contact to the first appearance of fibrin, and if it is prolonged there is a gross deficiency or inhibition of some essential factor. But it is very insensitive to delays in stages which normally occur rapidly, and it may not reveal a serious deficiency of factors such as fibrinogen, prothrombin, Factor V and the platelets. Even deficiency of antihæmophilic globulin (Factor VIII) and Christmas factor (IX) may be severe enough to produce dangerous bleeding without significantly lengthening the clotting time since, although fibrin formation may begin within the normal time it then proceeds slowly. The "prothrombin time" which records the clotting time of recalcified plasma with added tissue extract is a useful test which differentiates certain clotting defects. It is normal in hæmophilia and Christmas disease, but abnormal if there is a deficiency of Factors V, VII, or X, or prothrombin. It is used in the control of dicoumarin therapy, which causes a reduction of the last three factors and also Factor IX. The thromboplastin generation test measures the rate and amount of prothrombin activator production in a mixture of adsorbed plasma, platelets and serum. By deriving any one of these components from the patient's blood, and the remaining two from normal blood, faults in the early stages of the patient's clotting mechanism can be differentiated. In hæmophilia, the plasma component is inactive, while in Christmas disease it is the serum component and in certain other conditions the platelets may be at fault. Ideally, it is more satisfactory to assay individual factors since practical methods have now been developed for routine use.[26]

Defective Coagulation

A number of clotting defects occur in human beings. Any of the factors mentioned may be deficient for one reason or another, and cause inefficient clotting of the blood, with more or less serious hæmorrhagic symptoms. In most cases these deficiencies occur as hereditary defects. *Fibrinogen* may be completely or partially absent as a rare inherited defect, or as the result of disease processes which prevent its formation, or hasten its destruction in the circulation. Acute fibrinogen deficiency may develop with disastrous rapidity in certain obstetrical conditions, and during surgical operations on the lungs. This may be the result of increased fibrinolysis or of intravascular defibrination caused by the entry of thromboplastic tissue fragments into the vascular system from the placental or wound site, causing slow intravascular fibrin formation. *Prothrombin* may be deficient idiopathically, or reduced as the result of vitamin K deficiency, or liver disease, or following the administration of drugs of the dicoumarin group which are used therapeutically in the treatment of thrombosis. Such drugs, however, mainly reduce *Factor VII* and also *Factor X*. Reductions of these two factors occur as inherited defects. A reduction of these factors is not distinguished by the 1 stage prothrombin time test from a reduction of prothrombin, because in each case the clotting time with added tissue extracts (such as brain) will be longer than normal. This defect is usually referred to as a "long prothrombin time" though the basic defect may not be primarily prothrombin deficiency. *Factor V* may be deficient as a hereditary condition, and the effect is similar to that of prothrombin deficiency. *The platelets* are reduced in conditions which cause a destruction of the bone marrow in general, or of the megakaryocytes in particular, or in which antibodies develop causing platelet destruction and capillary damage. Thrombocytopenia involves a shortage of phospholipid available for prothrombin activation and thus reduces the amount of thrombin formed in a given time. There is not, as a rule, any great prolongation of the clotting time of the blood because the thrombin, though deficient in amount, first appears in approximately the normal time. There is, however, incomplete consumption of prothrombin which can be demonstrated in the serum.

The best known of the coagulation defects is hæmophilia, which is inherited as a sex-linked recessive condition causing a deficiency of *Factor VIII* (anti-hæmophilic globulin). Lack of this factor causes inefficient coagulation and a serious hæmorrhagic diathesis. In 1952 it was discovered that some cases previously diagnosed as hæmophilia were in reality examples of a condition distinct from it, the basic defect being a deficiency of *Factor IX* (Christmas factor), a separate component of the intrinsic prothrombin activator system[27]. Inherited deficiencies of *Factor XI* (PTA) and *Factor XII* (Hageman Factor) also occur.

In a small number of cases, defective coagulation has been shown to be due to an increase of inhibitors. The most interesting of these is a factor which inactivates anti-hæmophilic globulin, and which has some resemblance to an antibody of the immune type. It has been found in hæmophilic patients who have been repeatedly transfused and in some otherwise normal females shortly after delivery.

CLOT RETRACTION

About 10 to 15 minutes after the coagulation of whole blood or plasma takes place *in vitro*, the clot begins to retract away from the walls of its container and fluid serum is expressed. This contraction is usually complete in an hour at 37° C., and its extent is limited by the volume of the red cells retained in the clot, since relatively few escape through the fibrin mesh with the expressed serum. Thus the clot formed by normal whole blood contracts to about 45 per cent of its original volume, while in anæmia the shrinkage increases in proportion to the decrease in the volume of red cells, and in plasma devoid of red cells (but containing platelets) the fibrin clot shrinks by 95 per cent or more.

The Mechanism of Clot Retraction

The expulsion of serum through a fibrin mesh sufficiently fine to retain red cells must involve appreciable force, and the source of this had been investigated and discussed for many years. Indirect evidence suggested that the platelets were involved. Any decrease in the normal platelet content of the blood was associated with a corresponding decrease in retraction. Retraction is inhibited by a number of substances such as dyes and cocaine which inhibit platelet activity, by specific anti-platelet serum, or by prolonged storage, freezing and thawing, ultra-violet light or short-waves which destroy platelets. Direct evidence was obtained by Budtz-Olsen[28] who observed the formation of long projections from the platelets attached to fibrin strands in a clot, and their subsequent shortening. He suggested that this shortening of the fibrin, which would naturally produce contraction of the clot, was due to the active contraction of these platelet pseudopodia. This explanation is now generally accepted, and an underlying mechanism in the platelets has been found. The platelets have been shown to contain a contractile protein, resembling actomyosin, now known as "thrombosthenin".[29] The dependence of normal clot retraction on the presence of glucose,[30] and the breakdown of the ATP contained in the platelets following their exposure to thrombin[31] suggests the source of energy which might motivate such a contractile system.

The Significance of Clot Retraction

It is not clear that clot retraction is a significant hæmostatic factor, though it might be supposed that the contracted clot would be mechanically stronger, and it has been suggested that the force of contraction draws the walls of injured vessels together. In certain conditions, such as thrombocytopenia and thrombasthenia, in which the platelets are quantitatively or qualitatively deficient, abnormal bleeding and reduced clot retraction are found. But in other conditions, particularly those associated with an increased blood fibrinogen, clot retraction may be reduced without abnormal bleeding.

The Fibrinolytic Mechanism

The fibrin formed by normal blood *in vitro* usually remains intact for some days if bacterial contamination is avoided. The fate of fibrin *in vivo* is less easy to observe, but ordinary experience suggests that in traumatised areas it is broken down more quickly, being superseded by the process of organisation and repair. Under certain conditions fibrin destruction may be greatly accelerated. Local bacterial infection, particularly by hæmolytic streptoccoci, may cause rapid fibrinolysis and so-called "secondary" hæmorrhage. But certain general disturbances, such as extensive or painful injury, hæmorrhage, anoxia, fear, severe exercise and other forms of stress cause a greatly increased rate of fibrin breakdown which can be demonstrated by the rapid disappearance of blood clots even when these are formed *in vitro*. This is not due to increased proteolytic activity of the tissues or of blood cells but to the activation of an enzyme normally present as an inert precursor in the plasma.

The mechanism underlying this process has been brought to light by the study of agents which are capable of inducing fibrinolysis *in vitro*. Briefly the plasma contains the proenzyme "plasminogen" which can be activated to plasmin in various ways which have a curious similarity to the different pathways of prothrombin activation. Plasmin is a proteolytic enzyme with a selective action on fibrin, but is also capable of attacking other substrates such as fibrinogen, casein, and gelatine. Plasminogen and plasmin were identified as the result of a study of the fibrinolytic action of culture filtrates of hæmolytic streptoccoci by Christenson and McLeod[32] and Milstone,[33] who showed that these filtrates had no direct action on fibrin itself, but require another plasma component from which the fibrinolytic enzyme was derived. The agent in the streptoccocal filtrate has been isolated and is known as "streptokinase". It causes activation of plasminogen, though its mode of action is not yet established. It does not appear to be an enzyme itself, but it may potentiate the autocatalytic activation of plasminogen by plasmin. Streptokinase is highly active with human plasminogen, but not bovine unless a trace of human plasma is also added. This led to the supposition that streptokinase does not act on plasminogen directly, but through a "pro-activator" which, it was postulated, was present in human but not bovine plasma. But attempts to isolate this pro-activator have not succeeded, and it is suggested that "pro-activator" may not exist. The lack of response of bovine plasminogen may thus be due to a species difference in autocatalytic activation which can be overcome if the reaction is started by the presence of a trace of human plasminogen. Streptokinase is of practical importance because of its use as a therapeutic agent in cases of thrombosis. Other bacteria, notably *Staphylococcus aureus*, also produce fibrinolytic kinases.

Another agent which activates plasminogen both *in vivo* and *in vitro*, is "urokinase" which is present in normal human urine and is apparently produced by the kidneys. This has been isolated in a relatively pure form and is in use as a therapeutic agent. Urokinase is an enzyme, with esterase and some proteolytic activity, which appears to activate plasminogen directly. Many tissue and organ extracts, and various other body fluids have also been shown to contain plasminogen activator. Astrup[34] and his colleagues, who have made an extensive study of this field have called these agents "lysokinases". Todd,[35] and Warren,[36] by an ingenious histological technique have shown that vascular endothelium, particularly of veins, is rich in plasminogen activator. (See Chapter 3, p. 52.)

Fibrinolysis in the Body

Local fibrinolysis is probably induced by plasminogen activator released by damaged tissues and by leucocytes, and there is some evidence that the clotting Factors XII and XI activated by surface contact also promote plasminogen activation. Thus both tissue damage and surface contact are initiators of plasmin production, as they are of thrombin production.

General activation of the fibrinolytic mechanism, as shown by rapid liquefaction of clots, or the presence of fluid blood in the vessels after death, is an occasional phenomenon which has been recognised for many years. Morgani[37] remarked on the absence of post-mortem clots in cases of sudden death, and this was shown by Morawitz[38] to be due to fibrinolysis. Later studies showed that post-mortem fibrinolysis was due to an enzyme apparently activated during death from asphyxia, hæmorrhage or electrocution.

Though less dramatic than this post-mortem lysis, increased activity also occurs in the blood of the living subject in conditions associated with stress. Investigation of the increased fibrinolytic activity demonstrable after injury or surgery showed that apprehension was a factor. Severe exercise or the injection of adrenalin will also produce this activity.[39] In some cases the clots produced by whole blood will re-liquefy within an hour or two of their formation, but lesser fibrinolytic activity requires special methods to demonstrate it. Simple dilution of the blood or plasma before clotting renders the fibrin formed more susceptible to lysis, and the globulin fraction when separated from the albumin often has more fibrinolytic activity than that demonstrable in the whole plasma.

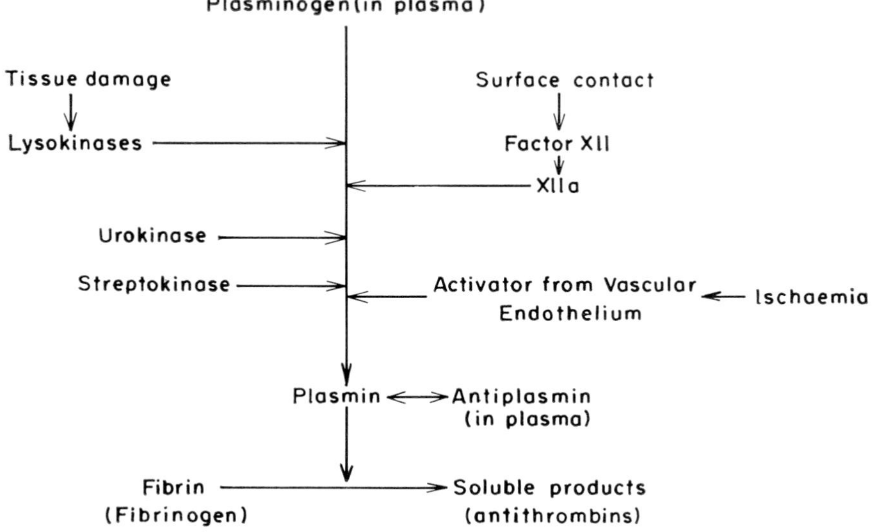

7/Fig. 3.—Some pathways for plasminogen activation.

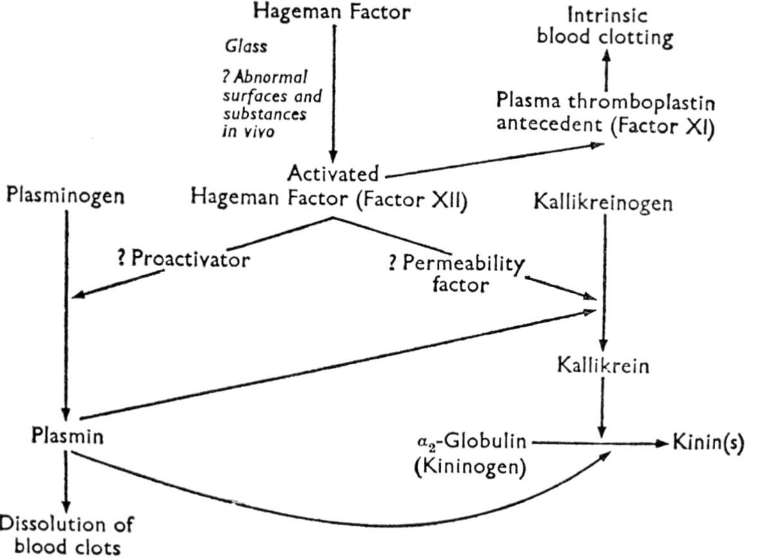

7/Fig. 4.—A scheme for the interaction of the factors concerned with kinin formation (From Eisen.[42])

Plasmin activity can also be detected, and measured, by its effect on pre-formed fibrin, usually prepared as a layer in a petri dish. A measured quantity of the material to be tested is placed in a well in the surface of the plate and the area of lysis produced in a given time is measured. These fibrin plates can be prepared with and without plasminogen, thus allowing plasmin to be differentiated from plasminogen activator, in a given sample of active material.

The Mechanism of Fibrinolysis

Analysis of the findings described above and the results of many fractionation experiments has led to a general hypothesis of the mechanism of fibrinolysis, and the ways in which it is activated. Normal plasma contains plasminogen, present in the globulin fraction, and antiplasmin, an α- globulin which is present in the crude albumin fraction.

In the circulating blood, any plasmin which may be formed is inactivated by antiplasmin, and no proteolysis occurs. During coagulation, however, both plasmin and plasminogen are adsorbed to fibrin, and are removed from the immediate effect of antiplasmin. If the plasmin is sufficiently active, fibrinolysis soon results, and if plasminogen activator is present more plasmin is activated in close association with the fibrin surface. Thus proteolysis is largely restricted to the destruction of fibrin,[40] and only in exceptional circumstances is there a plasminæmia in the circulating blood sufficient to cause destruction of fibrinogen and other soluble proteins.

In vitro, dilution favours the action of plasmin by reducing the concentration of antiplasmin, and it may also cause dissociation of a plasmin-antiplasmin complex. Fibrinolytic activity can be induced, also *in vitro*, by solvents such as chloroform, or ether, which destroy antiplasmin. *In vivo*, fibrinolysis can be promoted by the entry of plasminogen activator into the blood. This may be in the form of tissue kinase released from areas of injury, or in certain obstetrical conditions in which amniotic fluid, or placental fragments may enter the maternal blood stream. More frequently it is due to the release of activator from vascular endothelium, and, as already mentioned, from venous endothelium in particular. This release seems to be triggered by anoxia. The action of adrenalin and certain other vaso-active drugs has been explained by supposing that their constricting effect on the vasa vasorum causes ischæmia of the vessel wall.[41] The current hypothesis of the mechanism of fibrinolysis, and the ways in which it can be activated is summarised in FIG. 3.

THE KININ SYSTEM

Local injury leads to the activation of other enzyme systems in the blood besides those involved in coagulation and fibrinolysis. The familiar manifestations of inflammation: redness, pain, heat and swelling (rubor, dolor, calor, and tumor) are due to some extent to the effect of certain peptides, or kinins, of which bradykin is an example. These peptides have complex actions on the small blood vessels, but, in general, they produce increased vascular permeability with a consequent loss of plasma through the vessel walls causing tissue œdema and a slowing of the blood flow through increased viscosity. These substances also have an action on nerve endings, and cause pain. Inflammation itself is described in detail in Chapter 3, and the kinin system can be only briefly mentioned here. There is a considerable literature on this subject, and Eisen[42] has reviewed the relationship of the kinin forming mechanism to coagulation and fibrinolysis.

Bradykin is formed by the proteolytic breakdown of a precursor substance present in the plasma, an α globulin known as "kininogen". Proteolytic enzymes, such as trypsin and plasmin, and various tissue extracts, have the ability to convert kininogen into kinin. Tissue extracts active in this respect are said to contain "kallikreins", with protease and esterase activity. Kallikrein activity can also be derived from the plasma, by the activation of an inert precursor, "kallikreininogen". This activation can be brought about by activated Hageman Factor (Clotting Factor XII) and also by plasmin (see FIG. 4). There are thus striking similarities between the clotting mechanism, fibrinolysis and the kinin system, and cross-connections between them. It is tempting to suggest that a cascade type of amplification also operates in all three systems, and that the multiplicity of stages contributes to the final "gain" in activity, and thus to their efficiency.

REFERENCES

1. MORAWITZ, P. (1905). *Ergebn. Physiol.*, **4,** 307.
   The classical theory of blood clotting.
2. LISTER, J. (1863). *Proc. roy. Soc. B*, **12,** 580.
   Contact activation of blood clotting.
3. ESNOUF, M. P., and MACFARLANE, R. G. (1968). *Advanc. Enzymol.*, **30,** 255.
   Action of thromboplastin.
4. LORAND, L. (1954). *Physiol. Rev.*, **34,** 742.
   Mechanism of the thrombin—fibrinogen reaction.
5. BAILEY, K., and BETTELHEIM, R. R. (1955). *Brit. med. Bull.*, **11,** 50.
   Mechanism of the thrombin—fibrinogen reaction.
6. LORAND, L. and JACOBSEN, A. (1958). *J. biol. Chem.*, **230,** 420.
   Fibrin stabilising factor.
7. SEEGERS, W. H. (1962). *Prothrombin.* Cambridge, Mass.: Harvard Univ. Press.
8. QUICK, A. J. (1935). *J. biol. Chem.*, **109,** 73.
   The prothrombin-time test.
9. QUICK, A. J. (1957). *Hemorrhagic Diseases.* Philadelphia: Lea & Febiger.
10. OWREN, P. A. (1947). *Acta med. scand.*, Suppl. 194. Factor V.
11. MACFARLANE, R. G. (1961). *Brit. J. Hæmat.*, **7,** 496.
    The coagulant action of Russell's Viper venom.
12. ESNOUF, M. P., and WILLIAMS, W. J. (1962). *Biochem. J.*, **84,** 62.
    The activation of Factor X by Russell's Viper venom.
13. BIGGS, R., and MACFARLANE, R. G. (1962). *Human Blood Coagulation and its Disorders.* Oxford: Blackwell Scientific Publications.
14. BIGGS, R., and DOUGLAS, A. S. (1953). *J. clin. Path.*, **6,** 23.
    The thromboplastin generation test.
15. RATNOFF, O. D., DAVIE, E. W., and MALLETT, D. L. (1961). *J. clin. Invest.*, **40,** 803.
    Activation of Factors XII and XI.
16. MACFARLANE, R. G., and ASH, B. J. (1964). *Brit. J. Hæmat.*, **10,** 217.
    The activation of Factor X by plasma factors.
17. HALL, C. E., and SLAYTER, H. S. (1959). *J. biophys. biochem. Cytol.*, **5,** 11.
    The size, and shape of the fibrinogen molecule.
18. MICHAEL, S. E., and TUNNAH, G. W. (1966). *Brit. J. Hæmat.*, **12,** 115.
    The purification and properties of Factor VIII.

19. Schoenmakers, J. G. G., Matze, R., Hannen, C., and Zilliken, F. (1965). *Biochim. Biophys. Acta (Amst.)*, **101,** 166.
Nature of Factor XII.
20. Milstone, J. H. (1960). *Proc. Soc. exp. Biol. (N.Y.)*, **103,** 361.
Esterase activity of thrombokinase.
21. Macfarlane, R. G. (1966). *Thrombos. Diathes. hæmorrh. (Stuttg.)*, **15,** 591.
The cascade hypothesis of blood clotting.
22. Sawyer, P. N., Pate, J. W., and Weldon, C. S. (1953). *Amer. J. Physiol.*, **175,** 108.
The effect of electric potential of vascular surfaces on clotting.
23. Connor, W. E., Hoak, J. C., and Warner, E. D. (1963). *J. clin. Invest.*, **42,** 860.
Massive thrombosis produced by fatty acid infusion.
24. McGovern, V. J. (1955). *J. Path., Bact.*, **69,** 283.
The presence of heparin-like substances in vascular endothelium.
25. Biggs, R., Macfarlane, R. G., Denson, K. W. E., and Ash, B. J. (1965). *Brit. J. Hæmat.*, **11,** 276.
Thrombin action on Factor VIII.
26. Biggs, R., and Macfarlane, R. G. (eds.). (1966). *Treatment of Hæmophilia and Other Coagulation Defects.* Oxford: Blackwell Scientific Publications.
27. Biggs, R., Douglas, A. S., Macfarlane, F. G., Dacie, J. V., Pitney, W. R., Merskey, C., and O'Brien, J. R. (1952). *Brit. med. J.*, **2,** 1378.
Christmas disease.
28. Budtz-Olsen, O. E. (1951). *Clot Retraction.* Oxford: Blackwell Scientific Publications.
29. Bettex-Galland, M., and Lüscher, E. F. (1961). *Biochem. biophys. Acta (Amst.)*, **49,** 536.
Thrombosthenin.
30. Lüscher, E. F. (1956). *Vox Sang. (Basel)*, **1,** 133.
Platelets and clot retraction.
31. Bettex-Galland, M., and Lüscher, E. F. (1960). *Thrombos. Diathes. hæmorrh. (Stuttg.)*, **4,** 178.
Clot retraction, platelets, and ATP.
32. Christenson, L. R., and McLeod, C. M. (1945). *J. gen. Physiol.*, **28,** 559.
Streptococcal fibrinolysis.
33. Milstone, J. H. (1941). *J. Immunol.*, **42,** 109.
Streptococcal fibrinolysis.
34. Astrup, T. (1956). *Blood*, **11,** 781.
The fibrinolytic enzyme system.
35. Todd, A. S. (1959). *J. Path. Bact.*, **78,** 281.
Plasminogen activator in vascular tissue.
36. Warren, B. A. (1964). *Brit. med. Bull.*, **20,** 213.
Plasminogen activator in vascular endothelium.
37. Morgani, G. B. (1769). *The Seats and Causes of Disease*, Vol. 3, Book 4. The fluidity of post-mortem blood.
38. Morawitz, P. (1906). *Beitr. chem. Physiol. Path.*, **8,** 1.
39. Macfarlane, R. G., and Biggs, R. (1948). *Blood*, **3,** 1167.
Fibrinolysis and stress.
40. Fletcher, A. P., Aekjaesrig, N., and Sherry, S. (1959). *J. clin. Invest.*, **38,** 1096.
Local action of fibrinolytic agents on fibrin.
41. Kwaan, H. C., and McFadzean, A. J. S. (1956). *Clin. Sci.*, **15,** 245. Fibrinolysis and vascular ischæmia.
42. Eisen, V. (1964). *Brit. med. Bull.*, **20,** 205.
The kinin system.

Chapter 8

THE REACTIONS OF THE BLOOD TO INJURY

2. Cellular Reactions

BY J. E. FRENCH and R. G. MACFARLANE

Introduction

Defensive and reparative mechanisms activated by tissue injury are essential to the survival of a living organism in a potentially hostile world. In the previous chapter, attention has been paid to enzyme systems in the plasma which are activated by injury, and to their defensive role in limiting blood loss from disrupted blood vessels. In the present chapter the reactions of the cells of the blood will be dealt with, though such a separation is arbitrary, since plasma and cellular reactions are closely interlinked.

All the cellular components of the blood respond to, or are affected by injury in ways which tend to limit or minimise the damage and ultimately to assist repair. These cellular components consist of the leucocytes, platelets and red cells. The leucocytes and platelets have a predominantly defensive function, and their reactions to injury are active and complex. In the leucocyte reactions both the local pattern of events at the site of injury, and the general effect of injury on the cell populations of the blood as a whole must be considered. The involvement of polymorphonuclear leucocytes at a site of acute bacterial invasion for example will usually produce a rapid rise in the number of such cells in the circulating blood. These responses are so regular that their occurrence is of diagnostic help, changes in the number or morphology of the leucocytes giving a clue to the nature of an infection or tissue-damaging disease. The subject is, however, very extensive, and only a brief outline can be given here; full accounts will be found in textbooks and reviews on hæmatology.[1] As regards the platelets considerable advances have been made within the past few years, and a rather more detailed description will be given of their structure and properties, and of the correlation of their physical behaviour with certain biochemical events which have been recently discovered. The red cells, mainly concerned with gas transport, are usually considered as inert containers of hæmoglobin, but their behaviour may have an effect on blood viscosity and thus on flow patterns in the injured area and even remote from it.

THE LEUCOCYTES

In normal people the circulating blood contains from 4,000 to 10,000 leucocytes per c.mm., figures above or below these limits would be referred to as "leucocytosis" or a "leucopenia" respectively. The routine methods used for sampling and counting involve a large error, and a number of disturbing factors (such as fear of having blood taken) may cause wide variations even in normal people, so that only large changes can be regarded as significant. Leucocytes are of three main sorts; granulocytes, lymphocytes and monocytes.

The Granulocytes

The granulocytes are subdivided into the neutrophils, eosinophils and basophils, depending on the staining reaction of their granules. They are also graded into arbitrary stages of maturity. The most mature is the segmented form in which the nucleus is divided into 2, 3 or more lobes connected by thin strands of nuclear material; this segmented form is preceded by the band-form, which has an unsegmented, but elongated, nucleus, and by the myelocyte, with a round or oval nucleus. All of them have the distinctive neutrophil, eosinophil or basophil granules. Segmented and band-form cells are normally found in circulating blood, but myelocytes only appear there in response to very active leucocyte production, or certain diseases of the bone marrow. Still earlier forms, promyelocytes and myeloblasts, characterised by nucleoli in the nucleus and undifferentiation or absence of the specific granules, are normally only found in the bone marrow, but may appear in the blood stream in cases of leukæmia and some other marrow diseases.

The production of granulocytes is from the myeloid tissue which in the adult, is mainly situated in the flat bones and upper ends of the long bones. The normal rate of cell production is about 3×10^{11} cells per day, or about 25 ml. of packed cells. The average life span in the circulation is about 9 days.[2] This rate of production can be greatly increased, and the number of granulocytes circulating can be maintained at 20,000 or more in response to injury. Rapid short-term increases in the number circulating probably represent the mobilisation of cells from the reserves of the marrow and other tissues, since it has been computed that only 1 in 8 of the total number of leucocytes in the body is normally present in the blood stream at any one time.

The granulocytes seem to have an almost exclusively defensive role, particularly directed against invading bacteria, through their most characteristic activity, that of phagocytosis. They contain a number of enzymes and the release of these at a site of injury may have functions in the dissolution of dead tissue, the promotion of vascular responses, and in the stimulation of faster granulocyte production by the bone marrow and local healing. Phagocytosis, and the apparent attraction of the granulocyte towards certain bacteria and foreign material ("chemotaxis") is described in Chapter 4. These functions, though useful in the blood itself, are primarily required in extravascular tissue spaces invaded by bacteria or which have been physically or chemically injured. This extravascular role is achieved by the extraordinary phenomenon of leucocyte migration, the cells passing through the walls of inflamed capillaries and venules. This process can be studied and photographed with comparative ease in transparent vascular preparations such as the mesentery of various animals, the hamster cheek pouch or by means of windows inserted into the ears of rabbits. The first sign of impending inflammation is often a change in the flow pattern of the leucocytes. Instead of travelling freely with the circulation they begin to roll along the wall of the vessel with an obvious reluctance, as if their surface or that of the endothelium had become sticky. Finally, they come to a halt, joined by other cells until the affected vessel has a complete internal cuff of leucocytes. The blood flow slows or may stop as plasma fluid leaks into the surrounding tissues, and then, slowly at first but with increasing frequency the leucocytes insinuate pseudopodia apparently through the endothelial junctions and literally flow through the minute openings so formed, and escape into the extravascular space. In this way large numbers of these cells accumulate, adding to the infiltration of already œdematous and swollen tissues, and, if present in sufficient numbers, they constitute the pus characteristic of abscess formation. It is of interest that red cells seldom escape in large numbers with the leucoytes, and that the platelets, which so readily adhere to vascular surfaces damaged by physical trauma seldom adhere to the endothelium of an intact but inflamed vessel. The factors determining the different behaviour of these cells in different types of injury are still unknown. Many hypotheses have been advanced to explain white cell sticking, involving chemical or electro-chemical changes in the leucocytes, the endothelial cells, or both, or the deposition of some adhesive substance on the cell surfaces from the plasma, or its excretion by the cells themselves. But the nature of this process remains obscure. The matter is dealt with in detail in Chapters 3 and 4.

In these inflammatory reactions, it is the neutrophil granulocyte which is mainly implicated. In lesions involving antibody-antigen reactions, however, the pattern is more complex. In special cases, as for example in the Arthus phenomenon (see Chapter 38) both leucocytes and platelets may clump within the affected vessels. In other local antibody-antigen reactions, the eosinophil leucocytes are selectively involved, and an increase in circulating eosinophils is a feature of most hypersensitivity and allergic states. Eosinophil granules are rich in enzymes, and seem to be lysosomal structures. The functions of these cells, particularly their tendency to congregate in areas of antigenic reactions, has been linked with histamine which at one time they were supposed to carry. More recent work[3] has suggested that eosinophils possibly inactivate histamine, serotonin, and bradykinin, and may have an anti-inflammatory action.

The function of the basophils is unknown. The histochemical similarity of their granules to those of the tissue mast cells has led to the suggestion that the blood basophils may carry heparin, which has been shown to be an important functional constituent of the tissue mast cell.[4]

The Lymphocytes and Monocytes

These cells are dealt with in detail in Chapters 4 and 5.

Changes in the Leucocyte Numbers in the Blood

The normal blood levels of the different cells described are shown in Table I but even under normal conditions various circumstances may cause wide variations. There is a diurnal variation, leucocyte numbers being lower in the early morning and reaching a maximum in the afternoon. Strenuous exercise produces a definite leucocytosis, which may reach 20,000 per c.mm., the increase being mainly in the neutrophils. A similar leucocytosis may occur in a normal subject exposed to any form of stress, such as acute fear, pain, hæmorrhage, trauma, burns, or exposure to cold. The administration of adrenaline, ACTH, or cortisone has a similar effect in producing a neutrophil leucocytosis, and also eosinopenia, and slight lymphopenia. This latter pattern is less clearly marked, but often discernable in the conditions previously mentioned. It might be supposed, therefore, that most of these stressful conditions lead to the liberation of adrenaline, followed by the production of "glucocorticoids" which affect

8/Table I

The normal range of relative frequencies and absolute numbers of the different types of leucocyte

Cell Type	*Per Cent*	*Absolute Numbers per c.mm.*
All types	100	5,000–10,000
Band cells	3–5	150–400
Segmented neutrophils	54–62	3,000–5,800
Eosinophils	1–3	50–250
Basophils	0–0·75	15–50
Lymphocytes	25–33	1,500–3,000
Monocytes	3–7	285–500

(*From Wintrobe*[1])

leucocyte regulation and may be responsible for the eosinopenia and lymphopenia. A direct effect of adrenaline stimulates the release of neutrophils from the bone marrow and spleen.

Leucocyte Changes in Pathological States

In many pathological conditions involving tissue damage the changes in the leucocytes are due to other factors besides the adrenal-pituitary mechanism. The main conditions affecting leucocyte numbers are exposure to radiation, intoxication by a variety of drugs and chemicals, allergic states, the invasion of the body by micro-organisms or parasites, and metabolic or neoplastic disorders damaging the leucopoietic tissues.

Ionising radiation has effects depending on the dosage and duration of exposure, type of radiation, and the tissues involved. Details cannot be given here but the subject of radiation injury is dealt with in Chapters 25 and 26, and a number of reviews have been published. A small exposure causes a rise in neutrophil and lymphocyte counts followed by a fall to normal within a few days. Repeated small exposures cause a lymphopenia, followed by a neutropenia and an increase in eosinophils, and may lead on to a reduction of all leucocytes and to aplastic anæmia due to marrow destruction. Acute exposure may cause a leucopenia followed in a few hours by a leucocytosis and later by a progressive fall in the lymphocytes, neutrophils and platelets, in that order, until the blood is almost devoid of cells other than red cells. Death usually occurs within a month from hæmorrhage, infection and anæmia. These complex changes are probably due to the variable degree of stimulation produced by tissue injury opposed by destruction of the leucopoietic tissues.

Toxic drugs and chemicals causing changes in the white cells are legion. In small doses, stimulation of the marrow may produce an increase in cells and the appearance of immature forms, but, as in the case of radiation, larger doses may be destructive. The most important agents of this sort, which may be used in industry, are benzol, toluol, aniline and their compounds, and, of those used in medicine, the sulpha-drugs, gold, arsenic, thiourea, amidopyrine, and chloramphenicol among many others. It is no exaggeration to say that almost any drug or chemical may produce adverse effects, since personal idiosyncrasies may render individuals vulnerable to agents apparently harmless to the majority of people. A lack of realisation of the potential danger of these substances, or of proper control in their usage, has caused many fatal cases of aplastic anæmia or agranulocytosis.

Infections

The recognition that certain infections cause marked changes in the leucocyte count goes back to the time of Virchow.[5] These changes are sufficiently specific to give considerable diagnostic help to the clinician, being related closely to the type of infection.

Infection by the pyogenic cocci (streptococci, staphylococci, pneumococci, meningococci and gonococci) and by certain bacteria (*Esch. coli*, *Ps. pyocyanea*, *C. diphtheriæ*) and fungi (Actinomyces) causes a rapid and considerable rise in the neutrophil count. The degree of this rise is related to the extent and severity of the infection, and it may reach 50,000, though 15,000–25,000 per c.mm. are more usual levels. Local but intense tissue destruction with the formation of pus under pressure may have a greater effect than a more extensive infection in which drainage of pus is adequate. The other cells of the blood are usually not greatly affected during the first (invasion) stage of the infection. Later, as the defences of the tissues are built up, there is a rise in the monocyte count, followed (during the recovery phase) by an increase in eosinophils and lymphocytes, and a decline in the neutrophils. Should the infection prove overwhelming, a leucopenia may occur and is a grave prognostic sign. These changes are considerably modified by the use of antibacterial or antibiotic drugs, which may suppress the leucocytic reaction not only by destroying bacteria but also by depressing the bone marrow.

In some non-pyogenic infections a similar sequence of events may occur. For example, in rheumatic and scarlet fever, and in some virus infections, including poliomyelitis, rabies and herpes zoster, and the later stages of smallpox, a pronounced neutrophil leucocytosis occurs.

On the other hand, a number of infections are characterised by a neutropenia, at least in the earlier stages of the disease. These include typhoid, paratyphoid and brucella infections, and certain virus diseases, including influenza, measles, rubella and, in its early stages, smallpox. In such conditions the lymphocyte count may be normal or increased. In tuberculosis there is usually an increase both in the lymphocytes and monocytes, but not in the neutrophils unless pyogenic infection is super-added. In glandular fever and possibly in other similar virus diseases there is a great increase in the lymphocyte count, these cells also having a characteristic and abnormal morphology. In whooping cough there is a considerable increase of morphologically normal lymphocytes. In both these conditions the blood picture may be an important diagnostic feature.

Finally, there must be mentioned the eosinophilia which is characteristic of allergic states. When a subject becomes sensitised to some allergen and is subsequently exposed to it, as in sufferers from asthma, hay-fever, urticaria, or certain skin diseases, or in parasitic infestation with absorption of foreign protein, there is usually an eosinophilia, reaching in extreme cases (e.g. in trichiniasis) 20,000–30,000 cells per c.mm.

The Mechanism of Pathological Leucocytosis

The mechanism of leucocytosis in the pyogenic infections has been the object of much speculation and experiment. Many consider that the products of cell breakdown directly stimulate marrow leucocyte production. The injection of nucleo-proteins produces a leucocytosis and a preparation known as "pentnucleotide" was for many years used as a marrow stimulant in cases of neutropenia. Menkin[6] has studied a number of α-globulins and polypeptide fractions derived from inflammatory exudates and which stimulate or depress leucocyte production. He believes that the release of such substances by damaged tissues can account for the changes in the leucocyte population of the blood which accompany the different stages of an inflammatory process. On the other hand, Rosenow[7] shows that a considerable leucocytosis can be produced in rabbits by the injection of bacterial protein, and that this effect can be inhibited by the administration of narcotics such as barbiturates which act on the brain stem. The leucocytosis-promoting effect of such protein might therefore act through the splanchnic-adrenal mechanism already described.

The more specific stimulation of eosinophils, monocytes and lymphocytes in allergy, tuberculosis, whooping cough and glandular fever respectively is unexplained.

THE PLATELETS

In some of the lower classes of animals, in which the plasma clotting mechanisms described in the previous chapter have not evolved, solidification of blood at a site of injury depends on the ability of certain specialised cells, called amœbocytes, to adhere together to form a solid aggregate.[8] In mammals, the blood platelets share many of the properties of these cells, but since the formation of a fibrin clot is such a striking event when mammalian blood is studied *in vitro*, the platelet changes may appear to be of minor significance. There are circumstances, however, in the living animal in which the reactions of the platelets are of primary importance and the formation of fibrin may be relegated to a secondary role. These reactions are primarily defensive as in the formation of solid hæmostatic plugs in disrupted vessels but they may be harmful as in thrombosis or in the blockage of vessels which occurs with certain immunological stimuli. A general account of the properties of the platelets is given in this section; their role in the mechanisms of hæmostasis and thrombosis is discussed in greater detail in Chapter 9.

Structure and Composition

The platelets, with a diameter of 2–5μ, are the smallest of the formed elements and, unless precautions are taken, they readily undergo rapid changes in shed blood. It is not surprising that their discovery awaited the perfection of the optical microscope in the last century[9] and that for many years there was much controversy as to whether they were a distinct class or were fragments of other cells, micro-organisms or even lipid droplets.[10] They can remain unnoticed in the blood vessels in tissue sections but are seen at high magnification in the transparent preparations used for studying the micro-circulation, and in a well-prepared blood film stained by the Romanowsky methods they are characterised by their small, often centrally-grouped azurophil granules.

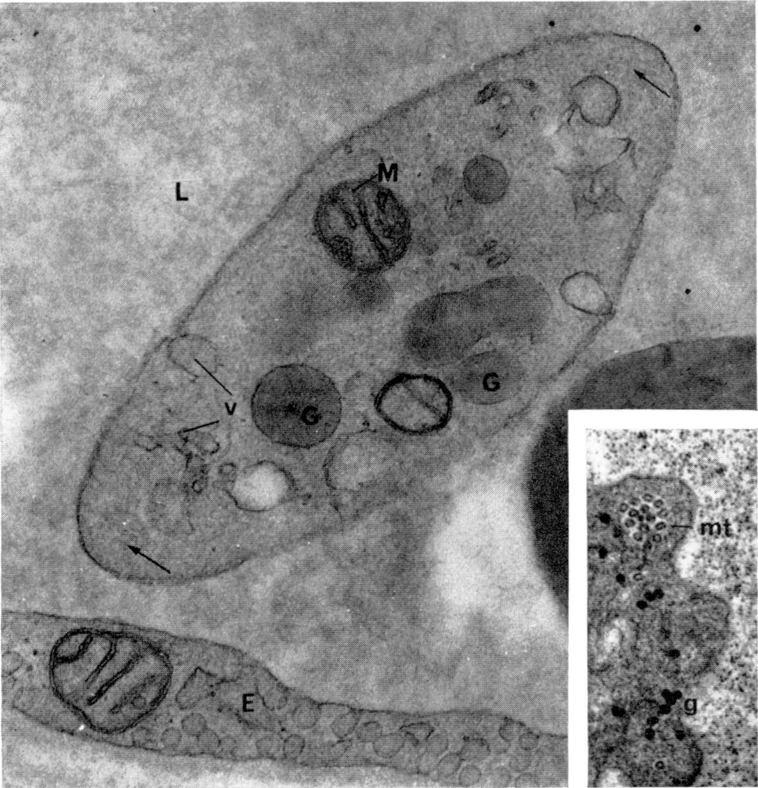

8/FIG. 1.—A platelet in the lumen (L) of a blood capillary in a rat is bounded by a plasma membrane and contains dense granules (G), mitochondria (M) and vesicular elements (v). The arrows indicate the position of the microtubules. Capillary endothelium (E) is seen in the lower part of the picture. (×48,000.) Another platelet (inset) shows the microtubules (mt) in greater detail and glycogen particles (g). (×60,000.)

A much more detailed picture of platelet structure is now available from electron microscopy which lends itself particularly well to the study of these small objects.[11] As seen in thin section in a blood vessel (FIG. 1) they usually show an elliptical profile representing a slice through a convex disc; they are bounded by a well-defined plasma membrane and contain a number of characteristic organelles: dense granules (0·2–0·3μ diam.), also membrane-bound, correspond to the azurophil granules of the light microscope; small mitochondria (0·15–0·2μ diam.); a variety of vesicles or vacuoles; other small dense inclusions of which the most constant are glycogen particles. When glutaraldehyde rather than osmium tetroxide is used as the fixative, other features may be revealed which include a system of microtubules orientated peripherally, and dense bodies within vacuoles which are thought to represent the 5-hydroxytryptamine content.[12] There is, however, a notable lack of some of the constituents found in other living cells; the platelets have no nucleus and although they may occasionally contain ribosomes these are invariably scanty and there is no organised rough-surfaced endoplasmic reticulum.

Details of the chemical composition and biochemical properties of the platelets will be found in a comprehensive review by Marcus and Zucker.[13] Like other living cells, platelets contain simple inorganic constituents and organic molecules of varying weight and complexity. On a dry weight basis they contain about 60 per cent protein, 15–20 per cent lipid and about 10 per cent carbohydrate. Plasma proteins, albumin, globulins and fibrinogen, occur in platelet extracts. While it is probable that these molecules can be adsorbed to the platelet surface or taken up secondarily from the plasma there is evidence that at least some of the platelet fibrinogen has distinctive properties and may be a true intracellular component. A specific platelet protein of particular interest in relation to clot retraction has been isolated and found to have similar properties to muscle actomyosin in that it will contract in the presence of ATP and magnesium and will act as an ATPase. This substance, termed "thrombosthenin", represents approximately 15 per cent of the total platelet protein. Immunochemical analysis of the antigens present in platelets have shown that, in addition to plasma protein components which as already mentioned may be adsorbed, there are other antigens which appear to be specific, producing antibodies which react only with the platelets or the parent megakaryocyte.[14]

The lipid component is probably very largely associated with protein as lipoprotein complexes of the cell membranes. Phospholipids, which make up 70–80 per cent of the total lipid, include phosphatidyl choline (25 per cent), phosphatidyl ethanolamine (25 per cent), phosphatidyl serine (10 per cent) and sphingomyelin (15–20 per cent). The total amount of phospholipid is slightly higher than in other blood cells (red cells and lymphocytes) but does not differ markedly in overall composition or fatty acid constituents from other tissues. Cholesterol makes up about 15 per cent of the total and is mainly in the free (non-esterified) form with only trace amounts of cholesterol esters. Other components include triglycerides, partial glycerides and non-esterified fatty acids.

The platelets carry a number of factors concerned with plasma coagulation. Some of these can be identified with plasma clotting factors adsorbed to the platelet surface, but "Platelet Factor 3" is an important component of the intrinsic clotting mechanism (see Chapter 7) which is specific to the platelets. Its activity is associated with phosphatidyl serine and phosphatidyl ethanolamine, but its composition in the natural state is unknown, and it may be a protein-phospholipid complex. Platelet Factor 3 activity is found in the cell membrane, and the cytoplasmic granules and organelles. The clotting activity becomes available during the coagulation process, since in fact, native platelets appear to be inert. Following damage, surface contact, or aggregation by thrombin or other agents, platelet Factor 3 activity becomes apparent, and is mainly associated with the cell membrane.[15]

Of the platelet carbohydrates only glucose and ribose have been detected as the simple monomers. The neutral hexoses (glucose, galactose, mannose and fucose), amino-sugars (galactosamine, glucosamine), and acidic carbohydrates (glucuronic and sialic acids) are bound together in a definite order to form a series of oligosaccharide units which are linked to protein, probably in the cell membranes. A proportion of these oligosaccharide prosthetic groups are terminated by sialic acid which is largely responsible for the negative charge at the cell surface. It has been calculated that there is eleven times more sialic acid per unit area of surface in platelets than there is in red cells. A sulphated mucopolysaccharide, with properties resembling chondroitin sulphate has been isolated from a granule fraction and is thought to be associated with the platelet 5-hydroxytryptamine.

The greater part of the 5-hydroxytryptamine content of whole blood is normally present in the platelets. This is not synthesised by platelets or megakaryocytes but is taken up against a concentration gradient by an active transport mechanism which can be inhibited by metabolic antagonists. A storage mechanism as distinct from transport can be blocked by reserpine.[12] Adrenaline and noradrenaline can also be taken up. Histamine is found in high concentration in platelets in the rabbit, but not in other species. In contrast to the other vasoactive amines, the histamine of the platelets is synthesised *in situ* by decarboxylation of histidine.

Platelets have been shown to contain a higher concentration of ATP than most tissues and this provides the source for the energy expended during clot retraction. It is generally considered that the glycolytic pathway is more active than the tricarboxylic acid cycle in the generation of these high-energy phosphate bonds. Platelets are now known to contain mitochondria and enzyme systems characteristic of ærobic intermediary metabolism; this alternative and more efficient mechanism may be responsible for producing a considerable proportion of the energy required for platelet activity.

Various hydrolytic enzymes have been detected in platelets, in particular acid phosphatase, β-glucuronidase and cathepsin. The major part of the acid phosphatase of serum is derived from the platelets. Since in other tissues this group of enzymes is characteristic of lysosomal activity it has been suggested that some of the platelet granules may fall into this category. The platelets appear to be ill-equipped for the synthesis of protein, and no doubt many of their components are furnished by the parent megakaryocyte, but there are many aspects of this question which require further investigation.

Origin and Life Span

The origin of these non-nucleated cells was for a long time a matter of speculation, but the view, put forward by Wright (1910),[16] that they were formed by fragmentation of the cytoplasm of the megakaryocyte has been fully confirmed by later studies. This very large cell, up to 160 μ diam. (FIG. 2), occurs in the bone marrow and in some species also in the spleen. It develops a polyploid nucleus with up to 32 times the usual complement of chromosomes before the cytoplasm breaks up into fragments representing individual platelets. This fragmentation of the cytoplasm is brought about by the development of a network of paired membranes in the cytoplasm, termed the demarcation membranes[17] (FIG. 3); it has been calculated that a single megakaryocyte can in this way release 3,000–4,000 platelets into the circulation.

Labelling experiments have shown that under normal conditions platelets survive for only 6–14 days but it is still not entirely clear whether this represents a life span which is limited by an aging process or whether platelets are used up in a random way as they fulfil one or other of their various functions. When

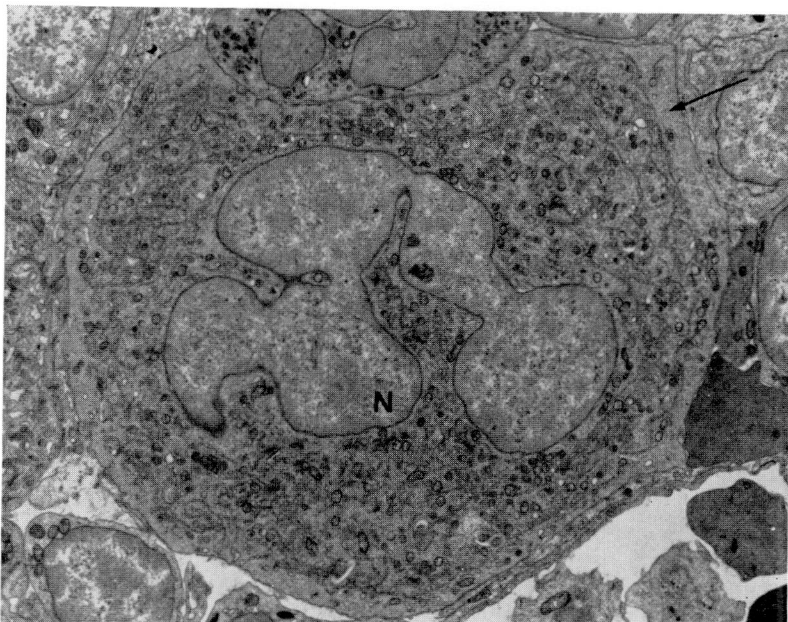

8/FIG. 2.—A megakaryocyte in bone marrow of a rat. It has a large folded nucleus (N). The cytoplasm is rich in granules, small mitochondria, and smooth-surfaced membranes and vesicles. The peripheral border of the cell is relatively clear (arrow). (× 5,250.)

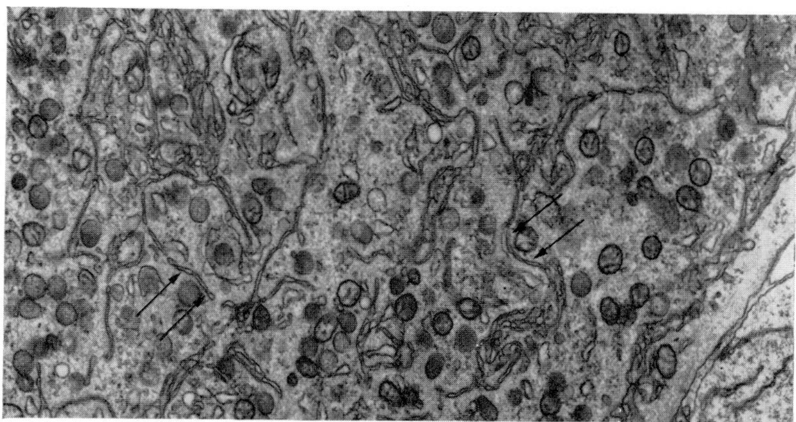

8/FIG. 3.—Part of the cytoplasm of a megakaryocyte at higher magnification to show the system of paired demarcation membranes (arrows). (× 11,000.)

circulating platelets become effete through old age or other cause they are probably removed by reticulo-endothelial cells, particularly in the spleen, but decisive evidence on this point is still lacking.[18]

In normal subjects, the number of circulating platelets may vary rather widely between individuals and from time to time in the same individual, as in the case of the leucocyte count. The mean normal figure is about 240,000 per c.mm. with a range of 140,000 to 340,000. Severe exercise, or the injection of adrenaline raises the platelet count in normal subjects by a factor of 2 or 3. The platelet count is raised following trauma or hæmorrhage, or surgical operations, particularly splenectomy. Persistently increased platelet levels are termed "thrombocythæmia", and occur in polycythæmia, chronic myelocytic leukæmia and other diseases affecting the bone marrow. Thrombocytopenia may occur in any condition in which the platelets are destroyed with abnormal rapidity, or in which their production in inhibited. Abnormal platelet destruction may be caused by a variety of chemicals or toxins, or by specific platelet antibodies. Production may also be inhibited by the same agents acting on the megakaryocytes in the bone marrow. The marrow itself may be destroyed giving rise to aplastic anæmia, as in radiation injury, leukæmia, the invasion of the marrow by neoplastic disease, and in some deficiency anæmias.[1] In many cases of thrombocytopenia, however, no specific cause can be found, and the beneficial effects of steroid therapy or splenectomy provide only presumptive evidence that they may be due to some auto-immune process.

Functional Properties

In the earliest studies on the platelets it was recognised that they had the ability to undergo morphological changes as blood clotted *in vitro*. The series of changes, to which the rather imprecise term "viscous metamorphosis" has been applied, can be seen quite readily by dark ground or phase contrast microscopy and further points of detail can be filled in from studies with the electron microscope. When whole blood, or recalcified plasma containing platelets, is placed on a glass slide the platelets swell up within a few seconds and appear to throw out small blebs and club-like excrescences from their surface. As this happens they become sticky and adhere readily to the surface of the glass and, when the preparation is agitated, to other platelets with which they happen to collide. It used to be thought on the basis of light microscopy that the platelets, having clumped, could fuse together into an amorphous mass, but electron microscopy has shown that the appearance is due to the formation of a very tight aggregate in which, although many of the platelets have lost their content of granules their plasma membranes are preserved.

In the clotting of whole blood or recalcified plasma the clumping of platelets and the morphological changes in them precede the formation of fibrin by an appreciable interval so that the events described can be said to be occurring *pari passu* with the sequence of plasma reactions discussed in Chapter 7. There are several clear indications that the two processes are interlinked: both are initiated by contact of the blood with a particular type of surface, both require the presence of ionised calcium, platelets furnish phospholipid required in blood coagulation, and thrombin generated during coagulation has important effects on platelet behaviour. Nevertheless there are points of difference which make it possible to study the two processes separately *in vitro* and, as we shall see later, there are circumstances *in vivo* where the platelet changes appear to be dominant while fibrin formation plays a secondary role in solidification of the blood.

When the properties of platelets are to be examined *in vitro* it is usual to withdraw the blood into siliconised glassware, thus reducing the stimulus of surface contact, and to avoid spontaneous aggregation by adding the anticoagulants sodium citrate or EDTA which reduce or abolish the concentration of free calcium ions. If the blood is then centrifuged at a sufficiently low speed (125 g.), red cells and leucocytes sediment more rapidly than the platelets which are retained in the supernatant to yield a so-called platelet-rich plasma. If the PRP is now taken off and recentrifuged at 750 g., a platelet pellet is obtained which can be resuspended in appropriate saline media. When necessary the platelets can be washed free from residual plasma components by further centrifugations.

Platelet adhesion.—The ability of platelets to adhere to surfaces of glass or metal, to certain tissue cells, and to connective tissue fibres, particularly collagen, can be demonstrated *in vitro* using whole blood, citrated platelet-rich plasma or saline suspensions containing calcium. Adhesion takes place within 1–2 seconds of contact of the platelet with the surface and will occur readily at 0° C., suggesting that the process is not energy-dependent and does not involve time-consuming reactions as does the clotting mechanism. However, very little is known about the forces involved or about the physical or chemical properties of a surface which make it recognisable as "foreign". As usually demonstrated, platelet adhesion is followed by aggregation and by release of platelet constituents but there are differences in these phenomena with regard to temperature and the requirement for calcium and protein factors which suggest that they can operate independently.[19] Measurements of platelet adhesiveness as usually carried out employ a glass surface. The number of platelets in a sample of blood or plasma is counted before and after rotating the sample in a glass cylinder or passing it through a column of glass beads. The missing platelets are presumed to be stuck to the glass, but it should be pointed out that these methods do not discriminate clearly between adhesion and aggregation.

In the living animal, adhesion of platelets is seen particularly in damaged vessels when injury leads to the exposure of sub-endothelial tissue including collagen fibres to the blood (Chapter 9). It will also occur when a "foreign surface" is placed deliberately in contact with the circulating blood, as may happen when a suture of catgut or silk is passed through the vascular lumen or when a graft of synthetic fabric is used to replace a segment of a vessel.

Phagocytosis.—The ability of platelets to ingest foreign particles which was first suggested from studies with the light microscope,[20] has now been clearly demonstrated by electron microscopy.[21] When particles of carbon or polystyrene latex are added to platelet-rich plasma the materials are taken up readily and are seen enclosed within vacuoles in the platelet cytoplasm (FIG. 4). Phagocytosis by platelets also occurs *in vivo* when particles of colloidal carbon or thorium dioxide are injected into the circulation. The property may extend to naturally occurring substances since lipid droplets, virus particles and antigen-antibody complexes have been identified by electron microscopy within cytoplasmic vacuoles.

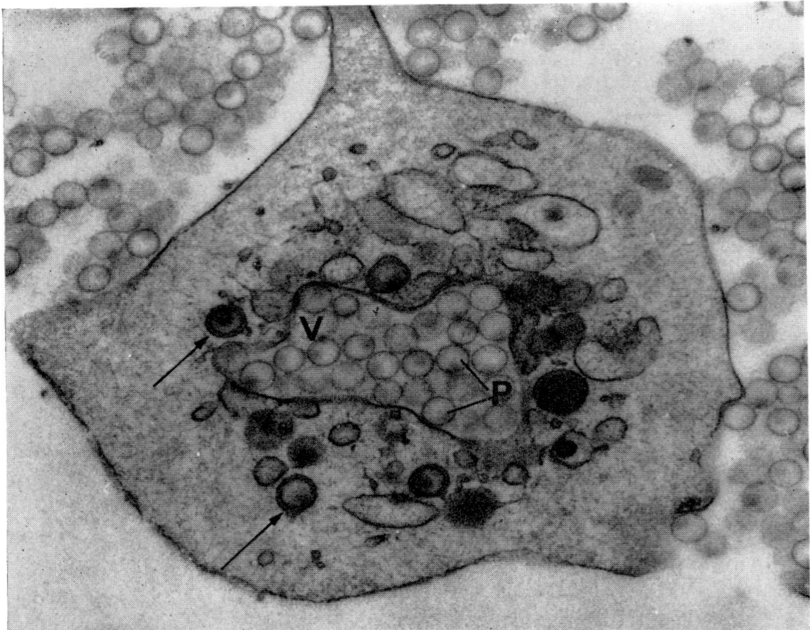

8/Fig. 4.—A platelet in platelet-rich plasma to which a suspension of polystyrene particles had been added. A group of particles (P) is enclosed within a vacuole (v). Other single particles (arrows) are seen within smaller vacuoles. (× 38,000.)

Phagocytosis by platelets is probably related to adhesion. Particles which are taken up in this way must first make contact with the platelet plasma membrane, but whereas the platelet may be stimulated to spread over a larger surface the smaller particle will be engulfed.

Aggregation

For many years it was supposed that the aggregation of platelets was directly related to the clotting process. A simple explanation would be that fibrin sticks the platelets together, but this appears to be no longer tenable. As mentioned previously, aggregation precedes the obvious formation of fibrin in clotting blood; it also occurs quite readily in the blood of patients with a constitutional lack of fibrinogen. Thrombin will undoubtedly cause platelets to aggregate (see below) but there is no evidence that it is always necessary. Aggregation occurs in the presence of sufficient heparin to prevent thrombin formation and also in artificial systems where no thrombin is present.

Within the last few years a new line of investigation has been opened up by the discovery that adenosine diphosphate (ADP) has an apparently specific role in causing platelet aggregation. It is effective in very low concentrations when added to platelet-rich citrated plasma. Moreover, other agents (collagen fibres, foreign particles and certain fatty acids) which will induce aggregation *in vitro* are now known to release ADP from the platelets themselves and it is probably this released ADP which causes the aggregation. These phenomena can apparently operate independently of the clotting process and may be of considerable importance in relation to the behaviour of platelets at sites of injury in the living animal.

Since aggregation of platelets can occur without adhesion to a fixed surface it can be investigated quite simply in platelet-rich plasma or platelet suspensions. The rate and extent of aggregation which follows the addition of a particular agent can be measured by recording continuously the transmission of light through the specimen.[22] As the aggregates form the transmission increases but returns to the initial value if the aggregates break up again. Some form of agitation is necessary to bring the platelets together and this is usually achieved by use of a mechanical stirrer.

Aggregating agents

(i) *Adenosine diphosphate.*—In 1960 Hellem[23] discovered a factor present in erythrocytes which markedly increased the "stickiness" of platelets. This was later identified as adenosine diphosphate,[24] and it has since been shown that this substance will aggregate platelets rapidly in all mammalian species so far tested.

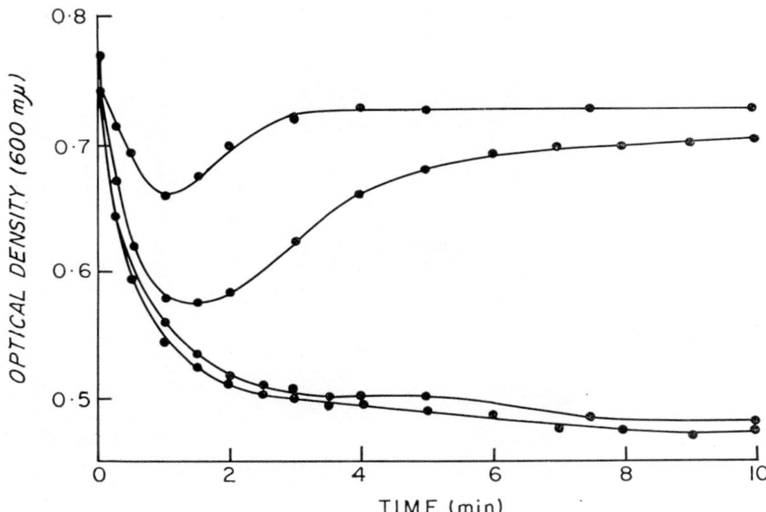

8/FIG. 5.—Effect of adding ADP on the optical density of plasma containing $4{\cdot}75 \times 10^{8}$ platelets/ml. ADP was added at zero time to give the following concentrations: A, $2{\cdot}5 \times 10^{-7}$ M; B, 5×10^{-7} M; C, 1×10^{-6} M; D, $2{\cdot}5 \times 10^{-6}$ M. (From Born.[25])

On addition of ADP to platelet-rich citrated plasma the aggregation begins immediately when the specimen is stirred and reaches a maximum after a few minutes. Unless high concentrations of ADP are used the aggregates then begin to break up again, presumably because the ADP is inactivated or destroyed by plasma or platelet enzymes. FIGURE 5 shows the changes in the optical density of the plasma which occur. If the aggregates from such a test are examined in the electron microscope most of the platelets appear still to be intact, but they are

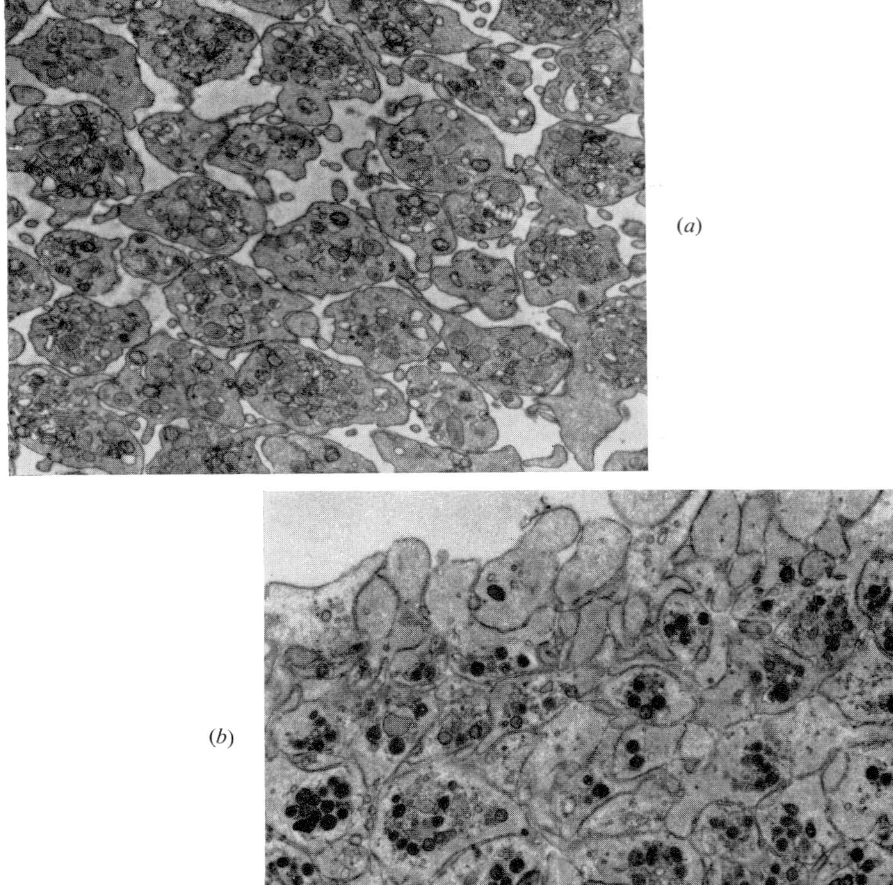

8/FIG. 6.—(*a*) Section through a pellet prepared from platelet-rich citrated plasma (PRP). The platelets are more irregular in shape than they are in the bloodstream but have remained discrete. (× 7,000.) (*b*) Part of a platelet aggregate from PRP to which ADP had been added. The platelets are closely packed together. They appear intact though a few have formed outward projections. (× 6,500.)

tightly packed together in a mosaic arrangement as seen in section, with a fairly regular spacing of 200–300 A° between the adjacent plasma membranes which is too narrow to be resolved with the light microscope (FIG. 6). The nature of the apparent gap between adjacent plasma membranes is not known, but it may represent an outer coating which is not shown up by conventional electron microscopic techniques. There is no fibrin formation and when the aggregates break up again, microscopy shows only discrete individual platelets.

Metabolic derivatives of ADP and a few other closely related substances will act as inhibitors of aggregation if they are added to the plasma before the ADP. Inhibition by AMP was the first to be observed but adenosine and several of its analogues, for example, 2-chloroadenosine, are also effective.[25] The aggregation phenomenon can be demonstrated in suspensions of platelets in artificial media but under these circumstances it is possible to show that there is an absolute requirement for calcium, though in a lower concentration than is needed for clotting, and for a plasma protein which is either fibrinogen or one very closely associated with it.

The mechanism of the action of ADP on platelets is still not clear. The most favoured view is that there are specific binding sites for ADP on the platelet surface which can be blocked by the inhibitors mentioned.[26] Bridges between adjacent platelets may be formed by bound ADP with calcium and the protein component, or alternatively, ADP may produce changes in molecular configuration at the platelet surface which enable disulphide bonds to be formed between the platelets and the protein component. The possibility has also to be considered that ADP is acting as a specific energy source for chemical reactions at the platelet surface which have yet to be defined. Although fibrinogen may be the protein molecule involved there is no other obvious link between the ADP-induced aggregation and the coagulation factors.

(ii) *Agents which release ADP from platelets.*—Platelets contain ADP, and a high concentration of ATP which can rapidly break down. It is therefore possible that aggregation may be caused by ADP, not only derived from an extrinsic source, but from the platelets themselves following certain stimuli. Agents which appear to promote aggregation *in vitro* in this way include "extracts" of collagen fibres, particles of carbon or latex, long chain saturated fatty acids, and immune complexes. In some situations the stimulus for ADP release is probably adhesion. Thus, the aggregation of platelets which follows the adherence of platelets to collagen fibres,[27] or the phagocytosis by platelets of foreign particles, which as mentioned above is related to adhesion, is associated with the appearance of ADP in the medium. It is suggested that this ADP can itself release more ADP from other platelets, so that a chain reaction results.[25] Of particular interest in relation to immunological reactions is the finding that antigen:antibody complexes can cause platelets to aggregate and that when they do so ADP is released.[28] With other agents, not clearly involving adhesion or phagocytosis, the ADP mechanism may nevertheless underlie the aggregating action. It has been found that the aggregation of platelets caused by thrombin (see below) and by certain long chain fatty acids is prevented by the presence of a substrate enzyme system (phospho-enol-pyruvate and pyruvate kinase) which causes the rapid removal of ADP as it is released.[29]

The aggregates promoted by the above agents have more or less the same structural features as those induced by extrinsic ADP, though there is a time lag before they are formed and rather more of the platelets appear to have projections or to have lost some of their organelles, which would be consistent with the release of some of their contents (Fig. 7*a*).

(iii) *Thrombin.*—The addition of small amounts of thrombin to platelet-rich plasma causes the formation of tightly packed aggregates in which platelets at the edges show loss of granules. In this case, fibrin appears later at the edges of

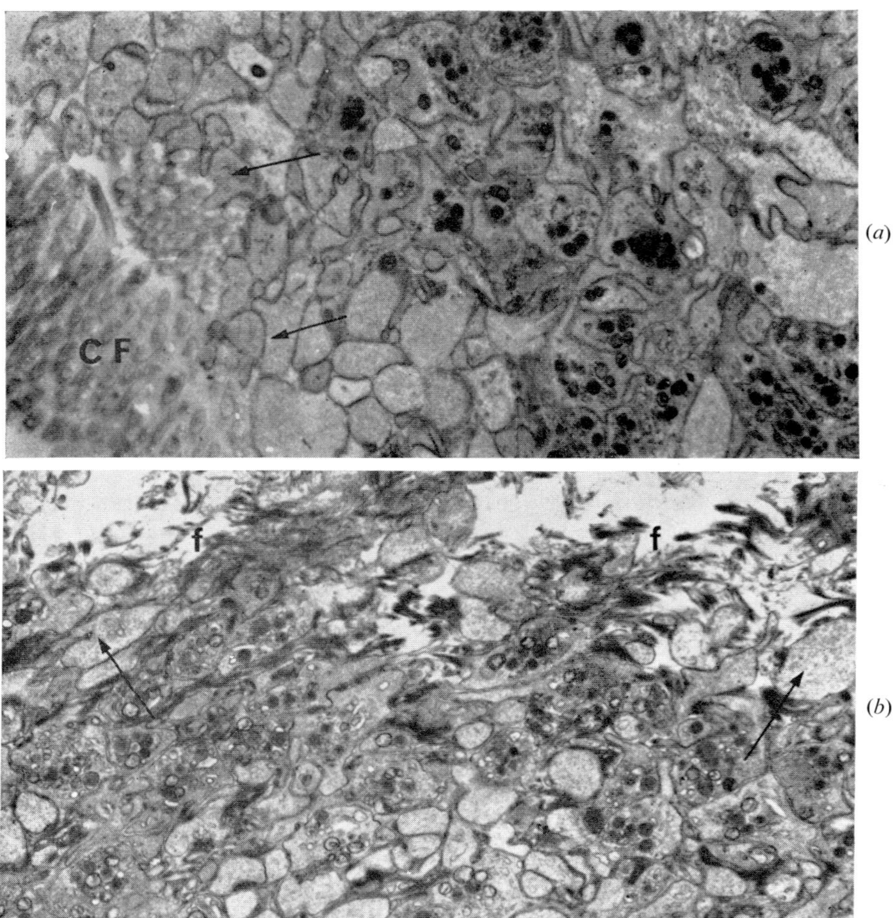

8/Fig. 7.—(*a*) Tightly packed platelet aggregate in PRP to which a collagen suspension had been added. Platelets in contact with collagen fibres (CF) appear to have lost their organelles (arrows). (× 8,500.) (*b*) Platelet aggregate formed in PRP following addition of thrombin. Platelets at the periphery (arrows) have lost their granules or formed outward projections. Strands of fibrin (f) are seen around the aggregate. (× 7,000.)

the aggregates as it does in clotting blood (Fig. 7*b*). Aggregation can also be caused by thrombin in platelet suspensions in which there is no obvious fibrin formation and this suggests that the action of thrombin on platelets may be independent of coagulation under some circumstances. It is therefore of interest that thrombin is a very effective agent in the release of platelet nucleotides and that its aggregating effect on platelet suspensions can be prevented by the substrate-enzyme system mentioned above which removes ADP as it is released.

(iv) *Other agents.*—A number of other agents which may be involved in reactions to injury can induce platelet aggregation *in vitro* though their effects show greater species differences and do not clearly involve the ADP mechanism. Adrenaline and noradrenaline cause aggregation of platelets in man but not in the rabbit; adrenaline and noradrenaline also potentiate the effectiveness of ADP in causing aggregation in man; [30] 5-hydroxytryptamine can cause aggregation, but again is more effective with human than with rabbit platelets.

The effect of aggregating agents *in vivo*.—Many of the agents described in this section will also cause platelet aggregation when injected into the circulation of animals. The infusion of ADP leads to the formation of intravascular platelet aggregates with the same structural features as those described *in vitro*. The aggregates are trapped temporarily in small vessels in the lung and elsewhere so that there is at first a fall in the circulating platelet count, but after a few minutes the aggregates break up again and the count returns to normal. A relatively high dose of ADP is required for the induction of aggregates *in vivo*, but this is probably explained by the rapid inactivation of ADP that occurs in the circulation.[31] Since ADP is a constituent of all cells in the body, and its concentration is increased in injured cells, its release at sites of injury may well be an important factor in causing platelet aggregation in injured vessels (Chapter 9).

Infusion of the other agents may activate coagulation in whole blood so that the aggregates which form *in vivo* are often associated with fibrin and are more stable than those induced by infusion of ADP. Infusion of thrombin in sufficient concentration to overcome the natural inhibitors causes a fall in the platelet count and the formation of platelet-fibrin aggregates in small vessels. These aggregates remain *in situ* for several hours but then break up again presumably as a result of fibrinolytic activity.[32] A striking effect is obtained by infusion of certain long chain fatty acids. In mice, for example, quite small amounts of sodium stearate will cause massive intravascular platelet aggregation and fibrin formation with rapid death of the animal.[33] Intravenous injection of various types of particle, including bacteria, also causes a fall in the platelet count and the formation of platelet clumps which lodge at least temporarily in small vessels in the lung and elsewhere.[34] (FIG. 8). In the past this phenomenon attracted considerable attention from its possible role in the defense against circulating organisms.[10] Possibly organisms trapped in this way are more susceptible to phagocytosis by other cells; though, as we have seen, platelets may ingest foreign material, there is still no clear evidence that they themselves play an important part in its disposal.

Release of platelet constituents.—The release of platelet ADP has already been discussed in relation to aggregation. It can be seen, however, that the platelets have a number of other active constituents which have potential pharmacological or pathological effects, should they escape from their limiting membranes. The mechanism by which platelets release their constituents, termed the "*release reaction*", is poorly understood, but it is known that it is stimulated by thrombin, certain other proteolytic enzymes, and may form a part of the response to other aggregating agents.

When thrombin acts on platelets in low concentration it not only leads to aggregation but causes the release of large amounts of adenine nucleotide and 5-hydroxytryptamine into the extracellular medium. Inorganic phosphate, potassium and some free amino-acids and protein are also liberated, but the amount of the latter is small, suggesting that there is not complete disruption of the cell.[36] This is borne out by electron microscope examination of the thrombin induced aggregates which shows the preservation of apparently intact plasma membranes. The appearance of the platelets is changed, however. Many appear more spherical in shape or have formed outward projections and there is a striking loss of platelet granules particularly at the edges of the aggregates (FIG. 7*b*). Probably when the platelets undergo these changes the platelet factors concerned in blood coagulation also become more readily available as is indicated by the first appearance of fibrin at the edges of altered platelets in clotting PRP. The release reaction is also stimulated *in vitro* by contact of platelets with collagen fibres and, in platelet-rich plasma, by foreign surfaces.

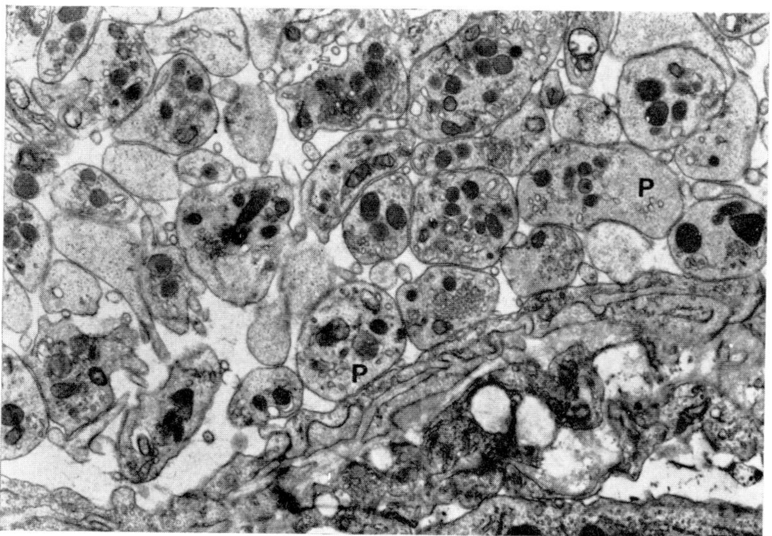

8/FIG. 8.—Aggregated platelets (P) in the lumen of a small vessel in the lung of a mouse injected intravenously with lipid particles. (× 8,250.) (From French.[35])

A number of observations have indicated that the platelet release reaction may be involved in certain immunological phenomena. The details are complex since there are differences in the behaviour of platelets from different species and uncertainties about the role of complement, but there is evidence that under appropriate conditions, antigen: antibody complexes, aggregates of γ-globulin, or endotoxin can bring about the release of platelet constituents.[13] Foreign surfaces coated with γ-globulin will stimulate release in the absence of other plasma components.[37]

There is at present little decisive evidence about the significance of the platelet release reaction in the response to injury in the living animal. The release of platelet amines has been implicated in the vasoconstriction which occurs in the hæmostatic mechanism but little attention has been given to the potential role of these platelet factors in causing permeability changes at a site of injury. Lysosomal enzymes in the platelets may be activated in the course of the reaction but it is not known how they might be liberated or what effects they would have on the tissues with which they came in contact. In immunological reactions, the release of histamine and 5-hydroxytryptamine from platelets during anaphylaxis has been established in the rabbit, but is not clearly involved in anaphylaxis in other species (Chapter 38). It is possible that the platelets which accumulate at sites of local antigen-antibody reaction—e.g. in the Arthus phenomenon—may play a part in the tissue changes which ensue. The destruction of platelets in the presence of complement by antibodies specific to antigens carried by the platelets themselves is discussed in relation to thrombocytopenic purpura in Chapter 40. Capillary hæmorrhages which occur in this condition appear to be due in part to an impairment of normal hæmostatic function through loss of platelets. Release of damaging agents from the platelets which are destroyed is not known to be a factor in this condition.

THE RED CELLS

Changes in the number or character of the circulating red cells following bodily injury are determined by the nature of the injury and by other and often opposing factors. Hæmorrhage will always cause a reduction of the total red cell population, but the number of cells in a given volume of blood depends upon the severity and duration of the bleeding. Serious hæmorrhage causes shock, with a greatly reduced blood volume and little compensatory hæmodilution, and in this condition the red cell count and hæmoglobin content of a sample of blood may be within normal limits. It is only during the recovery phase, when the blood volume is restored by hæmodilution that the true state of anæmia is revealed by a reduction of the red cell count and hæmoglobin concentration. Within about 24 hours of a severe hæmorrhage, active regeneration normally begins and is indicated by a reticulocytosis. Changes in the red cells produced by injury are thus the resultant of the direct effects of shock, blood loss, and regeneration and also of other and less explicable factors. For instance, a fairly constant result is a degree of anæmia which cannot be explained by hæmorrhage alone. In severely burnt patients, in whom there is no direct loss of blood, anæmia may be a striking feature following an initial period of hæmoconcentration. This anæmia has been attributed to toxic inhibition of red cell production and to increased intravascular destruction of red cells which have been damaged directly by heat or indirectly by the products of tissue destruction. In simple traumatic injuries such as fractures, there is also an anæmia which cannot be explained by the blood lost into the injured area and again it is believed that a combination of increased red cell destruction is responsible. A common effect of injury is a tendency for the cells of the blood to form aggregates in the capillary circulation, due to a loss of "suspension stability" which is discussed below. Such aggregation, if severe, may result in considerable slowing of the capillary circulation and an increased tendency for the red cells to hæmolyse. Gelin,[38] who has studied this phenomenon in human subjects and experimentally in animals, and has reviewed the whole problem of anæmia following injury, believes that intravascular aggregation leading to hæmolysis may be an important factor.

The Suspension Stability of the Blood

In the normal circulation the formed elements of the blood remain discrete, showing no tendency to adhere to each other or to the walls of the vessels. This suspension stability is lost in the local circulation in inflamed or traumatised areas of tissue and may be generally reduced throughout the blood stream in cases of severe or long continued damage. A manifestation of such a change is an increase in the sedimentation rate of the red cells in blood withdrawn from the body.

If normal blood is run into a glass vessel it clots homogeneously. But in certain pathological conditions the red cells sink so rapidly that before coagulation is complete a clear layer of plasma is formed at the top of the tube and the clot, when finally produced, is composed of a lower, red part, and an upper, yellow part. The observation of this phenomenon goes back into antiquity. The Greeks related their theory of disease to the fact that the blood separated into layers when obtained from sick patients, the four "humors" being represented by these separated parts of the blood. The sedimented red cells can be divided into a dark or "melancholic" humor and a red or "sanguine" humor, depending on the degree of oxygenation, while the upper cell-free fibrin clot constituted the phlegmatic and the supernatant serum the choleric humor. It was not unnatural to suppose that this separation, apparently due to an abnormal increase of one of the humors, was the cause rather than the result of illness, and hence that removal of the abnormal humor by bleeding would be likely to restore health. Hewson in 1772[39] was apparently the first to recognise that it was the increased rate of sinking of the red cells which produced the appearance of an excessive "buffy coat" or phlegm (plasma clot and leucocytes) seen in illness. In 1827 Hodgkin and Lister[40] watched the red cells in such abnormal blood "apply themselves to each other by their broad surfaces, and form piles" like piles of coins or rouleaux. This increased rouleaux formation, which was clearly associated with the increased rate of sedimentation, was thought by Norris[41] to be due to an increased stickiness of the cells. The first practical application of the phenomenon of sedimentation as an index of disease is described by Fåhræus[42] in his comprehensive review of the whole subject.

The Mechanism of Sedimentation

The rate at which red cells sink in plasma is controlled by a number of factors. The cells have a relative density of about 1·09 as compared with the corresponding figure of 1·03 for plasma. Gravity therefore tends to make them sink, the actual driving force being determined by the density difference. The speed of fall is the resultant of this force and the opposing resistance offered by the viscous plasma. This resistance is proportional (for spherical particles) to the radius of the falling particles, whereas the weight, or driving force, is proportional to the cube of their radius. Thus larger particles tend to sediment more rapidly than smaller ones of the same composition, since the driving force increases more rapidly with size than the resistance. This phenomenon is familiar from everyday experience; stones sink more rapidly in water than fine sand. If red cells remain separated they sink relatively slowly, but if they become aggregated into rouleaux, which are masses larger than individual red cells, they sink more rapidly. The increased sedimentation rate in disease is, in almost every instance, merely a measure of the degree of rouleaux formation.

Rouleaux Formation

Rouleaux formation thus becomes the centre of interest in any investigation of the sedimentation phenomenon. The reasons why the cells remain discrete in normal, but form rouleaux in abnormal, blood are obscure. Discs such as red cells would, in fact, be expected to form rouleaux if they come into contact with one another, unless there is some positive force which prevents contact and adhesion. Norris[41] in 1869 showed that discs of cork coated with oil and immersed in water came together and formed into perfect rouleaux by the action of surface tension (FIG. 9). As the discs touched they slid over one another under the influence of surface tension to form cylinders. To explain the absence of rouleaux in normal blood it was suggested that red cells carry an

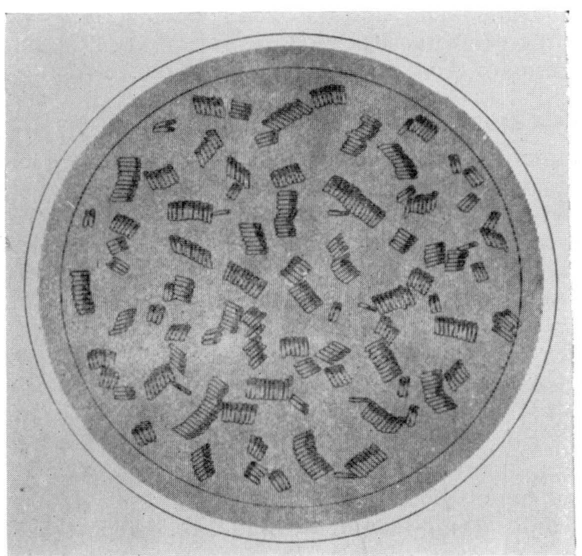

8/FIG. 9.—Artificial rouleaux formed spontaneously by discs of cork previously wetted with some liquid which is immiscible with the one in which they are submerged. Reproduced from an experiment carried out by Norris[41] in 1869.

electric charge, so that they exert a mutually repulsive force preventing close contact. A hypothetical reduction in this charge produced by disease would then allow rouleaux formation to take place. But no direct evidence of any electrical difference between the cells in normal and abnormal blood has been obtained. Another unproved hypothesis is that an increased stickiness of the red cell envelope causes sufficient adhesion of cells which come into chance contact to allow surface tension to produce rouleaux.

Positive advances in the investigation of the phenomenon have come not from the study of the red cells but of the plasma. The cells from a blood sample showing rapid sedimentation, sediment normally in normal plasma, whereas normal cells will sediment rapidly in abnormal plasma. No specific substance analogous to an agglutinin can be isolated from the abnormal plasma and the activity is not reduced in the process of forming rouleaux. The activity seems to be related to a physical state of the plasma rather than to a definite agent, and this state is itself related to the proportion and character of the plasma proteins. In general it is found that the greater the concentration of the large molecule proteins such as fibrinogen and globulin, the greater is the rouleaux formation. Many macro-molecules foreign to the plasma, such as hyaluronic acid,[43] dextran, gelatin, gum acacia and polyvinyl pyrrolidine,[44] have an effect proportional to their concentration and molecular weight. Hardwicke and Squire[44] found that elevated fibrinogen values do not account completely for the rise of the sedimentation rate in disease, since in pathological cases the red cells sediment more rapidly in the patient's serum than in the normal serum. This increased serum sedimentation rate was related to the concentration of *alpha* and *gamma* globulin, and was closely parallel to its viscosity. Estimations of plasma or serum viscosity therefore probably give the same information as the determination of the sedimentation rate of red cells.

The Estimation of the Sedimentation Rate

The application of the phenomenon of sedimentation to clinical medicine involves a reasonably accurate determination of the rate of sinking. The usual practice is to add an anticoagulant to the blood, and then to measure the rate of fall of the upper layer of red cells in a long column of blood contained in a graduated tube. At the end of a specified time the upper level of the red cells is read against a scale and the number of mm. traversed in the specified time determined. Analysis of the behaviour of the falling cells shows that for the first few minutes after setting up the tube there is little sedimentation since rouleaux formation is incomplete. With the completion of aggregation a more or less linear rate of fall of the red cells takes place, until they are brought to a standstill by the packing of the cells at the bottom of the tube. The tube must be long enough, therefore, to prevent this event curtailing rapid sedimentation before the specified time has elapsed.

A number of disturbing factors are found to influence the sedimentation rate. The most important of these is anæmia. Simple dilution of normal blood with its own plasma increases the sedimentation rate, both because this promotes rouleaux formation and because, there being fewer cells to sink through a given volume of plasma, there is less upward displacement of the plasma and hence less resistance to sedimentation. Many patients in whom sedimentation is to be measured are anæmic, and there have been a number of attempts to control this complicating factor by the use of correction charts and other devices. In almost every case the "corrections" have introduced insoluble problems of their own, and it can be said that none is satisfactory.[45] Other, and avoidable, complicating factors include the accidental inclination of the tube from the vertical, which hastens the sedimentation rate, since the cells slide down the lower wall of the inclined tube and the plasma rises along the upper one; the use of dirty apparatus, since dried protein from previous blood samples may increase the sedimentation rate of subsequent blood samples; and delay in setting up the test, since the ability of cells to form rouleaux diminishes with time.

The Significance of Sedimentation

In normal people, the sedimentation rate is usually only a few millimetres per hour. The upper limits of normal vary with the method used, and with the sex of the patient. By the Westergren method the upper limits are 5 mm./hr. for men, and 7 mm./hr. for women, and by the Wintrobe method 9 mm. and 20 mm. respectively.

An increased sedimentation rate is observed in most conditions in which there is an increased tissue breakdown, which in turn causes an increased fibrinogen and globulin level in the plasma. It is raised therefore in cases of traumatic damage, in general infections and in localised inflammatory conditions depending on their severity and nature. High sedimentation rates are observed in rheumatoid arthritis, tuberculosis and pneumonia. It is raised in normal pregnancy, and is said to be increased by exercise and conditions which stimulate adrenal activity. The mechanism by which the concentration of fibrinogen and globulin is increased in these states associated with an increased sedimentation rate is not known. In certain diseases unassociated with infection, such as myelomatosis, Hodgkin's disease, carcinomatosis, and some cases of leukæmia, the presence of abnormal proteins of high molecular weight in the plasma may cause sedimentation rates of 100 mm. per hour or more, despite a great increase of plasma viscosity.

BLOOD SLUDGING

A series of curious and rather indeterminate observations on alterations in the intravascular blood flow produced by trauma or infection have recently attracted considerable attention and seem to be related most closely to the sedimentation rate. The increased rouleaux formation observed *in vitro* is known also to affect the red cells *in vivo*. FIGURE 10, for instance, shows rouleaux in a capillary of a living rabbit's ear. In 1869 Norris[41] observed red cell clumping in inflamed capillaries, and Hüter[46] made a similar observation in the conjunctival capillaries in dogs suffering from bacterial infection. Ploman[47] and Fåhræus[42] were able to correlate variations in the sedimentation rate with the degree of clumping of cells in retinal and nail-bed capillaries in human beings. The significance of such intravascular clumping was not at once apparent, although it might be expected to interfere with blood flow, as Norris had suggested. Considerable interest in the subject was aroused by the numerous publications of Knisely and his co-workers.[48] Their first contribution was the observation of agglutinated masses of cells in the mesenteric vessels of monkeys infected by malaria. Their description of the transformation of normal blood to a "thick muck-like sludge" was responsible for the coining of the term "sludged blood" to describe the change. From this they went on to describe sludging and consequent stasis of the blood flow in the immediate region of infected or damaged tissues, and even in the general circulation, in a wide variety of pathological states in human beings. Other authors have described similar findings in pregnancy, skin diseases, allergy, hypertension and other conditions. The formation of red cell masses as the result of injury was thought to be responsible, by causing blockage of important vessels, for the pathological changes of traumatic shock, the anuria of the crush syndrome,[49] and the formation of peptic ulcers.[50]

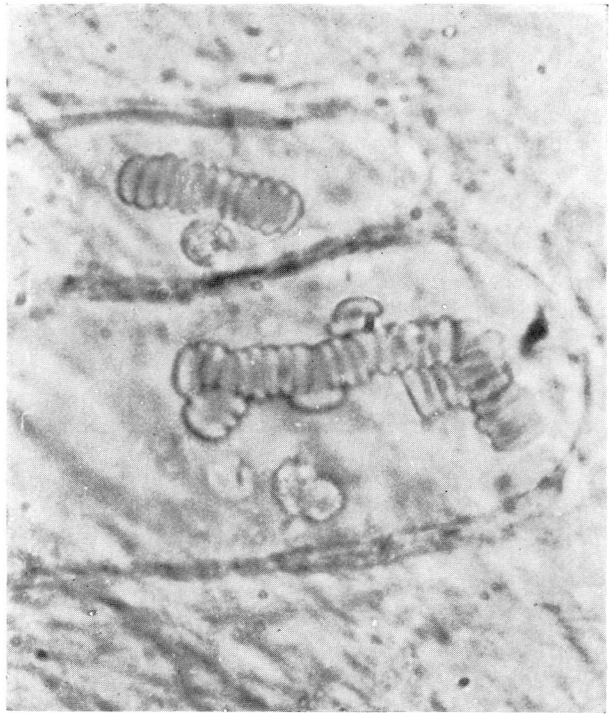

8/Fig. 10.—Rouleaux formation *in vivo*. Red cells in the growing capillaries of a rabbit's ear.

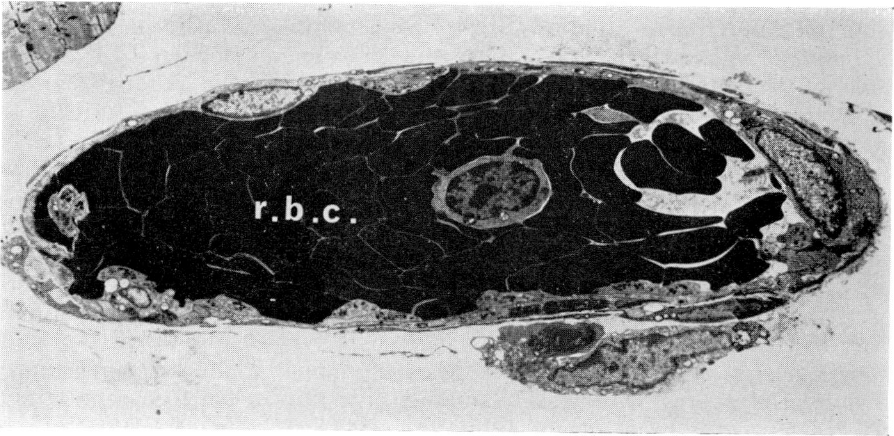

8/Fig. 11.—Closely packed red cells (rbc) in the lumen of a venule in a rat at a site where vascular permeability had been increased by local application of histamine. (× 2,300.)

The matter has been reviewed by Lutz,[51] who believes that blood sludging is relatively unimportant since the pathological conditions which it is supposed to produce can occur in its absence, and the reputed occurrence of blood sludging in a large proportion of the population often has no obvious effect. Gelin, however, has shown[38] that the formation of intravascular aggregates which takes place after trauma or the injection of high molecular weight dextran, is closely correlated with the development of anæmia, and he believes that the mechanical trapping of red cells in the capillary circulation favours their hæmolysis. The underlying mechanism of sludging is unexplained. It has been found that stimulation of the sympathetic system or the injection of adrenaline will produce it.[52] In part it is due to an increase of the "stickiness" of the cells of the blood, but the nature of this change is obscure. It is not strictly correlated with rouleaux formation, since after injury sludging occurs before there is a significant rise in the sedimentation rate[38]; it does not seem to be related to the clotting mechanism, since sludging can occur in animals receiving anticoagulants such as heparin and dicoumarol.[53] Lutz[51] considers that the primary cause of slowing of the capillary circulation is contraction of the pre-capillary sphincters, and that sludging is the result rather than the cause of stasis.

An undoubted cause of compaction of the red cells in the micro-circulation is the loss of plasma fluid through vascular walls made more permeable by an inflammatory process or the products of cellular damage. The red cells packed together in this way form viscous and coherent masses which can be seen to preserve some cohesion when they escape into larger vessels. FIGURE 11 shows such a mass of packed red cells in a vessel made more permeable by an injection of histamine. It is possible, therefore, that one of the factors involved in "blood sludging" may be the mechanical one of fluid loss from abnormally permeable vessels.

True intravascular agglutination due to specific agglutinins may occur in certain conditions. The development of "cold agglutinins", which are inoperative at normal body temperature, may result in the formation of agglutinated masses of red cells in the cooler peripheral capillaries, particularly in the hands and feet in cold weather. Capillary blockage by such agglutinated red cells is one of the causes of Raynaud's disease. The subject is well reviewed by Forbes.[54]

REFERENCES

1. WINTROBE, M. M. (1951). *Clinical Hæmatology*, 3rd edit. Philadelphia: Lea & Febiger. Normal range of leucocytes.
2. BIERMAN, H. R. (1961). In *Functions of the Blood*, p. 349. Eds. MACFARLANE, R. G., and A. H. T. ROBB-SMITH. Oxford: Blackwell Scientific Publications. Homeostasis of the blood cell elements.
3. ARCHER, R. K., and BROOME, J. (1963). *Nature* (*Lond.*), **198,** 893.
   The function of the eosinophils.
4. RILEY, J. F. (1963). *Ann. N.Y. Acad. Sci.*, **103,** 151.
   Heparin and the mast cells.
5. VIRCHOW, R. (1871). *Die Cellularpathologie in ihrer Begründung auf physiologische und pathologische Gewebelehre. Vorlesungen über Pathologie.* 4th edit. Berlin: A. Hirschwald.
   Leucocytosis in disease.

6. Menkin, V. (1955). *Ann. N.Y. Acad. Sci.*, **59,** 956.
A leucocytosis-producing factor from inflamed tissues.
7. Rosenow, G. (1951). *Acta. hæmat. (Basel)*, **5,** 1.
The nervous control of the leucocytes.
8. Silberberg, M. (1938). *Physiol. Rev.*, **18,** 197.
The causes and mechanism of thrombosis.
9. Robb-Smith, A. H. T. (1967). *Brit. J. Hæmat.*, **13,** 618.
Why the platelets were discovered.
10. Tocantins, L. M. (1938). *Medicine (Baltimore)*, **17,** 155.
Mammalian blood platelets in health and disease.
11. David-Ferreira, J. F. (1964). *Int. Rev. Cytol.*, **17,** 99.
The blood platelet: electron microscopic studies.
12. Pletscher, A. (1968). *Brit. J. Pharmacol.*, **32,** 1.
5-hydroxytryptamine in blood platelets.
13. Marcus, A. J., and Zucker, M. B. (1965). *The Physiology of Blood Platelets.* New York: Grune and Stratton.
14. Salmon, J. (1967). In *Biochemistry of Blood Platelets*, p. 47. Eds. Kowalski, E., and Nicwiarowski, S. New York: Academic Press. Platelet immunology.
15. Verstraete, M. (1966). In *Diffuse Intravascular Clotting*, p. 397. Transactions of a Conference of the International Committee on Hæmostasis and Thrombosis. Stuttgart: Schattauer-Verlag.
16. Wright, J. H. (1910). *J. Morph.*, **21,** 263.
The histogenesis of the blood platelets.
17. Yamada, E. (1957). *Acta anat. (Basel)*, **29,** 267.
The fine structure of the megakaryocyte.
18. Davey, M. G. (1966). *The Survival and Destruction of Human Platelets.* Basel: Karger Libri.
19. O'Brien, J. R. (1966). *Ann. Rev. Med.*, **17,** 275.
Platelet adhesiveness.
20. Tait, J. (1918). *Quart. J. exp. Physiol.*, **12,** 1.
Phagocytosis by platelets.
21. Movat, H. Z., Weiser, W. J., Glynn, M. F., and Mustard, J. F. (1965). *J. Cell Biol.*, **27,** 531.
Platelet phagocytosis and aggregation.
22. Born, G. V. R., and Cross, M. J. (1963). *J. Physiol. (Lond.)*, **168,** 178.
The aggregation of blood platelets.
23. Hellem, A. J. (1960). *Scand. J. clin. Lab. Invest.*, **12,** Suppl. 51. The adhesiveness of human blood platelets *in vitro.*
24. Gaarder, A., Jonsen, J., Laland, S., Hellem, A., and Owren, P. A. (1961). *Nature (Lond.)*, **192,** 531.
Adenosine diphosphate in red cells as a factor in the adhesiveness of human blood platelets.
25. Born, G. V. R. (1962). *Nature (Lond.)*, **194,** 927. (1965). *Ann. roy. Coll. Surg. Engl.*, **36,** 200.
Aggregation of blood platelets by adenosine diphosphate and its reversal.
26. Born, G. V. R. (1967). *Fed. Proc.*, **26,** 115.
Mechanism of platelet aggregation.
27. Hovig, T. (1963). *Thrombos. Diathes. hæmorrh. (Stuttg.)*, **9,** 264.
Release of adenosine diphosphate from platelets by extract of tendons.
28. Movat, H. Z., Mustard, J. E., Taichman, N. S., and Uriuhara, T. (1965). *Proc. Soc. expl Biol., (N.Y.)*, **120,** 232.
Platelet aggregation and release reaction by antigen-antibody complexes.

29. HASLAM, R. J. (1964). *Nature* (*Lond.*), **202,** 765.
Aggregation of human blood platelets by thrombin and by fatty acids.
30. ARDLIE, N. G., GLEW, G., and SCHWARTZ, C. J. (1966). *Nature* (*Lond.*), **212,** 415.
Influence of catecholamines on nucleotide-induced platelet aggregation.
31. NORDOY, A., and CHANDLER, A. B. (1964). *Scand. J. Hæmat.*, **1,** 16.
Platelet thrombosis induced by adenosine diphosphate.
32. MUSTARD, J. F., JORGENSEN, L., HOVIG, T., GLYNN, M. F., and ROWSELL, H. C. (1966). In *Pathogenesis and Treatment of Thrombœmbolic Diseases*, p. 131. Eds. DUCKERT, F., and STREULI, F. Stuttgart: Schattauer-Verlag. Role of platelets in thrombosis.
33. CONNOR, W. E., HOAK, J. C., and WARNER, E. D. (1966).In *Pathogenesis and Treatment of Thrombœmbolic Diseases*, p. 193. Eds. DUCKERT, F., and STREULI, F. Stuttgart: Schattauer-Verlag.
The role of lipids in thrombosis.
34. DUDGEON, L. S., and GOADBY, H. K. (1931). *J. Hyg.* (*Lond.*), **31,** 247.
Platelets after intravenous inoculations of *Staphylococcus aureus* and indian ink.
35. FRENCH, J. E. (1967). *Brit. J. Hæmat.*, **13,** 595.
Blood platelets: morphological studies on their properties and life cycle.
36. GRETTE, K. (1962). *Acta physiol. scand.*, **56,** Suppl. 195.
The mechanism of thrombin-catalysed release reaction in platelets.
37. MUSTARD, J. F., GLYNN, M. F., NISHIZAWA, E. E., and PACKHAM, M. A. (1967). *Fed. Proc.*, **26,** 106.
Platelet-surface interactions.
38. GELIN, L-E. (1956). *Acta chir. scand.*, Suppl. 210.
Anæmia following injury.
39. HEWSON, W. (1772). Works ed. by GULLIVER. London (1846).
The increased sedimentation rate in inflammation.
40. HODGKIN, T., and LISTER, J. (1827). *Phil. Mag.*, **2,** 130.
Rouleaux formation.
41. NORRIS, R. (1869). *Proc. roy. Soc.*, **17,** 429.
Artificial rouleaux-forming systems.
42. FÅHRÆUS, R. (1921). *Acta med. scand.* **LV,** 1.
The suspension-stability of the blood.
43. MEYER, K., HAHNEL, E., and FEINER, R. R. (1945). *Proc. Soc. exp. Biol.* (*N.Y.*), **58,** 36.
Hyaluronic acid increases sedimentation.
44. HARDWICKE, J., and SQUIRE, J. R. (1952). *Clin. Sci.*, **11,** 333.
Macro-molecules accelerate red cell sedimentation.
45. POOLE, J. C. F., and SUMMERS, G. A. C. (1952). *Brit. med. J.*, **1,** 353.
The correction of the sedimentation rate for anæmia.
46. HÜTER, C. (1876). *Zbl. med. Wiss.*, **14,** 505.
Clumping of red cells *in vivo*.
47. PLOMAN, M. G. (1920). *Ann. Ocul.*, **157,** 569.
Clumping of red cells *in vivo* correlated with sedimentation rate.
48. KNISELY, M. H., STRATMAN-THOMAS, W. K., and ELIOT, T. S. (1941). *Anat. Rec.*, **79,** 90.
BLOCH, E. H. (1945). *J. nat. Malar. Soc.*, **4,** 287.
Sludging in malaria-infected monkeys.
KNISELY, M. H., and BLOCH, E. H. (1942). *Anat. Rec.*, **82,** 426.
Sludging in human diseases.
KNISELY, M. H., BLOCH, E. H., ELIOT, T. S., and WARNER, L. (1947). *Science*, **106,** 431.
Sludged blood.

49. Fleming, J. F. R., and Bigelow, W. G. (1951). *Surgery*, **30,** 994.
Intravascular agglutination as a cause of stasis in crush syndrome.
50. Key, J. A. (1952). *Ann. Surg.*, **135,** 470.
Intravascular agglutination in peptic ulceration.
51. Lutz, B. R. (1951). *Physiol. Rev.*, **31,** 107.
Criticism of the concept of "sludged blood".
52. Fowler, E. P. (1949). *Proc. Soc. exp. Biol.* (*N.Y.*), **72,** 592.
Blood sludging produced by sympathetic stimulation.
53. Laufman, H., Martin, W. B., and Tanturi, C. (1948). *Science*, **108,** 283.
Blood sludging not prevented by anticoagulants.
54. Forbes, G. B. (1947). *Brit. med. J.*, **1,** 598.
Review of intravascular cold agglutination.

Chapter 9

HÆMOSTASIS AND THROMBOSIS

By J. E. French and R. G. Macfarlane

The evolution of a high-pressure circulatory system entails the danger of loss of blood in the event of damage to even the smallest vessels. An essential parallel development, therefore, has been a system of automatic safeguards which quickly controls bleeding from all but the major blood vessels. The term *hæmostasis* refers to this system of safeguards and can be defined as "the spontaneous arrest of hæmorrhage by a physiological process based on the reactions of the blood and tissues to injury"[1]. In discussing the events in hæmostasis we can divide them into two parts—the formation of the *hæmostatic plug*, which is built up entirely from constituents of the blood and which occludes the opening in the severed vessel; and the complex pattern of *vascular reactions* which reduce the flow pressure at the site of injury.

We shall also need to consider how alterations in the normal functioning of the hæmostatic mechanism may lead to disease states. Various hæmorrhagic disorders occur in which there is a defect in one or other of the hæmostatic factors. A more common pathological event, however, is an apparent misplacement of the hæmostatic mechanism, by which a mass, resembling the hæmostatic plug, forms within the lumen of a vessel which is not externally ruptured. This process is called *thrombosis*, and the mass which is formed under these conditions is called a *thrombus*. To avoid confusion with other solid objects, for example tumour fragments, which may appear in the lumen of vessels, and the clots which may form in the vessels after death, a thrombus is defined more precisely as a solid mass or plug formed in the living heart or vessels from constituents of the blood[2].

In the preceding chapters many properties of blood have been discussed that are relevant to hæmostasis and thrombosis, but before applying them in the present context, there is one fundamental point which needs to be emphasised. The effect of hæmostasis or thrombosis—advantageous in one but disadvantageous in the other—is to stop or impair the flow of blood. This means that the processes with which we are concerned must be able to operate in flowing blood: arrest of flow is achieved only *after* these processes have had their effect. The following experiment[3] illustrates how the introduction of this additional factor of flow may influence the processes of blood coagulation and platelet aggregation. Fresh blood is introduced into a length of plastic tubing until it is half filled. The ends of the tubing are then fixed together to form a circular loop which is immediately placed on a revolving wheel so that, in effect, the blood is made to flow round the tube. Blood coagulation and platelet changes are initiated by contact with the foreign surface as they would be in a test tube, and proceed in the same sequence, but the blood as a whole does not now form a clot. Instead a small solid object is formed at the leading edge of the column of blood (Fig. 1*a*). The object has a pale head consisting predominantly of large platelet aggregates

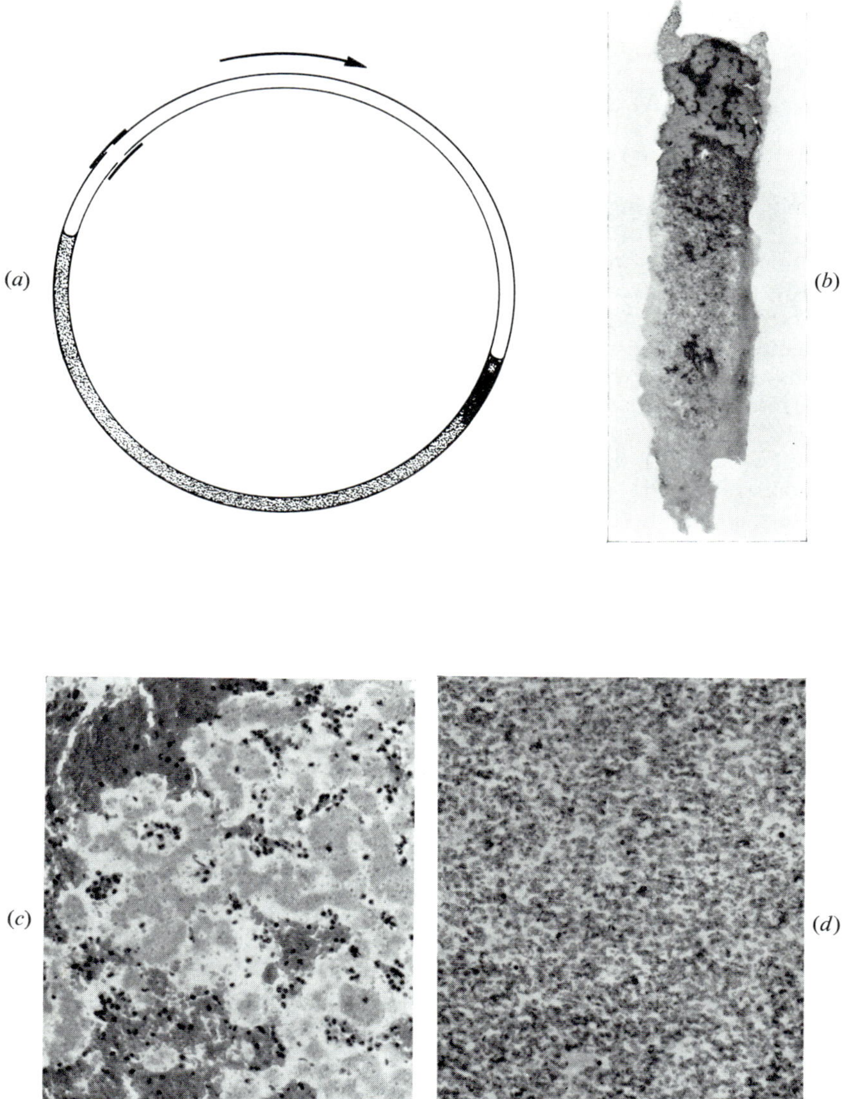

9/Fig. 1.—Formation of an "artificial thrombus" from blood in a rotating tube. (*a*) Diagram of the tube showing the small solid object at the leading edge. (*b*) Longitudinal section of the artificial thrombus × 7. (*c*) Section through the head. Pale grey areas, representing platelet aggregates, are surrounded by leucocytes shown as dark dots, and red cells. Hæmatoxylin and eosin × 145. (*d*) Section through a blood clot. Hæmatoxylin and eosin × 145.

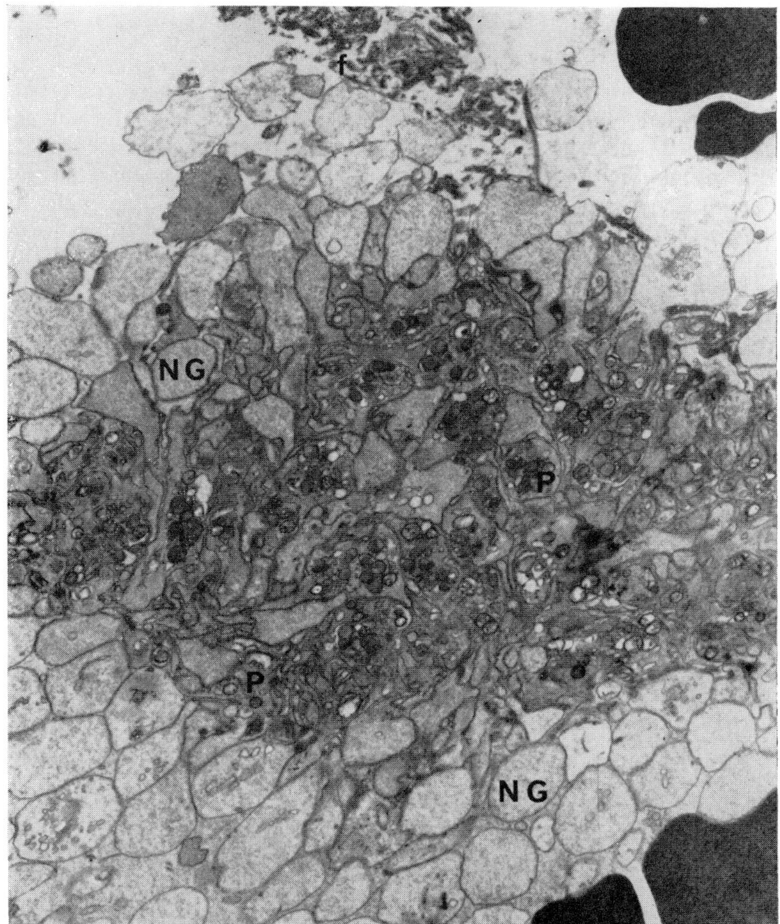

9/FIG. 2.—Electron micrograph of a platelet aggregate in the head of an "artificial thrombus". It shows close packing of platelets (P) at the centre and non-granular bodies (NG) towards the edge. Fibrin (f) and red cells are found outside the aggregates. (× 7,500.)

surrounded by leucocytes and linked together by a fibrin network in which red cells are entangled. Behind the pale head there is a red tail consisting of an extension of the fibrin network with randomly distributed red cells and occasional leucocytes (FIG. 1*b* and *c*). This simple change in the physical conditions under which blood reacts to a foreign surface has led to the formation of a solid object in which the platelet aggregates are much more prominent, and the distribution of leucocytes and fibrin strikingly different from the coagulum formed from static blood in a test tube (FIG. 1*d*). The appearance of the platelet aggregates as seen in the white head by electron microscopy[4] is illustrated in FIG. 2.

HÆMOSTASIS

Formation of the Hæmostatic Plug

The familiar observation that wounds which have ceased to bleed are usually filled with clotted blood may suggest that it is blood coagulation which has actually stopped the bleeding. This is reinforced by the fact that bleeding persists in conditions in which clotting is demonstrably impaired. But the relationship is more complex. As long ago as 1882, Hayem[5] observed that during the flow of blood from a small wound in a jugular vein in dogs, the mass which formed at the site of injury and eventually plugged the opening in the wall of the vein consisted of the blood platelets, then newly recognised by himself and by Bizzozero.[6] He concluded that in flowing blood the platelets had the primary role in the arrest of hæmorrhage and that the formation of fibrin was only a secondary phenomenon. In 1885 Lubnitzky[7] reached similar conclusions from a histological study of wounded arteries. A drawing from her paper, reproduced in FIG. 3, shows a part of the plug obviously consisting of platelets and a more homogeneous part in which she thought the platelets had fused together.

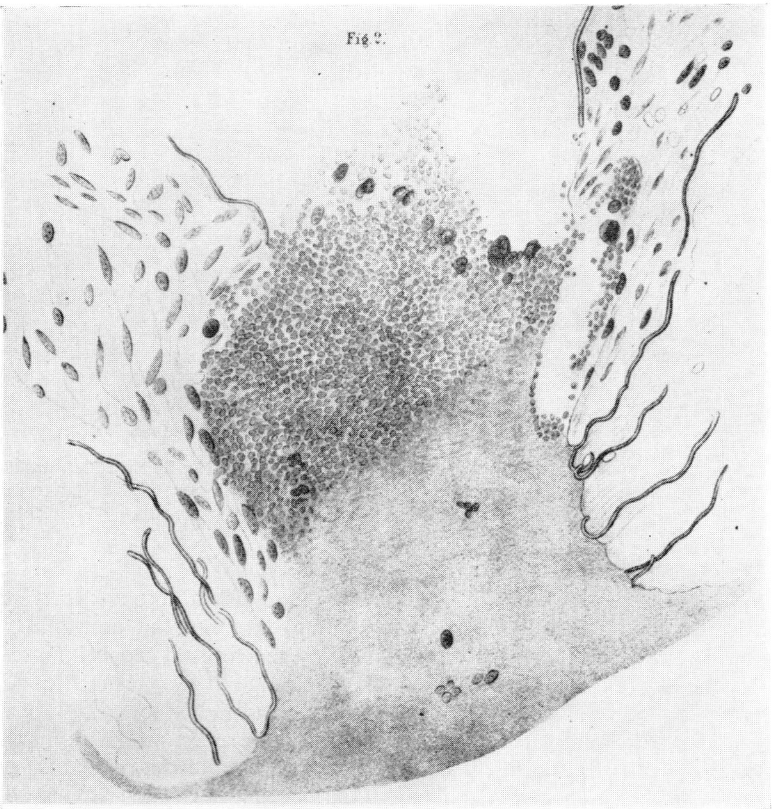

9/FIG. 3.—Drawing of a hæmostatic plug in an injured artery depicting the platelets as seen by light microscopy. (From Lubnitzky.[7])

Much of the experimental work which has followed has been related to plug formation in relatively small arteries and veins, where the effluent blood can be washed away until bleeding stops and the field of view for microscopy is not swamped by massive hæmorrhage. These experiments have been consistent in confirming the important role of the platelets but at the same time have shown that fibrin formation has an essential supplementary function. A fairly clear picture of the formation of the plug in these small vessels has now been built up with the aid of micro-cinematography and electron microscopy.[8, 9]

The sequence of events is generally as follows. Immediately after the vessel has been severed there is a period of hæmorrhage. The vessel may show constriction at or above the site of injury, but it is only occasionally that this constriction is sufficient to stop the bleeding. Platelets adhere within seconds to connective tissue at the rim of the opening and within a minute or two a mass of rather loosely arranged platelets begins to fill the opening, projecting outward into the wound and, to a lesser extent, backward into the lumen of the vessel. As this occurs the escape of blood becomes slower and the vessel may appear to contract around the mass, increasing its obstructive effect. Bleeding usually stops altogether in about three minutes but may be intermittent for a short time before ceasing permanently and plasma may continue to seep through the plug for some minutes after the red cells are retained. If the plug is examined by electron microscopy at the stage when bleeding has just stopped it is seen to consist largely of platelets, in places packed tightly together and in others more loosely aggregated. A few centrally placed red cells suggest that up to this moment there may have been some continuing flow through the centre of the plug. At the edges of the plug, platelets can be seen which are closely applied to collagen fibres but there is little change in the morphology of individual platelets and fibrin is inconspicuous, appearing only as a few strands at the edge of the platelet mass (FIG. 4*a* and *b*). This detailed structure of the platelet mass is very similar to that formed *in vitro* by adding ADP to platelet suspensions and it is reasonable to suppose that ADP has indeed been released from the damaged tissue or from the platelets which have adhered to collagen fibres (see Chapter 8).

With the passage of time (5–30 mins.) the plug becomes more compact and cohesive (FIG. 5). Platelets at the centre are very closely packed together and some are distorted in shape. At the edges there is a rim of non-granular bodies which may be degranulated platelets or projections from platelets situated more deeply. Fibrin is now much more conspicuous at the edges of the mass and, particularly near the margins of the cut wall, it appears to extend into the interstices in the fringe of degranulated platelets. It is probable that fibrin adds mechanical strength to the hæmostatic plug, reinforcing the rather friable platelet mass like the steel rods in ferroconcrete. Thus, though a platelet plug might be unable to withstand the blood pressure and might break down, the composite hæmostatic plug effectively seals an opening in these small vessels. This consolidation of the plug can be attributed to the local generation of thrombin which, as we have seen, causes similar platelet changes in the *in vitro* systems as well as fibrin formation.

At a still later stage (24 hours) the appearance of the plug undergoes a further change. By light microscopy it appears as a diffusely granular mass which takes a fibrin stain throughout.[10] Platelets or platelet remnants can, however,

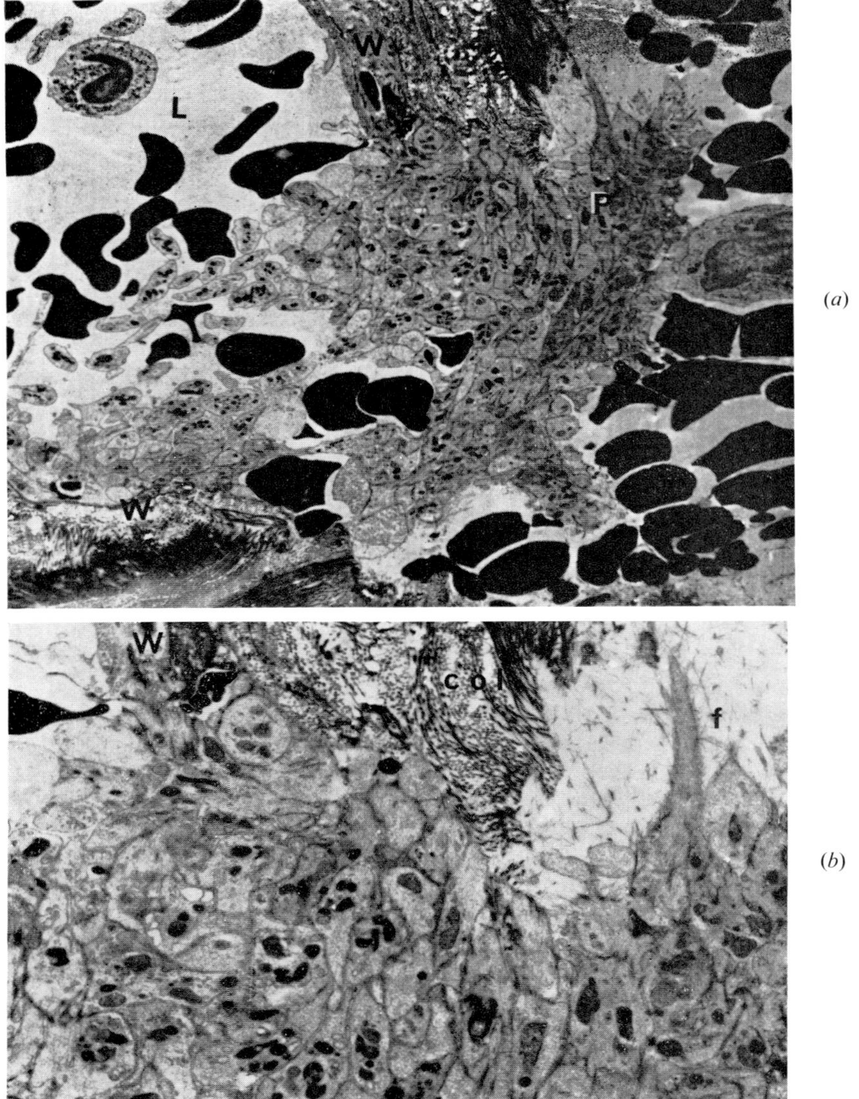

9/Fig. 4.—(*a*) Electron micrograph of a hæmostatic plug in a cut artery in a hamster cheek pouch. A compact mass of platelets (P) between the cut edges of the wall (W) is partly inside and partly outside the lumen. (× 3,500.) (*b*) Detail from the hæmostatic plug shown above. Platelets are closely associated with the damaged wall (W) and with extravascular collagen fibres (col). Fibrin strands (f) occur at the edge. (× 9,600.) (From French *et al.*[9])

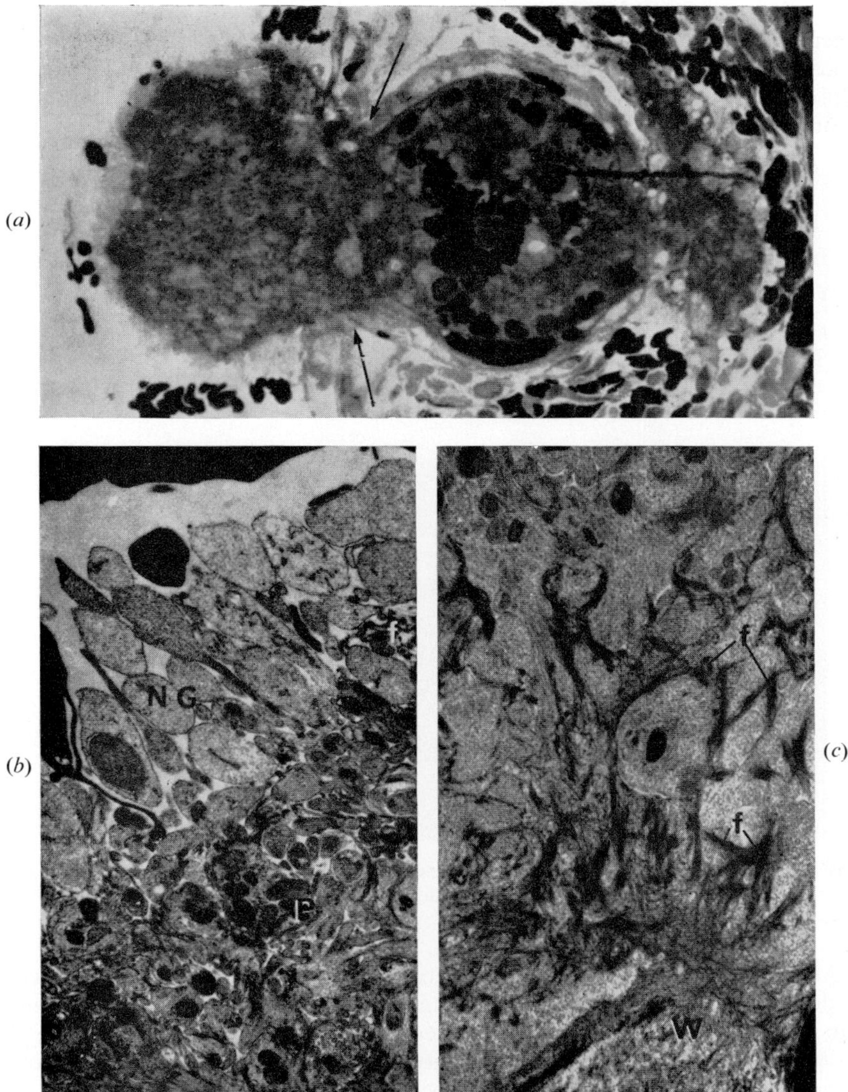

9/Fig. 5.—Hæmostatic plug in a small artery in a hamster, fixed 30 mins. after bleeding had ceased. (*a*) Cross section of the complete plug as seen with the light microscope. The position of the cut is indicated by the arrows. (× 650.) (*b*) The margin of the plug shows tightly packed platelets (P), a fringe of non-granular bodies (NG) and some strands of fibrin (f). Electron micrograph × 10,000. (*c*) At the cut edge of the wall (W), fibrin (f) extends into the fringe of non-granular bodies. (× 16,000.) (5*a* and *b* from French.[22])

still be identified by the electron microscope, but they are now more widely spaced and strands of fibrin extend between them (FIG. 6). The final stage is one of healing and repair. Concomitant with the resolution of the temporary seal, fibroblasts grow into the gap and by their synthetic activities effect a permanent closure by connective tissue.

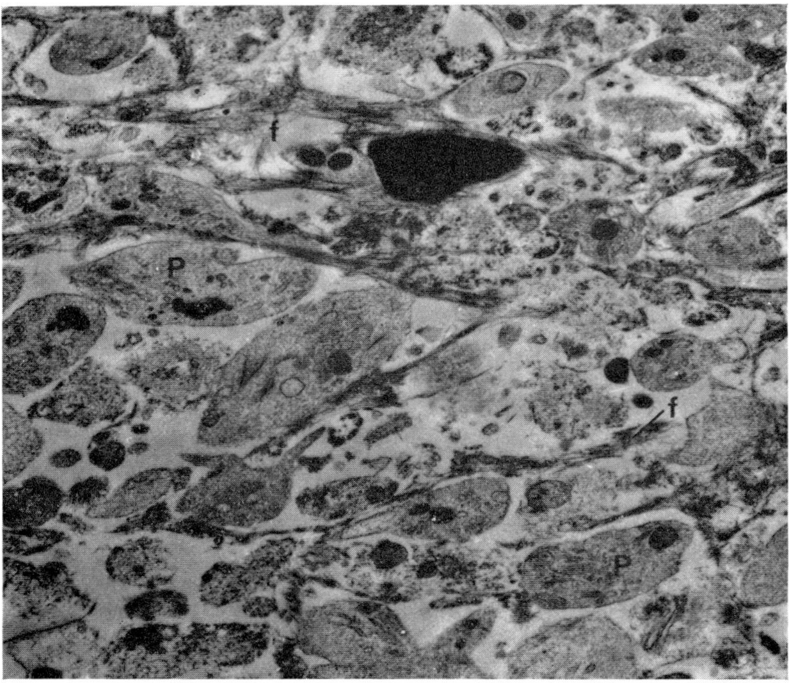

9/FIG. 6.—Part of a hæmostatic plug, 24 hours after its formation at the cut end of a small artery in a hamster. Platelets (P) can still be identified. They are separated by relatively wide spaces containing fibrin (f). (× 12,250.)

Although observations on small arteries and veins have been used to describe the development of the hæmostatic plug, it should be stressed that differences from this picture may occur which depend on the extent of injury and the size and type of vessel injured. In small incised arteries and veins the flow is not so strong that it disrupts the platelet plug before fibrin can form, but it nevertheless continues long enough for many platelets to be brought to the site; these conditions are not necessarily satisfied in other types of vessel.

In the larger arteries the formation of a hæmostatic plug is mechanically difficult in the face of a stream of blood issuing with considerable force. Even in such a situation, arterial constriction may reduce the flow to proportions which can be halted by platelet aggregation and fibrin formation, but often bleeding may continue to the point of exsanguination unless artificial aids such as pressure, dressings, tourniquets or ligatures are applied. Under conditions of flow where a plug can be formed, histological examination shows a laminated structure of platelet masses and layers of fibrin, deposited from the stream of issuing blood. Behind the plug, the lumen of the vessel, up to the first intersection, that is the region where the flow has been stopped, is usually filled with blood clot, consisting of fibrin, red cells and leucocytes distributed at random in contrast to the pronounced layered structure of the plug itself.

The manner in which bleeding from damaged capillaries is arrested has been a matter of controversy for many years. Platelet plugs were not found in severed human capillaries examined histologically by H. D. Zucker,[11] but, from their more recent studies, Jorgensen and Borchgrevink[10] considered that the formation of platelet plugs was an important factor in the arrest of capillary bleeding. Persistent capillary oozing is characteristic of conditions in which platelets are deficient either in number or function, and electron microscopy shows that platelets have the propensity to plug even the most minute gaps in the endothelial lining of small vessels (see Fig. 17). There is evidence, however, that the initial process of arresting flow may in some circumstances be served by other mechanisms in the capillaries.

Macfarlane[12] observed the disappearance of punctured human skin capillaries viewed microscopically and suggested that their lumen had been obliterated by contraction, but it is uncertain whether this could occur in all capillaries. Indeed the question whether true capillaries, which have no smooth muscle in their wall, can contract at all has still to be resolved. As another possibility, it has been suggested by Chen and Tsai[13] that endothelial adhesion may be a factor in preventing capillary bleeding. In cutting through tissue, capillary walls are forced together by pressure before they are severed and may adhere so that the lumen is obliterated. If this is the case, it must involve an almost instantaneous change in endothelial surface properties, since normal capillaries cannot be permanently obliterated by simple pressure in the absence of tissue damage.

Vascular Factors

The closure of disrupted vessels is often facilitated by reactions in the adjoining vasculature which bring about a reduction in the force and rate of flow. The blood vessels are not rigid pipes conveying a Newtonian fluid at steady rates of flow. They are elastic, contractile and, in the case of the minute vessels, of selective and variable permeability. In response to injury there are therefore complex changes involving not only the calibre of the vessels but also the viscosity of the blood which they contain.

In extensive injuries, shock or fainting may reduce the general blood pressure considerably and minimise the force against which the hæmostatic mechanism must operate. At the site of injury, constriction of vessels with muscular walls can often be observed; this is particularly important in the case of the larger vessels but can be seen also to occur in quite small ones when they are viewed with the microscope in such preparations as the cerebral cortex of the rabbit and cat, the web of a frog's foot, the mesentery in various animals, and the hamster cheek pouch. The microcirculation in the hamster cheek pouch is very labile and the blood flow can become static, or even reversed, as a result of injury. In consequence an area of damage may be virtually isolated from the circulation by the constriction of small feeding arteries and the opening up of shunts and by-passes, but the extent to which such factors are involved generally in the hæmostatic mechanism is not known.

The reactions of vascular smooth muscle have been extensively studied, but the chain of events linking the traumatic stimulus with the response of contraction is not clearly understood and it is probable that the pattern varies, not only from species to species but from one anatomical site to another. Smooth muscle cells may be stimulated directly by trauma, or via the innervation of the vessel wall, or by vaso-active substances which are released locally as the plug forms. As pointed out in Chapter 8, platelets contain 5-hydroxytryptamine, histamine, adrenaline and noradrenaline which are released by the action of thrombin. Vaso-active peptides of the kinin group are formed during the clotting of blood *in vitro* and presumably are also formed in the vicinity of the hæmostatic plug (Chapter 7).

The problem of whether the true capillaries can contract or not has already been mentioned but it is necessary to add that permeability changes in the smallest vessels (capillaries and venules) may under some circumstances be an important factor in the hæmostatic mechanism. On the one hand, a rising extravascular pressure due to œdema can reduce the pressure differential between blood and tissues; on the other, loss of fluid from more permeable vessels will lead to an increase in the viscosity of the blood and, when this is extreme, to compaction of the red cells in the vessel lumen (see 8/Fig. 11).

The Hæmostatic Mechanism as a Whole

Normal hæmostasis involves the integrated operation of at least three main factors: vascular constriction, platelet adhesion and aggregation, and blood coagulation. The three may have evolved from different primitive mechanisms. Co-ordinated vascular contractions are a feature of the circulatory mechanism in many lower animals; platelets are probably analogous to the so-called amœbocytes which bring about an almost exclusively cellular type of clotting in certain crustacea and insects; fibrin formation may be an adaptation of an even more primitive intracellular precipitation reaction to injury;[14] but in mammals these reactions have become interdependent and only under rather special conditions will one function adequately without the others.

Vasoconstriction is clearly an important factor in reducing the force of hæmorrhage, but its effect is transient and can at the best lead only to a temporary arrest of bleeding.

Platelet adhesion and aggregation occur rapidly and specifically at the site of injury, if the force of flow is not too great. As the aggregate grows in size it further restricts flow, rather as a sponge would do, and since it later becomes more compact is a potential seal. However, acting by itself this mechanism has an inherent instability; the platelet aggregate could break up spontaneously or be dislodged if the vessel were to dilate again, making it inadequate for complete arrest of hæmorrhage except in the smallest vessels.

The coagulation mechanism serves to stabilise the platelet plug by the formation of thrombin and fibrin and includes a potential "feed-back" whereby thrombin promotes further platelet aggregation. If it were not for the earlier events, however, which reduce or stop flow, it can be seen that the coagulation mechanism would by itself be ineffective. The formation of thrombin is the end result of a series of regulated and time-consuming steps which ensure that in the living animal a sudden and catastrophic coagulation of the blood as a whole cannot occur. The necessary concentration of the coagulation factors can only be built up at the site of injury if the auxiliary hæmostatic mechanisms are functioning properly.

In *in vitro* systems the three components of the hæmostatic mechanism can be studied in isolation and this approach has led to great advancement of knowledge in this field. When the mechanism operates as a whole *in vivo* the different components have a variable contribution to make depending on the nature and extent of injury and on the vessel involved, so that any generalisation about the hæmostatic mechanism runs the risk of over-simplification. Nevertheless it cannot be too strongly stated that the closely integrated action of the three components, not coagulation, platelet behaviour or vasoconstriction individually, is the physiological basis of the hæmostatic mechanism. A scheme illustrating this integrated action is shown in FIG. 7.

Hæmostatic Defects

An increased tendency to bleed may be associated with an abnormality of the clotting mechanism, of the platelets or of the blood vessels. Occasionally there is more than one defect, and in such cases the hæmorrhagic tendency may be severe, even though the separate defects might not by themselves be sufficient to cause bleeding.

Coagulation defects characteristically cause abnormal bleeding following severe trauma. They may first be suspected when bleeding is excessive after accidental injuries or after surgical procedures such as tonsillectomy or the extraction of several teeth. The bleeding may be overt, but if confined within the tissues as a hæmatoma it can cause serious and sometimes permanent disability, particularly in muscles, joints and around nerves. Epistaxis, gastro-intestinal bleeding, and hæmaturia may occur without obvious trauma.

The main causes of defective coagulation have been mentioned in Chapter 7, but the fact that a particular clotting factor can be shown to be reduced in amount does not necessarily mean that there will be a hæmorrhagic tendency. The most common hereditary diseases associated with severe bleeding are hæmophilia (deficiency of Factor VIII) and Christmas disease (deficiency of Factor IX). Acquired coagulation defects associated with bleeding may be produced inadvertently by the therapeutic use of anticoagulants, but are otherwise uncommon. The most important of these is the acute defibrination syndrome, met with in obstetrical and occasionally in surgical practice. Other rare defects of coagulation associated with bleeding include the development of inhibitors, perhaps of an antibody type, against various clotting factors.

Platelet defects may be quantitative or qualitative and when they are associated with bleeding this usually differs in type from that occurring in the coagulation defects. The type of bleeding is called purpuric and takes the form of small hæmorrhages in the skin, termed petechiæ and ecchymoses, and oozing of blood from apparently intact mucus membranes of the nose and gums. Gastro-intestinal and uterine bleeding are common. It is characteristic of these conditions that the bleeding time is prolonged when a small stab wound is made in the skin which damages the superficial network of small vessels. This is in con-

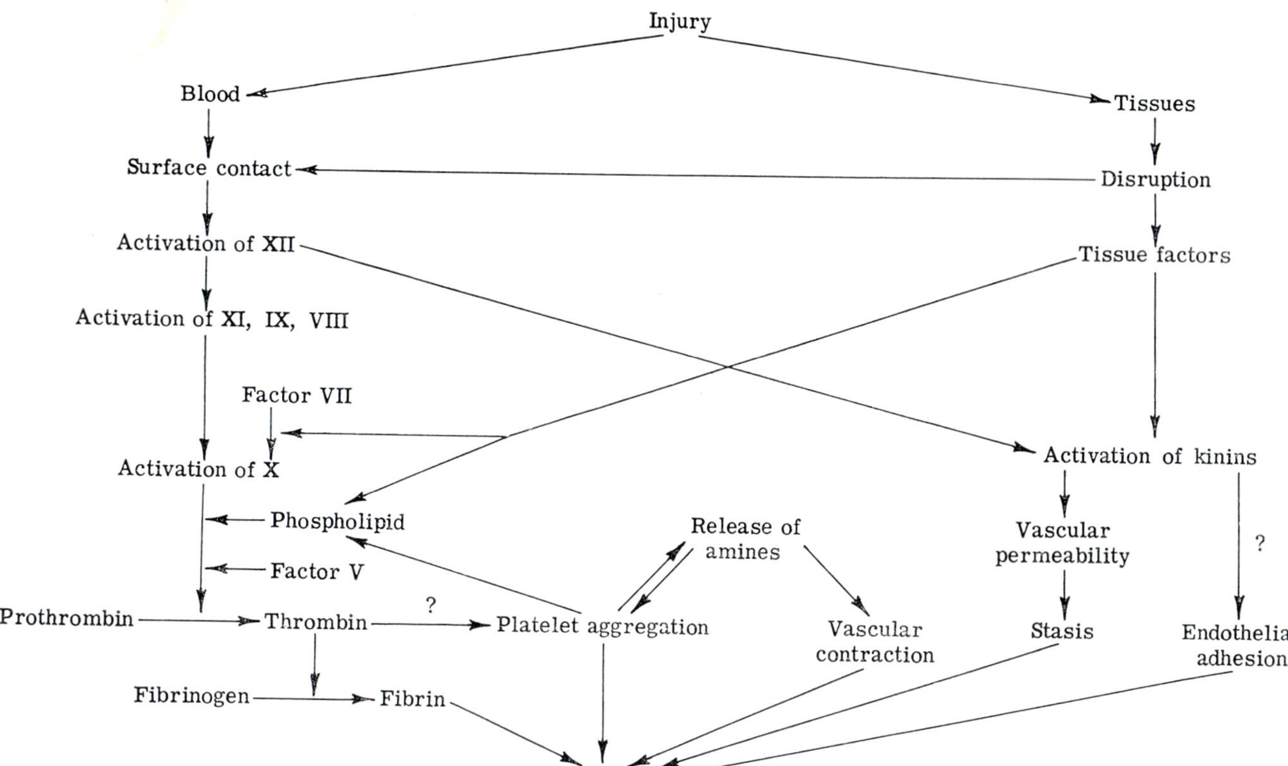

9/Fig. 7.—Scheme showing some of the factors concerned with hæmostasis, and their interactions. (From Macfarlane.[1])

trast to the cases of defective coagulation where the bleeding time measured in this way is within normal limits. The platelet defects are also characterised by an increase in the number of petechial hæmorrhages which appear in the skin of the forearm when the venous pressure is raised by compressing the upper arm with a sphygmomanometer cuff inflated to 80 mm. Hg (tourniquet test).

Thrombocytopenia is the commonest quantitative abnormality of the platelets associated with abnormal bleeding. Paradoxically, essential thrombocythæmia, a condition in which the platelet count may be over 1 million per c.mm., is also often associated with abnormal bleeding. Release of abnormally large amounts of platelet factor 3 which, in excess, acts as an inhibitor of coagulation *in vitro* is thought to be significant in this condition, but the bleeding is nevertheless of the purpuric type. Reduction of the number of circulating platelets by treatment with P^{32} usually restores normal hæmostasis.

Qualitative platelet defects associated with hæmorrhage of the purpuric type are uncommon. Thrombasthenia is a hereditary condition in which there is deficient clot retraction, due to the inability of the platelets to utilise ATP, and a failure of platelet aggregation on the addition of ADP. Thrombocytopathia is an inherited defect in which there is a failure to release platelet factor 3.

Vascular defects can cause abnormal bleeding. Hæmorrhagic telangiectasia is inherited as a simple dominant character. The lesions appear in adult life in the form of localised groups of greatly dilated capillaries, producing small red spots resembling petechiæ, but disappearing on pressure. These telangiectases may occur on the skin, lips, inside the mouth and nose, and in the gastro-intestinal, pulmonary and renal tracts. When injured they bleed profusely and persistently despite the fact that clotting and platelet function are usually normal. Gastro-intestinal bleeding, hæmaturia and hæmoptysis may also occur with such severity that serious anæmia develops.

Von Willebrand's disease is a hæmorrhagic state which is difficult to classify, since it seems to involve defects in all three components of the hæmostatic mechanism. It is inherited as a simple dominant, and may be very severe. The bleeding is of the purpuric type and it is a feature of this condition that a skin puncture wound not only bleeds for longer than normal but also bleeds at an increased rate. However, the platelet count is normal, and platelet function has been described as normal by many investigators, although, by special techniques, it has been shown that platelet adhesion to glass is impaired. The skin capillaries are often irregularly shaped and dilated, so that a capillary abnormality may be involved. Finally, it has become established within the past few years that Factor VIII is reduced to as little as 10–20 per cent of normal in a high proportion of cases, indicating that there is also a coagulation defect.

For further details of these various hæmorrhagic states, see Biggs and Macfarlane.[15]

THROMBOSIS

The ability of flowing blood to form a solid mass or plug from its constituents, though an essential part of the hæmostatic mechanism, becomes a pathological process when it occurs *within* the vascular system. This process of thrombosis will be discussed in detail in this section. It will be seen that many of the features have their counterpart in hæmostasis, but in this case the mechanism

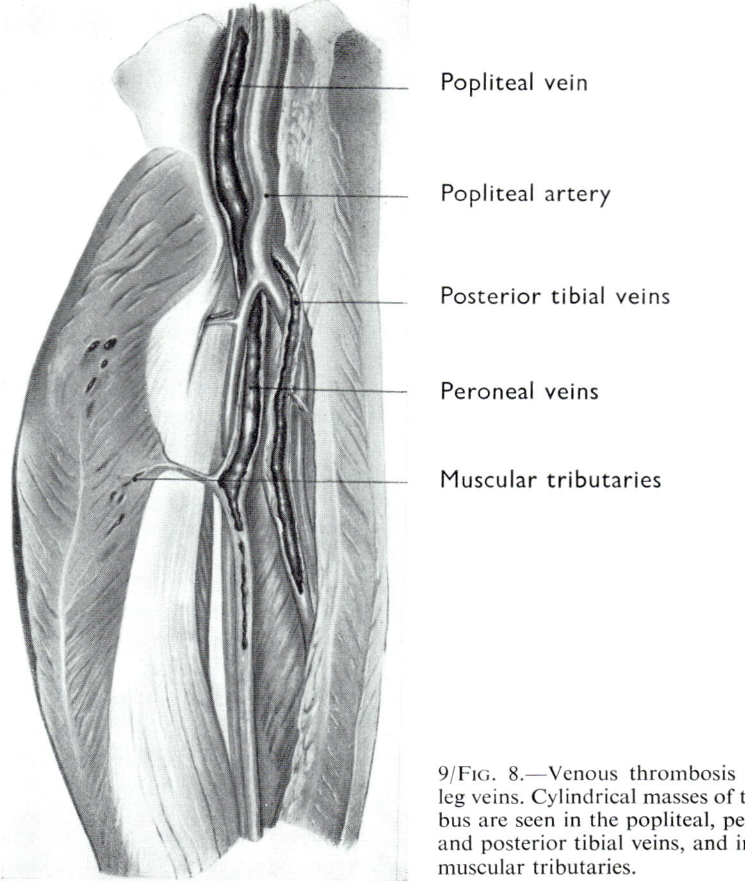

9/FIG. 8.—Venous thrombosis in the leg veins. Cylindrical masses of thrombus are seen in the popliteal, peroneal and posterior tibial veins, and in their muscular tributaries.

is misplaced and involves to a varying degree a change in those factors which normally preserve the fluidity of the circulating blood.

The Gross Appearance of Thrombi

Thrombi may occur anywhere in the circulation: in the chambers of the heart, in the arteries and veins and in the capillaries. They are usually attached in one or more places to the vessel wall. *Occluding thrombi* occupy the whole lumen of the vessel and obstruct the blood flow. *Mural* or *parietal thrombi* are attached only at one side and the blood continues to flow past their free border; thrombi of this type may appear flattened against the wall of the vessel or project as polypoid masses into the lumen.

In capillaries, thrombi occur when there is severe tissue injury or necrosis but they are otherwise uncommon and will not be discussed further. In the veins they may occur as small polypoid mural thrombi or as long cylindrical masses which completely fill the lumen over a considerable length of the vessel (FIG. 8).

They have a rather dry granular appearance which, when it has become familiar, distinguishes them from the more gelatinous-looking blood clots which may form in the vessels after death. Venous thrombi have a predominantly dark red colour, but when they are examined carefully it is usually possible to distinguish a pale *head* at the point of attachment to the vessel wall, a *neck* with pale rib-like markings on the surface—the so-called *striæ of Zahn*—and a red *tail* which usually makes up the greater part of the total bulk. Thrombi sometimes form in veins when there is an obvious inflammatory process affecting the wall, for example in the uterine veins in puerperal sepsis or in the sigmoid sinus following an infection of the middle ear. In the veins of the legs, they occur commonly when the walls are apparently healthy, and in these cases a sluggish blood flow is the more obvious predisposing factor. There is recent statistical evidence that in women the hormones taken as oral contraceptives may predispose to this type of thrombosis.[16]

In arteries, thrombi have a more compact structure. The mural variety is usually flat against the arterial wall and when occluding thrombi occur they often occupy only a relatively short segment of the vessel. Arterial thrombi are pale or show alternating laminæ of pale and dark red material, without an

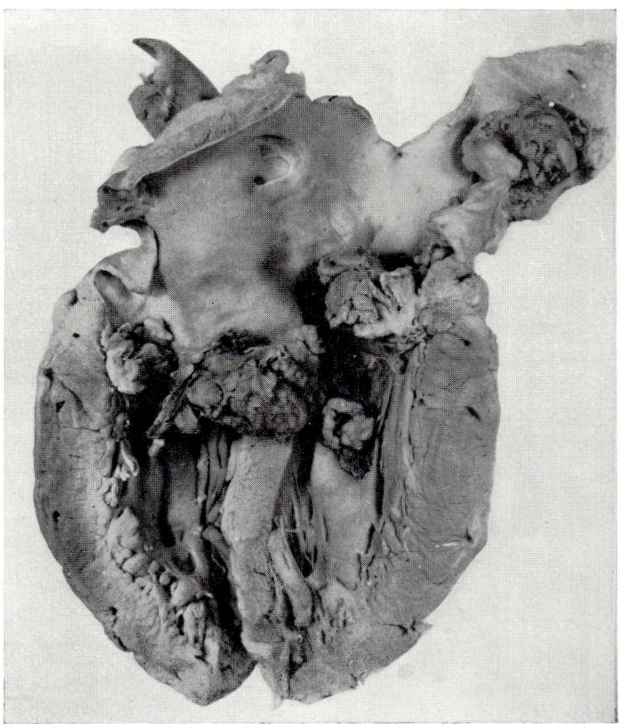

9/Fig. 9.—Bacterial endocarditis. The heart has been opened to display the mitral valve. The valve cusps are covered with bulky, crumbling vegetations (thrombi) which extend downwards along the chordæ tendinæ and also upwards over the wall of the left atrium.

obvious distinction between 'head' and 'tail'. Thrombi may be formed in arteries when there is an infection or an injury of the wall, but they are much more commonly associated with atherosclerosis—a chronic disease of the intima of the arteries which will be discussed in Chapter 18.

In the heart, thrombi take a variety of forms. Mural thrombi occurring on the surface of inflamed heart valves are known as "vegetations" and take the form of small compact nodules in rheumatic fever or larger polypoid masses in bacterial endocarditis (FIG. 9). Large thrombus masses may be attached to the wall of the ventricles when there is necrosis of the underlying endocardium, or may fill an auricular appendix in cases of cardiac disease with gross distension of the atria.

The Microscopic Structure of Thrombi

A longitudinal section taken through the attached head of a thrombus shows a framework of pale granular material partly surrounded by a fibrin coagulum containing red cells and leucocytes. The framework may have a complicated

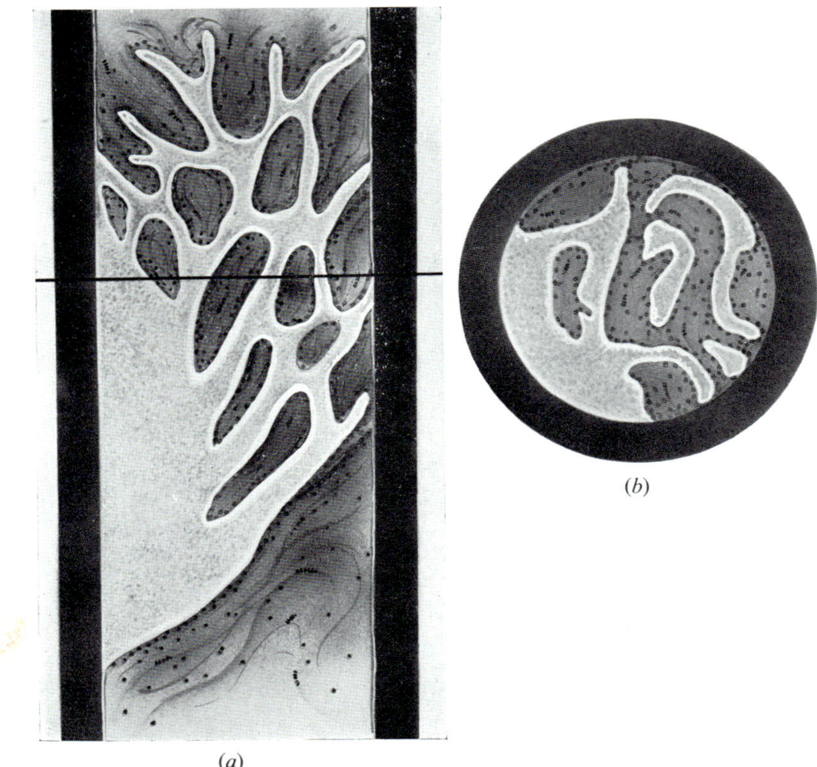

9/FIG. 10.—A diagram showing the basic structure of a thrombus. A coral-like framework of conglutinated platelets is covered over by a condensed layer of fibrin containing leucocytes. The spaces between the framework are filled by blood clot. (*a*) Longitudinal section; (*b*) Transverse section.

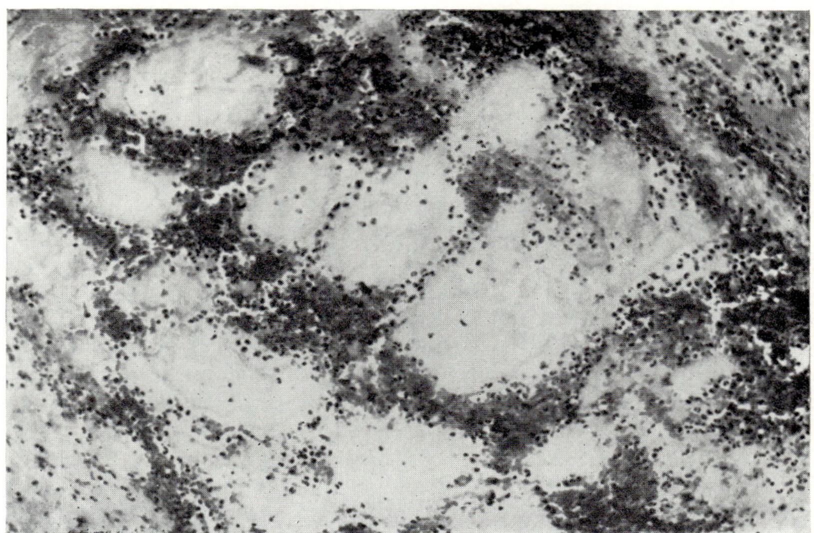

9/FIG. 11.—Microscopic appearance of a thrombus. The pale areas show the platelet framework cut across at various angles. The darker areas between consist of fibrin and red and white blood cells. Hæmatoxylin and eosin. (× 220.)

branching structure with its base at the point of attachment to the vessel wall. In veins it often forms a coral-like system in which the striæ of Zahn are formed by the extremities of the branches where they reach the free surface. The framework consists of a mass of more or less altered platelets covered over by a layer of condensed fibrin strands containing numerous leucocytes. Filling up the spaces between the branches of this structure is a looser network of fibrin with red and white cells in the proportions found in normal blood (FIG. 10). It is unlikely that an axial view of a thrombus will be seen in a single section; more commonly the framework will be cut obliquely or transversely so that islands or strands of granular material will be seen, often with leucocytes packed around them, and with fibrin and red blood corpuscles filling the intervening spaces (FIG. 11). The parts of the thrombus furthest from the attached head may show none of the platelet framework

The Stages in the Development of a Thrombus

The natural thrombi which are seen *post-mortem* or in surgical material are usually at a late stage in their development and, since they may have been *in situ* for days or weeks before being examined they have often undergone degenerative changes which make their components difficult to identify. Information about the early stages of thrombus formation and about the way in which the mass grows in the circulation has been obtained very largely from observations on experimental animals in which events can be observed directly in living vessels or in which the tissues can be fixed at chosen intervals for histological examination.

The first direct observations on thrombus formation in living vessels were made in the frog in which species the web of the foot, the mesentery, or the tongue are suitable for microscopic examination. In 1851, Wharton-Jones[17] had seen an artery in the injured web "become blocked by a mass composed apparently of colourless corpuscles and fibrin . . . so that the blood was arrested in its course, and passed off by the first considerable branch above the obstruction". He also saw "similar masses adhering to the wall of the vessel, but not entirely stopping it up". In 1875 Zahn[18] carried out a systematic study of the problem using a frog's mesentery for direct observation. When the vessels were injured by pressure or by applying a crystal of common salt, he noticed that cells were deposited on the inner wall and continued to accumulate in layers from the flowing blood (FIG. 12*a*) until the lumen became completely occluded. Zahn thought that the cells then underwent rapid degeneration to form a mass of granular material, but with the greater resolving power of the electron microscope it is now possible to see that the cells in this small thrombus in the frog still retain their identity in the initial stages but become very tightly packed together (FIG. 12*b*).

The cells (thromboyctes) in frog's blood which correspond to the mammalian platelets have nuclei, and Zahn, like Wharton-Jones, regarded them as leucocytes. However, in the year 1882 when Hayem first described the role of platelets in hæmostasis, Bizzozero[6], in the course of observations on the appearance of platelets in living vessels, repeated Zahn's experiment, using this time the mesentery of guinea-pigs or young rabbits. When he injured a small vessel by pressure with a needle he was able to distinguish that it was the platelets which were first arrested at the site of injury, and which accumulated rapidly to form an adherent mass on the wall (FIG. 13). This mass progressively impeded the flow of blood, but it was often disrupted by the force of the stream and the fragments were carried off. When this happened the mass began to grow again and the cycle of breakdown and regrowth might be repeated three or four times within the first fifteen minutes following injury. Similar deposits of platelets occurred on the surface of threads which were inserted into the jugular vein of rabbits or dogs. These observations were confirmed and extended a few years later by Eberth and Schimmelbusch[19] and by Welch[20]. The former, using living preparations, showed clearly that the growth of a platelet mass was the first event in experimental thrombosis, and that a fibrin coagulum did not appear until later when the blood flow was greatly reduced or stopped. Welch examined newly formed experimental thrombi by histological methods at intervals of up to one hour from their beginning. The first deposit consisted of gray, viscid, translucent material made up of platelets alone. At a later stage, which coincided with the reduction of the blood flow in the living preparations, polymorphonuclear leucocytes collected on the surfaces of the platelet masses, and fibrillary fibrin made its appearance for the first time on the surfaces but not within the platelet framework. Finally, as the circulation stopped, a fibrin coagulum filled the interstices of the platelet framework.

It was still a controversial question whether these observations on small vessels in experimental animals were relevant to the situation in man where fibrin and leucocytes are often conspicuous components of the thrombus and the granular component is by no means always clearly of platelet origin. Welch discussed this question in detail and based his conclusion that natural and

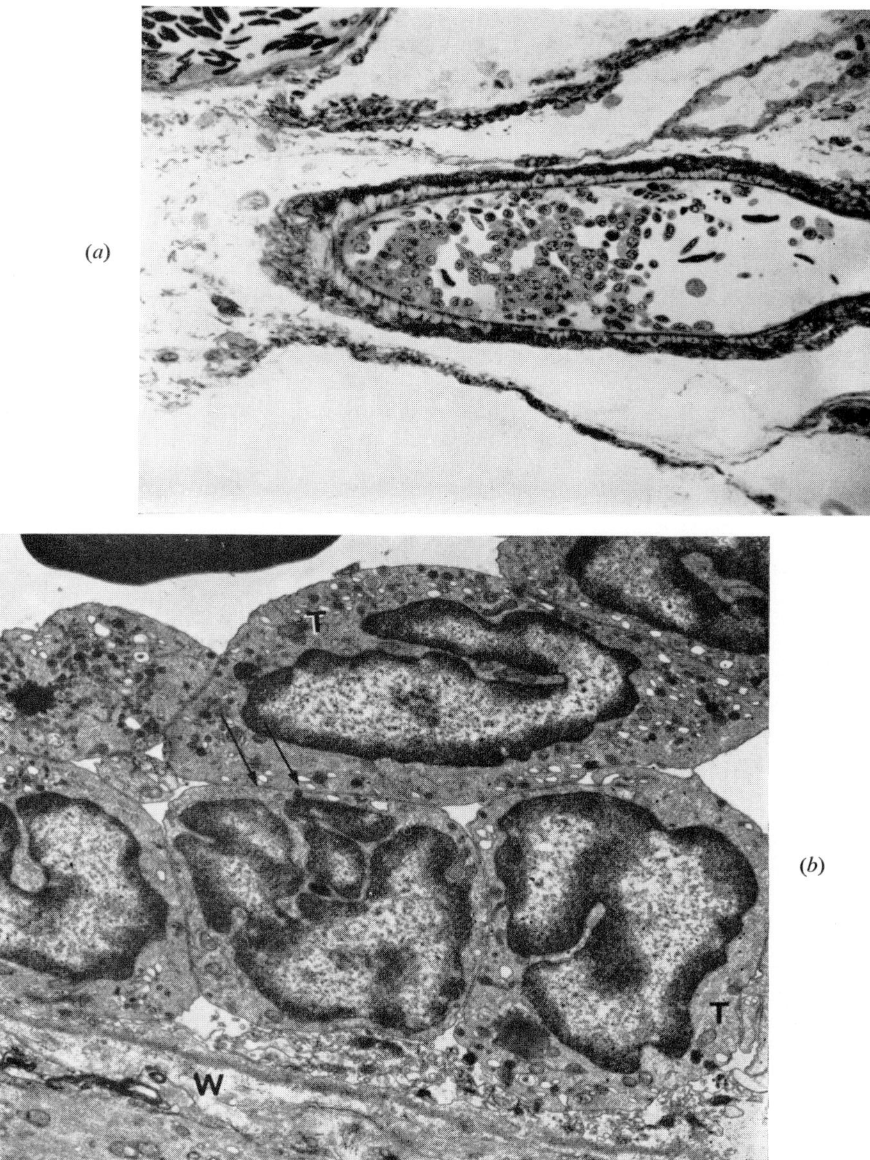

9/FIG. 12.—(*a*) Accumulation of thrombocytes in an artery in the tongue of a frog at a site injured by crushing—photomicrograph × 245. (*b*) Thrombocytes (T) adhering to the damaged wall (W) are very closely packed together (arrows)—electron micrograph × 9,600.

experimental thrombi were formed in the same way on the following evidence. First, he was able to show that when experimental thrombi were examined at later intervals the number of leucocytes and the amount of fibrin increased so that with time they acquired the characteristics of natural thrombi. Secondly, when he could obtain recently formed natural thrombi he was able to satisfy himself that the granular material did indeed consist of more or less altered platelets.

It was necessary to note one further effect of the primary occlusion before the elongated structure of natural venous thrombi could be understood. When the lumen is blocked, the column of blood extending to the nearest confluence of two veins is brought to a standstill and coagulates. The extremity of this clot may now come into contact with flowing blood where it enters from the branch, and act as the stimulus for the formation of another platelet thrombus at this point. If a second occlusion forms, the process can spread progressively from smaller to larger vessels. When a thrombus grows in this way by *propagation* it usually shows small pale platelet masses alternating in a longitudinal direction with longer dark red zones of coagulation.[2]

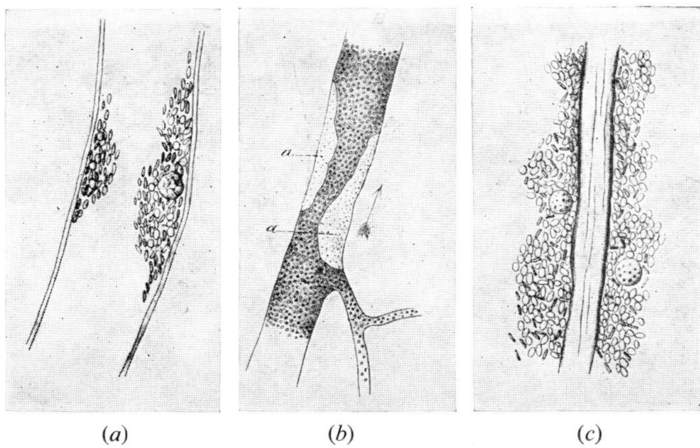

(*a*) (*b*) (*c*)

9/Fig. 13.—Platelets in experimental thrombi: (*a*) platelets adhering to the wall of a small artery in the mesentery of a guinea-pig; (*b*) a small venule with two mural thrombi (*a*), consisting only of blood platelets, in the mesentery of a guinea-pig; (*c*) platelets adhering to a fibre of linen thread with which dog's blood has been beaten for 45 seconds. (From Bizzozero.[6])

In the work which has followed these early studies, other experimental models have been used[21] and in recent years the appearances have been illustrated in greater detail with the electron microscope,[22] but although some further points have been added they have not changed our views about the basic pattern of events.

Thrombosis in injured vessels begins with the accumulation of platelets to form a visible mass or "white body". The platelets may be loosely arranged at first but become closely packed together in a characteristic mosaic pattern as seen in section by electron microscopy (Figs. 14 and 15). Individual platelets appear to be intact at this stage, but the apposition of their adjacent plasma membranes is so close (~200 A°) that by light microscopy they seem to have undergone fusion, and indeed this was formerly thought to occur. Nevertheless the mass is inherently unstable, so that small or larger fragments may be repeatedly detached from it and swept away by the bloodstream, sometimes over quite prolonged periods.

Usually no fibrin can be detected in the platelet mass when it is first formed and, since in this and other respects it resembles the platelet aggregates induced by ADP *in vitro* (see Chapter 8), it is thought that a local release of ADP could be the effector mechanism. It would be difficult to detect chemically the small amounts of ADP which may be involved but two lines of indirect evidence are consistent with such a mechanism. First, infusion of inhibitors of ADP aggrega-

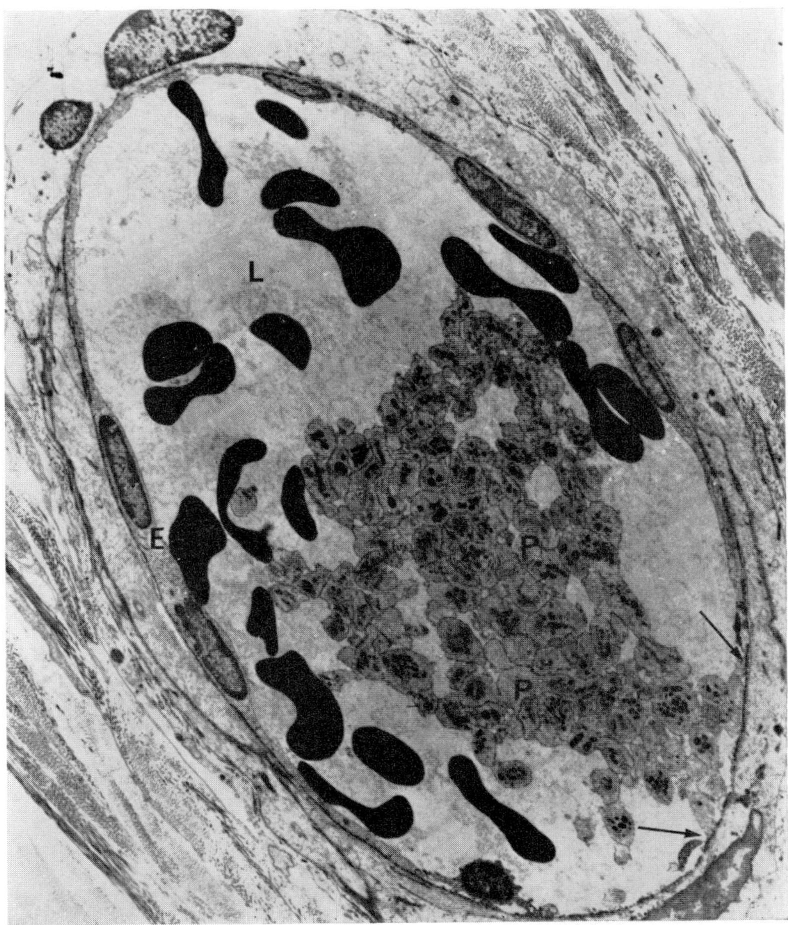

9/Fig. 14.—A mass of platelets (P) in an injured artery in the cheek pouch of a hamster is attached to the wall at the point (arrows) where the endothelium (E) has been destroyed. (× 3,000.) (From French *et al.*[9])

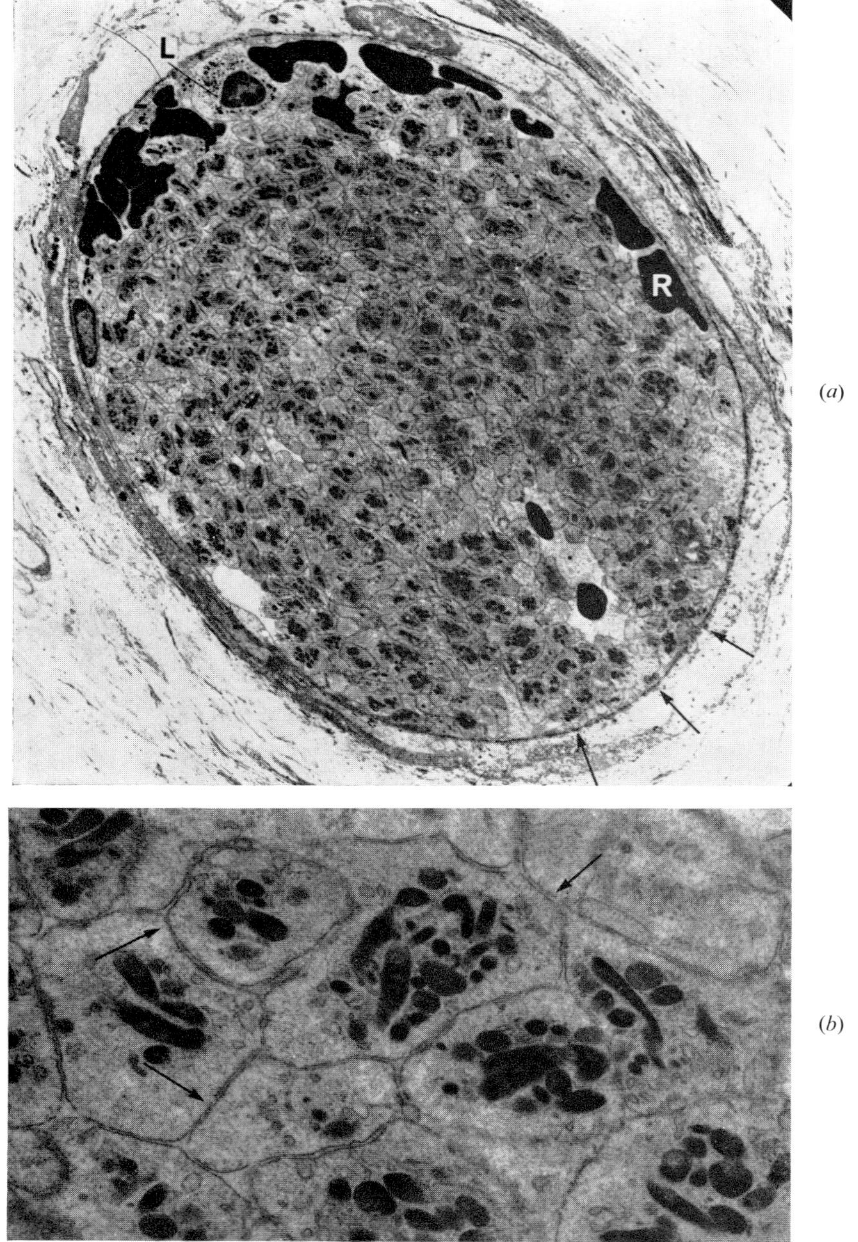

9/Fig. 15.—(*a*) A mass of platelets occupies the lumen of an artery injured at bottom right (arrows). A few red cells (R) and a leucocyte (L) are seen at the edges of the mass. (× 3,500.) (From French *et al.*[9]) (*b*) Centre of the mass (above) to show the very close packing (arrows) of apparently intact platelets. (× 17,500.)

tion (adenosine and 2-chloroadenosine) will suppress the formation of the platelet mass at a site of injury.[23] Second, application of ADP to vessels which have been mildly injured, but not to such a degree that aggregates form spontaneously, will provoke the aggregates to form.[24]

Under conditions where the platelet mass can grow to sufficient size to impede blood flow without being dislodged, it undergoes a series of changes beginning at the edges which apparently increase its stability. These changes appear to be identical with those already described at the edges of the hæmostatic plug (FIG. 5*b*), or at the edges of the platelet aggregates in the Chandler tube (FIG. 2); they include loss of platelet granules, formation of projections from the platelet surface and the first appearance of fibrin. They can be attributed to the action of thrombin which is probably first formed in pockets within the interstices of the platelet mass. Leucocytes then adhere to the altered platelets and fibrin fills in the spaces between the platelet aggregates and binds them together. As the flow is further reduced or stopped, coagulation extends into the stagnating column of blood so that the part of the thrombus which is formed last may have the same structure as a blood clot formed *in vitro*. However, since blood flow does not necessarily stop altogether before coagulation can occur, the fibrin in this part of the thrombus may be arranged as dense bands in a streamline pattern.[21]

In summary, most fully formed occluding thrombi consist of two more or less different parts. One part, corresponding to the *head* in venous thrombi, has a pale appearance and consists very largely of aggregated platelets. It is formed in flowing blood and has the effect of reducing flow. The other part is usually red and is formed by the clotting of stagnant blood. It may extend to the next patent branch in an occluded vessel, and may form the larger portion of the total bulk, particularly in veins.

Predisposing Factors in Thrombosis

It has been customary since the time of Virchow[25] to recognise three groups of predisposing factors in the pathogenesis of thrombosis, often known as *Virchow's triad*; (1) changes in the vessel wall; (2) changes in the local pattern of blood flow; (3) changes in the constituents of the blood. In relating these factors to the events described in the previous section it can be stated in general terms that the change in the wall, usually a mechanical injury in the animal experiments, provides the initial stimulus and the focus for platelet adhesion and aggregation. The local pattern of blood flow determines the accessibility of platelets at the site and whether a threshold concentration of thrombin can be built up to consolidate the platelet mass before it is washed away. Changes in the blood itself, such as increased platelet numbers or adhesiveness, or increased blood coagulability, can exaggerate the rate or extent of response to the other factors.

1. Changes in the vessel wall.—(*a*) *The role of abnormal surfaces.* The entire surface of the vascular system is normally covered by a thin pavement of endothelium, which when viewed *en face* is seen to consist of a mosaic of closely set polygonal cells (see 3/FIG. 1). It has frequently been pointed out that the nature of the surface is such that it does not normally activate either blood coagulation or the adhesion of platelets, but the explanation of this is still not clear. It has been proposed that the surface of the endothelium is covered by a layer of adsorbed protein, or that there is a surface film of mucoprotein with anticoagulant properties which may be secreted by the endothelial cells, but so far no extracellular material which might correspond to such a surface layer or film has been identified by standard methods of electron microscopy. However, it is possible that the plasma membrane of the endothelial cell itself has special properties, perhaps depending on an extraneous coat of polysaccharide.[26]

The changes in the vessel wall which lead to thrombosis may involve an actual destruction of the endothelium. This is clearly the case in experiments where the wall is deliberately denuded of its inner lining by scraping, but it has been shown that crushing, or injection of chemical irritants, can lead to desquamation of endothelial cells leaving bare areas on the inner surface in contact with the circulating blood. Another effective way of inducing thrombosis is to place a "foreign" surface in contact with the blood, for example, by passing a suture of catgut, silk or collagen through the wall and lumen of a vessel. Such regions of endothelial loss, or the foreign surface, provide the focus for the initial adhesion and aggregation of platelets. This can be seen in injured arteries or veins when the luminal surface is viewed *en face* with the light miscroscope[27, 28] and more clearly in transverse sections by electron microscopy. FIGURE 16 shows the site of attachment of a small platelet thrombus induced by an electrical injury in an artery in a hamster. The endothelium is missing and the first layer of platelets is in contact with exposed subendothelial fibres.

It seems probable that the adhesion and aggregation of platelets are activated by contact with the subendothelial tissue. The aggregation which follows adhesion of platelets to collagen fibres *in vitro* and to *extravascular* collagen fibres in the hæmostatic plug suggests that a similar mechanism is operating in thrombosis, but it is not certain that this is specific to collagen; exposed elastic fibres, components of the intimal ground substance or abnormal components in diseased intima could possibly have a similar effect.

In man, loss of endothelium from the inner surface of the vessels is probably an important predisposing factor in thrombosis, particularly in diseased arteries. In severe atherosclerosis the surface of the lesions is often ulcerated or broken so that blood comes directly into contact with necrotic material in the intima. In the veins, the gross abnormalities in the vessel wall which predispose to thrombosis are usually inflammatory, and when severe are associated with necrosis or desquamation of endothelium.

In the more common type of thrombosis in the veins of the legs it is often not possible to demonstrate, by conventional histological methods, that there has been any change in the endothelium. This raises the question whether a failure on the part of endothelium to maintain its normal surface characteristics can be a sufficient stimulus to thrombosis without there being an actual loss of cells. Microscopic examination of a vein *en face* makes it possible to see the structure of the endothelial cells in greater detail, and this technique has been used in several experimental investigations to observe the effects of relatively mild injury. It has been reported that changes in the pattern and staining properties of the so-called cement lines occur and that platelets first adhere in these regions.[27, 29] The suggestion has therefore been made that in response to mild injury there is a change in the amount and consistency of the intercellular substance which favours the adhesion of platelets.

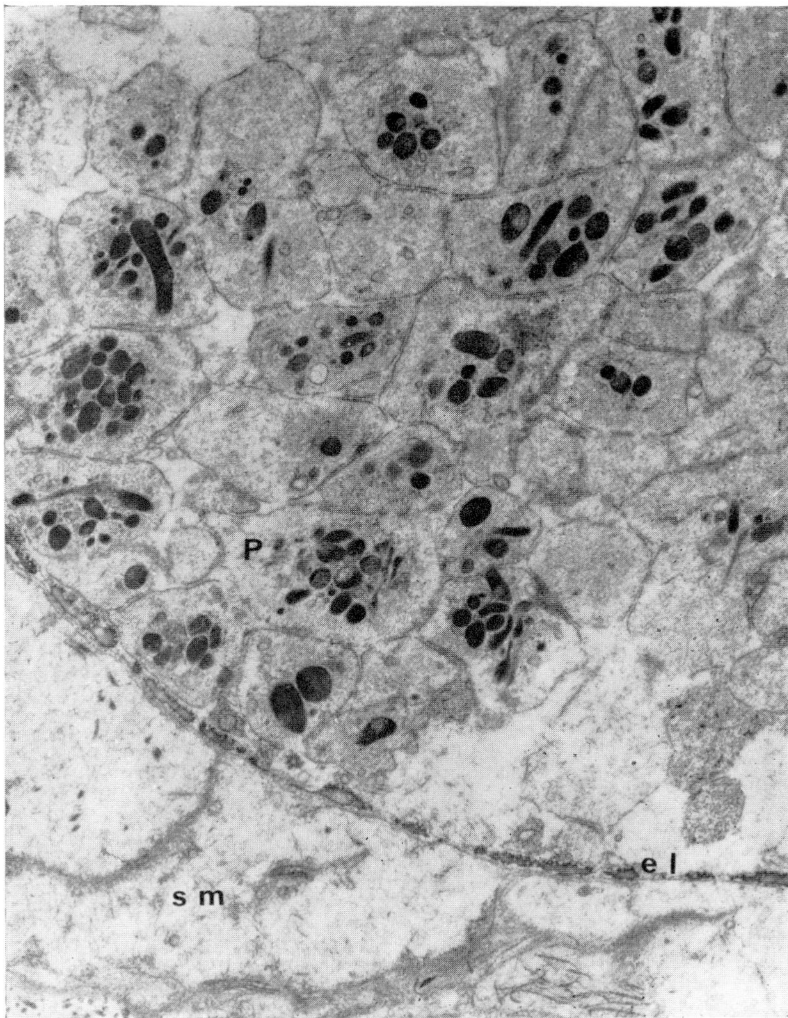

9/FIG. 16.—Attached edge of a platelet thrombus in a small artery in a hamster. A part of the wall shows injured smooth muscle cells (sm) and exposed elastic fibres (el); the endothelium is missing. (× 12,000.) (From French *et al.*[9])

Examination of mildly injured veins by electron microscopy has indicated one explanation of this apparent predilection of platelets for the region of the intercellular lines. It can sometimes be seen that small gaps have formed between otherwise undamaged endothelial cells which allow platelets to become interposed and so make contact with the subendothelial tissue (FIG. 17). When in a particular section platelets appear to be sticking to intact endothelium it is usually not possible to see any extracellular substance which would account for this but an endothelial defect may be found nearby if serial sections are taken.[30]

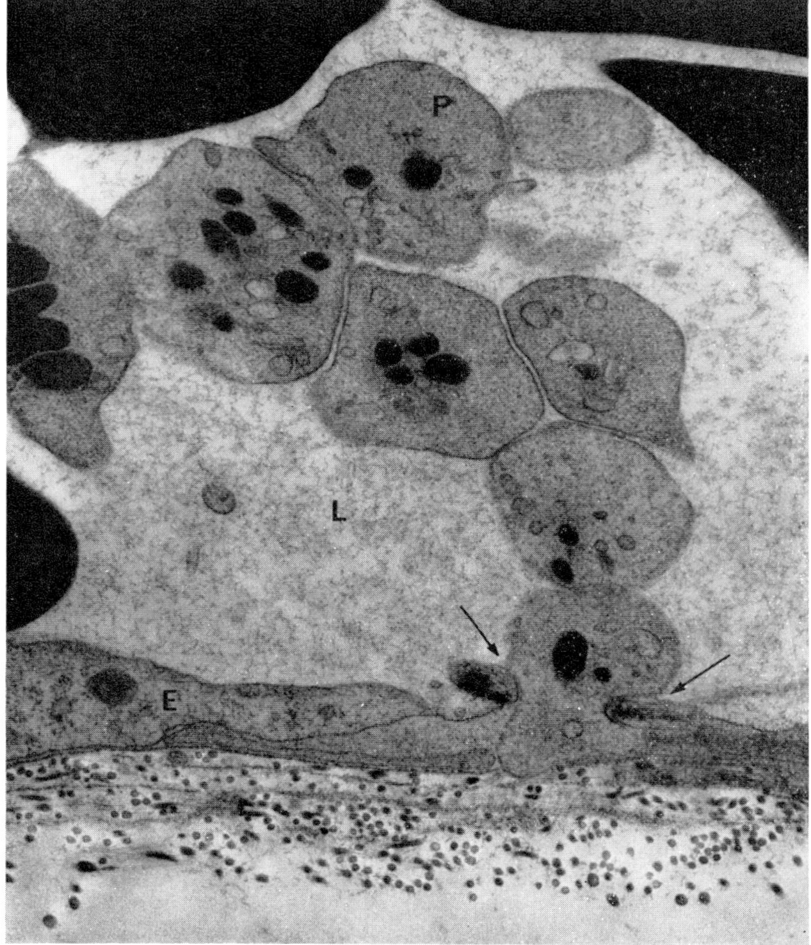

9/FIG. 17.—Part of the wall of a small vein in a hamster shows a group of platelets (P) in the lumen (L). One platelet occupies an intercellular gap (arrows) in the endothelium (E). (× 24,000.) (From French *et al.*[9])

Intact endothelium can develop a property of stickiness to leucocytes, but it is doubtful if platelets respond to this change in the same way as the leucocytes and on the basis of present evidence it seems likely that tenacious adhesion of platelets to a vessel wall requires a loss of endothelial continuity, even though this may be on a sub-microscopic scale.

The types of mild injury which are thought to produce endothelial changes in the veins in man are anoxia resulting from venous stasis, or prolonged pressure, such as may be caused, for example, by contact with the mattress when patients are immobilised for a long time in bed. In arteries, the possibility has to be considered that defects may occur at sites subjected to particular mechanical stresses if the normal replacement of effete endothelial cells by mitosis should become inadequate.

(*b*) *Other changes in the wall.*—In many types of experimental thrombosis it is probable that injury is not confined to the endothelium but that other cells in the wall are damaged or destroyed. The discovery of the role of ADP in platelet aggregation was made from observations on the effect of damaged red cells, but it is known that when other cells are injured some of their ATP is broken down. It is therefore possible that release of ADP from injured cells in the vessel wall is concerned in promoting platelet aggregation. This is supported by the finding that enzyme poisons which suppress the metabolism of injured tissue will prevent the formation of visible platelet aggregates in severely injured vessels.[24] Changes in the vessel wall may also be concerned in the formation of thrombin if the intrinsic coagulation mechanism is set in motion by contact of the blood with the abnormal surfaces, or if the extrinsic mechanism is activated by release of tissue thromboplastins known to be present in the vessel wall.

2. Changes in the local pattern of blood flow.—The initiation of thrombosis can usually be attributed to changes in the vessel wall, but the early events are potentially reversible and it is unlikely that a stable mass will be built up unless other circulatory factors favour the accumulation of platelets and the generation of thrombin. It has been found repeatedly in animal experiments that it is difficult to induce an occluding thrombus in arteries simply by damaging the vessel wall. No more than a thin deposit of platelets may form on the damaged surface of the vessels unless there is a simultaneous disturbance of blood flow. It is this fact which allows the operation of thrombo-endarterectomy or the insertion of arterial grafts to be carried out successfully in man. These surgical procedures involve the destruction of the inner part of the wall of an artery, or leave an area denuded of endothelium, but they are not usually followed by occluding thrombosis provided that a rapid blood flow is restored.[31] It will be obvious, too, that the milder types of injury to the endothelium of veins must occur frequently, and yet it is only in a few individuals that they are followed by the formation of an occluding thrombus.

When blood flow is rapid and linear, platelet aggregates may break up and be washed away before there has been time for consolidation to occur. This dissemination of the platelet aggregates was observed in the earliest experiments on living vessels; it applies particularly in arteries and may indicate that many incipient thrombi never progress beyond this early stage. On the other hand when the flow is slower, not only is the mass less likely to break up, but fresh platelets borne by the passing blood are more accessible to the altered surface. During the course of direct observations on the circulation in the dog's omentum, Eberth and Schimmelbusch[19] noted that when the flow was retarded the platelets left the axial stream and moved into the outer, more slowly moving plasma zone. These authors considered that only when this occurred could the platelets come into contact with the vessel wall. Gravitational forces may accentuate this settling out of the formed elements of the blood in a slowly moving stream.

Irregular patterns of flow such as whirling or eddying movements may also favour the deposition of platelets (Fig. 18), and at some sites in the body are probably of greater significance than slowing of the stream. Aschoff[32] compared

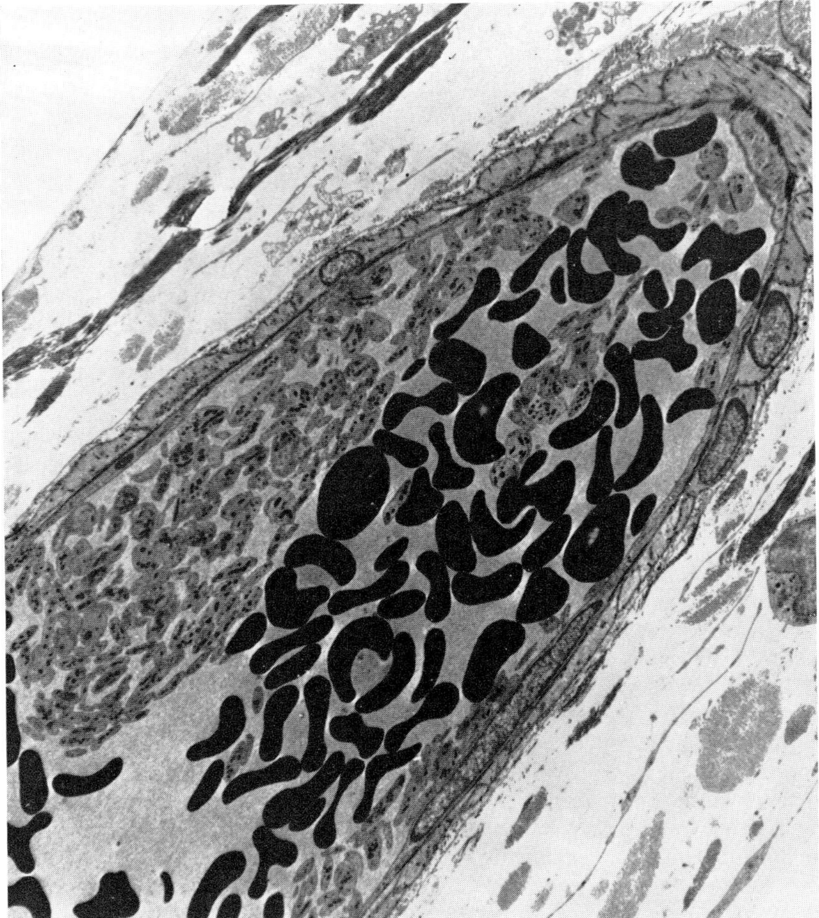

9/Fig. 18.—Accumulation of platelets at the mouth of a side branch in an artery in a hamster cheek pouch following a distal occlusion of the main vessel. Eddies could be observed in this region with the dissecting microscope. Electron micrograph × 2,400.

the process to the silting-up which occurs in rivers at places where the river bed widens or deepens, and pointed to the common occurrence of thrombi in the ampullæ of venous valves and in aneurysmal sacs in arteries, where eddies must occur.

In arteries, the deposition of platelets is favoured by the flow patterns which occur at sites of branching. Mustard and his colleagues[33] have used extracorporeal shunts as models of the arterial tree to show that deposition of platelets does not occur diffusely over the inner surface of the model but is localised at bifurcations and around the orifice of right-angle branches. They also found that thrombosis of the aorta could be induced more readily in experimental animals if the endothelial surface was damaged in the region of the bifurcation rather than at sites of undisturbed flow. It is an old observation that gross thrombosis can be induced more easily in relatively large arteries if an injury is so severe that it distorts the local flow pattern. One method which has been used is to tie a ligature tightly round the wall and then to release it again. Under these circumstances the wall is disrupted and fragments of damaged tissue project into the lumen of the vessel.

In addition to their effect on the behaviour of platelets, changes in the rate or pattern of flow have an important effect on the coagulation phase of thrombosis. The coagulation mechanism is probably set in motion by changes in the wall and may be accelerated by the formation of the platelet aggregates, but since there is a time lag between the initiation of coagulation and the formation of thrombin the mechanism is at a disadvantage in free flowing blood. Activated clotting factors will be widely dispersed as they are formed and also inhibited by the various mechanisms discussed in Chapter 7. The changes in flow which allow an effective local concentration of thrombin to be built up can generally be considered secondary to the growth of the platelet mass but in any particular situation the overall rate at which this occurs and the extent to which coagulation spreads must depend on the pattern of flow which already pertains at the site.

In man, slowing or stagnation of flow is seen most clearly as a predisposing factor in venous thrombosis. Thrombosis occurs frequently in the leg veins of patients who have cardiac disease or are confined to bed for long periods, particularly following abdominal operations.[34] Under these circumstances it has been shown, by injecting tracer substances into the circulation, that there is a considerable delay in the venous return from the legs.[35] Blood flow in veins can also be studied by cine-radiography after injecting the veins with a dye which is opaque to X-rays. It has been found that there is stagnation of blood in veins of the legs and particularly in the valve pockets even when a normal subject remains immobile in the supine position.[36] In arteries, with their more rapid flow, hæmodynamic factors other than slowing have usually to be considered. In atherosclerosis, for example, eddy currents may be set up in arteries which are irregularly narrowed, or thickened plaques may project from the walls into the axial stream, particularly at sites of branching. The circulation in the coronary arteries, where thrombosis is a frequent complication of atherosclerosis, has certain special features. The flow in these vessels is periodically reduced by the contraction of the ventricles, and is probably halted or reversed in early systole.[37]

3. Changes in the constituents of the blood.—The ability of changes in the constituents of the blood to modify the course of events in thrombosis has important implications in clinical medicine. It often appears that although changes in the vessel wall and in local hæmodynamics have established conditions which can lead to thrombosis, this does not necessarily develop, at least on a clinical scale, unless there is an increased "thrombotic tendency" in the blood as a whole.

In spite of the undoubted importance of this component of "Virchow's triad", the amount of precise information is surprisingly meagre. Animal experiments have so far provided relatively little information. In man, it has proved difficult to interpret the significance of *in vitro* tests which indicate an increased coagulability of the blood or altered platelet function. Changes in the blood which predispose to thrombosis might be effective even though they were only transient, and in this case they could easily be missed in a particular test. On the other hand, changes which are revealed by *in vitro* tests may be ineffective in the living animal when they can be opposed by protective mechanisms. It is convenient to consider the changes as they affect the platelets and the coagulation mechanism separately, but it should be remembered that in the development of a thrombus platelet behaviour and coagulation are closely interlinked and that changes in the one frequently affect the other.

Changes in the platelets which predispose to thrombosis may be quantitative or qualitative. The importance of an increase in platelet number has been suggested by the finding that following parturition or surgical operations, when there is a predisposition to venous thrombosis, the platelet count in the blood frequently rises. The size of the increase and the time at which it occurs is variable in different individuals, but the averaged results indicate a maximum on about the tenth day after parturition or a surgical operation and this coincides with the time when thrombosis is most likely to occur.[38] A rise in the platelet count may also occur during the actual course of an extensive surgical operation and this is possibly a significant factor when thrombosis is detected earlier in the post-operative period.[39] The increase in the platelet count which follows various forms of trauma or stress in experimental animals may be relevant, though the tendency for such animals to develop thrombosis has not been investigated. An increase in the number of circulating platelets may be one of the factors associated with an increased tendency to thrombosis in patients with polycythæmia vera. Quantitative changes in the platelets have not been correlated with a predisposition to thrombosis in other clinical conditions.

The possibility that qualitative changes can occur in platelets which predispose to thrombosis has been widely considered. Attempts have been made to correlate various tests of platelet function (adhesiveness to glass, rate of aggregation by ADP, electrophoretic mobility and survival time of labelled platelets in the circulation) with a clinical tendency to thrombosis,[40] but the results are not clear cut and in many cases difficult to interpret; indeed it remains uncertain whether a suitable way of assessing platelet function in relation to thrombosis has yet been devised. Increased adhesiveness of platelets to glass has been observed in conditions where the platelet count in the blood is increased, suggesting a functional difference in platelets which are released prematurely into the circulation.[38] Increased platelet adhesiveness has also been observed in some patients who have had a recent thrombosis but this change may be an effect of the thrombosis rather than a potential cause. Decreased platelet survival time, indicating an increased platelet turnover, is thought to reflect an increased tendency for platelets to form aggregates *in vivo*. It has been observed in patients on high fat diets and suggests a possible way in which this condition may be linked with thrombosis.[33]

A number of the chemical agents which induce platelet aggregation *in vitro* (ADP, thrombin and certain unesterified fatty acids) also cause platelets to aggregate when injected into the circulation. If such agents should be present in the blood, if only temporarily, under natural conditions, it can be presumed that they would have an important influence on thrombus formation. Unesterified fatty acids are normally carried in the blood as a complex with albumin and in this form do not promote platelet aggregation, but they might on occasions enter the blood in excess of the albumin binding capacity.[41] As a further indication that lipæmia may have an effect on platelet behaviour it has been shown that injection of lipid particles causes intravascular platelet aggregation (see 8/FIG. 8) and that platelet thrombi form more readily in injured vessels in experimental animals when lipæmia has been established by feeding fat.[42]

An increased coagulability of the blood might be expected to favour thrombosis by increasing the rate at which the platelet mass was stabilised and the extent to which coagulation could spread into neighbouring zones of stasis. It has been shown experimentally that increased coagulability *in vivo*, induced, for example, by infusion of serum, is not by itself a sufficient stimulus to thrombosis in circulating blood. However, if in addition stasis is induced by occluding a segment of a vein, the contents of the occluded segment will clot; this does not happen in an occluded segment in an untreated animal.[43]

Much effort has gone into an attempt to define a thrombotic tendency as indicated by an increase of clotting activity *in vitro*. No clear picture has so far emerged, which may in part be explained by the technical difficulties involved. Most of the standard clotting tests are more sensitive to deficiencies than to excesses of clotting factors; moreover when changes are observed *in vitro* it is not certain that they would function in the living animal where they may be balanced by inhibitory and clearance mechanisms. With these reservations in mind it can be stated that there is some evidence of increased coagulant activity in the blood of patients who have already had a thrombotic episode.[44] There is also little doubt that lipæmia can increase the coagulability of the blood as shown by *in vitro* tests and that if saturated long chain fatty acids are present in the free form *in vivo* they can cause clotting in a stagnant column of blood.[41, 45]

The production of changes in the blood which *reduce* the thrombotic tendency appears the most practicable method available at present for preventing or controlling thrombotic disease. The use of anticoagulant drugs seems an obvious choice but it has been shown that neither the administration of heparin in therapeutic doses, nor treatment with the coumarin group of drugs can prevent the accumulation of platelets in the initial stages of thrombosis.[46] In an attempt to control this step attention is therefore being given to the development of drugs which would interfere with platelet aggregation *in vivo*, but would not upset the normal hæmostatic mechanism or have other adverse effects.[47] Anticoagulants can be expected to interfere with the stabilisation of the platelet mass by fibrin and to limit the extension of clotting into neighbouring segments of the vessel. This argument is the basis for the use of heparin and coumarin drugs in the treatment and prophylaxis of thrombosis and embolism. Since the coagulation component often forms the major part of the total bulk of venous thrombi in the legs and of the consequent pulmonary emboli it is not surprising that it is in this group of conditions where anticoagulant therapy has most clearly been shown to be successful.[48] In coronary thrombosis, where the platelet component tends to be predominant, results with anticoagulant therapy have been disappointing.[49]

Subsequent Changes in Thrombi

The appearances described so far are seen in a freshly formed thrombus. Once formed, however, a thrombus may undergo changes which alter its structure and modify the effects which it has on the circulation. These changes can be classified as resolution, organisation and embolism.

Resolution.—Not all the thrombi which begin to form persist for any length of time in the vessels. At each stage in the development of a thrombus there may be protective mechanisms which need to be overcome before the thrombus can progress further. Thus the breakup of platelet aggregates of the type induced by ADP, may be facilitated by the action of phosphatases present in the plasma or vessel wall. Even the more stable fibrin-platelet deposits could presumably be dispersed by fibrinolytic activity if the plasminogen activator, known to be present in endothelial cells (see Chapter 7), were made available at this stage.

Thrombi which do persist beyond the initial stages undergo a series of changes which reduce their bulk. The early increase in fibrin and leucocytes and the alterations in platelets have already been mentioned. During this period the thrombus shrinks by a process which probably corresponds to clot retraction *in vitro*. Mural thrombi become more compact; occluding thrombi develop clefts or are drawn away from the wall at points where they are not firmly adherent. Release of autolytic enzymes, by degenerating platelets or by leucocytes trapped within the mass, then leads to a partial digestion of the thrombus. This change is seen particularly in large thrombi where the centre often undergoes softening and liquefaction. During the process of organisation described below, macrophages enter the thrombus and ingest with other debris, free hæmoglobin, trapped red cells and platelets[50] (FIG. 19). Hæmosiderin, formed from hæmoglobin by these macrophages, is responsible for the brown colour and the staining reaction for iron, which are frequently observed in older thrombi. Macrophages which have ingested platelets subsequently show stainable lipid in their cytoplasm and so may be the source of the foam cells seen in some organising thrombi.[51]

The eventual removal of fibrin may depend partly on phagocytosis and partly on fibrinolytic enzymes released by the leucocytes. The plasma fibrinolytic mechanism, described in Chapter 7, may also have a role if it is activated, for example, by local ischæmia. Intravenous administration of plasminogen activators will hasten the resorption of newly formed coagulation thrombi in experimental animals and these agents are being used therapeutically in an attempt to aid resolution of thrombi in man.[52] The phenomenon of post-mortem fibrinolysis, also discussed in Chapter 7, might lead to the disappearance or dislodgement of thrombi which were present at the time of death, and should therefore be considered in the interpretation of post-mortem findings.

Some of the factors which effect the rate of resolution of thrombi may possibly operate through the fibrinolytic mechanism. For example, Wright and Kubik[53] have shown that the administration of anticoagulant drugs of the coumarin group to rabbits may facilitate the resorption of coagulation thrombi. To explain this effect, the authors suggest that fibrin is continually being deposited on the surfaces of formed thrombi, and that the anticoagulant, by preventing this, allows the fibrin already present to be removed by fibrinolysis.

It is also possible that inhibitors of the fibrinolytic mechanism might delay the resorption of thrombi or lead to the persistence of small thrombi which would otherwise be resolved. Administration of the inhibitor ε-amino caproic acid will certainly delay the spontaneous resorption of fibrin. Under some circumstances, the inhibition of fibrinolysis which appears to be associated with lipæmic states might possibly be significant[52].

Organisation.—At the same time as the thrombus is undergoing partial resolution, reactive changes occur in the vessel wall and gradually transform the mass, in whole or in part, into vascular connective tissue. The process of healing, whereby fibrin and tissue debris are gradually replaced by organised connective tissue, is discussed in detail in Chapter 17. The organisation of a thrombus follows a similar pattern but has certain special features which require further comment. These concern the vascularisation of the new tissue and the rôle of smooth muscle cells in its histogenesis.

Endothelium can cover the surface of mural thrombi by ingrowth of cells from the edges.[54] Endothelium also proliferates and lines any accessible clefts or spaces in an occluding thrombus. It has been proposed by a number of investigators that this new endothelium, which often appears to cover the surfaces of a thrombus within a few days, is derived in part from blood-borne cells. There is no doubt that a temporary lining may be formed by blood monocytes which spread out on the surface, but it has yet to be established that a true endothelium can be formed in this way.

Endothelium from the surface may invade the substance of a thrombus, much as capillary buds invade during organisation elsewhere, to form small vascular channels in continuity with the main lumen. In addition, capillaries derived from the vasa vasorum may grow into the thrombus at its points of attachment to the wall. In a vein these new vessels develop from a vascular plexus which lies just outside the internal elastic lamina.[55] In arteries, the nearest vessels are situated more deeply in the media, so that vascularisation of the inner part of the wall has to precede the penetration of the thrombus by new vessels from the vasa vasorum. In some organising arterial thrombi this transmedial vascularisation is not achieved.[56]

As the thrombus becomes vascularised there is a migration of cells from contiguous parts of the wall which begin to elaborate the ground substance and fibres of the new connective tissue. In contrast to the typical appearance of fibroblasts in healing tissue at other sites, the cells which take part in healing reactions in the arterial wall have the morphological features of vascular smooth muscle and apparently have the ability to synthesise elastin as well as collagen.[30] Thus the organising thrombus is eventually transformed into tissue which is rich in collagen and elastin fibres and in which smooth muscle cells are the predominant cell type (FIG. 20).

The blood vessels which enter the thrombus provide the blood supply for the new connective tissue as in organisation at other sites, but in addition, as organisation proceeds, one or more vascular channels may develop which have the further function of re-establishing the blood flow through the substance of the thrombus. This special feature of the organisation of thrombi is called *re-canalisation.* The majority of the through channels are probably derived from the irregular clefts and spaces in the thrombus which at first are lined only by

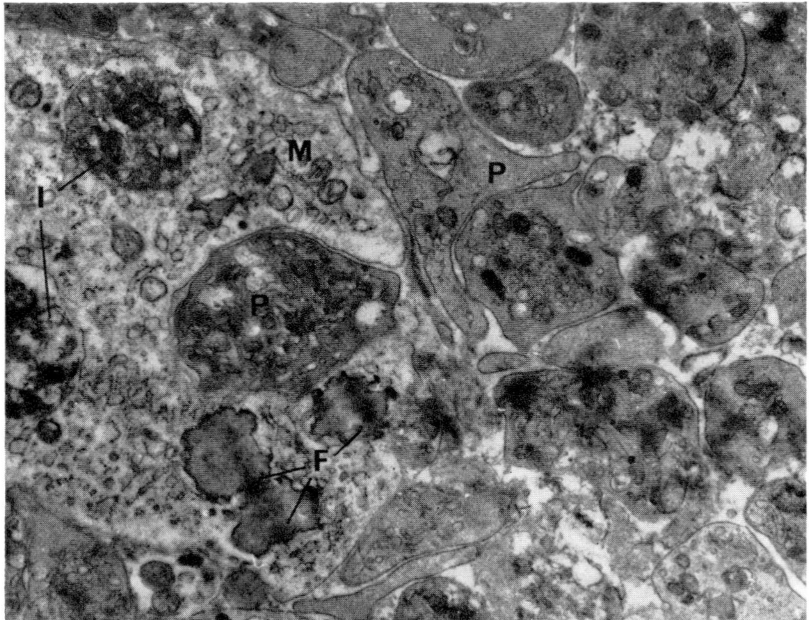

9/Fig. 19.—Section through a mural thrombus on the surface of a fabric graft inserted one week previously in the aorta of a baboon. It shows part of a monocyte (M) which has almost completely engulfed a platelet (P). Inclusions (I) in the cytoplasm of the monocyte probably represent partially disintegrated platelets. (× 10,500.)

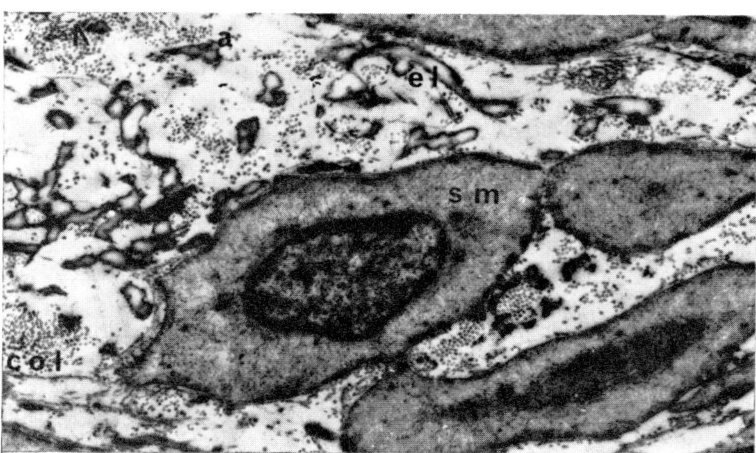

9/Fig. 20.—Section through a fully organised mural thrombus in a baboon's aorta shows two smooth muscle cells (sm), elastic tissue (el) and collagen fibres (col) cut transversely. (× 9,500.)

endothelium. Later, by a process of remoulding and growth of tissue in their walls, these channels become differentiated and appear as new arteries or veins inside the original vessel. The capillaries which grow in from the vasa vasorum are probably not directly concerned in recanalisation and, in the arteries at any rate, serve only to vascularise the substance of the new tissue.[56]

When the length of an occluding thrombus is short, recanalisation may restore the original pattern of blood flow. When a longer segment is occluded, a new lumen may not be established throughout the thrombus, but some new channels may still develop which are in continuity with patent side branches (FIG. 21). In occluded arteries of the legs, for example, it has been shown that

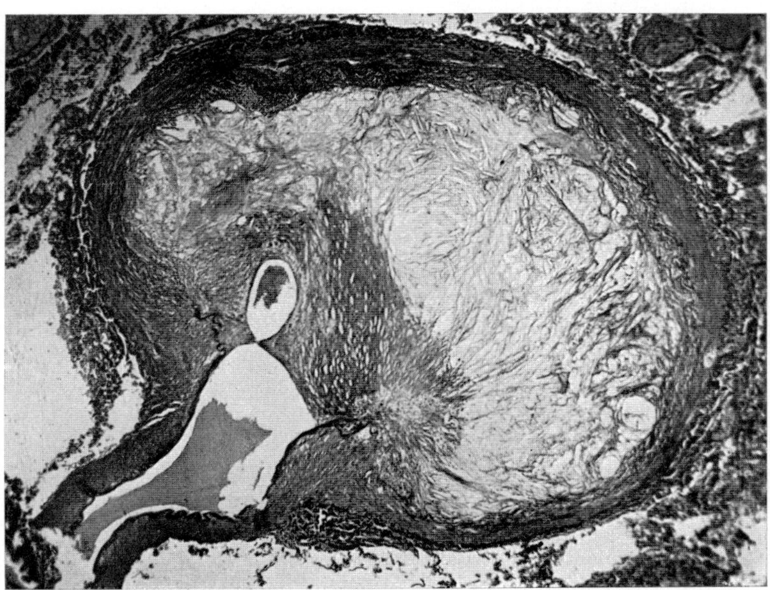

9/FIG. 21.—Recanalisation of an occluding thrombus in an artery. The newly formed blood channel communicates with a patent side branch. Weigert's elastic stain. (× 40.) (From Akrawi and Wilson.[57])

the newly formed arteries inside the organised thrombus form links between two side branches or between a side branch and the veins of the vasa vasorum. Blood enters these channels by reversal of the flow in the proximal branch and thus makes a detour which avoids the proximal part of the thrombus.[57]

Mural thrombi in arteries frequently organise less readily than other types. The superficial parts may be organised by cells which grow in from the edges and are nourished by diffusion from the lumen, or by "high pressure" capillaries in continuity with the lumen, but the centre of the thrombus is liable to remain unorganised and to undergo degenerative changes. This has been attributed to the effect of arterial pressure transmitted through the vessel wall in preventing the ingrowth of capillaries from the vasa vasorum.[58] It should also be pointed out that such mural thrombi often form on the surface of atherosclerotic plaques, where the intima already contains necrotic tissue likely to interfere with the free growth of capillaries.

Through these processes of organisation thrombi are converted into masses of musculo-elastic tissue, sometimes containing stainable lipid, which are firmly attached to the wall[59]. Organised occluding thrombi may obliterate the lumen completely or be traversed by new blood channels formed in the ways discussed. Mural thrombi contract against the wall and, since they are covered by endothelium, may appear as focal thickenings of the intima. The intimal thickenings which are found quite commonly in the veins of the legs may be formed in this way. In the arteries, mural thrombi which form on the surface of atherosclerotic plaques are incorporated in the thickened intima and are often the cause of the extreme narrowing of the lumen of the arteries which is found in this disease (see Chapter 18).

Embolism.—Embolism is defined as the impaction in some part of the vascular system of any undissolved material brought there by the blood stream. The transported material is known as an *embolus*.[2] Although a variety of substances, such as fat droplets, gas bubbles or fragments of tumour tissue, may enter the circulation, the most common cause of embolism is dislodgement of the whole or part of a thrombus, and, unless otherwise specified, the term embolism usually refers to this process.

The concept of embolism was developed by Virchow in a series of experimental and clinical studies between 1846 and 1856, and was a major advance in the understanding of many disease processes. However, as Welch[2] points out, once the idea has been accepted, it appears an obvious corollary of the discovery of the circulation of the blood, and indeed the mechanism of embolism may be largely deduced from a consideration of the anatomy of the heart and blood vessels. For this reason the distribution of emboli will not be discussed in detail, but it must be emphasised that embolism is one of the most important features of the pathology of thrombosis, and that emboli frequently have more serious effects than the thrombi from which they were formed.

Since emboli move down-stream it follows that those which originate from occluding thrombi can arise only in veins, in which the lumen widens progressively. By the same argument, emboli can become impacted only in the arterial circulations where there is progressive narrowing of the vessels. Emboli may originate from mural thrombi in any of the various positions which have been mentioned. When they arise from thrombi in the left side of the heart they become impacted in the systemic arteries, commonly in the kidney, spleen or brain. Mural thrombi in arteries can lead to embolism when fragments are detached and carried further into the arterial tree. For example, mural thrombosis in the internal carotid arteries may give rise to multiple small emboli which are arrested at least temporarily in small arteries in the brain or retina.[60] Similar events may occur also in the coronary circulation and in the arteries of the legs.

The embolism most often met with in practice is that which occurs as a sequel to thrombosis in the systemic veins. In this case the emboli become impacted in the pulmonary circulation.[61] The propagated thrombi which form in the veins of the legs may extend as "eel-like" formations into the femoral vein. When first formed they are firmly anchored at their lower end, far down in the leg, but the part in the femoral vein may be retracted from the wall and fragile as a result of autolytic changes. In the most serious form of pulmonary embolism a major part of the thrombus becomes detached. A sudden movement can cause a break, often at the level of the knee, and the mass in the femoral vein then floats away and becomes impacted as a coiled embolus, 40–50 cm. in length when unravelled, in the main branches of the pulmonary artery (FIG. 22). Smaller pulmonary emboli may pass unnoticed clinically, but post-mortem studies have indicated that the detachment of embolic fragments, often multiple, from thrombi in the leg veins is a common event.

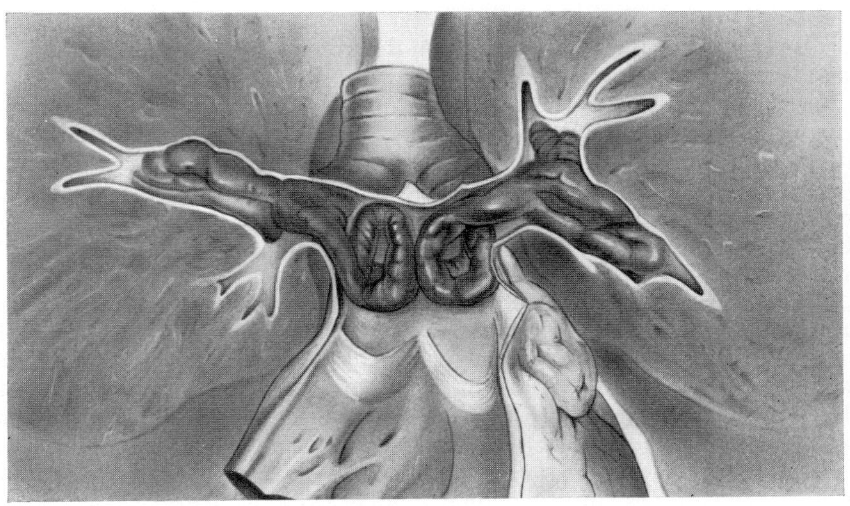

9/FIG. 22.—Fatal pulmonary embolism. A large thrombus, formed in the leg veins, has been impacted as a coiled mass at the bifurcation of the pulmonary artery.

Occasionally micro-emboli, consisting of platelets or platelets and fibrin, may be formed in the circulating blood without there being an obvious focal source. Multiple emboli of this type have been described in the lungs in man following severe injury or burns.[62] There is also a risk of micro-emboli entering the blood during surgical procedures which employ an extracorporeal circulation unless adequate precautionary measures are taken.

Some emboli, particularly the small ones consisting of recently formed platelet aggregates, may disperse spontaneously after lodging in an artery. Other more stable emboli may block the lumen completely or, if they do not do so, they may initiate the formation of a new thrombus which will close any remaining gaps. The subsequent course of events is then the same as for primary occluding thrombi in arteries.

THE EFFECTS OF THROMBOSIS AND EMBOLISM

The primary effect of a thrombus or embolus is on the local circulation. The partial or complete occlusion of the lumen of a vessel is followed, in general, by a reduction in the total blood flow in the area supplied. This *ischæmia*, as it is called, of the local tissues leads in turn to changes in their function and structure. There are, of course, considerable differences in the anatomy and physiology of the circulation at different sites in the body and also in the susceptibility of different tissues to deprivation of their blood supply. This means that thrombosis and embolism have a wide range of possible consequences. The details of these, as they affect the various organs, are outside the scope of general pathology, and only some of the more general principles will be considered here.

Effects on the Circulation

The immediate effects on the circulation of an occlusion of a vessel will depend largely on anatomical factors, i.e. on the type of vessel, whether artery or vein, on the size of the occlusion and on the availability of a collateral circulation to maintain the blood flow.

On the venous side of the circulation there are frequent cross anastomoses between one vein and another so that obstruction of a small vessel may have little or no effect on the local circulation as a whole. When venous thrombosis is extensive, or affects a major vessel, it may lead to an increase in capillary pressure behind the obstruction and consequent congestion and œdema. For example, thrombosis of the femoral vein is usually followed by œdematous swelling of the limb, a condition known as "white leg".

In the arteries there is a wide variation in the frequency of cross anastomoses between the branches in different parts of the body. In the limbs, for example, the terminal branches of the arteries communicate freely with one another and the occlusion of one of them, like the occlusion of a small vein, may have little effect. At the other extreme, there are distributing arteries which have either no connections with neighbouring arteries or merely capillary anastomoses which are quite inadequate to carry on the circulation in the area. Such arteries may be called "end arteries" in a functional, if not in a strictly anatomical, sense, and occlusion of one of them leads to a complete ischæmia in the area normally supplied by the artery. The central artery of the retina is the best example of this type, but from the practical point of view many of the small arteries in the brain, kidney and spleen come into the same category. In the normal heart there are small communicating arteries, up to 350μ in diameter, which join branches of the same coronary artery and branches of the two coronary arteries with one another.[63] In this case there is a potential collateral circulation but one which is usually incapable of preventing ischæmia in the heart when the normal blood supply is stopped by occlusion of a coronary artery.

Thrombosis and embolism sometimes have an immediate widespread effect on the circulation which is not explicable simply in terms of direct obstruction to blood flow. This is most striking in some cases of pulmonary embolism when the degree of circulatory collapse is much greater than would be expected from the size of the obstructed artery. There is some evidence that the impaction of an embolus in the lungs causes a reflex spasm in other branches of the pulmonary arteries.[64] It is also possible that pharmacologically active substances could be released at the site of embolism and excite chemoreflexes which would lead to hypotension and bradycardia.[65] 5-hydroxytryptamine is present in high concentration in circulating platelets but it is not yet known if it could be released rapidly enough from the platelets in a thrombus to produce pharmacological effects. It is also possible that the peripheral circulatory collapse which is frequently seen after coronary occlusion is partly reflex in origin.

So far only the immediate effects on the circulation of occlusion of an artery or vein have been considered. With time, adaptive changes occur in the collateral vessels and tend to restore, more or less, an adequate circulation in the affected part. The earliest change is probably a relaxation of muscle tone in the collateral vessels, but this is soon followed by growth, both in circumference and length, so that previously inconspicuous vessels appear dilated and tortuous (FIG. 23).

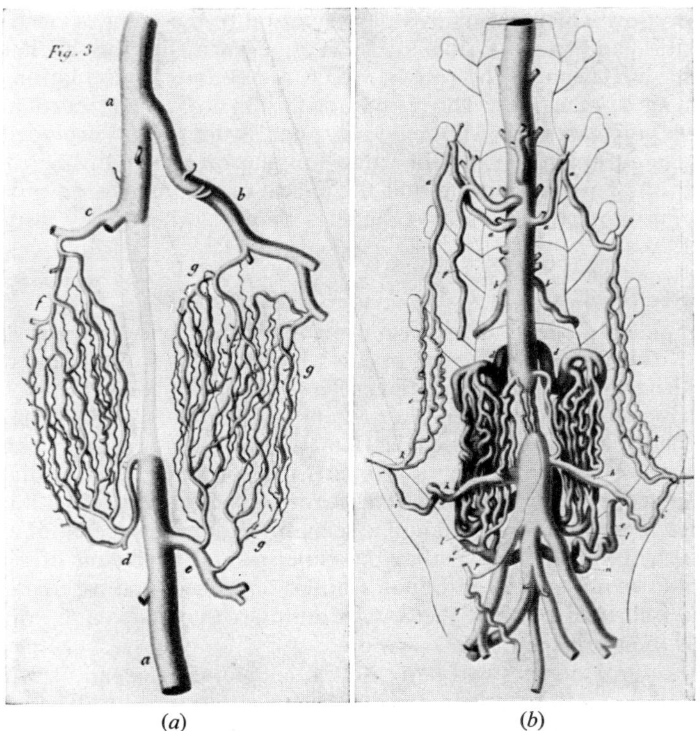

(*a*) (*b*)

9/FIG. 23.—The development of a collateral circulation (*a*) 3 months after ligating the femoral artery of a dog, (*b*) 15 months after ligating the aorta of a dog. (From Luigi Porta, 1845, *Delle Alterazioni patologiche delle Arterie*. Bernardoni di Gio, Milan.)

When the femoral artery in a rabbit is occluded by a thrombus, for example, enlargement of collaterals, which join branches of the femoral artery above and below the obstruction, can be demonstrated within a few days.[66] Similarly in the heart, the experimental occlusion of a coronary artery in a dog is followed by enlargement of the collateral vessels up to ten times their normal diameter.[37]

The development of a collateral circulation may be stimulated by partial as well as complete occlusion of an artery. In pigs, the reduction of the lumen of a major coronary artery by a restricting ligature stimulates the growth of collateral vessels. If animals survive this procedure for 12 days or more, the major artery can then be completely occluded without causing death, as it would do when there has been no previous collateral development.[67] In man, the development of a collateral circulation may be stimulated by the partial occlusion of the coronary arteries which occurs in atherosclerosis.[63] It can be seen that this may be an important factor in determining the extent of the ischæmia which follows a subsequent complete occlusion.

The duration of ischæmia following occlusion of an artery will depend on the rate at which the collateral circulation develops. This can be followed in experimental animals by observing the rise in pressure and in the rate of retrograde blood flow which occurs in an artery distal to the point of obstruction as the circulation improves. Using this technique it can be shown that there is considerable variation in the rate at which the collateral circulation develops at different sites in the body. The retrograde flow in an occluded coronary artery, for example, increases much more slowly than it does in an occluded femoral artery and may not reach its full value for one or two months.[37] This is an important difference, indicating that the effects of thrombosis or embolism, as well as being more extensive at some sites than at others, may also be more prolonged.

Effects on the Tissues

The immediate effects of ischæmia on the tissues will be on their normal function. If this function is a vital one death may occur without any detectable structural change in the tissues themselves. For example, when a thrombus occludes a major coronary artery the first effect is probably to make the ischæmic muscle hyperexcitable and sudden death may occur from ventricular fibrillation. Less extensive ischæmia in the vital organs may produce an immediate loss of function, but one which is compatible, for a while at any rate, with continued life. Sudden loss of cerebral function is seen, for example, in cerebral embolism. In the heart, it can be shown that the experimental occlusion of a coronary artery, if it does not excite ventricular fibrillation, causes an immediate weakening of the ischæmic part of the myocardium so that it expands rather than shortens with each heart beat.[37]

The structural changes within an ischæmic area will depend on whether the cells can survive until an adequate collateral circulation is established. If there is no collateral circulation all the cells in the area supplied by an occluded artery will eventually undergo necrosis. This is seen following embolism of one of the functional end arteries in the kidney or spleen, for example. When the area has a partial but inadequate collateral circulation, necrosis may occur in the central part but be less extensive than the distribution of the artery. A necrotic area of tissue formed under one or other of these circumstances is called an *infarct*. Its shape, corresponding more or less to the distribution of a particular artery, is usually conical with the base of the cone towards the periphery of the organ. Its colour may be pale or dark red, depending on whether blood can seep into the stagnant vessels of the infarct from neighbouring capillaries or from other collateral vessels (FIGS. 24 and 25).

In general the ability of various tissues to survive a period of ischæmia depends on the metabolic requirements of the individual cells and on the capacity of surviving cells to regenerate if conditions improve. The cerebral neurones are the most susceptible cells and, since they cannot regenerate, even a few minutes of complete ischæmia in the brain may cause permanent damage. In the heart, the connective tissue is less susceptible to ischæmia than the muscle fibres. Thus, if ischæmia is only partial or of short duration, it may lead to a selective change in which the muscle fibres die and are replaced by an overgrowth of the surviving fibrous tissue. When all the cells die, as they commonly do in the centre

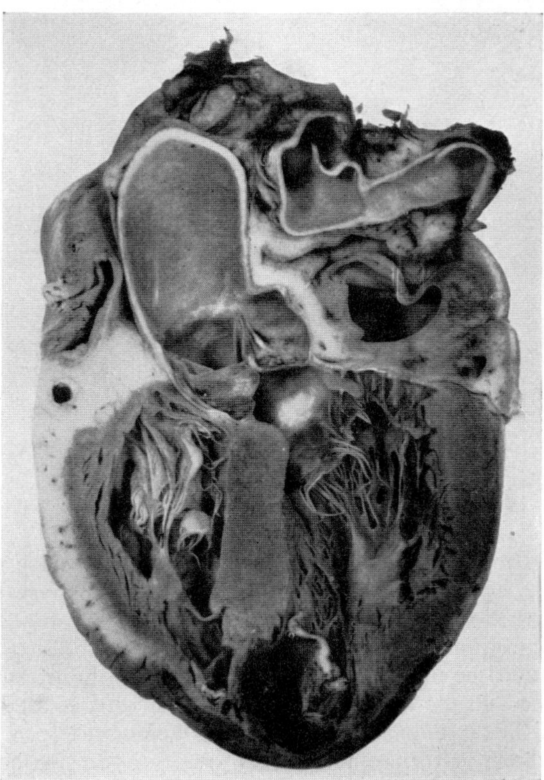

9/FIG. 24.—Myocardial infarct. The dark area in the muscle at the apex of the heart and in the lower part of the interventricular septum shows the position of the infarct. There is a mural thrombosis in the left ventricle overlying the infarcted tissue.

of a cardiac infarct, subsequent improvement of the circulation can lead only to growth of connective tissue from the edges of the infarct since cardiac muscle fibres cannot regenerate. The infarcted area therefore ultimately becomes a fibrous scar. In the skeletal muscles, on the other hand, where the specialised cells can regenerate from the edges following infarction, an improvement of the collateral circulation may lead eventually to a restoration of structure and function.

Reference has already been made to structural changes in the vessels themselves, particularly the thickening of the intima of the arteries, which may result

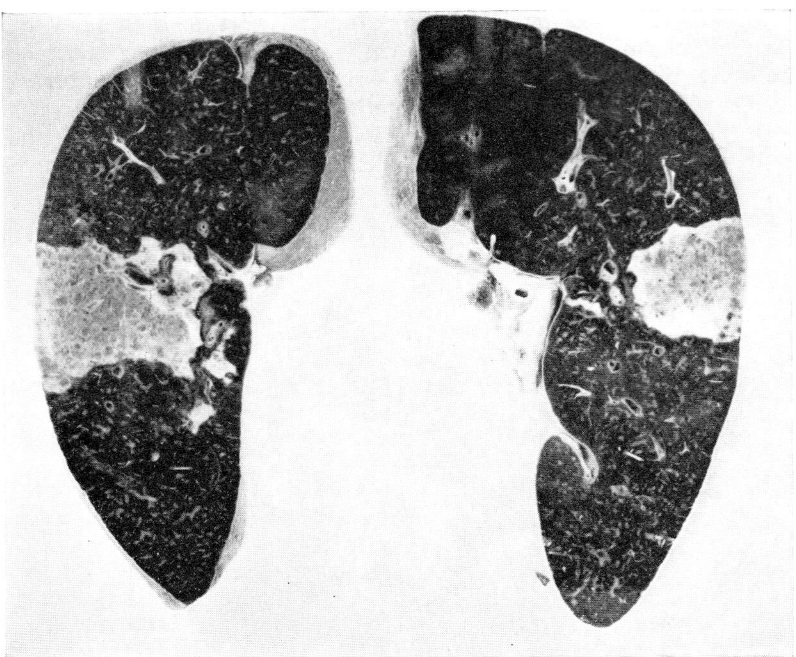

9/Fig. 25.—Pale infarcts in the spleen. These were caused by emboli which had arisen from a thrombus in the left auricular appendix in a patient with mitral stenosis.

from the organisation of thrombi; this effect is discussed more fully in relation to atherosclerosis in Chapter 18. Sclerosis of the pulmonary arteries can be caused by organisation of multiple emboli and may be associated with the development of pulmonary hypertension in man.[68]

Finally, it should be mentioned that infected thrombi or emboli have additional consequences in the tissues which are not directly related to obstruction of a blood vessel. Thus, for example, the emboli which arise from the vegetations in acute bacterial endocarditis, though they are often too small to be important mechanically, may nevertheless have significant effects, causing metastatic abscesses where they become impacted in the tissues.

REFERENCES

1. Macfarlane, R. G. (1965). In *The Inflammatory Process*, p. 465. Eds. Zweifach, B. W., Grant, L., and McCluskey, R. T. New York: Academic Press.
   Hæmostatic mechanism.
2. Welch, W. H. (1899). In *Allbutt: System of Medicine*, Vol. 6, p. 155. London: Macmillan & Co.
   Thrombosis.
3. Poole, J. C. F. (1959). *Quart. J. exp. Physiol.*, **44**, 377.
   A study of artificial thrombi produced by a modification of Chandler's method.
4. French, J. E., and Poole, J. C. F. (1963). *Proc. roy. Soc. B*, **157**, 170.
   Electron microscopy of the platelets in artificial thrombi.

5. HAYEM, G. (1882). *C.R. Acad. Sci.* (*Paris*), **95,** 18.
The mechanism of the arrest of hæmorrhage.
6. BIZZOZERO, J. (1882). *Virchows Arch. path. Anat.*, **90,** 261.
Description of blood platelets.
7. LUBNITZKY, S. (1885). *Arch. exp. path. Pharmak.*, **19,** 185.
Structure of hæmostatic plug in arteries.
8. KJAERHEIM, A., and HOVIG, T. (1962). *Thrombos. Diathes. hæmorrh.* (*Stuttg.*), **7,** 1.
The ultrastructure of hæmostatic blood platelet plugs in rabbit mesenterium.
9. FRENCH, J. E., MACFARLANE, R. G., and SANDERS, A. G. (1964). *Brit. J. exp. Path.*, **45,** 467.
The structure of hæmostatic plugs and experimental thrombi in small arteries.
10. JORGENSEN, L., and BORCHGREVINK, C. F. (1963). *Acta path. microbiol. scand.*, **57,** 40.
The structure of platelet plugs.
11. ZUCKER, H. D. (1949). *Blood,* **4,** 631.
Platelet plugs in human hæmostasis.
12. MACFARLANE, R. G. (1941). *Quart. J. Med.*, **10,** 1.
The mechanism of hæmostasis.
13. CHEN, T. I., and TSAI, C. (1948). *J. Physiol.* (*Lond.*), **107,** 280.
The mechanism of hæmostasis.
14. HEILBRUNN, L. V. (1961). In *Functions of the Blood*, p. 283. Eds. MACFARLANE, R. G., and ROBB-SMITH, A. H. T. Oxford: Blackwell Scientific Publications.
15. BIGGS, R., and MACFARLANE, R. G. (1966). Eds. *The Treatment of Hæmophilia and Related Conditions.* Oxford: Blackwell Scientific Publications.
16. VESSEY, M. P., and DOLL, R. (1968). *Brit. med. J.*, **2,** 199.
Oral contraceptives and thrombosis.
17. WHARTON-JONES, T. (1851). *Guy's Hosp. Rep. 2nd ser.*, **7,** 1.
Thrombosis in the frog.
18. ZAHN, F. W. (1875). *Virchows Arch. path. Anat.*, **62,** 81.
Thrombosis in the frog.
19. EBERTH, C. J., and SCHIMMELBUSCH, C. (1888). *Thrombose nach Versuchen und Leichenbefunden.* Stuttgart: Enke.
20. WELCH, W. H. (1887). Reprinted in *William Henry Welch, Papers and Addresses*, Vol. 1, p. 47. Baltimore: Johns Hopkins Press.
The structure of white thrombi.
21. HONOUR, A. J., and ROSS RUSSELL, R. W. (1962). *Brit. J. exp. Path.*, **43,** 350.
Experimental platelet embolism.
JORGENSEN, L. (1964). *Acta path. microbiol. scand.*, **62,** 189.
Histological study of experimental thrombi.
22. FRENCH, J. E. (1967). In *Modern Trends in Pathology*, 2, p. 208. Ed. CRAWFORD, T. London: Butterworth & Co.
Electron microscopy of thrombus formation.
23. BORN, G. V. R., HONOUR, A. J., and MITCHELL, J. R. A. (1964). *Nature* (*Lond.*), **202,** 761.
Inhibition of the formation and embolization of platelet thrombi.
24. HONOUR, A. J., and MITCHELL, J. R. A. (1964). *Brit, J. exp. Path.*, **45,** 75.
Platelet clumping in injured vessels.
25. VIRCHOW, R. (1856). *Gesammelte Abhandlungen zur Wissenschaftlichen Medicin,* pp. 458–636. Frankfurt: Meidinger Sohn & Co.
26. LUFT, J. H. (1965). In *The Inflammatory Process*, p. 121. Eds. ZWEIFACH, B. W., GRANT, L., and MCCLUSKEY, R. T. New York: Academic Press.
Endothelial ultrastructure.
27. SAMUELS, P. B., and WEBSTER, D. R. (1952). *Ann. Surg.*, **136,** 422.
The role of venous endothelium in the inception of thrombosis.

28. Poole, J. C. F., Sanders, A. G., and Florey, H. W. (1958). *J. Path. Bact.*, **75,** 133.
The regeneration of aortic endothelium.
29. Gottlob, R., and Zinner, G. (1962). *Virchows Arch. path. Anat.*, **336,** 16.
Endothelium after hard and soft trauma.
30. French, J. E. (1966). *Int. Rev. exp. Path.*, **5,** 301.
Endothelium and thrombosis.
31. Sabiston, D. C., Smith, G. W., and Talbert, J. L. (1960). *Surg. Gynec. Obstet.*, **110,** 563.
Experimental endarterectomy.
32. Aschoff, L. (1924). *Lectures on Pathology.* New York: Hoeber.
33. Mustard, J. F., Rowsell, H. C., Murphy, E. A., and Downie, H. G. (1963). In Evolution of the Atherosclerotic Plaque, p. 183. Ed. Jones, R. J. Chicago, Ill.: Univ. of Chicago Press.
Intimal thrombosis in atherosclerosis.
34. Gibbs, N. M. (1957). *Brit. J. Surg.*, **126,** 270.
Venous thrombosis of the lower limbs.
35. Wright, H. P., Osborn, S. B., and Edmonds, D. G. (1951). *Lancet*, **1,** 22.
Rate of venous blood flow.
36. McLachlin, A. D., McLachlin, J. A., Jory, T. A., and Rawling, E. G. (1960). *Ann. Surg.*, **152,** 678.
Venous stasis in the lower extremities.
37. Gregg, D. E. (1950). *Coronary Circulation in Health and Disease.* Philadelphia: Lea & Febiger.
38. Wright, H. P. (1942). *J. Path. Bact.*, **54,** 461.
Changes in the adhesiveness of blood platelets following parturition and surgical operations.
39. Sharnoff, J. G., Bagg, J. F., Breen, S. R., Rogliano, A. G., Walsh, A. R., and Scardino, V. (1960). *Surg. Gynec. Obstet.*, **111,** 469.
Postoperative platelet counts and coagulation studies.
40. McDonald, L. (1968). *Brit. Heart. J.*, **30,** 151.
Platelets in coronary heart disease.
41. Connor, W. E., Hoak, J. C., and Warner, E. D. (1966). In *Pathogenesis and Treatment of Thrombo-embolic Diseases,*, p. 193. Eds. Duckert, F., and Streuli, F. Stuttgart: Schattauer-Verlag.
The role of lipids in thrombosis.
42. Born, G. V. R., and Philp, R. B. (1965). *Brit. J. exp. Path.*, **46,** 569.
Platelet thrombi in non-lipæmic and lipæmic rats.
43. Wessler, S. (1963). *Fed. Proc.*, **22,** 1366.
Stasis, hypercoagulability and thrombosis.
44. Erichson, R. B. (1965). *N.Y. St. J. Med.*, **65,** 1091.
The hypercoagulable state.
45. Poole, J. C. F. (1962). *Fed. Proc.*, **21,** 20.
Effect of diet and lipæmia on coagulation and thrombosis.
46. Studer, A. (1966). In *Pathogenesis and Treatment of Thrombo-embolic Diseases,* p. 109. Eds. Duckert, F., and Streuli, F. Stuttgart: Schattauer-Verlag.
Experimental platelet thrombus.
47. Born, G. V. R. (1966). In *Pathogenesis and Treatment of Thrombo-embolic Diseases,* p. 159. Eds. Duckert, F., and Streuli, F. Stuttgart: Schattauer-Verlag.
Inhibition of thrombogenesis by inhibition of platelet aggregation.
48. Sevitt, S. (1966). In *Pathogenesis and Treatment of Thrombo-embolic Diseases,* p. 287. Eds. Duckert, F., and Streuli, F. Stuttgart: Schattauer-Verlag.
Anticoagulant prophylaxis against venous thrombosis and pulmonary embolism after injury.

49. Report to the Medical Research Council (1964). *Brit. med. J.*, **2,** 837.
An assessment of long-term anticoagulant administration after cardiac infarction.
50. Poole, J. C. F. (1966). *Quart. J. exp. Physiol.*, **51,** 54.
Phagocytosis of platelets in organising thrombi.
51. Hand, R. A., and Chandler, A. B. (1962). *Amer. J. Path.*, **40,** 469.
Atherosclerotic metamorphosis of thrombo-emboli.
52. Macfarlane, R. G. Ed. (1964). *Brit. med. Bull.*, **20,** No. 3.
Fibrinolysis.
53. Wright, H. P., and Kubik, M. M. (1953). *Brit. med. J.*, **1,** 1021.
Recanalization of thrombosed arteries under anticoagulant therapy.
54. Florey, H. W., Greer, S. J., Kiser, J., Poole, J. C. F., Telander, R., and Werthessen, N. T. (1962). *Brit. J. exp. Path.*, **43,** 655.
Growth of endothelium over surface deposits.
55. Short, R. H. D. (1940). *J. Path. Bact.*, **50,** 419.
The vasa vasorum of the femoral vein.
56. Dible, J. H. (1966). *The Pathology of Limb Ischæmia.* Edinburgh: Oliver & Boyd.
57. Akrawi, Y. Y., and Wilson, G. M. (1950). *J. Path. Bact.*, **62,** 69.
Vascular channels in occluded arteries.
58. Crawford, T., and Levene, C. I. (1952). *J. Path. Bact.*, **64,** 523.
Organisation of mural thrombi in aorta.
59. Filshie, I., and Scott, G. B. D. (1958). *J. Path. Bact.*, **76,** 71.
Organisation of venous thrombi.
60. Gunning, A. J., Pickering, G. W., Robb-Smith, A. H. T., and Ross Russell, R. (1964). *Quart. J. Med.*, **33,** 155.
Mural thrombosis of the internal carotid artery and subsequent embolism.
61. Marshall R. (1965). *Pulmonary Embolism.* Springfield, Ill.: Charles C. Thomas.
62. Eeles, G. H., and Sevitt, S. (1967). *J. Path. Bact.*, **93,** 275.
Microthrombosis in injured and burned patients.
63. Baroldi, G., Mantero, O., and Scomazzoni, G. (1956). *Circulat. Res.*, **4,** 223.
The collaterals of the coronary arteries in normal and pathologic hearts.
64. Aviado, D. M., and Schmidt, C. F. (1955). *Physiol. Rev.*, **35,** 247.
Reflexes from stretch receptors in blood vessels, heart and lungs.
65. Dawes, G. S., and Comroe, J. H. (1954). *Physiol. Rev.*, **34,** 167.
Chemo-reflexes from the heart and lungs.
66. Longland, C. J. (1953). *Ann. roy. Coll. Surg. Engl.*, **13,** 161.
The collateral circulation of the limb.
67. Blumgart, H. L., Zoll, P. M., Fredburg, A. S., and Gilligan, D. R. (1950). *Circulation*, **1,** 10.
Experimental production of intercoronary arterial anastomoses.
68. Goodwin, J. F., Harrison, C. V., and Wilcken, D. E. L. (1963). *Brit. med. J.*, **1,** 701, 777.
Obliterative pulmonary hypertension and thromboembolism.

Chapter 10

HÆMORRHAGE AND SHOCK

By K. B. Roberts

No problem in medicine can have excited so much interest throughout the ages as loss of blood. From earliest times human beings must have known of the dangers of severe hæmorrhage from wounds; acquaintance with minor injuries, with menstruation and with the inevitable loss during normal childbirth must have taught them that small hæmorrhages, however, have little effect on health. Some such observations probably encouraged the deliberate adoption of blood removal in the treatment of illness; undoubtedly in some cases, venesection improved the patient's condition—in congestive cardiac failure, for instance. At any rate, the practice of blood-letting can be traced back to about 2500 B.C.; by this time, man must have learnt that veins, in contrast to arteries, can be opened with safety. Hippocrates bled patients extensively and wrote a treatise on blood-letting. Galen specified the proper quantities to be removed under various conditions; his figures—$\frac{1}{2}$–$1\frac{1}{2}$ pints—agree quite well with modern practice. In late mediæval and early modern times people went, without medical advice, to the barber's to be bled. No doubt the treatment was sometimes of assistance, or at least harmless, but invalids lost their lives through over-enthusiastic venesection. A little over a century ago Marshall Hall[1] wrote, "of the remedies of medicine blood-letting ranks pre-eminently as first. . . . Place the patient upright and looking upwards, and bleed till incipient syncope"; a limit is to be placed upon bleeding because of syncope or fainting.

Many centuries before, the effects of serious hæmorrhage had been recognised, "Now when the heart is penetrated, much blood issues, the pulse fades away, the colour is extremely pallid, cold and malodorous sweats burst out as if the body had been wetted by dew, the extremities become cold and death quickly follows" (Celsus, fl. 20 A.D.). Compare this description with one given in 1932 by Thomas Lewis[2] in which the orderly progress of symptoms is followed from premonitory feelings of instability or uncertainty, dimming of the vision and a feeling of giddiness, through a sensation of nausea, sometimes retching, pallor of skin and mucous membranes, deep sighing respiration, sweating of lips and forehead spreading to all parts of the body, to loss of consciousness without any feeling of alarm. With these subjective features go a progressive lowering of the blood pressure.

THE EXPERIMENTAL STUDY OF BLOOD LOSS

In clinical practice hæmorrhage is frequently a complication of traumatic injury or accidents occurring, for example, during childbirth. Severe blood loss has often been the terminal event in conditions such as pulmonary tuberculosis. However, if we wish to study the physiological reponses to hæmorrhage then we must include observations on blood loss on the previously normal. There have been many excellent studies of controlled, uncomplicated hæmorrhage in healthy human beings, studies on blood donors, for example. Much of our knowledge however, comes from experiments on animals, particularly on the dog, which tolerates blood-letting well, can be trained to put up with the manipulations required in serial studies, and is large enough to allow repeated small sampling of blood.

In such investigations, the plan is simple. Known quantities of blood are removed, from a large vein or an accessible artery. More recently a useful technique has been adopted whereby bleeding can be so controlled that any systemic arterial blood pressure is maintained.[3] A major artery is cannulated and the cannula connected to a large reservoir vessel; the animal will bleed into it until the level of the blood in the reservoir balances arterial pressure. In this way, mean arterial pressures of say 60 mm. Hg may be rapidly reached and kept for varying periods of time; if the pressure in the animal falls, blood will pass from reservoir into the artery, and *vice versa*. Transfusions may be easily effected by raising the reservoir.

Before the blood is removed, studies can be made of the total blood, plasma and red cell volumes, the plasma protein and electrolyte concentrations of the blood and an assessment attempted of cardiovascular function. The latter includes estimations of arterial and central venous pressures, cardiac output, total peripheral resistance and blood flow in various organs and tissues.

Animals smaller than dogs, particularly rats and mice, may also be used in experiments on the effects of blood loss; quantitative evaluation is made easier by greater uniformity in size and the use of larger numbers.

Hæmostatic Mechanisms and Hæmorrhage

Before considering cardiovascular and other responses of experimental animals and man to blood loss, it is relevant to refer to processes of hæmostasis, whereby further blood loss is prevented. This is the subject matter of Chapter 7. One aspect of hæmostasis, however, can be mentioned here; it is an unusual control mechanism.

Table 1 is based on experiments in which a rabbit was bled known fractions of its blood volume and the speed at which its blood coagulated in a capillary tube was estimated at intervals during and after bleeding. As bleeding continued, the blood was found to clot more and more rapidly. In man, too, coagu-

10/TABLE I

HEWSON'S EXPERIMENT, AS REPEATED BY T. HUSAIN

Time interval	*Coagulation time (minutes)*
ZERO	2·5
Bled 20 ml., i.e. 15·4 per cent blood volume	1·75
Bled 15 ml., i.e. 11·6 per cent blood volume	1·45
Bled 5 ml., i.e. 3·9 per cent blood volume	1·0
2 hours later	2·1
5 hours later	2·0
24 hours later	2·5

Rabbit 2 kg. B.W. Blood volume 130 ml.

lation is hastened during the course of the hæmorrhage. In 1772, William Hewson[4] described this remarkable response:

"Believing it would be sufficient for this purpose, to attend to the properties of the blood, as it flows at different times from an animal that is bleeding to death, I therefore went to the markets, and attended the killing of sheep; and having received the blood into cups, I found my notion verified. For I observed, that the blood which came from the vessels immediately on withdrawing the knife was about two minutes in beginning to coagulate; and that the blood taken later on, or as the animal became weaker, coagulated in less and less time; till at last, when the animal became very weak, the blood, though quite fluid as it came from the vessels, yet had hardly been received into the cup before it congealed. I have also repeated the experiment, by receiving blood into different cups at different times, whilst the animal was bleeding to death; and though the time taken up in killing the animal was not commonly more than two minutes, yet I observed, on comparing the cups, that the blood which issued last coagulated first."

In other experiments it has been shown that when dogs, cats and rabbits are bled, coagulation of the blood is hurried up and intravascular deposition of fibrin may even occur. There is a rise in plasma thromboplastin and an appearance of a clot-accelerating factor. Similar changes occur during fear, and it is probable that the release of catecholamines initiates these changes. If bleeding continues, there is a later stage, after a few hours, when the hæmostatic mechanisms may completely break down, with platelets, fibrinogen and other coagulation factors depleted; fibrinolysis may occur at this stage. These findings[5] in experimental animals are similar in some respects to alterations in hæmostasis that happen in cases of obstetrical accidents[6] or whenever severe bleeding continues. In both situations there are very low levels of fibrinogen in the blood. It may be that fibrinogen and platelets are lost by concealed or frank hæmorrhage, with some degree of loss by extra- or intravascular fibrin deposition; recovery occurs when these and other factors are regenerated in the liver and bone marrow.

Depletion of Blood Volume

Hæmorrhage disturbs the usual relationships that exist between blood volume and the capacity of the circulation. Restoration of the lost blood is the most effective and satisfactory treatment, and man has, after centuries of disastrous attempts, finally learnt how to transfuse blood safely from healthy donor to blood-depleted recipient. Many animals make use of a similar dodge, although this time the transfusion is provided from their own blood reservoirs. Joseph Barcraft and his co-workers have demonstrated that one such reservoir exists within the spleen. They showed that hæmorrhage induces contractions in the exteriorised spleen of the cat.[7] As a result, blood from the splenic sinuses, with a hæmatocrit level about 50 per cent greater than venous blood, is squirted into the portal circulation. A total of from 14 to 28 ml. blood has been estimated to be added in this way, an amount not to be despised in the hunting animal. The position in man is, however, not so favourable, for the spleen is a relatively smaller organ and there is no evidence that its contraction influences the blood volume to any significant extent.

There are other ways of compensating for a diminished blood volume following hæmorrhage, some coming into effect promptly, others more gradually. These reactions will first be described in the experimental animal and then in man.

Cardiovascular Responses in Experimental Animals

With increasing blood loss, the cardiac output declines, the arterial blood pressure begins to fall and the heart rate becomes rapid; the total peripheral resistance may at first increase. Some data are set out in Table II modified from John and Blalock.[8]

10/Table II

The Effects of Hæmorrhage on the Cardiac Output, Pulse Rate, Blood Pressure and Oxygen Consumption of a Dog

Time (minutes)	*Blood lost (per cent B.W.)*	*Pulse rate per min.*	*B.P. (mm. Hg)*	*Cardiac output (ml. per min.)*	*Oxygen consumption (ml. per min.)*
Zero	—	129	162	3412	131·00
Z + 100	0·5	120	159	3335	156·09
Z + 160	1·0	150	140	3588	142·07
Z + 220	1·5	156	139	2402	138·38
Z + 280	2·0	164	137	2149	144·46
Z + 340	2·5	160	120	2516	166·05
Z + 400	3·0	167	117	1899	168·63

(*Modified from Johnson and Blalock.*[8])

When a certain amount of blood is lost and the total blood volume falls below a level which varies from animal to animal, the filling pressure of the heart falls off, as shown by direct measurements of right auricular pressure; the cardiac output therefore decreases and the arterial blood pressure falls. It will be remembered that the blood pressure in the larger arteries is determined by cardiac output and total peripheral resistance. For a time after hæmorrhage peripheral resistance keeps up or may rise; arterial blood pressure is maintained. With increasing blood loss all three factors decline and serious impairment of cardiovascular function sets in and the animal passes into the condition often called hæmorrhagic shock.

We know from the investigations of Heymans and others[9] that a fall in pressure in the carotid sinus decreases the afferent discharge of impulses along the carotid sinus nerve from pressure receptors in that sinus and that this in turn alters the discharge of impulses from the vasomotor and vagal centres in the medulla. Similar effects are produced in the baroreceptor areas of the aortic arch. With a fall in arterial pressure, reflexes are thus set going which bring about vasoconstriction in many organs and an increased heart rate due to removal of vagal restraint. We would like to know more about the reaction of hæmorrhage of the venous side of the circulation. Is there venoconstriction to reduce the capacity of these vessels?

As Cannon showed, a humoral factor contributes to the reactions; animals liberate effective doses of catecholamines from the adrenal medulla even after mild blood loss. Direct measurements of the adrenaline and nonadrenaline levels in the adrenal venous blood have confirmed this.[10] Adrenaline constricts many types of arterioles but dilates muscle arterioles. Noradrenaline constricts most vascular beds but dilates the coronary vessels. Thus an increased supply of blood to the cardiac muscle is produced; the metabolic activity of the heart is also raised. It is possible that the resulting increased delivery of oxygen is more than counterbalanced by catecholamine-induced rise on oxygen usage.

It is known that hæmorrhage induces vasoconstriction in the skin, salivary glands, intestines, liver, spleen and kidneys. In the cat the net (total) peripheral resistance may rise by 45 per cent during hæmorrhage and this may be sufficient at first to maintain arterial blood pressure.[11] A severe hæmorrhage may reduce hepatic blood flow in the dog from 43 to 20 ml. per kg. per min.[12] The blood service to these organs is restricted after hæmorrhage but is at first well maintained in essential organs such as the diaphragm, intercostal muscles, heart and brain. Thus it would appear that in the emergency arising out of a serious hæmorrhage the blood supply to the non-vital organs is reduced, while the supply to more essential tissues is initially maintained. However, further blood loss will reduce blood volume, cardiac output and blood pressure still further and a more serious condition develops leading to death.

The Effect of Hæmorrhage on the Tissues

So far it has been assumed that severe blood loss leads to deficient oxygen supply to the tissues. Some studies[13] on tissue oxygen partial pressure bring direct support for this view. For all animals tested, including monkey and man, the normal tissue oxygen partial pressures were found to lie between 20 and 40 mm. Hg; Pco_2 is usually about 40–50 mm. Hg. Bleeding markedly lowers tissue Po_2 in rabbits so that conditions are set for the injurious action of anoxia. Other investigations demonstrate that counter-measures against anoxia, such as increased dissociation of oxyhæmoglobin within the peripheral capillaries and hyperventilation of the lungs, are brought into play early in the course of the hæmorrhage. The biochemical changes following injury are considered in Chapter 11.

Fluid Shifts following Hæmorrhage in Experimental Animals

Following a moderately severe blood loss, the plasma volume is restored to normal by fluid entering the blood vessels from the extravascular interstitial spaces and, indirectly, from the cells themselves. The factors determining the entry of tissue fluids into the circulation are those elucidated by Starling, by Landis and others (see Chapter 12). The hydrostatic pressure within the microcirculation falls for two reasons: first, because there is a fall in systemic arterial blood pressure, and secondly because arteriolar vasoconstriction frequently causes a further fall on the distal side. Immediately following a sudden hæmorrhage, blood with its plasma protein level still exerting a normal colloid osmotic pressure remains within the circulation. The net osmotic suck of fluid into the small vessels will exceed the net hydrostatic pressure forcing fluid out. Bulk flow of fluid into the circulation will occur and the concentration of hæmoglobin, red cell numbers, packed cell volume—and arterial oxygen content—

will be reduced. The blood is therefore diluted for some days, that is, until the bone marrow gains speed in its new production of red corpuscles. These responses may be seen in rats subjected to sudden removal of approximately 50 per cent of the blood (Table III).[14] Within a few hours, the *plasma* volume has been restored to normal, but the red cell mass is still at half its previous value, for there has as yet been no regeneration of erythrocytes. Consequently the total *blood* volume is only about 80 per cent of previous levels and the hæmatocrit is low. As can be seen from the Table, plasma proteins are already being made in increased quantities eight hours after hæmorrhage.

10/TABLE III

FLUID SHIFTS AFTER HÆMORRHAGE IN RATS

(Rats of similar weight subjected to rapid withdrawal of 2·5 ml. whole blood per 100 g. body weight, equivalent to *c.* 50 per cent blood volume)

	Measured Values			*Calculated Values*		
	Hæmatocrit	*Red Cell Mass ml./100 g.*	*Plasma Proteins g./100 ml.*	*Plasma Proteins g./100 g.*	*Total Blood Volume ml./100 g.*	*Plasma Volume ml./100 g.*
Control	48 (100%)	2·5 (100%)	6·3 (100%)	0·17 (100%)	5·2 (100%)	2·7 (100%)
2 hrs. after Bleeding	35 (72%)	1·4 (54%)	1·4 (77%)	0·13 (73%)	3·9 (75%)	2·6 (94%)
4 hrs. after Bleeding	32 (66%)	1·3 (52%)	4·6 (72%)	0·13 (73%)	4·1 (78%)	2·8 (103%)
8 hrs. after Bleeding	31 (64%)	1·3 (52%)	5·5 (87%)	0·16 (92%)	4·2 (81%)	2·9 (108%)

(Modified from Pareira *et al.*[14])

There are other factors relating to fluid balance following hæmorrhage. Thirst is usually intense after a large blood loss. Sites of water loss are closed down, particularly in the kidneys, the salivary glands and the vast secretory surfaces of the small intestine. Lymph flow diminishes. Some of these responses are discussed later.

Longer Term Restoration of Blood

As we have seen, the fluid added to the circulation in the first few hours following hæmorrhage comes from the tissue fluids and is poor in protein. Later plasma proteins are produced, by an unknown homeostatic mechanism, by the liver. The bone marrow also responds with an increased production of the various formed elements of the blood. In the case of those cells that have a quick turnover, that is, the platelets and the polymorphs, replacement is rapid. But erythrocyte replacement is a slower matter. The normal life expectancy of a red cell is 110 days or so, and this would be the period for complete restoration of the red cell mass if the marrow went on working at its ordinary rate. That, however, is not the case, for the bone marrow flares into activity and new foci of erythrocyte formation appear throughout extensive regions of the marrow cavity previously occupied by fat. The stimulus to the marrow that induces proliferation is the hormone, or growth factor, erythropoietin; this is a mucoprotein produced in the kidneys.[15] The life-span of these newly-formed red cells after hæmorrhage is shorter than usual.

There is therefore a lag period between the hæmorrhage and effective marrow proliferation in which little more than the normal quota of red cells is added to the circulating blood.

HAEMORRHAGE IN MAN

Fainting during Hæmorrhage

It is a matter of common experience that people may faint when they lose blood. Often enough this not related directly to the blood loss. Those of us who teach medical students how to obtain blood from each other by venepuncture know that a small proportion of the apprehensive men, or less commonly, women, will faint before any blood is taken. The fainter may be the man preparing to donate blood, the man with the syringe, or an onlooker. Fear turns to fainting when flight is impossible or inhibited by social or other considerations.[16] Poles and Boycott[17] when bleeding large numbers of donors found that 2·8 per cent fainted; most of these fainted however, after 400 ml. had been taken. During the faint the blood pressure falls, the heart rate slows to 30–40 beats per minute and becomes impalpable, breathing is slow and shallow, and marked pallor and sweating, particularly of the hands and face, appears. In Poles and Boycott's series the fainting rate was higher with the second or subsequent bleeding; there was no sex difference and obesity played no part.

A detailed study of what goes on in the cardiovascular system before and during fainting has been carried out by Barcroft *et al.*[18] One of their most interesting charts is given here (FIG. 1). The subject was bled 1020 ml. During venesection, the heart rate increased somewhat, the cardiac output, measured by means of the Fick principle and cardiac catheterisation, and the right auricular pressure, also directly measured by means of the cardiac catheter, fell steadily, but the arterial blood pressure was largely maintained in spite of the falling cardiac output. Now the mean arterial pressure is proportional to the resistance to flow imposed by arterial tone, i.e. the total peripheral resistance, and also to the volume of blood passing from the heart to the arteries in unit time, i.e. the cardiac output, so that from the values of the blood pressure and cardiac output we can calculate the total peripheral resistance. It will be seen from the chart that this increases throughout venesection, which means that vasoconstriction is occurring in the peripheral vascular system.

Contrast this with what happens when fainting occurs. The blood pressure falls suddenly, the pulse slows, but the cardiac output and right auricular pressure may rise slightly or remain unchanged. Meanwhile the peripheral resistance decreases greatly as peripheral vessels dilate. This phenomenon is responsible for the acute fall in blood pressure, for there is no further fall in cardiac output, and slowing of the heart rate is severe only during the faint and does not appear to initiate the faint. (In other experiments, in which cardiac slowing was prevented by adequate atropinisation, fainting still occurred.) The forearm blood flow has been measured by venous occlusion plethysmography in these cases and is found to be almost doubled. Since the blood pressure is about halved, the accelerated blood flow must mean that very considerable vasodilatation has occurred in the limb, principally in the muscles. If vasodilatation affects the whole body musculature a very considerable drop in blood pressure will occur as in fainting. Vasoconstriction takes place in the skin vessels of the face, and this may be a response to the increased amounts of A.D.H. (vasopressin) released during hæmorrhage.[19]

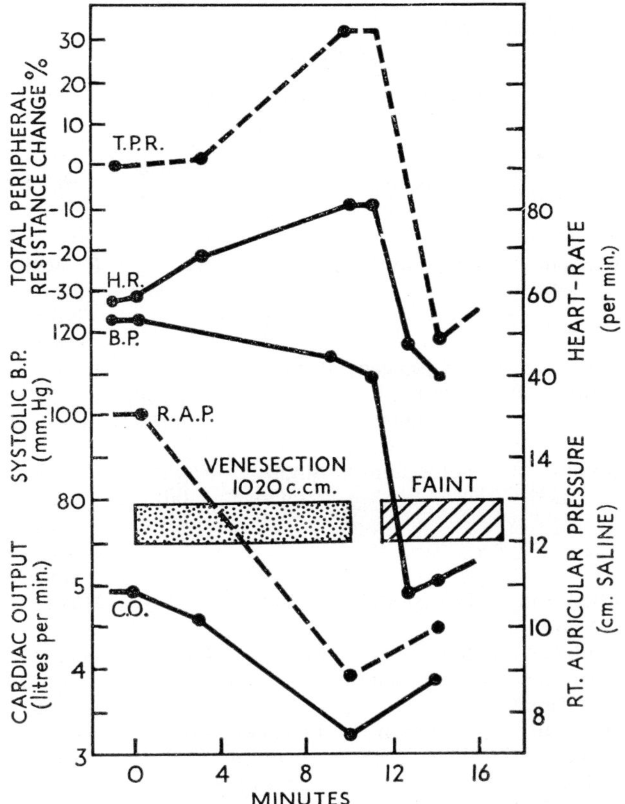

10/Fig. 1.—Faint induced by venesection, showing the behaviour of right auricular and systolic blood pressures, cardiac output, heart rate and total peripheral resistance. (After Barcroft *et al.*[18])

In the faint there is as a rule a vaso-vagal reaction from which recovery is rapid. The biological (evolutionary) advantage of fainting is, perhaps, that it causes the subject to fall to ground; in the horizontal position, the cerebral blood flow rapidly improves. If the subject is prevented from falling, as in a crowd, he will remain unconscious; after 20 seconds of syncope, convulsions may occur and the restoration in venous return may result in consciousness being regained. Following a simple faint, the subject's condition is soon normal and he is left with no after-effects. Should anything occur which prolongs the fainting unduly, or leads to a series of faints, then ill effects may arise since the blood flow to vital tissues may be seriously impaired, and the outcome may be fatal. In this case the subject's condition is very like that often described as shock.

Other Responses to Hæmorrhage in Man

Table IV summarises information from experiments on volunteers and observations on blood donors. The immediate effects of the loss of known quantities of blood are given.

10/Table IV

Blood Loss in Human Beings

Amount of blood lost (ml.)	*Source of information*	*Fainting*	*Pulse*	*Blood pressure*	*Other disturbances*
300–900	Warren *et al.*[41]	Occasionally	—	No change	R. auric. pressure fell 20–65 mm. H_2O No generalised vaso-constriction
440	Poles and Boycott[17]	2·8 per cent fainted (10,000 donors)	Slow	Low during faint	Pallor, sweating
500–1000	Shenkin *et al.*[42]	Some faint	Slight change	Slight fall	Changes slight when recumbent; rapid pulse and greater fall in B.P. when upright
700–1200	Ebert and Stead[20]	Occasionally	Slowing	—	Hæmodilution
1000–1200	Wallace and Sharpey-Schafer[43]	Not uncommon	Slow	Falls	Hæmodilution slow, complete after 40 hours
1500–2000	Howarth and Sharpey-Schafer[44]	Common	Increased (wound shock)	Low	Air-hunger, sweating, low cardiac output

Consideration of these studies indicates that depletion of the blood volume in man leads to a fall in venous pressure, diminished cardiac output, hypotension and slowing followed by increase in the pulse rate. It would appear that these phenomena may be explained in the same way as the animal results. So, too, there is plasma volume increase with dilution of the blood, followed in a more leisurely fashion by red cell and hæmoglobin regeneration. Table V gives some information about this matter.

10/TABLE V

REGENERATION OF BLOOD IN HUMAN DONORS AND SOLDIERS

Blood loss (ml.)	*Number of donors*	*Speed of red cell and plasma regeneration*	*Source of information*
1200–2000 lost within 1–23 days	50	Normal Hb. within 10 days	Jones *et al.*[38]
400–700	1076	Normal Hb. within 2 months	Brewer[39]
Mean 555·7	200	Mean recovery in 49·6 days (18–98 days) Daily Hb. average restoration 0·049 g./100 cc. blood	Fowler and Barer[40]
760–1220, i.e. 15·5–19·7 per cent blood volume	6	Plasma volume restored in 3–4 days	Ebert and Stead[20]
20 per cent blood volume	Soldiers	Hb. 95 per cent after 12 hours	Grant and Reeve[26]
21–40 per cent blood volume	Soldiers	Hb. 86 per cent after 12 hours	Grant and Reeve[26]
40 per cent blood volume	Soldiers	Hb. 74 per cent after 12 hours	Grant and Reeve[26]
50 per cent blood volume	Soldiers	Almost a litre plasma added in 12 hours	Grant and Reeve[26]

Restoration of plasma volume by an influx of tissue fluids into the circulation occurs in man as in rats and cats. Ebert and his colleagues,[20] for example, found that the plasma volume was raised within two hours by protein-poor fluid. Thereafter the liver increased its manufacture of plasma proteins so that by three days about a quarter of the circulating protein had been added since venesection. Hæmatocrit readings accurately reflected these changes. Unlike the findings in rats, the plasma volume was not completely restored after three or four days. Changes in renal function occur. There is vasoconstriction in the arterioles, both afferent and efferent, to the glomerulus, and this will with the lowered systemic arterial blood pressure produce a low glomerular filtration. There is increased production of A.D.H. which will further reduce urine flow. The changes in perfusion of the juxtaglomerular apparatus will lead to increased production of renin, which, activating the angiotensin system, will give rise to increased aldosterone formation and this will increase tubular reabsorption of salt and water. Hæmorrhage is a standard technique used experimentally to increase aldosterone formation.[21] With these mechanisms operating on the kidney the flow of urine is diminished and may, in severe cases, fall to zero. The relationship that Hewson discovered long ago between clotting time and extent of blood loss has already been mentioned. It appears, therefore, that with confidence we may apply animal results to the human problem.

Replacement Therapy after Blood Loss

It is obvious that replacement of spilt blood with compatible blood is a reasonable therapeutic measure. The necessary precautions against transfusion reactions, and the techniques of administration, are not discussed here but it should be emphasised that there are difficulties of obtaining blood, storing and distributing it and using it safely in human beings. Transfusion is a procedure carrying a small but definite mortality. Substitutes have, therefore, been looked for.

It has long been known that replacement of a volume of blood lost during hæmorrhage by an equal volume of isotonic salt solution is not retained in the blood in sufficient quantity to restore the plasma volume to normal; this has been observed repeatedly in animals and is also the case in man.[20] Solutions of many different substances have been given as *plasma expanders* in the hope of raising the blood volume for useful periods of time so that venous return, cardiac output and blood pressure will be restored towards more normal values. The plasma expanders have been those colloidal substances to which the capillary wall is relatively impermeable. Plasma itself is given, and—if it were not for the difficulties in obtaining it and the dangers of cross transmission of viral diseases from pooled plasma—would be the most satisfactory solution to give after blood. Dextrans, sulphonated polysaccharides that can be obtained in various molecular weights, are extensively used.

Recently the case for saline infusion after blood loss has been re-examined in the experimental animal.[22] Dogs have been subjected to severe hæmorrhage such that all untreated animals died. The treated animals received a balanced salt solution containing lactate. The solution was infused at pH 8·5 to counteract the acidæmia that develops following poor circulation through the tissues. Instead of replacing the lost blood, volume for volume, with this solution, four times its volume was infused as saline; half the animals survived. Work in man[22] shows that buffered saline infusions are an efficacious replacement therapy following acute hæmorrhage, providing the volume given is considerably greater than the volume of blood loss. About a third of the infused solution stays in the plasma when 2·5 times the volume is given.

Massive Blood Loss

The value of blood or plasma or plasma-substitute infusion in the treatment of severe hæmorrhage is not in dispute providing adequate volumes are given without delay. There is a case for treatment, at least when these fluids are not easily available, with very large volumes of buffered saline solutions. With therapy of this kind, the right auricular pressure and the cardiac output increase and arterial blood pressure return to normal or near normal within a short time. If, however, there has been a large loss of blood and the experimental animal or man has not been rapidly transfused, hypotension will persist and poor perfusion of tissues bring in its wake a number of dire consequences. In the most severe cases, failure of the circulation will not only affect the higher centres of the brain causing loss of consciousness but also the medulla with resultant respiratory failure. The perfusion of the coronary vessels may also fall to low levels and the heart may eventually not respond to increased venous return, following treatment by infusions, with an increased output. In such cases, the right atrial pressures will continue to rise if fluids are injected intravenously; there will be no improvement in the dynamics of the circulation and death may follow.

Inadequate circulation through other tissues may contribute to death. The kidney may stop secreting any urine, the liver may fail. Moreover, severe acidæmia may develop, associated with hypoxic conditions in the tissues. If attempts at restoring fluid balance have been made without appropriate amounts of electrolyte replacement, there may be sodium deficiency.

It can be seen that if profound hypotension following hæmorrhage persists for some time then treatment is likely to become less and less effective. Infusions will fail to raise the arterial blood pressure in face of circulatory collapse.

This phase, progressing to death, has been termed irreversible hæmorrhage shock. The word shock is used, in medicine and in general conversation in an imprecise way ("emotional shock" may mean a psychological upset, while newspaper headlines may read "wage negotiation shock"). However, the word is firmly entrenched in the literature of hæmorrhage and related topics. The meaning of the phrase 'irreversible hæmorrhagic shock' is, in this context, hypotension not responding to treatment and progressing towards death. It is therefore a diagnosis that can only be made after the individual has died and serves little purpose but to warn, quite correctly, that persistent hypotension following hæmorrhage is a disasterous condition unless treated promptly. "Therapy may vary markedly from case to case but if the initial supportive efforts fail to improve the circulatory dynamics and permit persistent hypotension to remain; these patients are in a precarious state and then survival may be in question."[23]

Hypotension following Injury (Traumatic Shock)

Following severe injuries, experimental animals and human patients may pass into a state clinically resembling the condition following severe hæmorrhage, and this, even when there has been little or no observable loss of blood. Controversy has raged round the ætiology of this condition for many years and theories have come and gone with great regularity.

In both traumatic and hæmorrhagic shock there is constantly a reduction in circulating blood volume leading to prolonged hypotension and its evil effects. In trauma, a reduction in blood volume follows loss of blood and exudation of fluid into and around the injured tissues. This has been demonstrated experimentally in dogs[24] and other species. Losses into injured area often amounted to some four or five per cent of body weight;[25] if a similar amount of blood is removed from an uninjured animal by controlled hæmorrhage, death usually results.

In humans too, the impression has been steadily growing that traumatic shock is basically similar to hæmorrhagic shock; at an Army symposium in Washington, Churchill stated that "The constant feature of wound-shock is a reduced circulating blood volume and this is initiated by, and to a major extent represents, the loss of blood volume from or into the site of injury". Grant and Reeve[26] who studied hæmorrhage and shock in battle casualties and civilian air-raid victims, decided that blood loss by hæmorrhage is far the most important factor in the illness associated with severe injuries. They point out that the mortality increases with increasing wound size, until with very large wounds over 50 per cent of patients die; with increasing wound size, the blood loss by hæmorrhage is clearly reflected in blood volume measurements. A useful indication of how far hæmorrhage has reduced blood volume is given by the systolic blood pressure, provided the patient has not been transfused. When the blood pressure is 100 mm. Hg or more the chances are very great that the blood volume is about 70 per cent normal or more, and when it is greater than 140 mm. Hg the chances are about 5:1 that the blood volume is at least 80 per cent of normal. A blood pressure less than 100 mm. Hg indicates that the blood volume is 70 per cent of normal or below. Emerson and Ebert[26] found that the blood volume had decreased by more than 25 per cent of predicted normal in all battle casualties with a systolic pressure below 85 mm. Hg. They stress the fact that arterial pressure is not greatly lowered until the blood volume deficit is large,

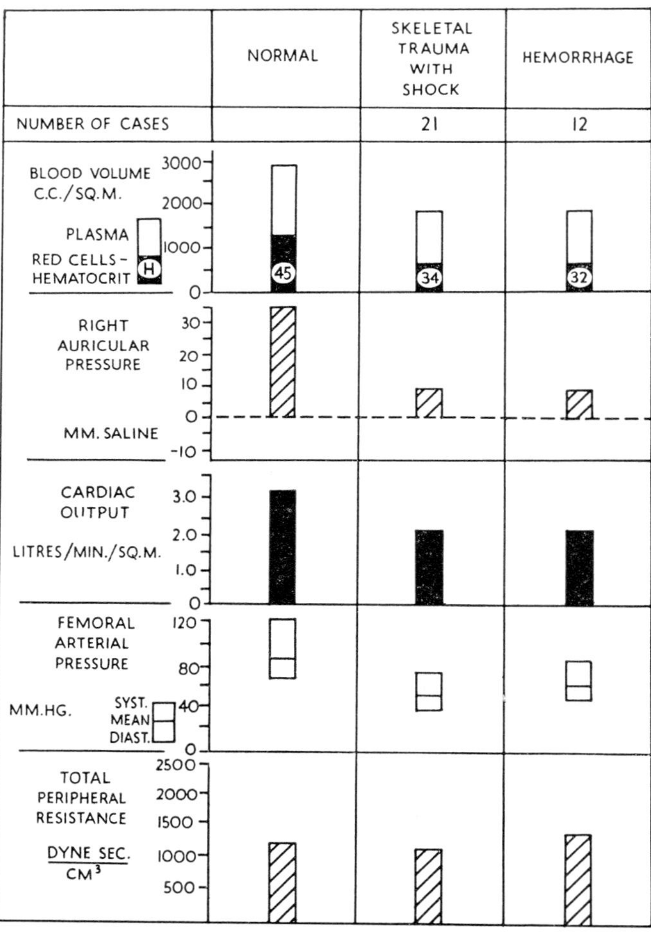

10/FIG. 2.—Comparison of normal human hæmodynamic findings with those in traumatic and hæmorrhagic shock. (After Richards.[37])

which suggests that the peripheral blood vessels are functioning normally. From such authortative statements based upon careful and extensive studies in the front line of battle and during air-raids, there can be little doubt that blood loss is a highly important factor in the causation of traumatic shock. The similarities are well shown in FIG. 2. Both with severe skeletal trauma and serious blood loss, Richards and his co-workers found a considerable decrease in the total blood volume, diminution in the cardiac output, fall in the right auricular and arterial pressures but no disturbances of peripheral resistance until the terminal stages. If the blood loss is severe, fluids will, as we have seen, gradually move into the microcirculation from the tissue spaces so diluting the blood that remains. In this way the extent of blood loss in traumatic accidents can be estimated, if the time of the injury is known, by the degree of hæmodilution. The hæmatocrit measurement can be an important investigation in shocked patients.[27]

The blood loss in trauma may be obvious, but in addition concealed bleeding into the tissues often occurs. A broken neck of the femur, for instance, may produce extravasation of 500 ml. or more of blood into the area round the fracture. To the blood loss is often added loss of fluid from the plasma; traumatised vessels will leak a protein-containing fluid; and if infection supervenes further loss will occur through inflammatory œdema. At one time, bacterial toxins from invading organisms or from the gut were implicated in the development of "irreversible" traumatic hypotension. However, mice and rats, reared under germ-free conditions following aseptic cæsarean delivery, develop hypotension as regularly as ordinary animals.[28]

If air or fat embolism occurs following trauma, this will add to the burden of the cardiovascular system by blocking important blood vessels, especially those of the pulmonary circulation. Another factor of practical importance is anæsthesia. Clinical observation shows how careful one must be in administering general anæsthetics to injured, hypotensive patients.[29]

Hypotension following Fluid Loss, including Burns

If a rabbit is suspended on a vertical frame with its head up, without anæsthesia, it becomes unconscious in 20–120 minutes, and it may die in a shock-like state within 24 hours with a very low blood pressure and suppression of urine, but no evidence of concentration of the blood. The rabbit is handicapped by a vast splanchnic circulation, and suspension leads, through the action of gravity, to pooling of much of the circulating blood within the splanchnic vessels.[30]

An anæsthetised dog vertically suspended with its feet down for 20–240 minutes goes into circulatory collapse[31] especially if it be bled small quantities of blood during suspension. In the rabbit, it is segregation of part of the circulating blood that precipitates a crisis because the remaining circulation cannot prevent the development of anoxia; the dog, however, loses much plasma through the microcirculation, develops hæmoconcentration and drifts into serious hypotension.

Towards the end of World War II Cameron and his colleagues[32] studied the effects of introducing hypertonic solutions into the subcutaneous tissues of animals. A 40 per cent aqueous glucose solution was used since this was tolerated well by rabbits and gives no pain while being injected subcutaneously. Massive œdema, generally free from hæmorrhage, developed around the site of injection. Within half an hour the rabbit displayed a rising hæmoglobin percentage, red cell count and packed cell volume, and direct estimation of the plasma volume of the blood showed that plasma was leaving the circulation. Here we are dealing with an uncomplicated anhydræmia and hæmoconcentration resulting from loss of fluid and protein. These rabbits became very ill in the later stages; they were cold and sat huddled up, their blood pressure fell to low levels, respiration and heart rate increased considerably and they excreted little urine. Finally, they often became comatose and died after some hours.

The resemblance to shock in human beings is close. Here we are dealing with an uncomplicated fluid loss and this has led to circulatory collapse, and frequently, death.

It has been known for a long time that the systemic effects of a burn are largely the result of fluid loss. When goats have 20 per cent of their total body

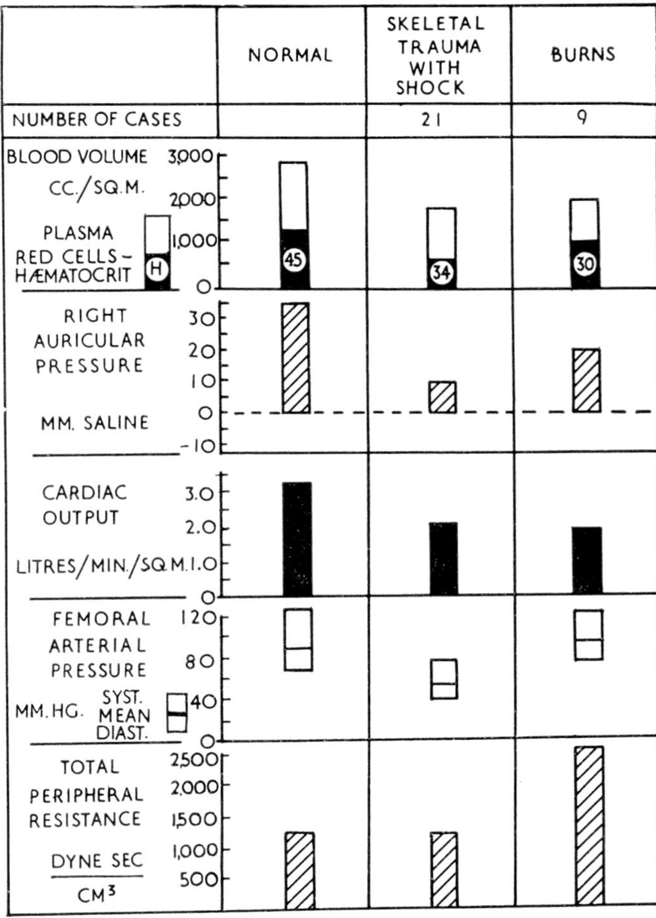

10/FIG. 3.—Hæmodynamic findings in human traumatic and burn shock. (After Richards.[37])

surface scalded, circulatory failure develops and the animal lapses into a comatose, shocked condition, from which it may not recover.

The fluid of œdematous burnt areas resembles plasma in its protein content.[33] Moncrief[34] has calculated that, if a lower extremity of a 70 kg. man suffers a second degree burn, and its diameter increases from 14 to 17 cm.—which can happen—then there is an increased volume of more than six litres of fluid in the tissues. Loss of fluid can occur also from the weeping surface of a burn and the whole area is easily infected with consequent further inflammatory œdema and exudation.

Replacement of lost plasma by transfusion lessens the risk of collapse and may even prevent it. Studies made in connection with the Peru burns project[35] show that saline solutions alone are effective as therapy during the shock period in man, provided adequate amounts are given. Plasma protein solutions, without adequate sodium content, were distinctly less effective.

FIGURE 3 from Richards, summarises a great deal of experience with human burns and shows that the cardiac output decreases considerably, though the peripheral resistance may be greatly increased so that the arterial pressure is maintained almost to the end. The blood volume falls, largely at the expense of the plasma volume. Indeed, the corpuscular volume may increase and the hæmatocrit may be high, indicating hæmoconcentration. The resemblance to traumatic shock and hæmorrhage shock is thus close, the greatest point of difference being hæmoconcentration in burns rather than hæmodilution.

HYPOTENSION FOLLOWING CORONARY OBSTRUCTION

Clinicians have been impressed for a long time by the serious symptoms and the extreme collapse that may persist when coronary obstruction leads to massive infarction of the left ventricle. The low blood pressure, rapid feeble pulse, diminished cardiac output, with respiratory distress and profound prostration, recall the circulatory disturbances in hæmorrhagic and traumatic shock. No doubt the determining factor is decreased cardiac output because of impaired myocardial contractility. So, too, pericardial tamponade, due to penetrating wounds and crushes with rapid bleeding into the pericardial sac, interferes with the adequate venous return to the heart so that it can no longer fill normally and passes into failure with profound hypotension. Massive pulmonary embolism, too, may bring about a similar condition because the venous return to the heart is obstructed in the lesser circulation. Many other examples might be added to these, but enough has been said to warrant their inclusion in a group of their own.

THE HYPOTENSION OF BACTERIAL ENDOTOXIN[36]

Pathogenic Gram-negative bacilli produce an endotoxin, a lipo-polysaccharide, which has remarkable cardiovascular effects when injected into experimental animals. Eventually these lead to a fall in cardiac output and hypotension and death. The way in which these end-results are brought about appears to vary from species to species. In dogs, there is a redistribution of blood by pooling in the liver—the result of hepatic venoconstriction. In other species, there is arteriolar vasoconstriction, especially in the lungs, gut and kidney. The bacterial endotoxin increases the liberation of adrenaline and noradrenaline and, possibly by reacting with leucocytes, promotes the formation of other vasoconstrictors. After a while there are further, less well understood, reactions whereby the precapillary arterioles and sphincters relax and blood then fills the dilated capillary beds. There are possibly other changes in the venous capacitance vessels allowing pooling of blood. Consequent on this redistribution of blood, the venous return and the cardiac output fall off and hypotension and death eventually follow.

Hydrocortisone in massive, pharmacological doses acts as an adrenergic blocking agent and may prevent death if given early enough after endotoxin administration.

Human patients, following operations on the gastro-intestinal tract to relieve obstruction, or following perforation of the bowel, or from other causes, sometimes develop a peritonitis and even a bacteræmia with Gram-negative organisms. Then patients will commonly pass into what has been called septic shock. There is a very high mortality for this condition, often greater than 70 per cent. There is no direct evidence that endotoxin is the cause of shock in these cases, but it is obvious that studies on the reactions of experimental animals to the endotoxin of Gram-negative organisms may prove to be directly relevant to the clinical conditions.

REFERENCES

1. HALL, Marshall (1839). *Med.-chir. Trans.*, **17**, 250.
2. LEWIS, Thomas (1932). *Brit. med. J.*, **1**, 873.
3. LAMSON, P. D., and DE TURK, W. E. (1945). *J. Pharmacol. exp. Ther.*, **83**, 250. (Method for accurate control of blood pressure during hæmorrhage).
4. HEWSON, W. (1846). *The Works of William Hewson, F.R.S.* Ed. GULLIVER, G. London: New Sydenham Soc.
5. TURPINI, R., and STEFANINI, M. (1959). *J. clin. Invest.*, **38**, 53. (Hæmostatic changes during hæmorrhage in the rabbit).
6. BIGGS, R., and MACFARLANE, R. G. (1962). *Human Blood Coagulation and its Disorders*, p. 190, 3rd edit. Oxford: Blackwell Scientific Publications. (Obstetrical fibrinogenopenia).
7. BARCROFT, J., HARRIS, H. A., ORAHOVATE, D., and WEISS, R. (1925). *J. Physiol. (Lond.)*, **60**, 443.
   BARCROFT, J., and STEPHENS, J. G. (1927). *J. Physiol. (Lond.)*, **64**, 1. (Splenic contraction in cats).
8. JOHNSON, E., and BLALOCK, A. (1931). *Arch. Surg. (Chicago)*, **23**, 848. (Effects of hæmorrhage on dogs).
9. HEYMANS, C., and NEIL, E. (1958). *Reflexogenic Areas of the Cardiovascular System.* London: J. & A. Churchill.
10. WALKER, W. F., ZILELI, M. S., REUTTER, F. W., SHOEMAKER, W. C., FRIEND, D., and MOORE, F. D. (1959). *Amer. J. Physiol.*, **197**, 773. (Adrenal medullary secretion after hæmorrhage).
11. GROOM, A. C., ROWLANDS, S., and THOMAS, H. W. (1965). *Quart. J. exp. Physiol.*, **50**, 35. (Response of cat to hæmorrhage).
12. SMYTHE, C. MCC. (1959). *Circulat. Res.*, **7**, 268. (Hepatic blood flow after hæmorrhage).
13. CAMPBELL, J. A. (1926). *J. Physiol. (Lond.)*, **61**, 249; and (1928). *J. Physiol. (Lond.)*, **65**, 255. (Oxygen partial pressures in the tissues).
14. PAREIRA, M. D., SERKES, K. D., and LANG, S. (1960). *Proc. Soc. exp. Biol. (N.Y.)*, **103**, 9. (Fluid shifts after 50% blood loss in rats).

15. HARRIS, J. (1962). *The Red Cell.* Oxford: Blackwell Scientific Publications. (Erythropoietin).
16. ENGEL, G. L. (1962). *Fainting*, 2nd edit. Springfield, Ill.: Charles C. Thomas.
17. POLES, F. C., and BOYCOTT, M. (1942). *Lancet*, **2**, 531. (Fainting in blood donors).
18. BARCROFT, H., EDHOLM, O. G., MCMICHAEL, J., and SHARPEY-SCHAFER, E. P. (1944). *Lancet*, **1**, 489. (Cardiovascular responses during fainting).
19. KERRIGAN, G. A., TALBOT, N. B., and CRAWFORD, J. D. (1955). *J. clin. Endocr.*, **15**, 265. (Vasopressin release).
20. EBERT, R. V., STEAD, E. A., and GIBSON, J. G. (1941). *Ann. intern. Med.*, **68**, 578. (Fluid shifts in humans after hæmorrhage).
21. BARTTER, F. C. *et al.* (1958). In *Aldosterone: Report of a Symposium.* London: J. & A. Churchill. (Aldosterone release during hæmorrhage).
22. DILLON, J. LYNCH, L. J., MYERS, R., and BUTCHER, H. R. (1966). *Surg. Gynec. Obstet.*, **122**, 967.
PRUITT, B. A., MONCRIEF, J. A., and MASON, A. D. (1967). *J. Trauma*, **7**, 767. (Treatment of hæmorrhage with large saline infusions).
23. POLLOCK, J. H. (1966). *A Survey of Surgical Shock.* Springfield, Ill.: Charles C. Thomas.
24. BLALOCK, A. (1931). *Arch. Surg.*, **22**, 598. (Experimental traumatic shock due to loss of fluid into injured tissues).
25. ROSENTHAL, S. M., and MILLICAN, R. C. (1954). *Pharmacol. Rev.*, **6**, 489. (Role of fluid loss in experimental traumatic hypotension).
26. GRANT, R. T., and REEVE, E. B. (1951). *Spec. Rep. Ser. med. Res. Coun.* (*Lond.*), No. **277.** London: H.M.S.O.
EMERSON, C. P., and EBERT, R. V. (1945). *Ann. Surg.*, **122**, 745. (Blood volume and hypotension after trauma).
27. MOORE, F. D. (1959). *Metabolic Care of the Surgical Patient.* Philadelphia:-W. B. Saunders. (Hæmatocrit measurements in shocked patients).
28. MCNULTY, W. P., and LINARES, R. (1960). *Amer. J. Physiol.*, **198**, 141.
EINHEBER, A., and WREN, R. E. (1967). *J. Trauma.*, **7**, 25. (Shock in germ-free animals).
29. MACINTOSH, R. R., and PRATT, F. B. (1939). *Brit. med. J.*, **2**, 1077. (Dangers of anaesthesia in shock patients).
30. COLE, W. H., ALLISON, J. B., MURRAY, T. J., BOYDEN, A. A., ANDERSON, J. A., and LEATHAM, J. H. (1944). *Amer. J. Physiol.*, **141**, 165. (Pooling of blood in suspended rabbits).
31. MAYERSON, H. S. (1944). *Amer. J. Physiol.*, **141**, 227. (Hypotension following suspension in dogs).
32. CAMERON, G. R., and COURTICE, F. C. (1947). *Quart. J. exp. Physiol.*, **34**, 165. (Hypertonic solutions subcutaneously).
33. UNDERHILL, F. P., and FISK, M. E. (1930). *Amer. J. Physiol.*, **95**, 330. (Composition of œdema fluid after burns).
34. MONCRIEF, J. A. (1965). In *Burns: A Symposium*, Eds. GOLDMAN, L., and GARDNER, R. E. Springfield, Ill.: Charles C. Thomas.
35. MARKELY, K., BOCAMEGRA, M., CHIAPPORI, M., MORALES, G., and JOHN, D. (1960). *Surgery*, **49**, 161. (Saline infusions as effective therapy after burns).
36. STRAWITZ, J. G., and GROSSBLATT, N. (Eds.) (1965). *Septic Shock: Proceedings of a Workshop.* Washington, D.C.: Nat. Acad. Sciences, Nat Res. Council.
BOCK, K. D. (1962). *Shock: Pathogenesis & Therapy.* Berlin: Springer-Verlag.
37. RICHARDS, D. W. (1947). *Ann. N.Y. Acad. Sci.*, **49**, 534.
38. JONES, H. W., WIDING, H., and NELSON, L. (1931). *J. Amer. med. Ass.*, **96**, 1297.
39. BREWER, H. F. (1939). *Brit. med. J.*, **1**, 895.
40. FOWLER, W. M., and BARER, A. P. (1942). *J. Amer. med. Ass.*, **118**, 421.

41. Warren, J. V., Brannon, E. S., Stead, E. A., and Merrill, A. J. (1945). *J. clin. Invest.*, **24,** 337.
42. Shentin, H. A., Cheney, R. H., Covons, S. R., and Starr, I. (1943). *Amer. J. med. Sci.*, **206,** 806.
43. Wallace, J., and Sharpey-Schafer, E. P. (1941). *Lancet*, **2,** 293.
44. Howarth, S., and Sharpey-Schafer, E. P. (1947). *Lancet*, **1,** 18.

Chapter 11

SOME EFFECTS OF INJURY ON METABOLISM

By G. V. R. Born

In higher animals, including man, injury is followed not only by local reactions in damaged tissues, but also by a sequence of general reactions which affect the body as a whole. The general reactions constitute a pattern which is very much the same whatever the type of injury that causes them. Thus, trauma, hæmorrhage, burning, freezing, and even acute infectious diseases bring about a similar series of changes in the organism. Because of this only one basic pattern of metabolic reactions to injury need be described.

The aim of this chapter is to give a brief description of these reactions and then to relate, as far as possible, the physiological and clinical phenomena to the biochemical disturbances which appear at the same time.

The General Reactions to Injury

From the moment of injury the general condition of the animal changes continuously until it dies or until normal health is restored. Increasing evidence indicates that these changes form links in one continuous metabolic chain which is controlled hormonally. Nevertheless, in the sequence of reactions it is possible to recognise three distinct periods.

The *first period* includes immediate and early effects. Immediately after injury the animal shows all the classical signs which result from an emergency.[1] The pupils are dilated, the mouth is dry, and the heart rate is increased. All these effects can be attributed to the stimulation of the sympathetic nervous system accompanied by the release of adrenaline from the adrenal glands into the blood stream. If the injury is slight the animal's condition reverts to normal within a few minutes. After more severe injury, the immediate emergency reactions give way to other early effects which may last from one to several hours and the most characteristic of which is a progressive fall in body temperature accompanied by cooling of the skin. If the injury is not too severe, or with appropriate treatment, these effects disappear and the animal slowly reverts to normal; otherwise different reactions supervene which constitute the second period.

The *second period* is that of *traumatic shock*[2]. This is defined as a period of diminished metabolic activity associated with circulatory failure which begins within a few hours of injury. Cuthbertson has called this very appropriately the "ebb" period[3]. The physiological background to the clinical features of shock is discussed in Chapter 10. Here, we shall be concerned with the biochemical effects of the physiological changes in shock which cause a progressive fall of blood pressure, and with attempts to identify the reasons why shock is sometimes fatal and sometimes not.

The *third period* is that of *recovery*. This begins with the passing of the first or the second, usually within 24 hours of the injury, and ends only when disturbances in the general condition of the organism can no longer be detected; this may take several weeks. Soon after this period begins, the inflammatory reaction at the site of injury reaches its height and is followed by repair. The body as a whole reacts with the general signs of inflammation, viz. rises in temperature, heart rate, and basal metabolism, as well as a leucocytosis. Cutherbertson has aptly called this the "flow" period[3].

Difficulties in Assessing the Biochemical Observations

Before describing the biochemical disturbances which have been found, we must consider why observations made on injured animals are exceptionally difficult to interpret.

The first reason is, of course, that we are considering reactions which involve the organism as a whole and which are, therefore, exceedingly complex. A change in blood sugar concentration, for example, is due either to increased addition of glucose to the blood or to decreased removal, and may be the result of changes in many different tissues which are influenced directly or indirectly by the secretions of endocrine glands. Moreover, animals undergo cyclical, e.g. diurnal, rhythms in their metabolism; these cycles also influence the metabolic responses to injury. Advances in understanding the disturbance of metabolism after injury clearly depend upon advances in our knowledge of normal metabolism.

Secondly, there is a tendency to regard all the metabolic consequences of injury as being designed to aid recovery—in other words, biochemical observations are often given teleological interpretations. Thus it has been suggested that the excessive breakdown of protein which follows serious injury is designed to supply carbohydrate for use as a source of energy, and amino-acids for the re-synthesis of protein in the damaged tissues, at a time when the wounded animal is less efficient in its search for food[4]. This is a plausible idea which is supported by the observation that when wounded rats receive a diet poor in protein, more of their body protein is used for synthesising new protein in a wound than when they receive a diet rich in protein[5]. On the other hand, a great deal of nitrogen is lost in the urine during the period of excessive protein breakdown after injury. In one patient studied by Cuthbertson, this loss amounted to 7·7 per cent of the total nitrogen in the body, which was more than the nitrogen in the entire liver.l Such gross destruction of protein would seem a very wasteful way of assisting ocal repair. This comment is made merely to point out that arguments from teleological considerations may be misleading.

Thirdly, in the normal organism a metabolic process can often be observed under comparatively steady conditions, but this cannot be done in the injured animal because its metabolism changes continuously until healing is complete. For example, the rate of oxygen consumption first falls and then rises again. The interpretation of biochemical findings is complicated by such changes.

A fourth source of difficulty is that substances released from tissues damaged by trauma may have an effect on the general metabolism of the body. Damaged muscle is known to release potassium, phosphate, creatine and amino-nitrogen into the blood stream. Burnt skin releases proteolytic enzymes[6]. Injury causes an increase in lymph flow. The lymph contains intracellular enzymes the type and concentration of which depend on the severity of the injury. In anæsthetised cats, hind limbs were injured, their lymph was collected and its enzyme content determined[7]. The mildest injury, i.e. ischæmia for one hour, caused no change. More severe injury, i.e. scalding at 60° for one minute, caused increases in the concentrations of cytoplasmic enzymes; with the still more severe injury of scalding at 80° for 20 seconds, there was an increase of mitochondrial enzymes as well; and after the most severe injury, i.e. freezing solid, there was also an increase of lysosomal enzymes. These experiments show that injury must be severe indeed to cause serious breakdown of the protective barriers provided by the external and internal cell membranes. Nevertheless, it is probable that much else enters the lymph and blood streams from damaged tissues.

Much work has been done to find out whether the released substances can account for any of the clinical or metabolic disturbances caused by injury. It is possible that they may do so, because if the circulation between an injured limb and the rest of the body is interrupted the onset of shock may be delayed and death may be postponed or even avoided. However, this observation can be interpreted in other ways. In animals, such as dog and goat, which normally harbour the anærobic micro-organisms *Clostridium welchii* and *Cl. œdematiens*, these proliferate in damaged, ischæmic muscle; their toxic products enter the circulation and may produce symptoms of shock. The outcome of shock may also be influenced by the extent to which bacterial endotoxins are absorbed from the gut[8].

The last difficulty is that the intensity of reactions to injury varies greatly, depending not only on the type of injury but also on the species, age, sex and previous condition, nutritional and otherwise, of the animal as well as on the environmental temperature before and at the time of the injury.

The problem in experimental investigations of the metabolic disturbances is, therefore, this: what quantitative criteria can be used to assess and compare the severities of different injuries? The ideal criterion would be an easily measurable biochemical change which formed part of the pattern of changes found after all injuries, the extent of the change being proportional to objective clinical measures of the severity of the injury. No such single criterion exists and this has limited the value of experimental results. Injuries of different kinds may be of the same intensity as judged by a common metabolic change, e.g. the rise in blood sugar concentration. However, the same injury in different subjects may produce results of very different intensities; e.g. fracture of the femur may produce slight shock in one person and severe shock in another. Some useful correlations have been discovered; for example, in man the blood sugar concentration rises after injury in direct proportion to its clinical severity[9].

Experimental Production of Standard Injuries

In order to provide reproducible and interpretable results experimental models usually have to be simpler than human injuries. The effects of the different components, ischæmia, hæmorrhage, and infection which together produce the damage in most clinical injuries must be investigated separately as far as possible. A suitable injury must satisfy the following criteria[10]: its nature and site must be known; it must be reproducible; and its intensity must be controllable and measurable. Methods have been developed, therefore, for injuring animals under controlled conditions in attempts to discover quantitative correlations between the clinical and physiological effects on the one hand, and the metabolic effects on the other. Ethical considerations are of extraordinary importance in investigations of this kind and should never be forgotten.

A rotating drum has been used[11] in which small animals are thrown against fixed projections. When rats were injured in this way, time of survival, the percentage of animals which died and the hæmoconcentration were all proportional to the number of revolutions of the drum. Although the lesions produced were very widespread correlation was statistically significant.

Hæmorrhage causes shock the severity of which depends, amongst other things, on the amount and the rate of the blood loss. Since these variables are easily controlled in experimental animals, much work has been done on the metabolic consequences of removing a known proportion of the animal's blood in a given time. Rats[12] have been bled in this way and classified as being in good, fair or poor condition on the basis of their pallor or cyanosis and of the rate and depth of respiration. The metabolic effects of such hæmorrhages were influenced by a great number of other factors such as the environmental temperature to which the animal was accustomed as well as the temperature during hæmorrhage; the position and the amount of muscular activity of the rat during bleeding; its previous consumption of water; and the presence or absence of upper respiratory infections. The effects of bleeding were also more consistent when the extent of blood loss was based on the animal's surface area rather than on body weight. This work demonstrated the difficulties in causing a "standard injury", in that even hæmorrhage produces varying effects unless all conditions are rigorously controlled.

Scalding of anæsthetised mice[13] can be standardised by increasing the temperature of the scalding fluid until about 90 per cent of the animals die within a given time, e.g. 48 hours. When mice scalded at that temperature were killed after two hours, the extent of the biochemical abnormalities in various tissues were similar from one animal to the next. However, percentage mortality and average duration of survival are crude measures of the severity of an injury, and they were used when no better criteria were available.[14]

The best method so far devised appears to be the production, under strictly controlled conditions, of ischæmia of limbs by constricting them temporarily with a tourniquet. This causes local effects in the damaged limb as well as characteristic general effects in the rest of the body. The injury is reproducible and its intensity can be controlled by varying the amount of tissue damaged, the duration of ischæmia, or the temperature of the limb. Moreover, when the intensity of this type of injury is diminished sufficiently it merges imperceptibly into physiological reactive hyperæmia which can be regarded as an effect of minimal injury. The method also provides a realistic model of an analogous clinical condition because acute limb ischæmia can cause shock and death in man. The method goes far towards satisfying Stoner's criteria who, with his collaborators, has used it to throw much light on the effects of such injury on metabolism.

With these considerations in mind, we may now discuss the metabolic disturbances produced by injury.

The First Period: Early Effects of Injury

The Role of Catecholamines

Immediately after trauma or hæmorrhage, there is a sustained increase in the blood sugar concentration, an observation first made in 1877 by Claude Bernard; a diminution in the amount of glycogen in the muscles; and a temporary increase in the glycogen concentration in the liver. In man, the increase in the blood sugar concentration varies directly with the severity of the injury[9]. If an animal is kept without food until the liver is depleted of glycogen, injury or hæmorrhage no longer bring about a rise in the blood sugar. The concentrations of lactate and pyruvate in the blood may increase but there is no change in the ratio of one to the other which implies that the relative rate of the ærobic and anærobic breakdown of carbohydrate is unchanged. These effects are also observed when adrenaline is injected into a normal animal[15] (except in the rat) or when its sympathetic nervous system is stimulated and they do not occur in injured animals if the adrenal medullæ have been removed before injury. The immediate effects of injury on carbohydrate metabolism are, therefore, presumably due to the release of catecholamines.

There is more direct evidence that injury brings about an increase in the concentration of adrenaline in the blood[16]. During and after surgical operation the rates of excretion of adrenaline and noradrenaline both go up, and the concentration of adrenaline in the adrenal gland decreases greatly.

The increased activity of the sympathetic system causes the mobilisation of fat from adipose tissues. This increase in lipolysis is brought about by adrenaline through a complex mechanism which involves the corticosteroids in some ways[17] (see below). The lipids which exist in the tissues as triglyceride appear in the blood as glycerol and free fatty acids. After injury, provided that the flow of blood through the adipose tissues remains adequate, there is a rise in the concentration of free fatty acids in the blood. There the fatty acids are bound to plasma albumin which can become saturated with them. When this happens the free fatty acids, being polar-nonpolar substances, may damage the surface membranes of circulating cells making, for example, the thrombocytes more susceptible to aggregation[18]. From the blood, the fatty acids are taken up by the tissues and metabolised or reconverted to triglyceride fat. This in turn may produce deposits of fat in abnormal situations, e.g. in the cells of the liver, thereby aggravating the effects of the injury.

The Effect of Adrenaline on the Adrenal Cortex

As we shall see later, some of the profound metabolic disturbances caused by injury are mediated by the hormones of the adrenal cortex. Great importance, therefore, attaches to the experimental proof that adrenaline increases the rate of secretion of adrenal cortical hormones. Marthe Vogt[19] showed that when small doses of adrenaline are injected into dogs there is a rapid increase in the quantity of cortical hormone in the venous blood coming from the adrenal glands. Long and Fry[20] found that injection of adrenaline into normal animals causes a decrease in the concentrations of ascorbic acid and cholesterol in the adrenal cortex. Since a similar decrease can be brought about in normal animals by injecting the adrenocorticotrophic hormone of the anterior pituitary (corticotrophin), it is believed that the decrease observed when adrenaline is injected also indicates increased secretion of cortical hormones. Adrenaline does not produce these effects in hypophysectomised animals; so it appears that adrenaline acts by stimulating the secretion of corticotrophin. This work forged a link between the comparatively short-lived effects of adrenaline and the longer-lasting effects which are associated with the adrenal cortical secretions.

Not only adrenaline but also stimulation of the central nervous system causes secretion of corticotrophin. Vogt[21] devised a method capable of measuring minute concentrations of adrenaline in the blood (down to about 1 mμg/ml.). With this method she showed that rats from which the adrenal medullæ had been removed responded to stress as well as to stimulation of the nerves with a fall in ascorbic acid concentration in the adrenal cortex, although in these rats the concentration of adrenaline in the blood was too low to account for the fall.

Adrenaline apparently does not act directly in the pituitary gland to release corticotrophin. In rabbits and dogs, the hypothalamus must be intact if stress is to lead to the secretion of corticotrophin[22, 23]. When adrenaline is injected into rats in which the basal infundibular part of the hypothalamus has been damaged, the decrease in circulating eosinophils which is characteristic of corticotrophin secretion no longer occurs[24].

The mechanism connecting the release of adrenaline with the increased secretion of adrenal cortical hormones may, therefore, on present evidence be summarised as follows:

adrenaline → hypothalamus → anterior pituitary gland → corticotrophin → adrenal cortical secretion

Activation of the Adrenal Cortex by Injury

The term "activation" is used as an abbreviation for "increased rate of secretion". We have seen already that injury activates the adrenal medulla and that this should bring about an increased rate of secretion from the cortex. There is much evidence to show that this is so. For example, in rats injury is rapidly followed by the loss of ascorbic acid and of cholesterol from the adrenals[25]. In man, the stress of surgical operations increases the rate of excretion in the urine of adrenal cortical hormones 3 to 30-fold[26]. This has also been shown directly by cannulating an adrenal vein during operation and estimating the concentration of hydrocortisone which accounts for more than five-sixths of the corticosteroids secreted into the venous blood. In man both glands normally secrete from 13–34 mg. hydrocortisone per day; during surgical operations they secreted at the rate of 111–232 mg. per day[16]. Many forms of injury lead to enlargement of the adrenal cortex[25]. Either injury or injections of corticotrophin or adrenal cortical hormones decrease the number of circulating eosinophils and lymphocytes, and bring about atrophy of lymphoid tissue throughout the body; neither injury nor corticotrophin has these effects after adrenalectomy[27]. Finally, as we shall see, many of the metabolic changes found after injury are strikingly similar to the effects of treating animals with excessive doses of corticotrophin or of adrenal cortical hormone.

The activation of the adrenal cortex by injury is thus well established. After moderate injuries the activation and the resulting metabolic changes are short-lived; both the ascorbic acid and the cholesterol in the adrenals are back to their normal concentrations within 24 hours. After more severe injuries the activation of the adrenal cortex continues. In the normal organism, the negative feed-back system which controls the relation between the secretion of corticotrophin and hydrocortisone ensures that hypersecretion of the latter diminishes the output of the former. It has been found, however, that after surgical trauma the concentrations of both hormones in the plasma rise simultaneously[28]. This suggests that trauma diminishes the effectiveness of the feed-back mechanism. Indeed, it has been shown that injury inhibits the breakdown of cortical hormones by the liver.[29]

Decreased Production of Energy

The greatest recent advance in our understanding came with the realisation that an early and invariable sequel to all physical injuries is a diminution in the body's energy production which is independent of the circulatory failure that characterises shock. Something happens to energy metabolism before the commencement of circulatory failure, so that the *primary event is metabolic rather than hæmodynamic*. The only measures which provide continuous information about the condition of the organisms are those directly related to energy production, viz. heat production and total oxygen consumption; both of these are characteristically diminished after injury. Energy appears as work and as heat. Both mechanical work (muscular) and metabolic work (osmotic, electric, etc.) are accompanied by heat production. After injury metabolic work necessarily continues but mechanical work and the heat produced by it are reduced to a minimum. At the same time, the temperature of the body falls. These effects were described clinically by Fischer in 1870. He observed a young man, previously healthy, who was struck in the abdomen by the pole of a carriage drawn by runaway horses. The patient was "lying very quietly, without paying any attention to events around him"; he felt cold and his rectal temperature was 1° C. below normal. Injured animals show a similar fall in temperature which is particularly striking in small mammals such as rats and mice (FIG. 1). This similarity suggests that conclusions drawn from experiments with such animals should apply, at least qualitatively, to man.

Decrease in Heat Loss

The fall in temperature could be due either to an increase in the rate of heat loss or to a decrease in the rate of heat production or to both. Clinical observation established long ago that the rate of heat loss was diminished rather than increased. The skin of injured people feels cold because the cutaneous blood vessels are constricted; indeed, as Cohnheim showed in 1890, the circulation through and heat loss from the skin may be reduced to such an extent that there is a temporary rise in *oral* temperature[30]. The rate and depth of respiration are decreased which also helps to conserve heat in the body.

The diminution in the rate of heat loss after injury has been confirmed experimentally. Rats were conditioned to live in a calorimeter in which the rate of their total heat loss was measurable with an error of less than 3 per cent.

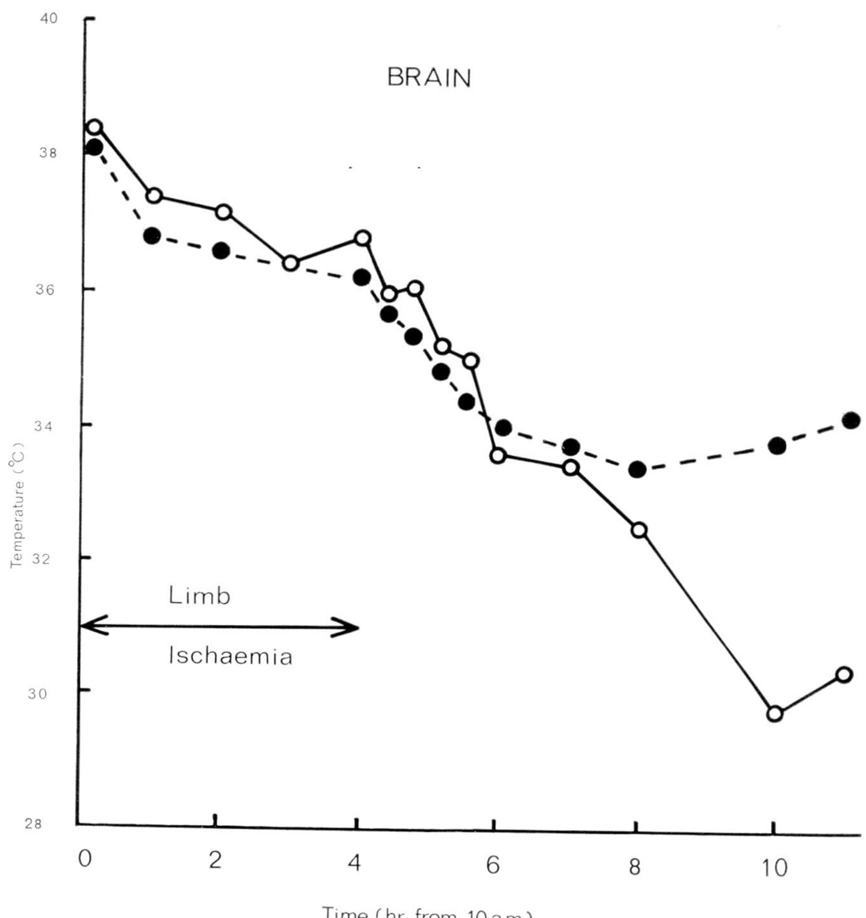

11/FIG. 1.—Mean brain and liver temperatures during and after 4 hr. bilateral hind limb schæmia in rats which subsequently died (○———○) and in those which recovered (●———●). Environmental temperature 18–22° C. (From Stoner.[10])

Ischæmic injury to their hindlimbs caused a decrease in heat loss which was most marked after the tourniquets were removed[31]. These facts indicate that the fall in temperature must be due to a fall in the rate of heat production.

Decrease in Heat Production

At rest, i.e. in the absence of muscular work, the main sources of body heat are liver and brain with a significant contribution also from the intestines[32]. To assess heat production it is necessary, therefore, to measure the temperature deep in the body, e.g. in the colon or in the liver. The fall in heat production and its independence from circulatory failure were established experimentally by simultaneous measurements of deep body temperature, blood pressure, and

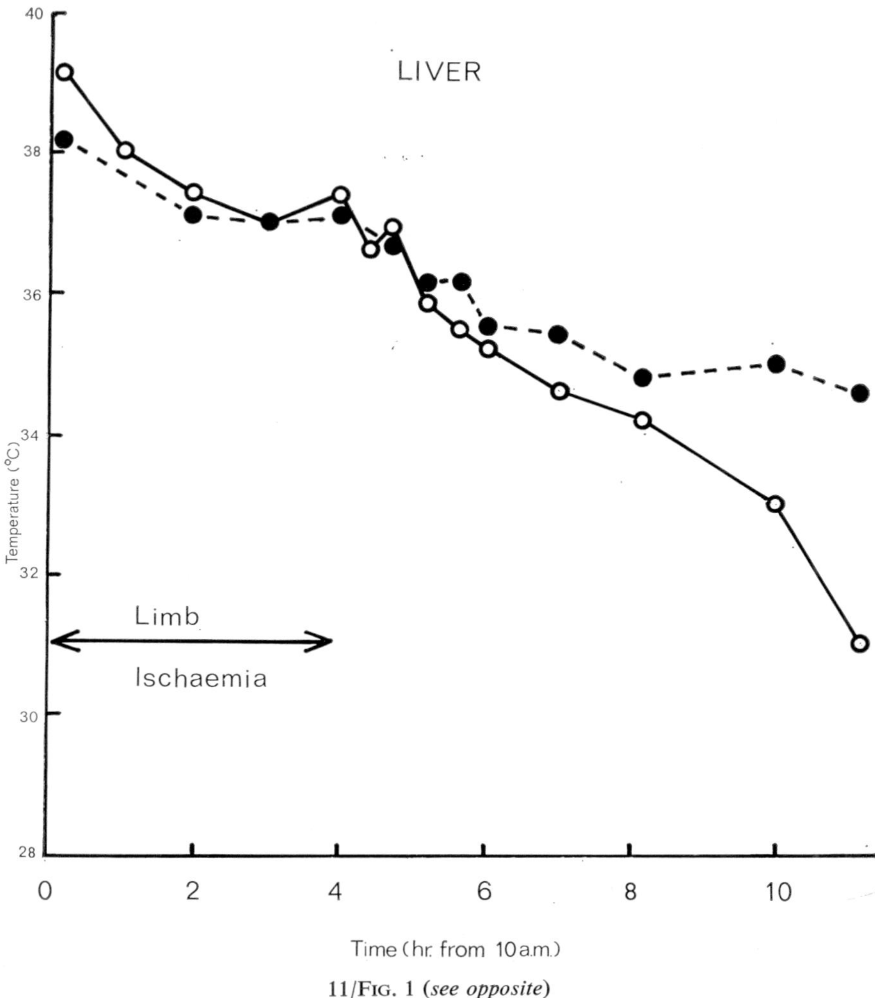

11/FIG. 1 (*see opposite*)

blood flow through vital organs, during and after bilateral hindlimb ischæmia in rats[33]. Soon after the tourniquets were applied the deep temperature began to fall and continued to do so after they were removed four hours later. While the tourniquets were in place, the blood pressure remained normal; after their removal the pressure remained only a little below normal for several hours until just before death. During this time the arterial oxygen saturation and the blood flow through liver and brain remained within normal limits.

At an environmental temperature of 18–22° C. the fall in colon temperature was proportional to the duration of limb ischæmia[33, 34]. The effect of the ischæmia on the deep temperature, measured in the liver, showed two phases (FIG. 1). In the first phase, the fall in temperature was similar in rats which died as in those which survived. In the second phase the temperature continued to fall in the animals which subsequently died but gradually returned to normal in those which survived. This showed that the changes in temperature as such did not determine the outcome of the injury which must depend therefore on other factors.

Decreased Consumption of Oxygen

The diminished rate of heat production is accompanied by a diminution in the rate of oxygen consumption. Experimentally, this was first shown in mice in which shock was produced, as in rats, by temporarily occluding the circulation to a limb by means of a tight rubber band. When the band was removed the rectal temperature fell almost as rapidly as after death, approaching the temperature of the environment within three hours; this was accompanied by a progressive diminution in oxygen consumption. The lower body temperature and the decreased rate of oxygen consumption were not due to an inadequate supply of oxygen to the tissues since neither could be increased by allowing the animals to breathe oxygen instead of air[35]. These results established that the tissues of injured animals do not use oxygen at the normal rate. This conclusion is supported by the following observations. When a normal mouse is transferred from an environmental temperature of 31°C. to one of 18° C. the animal increases its rate of oxygen consumption and then maintains it steadily at about 2·0 ml./min., the body temperature remaining at about 37° C. When an injured mouse is transferred from the higher to the lower environmental temperature the rate of oxygen consumption does not rise above 1·1 ml./min. and the body temperature falls. Thus, under these circumstances, injury has reduced the capacity of the animal to use oxygen by almost one-half.[35]

Recent experiments on the effect of altering the environmental temperature after ischæmic injury to rats have established that its main effect is on that part of the oxygen consumption which is concerned with the production of heat for the maintenance of body temperature. Thus, after injury the animals became poikilothermic and were unable to produce heat in response to environmental demands.[36]

Mechanism responsible for the Decrease in Energy Production

In the body energy is made available mainly through oxidative metabolism and trapped as high-energy phosphate compounds, i.e. adenosine triphosphate (ATP) and creatine phosphate. The efficiency of this process is less than complete and a constant fraction is dissipated as heat[37, 38]. Therefore, the only way in which heat production can be diminished is by a decrease in the rate of oxidative metabolism. Clearly, this could come about through a deficiency in the oxygen supply, but we have already seen that this cannot account for the early fall in heat production after injury. Other possible causes include:

(1) damage to the oxygen-utilisation structures of the cell;

(2) breakdown and depletion of labile phosphate esters, particularly of adenosine diphosphate (ADP) the concentration of which controls the rate of oxidative phosphorylation;

(3) exhaustion of the stores of carbohydrate which provide the principal immediate substrates for energy production;

(4) blocking of the tricarboxylic acid or glycolytic cycles which would cause carbohydrate breakdown to be interrupted; and

(5) decrease in the rate of carbohydrate catabolism as a result of the increased secretion of hormones from the adrenal cortex.

Damage to the oxygen-utilising systems.—Since oxidative phosphorylation is carried out by mitochondria, the metabolic capabilities of liver mitochondria prepared from normal animals have been compared *in vitro* with those from injured animals; no differences were found, suggesting that these mitochondria function normally in the injured animals.[39] However, mitochondria cannot be prepared for biochemical experiments *in vitro* without being deprived of oxygen for a least a few minutes; this may damage them to such an extent that any damage suffered previously *in vivo* may be insignificant by comparison and may therefore have eluded detection. All other work with isolated, surviving tissues has been equally inconclusive but perhaps only because the available methods are too crude to detect any changes.

Breakdown of labile phosphate esters.—After trauma or hæmorrhage there is always a large increase in the concentration of inorganic phosphate in the blood.[40] Although it has been suggested that this increase may be due in part to slowed excretion of phosphate in the urine, the chief cause seems to be a breakdown of unstable phosphate esters.

The concentration of creatine in the blood rises progressively and it is likely that the source of the creatine is striated muscle, which contains by far the highest concentrations of creatine and of creatine phosphate of all tissues.[41] In traumatised muscle creatine phosphate is released from damaged cells and rapidly hydrolysed. Experiments by Ord and Stocken[42] suggested a mechanism whereby creatine would be released also from non-traumatised muscle in shock. They perfused the hindlimbs of rats with diluted blood and found that, when the glucose concentration of the perfusing blood was reduced, increased amounts of creatine appeared in it. If sugar was added to the blood the extra creatine disappeared again. It seems, therefore, that one factor controlling the movement of creatine between muscles and blood is the blood sugar concentration, and when this is diminished in shock creatine leaves the muscles and appears in the blood. Ord and Stocken suggest that the liberated creatine comes from split creatine phosphate, because it is known that shortage of oxidisable substrate results in the rapid breakdown of creatine phosphate. In this breakdown inorganic phosphate is, of course, also set free and may account in part for the elevated phosphate concentration in the blood.

The other phosphorylated substance the fate of which in shock has been particularly carefully investigated is adenosine triphosphate (ATP), because of the mass of biochemical evidence which shows that ATP is in some ways necessary for providing energy for all kinds of cellular reactions and for maintaining the normal structure of cells and of their organelles such as mitochondria. The question arises whether breakdown of ATP in shock occurs only in traumatised tissues or in all the tissues throughout the body, since the destruction of ATP could presumably account for the failure of the energy-producing mechanism in shock.

In damaged tissues ATP is certainly destroyed. In ischæmic muscles of guinea-pigs and rabbits ATP was dephosphorylated and deaminated.[43, 44]

When the circulation was re-established after three hours ATP was resynthesised but, after five hours of ischæmia, the ATP concentration no longer returned to its normal value. Similarly, in rats, if limb ischæmia lasted for less than three hours the amount of total acid-soluble phosphorus in the ischæmic muscles was unchanged but if the circulation was re-established after more than three hours the muscles lost much inorganic phosphate to the blood.[45]

Apart from inorganic phosphate, are ATP and other adenine nucleotides released from traumatised tissues into the general circulation? The answer to this question became important in 1943, when Green[46] described a shock-like state that could be produced in experimental animals by the injection of large amounts of adenine nucleotides. Kalckar and Lowry[47] have shown convincingly that, although small quantities of adenine nucleotides can be demonstrated in the blood plasma coming from badly traumatised limbs, the concentration in the general circulation is far too low to account for the low blood pressure from which the animals suffer. Ischæmic muscles release into the blood not adenine nucleotides[45] but their breakdown product inosine monophosphate[48] which has no effect on the blood pressure. These results dispose of the possibility that free adenine nucleotides in the circulation are responsible for the symptoms of traumatic shock.

Are the *undamaged tissues* of the body depleted of adenine nucleotides? On the basis of work done during the war of 1939–1945, Potter and his colleagues claimed that this was, indeed, the case and they suggested that the arrest of energy production was due to the breakdown of the "energy-rich" phosphates, ATP and creatine phosphate, in those tissues which are of crucial metabolic importance to the animal. According to LePage[49], hæmorrhage in rats produced a great diminution of labile phosphate in the liver; less disappeared from the kidneys; and even less from the brain, heart and striated muscle, all of which retained considerable amounts of acid-labile phosphates at death. However, the methods employed were not specific for ATP, ADP or creatine phosphate, and others have not been able to repeat the observations. With more specific methods[50] no significant changes were found in the ATP concentrations in the brain, liver and undamaged muscles after injury; only the creatine phosphate in the latter was slightly diminished.

The wide-spread breakdown of ATP to ADP is, moreover, unlikely because of the following consideration: The system by which carbohydrate is oxidised and ATP simultaneously synthesised from ADP and inorganic phosphate is in the mitochondria where oxidation is coupled so tightly to phosphorylation that little oxygen is used so long as adenine nucleotide is mostly in the form of ATP. As soon as ATP is split into inorganic phosphate and ADP the consumption of oxygen is greatly increased. Thereafter the machinery of oxidative phosphorylation runs on at a high rate until most of the "phosphate acceptor", ADP, has been turned once more into ATP.[51] Now if injury caused the breakdown of ATP to ADP in many tissues at the same time, oxygen consumption should be increased whereas, in fact, it is decreased.

It does not seem, therefore, that the diminution in energy production can be explained on the basis of a widespread disappearance of "energy-rich" phosphate compounds from the tissues.

Depletion of carbohydrate.—The most complete, thorough and critical investigation of this possibility has been made by Stoner and his colleagues, using the technique of bilateral hindlimb ischæmia in rats.[33] The conclusion from this work is that the early fall in energy production cannot be accounted for by a concomitant disappearance in total body carbohydrate.

Stoner, Threlfall and Green[52] estimated the total amount of reducing sugar in whole rats, i.e. sugar present either free as glucose in blood and tissues or derived by acid hydrolysis from glycogen, glucose-1-phosphate, fructose-1-phosphate and fructose-1, 6-diphosphate; the estimations did not include glucose-6-phosphate. In injured animals the total amount of carbohydrate represented by these compounds rapidly diminished.

The carbohydrates which disappeared could be quantitatively accounted for as glucose-6-phosphate which accumulated in the undamaged muscles, on the assumption that muscle makes up about 40 per cent of the body weight.[53] Now the classical work of Cori established that adrenaline brings about the rapid breakdown of muscle glycogen which accumulates in the form of glucose-6-phosphate. Sutherland[54] showed that adrenaline increases the amount of active phosphorylase in liver and muscle. This enzyme catalyses the phosphorylytic breakdown of glycogen to glucose-1-phosphate, a process in which inorganic phosphate disappears from the blood plasma in amounts equivalent to the glucose-1-phosphate formed. Glucose-1-phosphate is in equilibrium with glucose-6-phosphate through the activity of the enzyme, phosphoglucomutase. Presumably, therefore, the accumulation of glucose-6-phosphate after injury is mediated by adrenaline.

Blocking of carbohydrate metabolism.—Recent experiments[55, 56] have clarified the cause of the hyperglycæmia that follows injury. The blood sugar rises not only because of the breakdown of liver glycogen mediated by adrenaline but also because of an inhibition of glucose utilisation by the tissues. The experiments were made with rats in the early period after standard ischæmic injury when the fall in temperature was not yet complicated by circulatory failure and oxygen deficiency. Glucose, fructose, and pyruvate, all labelled with C^{14}, were injected intravenously into uninjured and injured rats, and the rates of disappearance of the labelled substances from the blood were compared, as well as their interconversions and their excretion after oxidation as $C^{14}O_2$. Although the results varied considerably in the injured rats, the following conclusions were established.

After labelled glucose was injected, the specific activity of the plasma glucose fell more slowly in injured rats than in normal ones, and the injured rats excreted less $C^{14}O_2$. In the injured rats the amount of glucose entering metabolism was diminished and there was an even greater diminution in the amount of glucose oxidised (Table 1). When radioactive pyruvate was injected into an injured rat 1·5 hr. after removal of the tourniquets more of the label passed to glucose and less passed to CO_2 than in a normal rat. It appears that the oxidation of carbohydrate in the liver and kidneys is inhibited at some stage after the formation of pyruvate.

The ratios of the yields of C^{14}-glucose from pyruvates labelled in different positions were unchanged by injury, indicating that the mechanism of gluconeogenesis from pyruvate was unchanged. The yields were doubled by injury but not apparently by an increase in glucose formation from glycogen, the breakdown of which was almost unchanged, but by an inhibition of pyruvate oxidation which is the alternative major pathway of its metabolism. This accounted for the increase in pyruvate concentration in the liver and for the decreased excretion of CO_2 formed from labelled pyruvate. The changes in carbohydrate metabolism brought about by injury can, therefore, all be explained by the inhibition of pyruvate oxidation. The mechanism of this inhibition is still unknown.

11/Table I

Effect of bilateral hindlimb ischæmia for 4 hrs. in fed rats on the utilization of glucose, determined by the intravenous injection of C^{14}-glucose 1·5 hr. after removal of the tourniquets

	Control Mean ± S.E.M.	*Experimental*
Rate of conversion of glucose to metabolites (mg. glucose/min. 100 g. body wt.)	1·17 ± 0·04 (4)	1·07 ± 0·05 (5)
No. of rats in brackets.		
Rate of glucose oxidation (mg. glucose/ min. 100 g. body wt.)	0·71 ± 0·04	0·50 ± 0·04

Controls injected at the same time of day.
Environmental temperature 18–22°C.
(Results from Ashby *et al.*, 1965)[56]

After injury the oxidation of the products of lipolysis, i.e. glycerol and fatty acids, is diminished to about the same extent as that of carbohydrate. This suggests that the metabolic lesion responsible for the inhibition of oxidations lies beyond the junction of carbohydrate and fat metabolisms. The diminution of these oxidative processes is too great to be caused by the fall in body temperature. It can be concluded, therefore, that the converse is true and that the fall in temperature after injury is caused by the inhibition of oxidation reactions.[56]

Decrease in the rate of carbohydrate catabolism under the influence of increased secretion of adrenal cortical hormones.—The administration of adrenal cortical extract to animals fed on large amounts of carbohydrates causes hyperglycæmia, deposition of glycogen in the liver, and glycosuria. The amount of glucose lost in the urine may be far in excess of the quantity that can be derived from the increased breakdown of protein which also occurs. This leads to the conclusion that adrenal cortical hormones reduce the rate of utilisation of glucose by the tissues.[58] How this comes about is not known. Glucose is utilised in three main ways which are (1) breakdown via glycolysis and oxidation for the production of energy; (2) polymerisation to glycogen; and (3) transformation into fat. Chiu and Needham[58] have shown that adrenal cortical extracts when added *in vitro* to liver slices increase the production of glycogen and decrease the disappearance of total carbohydrate. This supports the conclusion that cortical hormones interfere with the catabolism of glucose. Although the relation between this effect and the inhibition of oxidative reactions remains obscure, it is likely that the accelerated secretion of cortical hormone after injury plays a part in slowing down the utilisation of glucose.

The Second Period: Metabolic Disturbances During Shock

We have defined shock as a period of progressive circulatory failure that follows injury. An enormous amount of work has been done in the endeavour to understand the cause of this particularly dangerous sequel to injury but so far without complete success.[59, 60] Clinically, shock is distinguishable from the periods that precede and follow it by a progressive fall in blood pressure. This is accompanied by general deterioration which is a source of difficulty in assessing experimental investigations when it is not clear to which stage of shock they apply. Results obtained with moribund animals tell us little about metabolic disturbances in patients who, if treated properly, can be expected to survive.

To account for the clinical features of shock an explanation is clearly required for the initiation and progression of the circulatory failure. In shock, therefore, the primary event that requires explanation is *hæmodynamic*, and the evidence incriminates loss of fluid from the circulation; toxic substances released from damaged tissues and from micro-organisms; altered activity of the autonomic nervous system; and diminished activity of the skeletal musculature. However, this chapter is not concerned with the causation of shock but with its effects on metabolism, so that the causative factors will be discussed only in so far as they may throw light on the metabolic disturbances particularly associated with shock. From this point of view, the most important causative factor is the loss of fluid from the circulation.

The resemblance between the effect of wound or traumatic shock and of simple hæmorrhage suggested long ago that the pathogenesis of shock involved the loss of blood or of plasma from the circulation. Indeed, it has been established that the circulatory failure of shock is usually associated with a rapid diminution in the volume of circulating blood. When there is hæmorrhage this is easy to understand, but when there is no obvious loss of blood the cause of the diminution in blood volume is less clear. Nevertheless, it has been established that, even if there is little actual bleeding, enough fluid may be lost from the blood into damaged tissues to produce shock. About half of this fluid comes directly from the blood; the other half comes from uninjured tissues elsewhere in the body. This loss is fatal if it amounts to more than about 5 per cent of the body weight.[61]

The importance of the loss of circulating fluid was confirmed by the therapeutic effectiveness of replacing the fluid by transfusion with blood, plasma, or plasma substitutes, which has saved the lives of innumerable wounded people. In experimental traumatic shock it has been shown that the circulatory failure can be reversed by administering sufficient fluids to the animals both to satisfy the capacity of the injured tissues to swell and to compensate for the diminution in blood volume. Such restitution may require large volumes, as much as 20 per cent of the body weight. Immediately after the end of limb ischæmia, plasma and physiological saline are equally effective and accumulate in damaged tissues to a similar extent; later, plasma is more effective than saline and remains longer in the circulation.

Successful treatment by transfusion does not prevent or reverse the early fall in body temperature already discussed.[62] Moreover, the effectiveness of such transfusions tends to diminish with time. Thus when, in the early stages, transfusion alone or with other treatment is able to bring about recovery shock is said to be in its reversible phase; this is followed by an irreversible phase during which neither transfusion nor any other treatment prevent deterioration and death.

Although shock can in many cases be accounted for by the loss of circulating fluid, this cannot be held responsible alone. Thus when, after bilateral hindlimb ischæmia, the tourniquets are removed the limbs swell rapidly and soon reach their maximum volume. If nothing further is done the animals deteriorate and die in irreversible shock; if, on the other hand, the tourniquets are rapidly reapplied the animals' condition improves and they survive.[63]

Metabolic Disturbances in Shock

During the progressive deterioration that is characteristic of shock, the metabolic disturbances become increasingly dominated by the effects of *oxygen deficiency*; this can account for most if not all of the abnormalities that have been described. The oxygen supply to the tissues is slowed because the loss of circulating blood or plasma has two effects. First, a decrease in the erythrocyte concentration diminishes the oxygen-carrying capacity of the blood through what Barcroft called "anæmic anoxæmia". Secondly, the fall in blood pressure is associated with a decrease in cardiac output and in circulation rate through the tissues. This "stagnant anoxæmia" is made worse by the loss of tone and the inactivity of the voluntary musculature. These diminish venous pumping and so the rate of return of blood to the heart. The resulting increase in venous pressure and in the loss of plasma from the circulation could indeed account for the progressive deterioration of shock. In early or moderate shock, the indications of oxygen deficiency may be less marked than the lowered blood pressure would lead one to expect. The explanation of this discrepancy lies in the diminished demand, already discussed, of the tissues for oxygen.

As shock begins, the metabolic picture is similar to that of the earlier, emergency period which is associated with the hypersecretions of both adrenaline and hydrocortisone. During experimental limb ischæmia in rats, while the tourniquets are on, the secretion of adrenaline raises the blood glucose concentration and causes the discharge of glycogen from muscle and an increase in liver glycogen via the Cori cycle. After removal of the tourniquet, the breakdown of glycogen in the undamaged muscles continues but glycogen diminishes also in the liver; these changes maintain for several hours the elevation of the glucose concentration in the blood as well as in other extracellular fluids. The reason for the fall in liver glycogen concentration is not known. It does not depend on the adrenal medulla but may be related to the uptake by the liver of amino-acids which have been released into the blood by proteolysis in the damaged muscles of the hindlimbs. This proposition is based on experiments[63a] which showed that when proteins or single amino-acids were fed to rats their blood sugar concentration fell rapidly with a large loss of glycogen from the liver but none from the muscles. Neither adrenaline nor insulin were involved in this effect, which was thought to be associated with the extra energy expended through the specific dynamic action of the amino-acids.

As shock progresses the blood sugar concentration falls, and the liver is depleted of glycogen. In 1941 Selye and Dosne[64] suggested that tissues which are injured in the production of traumatic shock utilise carbohydrate faster than normal tissues. If the circulation to the hindlimb of a cat was blocked for 3 hours and then restored, the difference in glucose concentration between arterial and venous blood was greater in the injured than in the normal hindlimb. The interpretation of these particular experiments remained doubtful since no measurement was made of the flow of blood through the limbs and glucose may merely have diffused out more rapidly into the ischæmic tissues. Russell, Long and Engel[65] showed that when a rat is eviscerated and the circulation of the liver is stopped, the subsequent rate of fall of the blood sugar concentration is greatly increased after hæmorrhage. In dogs, similar observations have been made, and they suggest that hæmorrhagic shock results in a heightened rate of utilisation of carbohydrate by muscles and other peripheral tissues.

In the rat but not in man shock is accompanied by a rise in the amino-nitrogen concentration in the blood. This occurs in all forms of clinical and experimental shock and has been carefully investigated by Engel and Long.[66] The rise in blood or plasma amino-nitrogen is roughly proportional to the fall in blood pressure and to the severity of the clinical signs of shock. Two causes have been found for the increased amino-nitrogen concentration. One is an increase in the rate of loss of amino-acids from striated muscles which contain more free amino-acids in shocked than in normal animals[67]; indeed, in dogs after hæmorrhage, increased amounts of amino-nitrogen are found in the venous blood coming from the limbs.[68] The other cause is the inability of the liver to deaminate amino-acids, and to form urea, at the normal rate; this happens whenever the oxygen supply to the liver is decreased.[12, 66]

In some forms of shock *the concentrations of enzymes increase in the plasma*. When shock is produced in dogs by bleeding or by injecting bacterial endotoxin the concentrations of glutamic oxaloacetic transaminase and of lactic dehydrogenase increase several-fold. It is thought that these enzymes come from the liver and from other tissues which are damaged sufficiently to release them into the blood. However, the release of enzymes does not necessarily mean that damage to tissues is extensive, for it has been calculated that in a 30 kg. dog the breakdown of 1–2 g. of tissue would be enough to account for the increase in plasma lactic dehydrogenase that is observed.[69]

In hæmorrhagic or traumatic shock, the tissues lose potassium into the plasma where its concentration increases. Some of this potassium is lost into the urine; but the potassium concentration may also increase in uninjured tissues, in erythrocytes, liver, pancreas and heart. Excess of potassium in the blood is more harmful to animals in shock than to normal animals;[70] this may be a factor in the progressive nature of shock.

Other disturbances to salt and water metabolism in shock are caused by hypersecretion of antidiuretic hormone from the posterior pituitary gland; as a result, water is retained in excess. The secretion of aldosterone is inhibited and the loss of sodium into the urine is accelerated. The plasma becomes markedly hypotonic. In reversible shock these disturbances soon disappear, as illustrated by the following case record:

A woman, aged 42, suffered from cholecystitis but was otherwise healthy. Her gall-bladder was removed by operation after which she was transfused with enough blood to replace what she had lost. Her blood pressure remained normal and her post-operative condition was as good as could be expected, but there was one striking feature: during the first 5 days after the operation the output of urine diminished progressively. At the same time her weight increased from 45 to 49 kg. and the concentration of sodium in the plasma fell from 142 to 118·5 mEq/1. After 5 days the volume of urine increased and by the seventh day the patient's weight and plasma sodium concentration were back to normal.

The Possible Involvement of Oxygen Deficiency in the Progress of Shock

It has been suggested that oxygen deficiency could account for the progressive deterioration in shock through the establishment of a vicious circle in the following way. After injury, the initial loss of blood or plasma into damaged tissues leads to a fall in blood pressure, which leads to a fall in blood flow through the tissues, which leads to oxygen deficiency of the vascular endothelium, which leads to accelerated outflow of proteins and fluid through the capillaries and venules, which leads to further reduction in blood volume; and so on. This suggestion raises two questions. First, does oxygen lack increase the permeability of capillaries; secondly, if so, does the required degree of oxygen deficiency ever occur in shock?

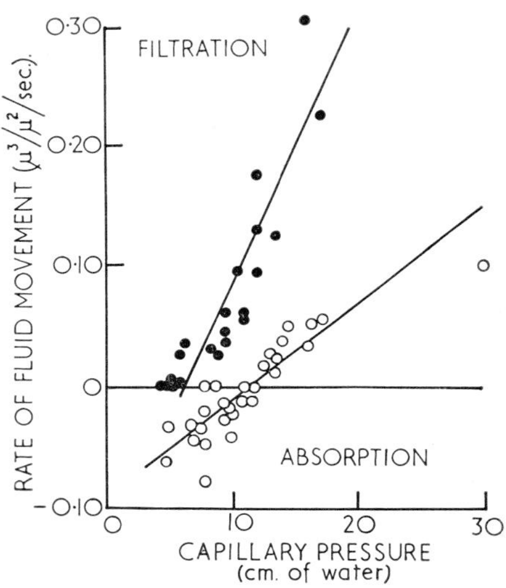

11/FIG. 2.—Chart showing rates of fluid movement across the wall of a mesenteric capillary in the frog, observed one minute (solid circles) and 15 minutes (open circles) after a 3-minute interruption of blood flow, while the mesentery was covered with boiled, oxygen-free Ringer's fluid. Abscissæ indicate the rate of fluid movement in cubic micra per square micron of capillary wall per second; ordinates the capillary pressure in centimetres of water. (After Landis.[71])

In 1928 Landis provided evidence that when capillaries are deprived of oxygen the rates of flow of water and plasma proteins through the capillary wall increases.[71] His results are shown in FIG. 2. The mesenteric capillaries of decerebrate frogs were observed under the microscope, and the lumen of one capillary was closed by gentle pressure with a blunt glass rod. The direction in which fluid moved across the walls of the closed capillary was followed by observing whether the red corpuscles moved towards or away from the closed end of the capillary; the rate of fluid movement was proportional to the initial rate at which the corpuscles moved after the capillary was occluded. Landis found that when the capillary circulation was interrupted for 3 minutes and then restored, fluid immediately filtered across the capillary wall at approximately four times the normal rate. At the same time protein moved out of the capillaries in increased amounts, thus reducing the effective osmotic pressure of the plasma proteins in the vessels to almost one-half of the normal value. With the return of the circulation the capillary wall rapidly recovered its comparative impermeability to protein and the rate of fluid movement was reduced practically to normal.

In most situations in the body the capillaries are so intimately associated with other tissue elements that it is impossible to find out how oxygen lack affects the metabolism of capillary endothelial cells. But in the lung the proportion of capillaries to other tissues is comparatively high, and experiments in which lungs were perfused with the metabolic inhibitor, 2, 4-dinitrophenol, have provided some evidence that the permeability of these capillaries at least begins to increase at about the time when almost all of the adenosine triphosphate (ATP) in the lungs has been broken.[72]

The work of Landis made it clear that complete though temporary interruption of the circulation can reduce the ability of the capillaries to retain the constituents of plasma in the blood. The presumption was that the change in the capillaries is due to oxygen deficiency. However, it may equally well be that interrupting the circulation leads to the release of substances which, like histamine, dilate the post-capillary venules and increase their permeability. The mildest handling of the skin of a guinea-pig is enough to increase the permeability of the superficial venules to the dye, pontamine blue.[73] It has often been suggested that shock in man is aggravated by the loss of fluid from the circulation into normal tissues through the walls of anoxic capillaries. This may be so but there is no direct evidence for it. The only relevant experiments were made with perfused hindlimbs of rats, and they suggest that moderate reductions in the oxygen content of the blood (down to 5–10 ml. 0_2/100 ml. blood) do not significantly increase the loss of fluid from the capillaries into the tissues.[74] It is not yet established that a man in traumatic shock ever suffers from oxygen deficiency so severe that it contributes to the loss of fluid from the failing circulation.

Another suggestion sometimes made is that in shock there is an excessive loss of plasma proteins into the tissues. Whipple has shown, however, that if dogs are bled continually and if the red cells only are restored to them in saline at the same rate, the concentration of circulating proteins may be reduced to 1 per cent without inducing the circulatory collapse of shock.[75]

Decreased Oxygen Supply as a Cause of Decreased Oxygen Consumption

The possibility has to be examined that the decrease in the oxygen supply may contribute to the decrease in oxygen consumption observed after injury. Stagnant anoxæmia is characterised by an increase in the difference in oxygen content between arterial and venous blood, while the saturation of the arterial blood is not greatly reduced. In dogs a normal arteriovenous oxygen difference of 3–7 ml./100 ml. blood is increased to 14–20 ml./100 ml. blood after trauma or hæmorrhage.[76]

In some interesting experiments by Tabor and Rosenthal[35] mice were bled at an environmental temperature of 26–29° C. and then transferred to one of 18° C. The rectal temperature fell rapidly as long as the mice breathed air, but when they were allowed to breathe pure oxygen the rectal temperature increased from 21–26° C. to the normal value of 37° C. The same reversal of the fall in body temperature was produced by re-injecting the blood intravenously, whereas the injection of similar volumes of saline was without effect. In these mice, therefore, the fall in body temperature appeared to be due primarily to tissue anoxia resulting from the diminished rate of oxygen supply after bleeding. This reaction is presumably closely related to the reversible fall in temperature which occurs in normal animals when they breathe low concentrations of oxygen.

When tissues are deprived of oxygen, their capacity to utilise oxygen becomes progressively less the longer the deprivation lasts. This is illustrated in FIG. 3 which represents results of experiments in which the arterial circulation through the liver of rats was arrested for increasing periods of time, after which the oxygen consumption of slices made from the livers was measured *in vitro*. Clearly, prolongation of anoxia was associated with increasing damage to the oxygen-utilising systems in the liver.[77]

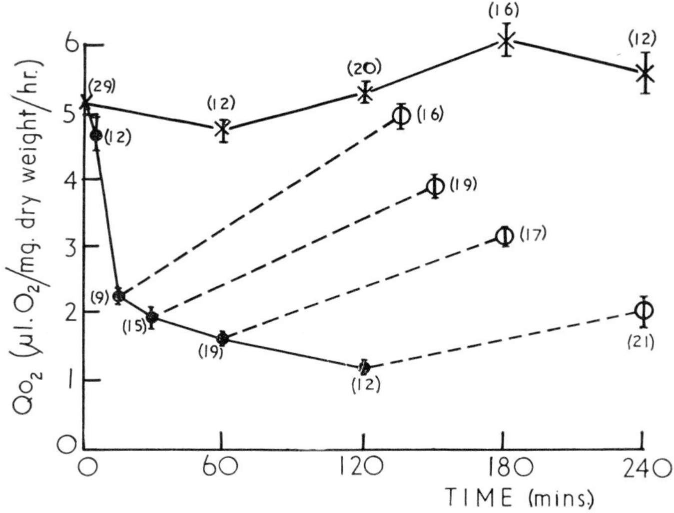

11/FIG. 3.—Effect of hepatic anoxia *in vivo* on respiration of rat liver slices *in vitro*. Crosses: control observations on liver samples from operated animals. Solid circles: samples from livers with hepatic artery clamped for 0, 5, 15, 30, 60 and 120 minutes. Open circles: samples taken two hours after restoration of circulation to the liver following 15, 30, 60 or 120 minutes of hepatic anoxia. Small figures at each point indicate number of observations. Vertical bars indicate standard error of the means. (After Wilhelmi *et al.*[77])

These observations link the decrease in oxygen supply with the decrease in oxygen consumption. However, the link has been forged only in experimental situations in which the supply of oxygen was cut off entirely. It is most unlikely that clinical shock is ever associated with oxygen deficiency of sufficient severity to cause irreversible damage to the vital organs except shortly before death.[59] Such deficiency, therefore, cannot by itself account for the conversion of reversible into irreversible shock.

Manifestations of Oxygen Deficiency in Clinical Shock

As the blood pressure continues to fall and the cardiac output to decrease, oxygen deficiency becomes increasingly evident. The oxygen content of the venous blood decreases while the concentrations of lactate, pyruvate and hydrogen ions increase. The lactate concentration rises more than that of pyruvate indicating that proportionately more cabohydrate is broken down by anærobic glycolysis. Really large changes in blood pH and lactate are observed only when profound or prolonged oxygen deficiency impairs the ability of the liver to remove lactate from the blood; this point was first established in hæmorrhagic shock and has been confirmed in other forms.

The inadequate supply of oxygen to the tissues manifests itself, therefore, as acidosis. This acidosis is partly metabolic as lactate accumulates and partly respiratory as the pulmonary ventilation decreases and carbon dioxide accumulates in the blood. The acidosis can be measured by the fall in the alkali reserve of the plasma or in the arterial pH. Experience has established that when the pH falls below 7·0 oxygen lack is so severe as to cause irreversible damage to the vital organs.

Conclusions about Shock

Clearly, we do not yet know the exact relationship of the circulatory to the metabolic disturbances in shock. It is conceivable that the latter are interlinked to such an extent that a primary defect can hardly be said to exist.

The Third Period: Metabolic Disturbances Associated with Recovery

The first two periods in the reaction to injury are generally over within twenty-four hours. The animal may die of shock; if it survives it enters the third or recovery period. In this period there are increases in pulse and respiration rates, body temperature and oxygen consumption, all—except the pulse rate—the opposite of what occurs during shock. These clinical features and the concomitant polymorphonuclear leucocytosis have provided the alternative name of "traumatic inflammation".[3] At the site of injury there is increased blood flow with emigration of leucocytes and the formation of inflammatory exudate, followed by other processes associated with healing. Traumatic inflammation occurs even after injuries too mild to give rise to shock. The changes which characterise this period are well illustrated in Fig. 4, taken from a paper by Cuthbertson[78]. Apart from the effects already enumerated, the chart shows a striking increase in the excretion of nitrogen. This is a highly characteristic response to injury which must be discussed in detail.

The Loss of Nitrogen after Injury

It has been known since 1872 that hæmorrhage is followed by an increase in the amount of nitrogen excreted in the urine.[79] A careful investigation of this phenomenon was made by Cuthbertson,[80] beginning in 1929. He found that every kind of injury led to the loss of nitrogen. In man this became noticeable as soon as the interruption of urine flow caused by the injury was over; the loss was maximal between the fourth and the eighth day after injury and then gradually diminished although in some cases, it was still measurable after six

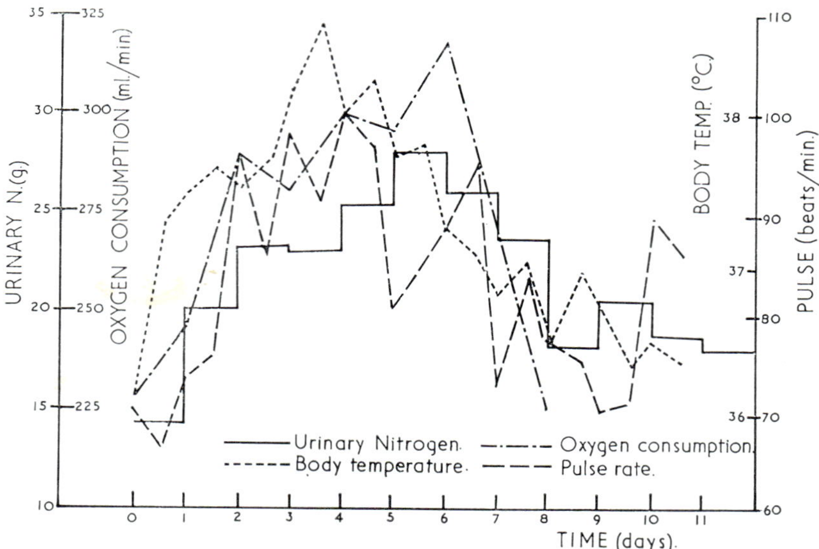

11/FIG. 4.—Changes in body temperature, heart rate, oxygen consumption and urinary nitrogen excretion after fracture of both bones of a leg in a man, aged 34 years. (After Cuthbertson.[78])

weeks. The phenomenon is illustrated in FIG. 4 which records disturbances in a man, aged 34 years, after he had been accidentally kicked on a football field and suffered fracture of both bones of one leg and bruising; shock was slight. The figure shows that the time course of the nitrogen loss was very similar to that of the increased oxygen consumption and to the rise and fall in the pulse and respiration rates and in the temperature.

Cuthbertson noticed that, even in the absence of injury, people who were partially immobilised in bed lost slightly more nitrogen than usual. Whenever the loss of nitrogen was increased there was also increased loss of phosphorus and sulphur in the urine. The ratio of sulphur to nitrogen, about 1 to 14, in the urine was similar to that found in muscle, and it was believed that the excessive nitrogen and sulphur came from muscle tissue, either through autolysis after trauma or through disuse atrophy in bed-ridden patients. However, the sulphur to nitrogen ratio of other tissues is much the same, and when the observations made on human accident cases were reproduced experimentally in injured rats, it soon became obvious that the excessive losses could not be accounted for by the loss of muscle substance at and around the site of injury. The injured man just mentioned lost 23 g. of nitrogen per day and the over-all loss over ten days was 137 g. which meant that the nitrogen content of the patient's body was reduced by as much as 7·7 per cent.

Apart from the loss of nitrogen, sulphur and phosphorus, the urine also contains excessive amounts of creatine. Moreover, the urinary excretion of potassium remains excessive for some time during which the excretion of sodium, is, if anything, diminished.

The Influence of the Nutritional State on the loss of Nitrogen

Cuthbertson[81] showed experimentally that the amount of nitrogen lost was influenced by the nutritional state of the animal at the time of injury and by the diet eaten while the loss was going on. If rats were fed on a diet containing very little protein and then injured, the subsequent loss of nitrogen was much reduced. The greater the proportion of protein in the diet before and after injury, the greater was the amount of nitrogen excreted, so that it seemed as if the nitrogen came from labile protein rather than from protein built into the tissues.

The catabolic response to injury is not peculiar in being affected by the intake of protein. In normal animals and people, the amount of nitrogen lost each day is also related to the amount of protein consumed. When a subject in nitrogen balance is put suddenly on a nitrogen-free diet, the rate of excretion of nitrogen falls approximately exponentially until a new, lower excretion rate is established. It seems that the rate of nitrogen excretion is roughly proportional to the mass of labile protein in the body. Borsook[82] proposed that most of the nitrogen excreted in the urine is derived immediately from labile protein of the tissues and only indirectly from ingested nitrogen of which the immediate fate must be, for the greater part, to be built up into tissue protein. The effect of injury appears to be to increase the rate of breakdown of labile protein, the actual rate of loss of nitrogen being proportional to this rate and to the total quantity of labile protein in the body.

If an animal eats carbohydrate after injury the loss of nitrogen is greatly diminished; this important effect will be discussed later. A diet with much protein in it does not prevent the wastage of body nitrogen to nearly the same extent; more nitrogen is still excreted than is taken in. If the animal fasts after injury, damaged tissues regenerate just about as rapidly as when the animal continues feeding: so it seems that tissues can be repaired by drawing on the animal's own resources.

The Source of the Lost Nitrogen

The excess nitrogen that is lost in the urine is in the form of urea. In the blood the concentration of urea is increased but not that of amino-nitrogen, showing that the liver is capable of metabolising amino-acids as rapidly as they reach it. In this, the recovery period differs from that of shock in which, as we have seen, the amino-nitrogen concentration is increased in the blood. The urea is presumably derived from proteins in the body by the usual processes of protein catabolism. The question is, from which proteins? Cuthbertson[83] showed that when human beings or rats fracture a long bone the excessive excretion of nitrogen cannot be accounted for by destruction of tissue at the site of the fracture or by wasting in the injured limb as a whole. Furthermore, when rats were fed a protein-free diet until the excretion of nitrogen had fallen to a steady value, fracture of the femur was not followed by the usual rise in nitrogen excretion.[81] It was concluded that the nitrogen came from the generalised breakdown of some kind of storage protein, i.e. protein without identifiable metabolic or structural function. What protein is storage protein? The plasma proteins might be so regarded, with reservations about their various known functions which are due to their osmotic, immunological, carrier, and other properties. However, injury produces only a slight lowering of the concentration of plasma albumin; plasma globulin and fibrinogen are, if anything, more concentrated despite the fact that the proteolytic activity of the plasma is increased (see Chapter 8). Moreover, it can be calculated that if after an injury to a healthy young man 10 per cent of the intravascular plasma proteins were broken down, they would give rise to no more than about 5 g. of additional nitrogen in the urine. This is little compared to the losses which have been recorded in many cases of injury in which there was actually no reason to believe that plasma proteins were destroyed.

Another possible source of the excreted nitrogen is the protein of lymphoid tissue, because injury brings about a reduction in the total quantity of lymphoid tissue and in the number of circulating lymphocytes.[84] Total lymphoid tissue makes up about 1 per cent of the body weight, corresponding to about 21 g. protein nitrogen in a man weighing 70 kg. Thus, even the complete destruction of lymphoid tissue would not nearly account for the amount of nitrogen which can be lost after injury.

The main protein masses in the body are the liver and the muscles. Liver protein is the most labile in the body, with muscle protein not far behind. Miller's experiments provide evidence against the view that some of the protein in liver is functionless storage protein; instead, it seems that the labile protein is "the working stuff of the cell".[85] In animals on a protein-free diet the activities of the enzymes catalase, alkaline phosphatase, cathepsin and arginase in the liver diminish in parallel with the loss of liver protein. If protein is then fed, the total enzyme content of the liver increases rapidly, again in parallel with the sharp rise in total liver protein.[86] It follows that if any of the nitrogen lost after injury comes from the liver, it is not derived from a protein store but from protein which must be presumed to take part in metabolic activities. Whether the nitrogen does originate in the liver is difficult to test, for the metabolic capacity of the liver is so great that its mass has to diminish to much less than half before any metabolic deficiency can be detected. There is no analogous information about striated muscle, which would be even more difficult to obtain.

Summarising, it can be said that the protein sources of the excess nitrogen excreted after injury are not known. The idea that the nitrogen originates in some form of protein store is probably too simple. It seems, rather, that some proteins, e.g. collagen, are much more stable than others, e.g. certain enzymes in the liver, and that presumably the more labile proteins contribute most. It is certain that destruction and atrophy of tissues at the site of injury do not account quantitatively for the loss of nitrogen, and, for various reasons, it seems unlikely that much is contributed by the plasma proteins, the proteins of lymphoid tissue, or those of the liver. It will be seen later the indirect evidence points to muscle as a major source.

Increased Turnover of Proteins

The excessive destruction of body proteins just described is only one aspect of protein metabolism at this time. The concentration of some proteins, such as fibrinogen, actually increases; and there is evidence that in the case of fibrinogen and of plasma albumin both the rate of synthesis and the rate of breakdown are enhanced. Whipple and his colleagues[87] injected turpentine under the skin of dogs to produce sterile abscesses. After 1 to 5 days plasma proteins labelled with lysine-C^{14} were injected intravenously into dogs with abscesses and into normal dogs, and the rates at which the labelled proteins disappeared from the blood were compared. In dogs with abscesses the half-life of labelled plasma albumin was about 2 days whereas in normal dogs it was 9 days. Since the concentration of albumin was not appreciably altered the results mean that the average rate at which the albumin molecules were made and unmade, the turnover rate, was sharply increased.

Only some proteins show an increased turnover rate; others are apparently affected in the opposite way. Whipple[87] found that in his dogs with sterile abscesses the rate at which hæmoglobin was synthesised was much reduced while the inflammation lasted. This observation may explain the hypochromic anæmia which frequently follows trauma in man.

Influence of Adrenal Cortical Hormones on Protein Catabolism

At this point it becomes necessary to discuss the evidence which relates the excessive destruction of proteins after injury to the activities of adrenal cortical hormones. We have already seen that injury immediately starts off a complex sequence of events which have the effect of increasing the secretion of these hormones. If the injury is severe but the animal survives, the adrenal cortices remain depleted of cholesterol and ascorbic acid well into the recovery period, which has been interpreted to mean that production and secretion of cortical hormones continue at a high rate.

This interpretation received support from the striking similarities in the changes in protein metabolism which are produced by injury, on the one hand, and by the injection of certain cortical steroids into fasted normal or adrenalectomised animals, on the other. Long, Katzin and Fry[88] showed in 1940 that such injections brought about a marked increase in nitrogen excretion and a simultaneous deposition of glycogen in the liver. Both the nitrogen and the glycogen were apparently derived from tissue protein by the processes which are called "gluconeogenesis". This classical report led to a great number of investigations in which the catabolic effect of adrenal cortical steroids on proteins was confirmed. The steroids which possess this type of activity have an oxygen atom in position 11 on their ring system; one of them is cortisone. FIGURE 5 shows that when a pellet containing cortisone was implanted under the skin of mice, their body weight decreased rapidly during the first 7 days; during this time nitrogen excretion increased sharply, the animals losing more nitrogen than they took in although they consumed 20 per cent more food[89].

The mechanism by which these hormones influence protein metabolism was investigated by Engel.[90] His method was to remove both kidneys from rats and to follow the rate at which urea accumulated in the blood. One of the assumptions upon which these experiments were based is that the blood urea is an end product of protein metabolism. Another is that an animal without kidneys is essentially normal with respect to nitrogen metabolism, at least for some hours. It is impossible to demonstrate whether this is true, but there cannot be much doubt that the kidney has a lively and idiosyncratic nitrogen metabolism of its own. In man about 10 g. of amino-nitrogen must be filtered by the glomeruli each day and over 90 per cent of this is reabsorbed. The reabsorption process differs for different amino-acids[91], so that the amino-acids must be involved in different metabolic transformations in the cells of the tubules. Even if such transformations affect only a fraction of the reabsorbed material, they could have a marked effect on nitrogen metabolism as a whole because the amount of amino-acid reabsorbed per day corresponds to about 100 g. of protein.

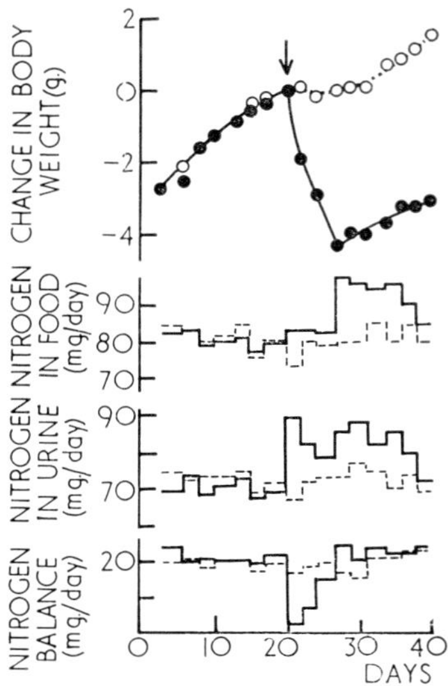

11/Fig. 5.—Effect of cortisone acetate on castrated mice. Cortisone acetate was implanted subcutaneously as a 13–15 mg. pellet at the time indicated by the arrow. The values for the control mice are indicated by the broken lines, and those of the mice treated with cortisone by the solid lines. Body weights of the control mice shown by open circles, those of cortisone-treated mice by solid circles. Ten mice in each group. The mean body weights of both groups before treatment were very similar. Therefore, the values for the control groups are masked in the graph. (After Kochakian *et al.*[89])

In the nephrectomised rats used by Engel the rate of accumulation of urea in the blood during the first few hours remained so constant that changes as small as 0·5 mg. urea nitrogen/100 g. body weight per hour were significant. Engel showed that the injection of adrenal cortical extract or cortisone increased the rate of urea formation. He then found that this increase was abolished when glucose was given—an experimental equivalent to the clinical observation that eating carbohydrate in the period of traumatic inflammation reduces the excessive loss of nitrogen from the body. In contrast, when insulin was injected and the blood sugar concentration thereby reduced, rats treated with cortical hormones showed a spectacular increase in the rate of urea production. It is clear, therefore, that the blood sugar concentration controls, at least in part, the effectiveness of the cortical hormones in nitrogen metabolism.

In a series of beautiful experiments Engel demonstrated further that the adrenal cortical hormones exert their effect on the breakdown of proteins rather than on that of amino-acids. Figure 6 summarises some of his results. When human serum albumin was injected into nephrectomised rats together with adrenal cortical extract, urea production increased and this increase was abolished by glucose. In contrast, although the injection of amino-acids also increased urea production, this increase was not abolished by glucose. When the liver was removed as well as the kidneys, amino-acids accumulated in the blood instead of urea; again, adrenal cortical extract increased the rate of accumulation

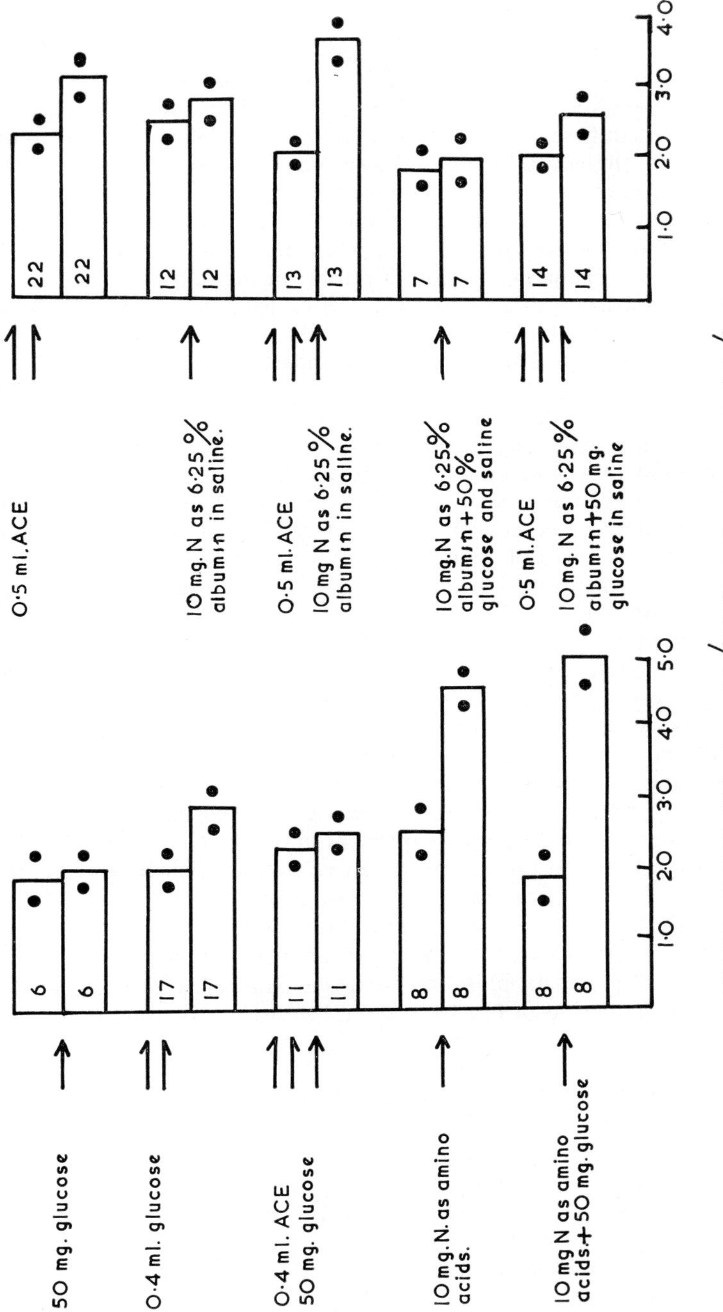

11/FIG. 6.—Rate of production of urea in rats 0–3 hr. (upper column of each pair) and 3–6 hr. (lower column) after nephrectomy. Numbers of rats shown in the columns, standard error by the dots. ACE means adrenal cortical extract. (After Engel.[90])

and glucose abolished this increase. This showed that the liver is not necessary for the inhibiting effect of glucose on the breakdown of body protein.

All this evidence is compatible with the view that the adrenal cortical hormones exert their effect on the control of protein breakdown in the tissues. Which tissues? The answer is not completely known. Mice under the influence of cortisone lose protein from muscle and lymphoid tissue. When corticotrophin is injected into dogs, the concentration of amino-acids in the plasma increases and the relative concentrations of the different amino-acids are smilar to those in striated muscle.[92] It seems probable, therefore, that proteins in several tissues contribute to the excessive loss of nitrogen, with muscle contributing most in absolute terms because of the great mass of muscle in the body.

Attempts to demonstrate that the cortical hormones increase the activity of proteolytic enzymes *in vitro* have been unsuccessful.

When corticotrophin or hydrocortisone is administered to patients for various clinical conditions, the expected excess of nitrogen excreted over nitrogen ingested is usually, but by no means always, observed. It seems that the magnitude of the nitrogen loss depends upon the patient's previous state of nutrition, his present diet, and upon the kind and severity of the disease for which he is being treated. These clinical findings concur with experimental work which shows that under some conditions excess of adrenal cortical hormones can actually *increase* the rates of protein synthesis, for instance in regenerating liver. These results are mentioned in order to point out that not only the excessive breakdown of protein but also the increased rate of protein turnover seen after injury may involve the adrenal cortical hormones.

In the recovery period the blood sugar concentration is usually raised, partly because glucose is produced from catabolised protein and partly because, as in the earlier periods, the utilisation of glucose is diminished, an effect also mediated by adrenal cortical hormones. Since carbohydrate inhibits the breakdown of protein, the increase in the blood sugar concentration may be thought of as a stabilising or homeostatic state for slowing the excessive destruction of protein. At the same time the respiratory quotient may fall. This is usually taken to mean that the oxidation of fat increases relative to that of carbohydrate. But this may be an over-simplification for the respiratory quotient would also decrease if less carbohydrate were converted to fat or if more fat were converted into carbohydrate. There is evidence that both conversions do, in fact, occur under the influence of corticotrophin and cortisone. Injured mice begin to lose body fat only after the period of intense protein breakdown is over.

The Mode of Action of the Adrenal Cortical Hormones

In the absence of both adrenal glands, these metabolic disturbances do not appear. We have seen that the changes in nitrogen metabolism produced by injury can be imitated experimentally by treating normal animals with certain cortical steroids and that the analysis of this effect strongly suggests that the accelerated protein breakdown following injury is due to the action of these hormones. We have given the evidence that injury leads to increased excretion of adrenal cortical steroids in the urine. In 1946 Selye discovered that injury causes hypertrophy of the adrenal glands as well as atrophy of the thymus and of other lymphoid tissues[27] which was later shown to be induceable by injecting corticotropin or cortisone-like steroids.

All this evidence led Selye to the hypothesis that the metabolic changes which follow every type of injury, or "stress" as he called it, were caused by an increase in the rate of secretion of adrenal cortical hormones into the blood stream. In 1947 Ingle, Ward and Kuizenga[93] obtained results which were inconsistent with this hypothesis. They removed the adrenal glands from rats and maintained them on a constant dose of adrenal cortical extract which, in itself, did not alter the excretion of nitrogen. When the leg bones of such a rat were fractured there was a marked increase in the non-protein nitrogen concentration in the urine. Here, evidently, the increased loss of nitrogen could not be related to increased amounts of cortical hormones in the blood, because there were no adrenal glands to secrete them.

On the basis of these experiments, Ingle proposed a different hypothesis, according to which the hormones of the adrenal cortex are necessary for but not quantitaively related to the increased nitrogen excretion after injury. The validity of this proposition has been established by a large amount of experimental and clinical evidence. Although adrenalectomised rats maintained on saline do not lose excess nitrogen after injury, they do so if maintained instead on small amounts of cortisone which by themselves are insufficient to increase nitrogen loss. Indeed, adrenalectomised animals maintained on a small but constant quantity of glucocorticoid hormone respond when injured with the same changes in carbohydrate metabolism and destruction of lymphoid tissue, as well as in nitrogen excretion, as do normal animals. The effect of injury on protein metabolism is almost entirely abolished by protein depletion; this does not diminish the loss of nitrogen provoked by cortisone.[94] Pellets containing 25 mg. of cortisone as the acetate were implanted under the skin of rats, while other rats suffered fracture of the femur. In both groups of animals the increase in the excretion of nitrogen was the same. The response to 50 mg. of implanted cortisone was greater than that to 25 mg., and almost identical to the response to 25 mg. plus fracture.[95] However, most of the response to fracture or to 25 mg. cortisone appeared to result simply from the incision through the skin and from subsequent manipulations. The additional response to a third 25 mg. pellet was very slight.

In man after uncomplicated surgery, the rise in the concentration of glucocorticoid hormones in the plasma is often over after one day whereas the increase in nitrogen loss reaches its maximum several days later.[28] A patient suffering from high blood pressure was treated by having first one and then the other of his suprarenal glands removed. For several days before and after the second operation he was given a constant amount (200 mg.) of cortisone acetate each day. FIGURE 7 shows that 2–4 days after removal of the second suprarenal gland the patient lost excessive amounts of nitrogen and potassium in the urine, but he retained sodium—all changes known to be mediated by adrenal cortical hormones but in this case obviously not due to their hypersecretion.[96]

Interpretations of the Effects of Injury which involve the Adrenal Cortical Hormones

As in all fields of research, the study of the metabolic effects of injury has been led from one experiment to the next by the use of working hypotheses, which are tentative explanations of experimental results. Apart from working hypotheses, some generalising propositions have been put forward which must now be briefly considered, bearing in mind that facts are still few and their interrelationships certainly complex.

The adrenal cortex is at the centre of both the interpretations to be considered. The reasons for this are, firstly, the long-established fact that when the

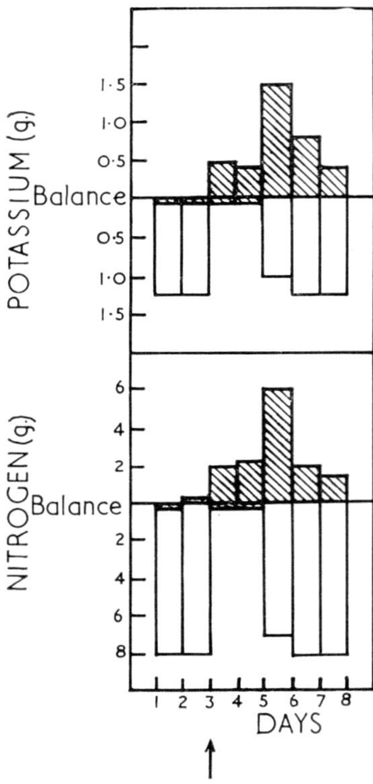

11/FIG. 7.—Balances of potassium and nitrogen before and after removal of the second suprarenal gland from a patient treated with 200 mg. of cortisone acetate per day. The arrow indicates the time of operation. Hatched areas represent loss. The areas below the balance line represent intake. In loss, urinary excretion is therefore indicated by the sum of the clear and hatched areas. (After Robson *et al.*[96])

adrenal glands are absent or diseased, the effects of injury are far worse than when the glands are functioning; and secondly, the mass of evidence already discussed which indicates that the metabolic effects of injury involve in some way the adrenal cortical hormones.

Selye[27] included the pattern of metabolic responses to injury in what he called the "alarm reaction", which is shown by every animal when subjected to "stress". He supposed that the alarm reaction was only the first stage of a sequence of generally recognisable reactions to which he gave the name of "general adaptation syndrome". Selye claimed that the metabolic responses of the alarm reaction were due to the excessive secretion of adrenal cortical hormones. However, as we have seen, this cannot be correct since the magnitude of the metabolic responses is not related directly to the amount of hormone available provided a certain minimum quantity is present.

Engel[90] has proposed an alternative interpretation which may be put as follows: He assumes that the function of the adrenal cortical hormones, like that of other hormones, is to maintain the steady states of normal metabolism, that is, to maintain homeostasis. The metabolic responses to injury are thought of as homeostatic reactions, in the sense that they are somehow necessary to bring back normal conditions. It seems, then, that the adrenal cortical hormones facilitate the homeostatic reactions which are brought about by the stimulus of injury. A certain minimum concentration of hormone is necessary for the facilitation to occur at all. An excess of hormone brings about an excessive response, such as, for example, a large loss of nitrogen after an injury so mild that in the presence of less hormone the nitrogen loss would have been minimal or absent. Such a complex relationship between the intensity of the injury, the amount of adrenal cortical hormone available and the magnitude of metabolic responses has to be postulated in order to account for the known facts.

Summary

The metabolic reactions to injury are, first, a brief hyperactivity associated with the release of adrenaline and possessing therefore the features of an emergency reaction; next, the metabolic depression associated with clinical shock, the cause of which is so far unknown and during which death frequently occurs; and finally, the prolonged hyperactivity occurring during the period of traumatic inflammation, in which damaged tissues undergo necrosis and autolysis after which the processes of repair begin. This period is marked by an extraordinary increase in protein metabolism which is mediated by the hormones of the adrenal cortex. More generally, the metabolic disturbances come about mainly through changes in the hormonal steady state which control metabolism in normal animals. The functional significance of these disturbances is not yet understood.

REFERENCES

1. Cannon, W. B. (1923). *Traumatic Shock.* New York: Appleton-Century.
2. Grant, R. T. and Reeves, E. B. (1951). *Spec. Rep. Ser. med. Res. Coun.* (*Lond.*), No. **277**.
3. Cuthbertson, D. P. (1942). *Lancet*, **1,** 433.
4. Cuthbertson, D. P. (1930). *Biochem. J.*, **24,** 1244.
5. Williamson, M. B., McCarthy, T., and Fromm, H. (1951). *Fed. Proc.*, **10,** 270.
6. Beloff, A., and Peters, R. A. (1945). *J. Physiol.* (*Lond.*), **103,** 461.
7. Lewis, G. P. (1967). *J. Physiol.* (*Lond.*), **191,** 591.
8. Fine, J. (1961). *Fed. Proc.*, **20,** 166.
9. Green, H. N., Stoner, H. B., Whitely, H. J., and Eglin, D. (1949). *Clin. Sci.*, **8,** 65.
10. Stoner, H. B. (1961). *Fed. Proc.*, **20,** 38.
11. Noble, R. L., and Collip, J. B. (1942). *Quart. J. exp. Physiol.*, **31,** 187.
12. Russell, J. A., Long, C. N. H., and Wilhelmi, A. E. (1944). *J. exp. Med.*, **79,** 23.
13. Rosenthal, S. M., and Tabor, H. (1945). *Arch. Surg.* (*Chicago*), **51,** 244.
14. Arturson, G. (1961). *Acta chir. scand.*, Supp.. 274.
15. Cori, C. F. (1931). *Physiol. Rev.*, **11,** 143.
16. Pekkarinen, A. (1960). In *The Biochemical Response to Injury*, p. 217, Oxford: Blackwell Scientific Publications.
17. Steinberg, G. (1966). *Pharmacol. Rev.*, **18,** 217 (see p. 231).

18. Born, G. V. R., and Philp, R. B. (1965). *Brit. J. exp. Path.*, **46**, 569.
19. Vogt, M. (1943). *J. Physiol. (Lond.)*, **102**, 341.
20. Long, C. N. H., and Fry, E. G. (1945). *Proc. Soc. exp. Biol. (N.Y.)*, **59**, 67.
21. Vogt, M. (1952). *J. Physiol. (Lond.)*, **118**, 588.
22. de Groot, J., and Harris, G. W. (1950). *J. Physiol. (Lond.)*, **111**, 335.
23. Hume, D. M., and Wittenstein, G. J. (1950). In *Proceedings of First Clinical ACTH Conference*, p. 134, Philadelphia: Blakiston.
24. McCann, W. M. (1953). *Amer. J. Physiol.*, **175**, 13.
25. Tepperman, J., Engel, F. L., and Long, C. N. H. (1943). *Endocrinology*, **32**, 373.
26. Venning, E. H., Hoffmann, M. M., and Browne, J. S. L. (1944). *Endocrinology*, **35**, 49.
27. Selye, J. (1946). *J. clin. Endocr.*, **6**, 117.
28. Cooper, C. E., and Nelson, D. H. (1962). *J. clin. Invest.*, **41**, 1599.
29. Wilson, G. M. (1955). *Proc. roy. Soc. Med.*, **48**, 819.
30. Cohnheim, J. (1890). *Lectures on General Pathology*, p. 1326. London: New Sydenham Society.
31. Stoner, H. B., and Pullar, J. D. (1963). *Brit. J. exp. Path.*, **44**, 586.
32. Grayson, J., and Mendel, D. (1956). *J. Physiol. (Lond.)*, **133**, 334.
33. Stoner, H. B. (1958). *Brit. J. exp. Path.*, **39**, 251.
34. Stoner, H. B. (1960). *The Biochemical Response to Injury*, p. 124. Eds. Stoner, H. B., and Threlfall, C. J. Oxford: Blackwell Scientific Publications.
35. Tabor, H., and Rosenthal, S. M. (1947), *Amer. J. Physiol.*, **149**, 449.
36. Stoner, H. B. (1968). *Ann. N.Y. Acad. Sci.* In the Press.
37. Krebs, H. A., and Kornberg, H. L. (1957). *Ergebn, Physiol.*, **49**, 212.
38. Lehninger, A. L. (1953). *Harvey Lect.*, **49**, 176,
39. Aldridge, W. N., and Stoner, H. B. (1960). *Biochem. J.*, **74**, 148.
40. Wilhelmi, A. E. (1948). *Ann. Rev. Physiol.*, **10**, 259.
41. Ennor, A. H., and Rosenberg, H. (1952). *Biochem. J.*, **59**, 272.
42. Ord, M. G., and Stocken, L. A. (1955). *Biochem. J.*, **50**, 272.
43. Bielschowsky, M., and Green, H. N. (1943). *Lancet*, **2**, 153.
44. Macfarlane, M. G., and Spooner, S. J. L. (1946). *Brit. J. exp. Path.*, **27**, 339.
45. Bollman, J. L., and Flock, E. V. (1944). *Amer. J. Physiol.*, **142**, 290.
46. Green, H. N. (1943). *Lancet*, **2**, 147.
47. Kalckar, H. M., and Lowry, O. H. (1947). *Amer. J. Physiol.*, **149**, 240.
48. Threlfall, C. J., and Stoner, H. B. (1957). *Brit. J. exp. Path.*, **38**, 339.
49. Lepage, G. A. (1946). *Amer. J. Physiol.*, **147**, 446.
50. Stoner, H. B., and Threlfall, C. J. (1954). *Biochem. J.*, **58**, 115.
51. Lardy, H. A. (1955). In *Conferences et Rapports of the Third International Congress of Biochemistry*, p. 287. Liege: Vaillant-Carmanne.
52. Stoner, H. B., Threlfall, C. J., and Green, H. N. (1952). *Brit. J. exp. Path.*, **33**, 131.
53. Threlfall, C. H., and Stoner, H. B. (1954). *Quart. J. exp. Physiol.*, **39**, 1.
54. Sutherland, E. W. (1951). *Ann. N.Y. Acad. Sci.*, **54**, 693.
55. Stoner, H. B., Heath, D. F., and Collins, O. M. (1960). *Biochem. J.*, **76**, 135.
56. Ashby, M. M., Heath, D. F., and Stoner, H. B. (1965). *J. Physiol. (Lond.)*, **179**, 193.
57. Engel, C. F. (1951). *Amer. J. Med.*, **10**, 556.
58. Chiu, C. Y., and Needham, D. M. (1950). *Biochem. J.*, **46**, 114.
59. Wiggers, C. J. (1950). *Physiology of Shock*. Cambridge, Mass: Harvard Univ. Press.
60. Levenson, S. M., Einheber, A., and Malm, O. J. (1961). *Fed. Proc.*, **20**, 99.
61. Millican, R. C. (1960). In *The Biochemical Response to Injury*, p. 269. Oxford: Blackwell Scientific Publications.

62. ROSENTHAL, S. M. (1960). *The Biochemical Response to Injury*, p. 397. Eds. STONER, H. B., and THRELFALL, C. J. Oxford: Blackwell Scientific Publications.
63. HAIST, R. E., and HAMILTON, J. (1944). *J. Physiol.* (*Lond.*), **102,** 471.
63*a*. MONRO, H. N., CLARK, C. M., and GOODLAD, G. A. J. (1961). *Biochem. J.*, **80,** 453.
64. SELYE, H., and DOSNE, C. (1941). *Proc. Soc. exp. Biol.* (*N.Y.*), **47,** 143.
65. RUSSELL, J. A., LONG, C. N. H., and ENGEL, F. L. (1944). *J. exp. Med.*, **79,** 1.
66. ENGEL, F. L., HARRISON, H. C., and LONG, C. N. H. (1944). *J. exp. Med.*, **79,** 9.
67. RUSSELL, J. A., and LONG, C. N. H. (1946). *Amer. J. Physiol.*, **147,** 175.
68. KLINE, D. L. (1946). *Amer. J. Physiol.*, **146,** 654.
69. SPINK, W. W. (1960). In *The Biochemical Response to Injury*, p. 361. Oxford: Blackwell Scientific Publications.
70. TABOR, H., and ROSENTHAL, W. M. (1945). *Pub. Hlth. Rep.*(*Wash.*), **60,** 401.
71. LANDIS, E. M. (1928). *Amer. J. Physiol.*, **83,** 528.
72. BORN, G. V. R. (1954). *J. Physiol.* (*Lond.*), **124,** 502.
73. MILES, A. A. (1951). *J. Physiol.* (*Lond.*), **114,** 34P.
74. HENDLEY, E. D., and SCHILLER, A. A. (1954). *Amer. J. Physiol.*, **179,** 216.
75. WHIPPLE, G. H., SMITH, H. P., and BELT, A. E. (1920). *Amer. J. Physiol.*, **52,** 72.
76. GREGERSEN, M. I. (1946). *Ann. Rev. Physiol.*, **8,** 335.
77. WILHELMI, A. E., RUSSEL, J. A., ENGEL, F. L., and LONG, C. N. H. (1945). *Amer. J. Physiol.*, **144,** 669.
78. CUTHBERTSON, D. P. (1932). *Quart. J. Med.*, **25,** 233.
79. BAUER, J. (1872). *Z. Biol.*, **8,** 567.
80. CUTHBERTSON, D. P. (1954). *Brit. med. Bull.*, **10,** 33.
81. MUNRO, H. N., and CUTHBERTSON, D. P. (1943). *Biochem. J.*, **37,** xii.
82. BORSOOK, H., and DUBNOFF, J. W. (1943). *Ann. Rev. Biochem.*, **12,** 183.
83. CUTHBERTSON, D. P , MCGIRR, J. L., and ROBERTSON, J. S. M. (1939). *Quart. J. exp. Physiol.*, **29,** 13.
84. SAYERS, G., SAYERS, M A., LIANG, T. Y., and LONG, C. N. H. (1945). *Endocrinology*, **37,** 96.
85. FISHER, R. B. (1954). *Protein Metabolism.* London: Methuen.
86. MILLER, L. L. (1948). *J. biol. Chem.*, **172,** 113; and (1950). *J. biol. Chem.*, **186,** 253.
87. YUILE, C. L., LUCAS, F. V., JONES, C. K., CHOPIN, S. J., and WHIPPLE, G. H. (1953). *J. exp. Med.*, **98,** 173.
88. LONG, C. N. H., KATZIN, B., and FRY, E. G. (1940). *Endocrinology*, **26,** 309.
89. KOCHAKIAN, C. D., and ROBERTSON, E. (1951). *J. biol. Chem.*, **190,** 481.
90. ENGEL, F. L. (1951). *Recent Progr. Hormone Res.*, **6,** 277.
91. SMITH, H. W. (1951). *The Kidney*, Chap. 5. New York: Oxford Univ. Press.
92. LOTSPEICH, W. D. (1950). *J. biol. Chem.*, **185,** 22.
93. INGLE, D. J., WARD, E. O., and KUIZENGA, M. H. (1947). *Amer. J. Physiol.*, **149,** 510.
94. GOODLAD, G. A. J., and MUNRO, H. N. (1959). *Biochem. J.*, **73,** 343.
95. CAMPBELL, R. N., SHARP, G. M. E., BOYNE, A. W., and CUTHBERTSON, D. P. (1953). *Nature* (*Lond.*), **172,** 158.
96. ROBSON, J. S., HORN, D. B., DUDLEY, H. A., and STEWART, C. P. (1955). *Lancet*, **2,** 325.

Chapter 12

ŒDEMA

By K. B. Roberts

When a part of the body is swollen by an accumulation of excess fluid in the intercellular tissue spaces, it is said to be œdematous. Hydrops and dropsy are other names occasionally used to describe œdema. When the excess fluid is found in the serous cavities it is specially named; as, hydrothorax, hydropericardium, or, if the fluid is in the peritoneal cavity, ascites. A generalised dropsical condition of the limbs together with ascites is called anasarca. The limbs may swell by as much as 10 per cent before the condition is clinically noticeable. Œdema is usually recognised by pressing firmly on a suspected part for several seconds when the excess fluid between the cells is pushed away leaving an indentation. This is called pitting œdema (Fig. 1).

Œdema may arise by a redistribution of the fluids available, with the

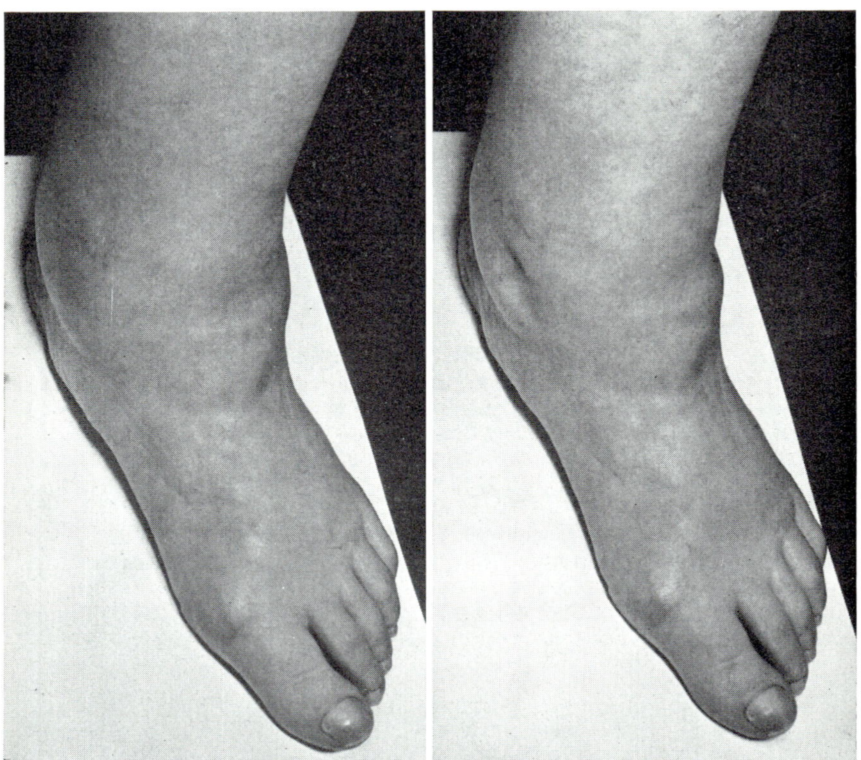

12/Fig. 1.—Pitting œdema. The ankle of an œdematous patient before and after pressing firmly with the thumb over the internal maleolus.

formation of a localised swelling. On the other hand, it may be associated with an increase in the total amount of fluid in the body. In this case renal and other factors which regulate total water and salt balance must be involved. A physician may be forewarned of a generalised œdema in such cases by a marked daily increase in weight caused by the retained fluid.

It is necessary to consider at first the physiological balances of fluid formation and absorption in normal tissue and then the regulation of the total extracellular volume in a normal individual. Against this background, an attempt can be made to present the functional derangements in various types of œdema.

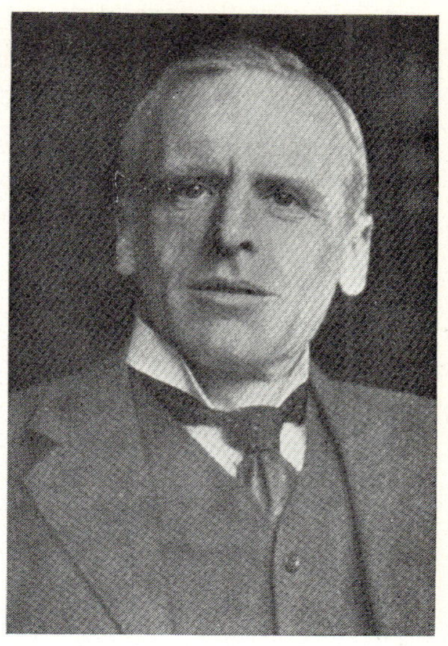

12/Fig. 2.—E. H. Starling.

Tissue Fluid Formation

Starling (Fig. 2) proposed, at the end of the last century, a hypothesis which now goes by his name. In 1895 he wrote a paper in the *Journal of Physiology* entitled "On the Absorption of Fluids from the Connective Tissue Spaces".[1] In this he suggested that, while water and salts would pass through the capillary wall with ease, the proteins of the plasma were retained within the capillary vessels in most tissues. The flow of water in and out of the capillary depends, he argued, on the hydrostatic pressure of the blood in the vessel forcing fluid out and the osmotic pressure of the plasma proteins drawing fluid in. The balance of these two forces was later thought to cause fluid to leave the capillary at the arterial end and to enter at the venous end. Direct measurement of those factors by Landis[2] in single capillaries of the frog's mesentery showed that this general statement is true (Fig. 3). It is to be noticed that at a hydrostatic pressure of 12 cm. of water, fluid neither enters nor escapes from the capillary. This is also the osmotic pressure of the frog's plasma proteins. That the same general condition also holds for mammals is shown in Table I. In each case the osmotic pressure of the plasma proteins lies between the capillary blood pressure at the arterial end and that at the venous

12/Table I

Colloid Osmotic Pressures of Plasma Proteins and Capillary Pressures of Three Mammals

		Rat	*Guinea-pig*	*Man*
Colloid Osmotic Pressure (cm. H_2O)		25	26·7	36
Cap. Pressure (cm. H_2O):	Arterial	30	38·5	43·5
	Venous	17	17	16·5

(*From H. Davson*[40]).

end. It should be stressed that these blood pressures are the mean of a number of determinations, and that the conditions essentially relate to the capillary bed of a tissue over a period of time and not necessarily to a particular capillary at a particular time.

The same generalisation applies to the experiments of Pappenheimer and Soto-Rivera.[3] They suspended isolated perfused hind limbs of dogs and cats from a sensitive recording balance. The venous pressure, arterial pressure and

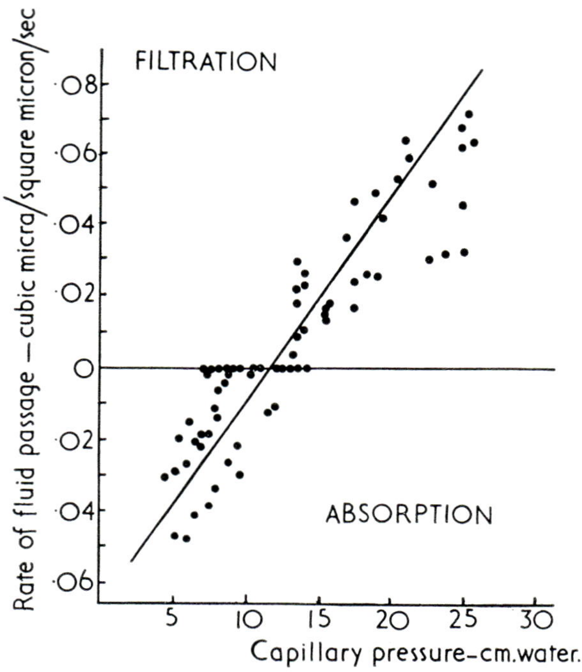

12/FIG. 3.—The influence of capillary hydrostatic pressure on the exchange of fluid across the capillary wall. (From Landis.[2])

protein osmotic pressure could be varied independently, while net filtration or absorption of fluid through the capillary bed was indicated by a gain or a loss in weight of the limb. They showed that Starling's principle might be applied with precision to such experimental conditions. When neither filtration nor absorption was occurring, that is with isogravimetric flow, the mean capillary pressure was found to approximate very closely (95 $\pm$ 5 per cent) to the colloid osmotic pressure as measured *in vitro*.

A net transport of water across the capillary membrane will occur in response to the factors outlined by Starling; with this water various solutes will move. However, water and dissolved substances may move not only under the influence of this filtration process, but also by processes which physiologists have called diffusion. It has been observed, for instance, that dyes may escape from a capillary along a concentration gradient even though a net absorption of fluid into that capillary was taking place. In the tissues, diffusion will move substances at a much faster rate than the "filtration-absorption" mechanism. If a rat is given water containing a small proportion of the tritium equivalent,[3] H_2O, to drink the label rises rapidly to a plateau in the plasma; by 15 minutes it has distributed itself throughout the entire body water.[4] From other studies it is apparent that three-quarters of the water in the plasma is moved every minute across the capillary membrane by diffusion without a net transport of water; only a minute faction of the plasma volume is moved with an actual change of volume by fluid leaving the capillaries.[5]

This discussion should be interrupted to ask what is the functional anatomy of the capillary bed, for it is here that the excess fluid of an œdematous person is eventually formed. At a first glance, as for example at the circulation seen in the web of a frog's foot, it would appear to be a uniformly distributed network. However, on closer examination some capillary beds are seen to be structurally orientated into a more precise arrangement.[6] Contraction or relaxation of those blood vessels which lead to the capillaries will obviously alter the pressure within; this probably occurs from time to time even in normal resting tissue of some animals, where it is called vasomotion. It is certain that, in an active area, the capillary bed opens widely. Conditions in a particular capillary, therefore, may favour transudation along its entire length, while reabsorption may be predominant in others. If the capillary bed retains the proteins of the plasma within the vessel, then according to the Starling hypothesis and the figures quoted from Landis and from Pappenheimer, little excess fluid will be formed. If, however, the permeability of the capillary wall is increased towards protein, this will pass into the tissue spaces and the effective osmotic pressure tending to draw fluid back into the blood will be reduced. In this way, excess fluid will begin to accumulate in the intercellular spaces and the process, if continued, will cause an œdema of the part.

Through what part of the capillary do substances leave the blood for the tissue fluids? It is apparent that the lipid-soluble and lipid-insoluble substances behave differently: the rate of movement of molecules soluble in lipid is very much faster than that of even small lipid-insoluble molecules.[7] It would seem that the whole of the capillary wall is permeable to fat-soluble substances. It has been suggested that the relative impermeability of lipid-insoluble substances is due to their passage through a restricted area of the capillary, possibly the intercellular area, and not through the cells themselves. The arguments in support of this are partly theoretical and partly derived from observation of ultrastructure in electron microscope pictures.

The capillary allows free passage of sodium and potassium ions, for example, at similar fast rates. But, as is well known, muscle cells, cells of the nervous system and even erythrocytes retain their functional integrity because of a highly selective permeability to these two ions. It would be strange if the living capillary endothelial cell differed from the cells which have been investigated. Pappenheimer and others[8] have calculated from data derived from experiments with perfused hind limbs, that the area available for filtration or diffusion of lipid-insoluble substances is only a small fraction of the total surface area of the capillary. He estimates that, of some 5,000 sq. feet of capillary surface in the body, only 10 or 11 sq. feet are apparently available. Thus the possibilities are that diffusion and filtration takes place through limited areas.

Electron microscopic evidence relevant to these arguments have been made on the smallest blood vessels of capillary beds (see Chapter 3). It has become apparent that the fine structure of these vessels varies from region to region. In the liver the endothelial wall is deficient and this is probably correlated with the high permeability to macromolecules so that liver lymph contains almost as much protein as plasma. In many sites however, for example in muscle, one endothelial cell abuts on its neighbour very much as other close-packed cells do with a gap of about 100 Å, This fine, intercellular cleft is apparently obstructed by tight junctions, or zona occludentes. If substances are to pass down this winding cleft they will have to do so in solution and the cleft must therefore be water-filled; moreover the tight junctions must not represent a complete barrier. There is evidence that a foreign marker protein—a peroxidase from horse-radish with a molecular weight of 40,000—makes its way down this cleft after intravenous injection and that the tight junctions allow the passage of molecules smaller than 45 Å.[9]

Two other properties of endothelial membranes of the micro-circulation have become apparent through electron microscopy. One is the functional importance of the basement membrane which proves to be a barrier to the movement of white cells during diapedesis. It may also restrict the movement of particles but seems to allow many smaller proteins to pass through unimpeded. Electron microscope pictures have also revealed that the endothelial cells of the capillary bed are capable of some degree of pinocytosis; this is a process in which droplets of the surrounding medium are taken into the cell. In the capillary these droplets may pass across the cell to be discharged at the tissue surface. The quantitative importance of the process has not been accurately estimated, and indeed it is difficult to measure dynamic processes from still pictures of fixed tissue. Pinocytosis may explain the presence of very high molecular weight substances in the tissue fluids and lymph.

With regard to permeability, the capillary is most easily thought of as a sieve with holes of a diameter small enough to exclude larger molecules. This conception, based essentially on a *statistical* evaluation of what goes through a whole capillary bed during a period of time, would seem to be a simplified and static explanation of what is probably a dynamic state. The permeability has been shown to vary with the degree of oxygenation of the blood and to some extent with the pressure inside the vessel. Remembering this qualification, an estimate of pore size has been arrived at by Pappenheimer and his colleagues.[8] An average pore radius of 30 Å would account for many of the observed properties of capillaries in the limbs of dogs and cats. This does not differ very much from the EM evidence relating to mouse muscle where the barrier seems to be the tight junction gap of 40 Å or so.

In a tissue such as muscle the volume of tissue fiuid is small compared with the volume of the cells. It is therefore difficult to obtain an unequivocal specimen. (Some critics indeed doubt whether free tissue fluid exists in the normal limb, suggesting that the fluid is held as a gel with mucoproteins.) Its supposed composition is inferred from lymph or from certain types of excess fluid. It is certain that in the limbs the vessel wall normally retains all but small amounts of protein, and it is thought that the total concentration in the extracellular fluid is about 0·3 g. per cent, most of which is albumin.[10] Liver lymph, as we have seen, contains a high proportion of protein. It has been estimated from studies on labelled protein[11] that 0·1 per cent of the plasma albumin leaves the vessels each minute to return to the blood, for the most part in the thoracic duct. This internal circulation of protein will play an important part in the economy of the tissue cells; in their nutrition and, in the case of protein hormones, their regulation by endocrine glands.

Ideally we should discuss the problems of fluid transfer between the tissue spaces and the cells themselves. The permeability of cell membranes is a problem engaging the attention of general physiologists; the information gained is now beginning to be applied to the pathology of mammalian tissues.

Lymphatic Drainage

The escape of fluid and its partial re-entry into the capillary bed has been considered. Some of the fluid, however, is taken up from the tissue spaces into lymphatics. These will carry away any protein, for such large molecules will not pass back across the capillary membrane against a diffusion gradient. Dissection in the anatomy room does not usually show lymph vessels; they are moreover inconspicuous in microscopical sections of normal tissue. In consequence, the importance of these vessels is neglected by the admirable student who trusts his eyes and not his textbooks. However, in living tissue, the lymphatics may be seen to form an extensive network permeating almost all tissues. This has been fully described in Chapter 3. In œdematous tissue, lymphatics are widely dilated, being kept open by their attachments to the surrounding connective tissue. In long-standing œdema, the valves of the lymphatics may become incompetent, thus disposing to an impaired clearing of tissue fluids.

General Fluid Balance

Lastly, from a physiological point of view, we would wish to know what regulates the total volume of extracellular fluid; that is, the volume of plasma and all the interstitial tissue fluids together. The Starling hypothesis well describes fluid exchange between plasma and tissues, but it gives no indication of the mechanisms which have as a specific function the regulation of the total amount of fluid in the body. These are of course primarily thirst, governing fluid intake, and the kidney, which varies the amount of fluid lost to the body. Secondarily, it involves the secretions of the posterior pituitary and the adrenal cortical hormones. The isolation of aldosterone,[12] the adrenal cortical hormone highly active in promoting the retention of sodium by the kidney, was an important advance in this field. Increased aldosterone formation occurs, for example, physiologically in salt-deprivation, after excessive sweating or after hæmorrhage. But the processes are incompletely known whereby the required amount of fluid is taken and the appropriate quantity lost in the urine, so that the volume of the extracellular fluid is normally kept within narrow limits. Variations in the ionic composition of the extracellular fluid, as appreciated by osmoreceptors, will account for water diuresis and the inhibition of urine flow in dehydration.[13] Œdema, however, is usually the result of a retention of a fluid of similar osmotic proportions to normal extracellular fluid. What is it that prevents us all becoming œdematous? This homeostatic mechanism may be mediated by receptors in the cardiovascular system. An increase or decrease in the extracellular fluid volume, and hence the blood volume, and perhaps the distribution of blood, may lead to a change in the rate of formation of aldosterone and consequently to changes in sodium and water excretion. In this way the excretion of salts by the kidney does not necessarily depend on the plasma concentrations. The adrenal nerves apparently play no part in such reactions for an increased aldosterone formation occurs with low sodium diets even from transplanted adrenal glands. The control of aldosterone release then is effectively brought about by a humoral substance. The hormone is not A.C.T.H. for this has little direct effect on the zone glomerulosa of the adrenal cortex where aldosterone is produced. The site of origin of the physiological aldosterone-releasing hormone is not known for sure, but there is evidence to suggest that the renin-angiotensin system is involved. Changes in blood flow through the juxtaglomerular apparatus in the kidney cause increased liberation of renin which, acting on the protein precursor normally present in plasma, produces angiotensin. This will cause an increased production of aldosterone.[14] Work is in progress in a number of laboratories to substantiate this working hypothesis.

In various types of dropsy the total extracellular fluid volume is enlarged, but the regulating mechanisms are not completely upset, for œdema does not increase indefinitely. Any consideration of œdema formation is incomplete unless those factors which limit the extent of that œdema are also described.

This introduction recalls only the outline of some relevant physiological matters; there will be an opportunity for further comment when considering particular types of œdema. Clinical œdema is rarely a simple matter. Starling used the following sentence when discussing the factors regulating the fluids of the body: "It is important to remember that probably under no circumstances can dropsy be ascribed to an abnormal change in one only of these processes."[15]

There are many clinically recognised types of œdema, but here we will consider inflammatory œdema, the œdema associated with cardiac and renal failure, the œdema of venous and lymphatic obstruction, famine œdema and pulmonary œdema.

INFLAMMATORY ŒDEMA

This has been discussed in Chapters 2 and 3. There is, in inflamed areas, an intensive hyperæmia. There is also local swelling of the part, due to an excessive production of tissue fluid containing a very high proportion of protein. This protein, and the breakdown of tissues to produce osmotically active smaller molecules, will abolish the osmotic suck of the plasma proteins. The lymph flow is increased and the lymph itself has a high protein content, but an excess of fluid accumulates and the part swells. The increase in tissue tension in the inflammatory area gives rise to much of the pain of inflammation. In this way, the "tumor" and the "dolor" of the classical tetrad are due to the same primary factor: an increased permeability of the capillary to protein. The rise in venous pressure locally will increase this exudate.

Increased permeability to protein, which is the basis of inflammatory œdema, is present in the small venules rather than in the capillaries themselves. This has been shown by correlative studies using light and electron microscopy in situations where the vessels are inflamed.[16] Such work emphasises that the phrase "capillary permeability" must be regarded as shorthand for "permeability of the vessels of the microcirculation".

ŒDEMA OF CARDIAC FAILURE

Patients suffering from circulatory disorders are commonly afflicted with œdema (FIG. 4). This may involve the legs if the patient is ambulant, or the sacral region if he is in bed; its position is determined largely by gravity. The œdema may extend to produce a general anasarca of severe degree. The condition is obviously associated with an increase in total body water. Another type of œdema seen in some cases of failure is one in which a rapid formation of

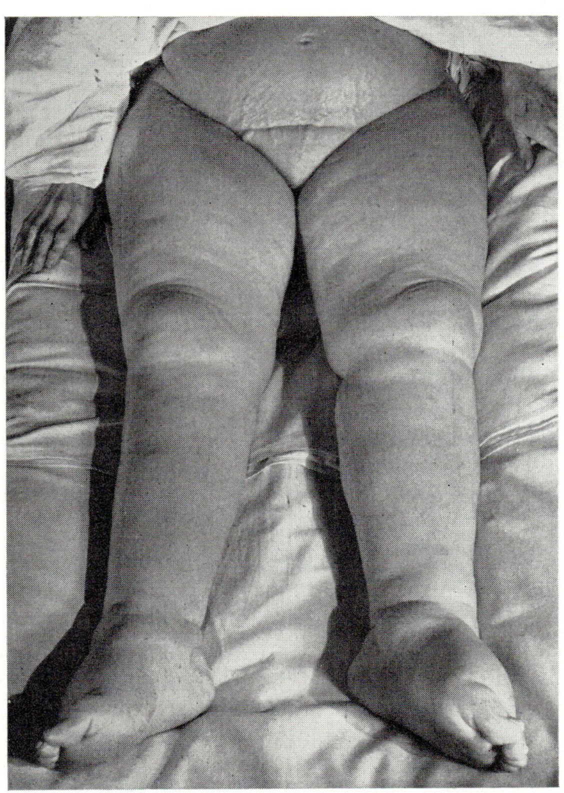

12/FIG. 4.—Gross œdema sometimes seen in cardiac failure.

excess fluid in the alveoli of the lungs leads to pulmonary œdema. There is in this condition a redistribution of body fluids without any significant increase in their total volume. This so-called "left-sided" failure will be considered later: the generalised œdema of congestive cardiac failure is dealt with now. The clinical picture of one type of heart failure commonly seen in Britain is this. After rheumatic fever in childhood or adolescence, a middle-aged man or woman notices breathlessness on exercise that was formerly undertaken with ease. The physician will find, on examination, changes in the heart: the mitral and aortic valves will commonly be damaged. He may find that the patient is breathless on slight exertion or even at rest, and there may be obvious cyanosis. The veins in the neck are engorged while the patient is sitting up, indicating an increased central venous pressure (FIG. 5). There is a diminution in the volume of urine and the quantity of chlorides excreted. If the patient has been active with these symptoms, he will complain that his feet are swollen. There is pitting œdema of the ankle and shin, the liver is engorged and there may be free fluid in the peritoneal cavity. This syndrome of congestive cardiac failure occurs in many types of heart disease.

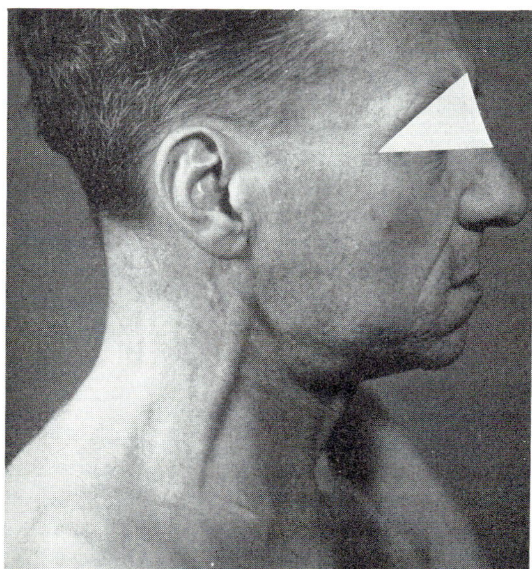

12/FIG. 5.—Heart failure. This picture shows the congested neck veins.

Classically the œdema was explained by a sequence of events embodying a concept of "backward failure". The failing ventricles are unable to deal with the normal venous inflow, and consequently dilate. There is a greater resistance to blood entering the heart. With the consequent rise in central venous pressure, there is a rise in pressure at the venous end of the capillary. This leads to increased transudation of fluid into the tissues and less reabsorption by the capillaries. Œdema follows. The passage of fluid out of the capillaries into the tissues should lead to a fall in the plasma volume and this will, it is said, in turn cause the kidney to conserve water and salt, and so account for the retention of these substances that is observed in cardiac patients.

Some authors, not content with this explanation, suggested a process of "forward failure", in which a diminution in cardiac output causes a tissue anoxia and an increased permeability of capillaries. This, it was said, produces the œdema.

Many who have written in the past on the subject of cardiac failure have attempted to synthesise these two theories of backward and forward failure.

It must be emphasised now that a substantial rise in venous pressure must be a contributing factor in the production of œdema in many cases of heart failure. The factors expressed by Starling are based on known physical principles and must of necessity operate in patients with heart disease as well as in normal persons. A rise in venous pressure is usual in congestive failure; increased transudation of fluid normally follows this, as we have seen already from the work of Landis and others. It has, however, become increasingly difficult to accept this *by itself* as an adequate explanation of the œdema seen in failure of the circulation. It can be shown, for example, that in some cases there is a gain in weight due to incipient œdema before there is any rise in venous pressure centrally.[19] Moreover, as far as can be seen, the œdema usually occurs in association with an increased plasma volume.[17] From the Starling hypothesis a diminution would be expected. In a series of cases there appears to be no consistent relationship between the height of venous pressure and œdema.[18] The ranges of venous pressure in œdematous and non-œdematous cardiac patients have a considerable overlap.

It would seem necessary to examine some factors which might possibly contribute to œdema formation in congestive cardiac failure, remembering Starling's dictum that no single one of these can be expected by itself to explain this œdema.

Plasma proteins.—The level of plasma proteins is low in some cases of cardiac failure, probably due to malnutrition, for in this condition there is frequently nausea and anorexia. But this is not an invariable association. When it occurs it will contribute to œdema formation.

The permeability of the capillaries to protein.—Changes in this property were suggested by earlier writers and embodied in a concept of forward failure, as has been explained. But direct measurement shows that the protein content of the excess fluid remains low.

The oxygen tension in congestive failure does not usually fall low enough to cause an increased capillary permeability. Moreover, any substantial increase in this property throughout the body would lead to a disastrous diminution in plasma volume long before enough fluid had accumulated in the tissues to produce pitting œdema. The concept is therefore untenable in this form.

Tissue pressure.—No reference has yet been made to this quantity.[19] The elasticity of the normal healthy skin and encircling fasciæ maintains the tissues under a measurable tension. This will reduce the effective pressure forcing fluid out of the capillaries; and Starling's first approximation must be modified accordingly. It can be shown by plethysmographic methods that, on standing, the feet and legs of a normal person will swell. Usually this swelling is slight. Increased tissue fluids have been formed, but the process is stopped short by a rapidly mounting tissue tension which opposes the increased capillary hydrostatic pressure. In congestive failure also, the tension in œdematous areas is high, but with a resolution of the œdema it falls. The connective tissue fibres have been stretched, and their elasticity partly destroyed. This will predispose to a recurrence of the œdematous condition. Using the plethysmograph on cardiac patients who have passed through œdematous episodes, it can be shown that, on standing, the swelling of the legs is progressive and not self-limiting as in the normal.

Lymph flow.—McMaster[20] has developed a method by which the lymph flow may be investigated in man. He uses an intracutaneous injection of dye; this finds its way into the local lymph plexus, and "streamers" of dye pass up the limb in the draining lymphatics. In œdematous cardiac patients the local plexuses filled without difficulty, but the absence of streamers suggested that there was a diminished drainage of lymph away from these areas. That this is not a necessary result of the œdema *per se* is shown by an increased drainage found in nephrotic œdema. However, as we have seen, lymphatics take away proteins of the tissue fluids. We would expect therefore, and indeed find, that in the œdema resulting from lymphatic obstruction, the excess fluid has a high protein content. In cardiac œdema, the protein content is low[21]; it is therefore unlikely that impairment of lymphatic drainage in this condition is of any considerable importance.

Venous pressure, extracellular fluid and blood volume.—In cardiac œdema there is an increase in the amount of extracellular fluid due to an increased retention of water and sodium by the kidney. Both compartments of the extracellular fluid (the tissue fluids and the plasma) are enlarged. In cardiac failure, therefore, conditions are favourable for the development of œdema; local factors will determine where the œdema will occur.

It is necessary to consider more carefully the relationship between venous pressure and extracellular fluid. Patients recovering from congestive cardiac failure can be put back into failure by stopping diuretics and adding salt to the diet. The development of œdema can then be followed. Weight and plasma volume rises before there is any increase in central venous pressure, and there is hæmodilution. This is in contradiction to the concept of backward failure, for the venous pressure should rise first to cause, secondarily, an œdema; the blood should become more concentrated. An alternative explanation agreeing with these observations is that the kidney retains sodium and water, the plasma volume rises and there is a consequent increase in venous pressure. It thus becomes important to examine more closely the function of the kidney in heart failure; it is necessary to remember from time to time however that heart failure occurs in patients with diseased hearts.[22]

Renal factors.—All observers agree that the kidney usually retains abnormal amounts of sodium and chloride during cardiac failure. Associated with this is an approximately equivalent volume of water. We have seen that this retention of sodium may be regarded as producing, of itself, the systemic and local conditions necessary for the development of an œdema of this type; namely, an increased extracellular fluid volume and an increased venous pressure.

Failure of the circulation may be considered as a condition in which the output of the heart is insufficient to meet the needs of the tissues. If the metabolic rate is increased, as in hyperthyroidism, the output may be raised and be still inadequate; in other types of heart disease where there is a normal or low metabolic rate, the cardiac output is lowered. How is this inadequacy of output appreciated in the body and what is the relationship between this and the retention of sodium by the kidney? Cardiac output is usually low, moreover the renal blood flow is further reduced by afferent and efferent arteriolar constriction in the glomeruli.[23] Consequently, when the heart fails as a pump, which is the only way in which it can fail, the amount of glomerular filtrate is reduced and sodium may be retained and, with this sodium, water. The resulting increase in extracellular fluid volume may cause both œdema and a rise in venous pressure.

However, it seems likely, though not certain, that any change in glomerular filtration rate is small. (It is not known what changes occur in the perfusion of the juxtaglomerular apparatus.) Abnormal reabsorption of sodium on the part of the tubular cells rather than any fall in glomerular filtration rate is probably responsible for the retention of this ion. It is as yet impossible to say how this is related to impaired cardiac function. There appears to be an increased level of aldosterone in many cases of œdema. The stimulus for this increased formation is not known. In experimental work on dogs, induced heart failure causes an increased production of aldosterone, through the renin-angiotensin system, and consequently an increased retention of sodium and water by the kidney.[24] These findings have formed the basis of the use of the spirolactone drugs in the treatment of some cases of persistent cardiac œdema.[25] The spirolactones have a close chemical similarity to aldosterone and probably act on the kidney as competitive inhibitors of this hormone. It should be noted that the excessive amount of circulating aldosterone that occurs with some tumours of the adrenal cortex may give rise to œdema but usually does not.

Studies on the blood flow through the juxtaglomerular apparatus and the activation of the renin-angiotensin system will probably provide relevant information as to the way in which the kidney is able to maintain approximately constant amounts of extracellular fluid in the normal individual. There will then be a better opportunity of finding out how these volume regulating mechanisms are readjusted in heart failure so that the extracellular fluid is allowed to increase by an abnormal tubular reabsorption of sodium and water.

ŒDEMA IN KIDNEY DISEASE

Œdema may be seen in three groups of patients with kidney disease: in acute glomerulonephritis, in a group of cases which we will consider under the term "nephrotic syndrome" and in chronic glomerulonephritis.

Acute Glomerulonephritis

The patient is usually a young adult or child with a recent history of an acute streptococcal infectious illness. When first seen, there is blood and albumin in a urine small in volume, frequently a raised arterial blood pressure and evidence of œdema. In the first place the œdema most commonly and typically involves the eyelids; it does not become extensive. Why does the excess fluid appear at first in the eyelids when this distribution is not seen in cardiac failure? The congested cardiac patient is often ambulant; if he is in bed, orthopnœa compels him to sit upright. Œdema is found in the legs or in the sacral region in these cases. On the other hand, the patient with acute nephritis is already in bed or will soon take to his bed after the sudden onset of hæmaturia and other symptoms; there he will rest lying flat on his back. Œdema is first formed in the loose tissues of the eyelids. Cases of heart failure who have no orthopnœa and are horizontal when œdema is formed will have a typical nephritic facies with eyes half closed by swollen lids. The experiments of Burch illustrate these points.[26] He found the tissue pressure to be normally low in the eyelids and not to rise significantly when small amounts of saline were injected into the local subcutaneous tissues; elsewhere in the body such amounts caused an appreciable rise in tissue pressure.

Even in nephritic œdema, the tissue pressure of the eyelids was low. The lymph flow was increased by blinking or on sitting up; swelling of the eyelids often appeared after a night's rest.

We have yet to explain why there is in this condition a tendency to œdema formation. Plasma proteins, particularly albumin, are lost in the urine. This with other unknown factors causes some fall in plasma protein level. In a series of cases, in which œdema was prominent, it was roughly proportional to the concentration of plasma proteins.[27] But lowering of the osmotic pressure of the blood cannot be a complete explanation, since œdema appears in the first few days of the disease; any change in plasma proteins occurs later.

A toxic factor increasing capillary permeability has often been invoked as an explanation, but the protein content of the œdema fluid is low (about 0·4 g. per cent in the legs, slightly higher in the sacral region).[28] In any case a generalised increase in permeability would rapidly lead to circulatory collapse well before œdema became clinically recognisable.

Many clinicians have noticed a rise in venous pressure and a dilatation of the heart in association with the hypertension seen in acute nephritis. Some think that œdema is the result of this associated congestive cardiac failure; however, cardiac output is often not reduced in such patients. Basically the functional disturbance is the same in the two types of œdema: an abnormal retention by the kidney of salt and water causing the extracellular fluid volume to expand. In heart disease, kidney function is involved in some unknown way secondarily to the circulatory disturbance, but in acute nephritis the actual lesion in the kidney is likely to be often a primary factor. Both glomerular filtration rate and tubular activity are abnormal, and in fact there may be a complete suppression of urine in the beginning of the disease. If fluids are given at this stage in excess of extrarenal losses, then they can only expand the extracellular fluid and œdema will appear. From this standpoint, heart failure and a fall in plasma proteins contribute to œdema formation in acute nephritis, but the most important cause is to be found in the renal disorder itself; local physical factors and the position of the patient will determine where œdema first shows itself.

Nephrotic Syndrome

Œdema is the presenting sign in these cases and it may extend until the patient is swollen with a severe anasarca. The ætiology in individual cases of the nephrotic syndrome is sometimes obscure; it may be associated with a variety of conditions affecting the kidney, e.g., it may occur following acute nephritis, renal vein thrombosis, amyloidosis.[29]

Albumin is always found in the urine, usually in large amounts, and this is undoubtedly the main reason for the low plasma protein level. Epstein,[30] applying Starling's hypothesis, suggested that this type of œdema was due to the diminished colloid osmotic pressure of the plasma. This pressure is indeed frequently below the critical levels at which œdema appears in dogs submitted to plasmapheresis. Certainly œdema is severe and irresponsive to treatment in most of those patients in whom the plasma proteins are below 4 g. per cent. But there are also changes in renal function, and the fact that a diuresis often clears the œdema without a rise in plasma proteins indicates that these renal factors may be predominant. It has long been known that sodium is abnormally retained in this condition and that a salt-free diet may prevent œdema extending.

A basic cause of the œdema in the nephrotic syndrome is thought to be the diminution of the plasma albumin level consequent on the selective leakage of the smaller plasma protein molecules through the kidney. Electron and light microscopic pictures have not yet revealed the pathognomonic lesion in the glomerulus that allows the escape of abnormal amounts of albumin. The retention of abnormal amounts of water and sodium is also of immediate importance in the cause of this type of œdema. The retention of sodium may be due to an excessive secretion of aldosterone but it is possible that the secretion of aldosterone in these cases is a response to the diminished plasma volume which accompanies the hypoalbuminæmia.

One of the most puzzling events in the clinical course of nephrotic cases is a diuresis which causes rapid lessening of œdema. There is, sometimes, an accompanying fall in the level of albuminuria, but the albumin level in the blood stays at its previous figure. There is as yet no definition of the balance of factors that at one time tilt towards œdema formation and a few days later tilt towards its resolution.

Chronic Glomerulonephritis

Œdema is not usually a marked feature in cases of chronic glomerulonephritis. If œdema appears, it seems to be due to the associated hypertensive heart failure.

HUNGER OR FAMINE ŒDEMA

Œdema cases not due to heart or kidney disease occur frequently in famine areas (FIG. 6). McCance[31] in a most scholarly and informative review has collected a number of historical references to the condition. He points out a probable reference in Nehemiah ix, 21 "Yea, forty years didst thou sustain them in the wilderness, so that they lacked nothing; their clothes waxed not old, and their feet swelled not". In Captain Bligh's diary during his voyage after the *Bounty* mutiny there is this comment "An extreme weakness, swelled legs, hollow and ghastly countenances, a more than common inclination to sleep, with an apparent debility of understanding, seemed to me the melancholy presages of an approaching dissolution". Clinical descriptions of the œdema of severe hunger appeared after the two great wars, and any third world war would be inevitably accompanied by famine in Europe and œdematous people would again be seen in the streets. The frequent famines in some areas of the Far East produce their numbers of famished people swollen with dropsy. The treatment of œdematous and non-œdematous starved persons is similar, but it is interesting to see what information is available as to the cause of œdema in this condition.

No particular vitamin or amino-acid seems to be lacking; the condition is a strict calorie deficiency disease. The depot body fats are exhausted and the starved person begins to live on his cell proteins. The body wastes and the plasma proteins may fall. This, when it occurs, enhances any tendency to œdema formation; but it has been reported many times that œdema may be unaccompanied by a fall in the proteins from their normal level in the blood. This was shown, for example, by the experiments conducted by Keys and others at the

University of Minnesota.[32] Human volunteers were kept on a deficient diet for six months and most developed pitting œdema. There was no significant fall in plasma proteins or colloid osmotic pressure in these cases. Conversely people in famine areas with very low protein levels are not always œdematous. There is no constant or direct relationship, therefore, between the œdema and the level of plasma proteins.

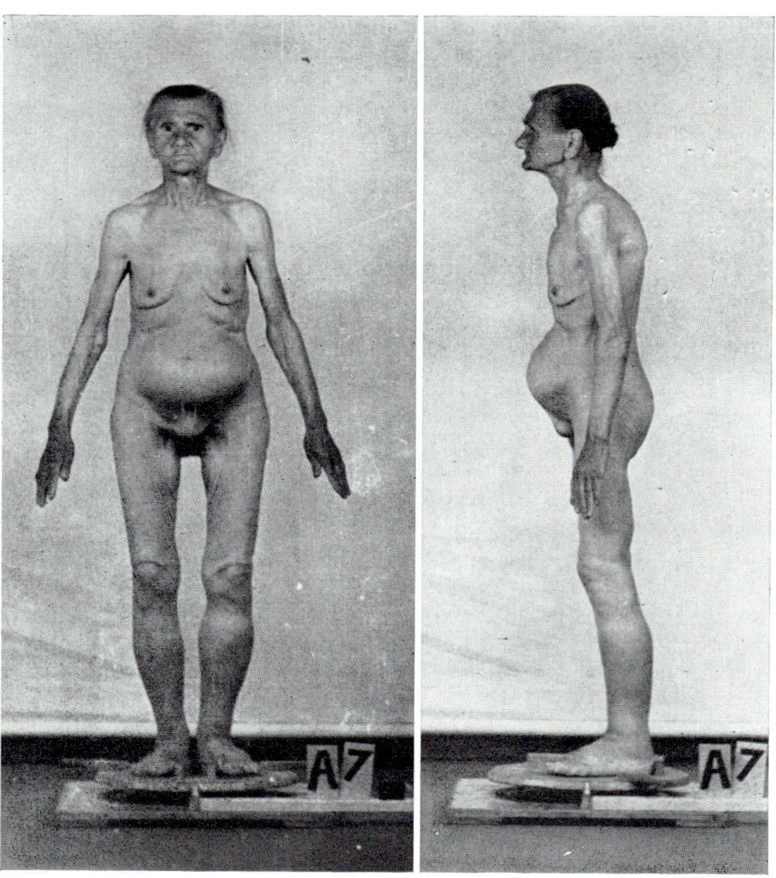

12/Fig. 6.—Hunger œdema. The swollen feet and ankles, and the ascites, contrast with the general emaciation.

One of the important causes must be that the body spaces formerly occupied by fat and muscle are replaced by fluid. This may move easily through the lax wasted tissues to appear as œdema in the dependent parts. All modern observers have noted that œdema disappears with rest in bed; this is accompanied by an increased flow of urine derived from tissue fluids.

In many cases of hunger œdema showing a normal plasma protein level, the extracellular fluid volume is not greatly raised; but in all undernourished people the ratio of this volume to the total cellular volume is increased. In the Minnesota experiment, for instance, the ratio doubled itself during the period of semi-starvation. Where there was once firm tissue, there is now only a watery fluid. When such a wasted man remains upright, urine flow is diminished and tissue fluid is increased further. Under the influence of gravity it seeps unimpeded to collect in the feet. The process may be repeated and œdema involve a greater and greater area, for tissue pressure does not rise and excess fluid formation is not self limiting. Low plasma proteins in some cases exaggerate this tendency to œdema.

OEDEMA WITH PROTEIN LOSS INTO THE GUT

Some plasma protein passes from the gastro-intestinal mucosa into the lumen of the gut where it is degraded by the proteolytic enzymes. This has not been precisely measured but it probably amounts to no more than a few grams a day in normal adults. In certain conditions the loss of protein increases greatly, and will cause eventually a fall in plasma protein levels in the blood. Œdema may follow.

There are many pathological lesions which can produce massive loss of protein via the gut lumen; the heterogenous collection are grouped together under the head of "protein-losing gastro-enteropathy".[33] The lesions may be local to the gut, for example the protruding surface of gut carcinomata may leak protein in large amounts. The cause may be at a distance as when the lymphatics draining the gastro-intestinal tract are obstructed in the thorax causing gross dilatation of the mucosal lymphatic vessels and a consequent loss of protein. Similar histological appearances of the gut lymphatics may occur apparently as a primary lesion unaccompanied by obstruction.

The existance of protein-losing gastro-enteropathy may be discovered by injecting a marker substance intravenously and estimating its loss into the fæces. The polymer, polyvinyl pyrrolidone (P.V.P.) has proved useful in this respect when tagged with radioiodine.

As in the nephrotic syndrome and in hunger œdema, and as we shall see in liver cirrhosis, the relation of plasma protein levels and the œdema is not a simple one, for œdema may resolve with little or no change in blood plasma proteins. However, when the plasma protein is low then œdema is very likely to occur and continued loss of protein will cause the œdema to persist or increase.

ŒDEMA OF VENOUS AND LYMPHATIC OBSTRUCTION

Œdema that is unilateral has rarely a general origin. It is commonly associated with obstruction of the veins or of the lymphatics draining the part (Fig. 7).

Veins may be obstructed by primary or secondary neoplasms, particularly when these involve the lymph nodes of the axilla or the groin, or by any other tumour. They may also be obstructed from within by thrombosis. The cause of œdema in such circumstances is the increased pressure in the small vessels draining into the obstructed veins.

Liver cirrhosis is frequently associated with extensive collections of fluid in the peritoneal cavity. There is an increased pressure in the portal veins because the outflow of blood is impeded by fibrosis in the liver; this must in turn

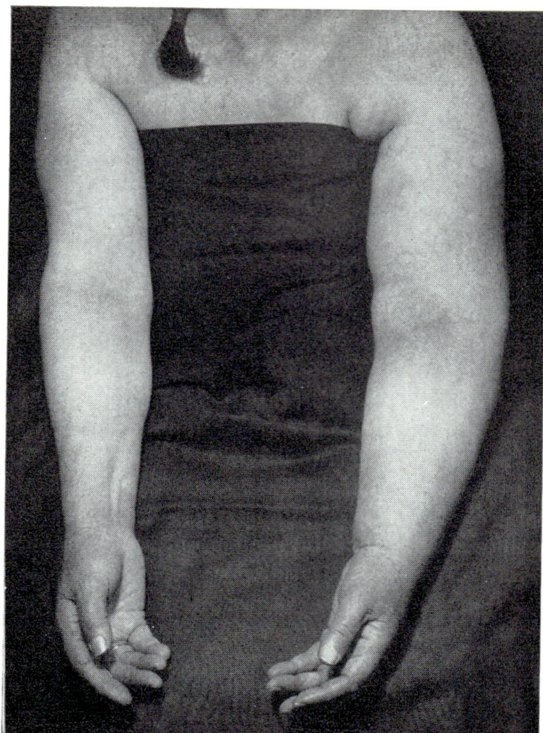

12/FIG. 7.—Unilateral œdema affecting the left arm after left radical mastectomy. The lymph nodes and lymphatics draining the breast have been removed on the left side, with the mammary gland.

increase fluid formation and pre-dispose to ascites. But the situation is complex for a low plasma protein level in the blood is often seen as a result of liver damage and malnutrition, moreover there is a continual loss of plasma protein into the peritoneal cavity. Changes in renal function occur by which sodium and water are retained in the body. There is an increased aldosterone blood level; this may be a response to a low blood volume or, alternatively, it may be a primary disturbance of unknown origin. A cirrhotic liver, moreover, cannot dispose in its usual way of steroids and there may possibly be an accumulation of salt-retaining hormones for this reason. The relative contributions of back-pressure, low plasma proteins and increased circulating aldosterone to the formation of the ascites have yet to be determined.

Lymphatic obstruction may occur in a number of inflammatory and non-inflammatory states but it is common in filariasis of long standing. This is a condition in which the parasitic worms of *Wuchereria bancrofti* develop in the regional lymphatics, particularly those of the pelvis. The resulting swelling and deformity are often very extensive; but the condition seen in the disease is not a simple œdema. Secondary infection of the swollen part and a reaction of tissues permeated with fluid of a high protein content cause fibrosis and induration of the affected area. This condition of elephantiasis has been produced experimentally. Acute lymphatic obstruction is always quickly relieved by the development of collateral channels. Even if the thoracic duct and the right lymph ducts are carefully tied, no permanent obstruction to lymph flow follows. However, Drinker and his colleagues[34] showed that when irritant fluids (they used a suspension of silica in a solution of quinine hydrochloride) were injected repeatedly into the lymphatics of a leg, a condition closely resembling elephantiasis developed. The extracellular fluid of the swollen tissues, both experimentally and clinical, contains a high proportion of protein and forms an excellent culture medium for the growth of pathogenic bacteria.

There are also a group of lymphatic œdemas which have a hereditary basis. This group is known as Milroy's disease after the clinician who gave the original description in 1892. It affects one or both legs, appears at birth or in childhood and lasts throughout life. The only complaint of the patient is the unsightliness of the abnormality. Milroy reports a family history of six generations in which 22 cases were seen in 97 members of that family.[35] Usually classified under the heading of lymphatic œdema, some have suggested that it may be more properly described as a congenital overgrowth of lymph vessels (congenital lymphangiectasis.[36] The subcutaneous fat is, in some cases, partly replaced by large quantities of such tissue.

PULMONARY ŒDEMA

Laennec described acute pulmonary œdema in association with heart disease and lung infections in his classic treatise on auscultation. Since then it has been noted as a terminal event in many cachectic illnesses. But pulmonary œdema seems to be specifically associated with heart disease (FIG. 8), uræmia, traumatic damage to the brain and intracranial hæmorrhage, and as a rare but dreaded event during the removal of effusions from the peritoneal or pleural cavities. A more obvious and direct association is observed in cases of pulmonary infection and in people who have inhaled poisonous gases as an industrial accident or in war. It also occurs in patients with obstruction to the pulmonary veins by neoplasms.

Even though pulmonary œdema is seen in such a bewildering variety of clinical conditions, it runs a similar course in each. This does not necessarily mean that it has always a similar immediate cause. What is apparent is that any excess fluid formed in the alveoli brings more fluid out of the lung capillaries. In this way œdema in one part of the lung has a tendency to extend. "In a fulminating form, the œdema occurs so rapidly and is so intense that, within a minute or two of crying out in fear, the patient is drowned by the copious bloodstained fluid that pours into the respiratory passages and overflows frothing from the mouth and nose" (Sir Thomas Lewis). The course of the disorder may be as short as this, it may however last for hours or days and is not necessarily fatal. In these more prolonged cases, the protein-containing fluid forms an excellent culture medium for the growth of bacteria. In this way infection and œdema are continuously reinforcing each other.

Drinker has described, in his short book on the subject,[37] the special characters of pulmonary structure and function that predispose to a rapid extension of œdematous processes in the lung. He gives particular attention to the permeability of the lung capillaries, pointing out that they receive their oxygen supply largely from the alveolar air and not from the venous blood that they contain.

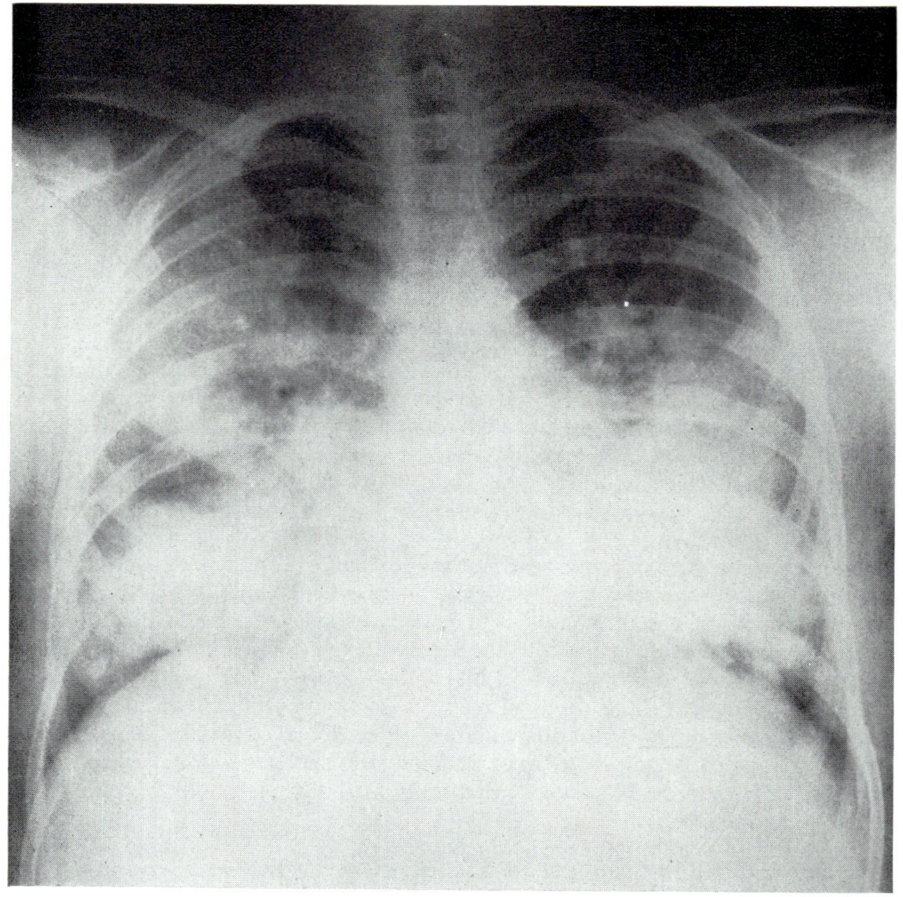

(*a*)

12/FIG. 8 (*opposite*).

Any fluid in the alveoli prevents adequate ventilation and leads to a low oxygen partial pressure in the alveolar capillaries. The consequent increase in permeability toward protein of those capillaries allows more œdema fluid to be formed. In this way a vicious circle is established. The fluid may spread through the lung segments by way of the interalveolar pores. Since the œdema fluid collects in the alveoli there is no effective tissue pressure to oppose its accumulation, as there would be, for example, in a limb.

Experimentally, the flow of lymph from the lung may be accurately measured in a proportion of dogs by cannulating the right lymph duct. An increased flow anticipates the actual development of œdema, but the lymph drainage is insufficient to prevent its occurrence. Applying Starling's principle to the circula-

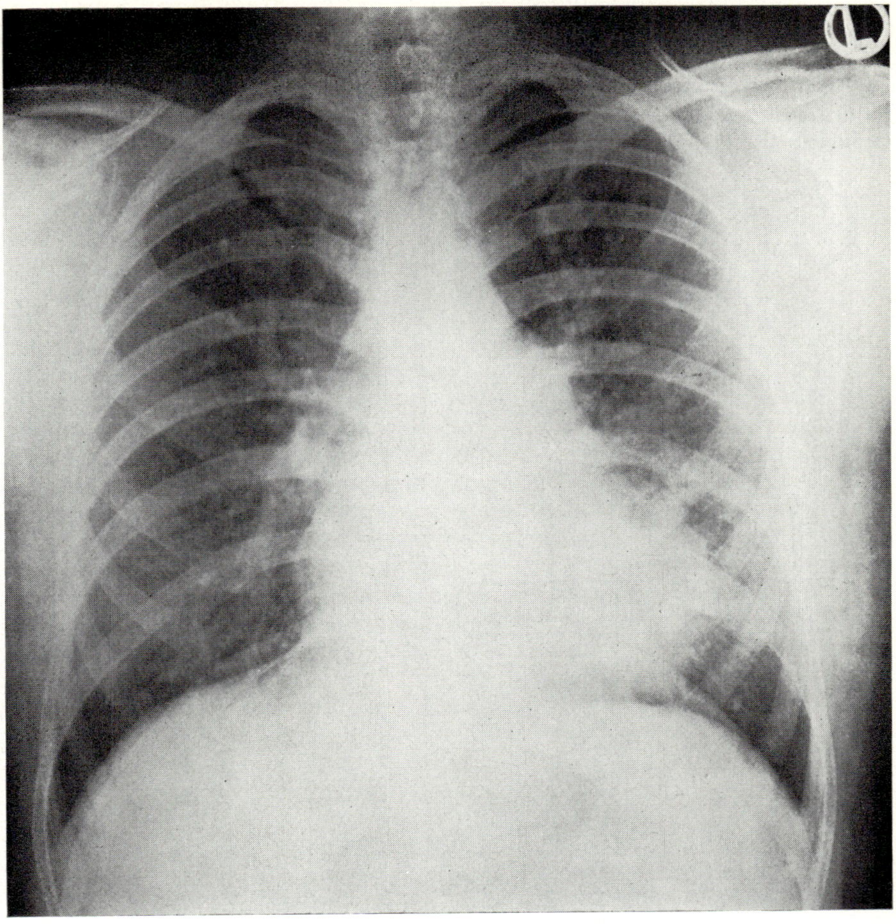

(*b*)

12/Fig. 8.—Pulmonary Œdema. X-ray Photographs of the Lung Fields of a Patient with Mitral Stenosis.

(*a*) During an attack of pulmonary œdema. (*b*) After recovery.

tory data, given in Fig. 9, it will be seen that conditions favour absorption of fluid since the colloid osmotic pressure of the plasma exceeds the hydrostatic pressure in the pulmonary capillaries at all points. Indeed, in experimental work on dogs, very large quantities of normal saline poured down the bronchial tree are rapidly cleared by way of the capillaries. However, if serum is used instead, it is slowly absorbed into the lymphatics over a period of days.[38] The fluid which escapes from the lung capillaries in most cases of œdema closely approaches serum in its protein content.[39]

The secondary factors predisposing to œdema formation in the lung do not, however, explain its initiation in the clinical states already listed. When considering the immediate causes, we may ignore renal and other factors concerned with water balance, for pulmonary œdema arises through a redistribution of the fluids available in the body. It is accompanied by a corresponding diminution of plasma volume and hæmoconcentration. We must look therefore to factors involving, directly or indirectly, the local circulation.

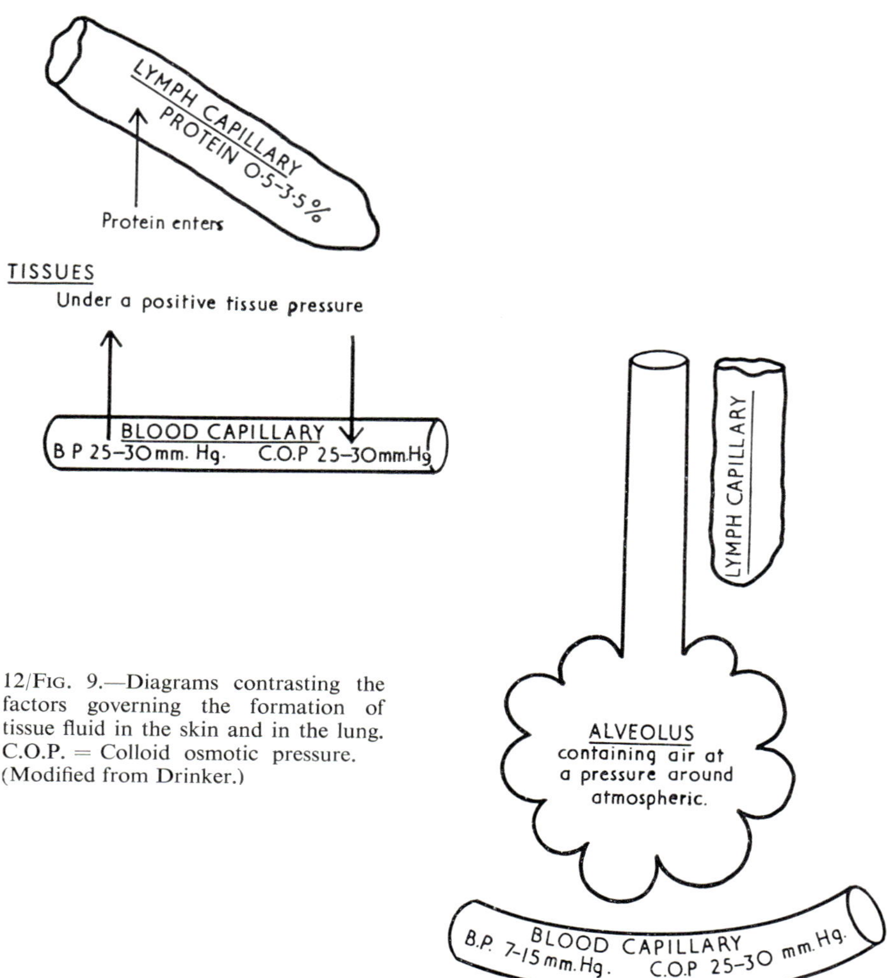

12/Fig. 9.—Diagrams contrasting the factors governing the formation of tissue fluid in the skin and in the lung. C.O.P. = Colloid osmotic pressure. (Modified from Drinker.)

That Starling's principle holds for the pulmonary circulation in the special case of the heart-lung preparation has been demonstrated by a number of workers. Arguing from this basis, pulmonary œdema arising in heart disease could be the result of an increased pulmonary capillary pressure. Moreover, it has been suggested that failure of the left ventricle to expel all blood it receives from the right side gives rise to pulmonary congestion, an increased capillary pressure and pulmonary œdema. Many clinical and experimental observations have been interpreted by this hypothesis of "left ventricular failure". The experimental studies have usually involved the production of œdema by severe damage to the left side of the heart; in some of these experiments the blood pressure in the pulmonary veins and, presumably, the pulmonary capillaries are observed to rise. But, in a number of well-controlled experiments, there has been a poor correlation of these factors; moreover, gross damage to the left ventricle affects the general, and not only the lesser, circulation. The bronchial and cerebral circulations, for example, are abnormal in these experiments. Damage to the *right* ventricle may also produce œdema in the lungs. Because of the confusing factors, the contribution that these studies make is limited.

A variety of experimental procedures will produce pulmonary œdema. Adrenalin given in large doses to some species can produce a rapidly fatal pulmonary œdema; toxic doses of the ammonium ion, prolonged hypoglycæmia, excessive partial pressures of oxygen and cranial trauma are other methods. Some of the thiourea derivatives, particularly ANTU (α-napthyl thiourea), that are used as rat poisons, kill by a seemingly specific effect on the permeability towards protein of the pulmonary capillaries. Phosgene probably acts in a similar way, for it is destroyed locally in the lung before it can enter the general circulation. A clottable mixture, containing fibrinogen, injected into the cisterna of the IVth ventricle gives rise to lung œdema.[39] In each of these experiments where the œdema fluid in the lungs has been analysed it has been found to contain a very high proportion of protein. Drugs having an inhibitory effect on sympathetic nerve endings and general cerebral depressants (anæsthetics, alcohol and morphia) will reduce the mortality in many of these experiments. So, even in phosgene and ANTU poisoning, the nervous system must play some role. How the nervous system affects the permeability of the capillaries is not known.

From these experiments, toxic, hæmodynamic and nervous factors have all been shown to cause lung œdema. It is not as yet possible to define these influences with any precision and one may only guess at their varying importance in each of the clinical types of the disorder.

REFERENCES

1. Starling, E. H. (1895). *J. Physiol. (Lond.)*, **19,** 312.
   Tissue fluid formation and absorption.
2. Landis, E. M. (1927). *Amer. J. Physiol.*, **82,** 217.
   Micro-injection studies of capillary permeability in the frog.
3. Pappenheimer, J. R., and Soto-Rivera, A. (1948). *Amer. J. Physiol.*, **152,** 471.
   Capillary permeability in mammals.
4. Barrowman, J., and Roberts, K. B. (1967). *Quart. J. exp. Physiol.*, **52,** 19.
   Distribution of tritiated water after drinking.
5. Flexner, L. B., Gellhorn, A., and Merrell, M. (1942). *J. biol. Chem.*, **144,** 35.
   Diffusion of water across the capillary wall.
6. Chambers, R., and Zweifach, B. W. (1947). *Physiol. Rev.*, **27,** 436.
   Intercellular cement and capillary permeability.
7. Renkin, E. M. (1952). *Amer. J. Physiol.*, **168,** 538.
   Capillary permeability of lipid-soluble molecules.

8. PAPPENHEIMER, J. R., RENKIN, E. M., and BORRERO, L. M. (1951). *Amer. J. Physiol.*, **167,** 13.
Capillary permeability theory.
9. KAMOVSKY, M. J. (1967). *J. Cell Biol.*, **35,** 213.
The ultrastructural basis of capillary permeability.
10. LANDIS, E. M., JONAS, L., ANGEVINE, M., and ERB, W. (1932). *J. clin. Invest.*, **11,** 717.
Capillary permeability during venous congestion.
11. WASSERMAN, K., and MAYERSON, H. S. (1951). *Amer. J. Physiol.*, **165,** 15.
Albumin in plasma and lymph.
12. SIMPSON, S. A., TAIT, J. F., WETTSTEIN, A., NEHER, R., VON EUW, J., and REICHSTEIN, T. (1953). *Experientia*, **9,** 333.
Aldosterone.
13. VERNEY, E. B. (1948). *Proc. roy. Soc. B.*, **135,** 25.
The antidiuretic hormone and osmoreceptors.
14. GROSS, F., BRUNNER, H., and ZIEGLER, M. (1965). *Recent Progr. Hormone Res.*, **21,** 119.
Renin, angiotensin and aldosterone.
15. STARLING, E. H. (1909). *The Fluids of the Body*, p. 157. London: Archibald Constable.
16. Majno, G., and PALADE, G. E. (1961). *J. biophys. biochem. Cytol.*, **11,** 571 and 607.
Light and EM studies on permeability of the microcirculation.
17. SCHREIBER, S. S., BAUMAN, A., YALOW, R. S., and BERSON, S. A. (1954). *J. clin. Invest.*, **33,** 578.
Blood volume in failure.
18. ALTSCHULE, M. D. (1938). *Medicine (Baltimore)*, **17,** 75.
Level of venous pressure and œdema not related.
19. BURCH, G. E., and SODEMAN, W. A. (1937). *J. clin. Invest.*, **16,** 845.
Tissue tension.
20. MCMASTER, P. D. (1937). *J. exp. Med.*, **65,** 373.
Lymph flow in œdematous skin.
21. STEAD, E. A., and WARREN, J. V. (1944). *J. clin. Invest.*, **23,** 283.
Protein content of œdema fluid.
22. STARR, I. (1949). *Ann. intern. Med.*, **30,** 1.
Congestive failure pathogenesis.
23. MAXWELL, M. H., BREED, E. S., and SCHWATZ, I. L. (1950). *J. clin. Invest.*, **29,** 342.
Renal circulation in congestive failure.
24. DAVIS, J. O. (1963). *Yale J. Biol. Med.*, **35,** 402.
Aldosterone in experimental heart failure.
25. FRIEDBERG, C. K. (1960). In *Edema: mechanisms and management*. Eds. MOYER, J. H., and FUCHS, M. Philadelphia: W. B. Saunders Co.
26. BURCH, G. E. (1940). *Arch. intern. Med.*, **65,** 477.
Formation of œdema in eyelids.
27. WRIGHT, G. P. (1950). *An Introduction to Pathology*, p. 333. London: Longmans, Green & Co.
Plasma proteins in acute nephritis.
28. WARREN, J. V., and STEAD, E. A. (1944). *Amer. J. med. Sci.*, **208,** 618.
Protein concentration of tissue fluids in acute nephritis.
29. SQUIRE, J. R., BLAINEY, J. D., and HARDWICKE, J. (1957). *Brit. med. Bull.*, **13,** 43.
The nephrotic syndrome.
30. EPSTEIN, A. A. (1917). *Amer. J. med. Sci.*, **154,** 638.
Plasma proteins in subacute nephritis.

31. McCance, R. A. (1951). *Spec. Rep. Ser. med. Res. Coun.* (*Lond.*), No. **275,** 21. Hunger œdema.
32. Keys, A., Brozek, J., Henschel, A., Mickelsen, O., and Taylor, H. L. (1950). *The Biology of Human Starvation.* Minneapolis: Univ. of Minn. Press.
33. Jarnum, S. (1963). *Protein-losing Gastroenteropathy.* Oxford: Blackwell.
34. Drinker, C. K., Field, M. E., and Homans, J. (1934). *Amer. J. Physiol.*, **108,** 509. Experimental elephantiasis.
35. Milroy, W. F. (1928). *J. Amer. med. Ass.*, **91,** 1172.
36. Allen, E. V., Barker, N. W., and Hines, E. A. (1946). *Peripheral Vascular Diseases.* Philadelphia: W. B. Saunders Co.
Milroy's disease.
37. Drinker, C. K. (1945). *Pulmonary Edema and Inflammation.* Cambridge, Mass.: Harvard Univ. Press.
38. Courtice, F. C., and Phipps, P. J. (1946). *J. Physiol* (*Lond.*), **105,** 186. Fluid absorption from the lung.
39. Cameron, G. R., and De, S. N. (1949). *J. Path. Bact.*, **61,** 375. Pulmonary œdema of nervous origin.
40. Davson, H. (1951). *A Textbook of General Physiology.* London: J. & A. Churchill.

Chapter 13

FEVER

BY G. W. PICKERING

FEVER IS a complex response of the body to infection by micro-organisms and to other disease processes. Its outstanding feature is a rise in body temperature produced by a disturbance in the mechanisms regulating it. It is one of the commonest manifestations of disease, and the measurement of temperature either in mouth, rectum or axilla is part of the routine examination of all sick people.

THE HISTORICAL BACKGROUND

The clinical condition of fever has been recognised since prehistoric times and many early writings contain specific reference to various fevers and careful descriptions of them. But the state recognised and named was the entire syndrome, including the elevated temperature of the patient, rather than this or that particular individual sign of a raised temperature. Nowadays the term fever, as distinct from specific fevers, means a pathologically elevated body temperature. This has not always been so, for Boerhaave in the eighteenth century thought an increased pulse rate to be the essential sign of fevers. Our changed attitude is due entirely to the careful use of the thermometer. It is, however, interesting to note that, while the clinical thermometer was introduced in the seventeenth century and perfected soon after, it was not until the middle of the nineteenth century that any substantial advance was made. Sanctorius (1561–1636), whose approach was essentially that of a biophysicist, is known for his protracted experiments in a weighing chair and for the invention of a clinical thermometer, in which the expansion of air moved a column of fluid along a scale. Already by 1684 the *Transactions of the Philosophical Society of Oxford* can record that, "Dr. Smith, takeing ye Chair, communicated an Abstract of a Letter from Paris, which sayes that there is a Thermometer, lately invented there by Monsr. du Val, . . . which serves to shew ye duration, increase, and Diminution of feavors, it is but 3 inches long; 4 or 5 lines in diameter; ye inner pipe, which contains ye refin'd quicksilver, is only half a line in diameter". Such mercury thermometers were perfected by Fahrenheit and measurement of temperature became an accurate technique; nevertheless, the study of temperature in patients was almost neglected for more than a hundred and fifty years. Some German clinics, however, began to use the thermometer routinely about 1850, and in 1868 C. R. A. Wunderlich (1815–1877) published a treatise on medical thermometry summarising his work of sixteen years.[1] During this time he had complete records of the temperature of many thousands of cases. He invented the familiar temperature chart for graphically recording his findings. As Garrison has said, "He found fever a disease and left it a symptom". A quotation from Wunderlich may be given to illustrate not only his modern approach but also the importance of fever as a diagnostic sign. "There are two well-ascertained facts, which not only justify us in endeavouring to determine the temperature of the body in diseases, and render the use of the thermometer both a duty and a valuable aid to diagnosis, but form the basis of all our investigations. The first fact is the constancy of the temperature in healthy persons, or, in other words, that healthy human beings of every age and condition, in all places and in all circumstances, and exposed to all kinds of influences, provided these do not impair health, have an almost identical temperature. The second fact is the variation of temperature in diseases, for in sick persons we are constantly meeting with deviations from the normal temperature of the healthy."

The Normal Body Temperature and its Regulation

The Normal Body Temperature

Many measurements of the body temperature were made in the last and the early years of this century, using mercury thermometers placed in mouth, axilla, groin or rectum. Of these the rectum consistently showed the highest readings, and it was generally believed that these were the best guide to arterial blood temperatures, since heat could be more easily lost to the environment from other sites. The mean daily temperature has been stated to be 98·2° F. (36·8° C.) and the range over which the temperature varies during the course of a day is from 99·3° F. (37·4° C.) to 97° F. (36·1° C.), giving a daily variation of 2·3° F. (1·3° C.) with a maximum about 6 p.m. and a minimum about 3 a.m.[2] In some, this daily rhythm is reversed if the subject sleeps by day and goes quietly about his business by night; in other subjects the rhythm persists.

As in other values, the concept of normality is a statistical one. Thus Ivy[3] measured the mouth temperature of 276 medical students seated in class in Chicago between 8 and 9 a.m. The mean was 98·1° F. . 68 per cent (within 1 standard deviation from the mean) were between 97·7 and 98·5° F. . 95 per cent (within 2 standard deviations from the mean) were between 97·3° F. and 98·9° F.

With the advent of the thermocouple it has been possible to measure the temperature accurately in other parts of the body. Many of the results would have been anticipated. Thus the temperature of the skin of the extremities varies greatly with environmental conditions, being sometimes close to that of the ambient air, sometimes close to that of the mouth. The deeper tissues of the limbs are usually warmer than the skin, but similarly vary with the environmental conditions; they are also affected by the state of activity of the muscles, muscle temperature rising during, and for a short while after, contraction. The skin and muscles of the trunk also vary in temperature but less widely than those of the limbs. Evidently the regulation of body temperature is not in the interests of these parts of the body. Temperatures measured simultaneously in the central arteries and veins do not differ by more than a fraction of a degree C. from one another or from those recorded in the mouth or rectum. What is surprising is that the rectal temperature is consistently the highest of these. Thus Eichna and others[4] found the following average mean deviations from rectal temperature:

Pulmonary artery:	—0·26° C.
Right ventricle:	—0·23° C.
Inferior vena cava:	—0·26° C.
Hepatic veins deep in the liver:	—0·03° C.

Cooper and Kenyon[5] also found the rectal temperature was up to 0·35° C. higher than the juxta-aortic temperature. The rectal temperature is also comparatively irresponsive to changes in arterial blood temperature (FIG. 1) and Cranston and others[6] conclude that the sublingual temperature, obtained with sealed lips, or the deep œsophageal temperature is ordinarily a better guide to changing arterial blood temperature than is the rectal.

The advantage to the body of this regulation of temperature has been fully discussed by Barcroft,[7] who points out that the complex series of chemical reactions, which are the basis of cellular activity, all have temperature coefficients and these temperature coefficients may differ. Observations in man show that at temperatures of 105° F. and above, many people become disorientated in time and space and may be maniacal; above 110° F. they are comatose; at temperatures of 82 to 86° F. and below they become unconscious. Temperature is one more illustration of Claude Bernard's dictum, "La fixité du milieu intérieur est la condition de la vie libre". In the case of temperature as in many other quantities, the brain is one of the most sensitive indices of a departure from "normality".

The Regulation of Body Temperature

Elementary physical principles teach us that the temperature of the body, taken as a whole, must depend on the balance struck between heat production and heat loss. In cold-blooded animals (poikilotherms) the body temperature is a little above that of the environment and varies directly with environmental temperature. In man and other warm-blooded animals (homoiotherms) the central body temperature in health tends to remain constant (within about 1° C.) despite changes in environmental temperature, provided of course that these are within certain limits. Evidently a mechanism or mechanisms exist that adjust heat production and heat loss in such a way that central temperature remains independent of environmental changes.

Heat production.—The heat production by the body is due to the metabolic activity of its various tissues. In a given subject, at complete mental and bodily rest, and in the post-absorptive state (i.e. fasting), heat production has a fairly constant value known as the Basal Metabolic Rate (B.M.R.). The B.M.R. ranges from about 1,400 to 1,800 calories per day in different individuals, being related to surface area. The B.M.R. is raised by over-activity of the thyroid gland and by raised body temperature, a rise of 1° C. producing an increase of about 13 per cent. The metabolic rate is increased by food, particularly by protein (specific dynamic action) and by alcohol. Light exercise, e.g. standing or dressing, raises metabolism by 25 to 60 per cent.; moderate exercise such as walking by 100 to 200 per cent; and severe exercise may increase it 10 to 15 times. If body temperature is to be regulated, these changes in heat production must be balanced by changes in heat loss. Thus, for example, the patient with thyrotoxicosis tends to have hot, moist hands in environments where normal hands would be cool and dry, and she dislikes hot weather. In such patients, therefore, obvious changes in skin circulation and in sweat secretion form part of the characteristic picture of the disease. The steam rising from the Rugby football scrum is a familiar sight to most University students.

Heat loss.—Heat loss can be divided into five categories, that of warming the inspired air (and food and drink) to the body temperature, insensible water loss from respiratory tract and skin, radiation from the skin, conduction from the skin and sweating. Some of these are more or less fixed. The heat lost to the air by breathing (which includes most of the insensible water loss) depends on external temperature and humidity, and the rate of breathing. It was thus an important factor on Everest. The body regulates heat loss chiefly by varying the remaining three factors. Heat loss by radiation is, in temperate climates and still air, the chief source of loss of body heat, its rate depending on the difference in temperature between the skin and the solid objects surrounding it. Heat loss by conduction and convection depends on the warming by conduction of the air film surrounding the skin, and its carrying away and renewal by convection; it is thus dependent not only on skin and environmental temperature but on air movement. Sweating cools the skin through heat lost in vaporisation, and heat loss is then dependent not only on the rate of sweating but also on external temperature, humidity and air movement. Dubois[8] found that in a naked man at rest in a chamber at 23 to 29°, more than half the heat loss is by radiation; as external temperature rises, radiation becomes progressively less important, until at temperature of 37° evaporation becomes the sole mode of heat loss. Heat loss by conduction and convection is ordinarily the smallest factor unless air movement is considerable.

Dubois found that in naked men there is a comfort zone at environmental temperatures of 28 to 30° C. where heat production and heat loss are practically identical, and where the skin vessels are moderately dilated and can easily balance heat loss by small changes in calibre. At temperatures a little above this zone the skin vessels dilate and there is a slight secretion of sweat. Just below this zone the vessels constrict. At about 27° the constriction is maximal. These relationships are of course much modified by clothing, the comfort zone being at a lower temperature the more efficient the protection given.

In adjusting heat production and heat loss, the body appears to have mechanisms of two orders of sensitivity that can be likened to the fine adjustment and the coarse adjustment of a microscope. The fine adjustment is that of skin blood flow, and hence of skin temperature, that regulates heat loss by radiation and by conduction and convection. The coarse adjustment is dual; at low environmental temperatures increased heat is produced by shivering, and at high environmental temperatures increased heat is lost through sweating.

The Regulating Mechanism

The efferent pathways for skin blood flow and sweating are the sympathetic nerves, and for shivering the motor nerves to muscle. That cold applied to the skin produces cutaneous vasoconstriction reflexly was first shown by François Franck.[9] It was supposed for many years that nerves from the temperature receptors of the skin were the only, or the chief, afferent pathways involved. However, I[10] was able to show in man that if an arm, whose circulation is arrested, is immersed in hot water, vasodilatation does not occur in the other hand until some three to five minutes after circulation to the immersed arm is released. If an arm with circulation occluded is immersed in cold water vasoconstriction occurs within a few second in the other hand but this wears off after some minutes and is succeeded by a more prolonged vasoconstriction when the circulation to the immersed arm is released. These observation showed clearly the existence of a central receptor responding to changes in blood temperature and reflexly regulating vasomotor tone to the skin. Gibbon and Landis[11] showed that immersion in hot water of the legs of a man with a transection of the cord produced vasodilatation in the hands. Snell[12] infused hot and cold saline intravenously and found hot infusions produced vasodilatation in the hand and cold ones vasoconstriction; furthermore he found the size of response was proportional to the size of the heat transfer. The heat transfers necessary to produce vasoconstriction and vasodilatation were of the same order of size in the experiments of Snell and myself. If the heat transfer were restricted to the circulating blood the temperature change necessary to excite the central receptor would be of the order of 0·25° C. This is a minimum estimate of the sensitivity of the receptor, but measurements of mouth temperature suggest that it is of the right order of size. Gerbrandy, Snell and Cranston[13] showed that in such experiments changes in sublingual temperature (with lips sealed) parallels the changes in vasomotor tone induced by hot infusions (FIG. 1), and that the two are quantitatively related (FIG. 2). Rectal temperature changes very little in such experiments.

Cooper and Kerslake[14, 15] have shown that there are also vasodilator re-

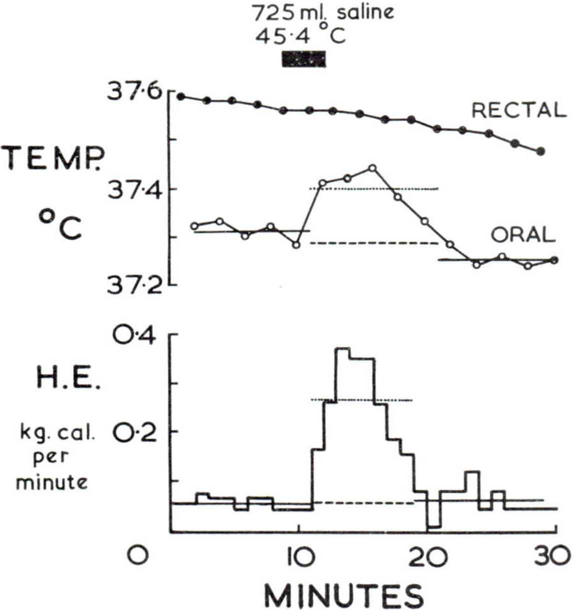

13/FIG. 1.—Shows rectal and sublingual temperature (obtained thermo-electrically with lips sealed) and heat elimination from one hand while an intravenous infusion of warm saline is given in the other arm. Note the quick rise of oral temperature and heat elimination. The rectal falls steadily throughout. The lines are drawn to show how the sizes of the responses were assessed. Continuous lines represent the mean temperature and heat elimination during the 10 minutes before and after response. The dotted lines represent the means before (lower line) and during the response: the size of response is the area between them. (Gerbrandy, Snell, and Cranston.[13])

flexes from the warm receptors of the skin, and have evidence that the afferent fibres travel with the sympathetic nerves.

Although not so extensively investigated, there is evidence that sweating is largely controlled by a central temperature-sensitive mechanism and that shivering is similarly controlled chiefly by a central mechanism, though reflexes from cold receptors in the skin play a part.

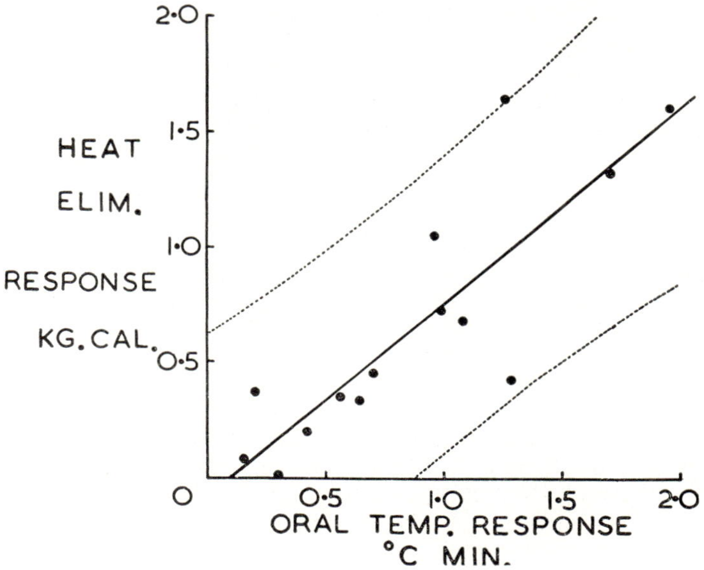

13/FIG. 2.—Relates response of hand vessels (heat elimination) to rise of oral temperature after infusion of warm saline, as obtained by experiments illustrated by FIG. 1. (Gerbrandy, Snell, and Cranston.[13])

To sum up it would seem that body temperature is regulated chiefly by reflexes induced from some central receptor sensitive to changes in blood temperature: the efferent impulses increase or decrease vasomotor tone in the skin and, should temperature rise above or fall below certain points, induce sweating or shivering respectively. This regulating mechanism is supplemented by reflexes from the skin, particularly from the cold, but also from the warm receptors, these reflexes having the same efferent pathways and presumably similar central connections.

The Central Mechanism

The mechanism regulating body temperature is very sensitive to anæsthetics, which are of course used primarily to suppress activity in the central nervous system. Thus the central mechanism must be studied in unanæsthetised animals; experiments under anæsthesia are irrelevant. The anterior hypothalamus seems to contain the thermoregulatory "centre", by which is meant (1) a focus of the synaptic connections between afferent and efferent tracts engaged in thermoregulation, (2) a focus responsive to changes in temperature, (3) a focus responsive to chemical agents with consequent changes in the level at which temperature is regulated. This conclusion is based on four lines of evidence (Cooper[16]). First, ablation experiments show that temperature regulation is lost by decerebration, by section below the midbrain and by destruction of specific areas in the hypothalamus. Second, electrical stimulation of certain parts of the hypothalamus will produce shivering, skin vasodilatation or sweating. Third, local heating of these areas will inhibit shivering and produce cutaneous vasodilatation and sweating. Fourth, the injection of minute amounts of "endogenous pyrogen" into the anterior hypothalamus will produce fever.

Snell's experiments (FIG. 1 and 2) suggest that the central thermoregulatory mechanism responds quantitatively to changes in temperature of the blood reaching it, whether these changes are up or down. A similar if more limited conclusion emerged from the experiments of Downey *et al.* (1964).[17] They recorded oxygen consumption in the conscious rabbit at constant ambient temperature while cold water was circulated through a silver chamber which could be placed around a given artery or vein. Rise in oxygen consumption was linearly related to heat abstracted from the blood. The regression coefficient, that is the increment in heat production for each calorie abstracted from the blood was much greater for the internal carotid than for any other artery or vein. The vertebral artery could not be tested.

The behaviour of the central mechanism in fever is discussed on page 406.

Feldberg and Myers[18] have shown that in the cat 5-hydroxytryptamine (5-HT) injected into the lateral ventricle or anterior hypothalamus caused the animal's body temperature to rise, while noradrenaline injected into these sites caused it to fall. Cooper *et al.* (1965) have shown that the reverse is true of the rabbit. The dog and monkey resemble the cat; the sheep and goat resemble the rabit. It is suggested that body temperature depends on the balance between the release of these two amines in the hypothalamus.

FEVER AND ITS MECHANISM

Fever may be defined as an elevated body temperature consequent on a disturbance of the regulating mechanism. A rise of body temperature accompanies physical exercise and in hard exercise such as running, football and squash rackets, the rectal temperature may reach 40° C. because heat production is so large that heat loss cannot keep pace, despite massive cutaneous vasodilatation and sweating. When exercise stops, heat production falls, increased heat loss continues and body temperature falls to normal. This is not usually termed fever. Nor does one usually term fever the rise of body temperature that occurs when the environmental temperature and humidity rise so high that some people, particularly those taking physical exercise, are unable to keep down their body temperature. In such circumstances the temperature may become high enough to produce loss of consciousness, usually with delirium, and finally death. Such an epidemic of "heat stroke" or "sun stroke" occurred in New York in August 1896 when the environmental temperature was between 80 and 98° F. for five consecutive days, the humidity was high and there were no breezes. In this epidemic Lambert[19] observed that all patients with a temperature of 110° F. or over were comatose; in them the skin was dry, hot and flushed, or pale and cool with clammy sweat. The blood showed a leucocytosis, hæmoconcentration and often free hæmoglobin in the plasma. Those patients who recovered from the very high temperatures showed conspicuous anæmia, headaches, weakness, numbness and tingling in hands and feet; three were left insane.

A condition rather like mild heat stroke or sunstroke used to be used extensively in treating syphilis and gonorrhœa. The body temperature was raised by wrapping the body in a kapok bag and passing a rapidly alternating current through the chest (diathermy). Body temperature rose, and when it had reached 104 to 105° F. (rectal) the electric current was switched off and the body temperature maintained at about the same value for four to six hours by varying the amount covered by the kapok bag. At the end of that time the covers were removed and body temperature fell rapidly. At the higher temperatures these patients often became disorientated in their minds and delirious and they often subsequently showed herpes labialis. It is very interesting that patients with lobar pneumonia if untreated develop similar temperatures, and also become disorientated and delirious in the same way and develop herpes; these symptoms of pneumonia may thus reasonably be ascribed simply to the high body temperature.

The rectal or mouth temperature is rarely found to be over 106° F. in fever. When it is 105 or more, the condition is termed hyperpyrexia, is recognised as dangerous; and is treated by tepid sponging and other methods to assist heat loss. It seems probable that the regulating mechanism breaks down over 106° partly because metabolism is so greatly increased by the high temperature and partly because the behaviour of the nervous system is affected.

The Causes of Fever

(1) By far the commonest cause of fever is infection by bacteria, viruses, protozoa or fungi. No attempt will be made to list all these. In tropical countries the commonest infections include malaria, typhoid and dysentery. In Western Europe and North America, the pyogenic cocci, the viruses and tuberculosis are some of the most frequent.

In infection, fever is usually accompanied by an increase in the erythrocyte sedimentation rate. Many infections also produce changes in the numbers of circulating white cells which have diagnostic value. The polymorphonuclear neutrophils are increased in infections with the pyogenic cocci (e.g. pneumonia) and in malaria, diminished in typhoid fever; the lymphocytes are often increased in whooping cough (pertussis); the eosinophils increased in infestation with parasitic worms (e.g. trichinella and ascaris).

The course of the fever is often characteristic of the infection. Thus in lobar pneumonia the onset is sudden, the temperature rising to about 104° F. in a few hours; the fever remains at about this level until the fifth to eleventh day when, usually within twelve hours, it falls to normal; this rapid fall is described as a fall by "crisis" as opposed to the slower fall by "lysis". In typhoid the temperature slowly rises over the course of four or five days to about 103°, remaining at this level for two or three weeks and then falling over the course of about a week to normal. In malaria the paroxysms of fever may recur on the third day in the benign and malignant tertian forms (*Plasmodium vivax* and *P. falciparum*) or on the fourth day in quartan malaria (*P. malariæ*), though the fever, particularly in falciparum infections, is often less regular in its form.

(2) Fever is common in conditions where tissue dies because its blood supply is interrupted. An example is infarction of the myocardium, where leucocytosis

and raised sedimentation rate are also found. The temperature seldom rises above 102° F.

(3) Fever is common in hæmorrhage. Thus a temperature up to 101° F. may occur in subarachnoid hæmorrhage, and after gastro-intestinal hæmorrhage.

(4) Fever may occur in malignant tumours, when the growth is extensive, and particularly when metastases occur in liver. The fever is usually not high.

(5) Fever occurs in many diseases of unknown ætiology, e.g. rheumatic fever, ulcerative colitis, rheumatoid arthritis, polyarteritis nodosa.

(6) Fever may also occur when certain areas of the brain are damaged, e.g. in cerebral hæmorrhage when the blood bursts into the cerebral ventricles. It is generally assumed in such cases that the fever results from a direct interference with the central mechanism regulating body temperature.

(7) Fever occurs in the severer attacks of gout, a disease in which sodium hydrogen urate is deposited in the joints.

(8) Fever occurs in hypersensitivity reactions such as serum sickness (p. 1129).

(9) Slight rises of temperature may occur in diseases where heat production is excessive or heat loss diminished, e.g. thyrotoxicosis and congestive heart failure.

Fever Producing Substances (Pyrogens)

Attempts to find a common factor in these diverse conditions have been made along three lines:

(1) It has been shown that some microbes, particularly Gram-negative bacilli, contain substances which when injected intravenously, intramuscularly or subcutaneously into mammals produce fever. To these substances Burdon-Sanderson, the first Professor of Physiology in Oxford, and Osler's immediate predecessor as Regius Professor of Medicine, gave the name pyrogens in 1875. Other micro-organisms such as pneumococci have not been demonstrated to contain pyrogens. In a general way it may be said that the pyrogenic properties of a variety of preparations introduced into therapeutics have been found to be due to the presence in them of living or dead micro-organisms. Nowadays much is done in therapeutics to replace lost blood, water and electrolytes, and to provide calories and vitamins by intravenous infusions; the removal of pyrogens from all apparatus used, and the prevention of bacterial contamination of the fluids at any stage is essential if the patient is to be spared the major upset which fever entails.

A good deal of work has lately been devoted to identifying chemically these pyrogens. An example is the chemical isolation of the pyrogen from *E. coli* by Westphal[20] and his colleagues and its identification as a lipo-polysaccharide of high molecular weight containing 74 per cent. of phosphorylated polysaccharide and 26 per cent of lipoid. The sugars obtained by hydrolysis of the polysaccharide include rhamnose, xylose, glucose, galactose and N. acetylhexosamine. 0·1 μg. of this substance injected intravenously is enough to induce fever in man. In general, bacterial pyrogens do not dialyse; they withstand boiling or autoclaving but are destroyed by dry heat at 160° C.

(2) Bennett and Beeson,[21] taking great care to avoid bacterial contamination, made saline extracts of all tissues in the rabbit and found only one pyrogenic, that from polymorphonuclear leucocytes, which they obtained either from the

buffy coat of the blood, or from peritoneal exudates induced by injecting sterile saline 4 hours before. The pyrogenic substance in leucocytes is quite different from that in bacteria. It is destroyed by boiling, but not by trypsin, chymotrypsin or ribonuclease. It does not dialyse. Snell and Atkins[22] have found a similar pyrogen is present in most, if not all, tissues, but in much smaller quantities.

(3) Menkin has sought a pyrogen in inflammatory exudates,[23] and has claimed to have obtained it in a high degree of purity. However, the sample of so-called "pyrexin" which Bennett and Beeson[21] tested resembled bacterial pyrogen much more than the substance present in normal leucocytes. The ubiquity of bacterial pyrogens and the extreme care that is needed to prevent contamination is a lesson only recently learned by most, and meanwhile the status of "pyrexin" remains uncertain.

The Phenomena Associated with Fever

The Course of Fever

There are three stages in fever: (1) the cold stage or period of rising temperature, which may be acute enough to constitute a chill, ague or rigor, (2) the hot stage, the period of sustained high temperature, the fastigium or flush, and (3) the sweating stage, the period of falling temperature or defervescence. The phenomena associated with these three phases are probably similar in most kinds of fever, but they are most conveniently studied when the whole cycle is short and when it is predictable. Sidney Ringer, the physician who discovered the importance of metallic ions for cardiac contraction, studied a case of malaria in which the chills occurred daily (quotidian malaria). Nowadays we generally use the fever produced by injecting intravenously a bacterial pyrogen.

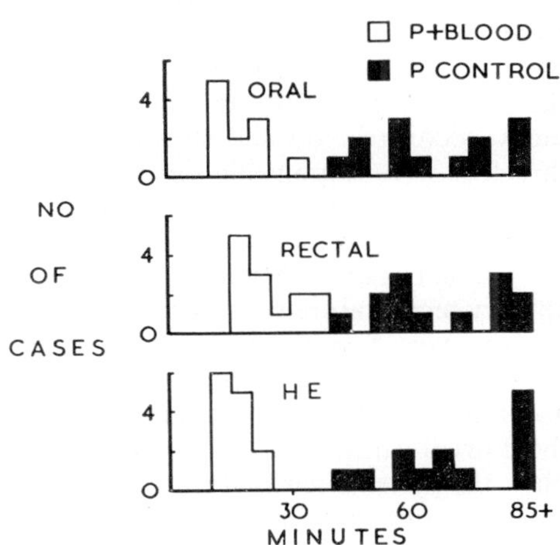

13/Fig. 3.—Latent periods between the intravenous injection in man of a bacterial pyrogen and the rise in oral and rectal temperatures and the fall in heat elimination. Open columns pyrogen incubated with the subject's blood; solid columns pyrogen incubated with saline. (Gerbrandy, Cranston, and Snell.[25])

The cold stage.—Ringer[24] observed in his patient that the temperature measured in the axilla rose before the subject began to feel cold. When, however, continuous measurements are made of blood flow through the hand as well as rectal and oral temperature, the hand flow falls before the oral temperature rises, and the rectal temperature rises last of all (Gerbrandy, Cranston and Snell)[25] (Fig. 3). Thus cutaneous vasoconstriction, which acts to diminish heat loss, is the first demonstrable change at the onset of fever, and this vasoconstriction remains until very nearly the end of the phase of rising temperature. When the temperature rise is large and abrupt, vasoconstriction is followed by an intense subjective sensation of cold; every current of cool air is noticed (this is partly the cause of the popular idea that sitting in a draught is a cause of fever); the subject puts on more clothes and often retires to bed with rugs and hot-water bottles; the pilo-erectors contract, the hairs stand up and goose-skin develops, he begins to shiver and the teeth chatter. The intense cutaneous vasoconstriction, the application of clothing and outside heat cut down heat loss to the minimum; shivering increases heat production through the energy used in the contractions of voluntary muscle. Dubois and his colleagues[8] showed by direct measurement that the most important factor in the rise of temperature in malaria or after injection of a bacterial pyrogen was increased heat production. The effect of these changes is to produce a rise in the central body temperature, including mouth, axillary and rectal, while the temperature of the skin, particularly of the extremities, may fall considerably.

The cutaneous vasoconstriction and the pilo-erection during the cold phase are mediated through the sympathetic nerves, and are said to be absent in a sympathectomised limb, which however participates in shivering. Shivering is mediated through the motor nerves. Fever can still occur after injection of bacterial pyrogens in totally sympathectomised animals, but not in those with high cervical section of the spinal cord; the effects of transections above this level have been variously interpreted and no clear statement can be made (for review see Bennett and Beeson[26]).

The extent to which cutaneous vasoconstriction and increased heat production each contribute to the rise of body temperature varies with species and, in a particular species, with the environment. Park and Palmer[27] injected bacterial pyrogen into human subjects exposed to hot and to cool environments. In each the temperature rise was the same, 2 to 3° C. But in the cool environment cutaneous vasoconstriction and shivering of sufficient degree to increase metabolism threefold were responsible for the rise, while in the hot environment a cessation of sweating and a slight cutaneous vasoconstriction sufficed and no increase in metabolism occurred.

The hot stage (fastigium).—Ringer noted that in his malarial patient the axillary temperature continued to rise after the cold stage had been replaced by the hot stage; how this happens is not yet clear. Essentially, however, the feature of the hot stage or fastigium is the maintenance of body temperature at a new and high level which in pneumonia or typhoid may be 104 or 103° F., though the diurnal variations are larger than in health. In the hot stage, as the name implies, the patient feels that his skin is hot, as indeed it is because of the cutaneous vasodilatation and the raised body temperature. Before the invention of the clinical thermometer, the experienced hand of the good clinician or the intelligent mother could recognise the increased skin temperature of the "fevered brow". In this phase, then, heat loss tends to be increased by cutaneous vasodilatation, though not usually by sweating. Heat production is also increased, not now by shivering but presumably because of the direct effect of temperature on the metabolic processes. FIGURE 4 shows the relationship between basal metabolism and body temperature in six different fevers.

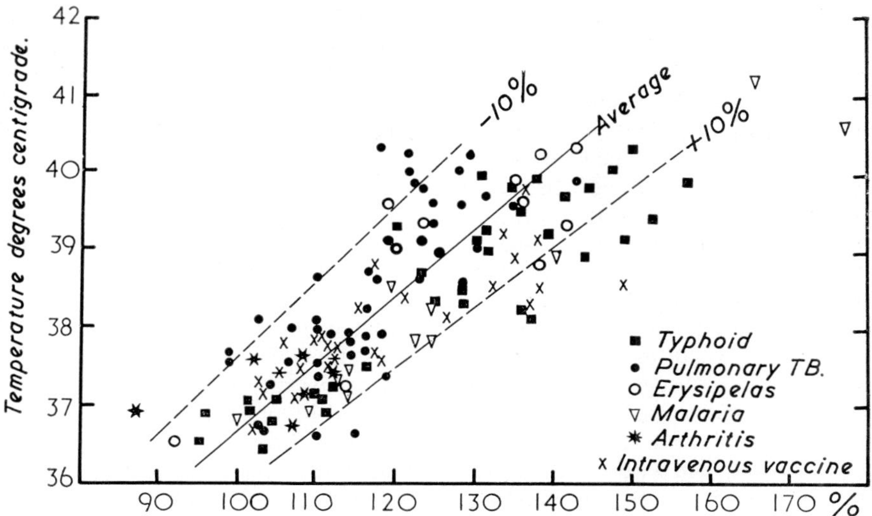

13/FIG. 4.—Relates basal metabolism (abscissa in per cent. of normal) and rectal temperature in six different fevers. The continuous line shows the average and the dotted line deviations from it of 10 per cent. (Dubois.[8])

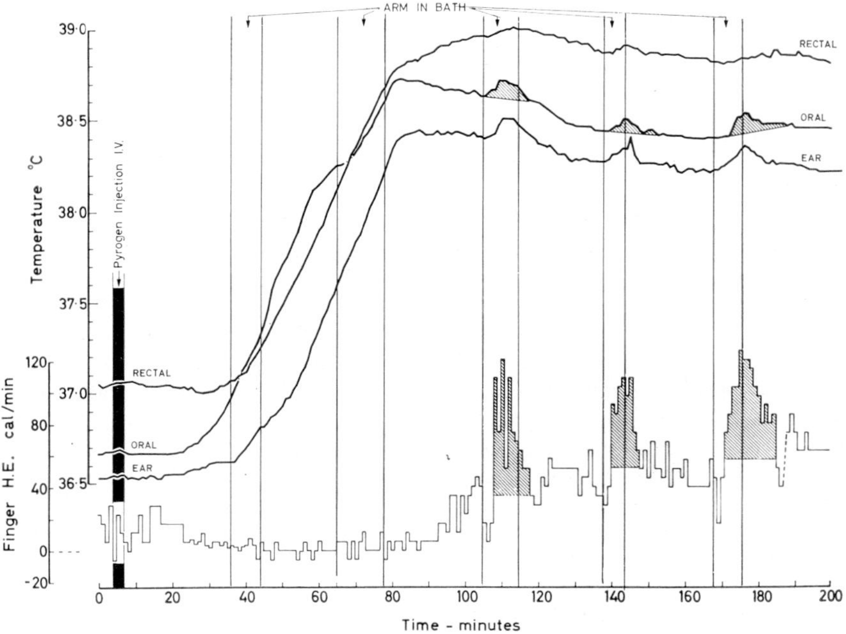

13/FIG. 5.—Responses of temperature and heat elimination in a normal subject injected with pyrogen. Responses of oral temperature and heat elimination, during stable temperature period, are shaded. (Cooper, Cranston and Snell.[30])

The central mechanism in fever.—Von Liebermeister[28] in 1875 suggested that fever was due to a "resetting" of the thermoregulatory mechanism at a higher level. Stern[29] and Cooper *et al.*[30] supported this by experimental evidence. FIGURE 5 shows the changes in heat elimination from the fingers of one hand in response to immersing the other arm in a hot bath during the febrile response to bacterial pyrogen. The response was absent during the period of rising mouth temperature, but returned when temperature was stable at a higher level. Moreover, the relationship between the change in mouth temperature and the extent of the vasomotor response in the fingers was the same before the injection of pyrogen and during the fastigium after it. It is the baseline, not the response, that has been changed by fever.

The sweating phase.—Ringer observed that in his patient with malaria the temperature began to fall before the onset of the sweating stage, but it was in this that the fall became rapid. In the abrupt paroxysms of fever that characterise malaria and septicæmia the onset of the sweating phase is often heralded by an intense subjective sensation of heat; the patient throws off all the bedclothes and he is drenched with sweat. Curiously enough the balance of heat production and heat loss has been little studied in this phase, but it would seem probable that the fall in body temperature is due to increased heat loss from the skin; in mild instances, perhaps, mainly by radiation, in severer instances mainly by sweating.

OTHER PHYSIOLOGICAL CHANGES IN FEVER

The Cardiovascular System

Some of the changes in the cardiovascular system may be ascribed to the rise in body temperature. Thus a quickening of the pulse by about 10 beats per minute per ° F. rise in temperature is common to most fevers, with the notable exception of typhoid and a few others in which the tachycardia is less. Again the rise in cardiac output that occurs in fever may be correlated with the increased metabolic rate.

But there are other changes that are totally unexpected and of great interest. The arterial blood pressure rises with the onset of the chill and falls during the hot phase. The fall during the hot phase may be considerable when the patient initially has a high arterial pressure; and the intravenous injection of pyrogenic agents was at one time used for the treatment of this condition. The hæmodynamics of this have been studied by Smith[31] and his co-workers. They have shown that the drop in arterial pressure is accompanied by a profound vasodilatation in the kidney. Amidopyrine prevents the rise of temperature following injection of a bacterial pyrogen, but does not prevent the fall in arterial pressure or renal vasodilatation; these vascular changes, then, are not consequences of the rise of temperature or indeed a part of the mechanism raising it. They represent another and as yet imperfectly understood aspect of the disturbance that is fever.

Other Functional Changes in Fever

It is common knowledge that the appetite is often lost in fevers. Faber showed that the gastric mucosa becomes invaded with inflammatory cells and that the secretion of HCl is diminished. As has been said, metabolism is increased in fever, and in high fevers greatly. The high metabolic rate together with reduced food intake probably account for the tendency of R.Q. to be low, the tendency to ketosis, the high excretion of nitrogen in the urine, and the rapid wasting of the body fat and muscles in prolonged fevers. These may all be corrected to some extent by feeding a high caloric diet.

Ringer[24] found in his patient with malaria that the urinary excretion of water, salt and urea rose throughout the cold stage to be most abundant at the termination of the cold and the beginning of the hot stage; excretion began to fall before the temperature reached its highest and continued to fall during the sweating stage. When the malarial paroxysms were stopped with quinine, the diurnal changes in urine flow persisted some days longer. The loss of water from the skin and respiratory tract is greatly increased during high fevers; when sweating is intense the loss of salt may be great. Thus dehydration and salt lack with their consequent tendencies to circulatory failure and renal failure are also common in fevers unless steps are taken to correct them.

The changes in mental function in fever have been mentioned as consequences of the high temperature; so are the increases in heart and respiratory rates.

Another curious disturbance is headache which occurs with many fevers and closely resembles that induced by histamine injection. In both cases the pain seems to arise from the meninges and, in both, pain is relieved by reducing arterial pressure, as by compressing with the finger one common carotid artery in the neck, or by raising intracranial pressure as by injecting physiological saline into the subarachnoid space. It is therefore suggested that in both, pain arises from the neighbourhood of the vessels of the circle of Willis or their main branches. How this happens in fever is quite obscure.

Injection of bacterial pyrogens produces a fall followed by an increase in circulating leucocytes and this is true even with pyrogens from bacteria such as *Salm. typhi.*, infection with which usually produces a fall in the leucocytes. The fall in the circulating white cells which occurs in the first stage of the action of pyrogens is generally attributed to their being trapped somewhere, such as in the spleen. The leucocytosis is ascribed to increased production by the bone marrow.

The Function of Fever

The preceding paragraphs have illustrated how profoundly the body mechanisms are disturbed in fever. A response to invasion of the body by microbes, that is so general and so widely distributed amongst mammalia, would, one might think, form part of the body's defence against infection. If so, then the precise part has never been clearly displayed. In many infections the temperatures reached in fever seem no more lethal to the invaders than they are to the host. In only two infections, gonorrhœa and syphilis, are the micro-organisms killed by the temperatures that can be reached in fever, and curiously enough in neither infection is the degree of fever actually induced in the disease enough to accomplish this purpose. But before the introduction of antibiotics, fever induced by malarial infection or a raised temperature produced by diathermy was one of the most effective methods of eradicating infection in these two diseases.

THE MECHANISM BY WHICH FEVER IS PRODUCED IN INFECTIONS

The foregoing account indicates that the raised central body temperature in bacterial infections is produced through the mechanism which regulates heat production and heat loss. The central mechanism controlling body temperature is probably situated in the anterior hypothalamus; it becomes reset in fever.

Proceeding now to the other end of the story, we know that some bacteria, e.g. *E. coli* and *Salm. typhi.*, contain substances which on intravenous injection produce fever. These substances are termed bacterial pyrogens or, and more loosely, "endotoxins". In the Gram-positive cocci pyrogens are more difficult to demonstrate and the fever may result from the cocci being particulate, or from hypersensitivity.

If a given dose of pyrogen is injected daily, the size of the fever (measured by the area of the curve of raised temperature) gradually lessens and after about a week or ten days becomes small and thereafter remains unchanged. The animal is now said to be tolerant. Left alone for 3 weeks and the pyrogen injected again, the response has returned to its original size. The tolerance has disappeared.[26] This tolerance is not due to the formation of specific antibodies for the following reasons: (1) Its rate of development during injection and its duration after injection are not parallel to the amount of immune antibodies in the blood, (2) it is not specific; an animal that has become tolerant to the pyrogen of one micro-organism gives a reduced response to related but not identical organisms.

In discussing how bacterial pyrogens produce fever it is necessary to consider separately the results obtained in the rabbit and in man, since they are, in some respects, different.

Fever produced by pyrogens in the rabbit.—If a purified bacterial pyrogen is injected into a rabbit in sufficient dose to produce fever, then as Grant and Whalen[32] showed, blood withdrawn from the heart 3 to 120 minutes later will produce fever when injected into another rabbit. However, the temperature curves given by blood taken at 5 minutes and 120 minutes differ. Blood at 5 minutes gives a rise of temperature that begins about 20 minutes after injection and has a secondary peak; this curve is similar to that given by the bacterial pyrogen itself. Blood removed at 2 hours gives a response beginning about 10 minutes after injection and having no or little delayed peak. Grant and Whalen further found that fever curves of this second or rapid type could be got by incubating the pyrogen with whole blood or citrated plasma. Grant[33] further showed that a given dose of pyrogen incubated with plasma from tolerant animals produced a reduced response, but when incubated with normal blood would produce a large fever in a tolerant animal. It thus seems probable that in the rabbit bacterial pyrogens react with a substance in plasma to produce an endogenous pyrogen which produces fever after a much shorter latency.

FIGURE 6 summarises an experiment in which a given dose of typhoid vaccine was injected into a rabbit with the consequent rise in rectal temperature in the upper curve (Atkins and Wood[34]). At intervals blood was withdrawn from this rabbit and injected into normal rabbits or rabbits made tolerant with the same typhoid vaccine, and the areas of the curves measured. Blood withdrawn 5 minutes after injection gave fever in the normal but not in the tolerant recipients. It clearly contained bacterial pyrogen whose concentration seems to have fallen

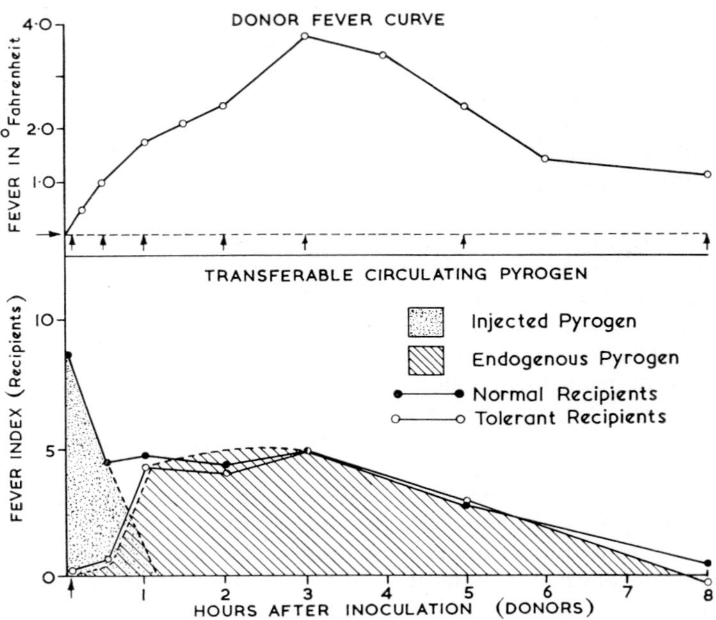

13/Fig. 6.—Relation of mean fever curve of donor rabbits receiving typhoid vaccine (upper chart) to the concentration of circulating endotoxin and endogenous pyrogen respectively, as measured by passive transfer to normal and tolerant recipients (lower chart). The donor rabbits received typhoid vaccine intravenously at zero time. Blood was removed at the arrows and the serum injected into normal rabbits and rabbits rendered tolerant by previous injection of typhoid vaccine. The points on the lower curves show the responses in the normal and tolerant recipients, and the shaded curves the concentrations of bacterial pyrogen and endogenous pyrogen deduced from these responses. (From Rafter, Collins and Wood.[37])

progressively in the first hour. Blood withdrawn later gave fever both in normal and tolerant recipients and clearly represented the effects of the second or endogenous pyrogen. The concentrations of bacterial and endogenous pyrogens are shown in the lower curve.

The fever producing substance circulating in the blood 2 hours after injection of bacterial pyrogen is destroyed by heating to 90° C. for 30 minutes. Rabbit leucocytes incubated in saline at 37° C., with and without bacterial pyrogen, release substances which are also destroyed by heat, and which produce fever of the rapid onset type in tolerant animals; the substances liberated from leucocytes by bacterial pyrogen may or may not be identical with that liberated in its absence. The substances liberated from leucocytes do not dialyse and can be separated from much of their protein and carbohydrate (Rafter *et al.*[37]).

The experiments of King and Wood[38] suggest that in the rabbit bacterial pyrogen acts by the release in the blood of endogenous pyrogen, which itself affects a centre in the brain. Their evidence comes from the time of onset and size of the febrile responses induced in rabbits by injecting material either into a carotid artery or an ear vein. Serum withdrawn 5 minutes after injection of bacterial pyrogen gave, in a given rabbit, responses at the same time and of the same size whether the injection was intravenous or intracarotid, provided sufficient time elapsed between them to prevent tolerance. On the other hand, 2-hour serum gave a response that was more rapid and larger when injected into the carotid rather than into a vein. The same was true of pyrogen prepared from leucocytes.

It is, however, uncertain whether the leucocytes are necessary for the formation of endogenous pyrogen in the rabbit. As we have seen, Grant and Whalen[32] noted that the quick acting heat-labile pyrogen could be produced by incubating bacterial pyrogen with serum, and this has been confirmed by Cooper and Cranston (unpublished). Bennett and Beeson[21] showed that animals deprived of polymorphonuclear leucocytes by treatment with nitrogen mustard respond with high fever to bacterial pyrogens, and that peritoneal exudates prepared in such animals contain a pyrogen with the usual properties of endogenous pyrogen, even though the exudates contain no polymorphonuclear leucocytes. Agranulocytosis in man is accompanied by liability to infections which also respond with fever.

The endogenous pyrogens are probably species specific since peritoneal exudates obtained from dogs produce fever when injected into dogs but not when injected into rabbits.[39]

Fever produced by pyrogens in man.—In man the position is slightly different, as Snell, Cranston and their colleagues have shown. Intravenous injection of purified polysaccharide produces a rise in mouth temperature after a latency of about 70 minutes; when the same dose of pyrogen is incubated with 50 ml. of the subject's blood for 3 hours and then injected, the mean latency is 20 minutes (FIG. 3). Clearly it would seem that the first stage in the body's response to a bacterial pyrogen takes place in the blood. However, in man the reaction seems to be between the pyrogen and white cells; plasma itself will not alter the response to pyrogen, while serum tends to destroy the response presumably because it destroys the lipopolysaccharide. The endogenous pyrogen, produced by the interaction of white cells and bacterial pyrogen, resembles the pyrogen extracted by Bennett and Beeson from rabbits' white cells, in that it is non-dialysable and destroyed by boiling. Tolerance to the bacterial pyrogen does not affect the response to the endogenous pyrogen. Thus Cranston and his colleagues incubated 1 μg. lipopolysaccharide with 100 ml. blood for 3 hours, injected 50 ml. into a patient and stored the remainder at 4° C. The patient now received 7 injections of 0·5 μg. polysaccharide at 2-day intervals, the response diminishing considerably. Two days after the last of these, the remaining 50 ml. of stored and incubated blood was injected to give a fever as large as the original one.[35]

Curiously enough, Cranston and his colleagues (unpublished) have failed to induce fever with sterile extracts of human leucocytes, however prepared.

Other Types of Fever

Hall and Atkins[40] have shown that during fever produced by tuberculin in sensitised rabbits, a transferable endogenous pyrogen is present in the serum. The same has been shown for the fever produced in rabbits by intravenous injection of influenzal virus.[41]

The fever of pneumococcal infections is of particular interest, since these infections produce some of the highest fevers in man, yet killed pneumococci are non-pyrogenic. Bennett[36] has studied the problem in the rabbit. He showed that intravenous injection of pneumococci produces fever after 6 to 8 hours. This was prevented by injection of 300,000 units of penicillin 30 minutes previously. Injection of pneumococci into the peritoneum produced a peritonitis with high fever. The exudates and thoracic duct lymph contained heat-labile pyrogens. However, none was obtained from the blood, though King and Wood[38] succeeded.

These experiments leave many questions to be answered. Are live pneumococci essential; do they act by causing the release of pyrogen from leucocytes or in some other way? Before the introduction of penicillin, the fever of pneumococcal pneumonia was one of the most dramatic. Osler, in his textbook, wrote "in no acute disease is the initial chill so constant and so severe". The temperature may rise to 104° to 105° within 12 hours. The temperature then remains constant for 5 to 9 days and then may fall, normally in from 5 to 12 hours. The pneumonic exudate is of course packed with enormous numbers of polymorphonuclear leucocytes, so that the stage is set for the release of leucocyte pyrogen. But the evidence is still lacking.

The action of pyrogens on the hypothalamus.—Cooper *et al.*[42] have injected bacterial pyrogen and leucocyte pyrogen bilaterally into circumscribed parts of the brain in rabbits. Only in the anterior hypothalamus and the preoptic region near the mid-line did pyrogens in small doses produce fever, bacterial pyrogen after 20–30 minutes, and leucocyte pyrogen after 6–10 minutes. The dose of leucocyte pyrogen was 1/50 to 1/100 of that required to produce fever by intravenous injection, while the dose of bacterial pyrogen was the same in the two instances. The minimum latent period for rise of temperature after bilateral injection of leucocyte pyrogen was 3 minutes, as compared with 1 minute for potassium chloride or noradrenaline. The difference could be due to the slower diffusion of leucocyte pyrogen (which is a large molecule) or to the release of appropriate amine, 5-HT in the cat or noradrenaline in the rabbit. These experiments provide powerful support for the idea that fever is due to the resetting of the anterior hypothalamic structure regulating body temperature as a result of the effect on it of "endogenous pyrogens" released particularly from leucocytes.

REFERENCES

1. Wunderlich, C. A. (1871). *On the Temperature in Diseases*, English translation of 2nd edit. by W. B. Woodman. London: New Sydenham Society.
2. Pembrey, M. S. (1905). *A System of Medicine*, ed. T. C. Allbutt, and H. D. Rolleston. Vol. **1**, p. 823. London: Macmillan.
3. Ivy, A. C. (1944). *Quart. Bull. Northw. Univ. med. Sch.*, **18**, 22.
4. Eichna, L. W., Berger, A. R., Rader, B., and Becker, W. H. (1951). *J. clin. Invest.*, **30**, 353.
5. Cooper, K. E., and Kenyon, J. R. (1957). *Brit. J. Surg.*, **44**, 616.
6. Cranston, W. I., Gerbrandy, J., and Snell, E. S. (1954). *J. Physiol. (Lond.)*, **126**, 347.
7. Barcroft, J. (1934). *Features in the Architecture of Physiological Function*. London: Cambridge Univ. Press.
8. Dubois, E. F. (1948). *Fever and the Regulation of Body Temperature*. Springfield, Ill.: Chas. C. Thomas.
9. Franck, François (1876). *Physiologie experimentelle travaux du Laboratoire du Marey*, **2**, 1.

10. Pickering, G. W. (1932). *Heart*, **16,** 115.
11. Gibbon, J. H., and Landis, E. M. (1932). *J. clin. Invest.*, **11,** 1019.
12. Snell, E. S. (1954). *J. Physiol.* (*Lond.*), **125,** 361.
13. Gerbrandy, J., Snell, E. S., and Cranston, W. I. (1954). *Clin. Sci.*, **13,** 615.
14. Kerslake, D. M., and Cooper, K. E. (1950). *Clin. Sci.*, **9,** 31.
15. Cooper, K. E., and Kerslake, D. M. (1953). *J. Physiol.* (*Lond.*), **119,** 18.
16. Cooper, K. E. (1966). *Brit. med. Bull.*, **22,** 238.
17. Downey, J. A., Mottram, R. F., and Pickering, G. W. (1964). *J. Physiol.* (*Lond.*), **170,** 415.
18. Feldberg, W., and Myers, R. D. (1965). *J. Physiol.* (*Lond.*), **177,** 239.
19. Lambert, A. (1897). *Med. News* (*N.Y.*), **71,** 97.
20. Ludnitz, O., and Westphal, O. (1952). *Z. Naturforsch.*, **76,** 148.
21. Bennett, I. L., and Beeson, P. B. (1953). *J. exp. Med.*, **98,** 477, 493.
22. Snell, E. S., and Atkins, E. (1965). *J. exp. Med.*, **121,** 1019.
23. Menkin, V. (1945). *Arch. Path.*, **39,** 28.
24. Ringer, Sydney (1859). *Med.-chir. Trans.*, **42,** 361.
25. Gerbrandy, J., Cranston, W. I., and Snell, E. S. (1954). *Clin. Sci.*, **13,** 453.
26. Bennett, I. L., and Beeson, P. B. (1950). *Medicine* (*Baltimore*), **29,** 365.
27. Reported by Hardy, J. D. (1950). *Ann. Rev. Physiol.*, **12,** 119.
28. Von Liebermeister, C. (1875). *Handbuch der Pathologies und Therapie des Fiebers.* Leipzig: Vogel.
29. Stern, R. (1892). *Z. klin. Med.*, **20,** 63.
30. Cooper, K. E., Cranston, W. I., and Snell, E. S. (1964). *Clin. Sci.*, **27,** 345.
31. Smith, H. W. (1951). *The Kidney.* New York: Oxford Univ. Press.
32. Grant, R., and Whalen, W. J. (1953). *Amer. J. Physiol.*, **173,** 47.
33. Grant, R. (1953). *Amer. J. Physiol.*, **173,** 246.
34. Atkins, E., and Wood, W. B. (1955). *J. exp. Med.*, **101,** 519.
35. Snell, E. S., Goodale, F., Wendt, F., and Cranston, W. I. (1957). *Clin. Sci.*, **16,** 615.
36. Bennett, I. L. (1956). *Bull. Johns Hopk. Hosp.*, **98,** 216.
37. Rafter, G. W., Collins, R. D., and Wood, W. B. (1959). *Trans. Ass. Amer. Phycns.*, **72,** 323.
38. King, M. K., and Wood, W. B. (1958). *J. exp. Med.*, **107,** 291.
39. Petersdorf, R. G., and Bennett, I. L. (1957). *Bull. Johns Hopk. Hosp.*, **100,** 277.
40. Hall, C. R., and Atkins, E. (1959). *J. exp. Med.*, **109,** 339.
41. Atkins, E., and Huang, W. C. (1958). *J. exp. Med.*, **107,** 383.
42. Cooper, K. E., Cranston, W. I., and Honour, A. J. (1966). *J. Physiol.* (*Lond.*), **186,** 22, P.

Chapter 14

DEGENERATIVE CHANGES AND SOME OF THEIR CONSEQUENCES

By E. P. Abraham and A. H. T. Robb-Smith

INTRODUCTION

Injury to the body is sometimes followed by a complex series of degenerative changes leading finally to the disappearance of the entire structure of the affected tissue. In this and the following chapter we shall consider the nature of some of these changes and the ways in which they are brought about.

The changes in structure and function which are first observed when the tissue cells are damaged, and which are often reversible when the source of the damage is removed, are known to pathologists as *degenerations* and *infiltrations*; the former term implies that there is an alteration in the tissue elements themselves, the latter that something is added to the tissues in the form of an unusual chemical substance or cellular unit. If the damage is prolonged or severe, irreversible changes may occur which are incompatible with cell function, and the resulting death of the tissue is called *necrosis*. These changes are sometimes accompanied by precipitation of calcium salts in the damaged area, which is a common form of *pathological calcification*.

What happens after necrosis depends on the nature of the tissue and the way in which its death is brought about. In some cases the subsequent changes are rather slow; in others the structural elements of the cells rapidly begin to dissolve and the tissue is said to undergo *autolysis*. If the dead tissue becomes infected with certain kinds of bacteria it undergoes a more extensive degradation which is known as *putrefaction*.

The appearance of tissue that has undergone various degenerative changes has been carefully described by morbid anatomists. It has been known for many years that organs are often swollen, heavy and pale in colour as the result of disease. Microscopic study has shown that the enlargement is often due to swelling of cells, which have become blown out with fluid, abnormal stores of fat, glycogen, mucus or other protein derivatives. In other cases, and this is often so with the infiltrations, abnormal products of cell activity are precipitated at cell surfaces or in intercellular spaces. Sometimes the appearance of the tissue indicates a mild departure from normal, whereas at other times the degeneration may impinge on cell death. The distinction often lies in nuclear behaviour, for certain morphological changes in the nucleus show quite clearly that the cells will die, and their absence indicates that recovery is possible.

If we are to understand the reasons for these changes, and for the more extensive ones which they sometimes portend, we must try to relate them to disturbances in the pattern of biochemical reactions on which the life of the cell depends. In 1931 Gavrilescu and Peters[1] introduced the term "biochemical lesion" to describe the initial change in tissue cells which precedes any damage that is visible with the microscope. This term has helped to focus attention on the relationship between pathological processes and the inactivation of enzyme systems; but we must remember that a whole series of reactions may link the primary lesion, or lesions, with the first change that we see and that the failure of a particular enzyme may be the consequence, rather than the cause, of injury to the cell. A comprehensive account of the complex changes associated with the degenerations cannot yet be given in biochemical terms. Nevertheless, we are beginning to form an idea of the kind of disturbance that can occur in the enzyme systems of the cell and what some of their consequences are likely to be. Krebs[2] has pointed out that the activity of certain enzymes may limit the overall rate of a long series of metabolic processes, and that the reactions catalysed by these enzymes, which are pace-makers, may be particularly vulnerable to toxic agents.

Enzymes and their substrates are not distributed at random in the cell but form highly organised systems whose integrity is essential if normal function is to be preserved.[3] In liver cells, for example, it has been shown that cytochrome oxidase, some of the enzymes of the citric acid cycle and the enzymes concerned with the oxidation of fatty acids are concentrated in the mitochondria. The enzymes involved in glycolysis, on the other hand, appear to be present in the soluble fraction of the cytoplasm and a major site of protein synthesis is the endoplasmic reticulum. In intestinal epithelial cells and cells of the proximal convoluted tubules of the kidney, alkaline phosphatase, which catalyses the hydrolysis of certain phosphate esters, is concentrated at the cell surface.

Since the cell takes in material from its environment and since the products of one enzymic reaction are commonly used by another, the passage of substances from one tissue to another and through cellular and intracellular membranes will clearly be one of the factors on which normal function depends. We now know that many substances do not penetrate these membranes by a process of simple diffusion, but are actively transported and sometimes maintained at quite different concentrations inside and outside the cell. Sodium and potassium ions provide one well known example. Although the mechanisms of active transport have not been finally settled, it is certain that they depend on a supply of energy from enzymic reactions and will only function when this energy is made available by respiration, or at least by glycolysis,[4] in the cell. Failure of active transport will lead to changes in ionic concentrations and osmotic pressure which will result, in turn, in the movement of water across cellular membranes. By thinking in these terms it is possible, as we shall see, to obtain some understanding of such degenerative changes as cloudy swelling.

In considering reversible changes in tissues we encounter the problem of how the cell is able to adapt itself to adverse changes in environment, for on this ability its survival may depend. Although cellular organisation in the higher animals is influenced by many factors which are as yet only dimly understood, insight has been gained into some of the ways in which systems of enzymic reactions are controlled. A mechanical analogy is provided by the principle of "feed-back", whereby an increase in the rate of one stage of a process is used to effect an automatic decrease in the rate of an earlier stage. In biochemical systems a rise in the products of one enzymic reaction may be instrumental in diminishing the rate at which a preceding reaction occurs.

In the processes of glycolysis and respiration, inorganic phosphate, adenosine diphosphate (ADP) and adenosine triphosphate (ATP) act as regulators in this way. For example, one of the reactions which form the pathway from glucose to lactic acid—the oxidation of 3-phosphoglyceraldehyde (triosephosphate) to 3-phosphoglyceric acid by nicotinamide-adenine dinucleotide (NAD)—involves the intermediate formation of 1:3-diphosphoglyceric acid and can only occur in the presence of free inorganic phosphate.

$$\text{3-Phosphoglyceraldehyde} + H_3PO_4 + NAD^+ \rightleftharpoons \text{1: 3-Diphosphoglyceric acid} + NADH + H^+$$

The oxidation of NADH through the cytochrome system, which occurs in respiration, is also coupled with phosphorylation. In this case the energy provided by the oxidative process enables phosphate to combine with ADP to form the high energy bond in ATP.

$$ADP + H_3PO_4 \rightarrow ATP$$

Hence, respiration will lower the concentration of inorganic phosphate, and by doing so will limit the rate of one of the reactions through which the breakdown of glucose takes place. Moreover, it appears that during respiration cells may be able to concentrate ATP in their mitochondria. Thus the first stage in the utilisation of glucose, which occurs in the cytoplasm and results in the formation of glucose-6-phosphate, may be affected by lack of ATP.

$$\text{Glucose} + ATP \xrightleftharpoons{\text{hexokinase}} \text{Glucose-6-phosphate} + ADP$$

Such considerations have enabled Johnson[5] and Lynen[6] to suggest a possible explanation of the well-known Pasteur effect. This is the phenomenon, first observed by Pasteur in his work on yeast and later shown by Warburg to occur in many animal tissues, that the breakdown of glucose occurs more rapidly under anærobic conditions than in the presence of oxygen. Thus the relatively low efficiency of glycolysis as an energy-producing process may be partly counterbalanced by an increase in the rate of glycolysis if respiration fails.

Many other examples are known of feedback control. Mitochondrial respiration is dependent on the availability of ADP and hence on the use of ATP[7]. The first enzyme involved in a sequence of reactions can frequently be inhibited by the end-product of the reactions, a phenomenon which has been named allosteric inhibition since the inhibitor is not a steric analogue of the substrate.[8] Moreover the synthesis of an enzyme may be repressed by the product of the action of the enzyme.[9]

Other changes in the enzyme pattern of the cell may stem from changes in the synthesis or structure of its ribonucleic acid (RNA) or desoxyribonucleic acid (DNA). Thus, thyroxine causes in turn a stimulation of RNA synthesis, a stimulation of protein synthesis and an increase in the basal metabolic rate. It appears that thyroxine, and perhaps other hormones, effect in a specific manner the transfer of information between the gene and the mechanisation for synthesis of protein.[10]

It seems that many degenerative changes could be associated with reversible alterations in the patterns of enzymic organization in the cell. But the ability to produce specific proteins is ultimately dependent on the structure of the DNA in the chromosomes. Thus, a genetic defect may result in the virtual absence of a particular enzyme. Damage to the nucleus which prevents self replication of DNA, or the synthesis of enzymes essential for the maintenance of cell structures, may clearly result in a disorganisation from which no recovery is possible. Other things being equal, cells that have a high rate of metabolism succumb more quickly than those that have not, and the parenchymatous cells of an organ may undergo necrosis while the connective tissue cells survive. This is not surprising, for a disturbance in the balance of enzymic reactions may be rapidly enlarged in a highly active cell.

What happens when the cell has died depends on the nature of the tissue and the way in which death has been brought about. If the degradative enzymes in the cell and its surroundings have been destroyed, no further rapid change is likely to be observed, but if these enzymes remain active they may cause a dissolution of the tissue structure.

DEGENERATIONS AND INFILTRATIONS

Among the degenerations are two which stand out from the rest because of their frequency of occurrence and the attention which has been devoted to their elucidation. They are cloudy swelling, including hydropic degeneration, and fatty change. The history of our knowledge of these important types has been described by Cameron[11] in some detail. Recent investigations have provided us with more precise information about their nature and also about the degenerations associated with glycogen and amyloid infiltration.

Cloudy Swelling and Hydropic Degeneration

These closely related conditions are commonly encountered in the heart muscle, liver and kidneys of persons suffering from relatively mild infections, intoxications, anæmia or circulatory disturbances. Diphtheritic and streptococcal infections, arsenical and phosphorus poisoning, pernicious anæmia and the cardiac failure changes in the liver and kidneys are the best-known examples. In cloudy swelling the cells are seen to be enlarged and their cytoplasm may be filled with granules, while in hydropic degeneration vacuoles appear in the cytoplasm. Generally speaking, both cloudy swelling and hydropic degeneration are mild changes and can be reversed completely, as when a patient recovers from an infection or a heart attack, but they may pass on to more severe and permanent damage, especially fatty change, and may even lead to death of the cells. However, the swelling of cells in response to mild injury is not necessarily accompanied by cloudiness and it has been suggested that cellular œdema is a more suitable term than cloudy swelling in many cases.

Many years ago, cytologists suggested that cloudy swelling resulted from a change in cell granules whereby the latter became swollen and vacuolated and might even break up into many more tiny bodies. They suggested, too, that disturbed water exchange between the cell sap and the granular substance might be the basis of this pathological process. Christie and Judah[12] used ultracentrifugation of liver homogenates in 0·25M sucrose to separate the characteristic globules from hydropic cells which are typical of the early stages of intoxication by chloroform or carbon tetrachloride. These fat-containing globules showed considerable succinoxidase activity and it was concluded that they were probably derived from mitochondria. But the relationship of the mitochondrial change to the swelling remained uncertain. Well-developed hydropic change was reported to be accompanied by other cellular changes, including nuclear swelling and irregular clumping of chromatin.

It has been realized for some time that cellular œdema is associated with a disturbance of active transport. Thus it can be shown with surviving slices of adult rat kidney and liver that the amount of water in the cells depends to a large extent upon their respiration. If the respiratory apparatus is poisoned by means of cyanide in certain concentrations, the water content increases; oxygen consumption increases and water content decreases again when cyanide is removed from the media in which the slices are suspended. 2:4-Dinitrophenol, which makes the energy released by oxidation unavailable for storage in adenosine triphosphate, causes the tissues to take up water, and this implies that energy is normally expended by the cells to prevent water distension. The situation is similar with liver mitochondria, which have been shown to maintain a low water content if incubated under conditions favourable to oxidative phosphorylation.[18]

Robinson[14] suggested that cell respiration governs the water balance of the tissue because some of the high energy phosphate bonds which it generates are involved in processes leading to the active extrusion of water from the cell. It was thought that intracellular fluids were normally hypertonic with respect to their environment, that swelling occurred when this hypertonicity was not maintained by active metabolic processes. However, Leaf[15] showed that the fluid entering the tissues in the process of swelling is not water alone but a solution approximately isotonic with the medium. He suggested that the dependence of fluid exchange of tissues on tissue metabolism could be explained by the requirements of metabolic energy for the maintenance of ionic gradients in tissues. The cell was considered to constitute a "double" Donnan system, its membrane separating a non-diffusible intracellular anion A^{n-} and an extracellular cation, Na^+, excluded from the cell. The osmotic effects of these two ions normally balance each other. But when the energy-yielding mechanism is disturbed sodium ions are no longer actively extruded from the cell, and enter it together with chloride ions. This leads to a temporary rise in osmotic pressure which is followed by tissue hydration. When metabolic activity is re-established Na^+ is again extruded and tissue hydration is reduced.

The work of Leaf indicated that it was unnecessary to assume that the osmotic pressure of the cell contents is higher than that of the extracellular fluid. Subsequent experiments, in which precautions were taken to avoid autolysis, provided direct evidence that extracts of liver and other tissues are iso-osmotic with plasma.[16, 17] It appears, therefore, that the active transport of water as a primary event does not occur and that cloudy swelling is a consequence of damage to a mechanism for the active transport of ions.

Fatty Change

We have known for some time now that fats accumulate within cells which have been damaged by a variety of agents. This leads to swelling and greasiness of certain organs, especially the heart, liver and kidneys. Chemical analysis shows that fat is indeed increased in such organs[21]; the commonest conditions found associated with fatty change in human beings are severe infections such as pneumonia and tuberculosis, prolonged anæmia or ischæmia and diseases like cancer where there is often serious nutritive disturbance and even starvation. A fatty liver is illustrated in FIG. 1. Sometimes there is a clear enough association with the storage of fluids and accordingly there has grown up a tradition, based upon morphological evidence, that cloudy swelling precedes fatty change in injured cells.

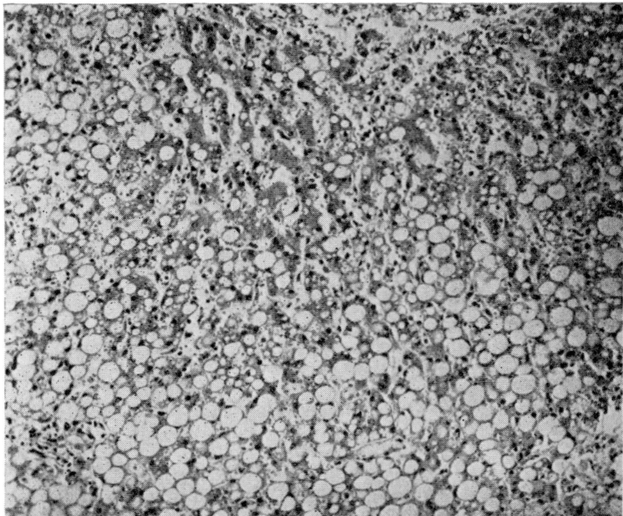

14/FIG. 1.—Fatty liver. Many of the liver cells show vacuoles from which fat has been removed during the preparation of the specimen.

It is clear, at least, that certain poisons, such as carbon tetrachloride and chloroform induce within cells both cloudy swelling, with hydropic degeneration, and fatty change. The liver from a human being suffering from chloroform poisoning as the result of prolonged anæsthesia, or the administration of quite moderate amounts of chloroform at the end of difficult and lengthy childbirth, may show all of these cell disturbances side by side with necrosis of many cells. In experimental animals, a fatty liver can be induced by a remarkable number of different agents. The fats which accumulate in the majority of cases are predominantly triglycerides.

Fatty acids are formed in the liver from carbohydrates and certain amino-acids, acetylcoenzyme A and malonyl coenzyme A being intermediates and the synthesis being catalysed by a cytoplasmic enzyme complex.[18] Fatty acids are also transported to the liver in consequence of the mobilisation of the triglycerides of adipose tissue, being carried in the blood in combination with albumin, and in the fasting animal they supply a major part of the energy needs of the body. Triglycerides from the diet are carried to the liver in chylomicra and are rapidly hydrolysed to free fatty acids. Some of the free fatty acid in the liver undergoes oxidation in the mitochondria, but much of it is esterified to triglyceride with L-α-glycerophosphate after activation to an acyl coenzyme A thiol ester. Triglyceride is transported from the liver to extrahepatic tissues and is carried in the plasma by lipoproteins of low density. It appears that esterification of fatty acids and synthesis of plasma lipoprotein occur in the endoplasmic reticulum of liver cells.[19, 20, 21]

The abnormal functioning of any one of a number of these processes could lead in theory to the accumulation of fat in the liver. When an experimental animal or human being is fed excessive amounts of fat the liver may receive more fat from the diet than it can dispose of. But fatty change may also accompany starvation or wasting disease provided that the fat depots have not been depleted of their lipids. Under these conditions the synthesis of fatty acids in liver is markedly depressed and the excess of fat in the liver comes from adipose tissue. An indication of how fat can accumulate when no abnormal amount of fat is fed has come from studies with animals given carbon tetrachloride, ethionine, and a diet deficient in choline respectively.[22]

The damage caused by carbon tetrachloride to the mitochondria of liver cells is accompanied by disorganisation of the chain of enzymes responsible for the control of the tricarboxylic acid cycle, by uncoupling of oxidative phosphorylation and by the appearance of a previously latent adenosine triphosphatase. It was suggested that such changes bring about the accumulation of fat in the liver because they render the oxidation of fat defective.[12, 23] However, this hypothesis could not be sustained. Recknagel and Anthony reported that the rise in liver fat precedes these changes in the mitochondria.[24] Other studies indicated that the endoplasmic reticulum, rather than the mitochondria, is damaged in the early stages of carbon tetrachloride poisoning.[25] FIGURE 2 shows electron micrographs of a normal rat liver cell and of a rat liver cell three hours after the animal had been treated with carbon tetrachloride.

Further progress came from the finding that the accumulation of triglycerides in the liver was accompanied by a decrease in the concentration of plasma triglycerides. Moreover, the non-ionic detergent Triton, which causes a rapid rise in the plasma triglycerides of normal animals by preventing their exit from the blood, failed to produce a comparable rise in animals which had received carbon tetrachloride orally three and a half hours previously.[26] In others it was found that after intravenous injection of [^{14}C] palmitic acid very little ^{14}C appeared in the plasma triglycerides of rats treated with carbon tetrachloride.

The results indicated that the release of triglycerides from the liver is blocked by carbon tetrachloride. Seakins and Robinson[29] found that the biosynthesis of the protein moiety of low density serum lipoprotein was rapidly inhibited by carbon tetrachloride. Since triglycerides are transported from the liver as lipoprotein it is likely that this represents an early stage in the process whereby carbon tetrachloride leads to the production of a fatty liver. This effect of carbon tetrachloride may be due to its action on cell membranes, but carbon tetrachloride is metabolised by dog and rat liver and the possibility arises that its toxicity is associated with the formation of a highly reactive metabolic product.[28]

Ethionine, the ethyl analogue of methionine, rapidly causes the development of fatty liver when given orally or parenterally to the rat. This is preceded by an inhibition of protein synthesis and is accompanied by a decrease in the level of plasma triglycerides and of low density lipoprotein. In the liver ethionine is converted, by reaction with ATP, to S-adenosylethionine, but the latter, unlike

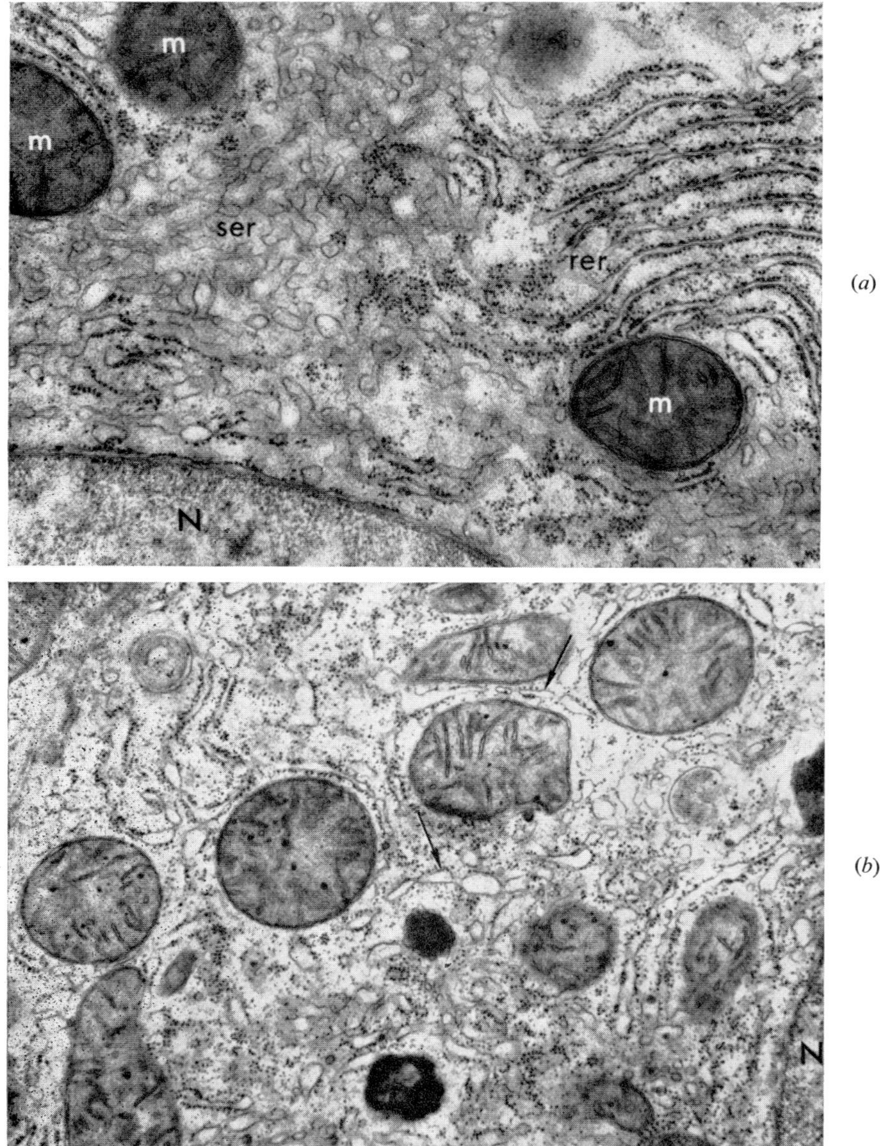

14/Fig. 2.—(*a*) Control liver cell. The membranes of the rough endoplasmic reticulum (rer) are aligned in almost parallel array at the right of the micrograph. An area of smooth endoplasmic reticulum (ser), mitochondria (m), and a portion of the nucleus (N) are indicated. (*b*) Portion of a liver cell of a rat three hours after treatment with carbon tetrachloride. The long profiles of the rough endoplasmic reticulum appear to be segmenting into smaller oval vesicles (arrows). A number of ribonucleoprotein particles are dispersed randomly in the cytoplasmic matrix. A portion of a nucleus (N) is at the lower right. (From Smuckler, Iseri and Benditt[25]).

S-adenosylmethionine, is not readily used for transalkylation and other metabolic processes and its adenine moiety is thus not available for the resynthesis of ATP. The resulting fall in the level of ATP appears to result in an inhibition of the synthesis of nuclear RNA, morphological changes in the endoplasmic reticulum and a failure of protein synthesis. All these changes, together with the accumulation of fat in the liver, can be prevented by the administration of methionine, ATP or adenosine.[29] It seems possible that an inhibition of the synthesis of low density lipoprotein, with a consequent failure in the release of triglycerides, is responsible for the fatty liver observed after the administration of ethionine.

Further studies of fatty change stemmed from the work of Best and his colleagues, who observed fatty livers in pancreatectomised dogs maintained on insulin, in which absorption of food from the intestine was seriously impaired.[30] This was found to be due to a lack of choline, and the latter was described as a lipotropic substance. Methionine was later shown to have lipotropic properties, but these may be due in part to its ability to provide methyl groups for the synthesis of choline.

More recent work has shown a two to three-fold increase in liver triglycerides occurs six to nine hours after a choline deficient diet has been offered to rats previously fasted overnight.[22] A progressive accumulation of fat in the liver was accompanied by a decline in the amount of phospholipid in the plasma, but both these changes could be halted by the oral administration of choline. Experiments with tritium-labelled palmitic acid showed that the fat deposited in the liver came from the fat in the diet and that the synthesis of plasma phospholipids was lower than that in control animals. The injection of [^{14}C] palmitic acid revealed that in choline-deficient animals there was a decrease in the incorporation of ^{14}C into plasma triglycerides. These results have led to the hypothesis that when the supply of choline is inadequate the synthesis of the phospholipid

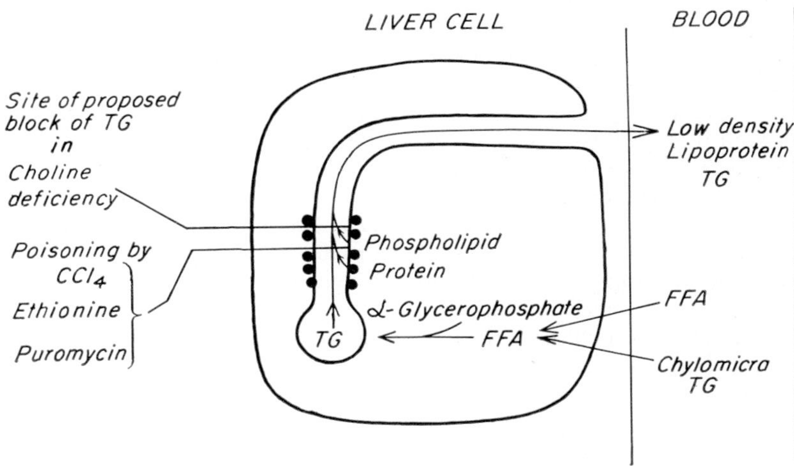

14/Fig. 3.—Hypothetical scheme indicating the role of the endoplasmic reticulum in the development of certain types of fatty liver. FFA denotes free fatty acid and TG denotes triglyceride. Data from ref. 22.

moiety of the low-density serum lipoprotein becomes progressively insufficient, so that an increasing amount of the fat from the diet is retained in the liver.

A significant amount of evidence has thus been obtained to support the view that fatty livers in carbon tetrachloride and ethionine poisoning and in choline deficiency are associated with a failure in the synthesis of low density lipoprotein and thus in the transport of fat from the liver. The accumulation of fat which occurs after the administration of puromycin, an inhibitor of protein synthesis, may be explained in a similar way. The ability of orotic acid to produce fatty liver appears to be associated with a defect in lipoprotein metabolism other than in the synthesis of the protein moiety.[31]

Electron micrographs have indicated that in the early stages of fat deposition in the liver lipid droplets may appear which are enclosed by a membrane in continuity with that of the endoplasmic reticulum.[22] Schemes of the type shown in Fig. 3 have been suggested for the role of the endoplasmic reticulum in some cases. However, not all types of fatty liver are associated with a fall in the concentration of plasma lipids.[32] In the cases of fatty liver induced by ethanol the release of triglyceride from the liver appears to be normal, and a depression of oxidation has been proposed as the significant factor.[33]

Glycogenic Infiltration

Glycogen, which consists of repeating 1:4-glucose residues interrupted by 1:6 branching points, is normally found in muscle and liver cells. In the normal animal it is largely distributed in the liver cell as particulate glycogen which is associated, together with important enzymes involved in its metabolism, with the smooth membrane of the endoplasmic reticulum. In starvation, glycogen depletion is accompanied by the appearance of the major proportion of these enzymes in the soluble fraction of the cell.[34]

Some of the enzymic pathways involved in the synthesis of glycogen are shown in Fig. 4. Glucose-6-phosphate may be formed from glucose, by phosphorylation with ATP, from phosphopyruvate in gluconeogenesis, or from glucose-1-phosphate produced by glycogenolysis with phosphorylase. The glucose-6-phosphate, however, may take part in several different reactions. It may be changed to glucose-1-phosphate, and the latter used in the production of glycogen by a process which appears to involve uridine diphosphate glucose (UDPG) as an intermediate, the presence of a polysaccharide primer, and the action of two enzymes, UDPG-glycogen glucosyl transferase and a branching enzyme, amylo (1, 4 $\rightarrow$ 1, 6) transglucosidase. Secondly it may be degraded by glycolysis or enter an alternative pathway of glucose metabolism. Thirdly it may be hydrolysed to glucose and phosphate by glucose-6-phosphatase, an enzyme normally present in liver and kidney.

During diabetes mellitus glycogenic infiltration is liable to occur in the cells of Henle's loops and an increased amount of glycogen may be found in heart muscle, but these conditions are now becoming rare in consequence of the treatment of diabetes with insulin. In the terminal stages of diabetes there is a great increase in gluconeogenesis in the liver, glucose being synthesized from amino-acids and glycerol in order to maintain a high blood sugar concentration. Severe ketosis may also occur and it appears that this is due to a fall in the rate of the tricarboxylic cycle so that some acetyl coenzyme A is not removed by

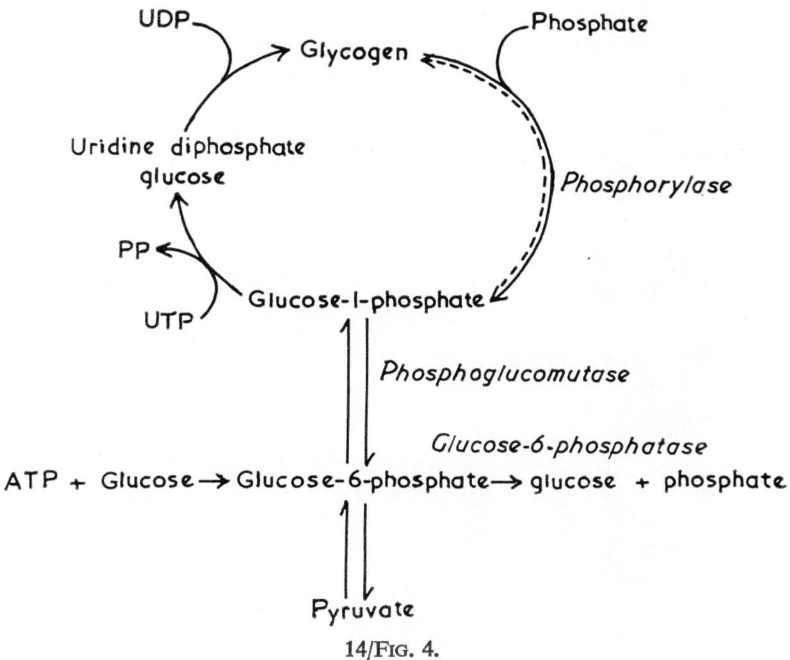

14/Fig. 4.

oxidation and in consequence condenses to acetoacetate. The effect on the tricarboxylic cycle has been attributed to a fall in the steady state level of oxaloacetate resulting from the conversion of the latter to phosphopyruvate at an increased rate during gluconeogenesis.[35]

The deposition of glycogen in the heart muscle during diabetes is associated with the high concentration of glucose in the blood. It would be misleading to suggest, however, that the situation is a simple one. Glycogen might be synthesized from glucose-6-phosphate produced in gluconeogenesis without free glucose being involved as an intermediate. Insulin appears to accelerate the first step in the utilisation of glucose by skeletal muscle or liver, and lack of this hormone hinders not only the breakdown of glucose in these tissues but also its conversion to glycogen. In heart muscle, on the other hand, the deposition of glycogen has been reported to be relatively independent of insulin. Cardiac glycogen in normal rats is increased during fasting and experiments with hypophysectomised rats have indicated that the increase is dependent on the action of the growth hormone.[36] In depancreatised cats and depancreatised-hypophysectomised cats (Houssay animals) the amount of cardiac glycogen has been correlated with the level of blood sugar.[37] It seems clear, therefore, that some of the factors responsible for glycogenic infiltration in heart muscle differ from those that govern glycogenesis and glycogenolysis in liver. But the biochemical reasons for these differences in behaviour remain to be determined.

Another condition that is associated with a derangement of carbohydrate metabolism is known as glycogen storage disease, in which liver cells, heart muscle cells and sometimes kidney cells may become ballooned out with massive glycogenic accumulations (Fig. 5). This condition appears to have a genetic basis; it is encountered mainly in young children and has been diagnosed so rarely during life that relatively few satisfactory studies of its nature have been possible. However, six types of glycogen storage disease can now be recognised.[38, 39] In the commonest type, von Gierke's disease (type I), there is a congenital absence of glucose-6-phosphatase in the liver and kidney and the ability to generate blood glucose from liver glycogen in response to epinephrine or

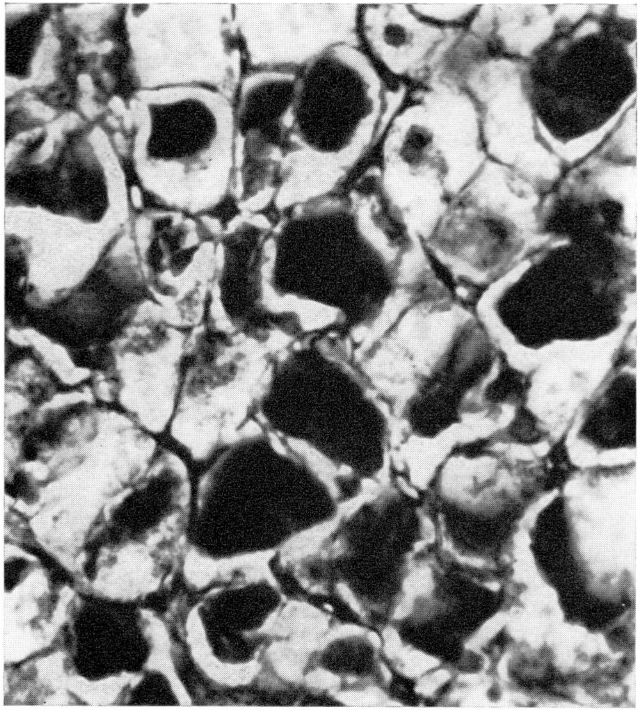

14/Fig. 5.—Liver with glycogen storage disease, stained by the periodic acid-Schiff method. The dark masses of material in the liver cells represent glycogen.

glucagon is completely lacking. This block in the pathway of glycogen metabolism should result in the availability of more glucose-6-phosphate for glycogen synthesis and could increase the rate of synthesis because glucose-6-phosphate activates the enzyme involved in the formation of glycogen from UDPG. Hence it may account for the accumulation of glycogen in liver and kidney. In Pompe's disease (type II) there is a generalized deposition of glycogen and the patients usually die during the first years of life. Children with this disease lack an enzyme (α-[1, 4]-glucosidase) which hydrolyses maltose and glycogen to glucose and which is normally present in liver, heart and skeletal muscles. This enzyme appears to be associated with the lysosomes of the cell (Chapter 15) and it has been suggested that it may catalyse the hydrolysis of glycogen in areas of the cytoplasm in which phosphorylase is inactive. In type III disease the glycogen is structurally abnormal, having relatively short outer chains. The specific debranching enzyme, amylo-1, 6-glucosidase, has been found to be absent from the liver and muscle of children with this disease. Hence, glycogen is degraded until a branching point is reached but further degradation is not possible. In a rare type IV disease the glycogen shows an abnormally low branching pattern and it appears likely that this is due to a deficiency of the branching enzyme, amylo-1, $4 \rightarrow 1$, 6-transglucosidase. In type VI disease the level of hepatic phosphorylase is unusually low and thus glycogenolysis does not occur at a normal rate. In another type (V), in which there is deposition of glycogen in muscle, an enzymic basis for the disease has not yet been found.

Amyloid Infiltration

Amyloid is an insoluble, faintly eosinophilic material which has an affinity for Congo red and is homogenous in the light microscope but shows positive birefringence.[40] Special colour tests have been described for its identification.[11] Amyloid infiltration was frequently encountered in the past with long-standing pulmonary tuberculosis complicated by secondary infection and with leprosy. In general it developed when there had been prolonged suppuration in the body, as with compound fractures, suppurative arthritis and secondary infection in tumours. Nowadays it is found in rheumatoid arthritis, renal infection in paraplegia, and in plasma cell myelomatosis, which have become the most common conditions associated with amyloidosis as methods for the treatment of sepsis have improved.

Amyloid forms around cells or on fibrils and is sometimes seen in the cell interior. In the worst cases many organs are involved in a deposition in the subendothelial tissues of capillaries and tiny arterioles. The spleen, liver (FIG. 6) and kidneys (FIG. 7) and small intestine are the chief sites of occurrence. Sometimes one organ alone is affected, or small lumps of amyloid develop in the upper respiratory passages or conjunctiva. The importance of amyloidosis lies in the secondary complications it adds to an already serious state of affairs, due mainly to the altered permeability of the vessels that accompanies it. Plasma proteins and water may thus be lost from the body through leakage from the kidneys and the small intestine, with proteinuria and diarrhœa.

The name amyloid was introduced by Virchow, following the discovery that the material showed a colour reaction with iodine similar to that shown by starch. But it subsequently emerged that amyloid and starch were not chemically related. Amyloid has been isolated from human and horse amyloid liver and from rabbit spleen by homogenization of the tissue and centrifugation under appropriate conditions. Electron microscopy has revealed that it contains fine fibrils, consisting of fibres about 75 Å in diameter and beaded at 100 Å intervals.[41, 42, 43] It is a protein and probably a glycoprotein with about 4·6 per cent carbohydrate. But it differs clearly from collagen, containing no hydroxyproline and no hydroxylysine.

Amyloidosis can be induced very easily, in some species, by prolonged administration of foreign proteins, such as casein. Mice fed unlimited amounts of cheese develop amyloid change. Horses used for the production of diphtheria antitoxin often show amyloid change in their organs and may even die from

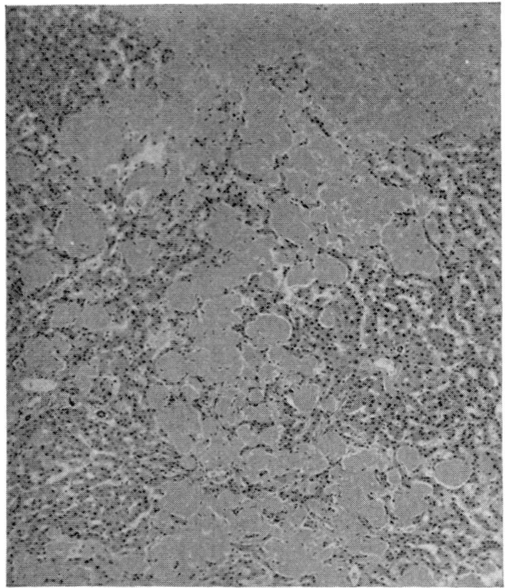

14/FIG. 6.—Amyloid liver. There is extensive replacement of normal structures by homogeneous, palely staining material.

severe liver infiltration. These findings, considered in conjunction with the development of amyloid change in plasma cell myelomatosis, suggest that a common factor involved in amyloidosis is a proliferation of protein-producing plasma cells.[44] In a solubilized form amyloid appears to be immunologically identical with a serum protein which is probably an α-globulin. It has been suggested that the amyloid protein is carried by the blood from its site of

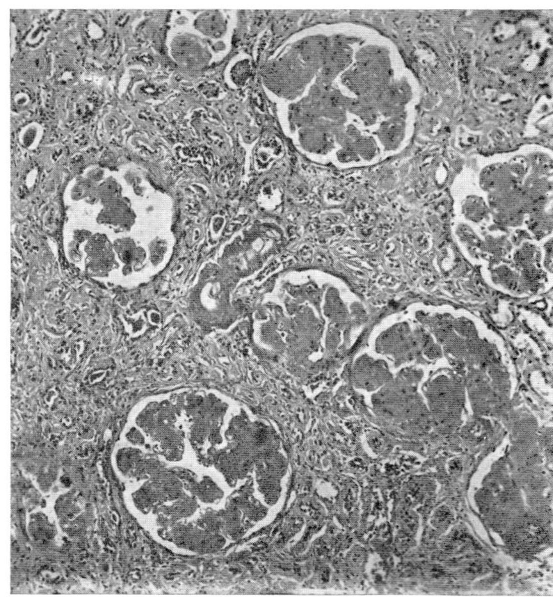

14/FIG. 7.—Amyloid kidney. Amyloid has been deposited in the walls of the afferent arterioles and glomerular capillaries.

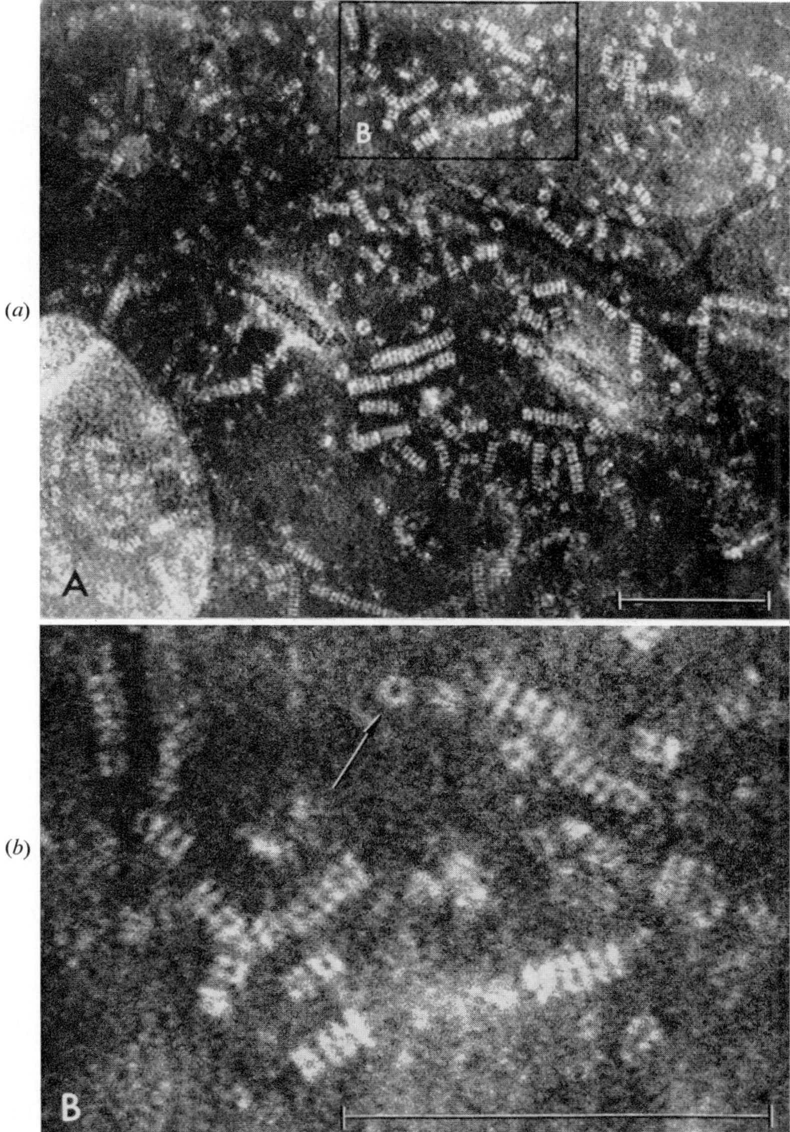

14/Fig. 8.—(*a*) Electron micrograph of isolated amlyoid material negatively stained with phosphotungstic acid. (*b*) The inset marked B in (*a*) at higher magnification. The bars = 1000 Å in both figures. Magnification (*a*) approximately × 196,875, (*b*) approximately × 564,375. (From Benditt and Eriksen.[43])

synthesis and leaks through vascular linings, and that the formation of deposits involves a change from a soluble to a fibril form.

Hyaline Degeneration

Hyaline degeneration is one of the commonest degenerative changes that occurs in the human body. It is usual to distinguish vascular hyaline, sclerotic hyaline and hyaline inclusions in epithelial cells.[45] In renal disease associated with gross proteinuria, the cells of the proximal convoluted tubules show cytoplasmic granules which are called hyaline droplets; these granules are distinct from the mitochondria which tend to become smaller, and it appears that the hyaline inclusions represent droplets of protein reabsorbed into the cell cytoplasm from the glomerular filtrate in the tubular lumen[46]. In certain forms of liver cirrhosis, the cells contain acidophil bodies known as alcoholic hyaline, consisting of a basic protein complex associated with bound phospholipid which is formed in dilated cisternæ of the endoplasmic reticulum of cells progressing to cell death.[47]

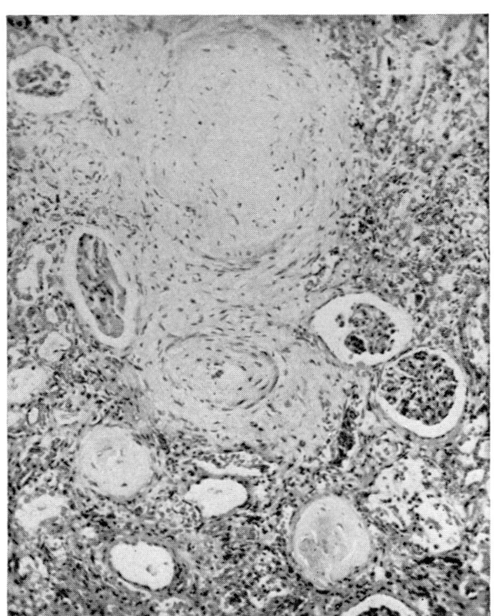

14/Fig. 9.—Kidney showing hyaline degeneration of the walls of arterioles.

Vascular hyaline is the deposition of a transparent acidophil material in the subendothelial region of medium sized arteries and arterioles and is often associated with hypertension and diabetes mellitus; it consists of glycoprotein, fat and fibrin in varying proportions and all the evidence would suggest that it is of hæmatogenous origin.[48, 49]. Sclerotic hyaline is a modification of connective tissue and would appear to be the resultant of a deposition of glycoprotein between collagen fibrils.

REFERENCES

1. Gavrilescu, N., and Peters, R. A. (1931). *Biochem. J.*, **25,** 2150.
2. Krebs, H. A. (1956). In *Ciba Foundation Symposium on Ionizing Radiations and Cell Metabolism.* London: J. & A. Churchill.
3. Schneider, W. C. (1955). In *Proceedings of the Third International Congress of Biochemistry.* New York: Academic Press.
4. Leaf, A., and Renshaw, A. (1957). *Biochem. J.*, **65,** 90.
5. Johnson, M. J. (1941). *Science*, **94,** 200.
6. Lynen, F. (1955). In *Proceedings of the Third International Congress of Biochemistry.* New York: Academic Press.
7. Chance, B., and Williams, G. R. (1955). *Nature (Lond.)*, **175,** 1120.
8. Monod, J., and Jacob, F. (1961). *Cold Spr. Harb. Symp. quant. Biol.*, **26,** 389.
9. Vogel, H. J. (1957). In *The Chemical Basis of Heredity.* Baltimore: Johns Hopkins Press.
10, Tata, J. R. (1964). *Biochim. biophys. Acta (Amst.)*, **87,** 528.
11. Cameron, G. R. (1952). *Pathology of the Cell.* Chapters 20 and 21. Edinburgh: Oliver & Boyd.
12. Christie, G. S., and Judah, J. D. (1954). *Proc. roy. Soc. B*, **142,** 241.
13. Price, C. A., Fonnesu, A., and Davies, R. E. (1956). *Biochem. J.*, **64,** 754.
14. Robinson, J. R. (1952). *Proc. roy. Soc. B*, **140,** 135.
15. Leaf A. (1956). *Biochem. J.*, **62,** 241.
16. Buckley, K. A., Conway, E. J., and Ryan, H. C. (1958). *J. Physiol. (Lond.)*, **143,** 236.
17. Maffy, R. H., and Leaf, A. (1959). *J. gen. Physiol.*, **42,** 1257.
18. Olson, J. A. (1966). *Ann. Rev. Biochem.*, **35,** 559.
19. Isselbacher, K. J. (1965). *Fed. Proc.*, **24,** 16.
20. Robinson, D. S. (1963). *Advances in Lipid Research*, **1,** 134.
21. Senior, J. R. (1964). *J. Lipid Res.*, **5,** 495.
22. Lombardi, B. (1965). *Fed. Proc.*, **24,** 1200.
23. Dianzani, M. U. (1957). *Biochem. J.*, **65,** 119.
24. Recknagel, R. O., and Anthony, D. D. (1959). *J. biol. Chem.*, **234,** 1052.
25. Smuckler, E. A., Iseri, O. A., and Benditt, E. P. (1962). *J. exp. Med.*, **116,** 55.
26. Recknagel, R. O., Lombardi, B., and Schotz, M. C. (1960). *Proc. soc. exp. Biol. (N.Y.)*, **104,** 608.
27. Seakins, A., and Robinson, D. S. (1963). *Biochem. J.*, **86,** 401.
28. Butler, T. C. (1961). *J. Pharmacol. exp. Ther.*, **134,** 311.
29. Farber, E., Shull, K. H., Villa-Trevino, S., Lombardi, B., and Thomas, M. (1964). *Nature (Lond.)*, **203,** 4940.
30. Best, C. H. (1941). *Science*, **94,** 523; Best, C. H., Lucas, C. C., and Ridout, J. H. (1956). *Brit. med. Bull.*, **12,** 9.
31. Roheim, R. S., Switzer, S., Girard, A., and Eder, H. A. (1966). *Lab. Invest.*, **15,** No. 1. p. 21.
32. Seakins, A., and Robinson, D. S. (1964). *Biochem. J.*, **92,** 308.
33. Di Luzio, N. R. (1966). *Lab. Invest.*, **15,** 50.
34. Tata, J. R. (1964). *Biochem. J.*, **90,** 284.
35. Krebs, H. (1965). Plenary Lecture, *Abstracts*, p. 351. 2nd Meeting Fed. European Biochem. Socs.
36. Russell, J. A., and Bloom, W. (1956). *Endocrinology*, **58,** 83.
37. Lukens, F. D. W. (1958). *Amer. J. Physiol.*, **192,** 485.
38. Cori, G. T. (1952–53). *Harvey Lect.*, **48,** 145.

39. Stetten D., jr., and Stetten, M. R. (1960). *Physiol. Rev.*, **40,** 505; Hers, H. G. (1963). *Biochem. J.*, **86,** 11.
40. Calkins, E., Cohen, A. S., and Larsen, B. (1960). *Ann. N.Y. Acad. Sci.*, **86,** 1033.
41. Cohen, A. S., and Calkins, E. (1959). *Nature* (*Lond.*), **183,** 1202.
42. Cohen, A. S. (1966). *Lab. Invest.*, **15,** 66.
43. Benditt, E. P., and Eriksen, N. (1966). *Proc. nat. Acad. Sci.* (*Wash.*), **55,** 308.
44. Azar, H. A. (1966). *Ann. Rev. Med.*, **17,** 49.
45. Delarue, J. (1961). *Path. et. Biol.*, **9,** 1917–1946.
46. Spector, W. G. (1954). *J. Path. Bact.*, **68,** 87, 196.
47. Reppart, J. T., Peter, R. L., Edmondson, H. A., and Barker, R. F. (1963). *Lab. Invest.*, **12,** 1138–1151.
48. Dustin, J. (1962). *Int. Rev. exp. Path.*, 1, 73–138.
49. Fisher, E. R., Perez-Stable, E., and Pardo, V. (1966). *Lab. Invest.*, **15,** 1409–1433

Chapter 15

NECROSIS, CALCIFICATION AND AUTOLYSIS

By E. P. Abraham

NECROSIS

Causes of Necrosis

In the previous chapter we discussed, in general terms, the kind of disturbances that could lead to the death of the cell. Human pathology provides many examples of necrosis caused by such disturbances. Mechanical injury may damage cell membranes and disturb the spatial arrangement of enzymes and their substrates. Blockage of the blood supply to a portion of the body tissue causes an infarct, in which the cells are deprived of oxygen and other substances that are necessary for the balance between synthesis and breakdown to be maintained. Heat denatures cell enzymes, and cold may destroy their organisation. Chemical substances may cause widespread damage to cell structures, or may merely prevent the function of one vital enzyme; or, like radiation, they may break or injure chromosomes.

Some of these factors are considered in Chapters 25, 26 and 30, but a few of them will be mentioned further here.

Heat and cold.—The first evidence of thermal injury to the surface of the body is usually œdema caused by an increased permeability of the capillaries. However, many animal cells die rather rapidly at temperatures higher than 45° C., probably owing to the denaturation of heat-sensitive proteins. Cohnheim showed in 1873 that immersion of a rabbit's ear in water at 52° C. for seven minutes produced necrosis. The earliest visible change in the damaged cells appears to be in the nuclei, which are swollen and show an abnormal distribution of chromatin.

All living cells are much less sensitive to cold than to heat. Unicellular organisms, such as bacteria, can often be subjected to extremely low temperatures without losing their viability. Nevertheless, animal cells can be killed by freezing. One of the factors responsible for their death is thought to be the increase in concentration of electrolytes in the surrounding medium which results from the separation of ice. Another may be mechanical damage produced by ice crystals. Death is less likely to occur if cells are frozen slowly in a medium containing 15 per cent glycerol, so that a relatively low temperature is reached before ice separates.[1] An increase in the concentration of electrolytes may cause damage to cell membranes and intracellular units. It is of interest that the enzyme system concerned with the oxidation of succinic acid, which is associated with the mitochondria, was found by Keilin and Hartree[2] to lose much of its activity on alternate freezing and thawing. The activity could be restored by the addition of an excess of cytochrome C, but since freezing and thawing had no effect on cytochrome C itself it was thought to alter the accessibility of this enzyme to the remainder of the system.

The higher animals are, of course, more sensitive than many tissue-cells to a lowering of temperature. This sensitivity is at least partly a result of the effects of cold on the circulatory system. Frostbite is associated with the formation of hyaline thrombi in the damaged blood vessels. In the notorious experiments carried out at Dachau during the war of 1939–45, it was found that immersion of clothed human subjects in water at 4° C. often proved fatal after one hour, when the rectal temperature was lowered to about 25° C. Death was due to heart failure, which was attributed to direct cold injury and to overloading caused by a great increase in the viscosity of the blood.[3] More recent studies have shown that there is a serious danger of ventricular fibrillation during hypothermia. However, by use of an artificial heart and by direct cooling of the blood, the nasopharyngeal temperature of patients requiring cardiac surgery has been reduced to 15° C. At this temperature circulatory standstill has been maintained for up to 50 minutes without evidence of damage to the brain.[3] Hamsters cooled at −5° C. have been resuscitated after 15 per cent (and in some cases as much as 50 per cent) of their body water was frozen.[1]

Chemical substances.—High concentrations of substances such as phenol, which denature almost all proteins, kill the cells of the tissues and completely inactivate their enzyme systems. Other substances, such as chloroform and carbon tetrachloride, which may act in part by disorganising the lipoid constituents of cell membranes and damaging the endoplasmic reticulum, can cause necrosis without inhibiting enzymes which are able to catalyse the breakdown of cellular structure. Changes in the endoplasmic reticulum also occur in liver poisoning caused by thioacetamide. But although this substance, like carbon tetrachloride, causes necrosis, it does not appear to produce a fatty liver.[4] Aflatoxin, which is considered in Chapter 24, causes liver necrosis and also the growth of tumours. The mode of action of this poison differs from that of a number of other agents which produce liver necrosis but resembles, in some respects, that of actinomycin D. It rapidly reaches the nucleus of liver cells where it combines with DNA and produces an inhibition of the synthesis of nuclear RNA, possibly by preventing the transcription of DNA by RNA polymerase. The suggestion has been made that it inhibits the production of messenger RNA and that this may block the formation of proteins required for the integrity of cellular membranes. An explanation would then be available for the appearance, at a relatively early stage, of hepatic enzymes in the serum.[5]

Among the substances which show a considerable degree of specificity in their toxic action on cells are a number which are alkylating agents and react, *inter alia*, with thiol groups. The question arises whether these substances act *in vivo* by damaging intracellular enzymes which contain free thiol groups that are essential for their activity. In some cases, at least, we have reason to believe that such reactions are important. But to account for the differences in toxicity between one substance and another we must assume that they do not all react equally well with the same enzymes and that some of them are transported more readily than others to sensitive points in the cell.

Lewisite (I), mustard gas (II) and the nitrogen mustards (III) provide examples of substances which react with thiol groups and which cause necrosis in concentrations that are too low to bring about a general denaturation of cell protein. Being soluble in lipoid solvents these substances quickly penetrate the epidermis and reach the aqueous medium of the cellular layer of the skin, where they act as powerful vesicants.

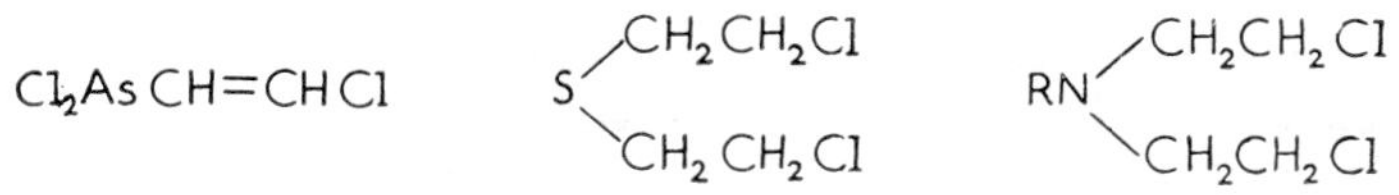

$$Cl_2AsCH{=}CHCl \qquad S\begin{matrix} CH_2CH_2Cl \\ CH_2CH_2Cl \end{matrix} \qquad RN\begin{matrix} CH_2CH_2Cl \\ CH_2CH_2Cl \end{matrix}$$

I II III

Lewisite reacts with simple monothiols, such as glutathione, in the following manner:

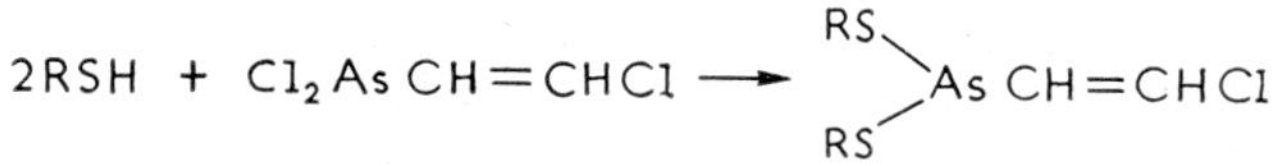

$$2RSH + Cl_2AsCH{=}CHCl \longrightarrow \begin{matrix} RS \\ RS \end{matrix}{>}AsCH{=}CHCl$$

It also reacts with proteins containing SH groups and has proved to be a particularly powerful inhibitor of an enzyme system in pigeon brain which brings about the oxidation of pyruvate. This system, unlike certain others, could not be protected by simple monothiols which might have been expected to compete with an SH enzyme for the toxic substance, but could be protected by the dithiol BAL (dimercaptopropanol, IV). The explanation was thought to be as follows: An enzyme of the pyruvate oxidase system contained two SH groups so placed that they reacted with lewisite to form a ring (V). This ring was more stable than the compound formed by lewisite and a monothiol, but it was less stable than the corresponding ring formed by lewisite and BAL (VI).

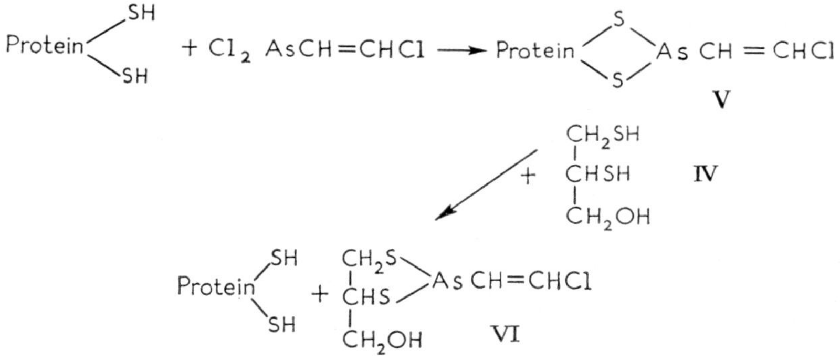

$$\text{Protein}\begin{matrix} SH \\ SH \end{matrix} + Cl_2AsCH{=}CHCl \longrightarrow \text{Protein}\begin{matrix} S \\ S \end{matrix}{>}AsCH{=}CHCl \quad \text{V}$$

$$+ \begin{matrix} CH_2SH \\ | \\ CHSH \\ | \\ CH_2OH \end{matrix} \quad \text{IV}$$

$$\text{Protein}\begin{matrix} SH \\ SH \end{matrix} + \begin{matrix} CH_2S \\ | \\ CHS \\ | \\ CH_2OH \end{matrix}{>}AsCH{=}CHCl \quad \text{VI}$$

BAL, unlike monothiols, was found to be an effective antidote to the toxic effect of lewisite on the tissues. It was therefore suggested that an inactivation of the pyruvate oxidase system was the initial biochemical lesion.[6] Lipoic acid (6 : 8-dithio-octanoic acid), which contains two potential thiol groups, has now been found to be a coenzyme for the oxidative decarboxylation of pyruvate and may well be the component of the enzyme system with which lewisite reacts.

Although this may be the lesion caused by lewisite it does not follow that it is the only lesion which initiates vesication. Other vesicants may act in different ways: an important effect of mustard gas on the enzyme systems of the skin appears to be the inactivation of hexokinase, an SH enzyme which catalyses the formation of glucose-6-phosphate from glucose and adenosine triphosphate.[7]

Although mustard and the nitrogen mustards are vesicants, it has been reported that in high dilutions their first observable action in the body is to inhibit the mitosis of dividing cells. Systemic mustard poisoning in the adult mammal may produce lesions in actively proliferating tissues, such as the bone marrow and intestinal mucosa, without comparable damage to the liver and the kidneys. With threshold doses the cells can subsequently recover, but with larger ones the damage leads to necrosis, and cell death is often accompanied by a fragmentation of the nucleus.[8] Various derivatives of nitrogen mustard have been used for the destruction of neoplastic cells, particularly those of malignant lymphatic tumours. One of the side-effects encountered has been necrosis of individual cells of the liver.[9] Among the cells that survive the action of these substances, some may be changed genetically. Exposure of the fruit fly *Drosophila melanogaster* to mustard gas vapour was found by Auerbach and Robson in 1942 to cause mutations in the sperm.

These changes in the dividing cell are analogous to some of those caused by radiation, but little is known of the way in which they are brought about. They appear to occur in concentrations of the toxic substances which are much lower than those required to produce the gross metabolic disturbances associated with vesication. One suggestion, based on the fact that the normal mustards contain two reactive groups, is that they form cross linkages between chromosomes; it seems unlikely, however, that this is an essential feature of their mode of action, because similar substances containing only one reactive group have proved to be mutagenic.

Appearance of Necrotic Tissue

The appearance of a necrotic area depends on the nature of the tissue, on how the necrosis was caused and in particular on which enzymes in the tissue remain active. Several main types of necrosis have long been distinguished.[10]

Coagulation necrosis.—This is the formation of necrotic tissue which is firm and dry. It is sometimes observed in areas from which the blood supply has been completely shut off, but whether a general coagulation of protein occurs in such tissues, and whether the conversion of plasma fibrinogen to fibrin plays an essential part in the phenomenon, appears to be uncertain. It is also observed in the mucosa of the respiratory passages in diphtheria. True coagulation necrosis is produced by poisons such as phenol, formaldehyde, or mercuric chloride, which denature and coagulate the proteins of the cell.

Caseation is a form of coagulation necrosis in which the dead tissue looks like cheese and contains a mixture of coagulated protein and fat. It occurs particularly in tuberculosis. The tubercle bacilli contain an outer layer of lipoid material, but it is not certain whether this is an important source of the fat in the caseous material, nor is it yet clear how the necrosis is brought about. Since caseous areas are often absorbed only very slowly, and thus appear to be devoid of autolytic enzymes, these enzymes have presumably been inactivated during the development of the lesion. It has been reported that carbohydrate and phosphatide fractions from the tubercle bacillus selectively inhibit intracellular proteinases of tuberculous tissue.[11]

Liquefaction necrosis.—In this condition, which is usually due to autolytic decomposition, the necrotic tissue is soft and surrounded by liquid. It occurs readily in the central nervous system and in tissue which is particularly rich in proteolytic enzymes, such as the gastro-intestinal mucosa and the pancreas. Suppuration is a form of liquefaction necrosis in which rapid digestion is brought about by the proteolytic enzymes from the leucocytes present in the area.

Fat necrosis.—This is a specific form of necrosis of fat tissue, in which the fat is split into free fatty acids and glycerol, the former being deposited as soaps and the latter diffusing away. Fat necrosis is nearly always a result of disease of the pancreas, which allows the lipase in the pancreatic juice to escape from the normal channels within the gland. It can be produced experimentally by injecting extracts of fresh pancreas into fat tissue.

PATHOLOGICAL CALCIFICATION

Dead or degenerating tissues in the body often become impregnated with deposits of calcium salts, which are only precipitated in the normal body in the formation of bone. Two main types of pathological calcification may be distinguished:

Dystrophic calcification, which is the type most often encountered, is the deposition of calcium salts in dead or dying tissues. It occurs in infarcts, in caseating tubercles, in areas of fat necrosis such as are found in pancreatic disease, and in blood vessels in arteriosclerosis. This type of calcification is not associated with an abnormal level of calcium in the serum.

Calcification in or under the skin, which has been termed calcinosis, should probably be regarded as a form of dystrophic calcification. In *calcinosis circumscripta* the deposits are usually in the skin of the fingers, and the patients are commonly found to have suffered from cold hands since early childhood. In *calcinosis universalis* the lesions are more widely distributed and there may be involvement of interstitial tissues.

Metastatic calcification is a rather rare pathological condition which was first described by Virchow in 1855. In this condition calcium salts are deposited in previously undamaged tissues, particularly in the kidneys, lungs, gastric mucosa and the media of blood vessels. Unlike dystrophic calcification and calcinosis, metastatic calcification is associated with an excess of calcium salts in the blood, and it is usually a result of destructive bone lesions and nephritis.

A number of preliminary questions must be answered before we can attempt to understand the reasons for pathological calcification. For example, what is the precise chemical nature of the deposits? How is the inorganic matter of which they are composed carried in the blood stream, and what factors govern its concentration in the blood and in the tissues?

So far as is known, the salts deposited in pathological calcification have a composition similar to those deposited in the normal calcification of bone. The main inorganic constituents of bone are calcium and phosphate, together with some carbonate and with small quantities of magnesium and sodium. The bone mineral is deposited, as minute hexagonal crystals, in an extracellular organic matrix which consists largely of collagen fibres and a ground substance containing mucopolysaccharides. The crystalline material shows an X-ray diffraction pattern similar to that of apatite and it is now thought to be a hydroxyapatite, $Ca_{10}(PO_4)_6(OH)_2$, on which varying quantities of other ions, such as carbonate, can be adsorbed.[12]

The Mechanism of Normal Calcification

The similarity in the composition of the deposits suggests that pathological calcification and normal ossification are processes which have a good deal in common, and that an understanding of the way in which calcium salts are deposited under normal conditions may be important for an understanding of the pathological processes.

Since basic calcium phosphate is the major constituent of calcium salt deposits, it would be expected that the concentrations of Ca^{++} and phosphate ions in the serum would have an important influence on calcification. These concentrations should determine, at least in part, the concentrations of the ions in the fluids bathing the tissues where salts are deposited.

The normal concentrations of calcium and phosphate in serum are dependent, *inter alia*, on the proper functioning of the parathyroid and thyroid glands, and on an adequate intake of vitamin D. Not all the calcium, however, is present in the form of free ions. McLean and Hastings,[13] who measured the concentration of ionic calcium from its effect on the amplitude of contraction of the frog's ventricle, reported that about 50 per cent of the total calcium of serum was bound to protein in a non-diffusible state. A small amount of diffusible but non-ionised calcium may also be present in combination with citrate. It is evident that a change in the ability of the body proteins to bind calcium, or in the concentration of citrate, could disturb the equilibrium between calcium ions in solution and calcium salts in the solid state.

The concentrations of calcium and phosphate in normal plasma are sufficient to bring about the deposition of mineral on dead bone at pH 7·4. However, MacGregor and Nordin[14] have reported that inorganic solutions of calcium and phosphate reach equilibrium with dead bone when the product $[Ca^{++}]^3 \times [PO_4^{\equiv}]^2$ is similar to that in normal plasma at pH 6·8. They suggest that Ca^{++} and $PO_4^{\equiv}$ (rather than $HPO_4^{=}$ as previously believed) govern the equilibrium between bone and the minerals in the tissue fluid and that the normal pH at the surface of living bone is 6·8. Nevertheless, the product of the concentrations of calcium and phosphate ions in normal plasma is below that at which spontaneous precipitation of calcium phosphate occurs in synthetic fluids.[15] Calcification may be initiated by a reaction, between the organic matrix and the ions to be deposited, which provides a nucleus for the formation of a crystal of hydroxyapatite; once formed, the crystal would be expected to grow at a rate which depended on the concentrations of calcium and phosphate. Similarly, resorption of bone is not merely a consequence of a fall in the concentrations of calcium and phosphate ions in the surrounding fluid: the bone mineral and the organic matrix are absorbed together and the process seems to be dependent on the activity of the osteoclast.[16]

Some light appeared to be thrown on the process of normal calcification when Robison[17] found in 1923 that the shaft and epiphyseal cartilage of the femur, tibia and humerus of young rats contained a phosphatase able to hydrolyse hexosemonophosphate with the formation of free phosphate. If calcium hexosemonophosphate was used as a substrate, calcium phosphate was precipitated from solution. This particular phosphomonoesterase—sometimes known as "alkaline phosphatase" because its pH optimum is at about pH 9—was always present in high concentration in ossifying cartilage but not in non-ossifying rib and trachea cartilage, and relatively small quantities appeared to be present in the other tissues examined except kidney and intestinal mucosa. It appears to be produced by osteoblasts. Robison showed that sections of rachitic bones underwent calcification when incubated with a solution of calcium hexosemonophosphate, and he suggested that the bone phosphatase played an important role in normal ossification, by liberating phosphate ions *in situ.*

Later work has confirmed the view that normal calcification in young animals is associated with phosphatase activity. A number of other facts, however, have made it clear that the presence of this enzyme is not sufficient in itself to account for the process. Why, for example, is calcium salt not deposited in other normal tissues which contain the phosphatase? And why is calcification *in vitro* inhibited by substances such as phlorizin, fluoride or iodoacetate in concentrations too low to have any effect on the phosphatase activity? Some property of hypertrophic cartilage in addition to its phosphatase activity seems to be important in ossification.

A constituent of cartilage which has been implicated in calcification is glycogen. The occurrence of glycogen in cartilage was first described by Rouget in 1859 and it was later discovered that cartilage cells accumulate large stores of this substance, prior to calcification, which disappear early in the course of calcium deposition. Marks and Shorr[18] reported that after glycogen had been removed from cartilage by incubation in Ringer solution, or treatment with saliva, calcification *in vitro* did not readily occur. In 1941 Gutman and Gutman[19] made the interesting observation that when glycogen and inorganic phosphate are incubated with ground epiphyses of young animals, the phosphate is rapidly esterified. The fact that the reaction is inhibited by phlorizin is in accordance with the assumption that it is catalysed by a phosphorylase: Glycogen $+$ phosphate$\rightleftharpoons$glucose-1-phosphate. This reaction supplies a mechanism whereby phosphate ions in the blood may be concentrated as organic phosphates in sites where calcification occurs. Its importance is confirmed by the fact that calcification which has been inhibited by phlorizin may be restored by the addition of glucose-1-phosphate. If an ester phosphate formed during the process of glycolysis were a substrate for the bone phosphatase it might be possible to understand why calcification is stopped *in vitro* by dilute solutions of iodoacetate and fluoride, as well as by phlorizin; among the glycolytic enzymes triosephosphate dehydrogenase is inhibited by iodoacetate and enolase by sodium fluoride. However, no such substrate for the bone phosphatase has yet been identified.

The theory that phosphatase brings about calcification of bone by raising the concentration of inorganic phosphate encountered some difficulties. Attention has therefore been focused on other aspects of the problem—the function of the organic matrix and pH changes produced by the metabolism of the bone cells. Boyd and Neuman[20] found that each of the sulphuric acid groups and glucuronic acid groups of chondroitin sulphate, which is present in the ground substance, can bind Ca^{++} and that subsequently phosphate can be taken up until the Ca/P ratio is that of a hydroxyapatite. Although the importance of these particular reactions *in vivo* is uncertain, there can be no doubt that specific structural features of the cartilage matrix confer on it the property of calcifiability. It has been suggested that phosphatase is concerned with the preparation of the matrix, by removal of ester phosphate, rather than with the process of calcification itself. Borle, Nichols and Nichols reported that samples of normal metaphyseal bone could metabolise glucose at rapid rate to form lactic acid.[21] They suggested that the solution or accretion of the bone mineral may be governed by local changes in pH which result from variations in the amount of lactic acid formed by the bone cells. During bone resorption lactic acid may be formed, in part, by metabolism of the organic matrix itself. The discovery that bone contains a variety of acid hydrolases which are latent in cell lysosomes suggests that the release of these enzymes in an acid environment contributes to the hydrolysis of the bone matrix[22].

Mechanisms of Pathological Calcification

Phosphatase, phosphorylase, glycolytic enzymes, structural characters of the organic matrix and local changes in pH have all been thought in turn to be concerned in making hypertrophic cartilage the site of normal calcification, but the precise roles that they play have not yet been determined. The local factors responsible for dystrophic calcification in necrotic tissues are at present even more obscure.

Dystrophic calcification.—Early observations of calcification in areas of pancreatic necrosis led to the idea that the deposition of calcium was connected in some way with the hydrolysis of fat. In 1905 Klotz maintained that fatty acids were formed in necrotic areas and combined with calcium, and that the calcium salts so produced were gradually replaced by calcium phosphate. There is no evidence, however, in support of this theory. Wells found that calcium soaps could not be extracted from tissues undergoing pathological calcification, and Wells and Mitchell showed that calcium soaps introduced into living tissue were absorbed, and not transformed into inorganic salts.

Another suggestion has been that necrotic tissues have an increased alkalinity, which is responsible for the deposition of calcium salts because the latter are soluble in acid, but this view, also, has no firm basis.

The work of Robison, which suggested that there was an association between phosphatase activity and the process of normal ossification, naturally raised the question whether dystrophic calcification was due to the presence of abnormal amounts of phosphatase in necrotic tissue. This question was studied by Gomori,[23] who devised a method whereby both phosphatase and preformed deposits of calcium salt could be detected in the same tissue slice. Calcium salt was detected by successive treatment with cobalt acetate and ammonium sulphide. Insoluble calcium phosphate and carbonate were converted to the corresponding cobalt salts which were subsequently transformed to black cobalt sulphide. The slice was then incubated with a solution of calcium glycerophosphate, and the calcium phosphate presumed to have been newly formed at sites of phosphatase activity was converted to lead phosphate by treatment with lead nitrate. Finally, the slice was stained with a mixture of methyl green and acridine red. After this procedure, preformed calcium salts appeared black, areas of phosphatase activity purplish red and nuclei blue-green.

Histochemical tests are seldom free from pitfalls and the reliability of this one for finding the precise locality of alkaline phosphatase has been questioned; it has been suggested that calcium phosphate may precipitate where there are cell structures favourable for its adsorption rather than at sites of enzyme action. However, by using the test, Gomori found that calcification in bone tumours, and in tubercles in rabbit lung, was invariably associated with phosphatase activity. The osteogenic sarcomata were strongly phosphatase-positive, especially in the most cellular peripheral portions. Deposits of calcium salts were formed in strands of connective tissue within the positive areas, and slowly coalesced. Early tuberculous granulation tissue was phosphatase-negative. As soon as necrosis set in, phosphatase appeared in the centre of the necrotic areas, but it subsequently disappeared from the centre and appeared in areas of fresh necrosis in the peripheral zone of spread. If calcification occurred, it always began at the centre of a phosphatase-positive area and often the deposits eventually formed concentric rings. In the rabbit, some phosphatase is normally present in the lining of the alveoli, the endothelium of the blood vessels and the leucocytes, but Gomori thought that the enzyme was too concentrated in areas of tuberculous necrosis to have come from purely local sources and he concluded that it was not brought in by the leucocytes because it appeared in necrotic tubercles from which leucocytes were absent. He suggested that it was adsorbed from the blood and tissue fluids by some compound of fresh necrotic tissue. This suggestion can be supported by analogy, for Gold and Gould showed that the presence of phosphatase on collagen fibres in healing wounds could be accounted for by the adsorption of the enzyme on collagen from surrounding tissue fluids.

Another possibility, however, is worth considering. Phosphatase may be present in such a form that it is not freely available under normal conditions but is liberated during damage to the tissue. Berthet and de Duve[24] showed that much of the acid phosphatase of rat liver was contained in intracellular particles, now known as lysosomes (see p. 446). When the cells were disintegrated in such a way that the lysosomes remained largely intact, the phosphatase was unavailable for catalysing the hydrolysis of organic phosphate. But the enzyme was liberated from the lysosomes when the latter were broken down by mechanical treatment, by freezing and thawing, by keeping in distilled water or by the action of lytic agents such as saponin and deoxycholate. An alkaline phosphatase in kidney and intestine is associated with a microsome fraction. Thus, phosphatase concerned with pathological calcification might be normally bound to cell constituents but liberated in certain types of necrosis.

While dystrophic calcification may sometimes be connected with an accumulation of free phosphatase, which increases the concentration of phosphate ions in a necrotic area, there is little doubt that it can be favoured by other local changes which are not yet understood. There appears to be no evidence that phosphatase is associated with calcification in human tubercles, and Gomori was unable to demonstrate that it was concerned with the calcification of the hyaline connective tissue which occurred in early arteriosclerosis of the aorta. If the mere accumulation of phosphatase were sufficient for calcium salts to be deposited, the question why calcification does not normally occur in tissues rich in alkaline phosphatase, such as the kidney and intestinal mucosa, would remain unanswered. Possibly the phosphate liberated in normal tissues is rapidly re-esterified by other enzyme systems. The formation of phosphate esters from inorganic phosphate is coupled, in most cases, with energy-producing reactions, and is likely to be greatly reduced by the general disorganisation of cell enzyme systems in necrotic areas. Moreover, a local increase in the concentration of free calcium ions, as well as in the concentration of phosphate, would help the formation of calcium salt deposits. Dystrophic calcification might therefore be favoured by the breakdown, in areas of necrosis, of substances able to bind calcium in a non-ionic form. It might also be favoured by the uncovering of cell structures that provide a suitable matrix for the initial deposition of calcium phosphate.

Metastatic calcification.—Unlike dystrophic calcification, which is caused by local changes, metastatic calcification is due to abnormal concentrations of calcium and phosphate in the blood. Thus, the parathyroid hormone, calcitonin, and vitamin D may play an important part in this phenomenon.

The importance of the parathyroid gland to calcium metabolism was shown by MacCallum and Voegtlin in 1909, who found that the tetany observed after parathyroidectomy was associated with low levels of calcium in the blood. In 1925 Collip prepared extracts from parathyroid tissue which were able to relieve the tetany of parathyroid deficiency and raise the blood calcium level in normal animals. Work by l'Heureux, Tepperman and Wilhelmi[25] indicated that the active material in these extracts consisted of polypeptide. Hawker, Glass and Rasmussen have isolated the hormone by chromatography on Sephadex G 100 and on carboxymethyl cellulose.[26] It appears to exist in the gland as a polypeptide with a molecular weight of about 10,000, but some fragment of this molecule may be split off when extraction of the gland is carried out under acidic conditions. It is closely associated with two other biologically active peptides.

The parenteral administration of parathyroid extract has effects on the serum calcium and phosphorus that are illustrated in Fig. 1. There is a rapid increase in the rate of phosphate excretion which is followed closely by a fall in serum phosphate. The serum calcium level begins to rise and much later the urinary calcium as well. When the extract is administered for a long time a net negative balance of calcium and phosphate develops, and the bone is depleted of its minerals.

Ellsworth assumed that the essential action of parathyroid extract was to lower the renal threshold for phosphate. The resulting fall in the level of serum phosphate was thought to disturb the equilibrium between Ca^{++}, phosphate ions, and insoluble calcium phosphate, so that fresh Ca^{++} from the body stores went into solution. This effect on phosphate excretion is important, but there is no doubt that the parathyroid also acts directly on bone. Parathyroid extract raises the level of serum calcium in nephrectomised animals and, when it is given to normal dogs, this level continues to rise even after the value of the ionic product $[Ca^{++}]^3 \times [PO_4^{\equiv}]^2$ has exceeded that required for the calcification of rachitic cartilage *in vitro*. Moreover, parathyroid transplants produce a local and specific resorption of bone in contact with them and inhibit collagen synthesis by the osteoblasts.[27] According to one theory, the hormone increases the production of citrate by the bone cells and the citrate carries calcium into the blood stream before being metabolised. Borle, Nichols and Nichols, however, reported that citrate production by the metaphyses of mice *in vitro* is not

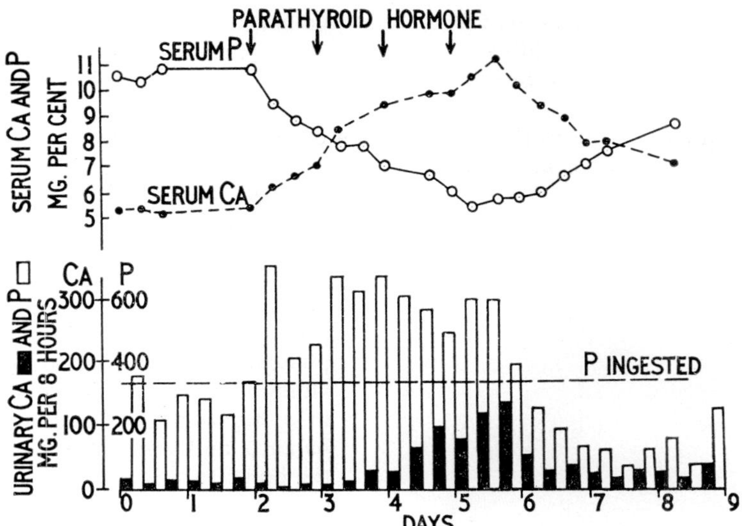

15/FIG. 1.—Effects of parathyroid hormone (50 units per day) in patient with ideopathic hypoparathyroidism. Food constant in amount and composition was given during each 8-hour period. Note immediate increase in excretion of phosphate (negative balance) accompanied by reversals of the high serum phosphate and low serum calcium levels, and much later increase in urinary calcium (as serum calcium rose above 8 mg. per cent). (After Albright and Ellsworth, *J. clin. Invest.*, 1929, **7**, 183, and after Fulton.[47])

significantly increased by prior administration of parathyroid extract to the animals, whereas lactic acid production in the presence of oxygen and glucose is increased substantially.[21] They suggested that the parathyroid hormone stimulates the metabolism of the organic matrix and that a fall in pH due to an increased production of lactic acid facilitates the solution of the bone mineral. This hypothesis appeared to be consistent with subsequent findings that the hormone exerted an effect on ionic fluxes across the mitochondrial membrane and that associated with this effect were changes in respiration and glycolysis.[28] However, assessment of the evidence for the theory of acid mobilization has been complicated by the fact that impure preparations of the hormone were used in some experiments, for these preparations are contaminated with peptides which affect glycolysis and the tricarboxylic acid cycle.

More recent work has directed attention to other possible effects of the parathyroid hormone on the organic matrix. Bone resorption induced by the hormone is inhibited by actinomycin D, perhaps because the latter blocks the mobilization of new osteolytic cells. After incubation of ascites cells with very low concentrations of hormone, a substance appeared in the extracellular fluid which caused the mobilization of carbon from dead bone.[29] Further studies in this field should lead to more precise information about the mode of action of the hormone at the cellular level.

In 1961 Copp obtained evidence that a second hormone, which he named calcitonin, was involved in the control of calcium levels in the blood.[30] Calcitonin is produced mainly by the thyroid gland and is a polypeptide.[31] In contrast to the hypercalcemic action of the parathyroid hormone it exerts a hypocalcemic effect and appears to inhibit resorption of bone. It leads to a decrease in the excretion of hydroxyproline in the urine, whereas the parathyroid hormone causes an increase.[32]

Vitamin D facilitates the absorption of calcium from the gut. A number of experiments have indicated that its action is dependent on RNA and protein synthesis and possibly on the synthesis of a protein which forms a complex with calcium.[33] Albright, Bloomberg, Drake, and Sulkowitch[34] found that in very large amounts it also increases the excretion of phosphate in the urine. Over-dosage with vitamin D may result, after a time, in a negative Ca^{++} and phosphate balance and loss of mineral from the bone. In this there is a similarity between the pharmacological effects of vitamin D and the parathyroid hormone, although the latter is ineffective in the treatment of vitamin D deficiency.

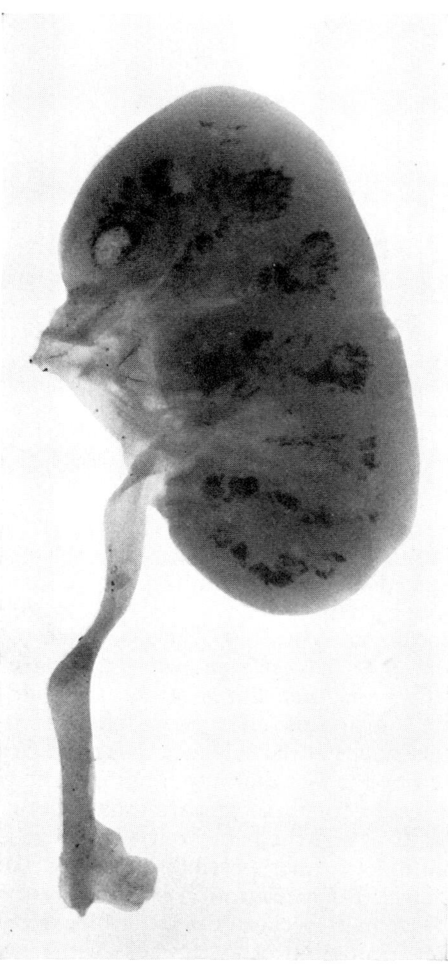

15/Fig. 2.—Radiograph of a human kidney in hyperparathyroidism showing the opacities of calcium deposited in the medullary region.

It is of interest that both hypoparathyroidism and hyperparathyroidism can result in abnormal calcification. Hypoparathyroidism is most commonly caused by accidental removal of the parathyroid glands in the course of a thyroid operation, but in rare cases it is idiopathic. In this condition symmetrical, bilateral calcification of the basal ganglia of the brain tissue is not uncommon. Albright and Reifenstein believe that the calcification is due to decreased excretion of phosphate, leading to increased serum phosphate and consequently to a tendency to supersaturation with calcium phosphate. This may be so, but the fact that calcium salts are selectively deposited in certain tissues requires an additional explanation.

Primary hyperparathyroidism may be due to an adenoma, or more rarely a carcinoma, of the parathyroid tissue. It gives rise to a condition known as osteitis fibrosa cystica, or von Recklinghausen's disease of bone. The disease may sometimes terminate in metastatic calcification, and the sequence of events is supposed to be as follows: a high serum calcium level; damage to the kidneys, possibly caused by a local precipitation of calcium salts; renal insufficiency which is responsible for a rise in serum phosphate; and finally precipitation of calcium phosphate in the tissues. The extensive calcification that may occur in

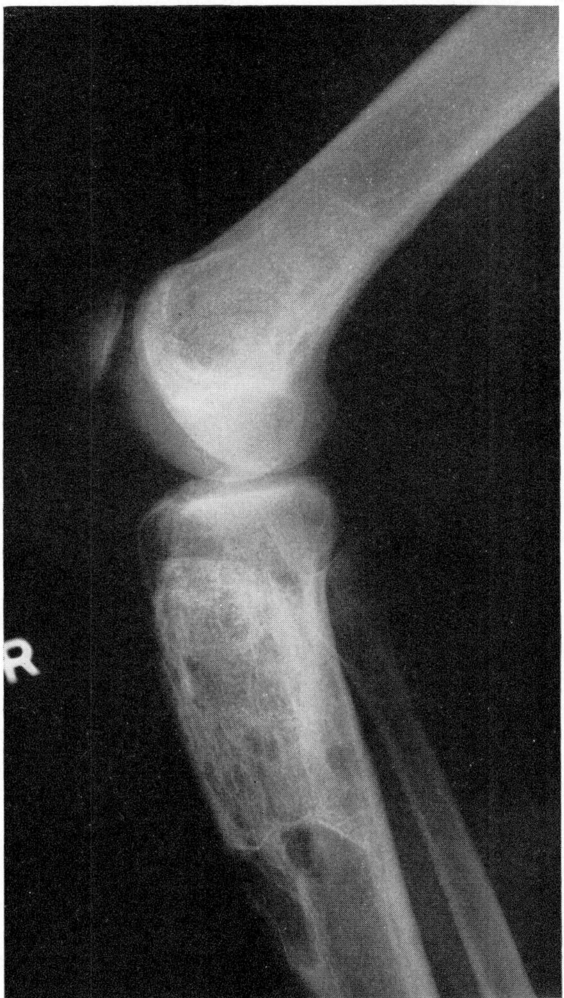

15/FIG. 3.—Radiograph of tibia showing well-marked rarefaction with cyst formation in a case of hyperparathyroidism.

the kidney is illustrated in FIG. 2, and the rarefaction of the bone in FIG. 3. Albright and Reifenstein[35] believe that in severe cases of osteitis fibrosa cystica a high calcium diet may be fatal and that this may have caused the death of "some of the patients with hyperparathyroidism in other clinics who died under rather mysterious circumstances shortly after entering the hospital".

Metastatic calcification can occur after the administration of excessive amounts of vitamin D. Gross overdosage of children with this vitamin has sometimes proved fatal. The effect is presumably a consequence of the ability of vitamin D to increase calcium absorption from the gut and to increase phosphate excretion in the urine. As in hyperparathyroidism, this may result in high serum calcium levels, renal failure, a consequent rise in serum phosphate and finally precipitation of calcium phosphate in the tissues. Whether pathological calcification is associated with calcitonin deficiency remains to be determined.

A series of events similar to those which follow parathyroid or vitamin D poisoning is probably responsible for the metastatic calcification which may accompany destructive bone lesions due to multiple myeloma, osteogenic sarcomata, or carcinomatous metastases in bone.

In all these cases of metastatic calcification it has been postulated that renal failure plays an important part, being responsible for bringing the serum phosphate to a level at which the product $[Ca^{++}]^3\,[PO_4^{\equiv}]^2$ exceeds that necessary for the deposition of calcium phosphate. Whatever the mechanism by which it is brought about, there is no doubt that renal damage almost always accompanies calcium metastases. This relationship was noticed by Virchow, who concluded that nephritis was a necessary second factor for the production of calcium deposits in skeletal disease. Since large doses of parathyroid hormone cause damage to the kidneys of experimental animals, the abnormal calcium and phosphate levels in the serum are probably themselves responsible for this phenomenon.

Metastatic calcification is usually localised in the kidneys, the alveoli of the lungs, the mucous membranes of the stomach, and the thyroid. In the kidney there is calcification of tubular epithelial cells and the formation of casts which plug the tubules. The formation of these calcium deposits in the kidney may be ascribed in part to a raised concentration of calcium and phosphate ions, but other local factors appear to be involved. To account for the calcification of the lungs and stomach, it has been suggested that the formation of deposits is facilitated by alkaline conditions resulting from the excretion of acid. However, this suggestion has no experimental support. In metastatic, as in other forms of calcification, much remains to be learned of the local mechanisms which facilitate the deposition of calcium phosphate.

AUTOLYSIS

In 1871 Hoppe-Seyler noted that dead tissue could liquefy in the body without undergoing putrefaction, as though it had been dissolved by digestive ferments. Salkowski showed later that the change was due to the digestion of the tissue by its intracellular enzymes, and in 1900 Jacoby named the process autolysis.

After death, practically all body tissues may undergo autolysis provided they have not been treated in such a way that their hydrolytic enzymes have been destroyed. The rate of autolysis, however, varies greatly. In connective tissues it takes place, if at all, only very slowly. In tissues such as the pancreas and gastric mucosa, which are exceptionally rich in proteolytic enzymes, it is very rapid. In liver, kidney, spleen, muscle or brain, it occurs at a moderate rate.

With most parenchymatous cells, one of the first morphological changes that occurs is in the nucleus. In a process known as pyknosis the chromatin strands, which contain desoxyribonucleic acid, condense to form a compact basophilic mass. This is followed by karyolysis, in which the nuclei lose their ability to be stained by basic dyes and all that appears to remain of the cell is a non-nucleated mass of cytoplasm. We are not yet able to give a detailed account of the biochemical reactions that are responsible for these histological changes. But we know that the enzyme desoxyribonuclease catalyses the depolymerisation into smaller units of the DNA obtained from the nucleus; and that nucleo-phosphatases can degrade these units further with the liberation of phosphoric acid. Mirsky[36] isolated chromosomes from thymus, pancreas, liver and kidney and reported that they consist of DNA, histone and a residual protein. The histone could be removed without any marked change in their appearance, but the combination of DNA with residual protein was essential for their morphological integrity. When DNA was removed from histone-free chromosomes by desoxyribonuclease, a mass of tiny coiled protein threads, which no longer stained like the original structures, remained behind. When the residual protein was disintegrated by a proteolytic enzyme, the DNA formed a viscous gel in which nothing could be seen under the microscope.

The chemical changes which occur during the autolysis of a tissue such as liver are too complex to be considered here in detail. If liver is minced immediately after death, one of the first recognisable changes is an increase in acidity, the pH falling from 7·2 to 6·8 in a few minutes and possibly to 6·2 within an hour. These changes reflect the liberation of phosphoric acid from nucleic acids and other substances by phosphatases, the liberation of fatty acids from fats by lipases, and the formation of acid by glycolysis. Proteolysis begins at once and can be detected by an increase in the amount of nitrogenous material that is soluble in trichloracetic acid. How far the breakdown of protein proceeds depends partly on the hydrogen ion concentration, for among the intracellular proteolytic enzymes, which are known as cathepsins, are some that show maximum activity on the acid side of neutrality. At pH 6·8 about 50 per cent of the liver protein is fragmented in a prolonged digestion, whereas if the pH is adjusted to 4·0 this percentage is raised to nearly 98.[37]

The question arises why autolysis occurs in dead but not in healthy tissue, since living cells of the body contain autolytic enzymes and some of these cells are also exposed to extracellular proteinases such as pepsin and trypsin.

Pepsin, trypsin and other extracellular proteolytic enzymes are not a source of internal danger to the cells from which they originate because they are secreted in an inactive form. For example, inactive trypsinogen is formed in the pancreas and converted to active trypsin by contact with enterokinase in the small intestine. However, the fact that the active enzymes do not dissolve cells of the digestive tract for long excited the curiosity of physiologists. Claude Bernard suggested that the cells were protected by a layer of mucus, and Wieland that they contained antienzymes. A trypsin-inhibitor, which combines with the enzyme to form an inactive complex, is present in certain worms able to live in the presence of trypsin in the intestine and is also found in the pancreas and the blood. But it is unlikely that such inhibitors are the main cause of the resistance of all living cells to proteolysis. Northrop[38] found that worms and certain unicellular organisms removed no trypsin from the surrounding medium while they were alive, whereas they took up large amounts of the enzyme—and were digested—once they had been killed by heat or mechanical injury. We must conclude that the outer layers of living cells, which appear to consist of muco- and lipoprotein, are resistant to digestion by common proteolytic enzymes, and that while these layers remain intact the enzymes are not able to enter the sensitive cytoplasm.

Some breakdown of complex molecules occurs continuously in living cells, but is balanced by synthesis. When cells die many of their synthetic activities are brought to an end. But whatever the way in which the autolytic process in dead cells begins, it is soon facilitated by factors other than the mere cessation of synthesis. The breakdown of intracellular membranes, which allows hydrolytic enzymes free access to their potential substates is probably of great importance. Thus de Duve has shown that certain animal cells contain a group of cytoplasmic particles, called lysosomes, which enclose a variety of hydrolytic enzymes. These enzymes show maximum activity at an acid pH and include acid phosphatase, cathepsins, a ribonuclease and a desoxyribonuclease. Lysosomes occur in liver and kidney and possibly in other tissues. They sediment somewhat more slowly than normal mitochondria in 0·25 M sucrose and appear to be bounded by a lipoprotein membrane. They are ruptured when placed in a medium of low osmotic pressure, when subjected to freezing and thawing, and when treated with surface active agents or with proteolytic enzymes, and their hydrolytic enzymes are then released into the surrounding medium.[39, 40]

In the early stages of liver injury caused by carbon tetrachloride or thioacetamide the lysosomes appear to remain largely intact.[41] But in the later stages of damage to the liver of rats, produced by ligature of the vascular pedicle of the left lobe or by injection of carbon tetrachloride into the animals, there was a considerable increase in the proportion of lysosomal enzymes found free in the homogenised liver tissue. It has thus been suggested that lysosomes are liable to be ruptured in dead or dying cells and that their hydrolytic enzymes then take part in tissue autolysis. The integrity of intracellular structures which contain substrates for these enzymes may also be preserved by barrier membranes. An analogy is provided by the T_2 bacteriophage which contains, like chromosomes, a high proportion of DNA, but is not susceptible to the action of desoxyribonuclease until the protein membrane that surrounds it has been damaged.[42]

The hydrolysis of proteins in necrotic tissue is favoured by two changes which increase the activity of the intracellular cathepsins. One is the fall in pH to which we have already referred. The other is the fall in the oxidation-reduction potential that follows a decrease or stoppage of the blood supply. Some of the cathepsins contain SH groups; they lose their activity when these groups are oxidised to -S-S- but are reactivated on reduction by, for example, glutathione: Enzyme-S-S-Enzyme $+$ 2RSH $\rightleftharpoons$ 2 Enzyme-SH $+$ R-S-S-R. A failure in the supply of oxygen thus favours the maintenance of the cathepsins in their active form. Moreover, the rupture of lysosomes occurs more readily in the absence than in the presence of oxygen and is favoured by a fall in pH. It may be that activation of cathepsins, following necrosis, enables these enzymes to attack the lysosomal membrane from within.

The relationship of the state of oxidation-reduction in tissue to the extent of autolysis was clearly illustrated in an experiment described by Voegtlin, Maver and Johnson in 1932, using rat tumour tissue.[43] Digestion was investigated first in an atmosphere of nitrogen, then under high oxygen-tension and finally for a second period under nitrogen, and cleavage was measured by the decrease in the amount of protein precipitated by trichloracetic acid. During the initial period of low oxygen-tension the total -SH remained constant and autolysis proceeded. In the period of high oxygen-tension the total -SH rapidly diminished and the amount of precipitable protein increased, indicating that protein synthesis more than compensated for protein cleavage. In the third period, when oxygen was replaced by nitrogen, autolysis was resumed.

Autolysis in Pathological Processes

Absorption of dead tissue in the body is commonly brought about by enzymic digestion. In some cases the digestion is accomplished entirely by the enzymes of the tissue itself, but in others it is greatly aided by the enzymes of leucocytes which have accumulated in the necrotic area.

Leucocytes contain a number of hydrolytic enzymes which vary with the type of cell and the species of animal from which it comes. Some of them, together with an antibacterial basic protein, appear to be localized in lysosomes.[39] In the living leucocyte these enzymes digest material that has been phagocytosed, but on the death of the cell they may escape into the surrounding tissue.[44] For example, a trypsin-like enzyme is liberated in considerable quantity from the polymorphonuclear leucocytes of man.[45] The serum, however, contains an inhibitor of this enzyme and the amount of proteolysis will therefore depend on the relative proportions of leucocytes and serous exudate in the area concerned. When necrosis is accompanied by the accumulation of large numbers of leucocytes the condition is known as suppuration, and the various cells and their degradation products, together with exuded blood plasma, constitute pus (see Chapter 4).

Pneumonia.—A remarkable example of autolysis is the stage of resolution in lobar pneumonia, now seen much less often than it used to be because the disease can usually be treated effectively with chemotherapeutic agents. During resolution there is a great and rapid digestion of the contents of the alveoli by the leucocytic enzymes, while the living lung-tissue, being immune to hydrolytic enzymes, remains unaffected.

Liver atrophy.—In a condition known as *acute yellow atrophy*, autolysis occurs in the liver. This condition appears to be caused by a variety of agents which can bring about massive necrosis of the liver without inactivating the autolytic enzymes of the parenchymatous cells.[46] It may be associated with infectious hepatitis, or with poisoning by chloroform, phosphorus, trinitrotoluene or arsenicals. The liver develops a yellow colour, possibly due to the formation of bilirubin from the blood pigment, and is reduced considerably in size, and large amounts of amino-acids appear in the blood and the urine.[48] If the process continues until death is caused by systemic poisoning, the liver may be found at autopsy to have lost from one-third to one-half of its volume.

PUTREFACTION

When necrotic tissue is invaded by certain bacteria, far-reaching putrefactive changes, catalysed by bacterial enzymes, are superimposed on the process of autolysis.

Among the most important bacteria that may infect necrotic tissue are some of the *Clostridia*. These anærobic organisms can bring about proteolysis and degrade the resulting amino acids to a variety of simpler and sometimes foul-smelling products. They can also break down lipoprotein by hydrolysing lecithin. When a wound is infected with the pathogenic *Cl. welchii*, *Cl. septicum* or *Cl. œdematiens*, the clinical condition is known as gas gangrene and is characterised by liquefaction of tissues around the wound and the appearance of bubbles of gas. Gas gangrene is now rare, at least in peace-time, but before the use of aseptic techniques it was a common sequel to surgery.

Some of the *Clostridia* contain enzyme systems which are able to bring about the deamination of amino acids with the liberation of ammonia and gaseous hydrogen. Many bacteria contain cysteine desulphurase, an enzyme which catalyses the decomposition of cysteine to hydrogen sulphide, ammonia and pyruvic acid. They also contain decarboxylases which convert amino acids into carbon dioxide and amines; lysine, for example, is decarboxylated to cadaverine in the following manner:

$$H_2NCH_2CH_2CH_2CH_2CHNH_2COOH \longrightarrow H_2NCH_2CH_2CH_2CH_2CH_2NH_2 + CO_2$$

Amines formed in this way are sometimes called ptomains and it was once thought that they were the main instruments by which bacteria caused disease. This view has long ceased to be tenable, but a few of the ptomains, such as histamine and tyramine, show considerable pharmacological activity.

CONCLUSION

In these two chapters on the degeneration, death and dissolution of body tissues emphasis has been given to the fact that the life of the cell depends on the integrity of highly organised systems of enzymes, separated, in some cases, from each other, and also from certain of their substrates by intracellular membranes. By considering the ways in which these systems may be damaged or disturbed it has been possible to obtain a general idea of the factors which are responsible for some of the changes in injured tissue. Nevertheless, changes are highly complex and our knowledge of most of them is yet only fragmentary. The various types of body cell differ greatly in their susceptibility to different kinds of injury, but the reasons for the differences are only dimly understood. The stability of a number of body tissues is partly controlled by hormones, but the mechanisms by which most hormones act are still undetermined. Even when the primary biochemical lesion in an injured tissue has been discovered, the problem remains of unravelling the thread of its numerous consequences. Here it is necessary to consider not only the organisation of enzymes within the cells, but also the organisation of the cells within the tissue, and the dependence of one tissue on another. A deeper understanding of such interrelationships in the normal animal may be one of the requirements for substantial progress in this field.

REFERENCES

1. Lovelock, J. E., and Smith, A. U. (1956). *Proc. roy. Soc. B*, **145**, 427.
2. Keilin, D., and Hartree, E. F. (1940). *Proc. roy. Soc. B*, **129**, 277.
3. Gagge, A. P., and Herrington, L. P. (1947). *Ann. Rev. Physiol.*, **9**, 409; Drew, C. E. (1961). *Brit. med. Bull.*, **17**, 37.

4. JUDAH, J. D., AHMED, K., and MCLEAN, A. E. M. (1965). *Fed. Proc.*, **24,** 1217.
5. CLIFFORD, J. I., and REES, K. R. (1967). *Biochem. J.*, **102,** 65; CLIFFORD, J. I., REES, K. R., and STEVENS, M. E. M. (1967). *Biochem. J.*, **103,** 258.
6. PETERS, R. A. (1948). *Brit. med. Bull.*, **5,** 313.
7. DIXON, M., and NEEDHAM, D. M. (1946). *Nature (Lond.)*, **158,** 432.
8. FRIEDENWALD, J. S. (1948–51). *Ann. N.Y. Acad. Sci.*, **51,** 1432.
9. SMITH, H. F. (1963). *Ann. N.Y. Acad. Sci.*, **104,** 821.
10. WELLS, H. G. (1920). *Chemical Pathology*, 4th edit. Philadelphia: W. B. Saunders Co.
11. WEISS, C., and HALLIDAY, N. (1944). *Proc. Soc. exp. Biol.* (*N.Y.*), **57,** 299.
12. CARLSTRÖM, D., and ENGSTRÖM, A. (1956). In *The Biochemistry and Physiology of Bone*. Ed. BOURNE, G. H. New York: Academic Press Inc.
13. MCLEAN, F. C., and HASTINGS, A. B. (1935). *J. biol. Chem.*, **108,** 285.
14. MACGREGOR, J., and NORDIN, B. E. C. (1960). *J. biol. Chem.*, **235,** 1215.
15. NEUMAN, W. F., and NEUMAN, M. W. (1953). *Chem. Rev.*, **53,** 1.
16. FOURMAN, P. (1960). *Calcium Metabolism and the Bone*. Oxford: Blackwell Scientific Publications.
17. ROBISON, R. (1923). *Biochem. J.*, **17,** 286.
18. MARKS, P. A., and SHORR, E. (1950). *Science*, **112,** 752.
19. GUTMAN, A. B., and GUTMAN, E. B. (1941). *Proc. Soc. exp. Biol.* (*N.Y.*), **48,** 687.
20. BOYD, E. S., and NEUMAN, W. F. (1951). *J. biol. Chem.*, **193,** 243.
21. BORLE, A. B., NICHOLS, N., and NICHOLS, G. (1960). *J. biol. Chem.*, **235,** 1206, 1211.
22. VAES, G. (1965). *Biochem. J.*, **97,** 393.
23. GOMORI, G. (1943). *Amer. J. Path.*, **19,** 197.
24. BERTHET, J., and DE DUVE, C. (1951). *Biochem. J.*, **50,** 174.
25. L'HEUREUX, M. V., TEPPERMAN, H. M., and WILHELMI, A. E. (1947). *J. biol. Chem.*, **168,** 1671
26. HAWKER, C. D., GLASS, J. D., and RASMUSSEN, H. (1966). *Biochemistry*, **5,** 344.
27. GAILLARD, P. J. (1961). In *The Parathyroids*, p. 20. Eds. GREEP, R. O., and TALMAGE, R. V. Springfield, Ill.: C. C. Thomas.
28. RASMUSSEN, H., FISCHER, J., and ARNOUD, C. (1964). *Proc. nat. Acad. Sci.* (*Wash.*), **52,** 1198.
29. TENENHOUSE, A., MEIER, R., and RASMUSSEN, H. (1966). *J. biol. Chem.*, **241,** 1314.
30. COPP, D. H., CAMERON, E. C., CHENEY, B. A., DAVIDSON, A. G. F., and HENZE, K. G. (1962). *Endocrinology*, **70,** 638.
31. GUDMUNDSSON, T. V., MACINTYRE, I., and SOLIMAN, H. A. (1966). *Proc. roy. Soc. B*, **164,** 460.
32. ARNAUD, C. D., TENENHOUSE, A. M., and RASMUSSEN, H. (1967). *Ann. Rev. Physiol.*, **29,** 349.
33. WASSERMAN, R. H., and TAYLOR, A. N. (1966). *Science*, **152,** 791.
34. ALBRIGHT, F., BLOOMBERG, E., DRAKE, T., and SULKOWITCH, H. W. (1938). *J. clin. Invest.*, **17,** 317.
35. ALBRIGHT, F., and REIFENSTEIN, E. C. (1948). *Parathyroid Glands and Metabolic Bone Disease*. Baltimore: Williams & Wilkins.
36. MIRSKY, A. E. (1950–51). *Harvey Lect.*, p. 98.
37. BRADLEY, H. C. (1938). *Physiol. Rev.*, **18,** 173.
38. NORTHROP, J. H. (1939). *Crystalline Enzymes*. New York: Columbia Univ. Press.
39. DE DUVE, C. (1959). In *Subcellular Partices*, p. 128. Washington: American Physiological Society.
40. BEAUFAY, H., and DE DUVE, C. (1959). *Biochem. J.*, **73,** 604.
41. SLATER, T. F., and GREENBAUM, A. L. (1965). *Biochem. J.*, **96,** 484.
42. HERSHEY, A. D., and CHASE, M. (1952). *J. gen. Physiol.*, **36,** 39.

43. Voegtlin, C., Maver, M. E., and Johnson, J. M. (1933). *J. Pharmacol. exp. Ther.*, **48,** 241.
44. Opie, E. L. (1922). *Physiol. Rev.*, **2,** 552; Zeya, H. I., and Spitznagel, J. K. (1963). *Science*, **142,** 1085.
45. Husfeldt, E. (1931). *Z. Physiol, Chem.*, **194,** 137.
46. Himsworth, H. P. (1947). *Lectures on the Liver and its Diseases.* Oxford: Blackwell Scientific Publications.
47. Fulton, J. F. (1949). *A Textbook of Physiology.* Philadelphia: W. B. Saunders Co.
48. Dent, C. E., and Walshe, J. M. (1954). *Brit. med. Bull.*, **10,** 247.

Chapter 16

THE FUNCTIONAL SIGNIFICANCE OF CONNECTIVE TISSUE

By A. H. T. Robb-Smith

Connective tissue is the most widely distributed of all the tissue elements in the body and is involved in most of its functional activities. It is only recently that this extracellular fabric has attracted attention because, for the last hundred years, interest had been focused on the cells rather than their surroundings.

History of the Fibre Concept

It would be tedious to trace the full historical evolution of the fibre concept, but briefly it may be said that until the Renaissance the idea of a fibre structure was restricted to those tissues such as tendons, muscles and vessels which have an obvious fibrillary pattern. It was Fernel who put forward the idea that all organs and tissues were built on a network of fibres, and the supporters of his theories were delighted to find, with the introduction of microscopy in the seventeenth century, that, in fact, the organs and tissues were made up of interlacing fibres and pores. For the next hundred and fifty years the fibre pattern was the basis of pathology, but this extreme mechanistic viewpoint was swept away by Boerhaave's chemical outlook, which introduced the idea that it was the tissue juices which were the source of the fibres. Albrecht von Haller, the founder of modern physiological thought, distinguished three properties of fibres: elasticity, contractility and sensibility, but this was still in the eighteenth century, and philosophic concepts, experimental findings and microscopic observations are intertwined; the clearer idea of the fibre pattern only held sway for a few years in the early nineteenth century. Woolf suggested the idea of a ground substance in which the fibres lay and from which globules were developed, and Bichat put forward the fundamental idea that there were only a limited number of tissues of which the organs were formed. Twelve years later, Amici and Lister perfected the achromatic objectives which were to alter the whole outlook of biology, for they enabled Schleiden and Schwann to see that the pores between the fibres, which the earlier microscopists had dimly seen, were more than pores; they were globules or cells, with a nucleus. Thus the cell theory was evolved; and with Virchow's *omnis cellula e cellula*, interest in the fibres of the tissues and the spaces between the cells waned, and the fibres came to be regarded as extensions of cells, if not formed within them.

The Modern Interest in Connective Tissue

The recent change in viewpoint with regard to connective tissue, so that it has become a field of active research and clinical misconceptions, has stemmed from a number of sources. Textile chemists have been deeply interested in the structure of natural and artificial fibres for years, and it was fortunate that this work was being done by men like Astbury, Schmitt[1] and Highberger, who were able to see beyond their immediate problems and develop the science of molecular biology. Their morphological studies were in the field of crystallography and X-ray diffraction analysis which for a proper understanding demanded a greater knowledge of physics than the average biologist then possessed. The electron microscope was the bridge, for its micrographs could be appreciated by histologists and provided confirmation of the mathematical deductions of the molecular biologists. In 1942 the first electron micrographs of collagen fibres were published and in that same year Klemperer, Pollak and Baehr published their historic paper on "Diffuse Collagen Disease". This was the other stimulus for the new approach—the revival of de Bordeu and Virchow's ideas that the extracellular tissue might be the seat of disease.

In the sphere of human pathology Klemperer[2] and his colleagues at the Mount Sinai Hospital, New York, had been interested for many years in an uncommon disorder called disseminated lupus erythematosus.

The importance of Klemperer's paper was not that he coined that much misused term "collagen disease", but that he put forward the concept of the extracellular tissue as a functional biological system, and pointed out that, in scleroderma and disseminated lupus, there were conspicuous and systemic alterations in the extracellular components of the connective tissue, so that, from the point of view of morphogenesis, they might be regarded as disorders of the connective tissue system. Comparatively little attention was paid to this masterly paper until the recognition that cortisone, an adrenal cortical hormone, appeared to be effective in the treatment of many disorders of connective tissue such as rheumatoid arthritis, disseminated lupus, etc.; then, as Klemperer said, "the impatience of clinical investigators and a peculiar worship of diagnostic terms have led to an exaggerated popularity of the diagnosis 'collagen disease'. There is a danger that it may become a catch-all term for maladies with puzzling clinical and anatomical features. It is not a term applicable to diagnosis and certainly does not define the morbid process of the diseases grouped together." It is too early to assess the true value of cortisone in these conditions, although it is clear that the initial claims were over-enthusiastic; however, there can be no doubt that the interest which has been aroused has facilitated fundamental research in the extracellular tissue and is providing most worthwhile results.

The Ubiquity and Unity of Connective Tissue

We may regard connective tissue as a continuous matrix varying in consistency from the limpid Wharton's jelly of the umbilical cord to the hardness of bone, in which lies an interlacing fabric of fibres of different sorts. The character and thickness of the connective tissue layer varies from organ to organ. In the lungs and endocrine glands it is extremely thin except for the capsule; in the liver and kidneys it is somewhat thicker; in the heart and muscular organs it forms a significant portion of the viscus, as it does in the intestinal tract and the skin; while the bones, joints and tendons are formed entirely of connective tissue. It is important to remember that the connective tissue is continuous throughout the body and represents about 30 per cent of the body's bulk, of which about a third is bone; when one recognises that all metabolites passing to or from a cell must pass through the extracellular tissue, its significance in health and disease begins to be apparent.

It is really immaterial which organ is selected to study the connective tissue n greater detail, but skin is a convenient example, though it will be necessary to discuss certain aspects of other organs.

The Connective Tissue of the Skin as a Type Example

Under moderate magnification (FIG. 1) it is possible to see that the surface epithelium is separated from the blood vessels and lymphatics by a loose zone

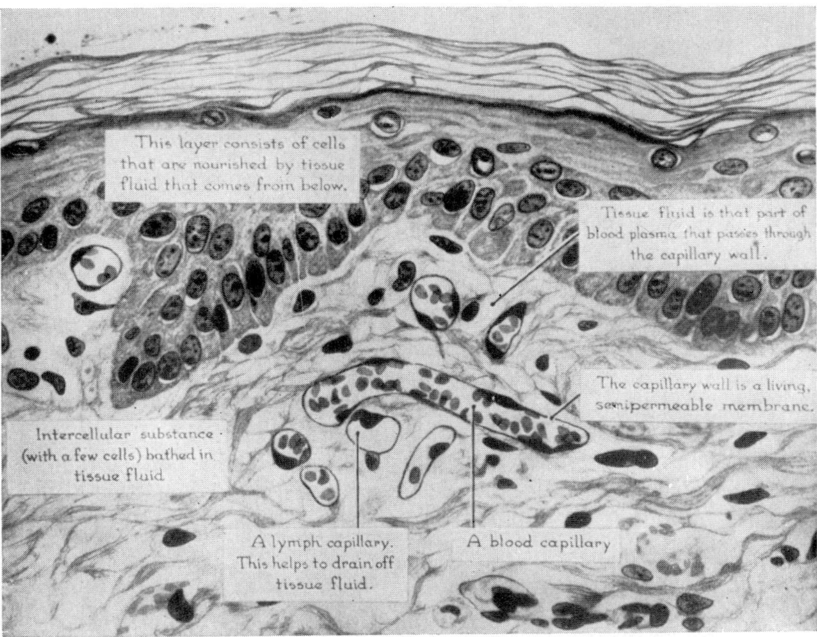

16/FIG. 1.—Section of skin showing the relationship between the connective tissue and the epidermis and blood and lymphatic capillaries. (From Ham.[3])

of fibrillary connective tissue in which there are a few cells. However, it is well to remember that a thin section is liable to be misleading in some respects; for instance, the blood supply appears very sparse whereas a thick injected section of the same sort of region (FIG. 2) reveals the rich blood supply that there is in the dermis. If the dermis is examined under polarised light (FIG. 3), an interlacing fabric of birefringent bundles can be seen. These are collagen, the principal fibrillary component of connective tissue, and the reaction under polarised light indicates that these bundles (1–100μ in diameter) are made up of orientated fibrils; the fibrils do not branch but the bundles branch dichotomously and anastomose; they take a straight or wavy course. A section, stained by orcein (FIG. 4), reveals the network of elastic fibres, another of the fibrillary components of connective tissue. Elastic fibres have a calibre of 0·2 to 1μ, are of a high

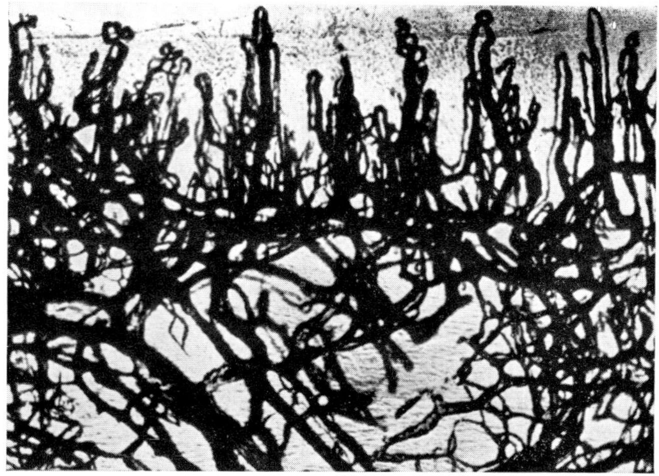

16/FIG. 2.—Section of skin with the capillaries injected, emphasising the complex blood supply lying in connective tissue.

refractive index, and although they branch freely, the individual fibres pursue a relatively straight course from one branch to the next. In certain sites, such as arteries, elastica may be condensed to form thick fibres or lamellæ.

If the dermis is examined under higher magnification when impregnated with silver salts (FIG. 5), the denser bundles of collagen, which were birefringent under polarised light, stain a light golden brown and are not so conspicuous in photomicrographs as the finer black fibrils, the so-called reticulin; these are of the same order of magnitude as elastica fibres and branch freely with one

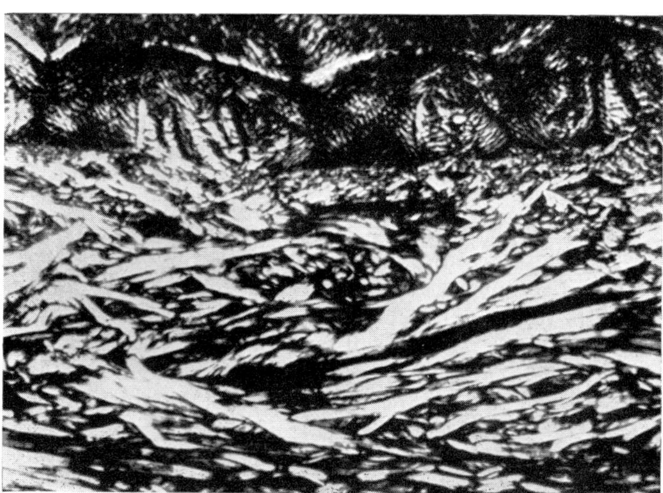

16/FIG. 3 —Section of skin under polarised light, showing the birefringent collagen bundles in the dermis.

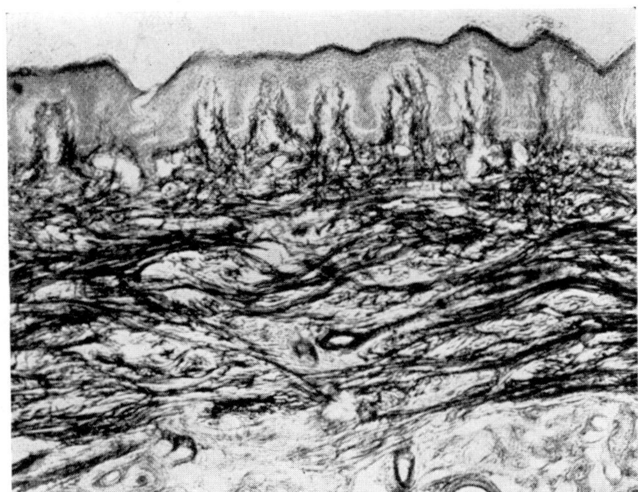

16/FIG. 4.—Section of skin stained with orcein to show the pattern of elastic fibres.

another and appear to merge with the collagen fibres; it can be seen how they are condensed at the dermic-epidermic junction and around the blood vessels forming the basement membrane. Now if a section is treated with periodic acid followed by Schiff's reagent—the "P.A.S." stain, which with certain limitations, will reveal the presence of carbohydrate—it can be seen that the spaces between the collagen fibres stain faintly, while those around the reticulin fibrils stain a more intense red. Thus, by the use of the microscope and simple staining methods, it is possible to get an idea of the nature of connective tissue—it consists of an interlacing network of collagen, reticulin and elastica fibres lying in a non-fibrillary matrix of ground substance which has a variable carbohydrate content.

Lying in the ground substance between the fibres are the connective tissue

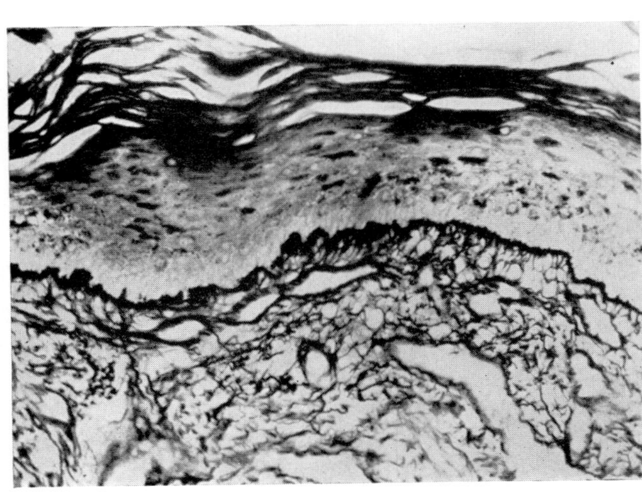

16/FIG. 5.—Section of skin impregnated with silver to reveal the collagen and reticulin fibres of connective tissue which are condensed at the basement membrane.

cells—fibroblasts, fat cells, histiocytes, reticulum cells and mast cells. In addition there may be blood leucocytes and plasma cells.

Reticulin and Collagen

If the coarse birefringent collagen bundles are examined with the electron microscope, they have a characteristic appearance with cross striations having a periodicity of 640 Å (Fig. 6). A great deal of work has been carried out on the structure of collagen fibre, and attempts have been made to determine, in the light of the characters that can be displayed by means of X-ray diffraction, electron microscopy and physiochemical analysis, just how the polypeptide chains are arranged and explain the banded appearance. The basic building unit or tropocollagen macromolecule is a long stiff rod 2,800 ×14Å, with a molecular weight in the vicinity of 360,000. Each macromolecule is composed of three polypeptide chains, one of which differs to some extent in amino-acid composition from the other two. These chains, each coiled in a left hand helix, are wound about each other in ropelike fashion in a right hand direction.

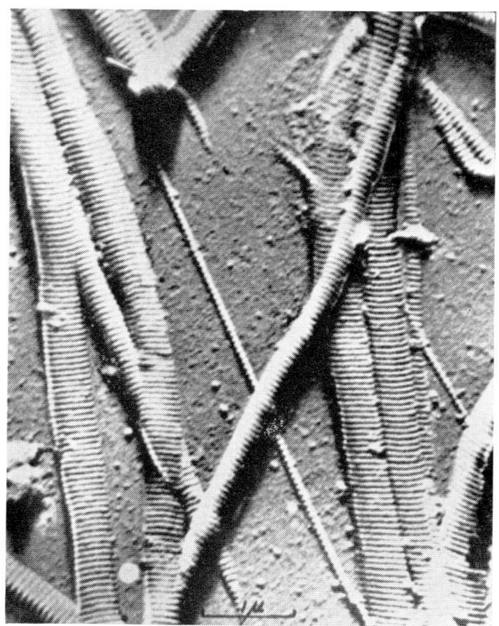

16/Fig. 6.—Electron micrograph of collagen fibres, showing the characteristic cross striations.

The molecule is stabilized by hydrogen bonds between the amino-acid residues, together with sterochemical restrictions which derive from the high content of pyrollidine rings (proline and hydroxyproline) in collagen. One of the most important consequences of this structure is that the polypeptide backbones are so tightly packed that every third position along the chains must be a glycine residue, as there is no room for a side chain; the amino-acid side chains are largely directed to the outside of the molecules, so their properties must be used for inter molecular interactions, which is exactly what would be expected, for the major function of collagen is to form fibrils.

It has been suggested by Hodge and Schmitt[4] that in native collagen the 640Å axial repeat could best be explained if the macromolecules were polymerised head to tail longitudinally and staggered one-quarter of their length laterally with respect to adjacent macromolecules. From the point of view of chemistry, collagen, which accounts for 70 per cent of the body's nitrogen, is a polypeptide, in which about a third of the amino-acid residues consists of proline and hydroxyproline, and another third consists of glycine, very small amounts of histidine, together with a small amount of carbohydrate. It is a protein with remarkable properties; in acid solutions it swells more than any other protein; it is insoluble in water but on heating is converted to a water soluble substance—gelatine, in which the superhelix has been unravelled, the individual chains separated and their helical structure randomized. In large bundles it has practically no extensibility and has a tensile strength up to 18,000 lb. to the square inch, about the same as cast iron. However, on heating to about 60° C. it contracts to about a quarter of its length and then develops a rubber-like elasticity which almost disappears on cooling. In discussing the nature of collagen, we have glibly moved from the magnification of the light microscope away beyond the limits of the electron microscope and the X-ray diffraction beam to the molecular level, and it is well to realise the orders of magnitude with which we are dealing, for it is all too common for confusion to arise owing to lack of clear thinking on this point (FIG. 7).

The nature of reticulin and its relationship to collagen has been a matter for discussion for the last fifty years or so, but Kramer and his colleagues[5, 6] have cleared away much of the confusion by examining with the electron microscope, X-ray diffraction, etc., material which histologically consisted of basement membrane reticulin almost free from collagen. Structurally, this reticulin consists of a network of very fine disorientated fibrils with the periodicity of collagen, lying in a matrix of polysaccharide and non-fibrillary material, probably only partially orientated. Chemical analysis of this reticulin showed that the amino-acid composition was almost identical with collagen, but that in addition it had 4·2 per cent of non-hexosamine carbohydrate, of which there is a negligible amount in collagen, and 10·9 per cent of bound fatty acids, none of which is present in collagen. These findings explain the difference in staining reactions and physical properties between basement membrane reticulin and collagen and may be of some importance in physiology and pathology.

We have now shown that the fibres which histologists have called reticulin are two distinct things—the immature collagen fibres, found in embryonic and regenerating tissue, which is a salt soluble collagen and the very stable basement membrane reticulin which is a lipo-mucoprotein; it could be that there are differences between basement membrane reticulin and the stromal reticulin present within the connective tissue.

ELASTICA

The nature of elastica is at the present time somewhat obscure. Chemically elastin is a polypeptide which resembles collagen in having a high content of glycine and proline but differs from it in having a high content of valine and a low content of residues with polar side-chains. It is remarkably stable and resists all the usual procedures for extracting protein from tissue; indeed, it has been defined as the fibrous material remaining in the débris after all else has been removed.

However, the summation of the evidence[6, 7] would suggest that elastic tissue consists of a core of fibres largely or entirely protein in nature lying in a homogeneous matrix either mucoprotein or mucopolysaccharide.

Electron microscopic studies would support this view,[8] and though elastic tissue is only found in association with collagen, it is always distinct from it and

5µ
5µ
1·0µ
1·0µ
a b1 b2 c d e
1000A
0·1µ
1000A
2800A
(i)
(ii)
(iii)
(iv)
2800A
100A
100A
8·5A
8·5 A
(v)
(vi)
(vii)
N
COH
HC
CH2
CH2
N
CH2
Proline
CO
CH2
N
Glycine
COH
RHC
N
Ammo Acid R
COH
HC
CH2
HCOH
N
CH2
Hydroxyprolin
CO
CH2
N
Glycine

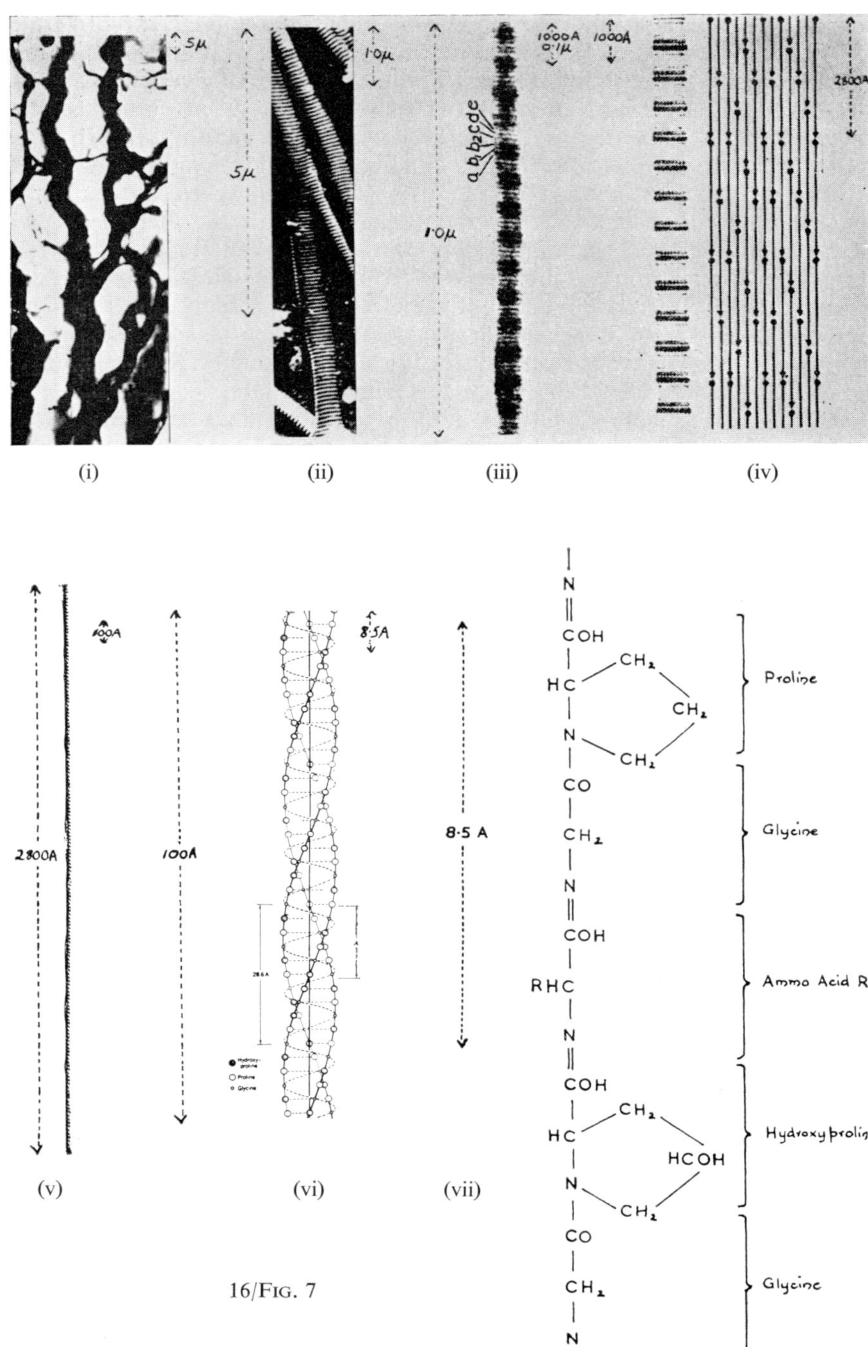

16/Fig. 7

mechanically appears to be complementary to it. It has much more elasticity than collagen but only about a tenth of its breaking strength; the essential characteristic of elastica is a long range reversible deformability similar to that of rubber.

Ground Substance

Lastly, what is the nature of the ground substance? In part it consists of extracellular fluid, derived largely from the blood plasma, and one should remember that the extravascular albumen pool is twice the mass of that within the vessels. In addition it has a high content of mucopolysaccharides, chiefly hyaluronic acid and chondroitin sulphate, and glycoproteins (which are mucopolysaccharide-protein complexes). Ordinarily it has a gel-like consistency and the histological evidence, for what it is worth, would suggest that the glycoproteins are least soluble at the basement membrane, where they are in close relationship to the reticulin and collagen fibres. In the inter-fibrillary spaces the glycoproteins are less condensed and may, under abnormal conditions, become more fluid, and finally water soluble.

THE STRUCTURAL VARIANTS OF CONNECTIVE TISSUE

There are structural variants of connective tissue. The limiting membrane of muscle, the basement membrane of gland tubules and Disse's space around the hepatic cords, consist of a thin membrane of polymerised mucoprotein in which course fine collagen fibrils. Tendon is characterised by a high proportion of coarse collagen fibre, with a variable admixture of elastica, embedded in mucopolysaccharide matrix.

The Formation of Cartilage

In the formation of cartilage, the metachromacy of the ground substance indicates a higher content of chondroitin sulphate, while the coarse collagen fibres are more widely separated (Fig. 8). The mesenchymal cells divide, become swollen with a high glycogen content in the cytoplasm, and then, as chondrocytes, become grouped but widely separated in the highly polymerised ground substance; their metabolic activities include glycolysis and oxidative phosphorylation. Cartilage is rich in orientated argyrophil fibrils resembling reticulin (Fig. 9); these fibrils show little branching, but their patterning is significant in relation to the shaping of cartilage. In addition there are collagen and elastic

16/Fig. 7 (*see opposite*).—Diagram illustrating the size relationship between collagen fibres as seen under the light and electron microscope and schematic representation of the tropocollagen macromolecule.

(i) Photomicrograph of collagen and reticulin, silver impregnation × 600.
(ii) Electron micrograph of collagen fibres shadowed with chromium × 8,000.
(iii) Electron micrograph of collagen fibre stained with phosphotungstic acid × 60,000.
(iv) Schema for the aggregation of the tropocollagen units in relation to the morphology of the collagen fibre × 60,000.
(v) Schema for the tropocollagen macromolecule × 3000,000.
(vi) Schema for the helical structure of the tropocollagen macromolecule × 6,500,000.
(vii) Schema for the molecular pattern of the polypeptide chain × 65,000,000.

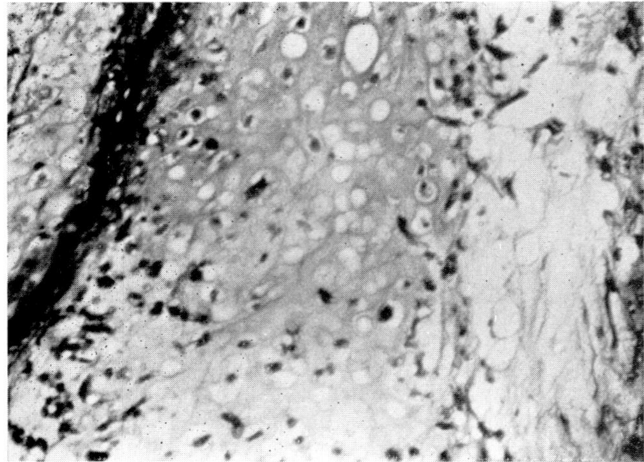

16/FIG. 8.—Formation of cartilage from fibrous tissue, showing the modification in the character of the connective tissue.

fibres, and in fibro-cartilage and elastic cartilage these are present in higher proportion. Precise chemical analysis of cartilage is lacking; it contains about 70 per cent water, and of the dried residue 80 per cent consists of collagen and chondroitin sulphate, in varying proportions according to the site from which it is obtained.

It should be appreciated that a joint is merely an area of connective tissue free from cells and fibres in which the ground substance—in the form of synovial fluid—consists of tissue fluids with a high content of hyaluronic acid. In the formation of a bursæ and ganglia we have the development of miniature joints in connective tissue.

The Formation of Bone

The formation of bone is essentially a patterned calcification of ground substance associated with increased vascularisation; and although, as a histo-

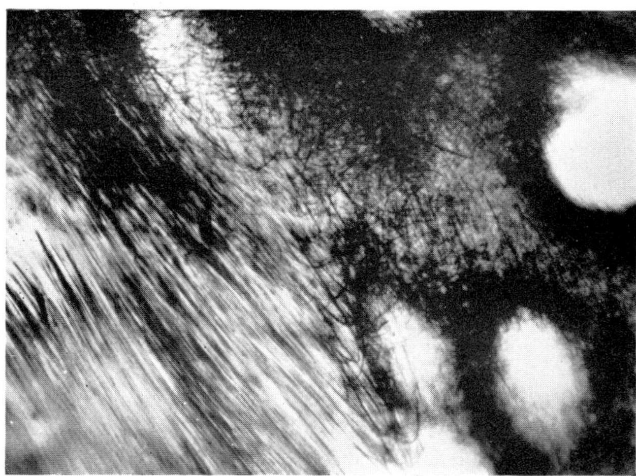

16/FIG. 9.—Section of cartilage stained to show the reticulin-like fibres in the stroma.

logist, one distinguishes between bone formation in fibre, bone formation by apposition and enchondral ossification, yet the changes in all three are really the same (FIGS. 10, 11 and 12). There is an increase of mucopolysaccharides in the ground substance with separation of the collagen fibres, and there is a morphological modification of the connective tissue cells. There is some dispute as to the stages that take place in calcification, but it is generally believed that Ca^{++} and $HPO4^{=}$ are first deposited on the organic matrix displacing water and that subsequent changes result in the formation of a crystalline hydroxyapatite $[Ca_7(PO4)_6\,(OH)_2]$ which can adsorb other ions, such as carbonate (Chapter 15). It would seem from the work of Glimcher[10] that it is only in native collagen that a configuration of the necessary reactive groups is achieved, which can initiate nucleation of apatite crystals from a solution of calcium and phosphate ions. In osteoid the bone salt crystals (400 × 25–50Å) (FIGS. 13 and 14) are laid down in relation to the bands of the collagen fibres, but in cartilage the crystals are laid down in the matrix between the fibrils and this raises the question as to whether it is the collagen molecule alone or the collagen-mucopolysaccharide complex which is concerned in the mechanism of calcification.[11]

In fibre bone collagen fibres are irregularly arranged, but in lamellar bone they lie in alternate layers at right angles to one another with other layers placed

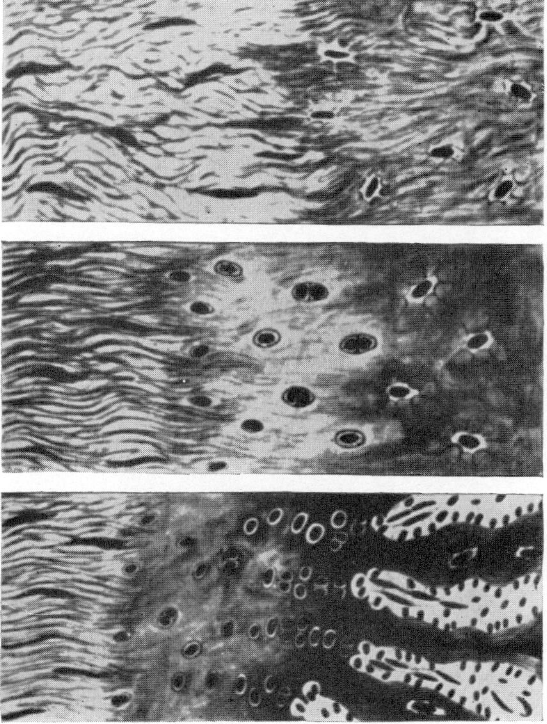

16/FIG. 10.—Diagram showing the characters of bone formation from fibre, by cartilaginous transformation and lamellar bone formation by vascularisation of cartilage. (From Hueck.[9])

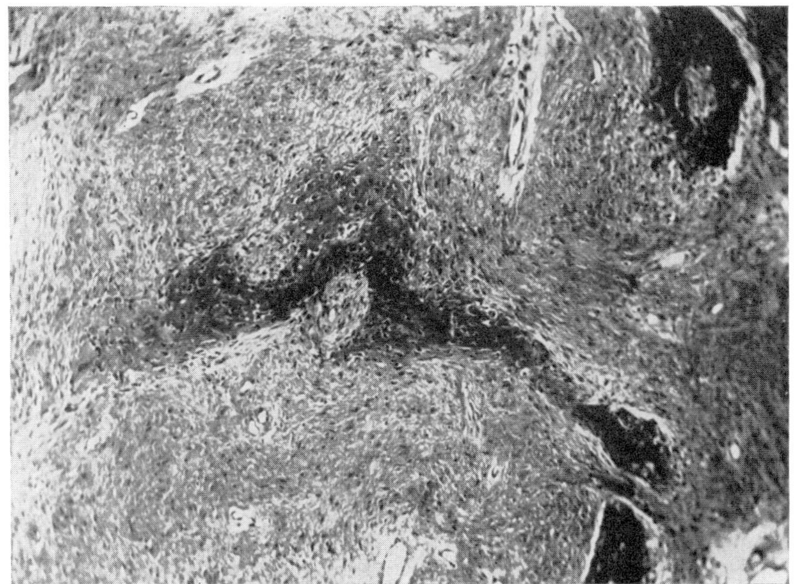

16/Fig. 11.

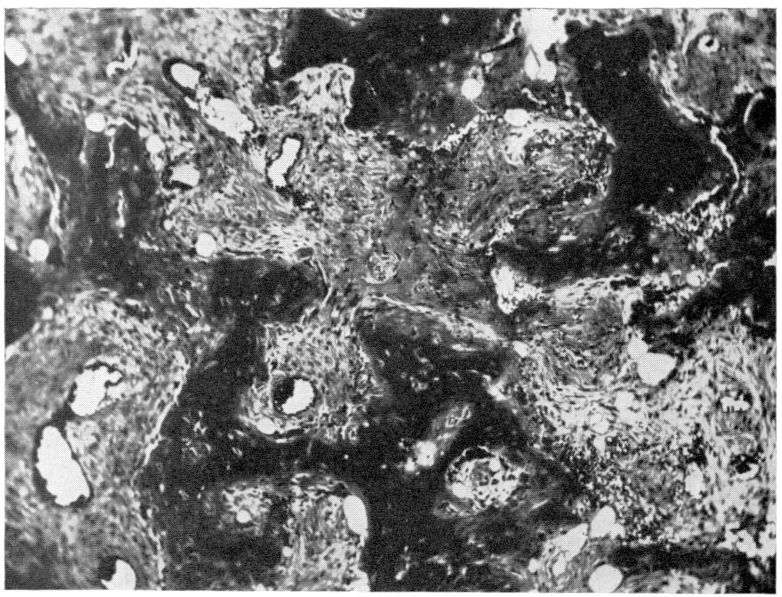

16/Fig. 12.

16/Figs. 11 and 12.—Stages in the formation of bone from fibrous tissue.

16/Fig. 13.

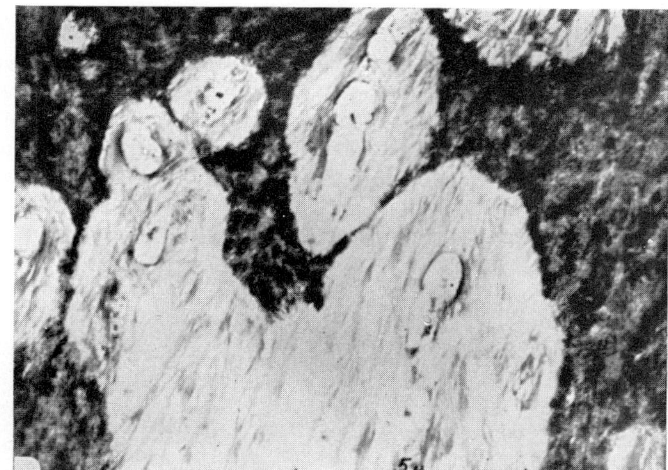

16/Fig. 14.

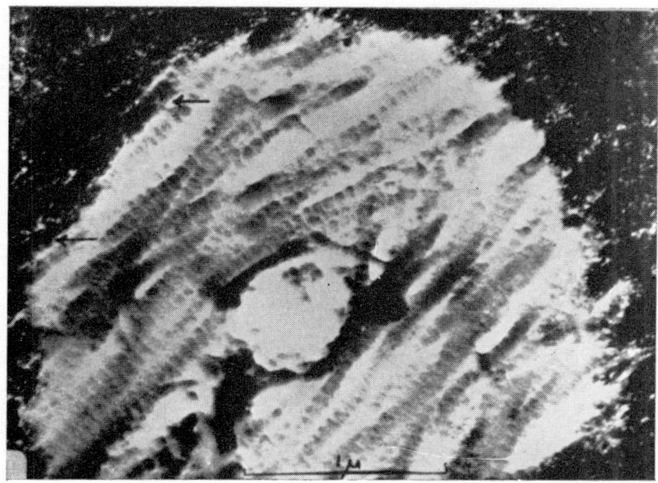

16/Figs. 13 and 14.—Electron micrograph of partially decalcified bone, showing the relationship between the bone salt crystals and the collagen fibres. In Fig. 14 the arrows call attention to the superimposition of the crystals on the doublet bands of the collagen fibres. (From Robinson and Watson.[17])

obliquely between them—the principle adopted in plywood and laminated plastics. The ultimate formation of bone, with its pattern of collagen and elastic fibres, and the appearance of the Haversian system is intimately related to the development of the vascular pattern, but Johnson[12] has emphasised that mechanical dynamics are the determining factors in the kinetics of skeletal remodelling.

THE FORMATION OF CONNECTIVE TISSUE

So much for the morphology and nature of connective tissue. Now, how is it formed? The answer, as is so often the case in biology, is that we do not really know. It is obvious that under ordinary circumstances the connective tissue cells that we call fibroblasts are the fibrogenic foci, and originally it was believed that fibrin fibres, as extensions of the fibroblast cytoplasm, were converted into collagen. This view can now be definitely excluded, although it may well be that when connective tissue fibres are forming, fibrin, by contraction, plays a part

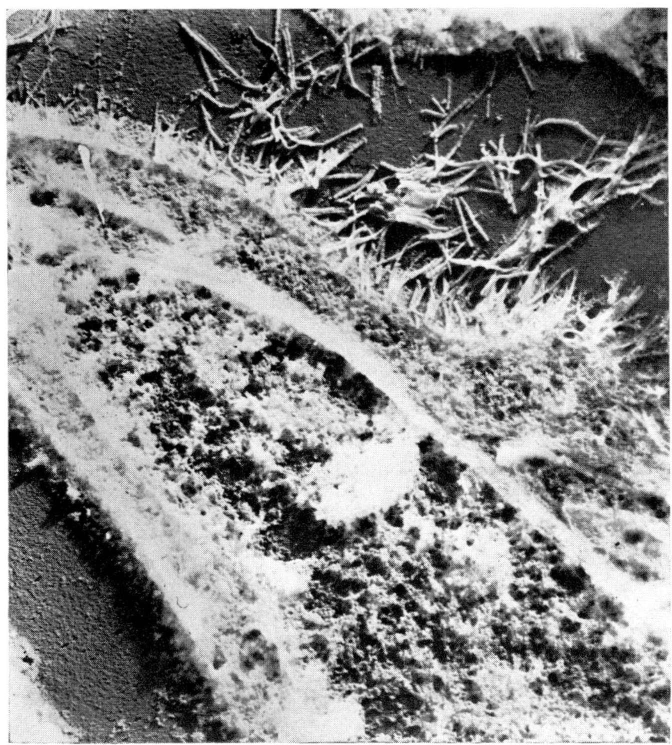

16/FIG. 15.—Electron micrograph of fibroblast, showing filaments of collagen seemingly developing from the surface of the cell. (From Wyckoff.[18])

in the orientation and alignment in a purely mechanical way. It has now been shown that the mode of collagen biosynthesis in the fibroblast is analogous to that which occurs in the synthesis of globular proteins, where the assembly of protein polypeptide chains occur on polysomes, clusters of ribosomes held together by what appears to be messenger RNA, in close relation to the endoplasmic reticulum. In collagen synthesis the initial phases appear to be the conversion of proline to hydroxyproline and aggregation of other aminoacids to form peptide sub-units which, under the influence of carbohydrate, are arrayed to form the triple helical tropocollagen molecule; the polyribosomes involved in collagen synthesis are much larger than those associated with the formation of globular proteins, the collagen accumulates in the endoplasmic reticulum as amorphous material and is transported to the cell surface in smooth vesicles, being discharged from the cell surface as a soluble protein, most of which precipitates as typical fibres between adjacent cells (FIG. 15); as yet it is uncertain whether the collagen particle extruded from the cell can be equated with the tropocollagen particle, is smaller or has already achieved some degree of macromolecular aggregation.

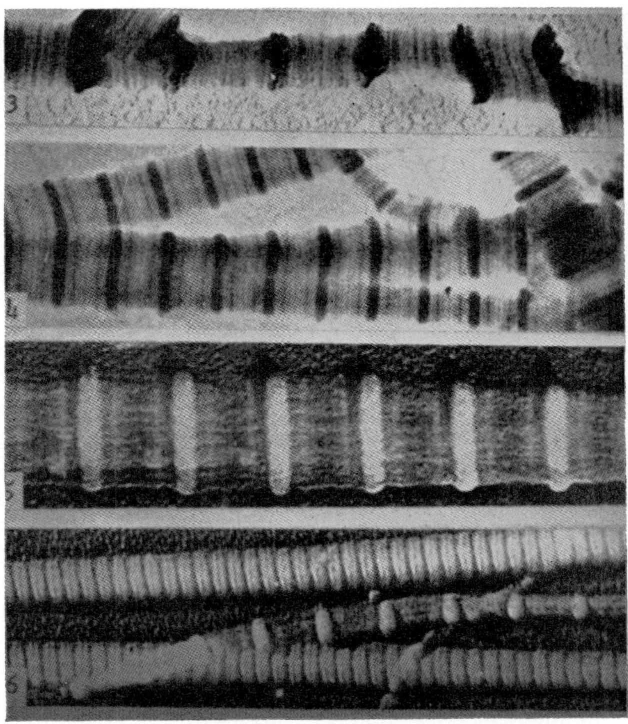

16/FIG. 16.—Electron micrographs of collagen fibres precipitated from admixture of procollagen and glycoproteins, showing normal and giant spacing fibres. (From Highberger, Gross and Schmitt.[19])

Goldberg and Green (1964) using fibroblast tissue cultures, found that while cells were actively growing, they appeared rather undifferentiated, rich in free ribosomes, but poor in endoplasmic reticulum, and synthesized very little collagen. When the number of cells becomes so dense that growth has virtually stopped, the morphology of the cells changes to a differentiated form and active collagen and hyaluronate synthesis proceeds, but the proportion varies in different cell lines. Fitton Jackson (1965) has studied the specificity of synthesis by comparing tissue cultures of embryonic osteoblasts and chondroblasts; each cell type showed difference in their general morphology and the chemical balance of their products. The osteogenic cells grew in sheets layer upon layer, the cells being aligned at right angles in succeeding layers whereas the chondroblasts tended to grow in whorls with considerable metachromasia. Collagen formation occurred early in the osteoblasts, was greater in amount and the fibrils were larger in diameter than in the chondroblasts, which on the other hand produced a much higher proportion of carbohydrate. How this environmental control is achieved in these connective tissue cells remains obscure.

The mechanism by which the extruded collagen particles are arrayed into collagen fibres has been determined in part by *in vitro* studies, in parts by analysing the sub-microscopic architecture of repair and embryonic development.

For more than fifty years it has been known that it was possible to dissolve certain forms of connective tissue in dilute acetic acid and this solution could be reconstituted into fibrils by the addition of salts or neutralisation and it has now been shown that these artifically formed fibrils have the electron-microscopic characters of native collagen. By various manœuvres it is possible to reconstitute collagen into structures with entirely different morphology, ranging from fibres without periods to those with axial periodicities of 220Å or 2,500Å (FIG. 16).

It has now been found that it is possible to extract collagen with weak acids, weak alkalis or with physiological saline and these various soluble collagens have differing metabolic activities.

It was then shown that a solution of salt extracted collagen could be converted to native collagen simply by warming the solution to 37° C. and at first this process could be reversed by cooling, but the longer the fibres remained at 37°, the more insoluble they became. Gross[15] has suggested that the major difference between the various soluble collagens might be their age and that, *in vivo*, the fibroblast, having secreted the collagen molecules into the ground substance, under the influence of physiological ionic atmosphere, temperature and perhaps certain rate regulating factors, the molecules would aggregate spontaneously to form fibrils. There would be an increasing perfection of fit between the molecules, as they gradually pack together into a more stable association in the striated fibrils, and the increasing formation of secondary cross links would make disruption of the fibril more difficult.

Although Gross has shown that this phenomenon can occur *in vitro* with preparations of highly purified collagen, the question still remains as to what part the mucopolysaccharides of the ground substance play in natural fibrogenesis. Wood[15] has suggested that they might be concerned with nucleation and growth and hence help to determine the rate of formation of fibrils and their ultimate size.

Paul Weiss[14] has described the stages of repair in amphibian basement membrane, which consists of a laminated fabric in which the collagen fibres of each layer are orientated at right angles to those of the adjacent layer. Initially the collagen sub-units lie randomly around the fibroblasts in the mucopolysaccharide matrix, then these sub-units polymerise into filaments which are bundled into fibrils without common orientation. Gradually layering appears, progressing from the outermost to the innermost layer and the fibrils assume the typical orientation of normal basement membrane, the final orientation again varying by 90° between adjacent layers. Fibril direction in each layer seems to be determined by the old fibre stumps at the wound edge and it would appear that the polar groups of the collagen chains can only be in equilibrium in this particular environment by assuming their unique positions, which then become 'nucleation' points for the fibres. This, Weiss says, "is an illustration of the general principle of progressive organisation, how a higher degree of patterning can arise from the especial interrelationship between two components of a composite system—in this case, mucopolysaccharide and collagen—neither of which would by itself produce the given pattern, but which when combined in a suitable environment establish a new degree of order."

Thus we have some evidence that mucopolysaccharides may play an essential part in collagen fibrillogenesis and that the fibroblast perhaps potentiates this, but it is clear that other factors are also involved in the formation of normal connective tissue. For instance, in the healing of wounds in scurvy, there is a deficiency of the formation of fibrillary collagen and reticulin and the ground substance contains a gelatinous fluid which is not metachromatic. There is a deficiency of phosphatase in the fibroblasts, which have the cytological characters associated with active formation of cytoplasmic protein, and there is an increase of glycoprotein in the serum. On administering ascorbic acid, the phosphatase content of the fibroblasts increases, the ground substance shows metachromasia, collagen is formed and the serum glycoproteins fall. This suggests that ascorbic acid is necessary for collagen fibril formation, although the biochemical lesion in ascorbic acid deficiency remains uncertain.

Ascorbic acid enhances the production of collagen in fibroblast tissue culture, probably by influencing the hydroxylation of proline to hydroxyproline, perhaps by catalyzing the formation of hydroxy radicals or acting as a donor and acceptor in microscomal electron transport. There is no good evidence that ascorbic acid has a direct effect on the stabilization of the collagen fibril, but in scurvy there is enhanced resorption of newly formed collagen, which could account for increased urinary excretion of hydroxyproline.

In addition ascorbic acid influences mucopolysaccharide production, acid mucopolysaccharides being replaced by neutral polysaccharides in scorbutic ground substance; this is apparently due to a block in the formation of galactosamine, resulting in a decrease in chondroitin sulphate, while there may be some increase of hyaluronic acid.

It is hardly surprising that tissue healing is poor in scurvy, and once again illustrates the interplay between fibrillogenesis and mucopolysaccharide.

Two further questions remain with regard to the formation of connective tissue: the source of elastica and of the mucopolysaccharide. Elastica formation is an enigma. In the embryo and in healing wounds, it appears much later than the collagen fibrils, and it would seem that collagen is a prerequisite for its formation. In tissue culture, elastic fibres are produced only by tissues which contain them *in vivo*; in heart muscle cultures they are most dense when subjected to the pull of the contracting muscle. It is generally agreed that elastica is formed extracellularly, and the impression that I have gained is that in an area of elastica formation there is usually an excess of metachromatic material; this takes on a beaded form and fine non-argyrophil metachromatic fibres appear, which gradually develop the staining reactions of elastica. At first the fibres are irregularly arranged in a fine meshwork, but later they develop into the fine branching and coiled refractile threads which are characteristic of elastica. Recent electron microscopic studies have shown that, at least in the aorta, elastica arises as small electron dense masses lying between collagen bundles and the basement membrane of smooth muscle cells.[20] Hass has suggested, on the basis of some interesting experiments, that elastica might be formed as a fibrillary membrane at fat-water interfaces in the tissues. We know from Lansing's work that the mature fibres are associated with lipoid and Tunbridge and his co-workers have shown an association with carbohydrate.

With regard to the origin of the mucopolysaccharides of the ground substance, there are different views. The presence in fibroblasts of granules and vacuoles having the histochemical reactions of mucopolysaccharides and the formation of large amounts of mucopolysaccharides in certain types of fibrosarcoma, and in fibroblasts in tissue culture, clearly indicate its importance in biosynthesis. On the other hand, the mast cell is known to store, if not to synthesise, heparin, and Asboe-Hansen,[6] has put forward much evidence to suggest that it is also the source of the connective tissue mucopolysaccharides; however, Ringertz[21] has shown that 80–100 per cent of the total polysaccharide in the mast cell is heparin and any non-sulphated polysaccharide is a heparin precursor. Not so very long ago the function of the mast cell was completely unknown, and now it is credited with the formation of heparin and connective tissue mucopolysaccharides, and is able to release histamine and 5-hydroxytryptamine.

Turning from biosynthesis to metabolism, we have even less information. There have been studies of collagen by Neuberger,[22] using C^{14} labelled glycine, which would indicate that in the growing animal the amino acid is taken up by the developing fibres and to a large extent retained there; in the adult animal very little is taken up. However it has been shown[23] that when animals are protein-deficient, mature collagen is broken down and takes part in the general protein metabolism; it may well be regarded as a protein reserve. With regard to the ground substance, Schiller and Dorfman[24] have shown that the turnover of hyaluronic acid is more rapid than chondroitin sulphate and that the rate of synthesis is influenced by insulin activity. There is indirect evidence that, with suitable stimuli, the degree of polymerisation of the glycoproteins alters with release of soluble products into the blood and urine, but farther than that we cannot go.

As yet I have considered the formation of connective tissue, but equally important is the mechanism for its removal. In development there is a constant remodelling of organs, seen in an extreme form in amphibian metamorphosis, when the tail of a tadpole is lost as it turns to a miniature frog, but a similar process occurs in the reshaping of a growing bone; the postpartum uterus rapidly returns to its ordinary size with much loss of collagen and, in some pathological states, such as hepatic fibrosis, if the toxic factor is withdrawn, there will be a restoration to near normality.

In amphibian metamorphosis Gross[14] has shown that the removal is selective, the older collagen disappears while that which is being laid down is spared, and that the process is achieved by a collagenolytic enzyme, secreted by epithelial cells under the influence of thyroxin; at the same time fibroblasts release a hyaluronidase which breaks down the ground substance causing a fraying of the already damaged fibre and proteases break these down into peptides which can be metabolized. In the remodelling of adult tissues, such as bone or the uterus, it seems probable that there is a different mechanism of collagenolysis, achieved by acid hydrolases mediated by lysosomes, which enter large digestive vacuoles of the mesenchymal cells, that disrupt and allow the extracellular attack. It is clear that there must be dynamic equilibrium between the synthesis and the degradation of connective tissue and a disturbance of such an equilibrium would result in disease, a return in a modern guise, to the ancient humoral hypothesis, which through the ages has alternated with the demoniac theory of disease, no matter whether the extrinsic cause was a witch's spell or a micro-organism.

THE FUNCTIONS OF CONNECTIVE TISSUE

Having outlined the nature and formation of connective tissue, one can proceed to consider its functions. Its mechanical function is generally accepted, though it inevitably leads us into teleology. D'Arcy Thompson studied the adaptation of the internal structure of bone to the stresses and strains to which it is subject. It has been shown that the tensile strength of bone is of the same order as cast iron. Cartilage provides a tissue which combines a certain amount of rigidity with considerable flexibility and resilience, and Matthews has recently suggested that there is a higher ratio of mucopolysaccharide to collagen in weight-bearing joints. Collagen has great tensile strength with flexibility, but negligible extensibility, and so in tendons transmits muscular contraction to the bones with a minimum loss of power. Elsewhere it maintains the shape of organs, and in its looser forms, combined with ground substance, forms an admirable flexible packing material. When loose collagen is combined with elastica it provides a tissue with great elasticity and resilience, as in blood vessels and the dermis. Hyaluronate is the only connective tissue mucopolysaccharide with a pronounced viscosity and its high content in synovial fluid results in an effective lubricating agent, while in the dermis it could act as a plasticizer, diminishing friction and wear between collagen fibres. A major function of connective tissue is the repair of physical trauma or the restoration of tissue after inflammatory reactions. However, newly formed collagenous tissue contracts and, in the absence of elastic tissue, stretches under tensile strain. Many of the chronic diseases and dysfunctions of the body are the result of these properties: hepatic or renal failure associated with scarring of the liver or kidney; cardiac failure due to mitral stenosis; intestinal obstruction due to a scirrhous carcinoma; an aneurysm of the aorta. The initial pathogenesis of these and many other conditions I could mention may be due to cellular dysfunction, but it is the collagen that strangles the organ or allows it to burst.

The Metabolic Function of Connective Tissue

We often ignore the metabolic function of connective tissue because we tend to think only of intracellular metabolism or general metabolism, but it should be realised that all metabolic processes, if transmitted, are transmitted and therefore modified by connective tissue; connective tissue has an intercommunicating system of protein fibrils whose surface is immense.

It is well known that if an animal is injected with a dye such as trypan blue and the tissues examined after a few days, the dye will be collected chiefly in the cells of the reticulo-endothelial system; yet the animal becomes blue in a matter of minutes. King showed that at this early stage, the dye is not in cells but is bound by connective tissue fibres all over the body, in collagen, reticulin and especially elastica, and that it is not absorbed into cells until 24 hours or more have elapsed. Barcroft[25] made similar observations with regard to the Wharton's jelly of the umbilical cord, and suggested that it might serve as a non-vascular conducting path of metabolites from the placenta to the embryo. A similar mechanism might apply in the nutrition of cartilage and the cornea. Ground substance is hydrophilic and may retain water and adsorb electrolytes, although it is possible that under normal conditions there is no free fluid and the electrolytes move through bound water. Opie and Rothbard[26] have shown that connective tissue takes up water by hydration, as does gelatin, and not by osmosis, as in the case of parenchymatous tissue. The extensibility of connective tissue in the living organism depends on its content of water, and when water content rises extensibility increases.

The storage of calcium and other metals in bone and their release from bone is generally accepted, but it is not always appreciated how rapid the resorption and reformation of bony stroma can be. Bloom,[27] for instance, has shown that much of the marrow trabeculæ of the long bones of active egg-laying birds disappears and reappears in cycle with the calcification of the egg-shell, that is to say, in a matter of hours. Gailard[28] has found that parathyroid can act directly on bone, producing a change in the ground substance, with a rise of serum glycoproteins. The depolymerisation results in a reduction of mineral binding capacity, and calcium and phosphate are liberated. There is an increased excretion of glycoprotein in the urine and, on occasions, mucoprotein phosphate carbonate casts are formed. Barnicot[29] found that vitamins A and D also have local osteolytic effects which is particularly significant in the light of Engstrom's findings that there is a disturbance of collagen fibre arrangement in rickets. It may well be that the proximate lytic effect is mediated through lysosomes, which have been shown to be activated by vitamin A.

Reaction of Connective Tissue to Hormones

The influence of hormones on connective tissue is also apparent in endocrine disorders, which one may look on as caricatures of normal hormonal balance and experimental procedures. In thyroid deficiency, the myxœdema is associated with a considerable increase in ground substance which is metachromatic, thus indicating some degree of depolymerisation. There is also an increase of tissue mast cells, and water retention. All these effects are reversed on thyroid medication. Now there are certain forms of nodular myxœdema in which there is no evidence of hypothyroidism, although the histology is identical; it may well be that the water retention is not a primary effect of thyroid deficiency but results from the altered metabolism of ground substance. Furthermore, the changes in connective tissue in myxœdema may not be due to a deficiency of thyroxin, but an excess of thyrotrophic pituitary hormone, as it has been found that a localised myxœdema is often associated with hyperthyroidism, and similar tissue changes can be induced experimentally by treatment with pituitary thyrotrophic hormone. In acromegaly, consequent on excess production of

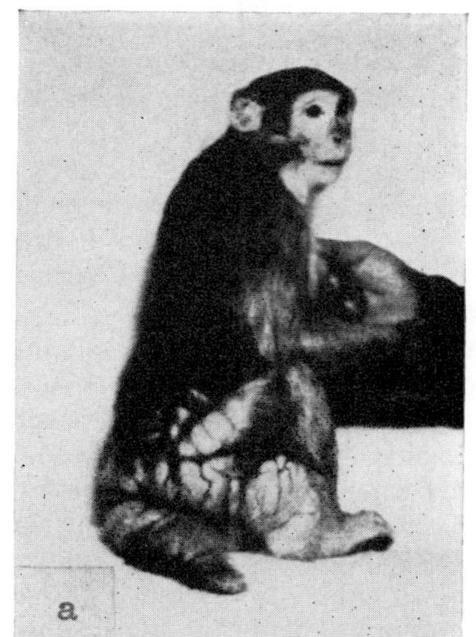

17/Fig. 17.—Swelling of Sex Skin of Rhesus Monkey

(*a*) Monkey, showing the swelling in the inguinal region.

(*b*) Biopsy of skin on the first day of the cycle.

(*c*) Biopsy of skin on the thirteenth day of the cycle; the collagen fibres are widely separated. (From Duran-Reynals, Bunting and Wagenen.[31])

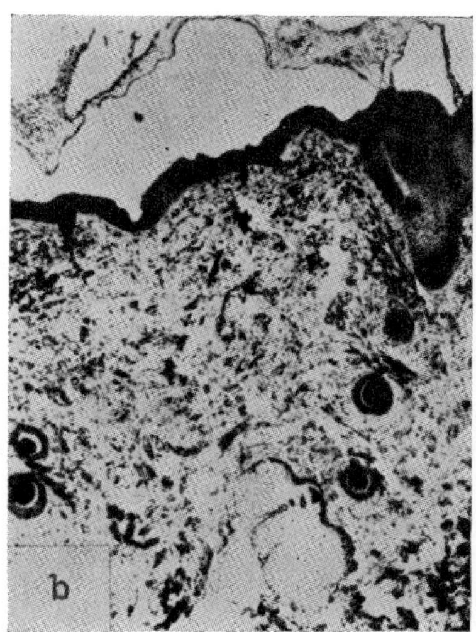

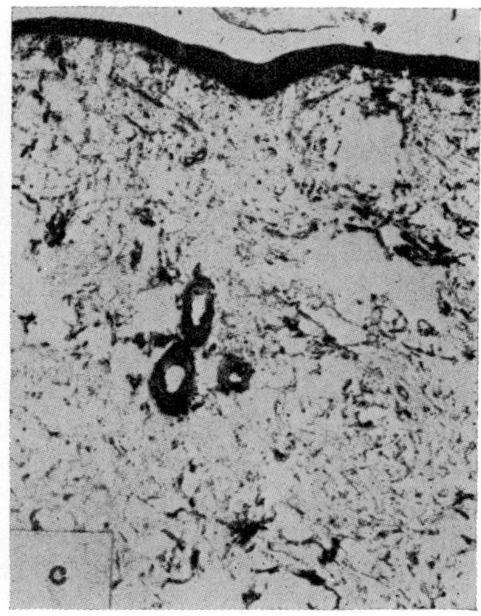

growth hormone by a pituitary adenoma, in addition to the generalised visceromegaly, there is a diffuse increase of connective tissue.

Focal reactions of connective tissue in response to hormonal stimulation are particularly well seen in the sex hormones. The alterations in the stroma of the breast and uterus in pregnancy are well known, and though the connective tissue changes may be secondary to the epithelial or muscular proliferations, there is experimental evidence that there is a direct effect on the connective tissue as well. In the uterus there is an increase of collagen during pregnancy which is reversible, returning to normal within a week of parturition. An even more localised reaction is the change in the symphysis pubis induced by the luteoid hormone, relaxin, which causes an absorption of bone and an increase of ground substance; in the ovary, a rhythmic remodelling of connective tissue is associated with the maturation of Graafian follicles at each œstrus cycle.[30] Analogous changes, though more general in distribution, are seen in the swelling of the sexual skin in monkeys (FIG. 17), which makes the mandrill such a colourful beast, and in the swelling of the cock's comb induced by testosterone. It would seem that œstrogens and testosterone induce synthesis of mucopolysaccharides, and an increase in their state of hydration, whereas gonadotrophins induce depolymerisation with increased permeability, an effect analogous to that of hyaluronidase.

The observation that there was impaired healing of wounds in cases under cortisone therapy stimulated work on the effect of adrenal cortical hormones on connective tissue. There has, however, been considerable confusion, as it was not recognised that there are marked differences in response in different species and that the guinea-pig is unhappily extremely resistant to cortisone. In general, it may be said that the effects of cortisone on connective tissue support the views expressed by Albright in 1942, seven years before Hench and Kendall introduced the drug to clinical medicine; that is to say, its action is anti-anabolic rather than katabolic. There is an increase in the urinary excretion of hydroxyproline, a failure to incorporate sulphate into chondroitin sulphate and a failure of fibroblast proliferation; but where fibroblasts are present, collagen and ground substances are normally laid down, and immature connective tissue becomes mature; by increasing the stability of lysosomes, there is a reduction in connective tissue breakdown. Mast cells lose their granules and appear degenerate, and this is true even of mast cell tumours of dogs. On the other hand, desoxycorticosterone has an opposite effect, stimulating fibroplasia and causing an increase of metachromatic ground substance. Adrenalectomy does not affect collagen fibres or their water absorption, but the ground substance is unable to retain water.

Ageing of Connective Tissue

It is logical now to consider the changes in connective tissue in ageing. Ageing has been defined as colloidal dehydration, and this process is well seen in connective tissue, which, in the embryo, has a very high water content and which gradually dries up with increasing years. As this occurs, the side chains of the polypeptides are probably drawn together with a loss of physical response and chemical reactivity; in this stable state there is an increased deposition of calcium, well seen in the aorta and in ageing cartilage.

PATHOLOGY OF CONNECTIVE TISSUE

It is possible to touch on only one or two aspects of the pathology of connective tissue, as it is a vast field which deals with functional and morphological changes in all organs and in all disease states. The response of connective tissue to injury has already been mentioned. It is well to realise, however, that in a parenchymatous organ such as the liver or kidney, one may have extensive cellular damage, but provided the connective tissue matrix has not been damaged, the organ will be restored to normal both morphologically and functionally, if cellular regeneration takes place. Furthermore, even when there has been fibrosis and scarring, this will at least in part be resorbed.

The Connective Tissue Response in Infections

In relation to infections, one considers principally the cellular and humoral defence mechanisms, but the part that connective tissue plays should not be forgotten. The polysaccharide gel will to some extent immobilise micro-organisms, and though it may be hydrolysed by enzymes of the hyaluronidase type formed by certain organisms, there is in connective tissue a non-specific hyaluronidase inhibitor; this is probably heparin. The coarse collagen membranes may thus encourage the localisation of an infective process, and although they may be broken down by the organism's proteases, the infection may be isolated by new formation of collagen. In the case of certain virus infections,

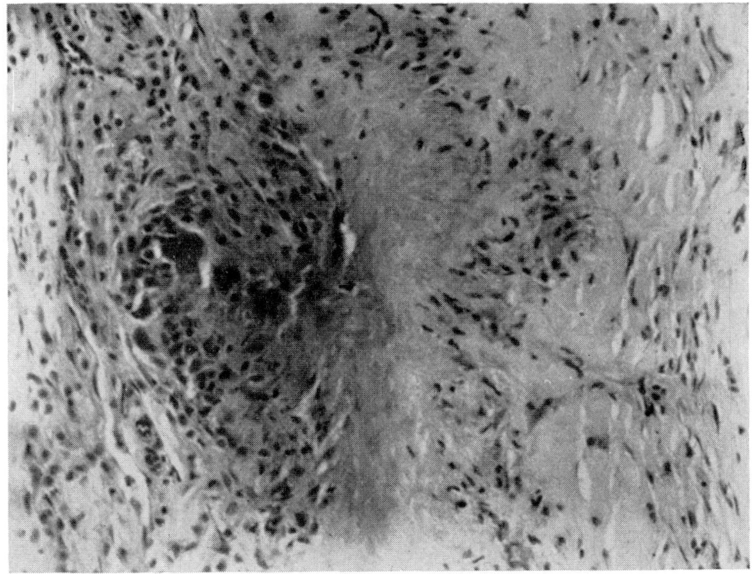

16/Fig. 18.—Connective tissue, showing fibrinoid change. There is an alteration in staining character as well as morphology of the fibres.

such as influenza, the entry of the virus into the cell is associated with the action of certain mucinases, probably having as their substrate mucoitin sulphate. A mucoprotein viral inhibitor is present in connective tissue and may well be a factor in the body's defences against virus infection.

In the immune response, antibodies are usually present extracellularly and react with parenterally introduced antigens. Hypersensitivity depends on the reaction of antigen with sessile antibody contained in or on cells, and although we have little or no knowledge of the proximate biochemical lesion, its effects on smooth muscle and capillary permeability are familiar enough. The ground substance becomes œdematous, and, in addition to the cellular reaction, a fibrinoid change (Fig. 18) may develop in the connective tissue. This is characterised by the appearance of a homogeneous, highly refractile, band-like material which histochemically appears to be of a variable nature according to the pathogenesis of the lesion; in some cases it is associated with the presence of fibrin, in others globulins are predominant.[32] Electron microscopy has confirmed that there is little change in the collagen fibres but a deposition of fibrillary material which is probably denatured fibrin.[33] There is good evidence that heparin and a histamine-like substance is released. It has been presumed to be derived from the damaged cells, but it seems more likely that the mast cell and platelets are the source.[34] Recently it has become popular to postulate that a whole range of general disorders of connective tissue are "auto-immune diseases", as the term provides the clinician, and perhaps the pathologist, with a sense of scientific security as did the misuse of Klemperer's "collagen disease" twenty-five years ago. It is of course true that auto-antibodies to a wide range of antigens can be detected in these diseases and that in many of them there are indications of abnormal immunological reactions, and the deposition of antigen-antibody complexes in the tissue, but the evidence that an auto-immune state is the cause of the disease is tenuous to a degree. Nevertheless this concept has stimulated much fundamental work on immunity which is proving as rewarding as the studies which resulted in the renaissance of connective tissue.

Serous Inflammation

Apart from these specific pathological reactions of connective tissue, there is the non-specific reaction—Eppinger's[35] serous inflammation. His idea was that, as a result of damage to capillary endothelium, cell membranes or ground substance, there is an accumulation of a protein-rich fluid in the connective tissue spaces. The consequent separation of the capillary from the parenchyma impairs the transport of nutritive materials and cellular metabolites, resulting in a secondary disturbance of cellular function (Fig. 19). This type of connective

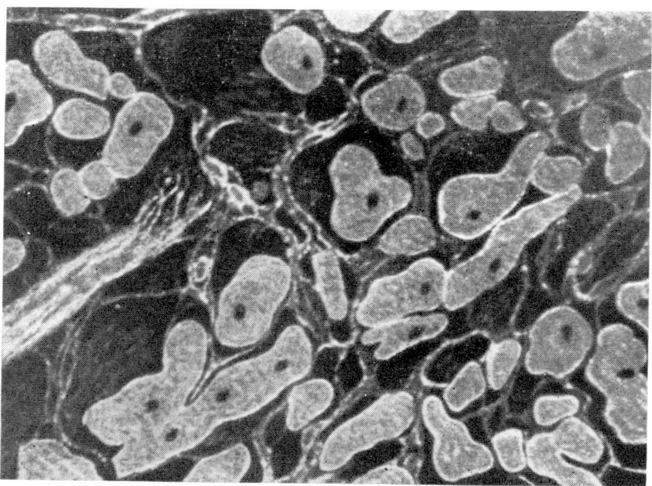

16/Fig. 19.—Serous inflammation. Section of myocardium examined with fluorescent microscopy, showing the wide separation of the basement membrane from the muscle fibres and blood vessels; the protein-rich exudate can be recognised as a faint blurring of the background. (From Eppinger.[35])

tissue changes is reversible if the damaging agent is removed or is low in activity. However, if the serous exudation persists, there will be an irreversible change in the ground substances with the occurrence, if conditions are suitable, of scarring or hyaline change, or the deposition of the fibrillary glycoprotein, amyloid. The conditions necessary for amyloid deposition are unknown, but it would seem that ascorbic acid deficiency associated with a high globulin content of the ground substance are underlying factors. The globulin may be antibody globulin or result from disturbance of protein metabolism which may be genetically determined.

Connective Tissue Reactions in Malignant Disease

One of the many problems in malignant disease is the mechanism of infiltration and of the development, rather than the transport, of metastases. This is clearly a problem of the reaction between the neoplastic cells and the connective tissue stroma. Conan has suggested that malignant cells show a decreased adhesiveness, amœboid movements and the presence of an enzyme of the hyaluronidase type. This work has not been confirmed, and the results may well have been due to bacterial contamination, as there is no increase of invasiveness if hyaluronidase is injected in the region of a tumour. Turning to the stroma, Cramer, and more recently Orr,[36] have shown that in the pre-malignant phase of experimental carcinogenesis, the connective tissue undergoes spectacular changes which occur only if the substance used is in fact carcinogenic; they are not simply a reaction to an irritant. Orr found that there was a marked increase of mast cells, increased elastic formation and a change in the connective tissue fibres, which were chiefly of the reticulin type. There was minimal cellular reaction. When malignant change occurred, breaks appeared in the elastica, and the mast cells disappeared. Gillman and his co-workers[37] have shown that much of the apparent increase of elastin is in reality an alteration in the character of the collagen ("elastotic degeneration") and they suggest that this may be of significance in the pathogenesis of skin cancers. The next stage, that of infiltration, has been studied by Gersh and Catchpole and by Sylven.[38] They found that in a rapidly growing tumour there was marked depolymerisation of the ground substance with increased serum glycoproteins, and the reverse was found in slow-growing tumours with a fibrous stromal reaction. The difficulty is that, given these morphological observations, one is uncertain how to interpret them. The answer may partially be resolved by the introduction of more critical methods for detecting depolymerising and proteolytic enzymes.

Diseases of Connective Tissue

As yet we have considered the reactions of the connective tissue in pathological states, but there are a considerable number of conditions in which there is an intrinsic disturbance of connective tissue, morphological or metabolic, some of which are genetically determined. A detailed account of these conditions would be out of place here, but it might be instructive to select one or two examples, not so much for their intrinsic importance, but because they are related to experimental models which offer clues to what Sir Rudolph Peters has called the biochemical lesion of disease.

In 1949 an Iowa orthopædic surgeon, Ignacio Ponseti, was interested in adolescent scoliosis and believed that a disturbance of protein metabolism was an important factor in its causation; he learnt that scoliosis had been induced in rats fed on a diet of sweet-pea meal. This had been done in an attempt to reproduce the effects of lathyrism in man, a disease characterised by muscular weakness and spasticity, which occurs in periods of famine when chick peas and other pulses have been eaten. (In fact, sweet peas have never been known to produce the neurological disorder in man.) Ponseti, in association with Baird, repeated the experiments, producing scoliosis and bone deformities with great success, but in addition he found that many of his rats developed hernias and dissecting aneurysms of the aorta; there was gross disturbance of cartilage and enchondral bone formation and in the aorta there was an excess of ground substance between the elastic fibres of the media with secondary rupture and consequent aneurysmal dissections. This naturally stimulated the interest of research workers in connective tissue and it was not long before the toxic factor in the pea meal was isolated as a β aminoproprionitrile and had been synthesised.

Various nitriles, as well as certain non-nitriles can induce the connective tissue changes in a range of experimental animals of which the rat and the chick are most popular. The chemicals act very quickly, in a matter of hours in the embryo, and there is an equally rapid reversion to normal development when it is withdrawn; partial protection is achieved by supplements of certain proteins and the toxic effects can be suppressed by thyroxin or cortisone. It only produces a significant effect in actively growing connective tissue and has no effect *in vitro*, on the calcification of normal cartilage cells or on the formation of fibrils from warm neutral solutions of collagen. In addition to the gross bony deformities, the tissues of affected animals are strikingly fragile. In adult animals, local changes comparable to those in the growing animals can be induced in the healing of wounds and fractures. In general there is a failure of growth in animals treated with lathyrogenic agents. The connective tissue cells (fibrocytes, chondrocytes) proliferate and there is an increase of intercellular material which has a raised content of hydroxyproline and mucopolysaccharide, and this is also increased in the serum; there is a decrease in certain enzymic activities. All the evidence would suggest that there is an inhibition of functional maturity of the connective tissue cells and though collagen is formed it is not condensed into large fibres, which may be due to inhibition or disruption of intermolecular cross links. However, the precise biochemical mechanism of experimental lathyrism remains to be defined.

It has been suggested that the aortic lesions resemble those seen in atherosclerosis in man, but this is not very sound as the changes in lathyrism are in the media whereas in atheroma it is the intima that is affected.

However, there is an aortic condition in man which morphologically closely resembles the lesions seen in pea-fed rats. It is cystic medial necrosis, the histological lesion usually associated with dissecting aneurysms. Here the first change is an increase of metachromatic material in the media with secondary rupture of the elastic laminæ.

Apart from the cystic medial necrosis seen in adults, there is a hereditary disorder—Marfan's disease, which has many affinities with experimental lathyrism. It is inherited as a simple mendelian dominant with a relatively high degree of penetrance, and the disorder is characterised by long slender bones with muscular weakness and hyperextensibility of the joints, so that the patient often suggests a figure in an El Greco painting; in addition there is a congenital dislocation of the lens associated with a stretching of the suspensory ligament of the iris.

In adult life, cardiovascular abnormalities become apparent with aortic dilatation and valvular lesions, while many of the patients die in their early twenties as a result of dissecting aneurysm. The pathology of the skeletal abnormalities has not been closely studied, but the aorta, in all cases in which it has been examined, whether or not dissection has taken place, shows cystic medial necrosis, and the valvular lesions, when present, are of a similar type; another interesting feature of this disorder is that there is an increase of acid mucopolysaccharide in the serum and considerable urinary excretion of hydroxyproline.

So it is that in experimental lathyrism we have an invaluable experimental tool in the study of connective tissue, which may also give a clue to this curious hereditary disorder, a serious form of vascular disease and incidentally may be of economic importance in husbandry, for a fatal disease breaks out from time to time in turkey farms which is very similar to experimental lathyrism.[39]

Another type of connective tissue disease was revealed with the chance observation in 1956 that when a rabbit receives an intravenous injection of crude papain, within a few hours, its ears collapsed. It was found that the cartilage had lost its rigidity, and its normal histological staining reaction and in fact the cartilaginous matrix throughout the body disappears so that chondroitin sulphate dissolves in the body fluids. After a single injection of papain the ears become erect again in two or three days, but the morphology of the cartilage may not recover for three weeks or so. The papain had broken down the chondroitin sulphate-protein complex, but this property is not peculiar to papain for it can be achieved by a whole range of proteases, including endogenous ones such as plasmin, and it has been suggested that an analogous process might be a factor in the development of arthritis.

If repeated injections of papain are given to growing animals, widespread deformities of the skeleton arise which have some resemblance to familial achondroplasia in dogs and some skeletal deformities in man are associated with a raised excretion of chondroitin sulphate.[40] In addition there are a distinct group of hereditary skeletal disorders in which there is an excess urinary excretion of chondroitin sulphate and heparitin sulphate, where there is a gene determined disorder of mucopolysaccharide metabolism, the deformities being in part due to failure of chondrification, in part due to accumulation of the mucopolysaccharide in the tissues and organs of the body, and there are other disorders in which there is a disturbance of collagen and elastica formation.[41]

It would not be difficult to instance many other conditions in which a disorder of connective tissue is of fundamental importance, but within the compass of this chapter these few examples must suffice to illustrate the ubiquity and significance of connective tissue in both physiological and pathological processes. In the controlled release of atomic energy, it is necessary to have a substance, known as a moderator, which slows down and to some extent controls the fast neutrons so that they are captured by the fissionable material, thus allowing the chain reaction to proceed. Korsshelt has described connective tissue as a temporal document on which the life history of the organism is indelibly inscribed. It is much more than that; it is the biological moderator of cellular energy.

REFERENCES

1. Schmitt, F. O. (1960). *Verhandl. IV Internat. Kongr. f. Electron Mikroscopie*, Band II, 1. Berlin: Springer-Verlag.
2. Klemperer, P. (1953/4). *Harvey Lect.* (Series 49). Springfield, Ill.: Charles C. Thomas.
3. Ham, A. W. (1953). *Histology*, 2nd Edit. Philadelphia: J. B. Lippincott Co.
4. Hodge, A. J., and Schmitt, F. O. (1960). *Proc. nat. Acad. Sci.* (*Wash.*), **46**, 186.
5. Randall, J. T., Editor (1953). *Nature and Structure of Collagen*. London: Butterworth and Co.
6. Tunbridge, R. E., Editor (1957). *Symposium on Connective Tissue*, (C.I.O.M.S.). Oxford: Blackwell Scientific Publications.
7. Ayer, J. P. (1964). *Int. Rev. Connective Tissue Res.*, **2**, 33.
8. Pease, D. C., and Molinari, S. (1960). *J. ultra-struct. Res.*, **3**, 447.
9. Hueck, W. (1937). *Morphologische Pathologie*. Leipzig: George Thieme.
10. Glimcher, M. J. (1960). *Amer. Ass. Adv. Sci. Symposium* No. 64, 421.
11. Neuman, W. F., and Neuman, M. W. (1958). *The Chemical Dynamics of Bone Mineral*. Chicago: Univ. Chicago Press.
12. Bergsma, D., Editor (1966). *Structural Organisation of the Skeleton*. Birth Defects, **2**, No. 1.
13. Goldberg, B., and Green, H. (1964). *J. Cell. Biol.*, **22**, 227.
14. Jackson, S. F., *et al* Editors. (1965). *Structure and Function of Connective and Skeletal Tissue*. London: Butterworth and Co.
15. Gross, J. (1958). *Bull. N.Y. Acad. Med.*, **34**, 701.
16. Wood, G. C. (1964). *Int. Rev. Connective Tissue Res.*, **2**, 1.
17. Robinson, R. A., and Watson, M. L. (1952). *Anat. Rec.*, **114**, 383.
18. Wyckoff, R. W. G. (1952). In *Transactions of the Third Conference on Connective Tissues*. New York: Josiah Macy, Jr. Foundation.
19. Highberger, J. H., Gross, J., and Schmitt, F. O. (1951). *Proc. nat. Acad. Sci.* (*Wash.*), **37**, 286.
20. Haust, M. D., More, R. H., Bencosme, S. A., and Balis, J. U. (1965). *Exp. molec. Path.*, **4**, 1965.
21. Ringertz, N. R. (1960). *Acid Polysaccharides of Mast Cell Tumours*. Uppsala: Almqvist and Wiksell.
22. Brown, R., and Danielli, J. F., Editors (1955). "Fibrous Proteins and their Biological Significance": *Symposia of the Society for Experimental Biology*, Number IX. London: Cambridge Univ. Press.
23. Harkness, M. L. R., Harkness, R. D., and James, D. W. (1958). *J. Physiol.* (*Lond.*), **144**, 307.
24. Schiller, S., Mathews, M. B., Goldfaber, L., Ludowieg, J., and Dorfman, H. (1955). *J. biol. Chem.*, **212**, 531.
25. Barcroft, J., Danielli, J. F., Harper, W. F., and Mitchell, P. D. (1944). *Nature* (*Lond.*), **154**, 667.
26. Opie, E. L., and Rothband, M. B. (1953). *J. exp. Med.*, **97**, 409.
27. Bloom, W., Bloom, M. A., and McClean, F. C. (1941). *Anat. Rec.*, **81**, 44.
28. Gailard, P. J. (1955). *Exp. Cell. Res.*, Suppl., **3**, 154.
29. Barnicot, N. A. (1948). *Nature* (*Lond.*), **162**, 848.
30. Harkness, R. D. (1964). *Int. Rev. Connective Tissue Res.*, **2**, 155.
31. Duran-Reynals, F., Bunting, H., and van Wagenen, G. (1950). *Ann. N.Y. Acad. Sci.*, **52**, 1010.
32. Vaquez, J. I., and Dixon, F. J. (1958). *Arch. Path.* (*Chicago*), **66**, 504.
33. Cochrane, W., Davies, D. V., Darling, J., and Bywaters, E. G. L. (1964). *Ann. rheum. Dis.*, **23**, 345.

34. MOTA, I. (1959). *J. Physiol. (Lond.)*, **147,** 425.
35. EPPINGER, H. (1949). *Die Permeabilitätspathologie*. Vienna: Springer.
36. ORR, J. W. (1938). *J. Path. Bact.*, **46,** 495.
37. GILLMAN, T., PENN, J., BRONKS, D., and ROUX, M. (1955). *Arch. Path. (Chicago)*, **59,** 733.
38. ASBOE-HANSEN, G., Editor (1954). *Connective Tissue in Health and Disease*. Copenhagen: Ejnar Munksgaard.
39. SELYE, H. (1957). *Rev. canad. Biol.*, **16,** 1; LEVENE, C. I., and GROSS, J. (1959). *J. exp. Med.*, **110,** 771; TANZER, M. L. (1965). *Int. Rev. Connective Tissue Res.*, **3,** 91.
40. MUIR, H. (1964). *Int. Rev. Connective Tissue Res.*, **3,** 101.
41. MCKUSICK, V. A. (1960). *Hereditable Disorders of Connective Tissue*. St. Louis: C. V. Mosby Co.

The following are reviews and symposia in which references to individual papers can be found:

ASHFORD, M., Editor (1952). *The Musculo-skeletal System*. New York: The Macmillan Co.

EMMRICH, R. (1959). *Chronische Krankheiten des Bindegewebes*. Leipzig: Georg Thieme.

RAGAN, C., Editor (1950/54). *Conferences on Connective Tissue*: New York: Josiah Macy, Jr. Foundation.

REIFENSTEIN, E. C., Editor (1949/53). *Conferences on Metabolic Interrelations*. New York: Josiah Macy, Jr. Foundation.

SPRINGER, G. F., Editor (1955/59). *Conferences on Polysaccharides in Biology*. New York: Josiah Macy, Jr. Foundation.

TALBOT, J. H., and FERRANDIS, R. M. (1956). *Collagen Diseases*. New York: Grune and Stratton.

FARBER, S. J., Editor (1964). *Connective Tissue: Intercellular Macromolecules*. London: J. & A. Churchill.

GARDNER, D. L. (1965). *Pathology of the Connective Tissue Diseases*. London: Arnold.

CHRAPIL, M. (1967). *Physiology of Connective Tissue*. London: Butterworth.

Chapter 17

HEALING

BY M. A. JENNINGS and H. W. FLOREY

WE have considered in some detail the immediate reactions of tissues to various forms of insult, such as mechanical violence and bacterial invasion, and have seen that changes, known as "acute inflammation", occur in the vascular system and its contained cells and in the cells of the tissue. These reactions tend to rid the body of noxious agents and to prepare the way for restoring normal structure and function to a damaged organ, if that is possible.

No hard-and-fast line can be drawn between what may be considered initial defensive reactions and those which are concerned with subsequent repair of damaged tissues, but for purposes of description it is easier to consider the events of healing as occurring later than the first stages of inflammation though, in fact, they may overlap. We will now concentrate on the cellular and vascular changes that take place in tissues that are being actively repaired. In mammals a body wound or any break in continuity of tissue is generally repaired by the formation of fibrous tissue which does not differ in essentials from that of the normal body. Let us see how such a scar is formed.

MICROSCOPICAL OBSERVATION OF HEALING TISSUE

As in so much that we have to study, the fundamental facts were elucidated by the classical methods of cutting sections of fixed material and reconstructing the march of events from them. Later it became possible to see the fascinating sight of living healing tissue and to follow in very considerable detail from day to day the complicated but co-ordinated changes that occur.

E. R. and E. L. Clark watched many of the changes following injury in the transparent tail of the tadpole, and with this background Sandison[1], working in the Clarks' laboratory, examined healing in mammalian tissues in the transparent rabbit ear chamber described in Chapter 3.

17/FIG. 1 (*opposite*).—THE DEVELOPMENT OF MACROPHAGES (STAINED BY INTRAVENOUS VITAL NEW RED) INTO HISTIOCYTES IN RABBIT EAR CHAMBERS

(*a*) A growing edge. The capillary loops are growing into a blood clot. The macrophages along the growing edge are stained with vital new red. (×75)

(*b*) Typical macrophages. Note the refractile granules and appearance of diffuse staining with vital new red: compare the size of the macrophages with that of the leucocytes in vessels. (× 515)

(*c*) Histiocytes in recently organised tissue. They are particularly numerous alongside vessels. (×105)

(*d*) Young histiocytes in new tissue. Note the discrete dye granules and the clear area where the nucleus lies. (×420)

(*e*) Old histiocytes lying next to a vessel. The cells are smaller and the dye is clumped. (×420)

(*f*) Giant cell. (×610) (From Ebert and Florey.[2])

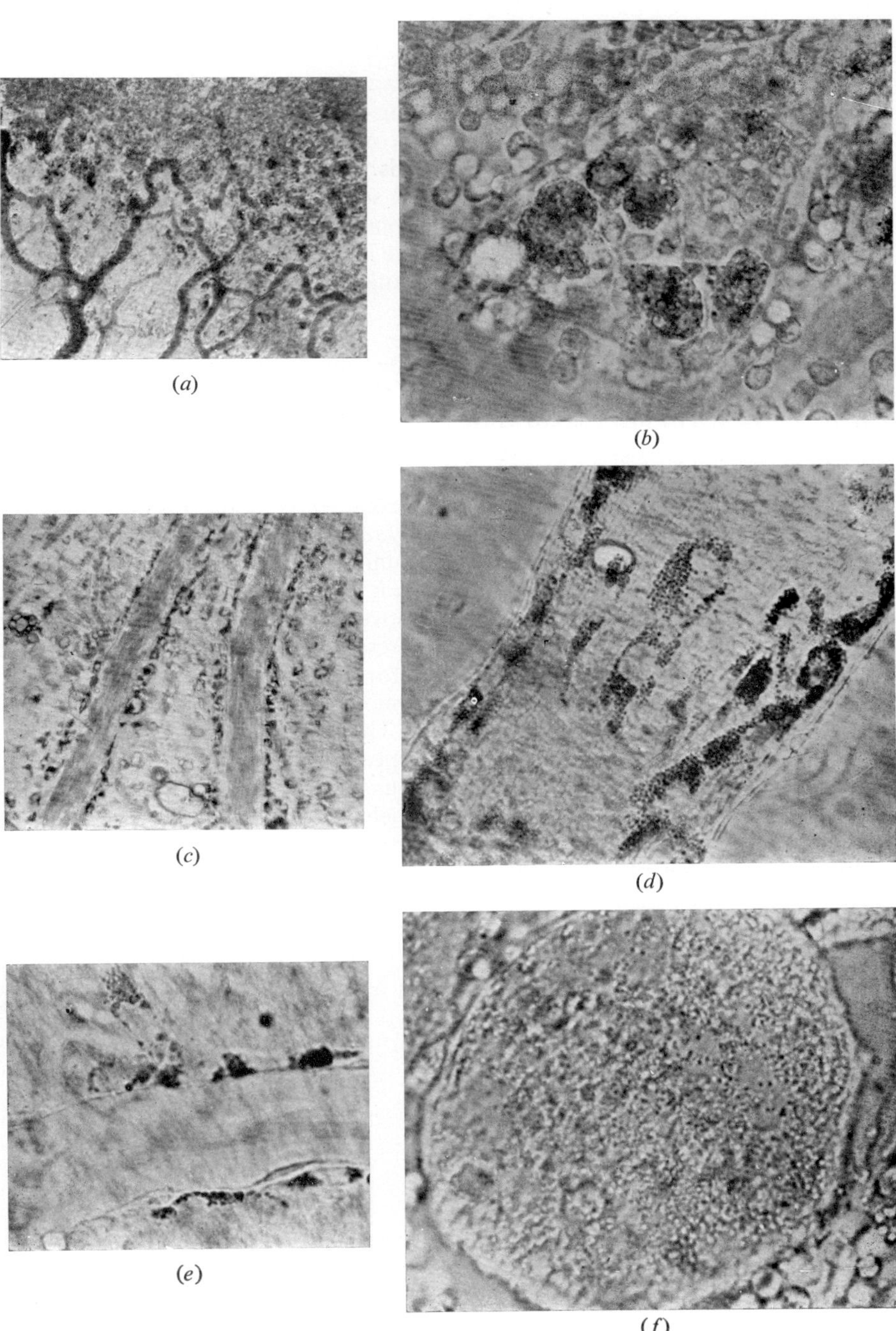

(*a*) (*b*) (*c*) (*d*) (*e*) (*f*)

17/Fig. 1.

The Clot

Immediately after insertion of a chamber the central table on which the observers will be able to follow the healing process, corresponding with the area from which tissue has been excised, is covered by a clot containing strands of fibrin, red cells and a few white blood cells. In the course of a day or two the fibrin strands, some of which are thick and some of extreme fineness, become more evident. The red blood cells lose their pink colour and become increasingly difficult to distinguish. In a few days the table is covered by a light brown granular mass in which fibrin strands can be identified.

Macrophages

While these changes are occurring in the area for observation the healing process gets under way at the periphery of the table, where pre-existing tissue adjoins the clot. The first cells to appear on the table are macrophages. They are seen as striking cells that normally contain numerous small refractile granules and move slowly by amœboid action. They are readily recognised, especially in thin chambers, and they stand out very prominently if the rabbit is given a number of intravenous injections of a vital dye such as trypan blue or, better still, vital new red. The dye appears at first to be uniformly distributed in the cell, but after a time it becomes concentrated in small, regularly disposed granules. The macrophages invade the clot and begin removing it. They ingest and digest red cells, fragments of fibrin and cellular debris present in the clot. These ingested and digested materials no doubt form nutriment for the macrophages, which increase in size and may reach a diameter of 30μ or more, and in some cases form multinucleated giant cells 100μ or so in diameter. The remains of the red cells furnish breakdown products of hæmoglobin that appear as yellow granules in the cells. They are composed of products known as hæmosiderin and hæmatoidin (bilirubin). Further, extracellular enzymes may help to digest the fibrin clot. Some of these may be secreted by macrophages, but probably they come mainly from the disintegration of polymorphs and other cells that die during their sojourn in the clot.

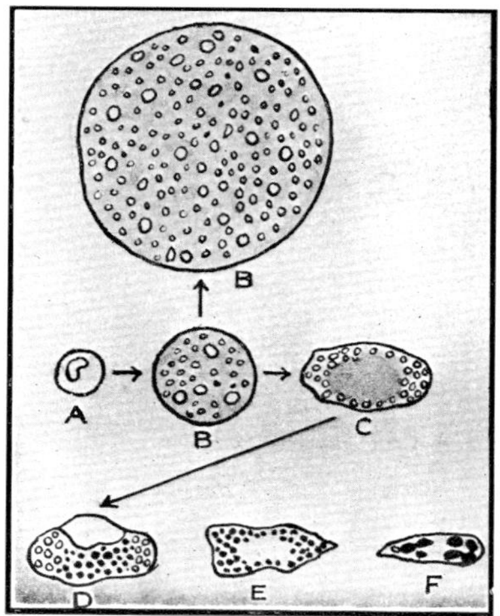

17/FIG. 2.—The series of changes from a monocyte to a histiocyte, shown diagrammatically. The monocyte (A) develops in the tissues into a macrophage (B, to the right). It can become a giant cell (B, above). More often it goes through transition forms between macrophage and histiocyte (C, D) to young histiocyte (E) and old histiocyte (F). (From Ebert and Florey.[2])

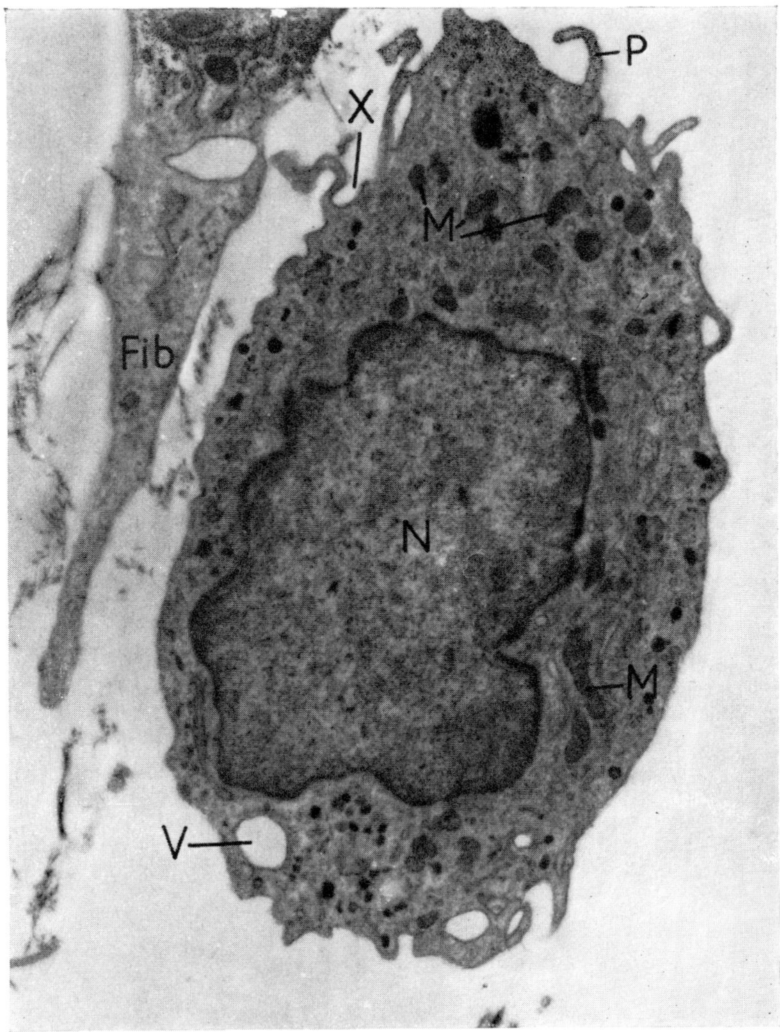

17/Fig. 3.—Electron micrograph of a young macrophage in growing connective tissue in a rabbit ear chamber. It contains some mitochondria (M) and some small very electron-dense granules and some of about the same size that are less dense. The endoplasmic reticulum is not conspicuous.

Whether the structures such as that marked at V are really vesicles cannot be determined; they may be indentations of the cytoplasm which connect freely with the surrounding medium as at X. A few cytoplasmic prolongations (P) which are almost certainly involved in the phagocytic activity of the cell can be seen. Fib = fibroblast; N = nucleus. (× 12,500)

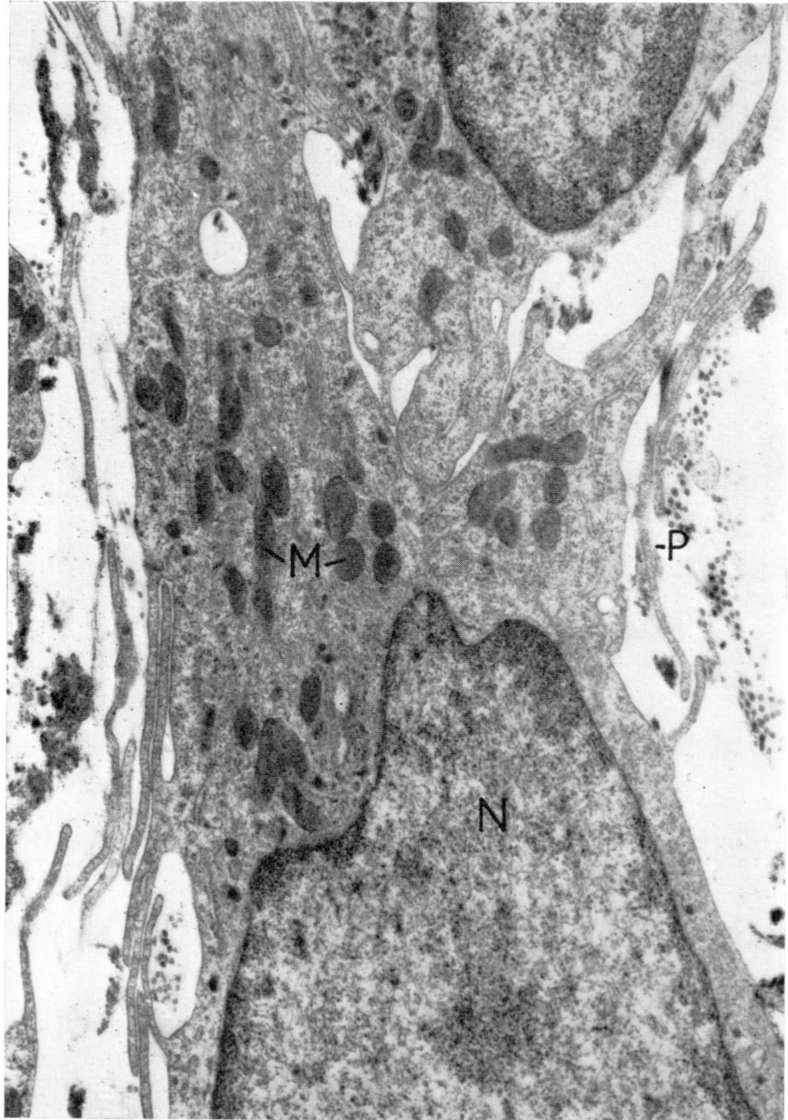

17/FIG. 4.—Electron micrograph of more mature macrophages than that shown in FIG. 3. There are numerous mitochondria but few granules of any size in the cytoplasm. The cytoplasmic prolongations (P) are numerous and extend some way from the cell. (× 20,500)

By injecting indian ink (a suspension of fine carbon) intravenously it proved possible to show that the tissue macrophages can originate in monocytes that come from the blood stream (see also Chapter 4). Some of the monocytes in the circulating blood take up the particles, and a few of these marked cells can be made to emerge from the vessels into the growing tissue by slightly damaging the vessels in the chamber. Thereafter the marked cells may be followed in the tissue for many weeks or months. They increase in size and occasionally divide. In the course of time they are transformed into "fixed" tissue phagocytes, now commonly called histiocytes, many of which are oriented along the newly formed blood vessels. These developments are illustrated in FIGS. 1 and 2.

Observations with the electron microscope of tissue from rabbit ear chambers show that young macrophages contain considerable cytoplasm in which occur some small electron-dense granules and numerous small vesicles, but only small amounts of endoplasmic reticulum. Numerous small mitochondria are present (FIG. 3). As the macrophages increase in age and size they show a striking feature in the long cytoplasmic extensions that project from the surface of the cell. These have been called "ruffles" by Palade.[3] It is probable that the cytoplasmic projections are structures which during life are in constant motion and to which the macrophage owes its capacity to engulf materials in its

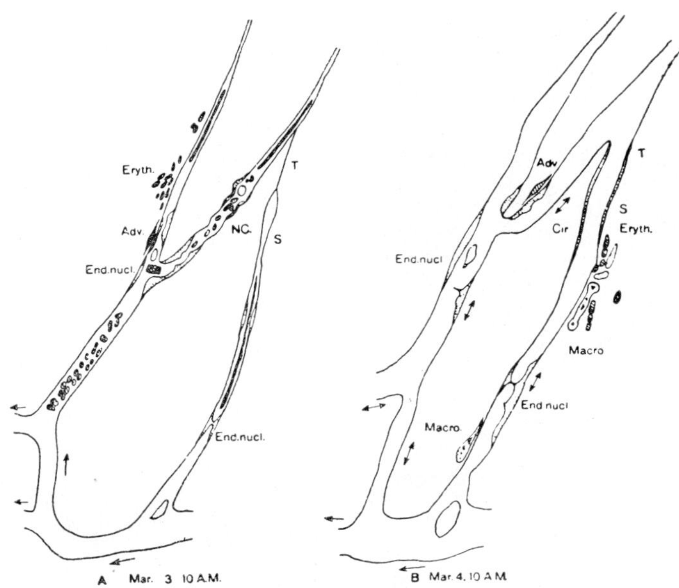

17/FIG. 5.—CAMERA LUCIDA DRAWINGS OF TWO STAGES IN THE DEVELOPMENT OF A CAPILLARY LOOP. (B was drawn 24 hours after A.) (×206)

Eryth. = erythrocytes; Adv. = adventitial cell; End. nucl. = endothelial nucleus; Macro. = macrophage.

In drawing A, S is a solid capillary sprout with a thread-like terminal prolongation T, which is attaching itself to another blind capillary sprout. In B these structures have developed into an open capillary loop. NC. in picture A indicates no circulation in the blind sprout, converted to Cir (circulation) in B. Arrows show site and direction of blood flow. (From Sandison.[1])

neighbourhood. Mitochondria are numerous in these older macrophages, but endoplasmic reticulum is still not conspicuous (FIG. 4).

Blood Vessels

Close behind the macrophages that are advancing into the clot appear capillaries that originate from blood vessels around the periphery of the table. Usually by about the seventh day after the insertion of the chamber blood vessels reach the edge of the table on to which they continue to advance, under favourable conditions, at from 0·1 to 0·6 mm. a day. This rate of advance is influenced by temperature, and is slower if the rabbit is kept in a cold room. The rate is also dependent on the consistency of the clot; if by accident it partially dries, it may form a mass which effectually prevents healing.

The first new blood vessels are formed by migration and mitosis of the endothelium of pre-existing blood vessels around the chamber. Whatever their final form, they first have the structure of capillaries. Sandison found that in the earliest stage the capillary sprout was a solid protuberance with a fine terminal prolongation. These sprouts can attach themselves to neighbouring sprouts or to capillary vessels already carrying blood. Within a few hours the solid capillaries

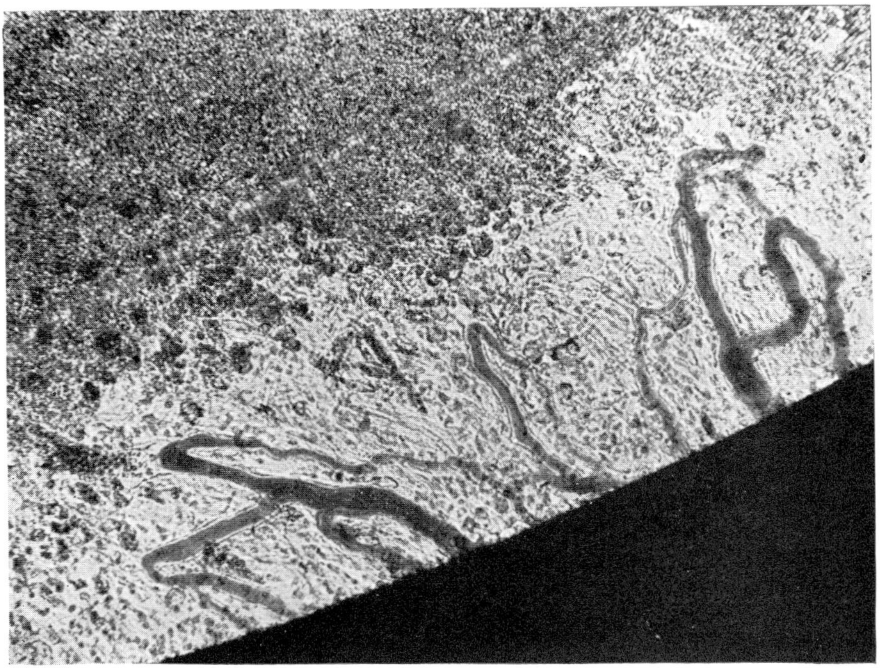

17/FIG. 6.—Shows capillary loops growing on to the edge of a round table. In the upper left-hand part of the picture the blood clot is being invaded by macrophages which, because of their content of debris, appear as large, rounded, dark granular structures. The beginning of differentiation of the capillaries into venules is taking place, and the cellular nature of the newly forming tissue can be appreciated. The new tissue is more translucent than the clot. (× 144).

develop a lumen, endothelial nuclei become clearly visible, and blood flows through what is now a capillary loop (FIG. 5).

Junction with another vessel does not always take place as described by Sandison. Tips of growing vessels in chambers often develop plump, blunt or even bulbous ends, into the lumen of which red corpuscles, platelets and an occasional white corpuscle are forced, but in which no fluid movement occurs, other than oscillations imparted by the heart beat and respiration. These capillary ends, shown in FIGS. 6 and 7, gradually extend into the areas cleared or softened by the action of macrophages and from time to time join one another or anastomose, forming capillary loops. In either way one of the characteristic features of the growing edge of healing tissue is produced: a series of arches of small vessels carrying a current of blood.

There is no evidence that blood capillaries form from anything but the endothelium of previously existing blood vessels.

The newly formed capillaries are very fragile and are more permeable than mature vessels. Red cells and fluid readily leak from them so that in an ear chamber the advancing edge of vessels is preceded by a bright red zone, easily seen by the naked eye, formed by freshly extruded erythrocytes. These red cells are phagocytosed and disposed of by the macrophages, so that the "thin red line" advances steadily in front of the blood vessels as they extend across the table. This zone frequently also contains free fluid in which cells oscillate to and

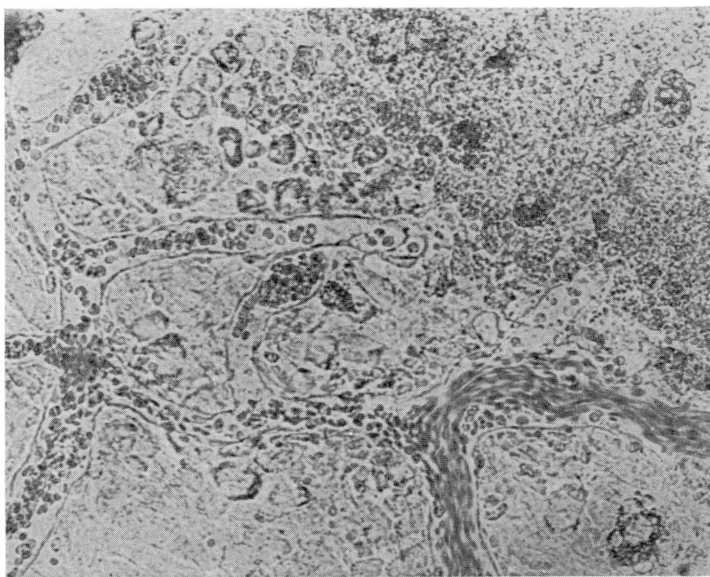

17/FIG. 7.—This is a photograph of a particularly thin portion of tissue in a chamber. At the right-hand top corner is an amorphous clot into which new vessels are growing from the left. Some of the tips of these new vessels have bulbous ends in which red corpuscles have concentrated. Many granular macrophages can be seen advancing into the clot ahead of the vessels. The flow of blood is brisk in the vessel at the bottom right-hand corner where the red corpuscles have moved during the taking of the photograph. ($\times$ 255).

fro synchronously with the heart beat. This fluid presumably arises from liquefaction of the clot by enzymes provided by disintegrating leucocytes and other cells, and from infiltration of the area with fluid from the leaky new vessels.

Fine Structure of Capillary Growth

There are still many obscurities in the precise mechanism by which the growing tips of the new blood vessels develop and anastomose to form loops. Mitoses are found not at the tips but about 0·5 mm. behind the tip. Cliff[4] has examined the tips by time lapse cinematography and with the electron microscope. FIGURE 8 shows an area at the growing edge of a healing chamber. In it a capillary can be seen which has a lumen admitting one red corpuscle. It is in a region where fibrin from the original clot is still present and where extravasated

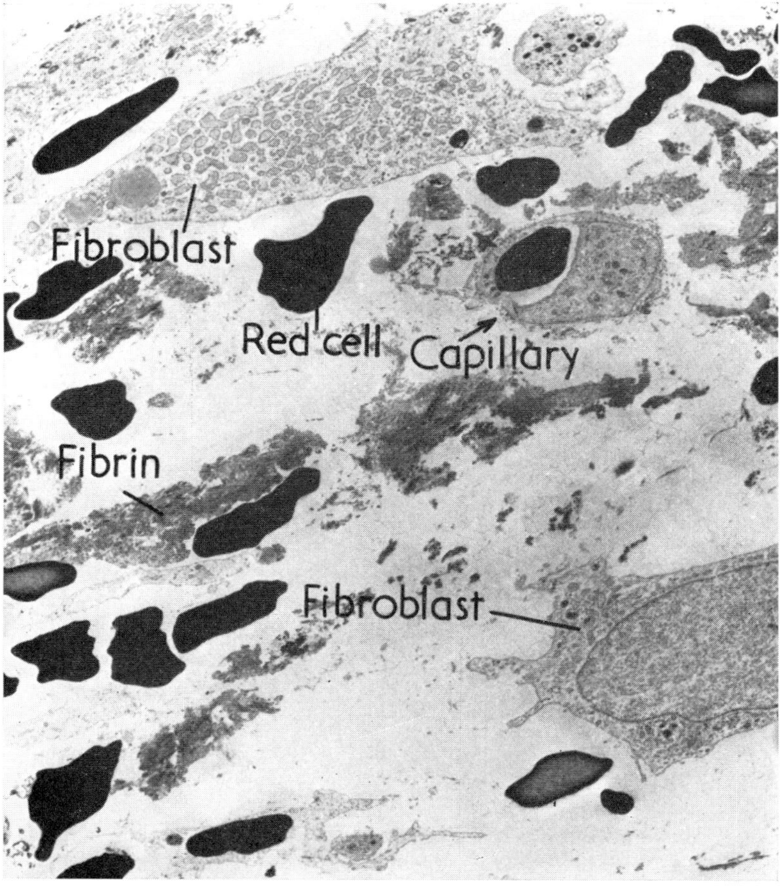

17/FIG. 8.—Electron micrograph near the growing edge of tissue in a rabbit ear chamber. It shows a capillary with a lumen accommodating a red cell. Fibroblasts, fibrin and extravasated red corpuscles are free in the newly forming tissue. (× 3,500)

red cells are abundant. FIGURE 9 shows a similar vessel at greater magnification. The endothelial cells are much thicker than those of mature capillaries. They possess pinocytic vesicles, and mitochondria and fine fibrils are seen in the cytoplasm. They contain relatively large amounts of endoplasmic reticulum similar

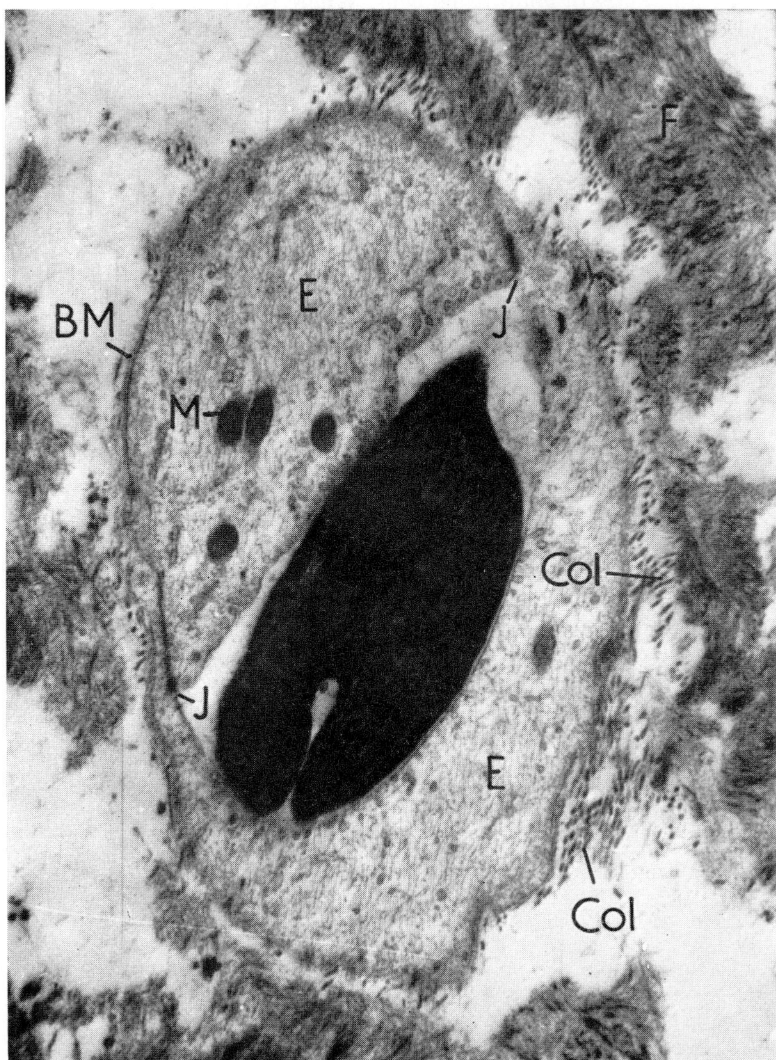

17/FIG. 9.—Electron micrograph of a capillary in healing tissue of a rabbit ear chamber. The two endothelial cells (E) are joined at junctions (J) which show electron-dense zones which are sometimes called "tight junctions". Pinocytic vesicles are visible especially along the luminal surface. Some mitochondria (M) are seen. The cytoplasm appears to contain numerous fine fibres. A basement membrane (BM) has formed and the external surface of the capillary is closely invested with collagen fibres (Col). The masses of dark material are fibrin (F). (× 17,500) (From Cliff.[4])

to that in fibroblasts. A basement membrane is present and collagen fibres have developed in close contact with the wall although the vessel is still embedded in much fibrin. Usually, however, a much more complicated picture is seen, as for example in FIG. 10. This shows a growing blood vessel in which spaces are forming between a number of endothelial cells. Where two cells adjoin one another, the usual kind of endothelial cell junction is developing complete with "tight" zone. As the spaces increase in size remodelling takes place, for example

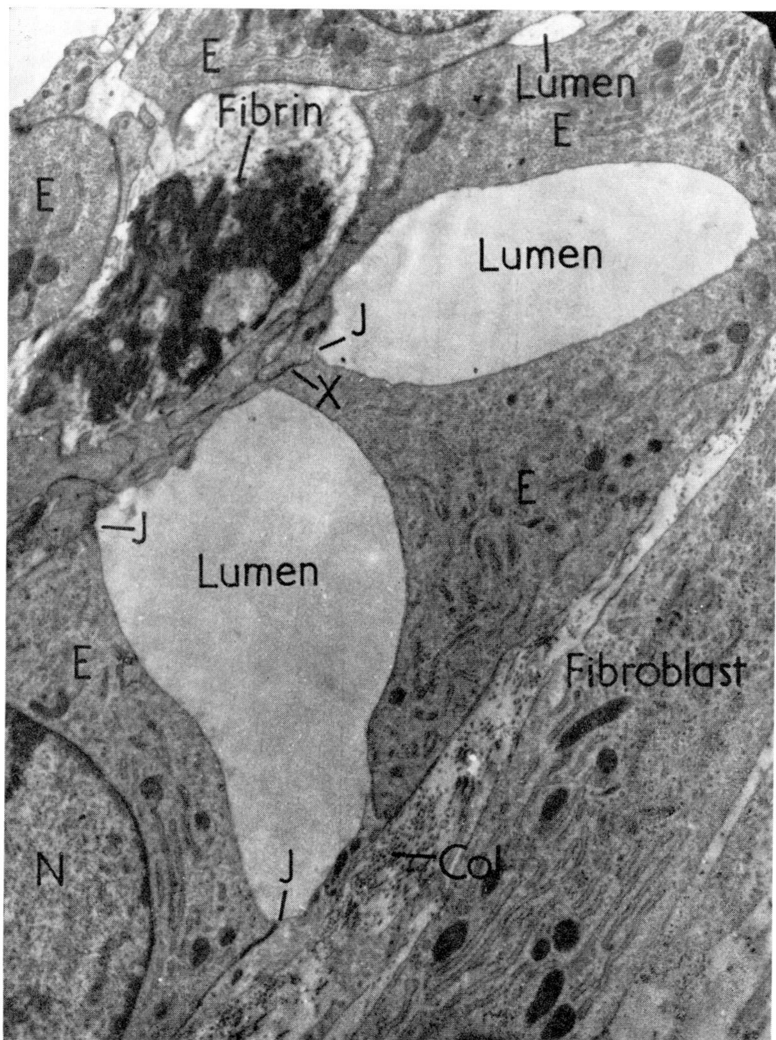

17/FIG. 10.—Electron micrograph of endothelium towards the tip of a growing vessel. A number of endothelial cells (E) are seen. Between them lumina are developing. The endothelial cells are joined at junctions (J) with the usual typical structure. They contain more endoplasmic reticulum than more mature endothelial cells. Possibly a junction will separate at X. (× 10,000)

the part of a junction marked X in FIG. 10 would probably separate with further growth and leave a single larger lumen, while the endothelial cells would become thinner.

Whether the fluid which fills the new lumen derives from surrounding tissue fluid or is a secretion of the endothelial cells is not certain. Cliff considered that the events which produce a channel in the vessel take place behind a solid tip of endothelial cells through the sliding of cells one upon another as the tip is pushed forward by endothelial proliferation. He believed also that as unwanted tips are resorbed their constituent cells slide into new positions and contribute to tips that are still growing.

Differentiation of Blood Vessels

The new vascular channels or capillaries at first consist only of endothelial cells. The blood flow within these fine tubes of endothelium changes direction from time to time. Their gradual development into one or other of the various parts of the vascular tree—arterioles, true capillaries, venules—begins within a few days and apparently depends on local conditions. It is thought that the straighter capillaries tend to turn into arteries, a view compatible with the doctrine of Thoma that the structure of a vessel wall is determined by the intravascular pressure and the amount of blood flow, and that where these are greatest an arteriole is formed.

Whatever the mechanism, it is an incontrovertible observation that arteries are formed by the endothelial tubes acquiring a muscle coat. At first this consists of single, circularly disposed muscle cells which manifest their true nature by contracting from time to time, and so producing isolated constrictions of the lumina of the young vessels. With increasing growth the vessel acquires a continuous circular coat of at least one layer of smooth muscle cells, and in the larger vessels two or three layers can sometimes be identified. It is still an unsolved problem where the muscle cells come from. Conceivably they could arise from differentiation of mesenchymal cells that have migrated into the matrix of the new tissue. Some colour is given at first glance to this idea by the fact that "adventitial" or fibroblast-like cells apply themselves longitudinally to the capillary walls at an early stage. Their function is unknown, but they do not appear to be contractile. Cliff watched the stages in which such a cell altered its orientation to encircle a capillary, which is the normal position of smooth muscle cells, and he thought that it became contractile. Another possibility is that new muscle cells arise from the muscle cells of pre-existing arterioles and migrate along the vessels, but this has never been clearly demonstrated.

What factors determine that a capillary channel shall become a venule is quite obscure, but observations show that some vessels undergo a change whereby they increase in diameter and drain off blood into larger venules. Muscle cells have never been described on the walls of venules in an ear chamber; as with the smallest venules in other situations, these vessels are apparently too small to require a muscle coat, but they can be recognised by their calibre and the direction of blood flow.

Most of the vessels connecting the arterioles and venules of the chamber remain simple endothelial tubes with adventitial cells and histiocytes applied to the walls, but direct anastomoses between arteries and veins also occur in the healing tissue of the rabbit's ear. These anastomoses are made by vessels with a muscle coat which can completely obliterate the lumen by its contraction. Such direct shunts from arteries to veins exist normally in a number of tissues, but whether they are present in all newly developing fibrous tissue is not known.

While the development of this differentiated vasculature is going on, there is a constant modelling and remodelling of the pattern, chiefly of the endothelial tubes, but, in the course of time, of the arterioles and venules as well. This modelling is brought about by the obliteration of many of the first formed capillaries. It appears that if the newly formed vessels do not carry any blood for about twenty-four hours their lumen begins to decrease in diameter and finally is obliterated. The solid cord thus produced breaks in two and the ends shrink back to the level of the next patent vessel. The process is illustrated in FIG. 11, The number of original capillaries that survive is variable, sometimes not more than 1 in 10, sometimes nearly all. Successive changes in the vascular pattern may be seen in FIG. 12.

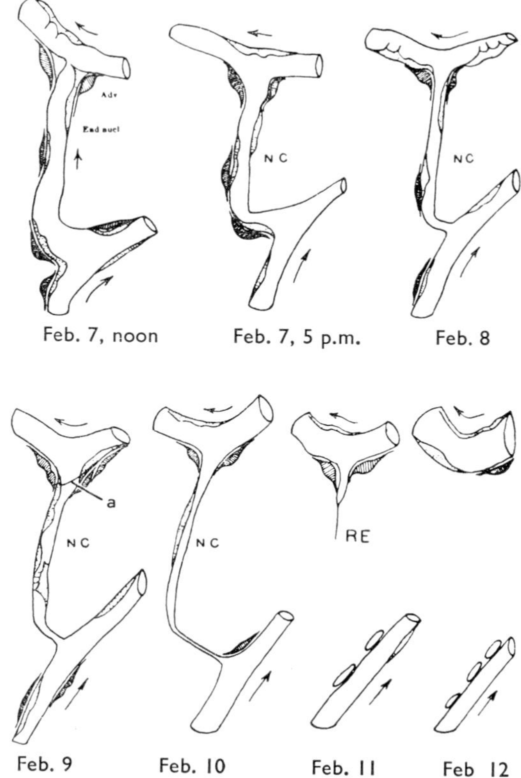

17/FIG. 11.– Successive camera lucida drawings showing closure and disappearance of a capillary following the cessation of blood flow through it. Arrows indicate presence and direction of blood flow. NC = no circulation; Adv = adventitial cell; End nucl = endothelial nucleus; RE = retracting end of vessel with an endothelial thread attached; a = a fine thread or strand of endothelium hanging across lumen of vessel. (×412.) (From Sandison.[1])

17/FIG. 12.—SERIES OF PHOTOMICROGRAPHS OF THE CENTRAL TABLE AREA OF A CHAMBER, SHOWING CHANGES DURING 6 MONTHS. The time interval after the operation is given for each figure. (From Clark, Hitschler, Kirby-Smith, Rex and Smith.[5])

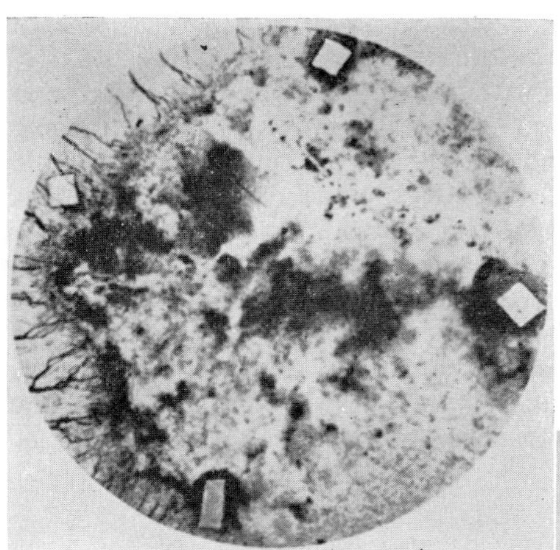

(*a*) 10 days. Shows new capillaries starting on to the table.

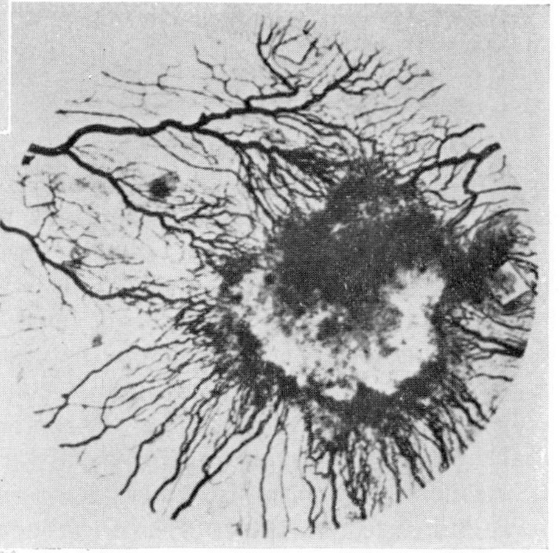

(*b*) 19 days. Shows vascular tissue invading blood clot.

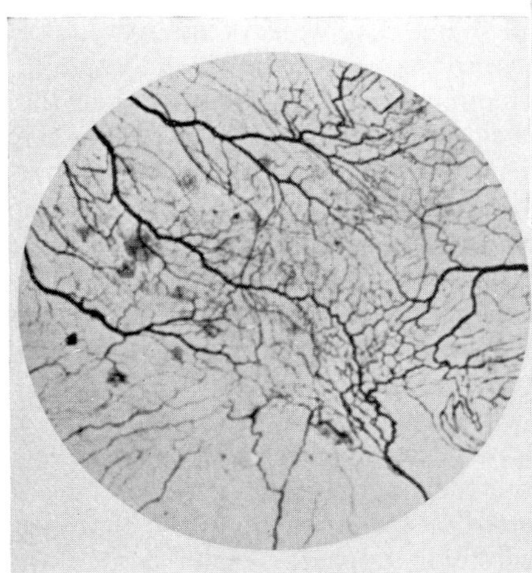

(*c*) 26 days. Shows table completely vascularised.

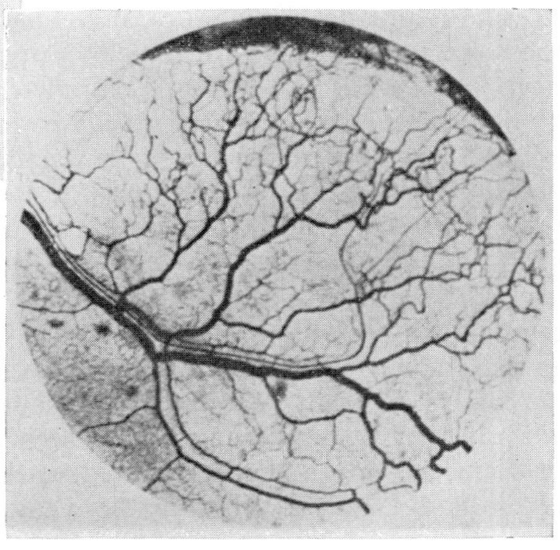

(*d*) 6 months. Shows a mature pattern which, however, can still change from time to time.

Vasomotor Nerves

Muscle cells begin to appear on the arterioles within two or three days of the formation of endothelial tubes, and with their appearance and increase in number the lumen of the vessel concerned becomes narrower. The muscle cells appear to give the vessels tone independently of active contraction. They do not contract unless and until a newly formed vasomotor nerve reaches them. The growth of such nerves has been followed in chambers by staining them from time to time with methylene blue, and has been deduced by watching new vessels for contraction. The earliest contractions were seen in a vessel that 10 days before had been an endothelial tube and the latest in an arteriole that was first seen to contract 7½ months after it had been formed. Some arterioles never acquire the capacity to contract and this is thought to be due to the fact that the ingrowing vasomotor nerves do not connect with all the newly formed muscle cells.

Lymphatics

The growth of the other important endothelial structures—the lymphatics—probably follows much the same course as that of the blood capillaries. The growing sprouts anastomose from time to time with one another or with already formed lymphatics, and by this means a network of lymphatic capillaries is developed (FIG. 13). They apparently grow more slowly and are less labile than blood capillaries, they send out fewer sprouts, and once formed show less tendency to retract or to change in size and shape. The walls of the lymphatics in a chamber, no matter what their size, are composed exclusively of endothelium.

The growth of lymphatics, as seen in chambers, is more irregular than that of the blood capillaries and nearly always begins later. In thin chambers, where the tissue is less than 40μ thick, lymphatics are rarely seen; in thick chambers they tend to follow the course of the larger blood vessels, growing inward along the clear space beside the vessel; if the tissue is loose they may form a plexus.

Though embryologically lymphatics probably spring from blood vascular endothelium, it is remarkable that the endothelial sprouts from blood capillaries unite only with other blood capillaries and lymphatic sprouts only with lymphatics. Thus no direct blood-lymph channels are formed.

The lymphatics contain clear fluid which appears to move hardly at all, if the behaviour of cells and particles suspended in the fluid is taken as an indication. Their walls are normally complete, but their contents may be forced out by light pressure such as can readily be exerted on the coverslip of the chamber. Minute openings made by slight damage remain open for many days if the vessel is surrounded by fluid, but if it is surrounded by the gelatinous matrix of newly formed tissue the holes close at once. It is possible that the formation of such openings is a usual occurrence during inflammation, enabling particles such as bacteria to find their way readily into the lymphatics and to drain to a regional lymph node

Clark,[7] basing his views on the extremely sluggish flow of lymph in the lymphatics of transparent chambers, and on the fact that regions in chambers without lymphatics appear to heal normally or at any rate to "show no evidence of disturbed physiology", doubted whether lymphatics in the peripheral parts of the body "play any useful role whatever". This seems to be going rather far

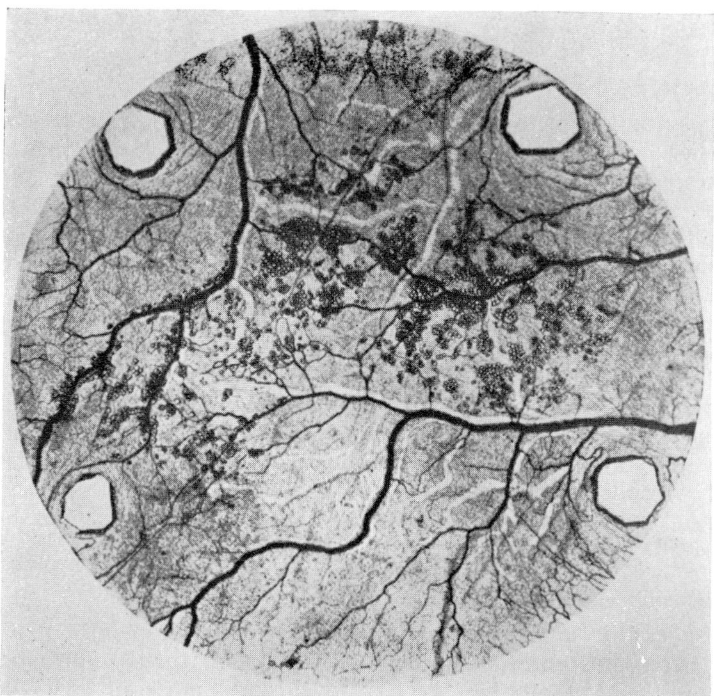

17/FIG. 13.—Table area of a chamber into which blood vessels started to grow at 5 days and lymphatics at 37 days after operation. The lymphatics, which appear as white lines, followed the arteriole and 2 venules for the greater part of their advance from the periphery where dense connective tissue had been formed. In the central region where connective tissue formation had been delayed they grew out as a plexus. This chamber also shows that fat cells develop in the connective tissue. (From Clark and Clark.[6])

and raises the question whether the behaviour of lymphatics in ear chambers is similar to that in other sites. The mouse's ear, though thin, is in every way a normal tissue, and it can be used for the study of normal lymphatics, as has been described in Chapter 3. Abscesses involving destruction of tissue were made in the ears of a series of mice by the injection of a small drop of turpentine. The mice were killed at intervals, the ear lymphatics having been injected with a fine suspension of carbon just before death. In this way it was shown that there was a very considerable proliferation of lymphatics in the healing edge of the abscess (FIG. 17). Great proliferation of lymphatics is also caused by painting tar on the ear or by inserting silica which causes the development of fibrous tissue. These findings support those previously made by many observers, and there can no longer be any doubt, such as some of the older pathologists entertained, that lymphatics proliferate freely in healing connective tissue. (Older work is discussed in some detail by Pullinger and Florey.[8])

As far as we are aware there are no studies on lymph flow from an aseptically healing wound, but in view of the considerable amount of fluid that probably passes through the delicate walls of young blood capillaries it would be extraordinary if there were not an increased flow of lymph into the lymphatic trunks draining the part.

Leucocytes

Leucocytes adhere to the walls of very young blood vessels apparently in the same way as to vessel walls in inflamed mature tissue. Having adhered, these leucocytes, mainly granulocytes, emerge from the vessels, especially at the growing edge. The granulocytes appear to wander about aimlessly in the extravascular tissue, and their rapid amœboid motions can be readily observed in ear chambers. With the passage of time they disappear, probably because they die and are then autolysed or ingested by macrophages. Though they do not apparently serve much useful purpose in life, when dead their granules are discharged and their proteolytic enzymes escape and probably help to liquefy the clot and any tissue debris.

Lymphocytes also emerge from the young capillaries and can be seen pursuing their apparently aimless and erratic course amongst the other cells.

Sometimes in the newly formed tissue of rabbit ear chambers plasma cells may be seen collected near a blood vessel (FIG. 14). These cells are characterised by a very abundant endoplasmic reticulum studded with ribosomes, indicating, it is believed, that they are engaged in elaborating protein.

Amorphous Matrix

It is evident in a chamber, and in healing wounds generally, that cells and growing structures are supported in an amorphous matrix after the formed elements of the blood clot have been removed. This matrix, or, as it is sometimes called, "ground substance", is semi-solid or gelatinous. During the first few days of healing one of its features is a relatively high content of mucopolysaccharide, though it is not clear whether this is chiefly derived from blood plasma or whether it is a secretion of cells in the healing area such as the fibroblasts.

The concentration of mucopolysaccharide begins to fall at about the time that the first young collagen fibrils appear. This may be no more than a coincidence. The part played by polysaccharides in the formation and maturation of collagen fibres is still somewhat obscure.

Fibrous Tissue

The essential material that heals wounds is the collagen laid down in the form of fibres in the terrain that has been cleared of clot and debris and supplied with nutriment by newly formed blood vessels.

There is little doubt that in such healing tissue the fibres are formed under the influence of the cells known as fibroblasts, whose movements can be watched in ear chambers just as can those of other cells. The fibroblasts arise from cells in neighbouring tissues which are stimulated to divide, probably from fibrocytes (the later form of the fibroblast) or from some less differentiated precursor. They seem to originate more readily in loose connective tissue, such as that round blood vessels, than in dense collagen layers like dermis or fascia in which the fibrocytes are very slender and "mature". They invade the clot just after the macrophages and at about the same time as the blood vessels. As they advance

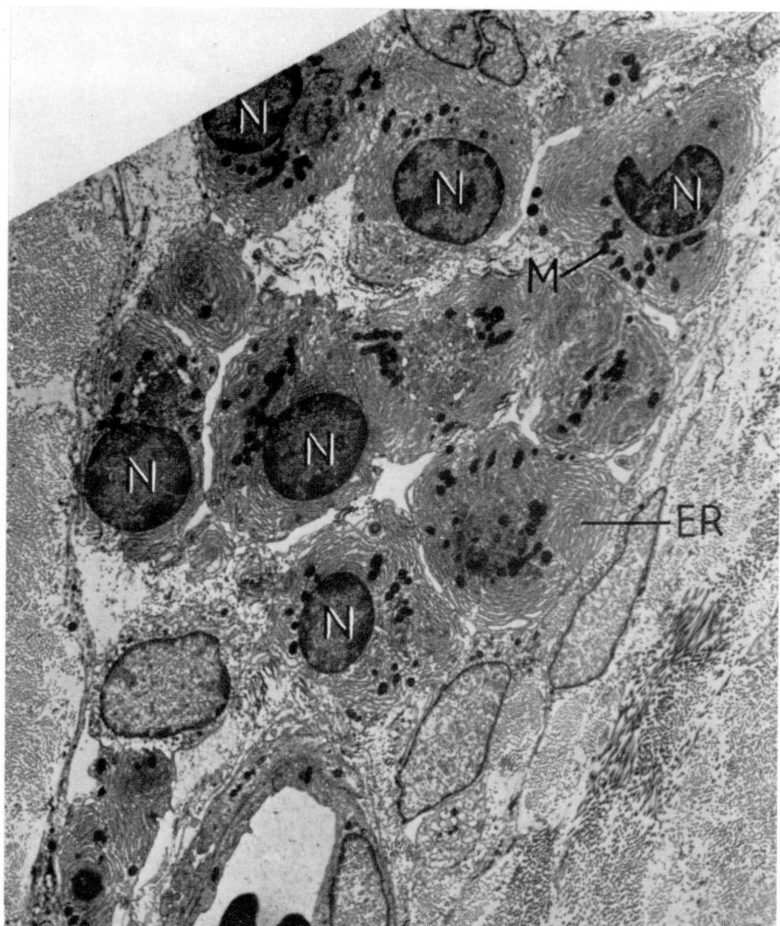

17/FIG. 14.—Electron micrograph of plasma cells in the newly formed tissue of an ear chamber. The nuclei of the plasma cells (N) are relatively electron-dense and the cytoplasm is occupied by closely packed whorls of endoplasmic reticulum (ER). M = mitochondria. (× 3,500)

into the chamber they are seen as stellate or more or less bipolar cells with fine processes protruding from them, but it should be emphasised that these processes are not the collagen fibres, which look quite different and appear at a later stage.

In electron micrographs fibroblasts can easily be distinguished from other cells such as macrophages by their very elongated cell bodies and by their large content of endoplasmic reticulum studded with ribosomes and with electron-dense material in the cisternæ (FIGS. 15 and 16). This indicates that the cell is metabolically very active and that it is probably producing protein. The fibroblasts do not have the cytoplasmic "ruffles" on the surface so characteristic of macrophages.

The fibroblasts migrate at the rate of about 0·2 mm. a day and progress

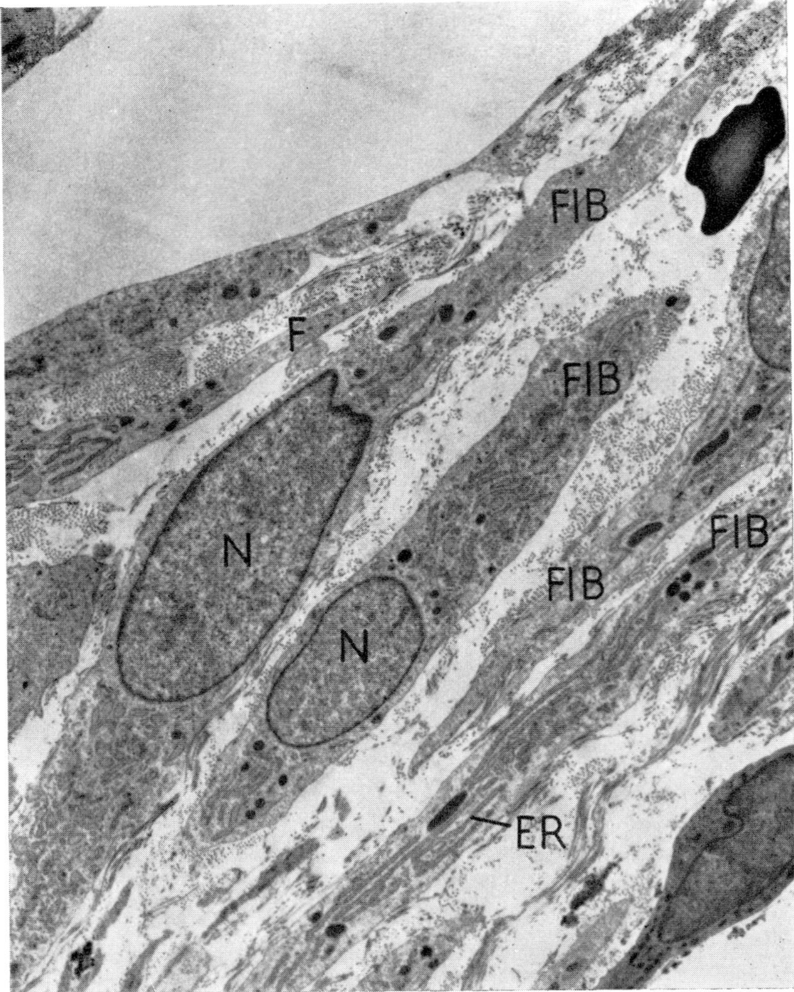

17/FIG. 15.—Electron micrograph to show fibroblasts (FIB) cut longitudinally. Some cells show their nuclei (N). In the cytoplasm can be seen much endoplasmic reticulum (ER) which contains in its interstices material more electron-dense than the surrounding cytoplasm. Between the fibroblasts are numerous collagen fibres, many of them cut transversely. (× 5,500.)

generally towards the centre of the table, though they may deviate to one side or the other of a direct line. Their number is constantly increased by fresh accretions from the surrounding tissue, and by mitotic division of the cells already on the table. The cells steadily advance into areas partially cleared of red cells and fibrin, now occupied by a transparent gelatinous matrix.

About six days after the fibroblasts appear the first collagen fibres, quite distinct from the fibres of fibrin in the clot, can be recognised by the light microscope near the periphery of the table. They advance towards the centre at

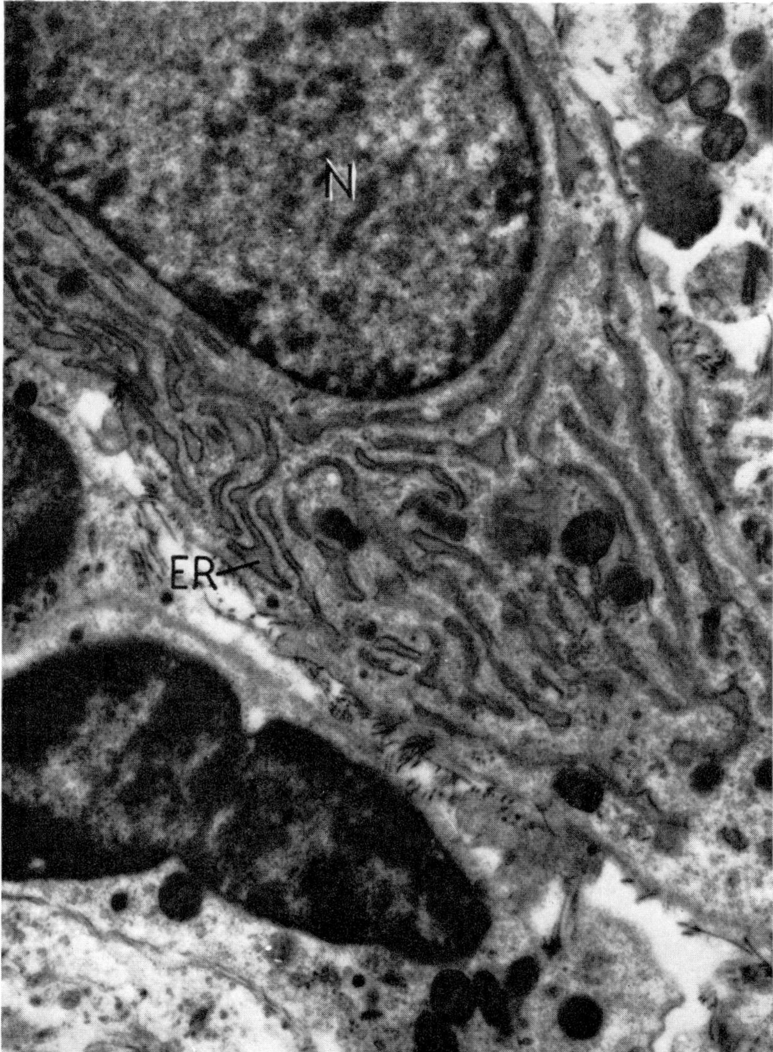

17/Fig. 16.—Electron micrograph of part of a fibroblast to show the abundant endoplasmic reticulum (ER) enclosing relatively electron-dense material in the cisternæ. (× 10,000)

about the same rate as the migrating fibroblasts. The fibroblasts have an intimate connection with the formation of these fibres, and what is known of this relationship, which now attracts very considerable interest, has been discussed in Chapter 16.

The fibres are at first oriented radially and are in one plane, but in the course of time, especially if the chamber becomes thicker during the growth of the tissue, other layers of fibres may appear. These are approximately at right

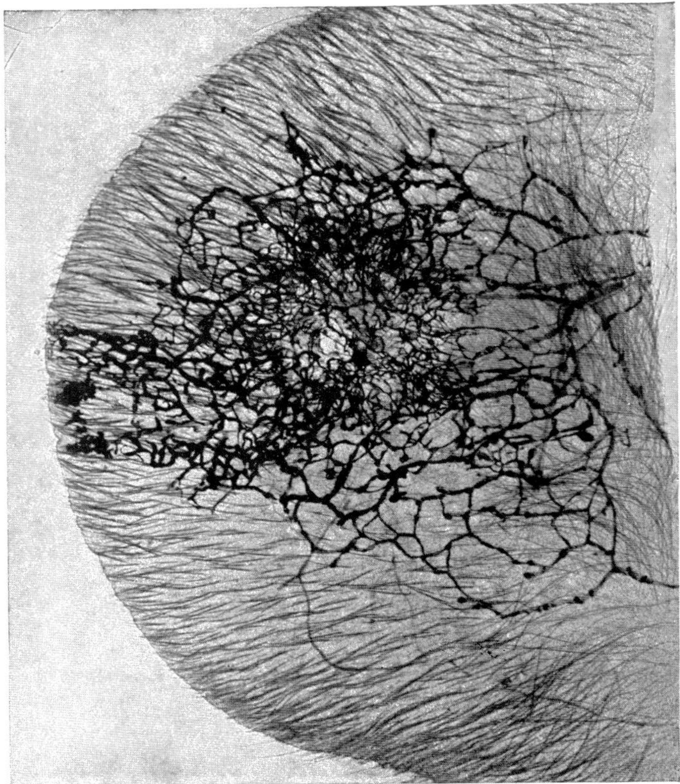

17/FIG. 17.—Lymphatics (shown up by hydrokollag) in a mouse's ear 21 days after turpentine injection. The abscess which formed perforated the ear. A dense network of new lymphatic capillaries surrounds the hole. (×20.) (From Pullinger and Florey.[8])

angles to those first formed. In this way a fairly uniform tough membrane of laminated collagen is developed. Tension on growing fibres apparently determines the direction in which they will lie and, if space permits, their abundance. This can be well seen in the neighbourhood of the buffers on the table. The Clarks' chambers tended to migrate towards the tip of the rabbit's ear and in so doing the fibres around the buffers were pulled on. Fibres then developed along the lines of tension, as can be well seen in FIG. 18.

Fat Cells

In old thick chambers fat cells are sometimes seen (FIG. 13). Adipose tissue is, in general, a special form of connective tissue, but the way in which new fat cells arise here or elsewhere has never been ascertained.

Healing of Wounds by First Intention

We have now seen how a gap cut through the soft tissues of a rabbit's ear is filled by a clot which is then replaced by new formation of vessels and fibrous

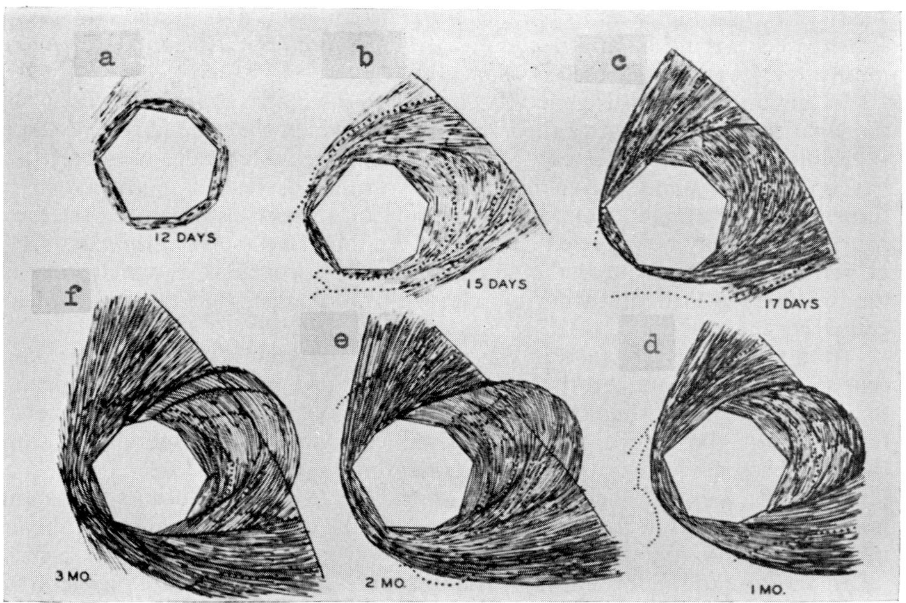

17/Fig. 18.—A series of camera lucida drawings of the development of collagen fibres around a buffer of an ear chamber. The fibres come to lie in bundles forming rings round the buffer, the response to the tension created by gradual shift of the chamber towards the tip of the ear. ($\times$30.) (From Stearns.[9])

tissue. Exactly similar processes occur following clean operation or accidental wounds in man or animals. Immediately after wounding there is an escape of blood from the cut blood vessels. Unless large arteries are involved, this soon ceases and the wound surface is covered with clotted blood and plasma that has exuded from damaged vessels. The sides of a clean wound are usually brought together by appropriately placed stitches so that there is the minimum of space between them. This small space is filled by clotted blood and exudate containing remains of cells damaged by the trauma, and in the first 24 hours large numbers of granulocytes, monocytes and lymphocytes migrate into the clot from surrounding vessels that are affected by inflammatory changes consequent on the mechanical damage. By the end of the first day after wounding new tissue formation begins, and mitoses are common in the connective tissue cells and endothelium by the end of the second day. On the third day capillary sprouts can be discerned. Reticulin fibres, probably the precursor of collagen, begin to appear by the fourth or fifth day, and soon after van Gieson-staining collagen fibres appear and increase rapidly in number by the process that we have followed in the rabbit's ear chamber. Electron microscopy during the first two weeks shows that the young collagen fibrils gradually get thicker.[10] Serial estimations of hydroxyproline in wound tissue give a quantitative picture of collagen formation and shows that the great bulk of the collagen is laid down during the second week of healing. Thereafter the process is largely one of slow consolidation of the fine van Gieson-staining fibres into coarser mature collagen.

Tensile strength increases in parallel with the collagen, and by the end of the second week should be approaching that of the uninjured tissue, though maximum strength is not regained for some time.

In human wounds it is generally considered justifiable to remove stitches by the eighth to tenth day after their insertion, by which time the fibrous tissue is sufficiently strong to resist any but unusual stresses. Generally a wound that has opened the abdomen—a laparotomy wound—is healed in from two to three weeks for all practical purposes. In plastic surgery, especially of the face, some stitches may be removed as early as the third day to avoid the possibility of permanent scars around the stitch holes. This procedure is satisfactory as long as there is little pull from muscles on wound edges that are still held together very tenuously.

At first, as we have seen in ear chambers, the young scar contains many cells and blood vessels so that, even when covered by epithelium, it appears red or, on cold days when the circulation is sluggish, bluish; but, as in all newly formed tissue, the number of vessels is reduced with the passage of time, and the scar becomes whiter than the surrounding tissues. Eventually the line of junction of a wound which had good apposition of its edges becomes less and less noticeable, and in the course of some months only a fine lamina of fibrous tissue marks the original site of the wound.

In addition to the formation of collagen fibres, elastic fibres are regenerated, though their time of appearance is variable—it is certainly much later than that of the fibrous tissue. Sensory nerves grow into healing wounds and may reach the new epidermis by the end of the third week, but specialised nerve endings are not reformed.

This form of repair is known as primary union or union by first intention and is the rule in wounds deliberately inflicted at operation. It is also frequent in small accidental injuries that are clean and are sutured within a few hours of their infliction.

Formation of Granulation Tissue. Healing by Second Intention

It is not always possible, nor if possible is it always desirable, to approximate the edges of a wound. In an open wound the base and edges become red and later swell from the accumulation of exudate and cells from the damaged blood vessels. From the surface of the wound a yellowish or light red, slightly turbid fluid exudes. This so-called secretion of the wound contains a considerable amount of protein including fibrinogen, which clots on the surface, thus covering the wound with a transparent fibrin layer containing leucocytes. Forty-eight hours to three days after the infliction of the wound its base appears red. Within the next few days the whole surface assumes a red and finely granular appearance. Each of the granules consists of a core of wide new capillaries, the growth of which raises the enveloping mantle of macrophages, fibroblasts and other cells into a small elevation. The granules being formed partly of new delicate blood vessels bleed very easily when touched. The granulation tissue gradually increases in thickness until the whole defect is filled; the growth of new tissue may even be excessive, so that "exuberant granulations" protrude from the wound. A section passing through a granulating wound discloses a thin superficial layer of cell debris, a layer of newly formed vessels among which granulocytes are conspicuous, and deeper layers containing maturing fibrous tissue produced by fibroblasts (FIGS. 19 and 20). In the course of time a contraction of the wound occurs which is due principally to shortening of the maturing fibrous tissue. This form of contraction, which is often known as contracture or cicatrisation, has in one way a beneficial action in that it causes a diminution of the size of the defect, but in some places it can bring with it undesirable consequences. Thus contracture of a wound of the cheek may cause the eversion of the lower eyelid, or the formation of much fibrous tissue in the angle of a joint following a severe burn may eventually cause considerable limitation of movement.

In some circumstances newly formed fibrous tissue subjected to tension may stretch; for example, the scar formed following opening of the abdomen may stretch so that some of the abdominal contents herniate into a sac bounded by fibrous tissue. The same phenomenon may be seen in the stretching of fibrous

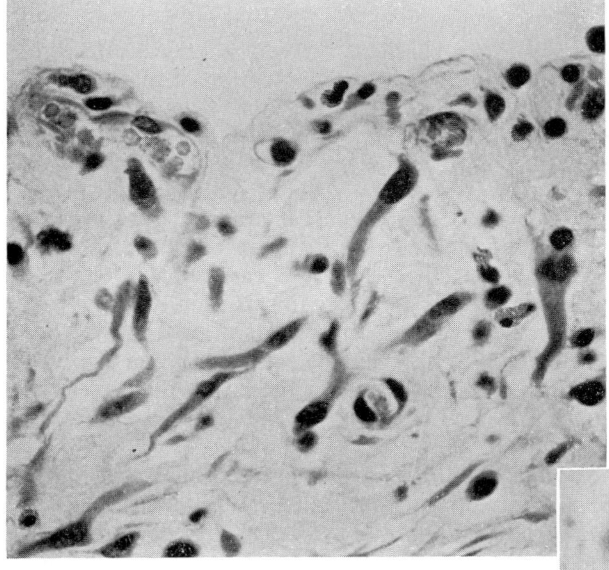

17/FIG. 19.—Fibroblasts and young blood vessels in granulation tissue forming in a clotted exudate on the surface of damaged tissue (rabbit). A few wandering cells, lymphocytes and polymorphs, are also present. Histological section stained hæmatoxylin and eosin.

17/FIG. 20.—Mitosis in a fibroblast of the preparation shown in FIG. 19.

tissue that has formed in the wall of the aorta as a consequence of syphilitic arterial disease. The stretched sac is here known as an aneurysm.

The maturation of the fibrous tissue takes many months, during which it becomes much less cellular than in the early stages, as we have seen in the ear chambers. The time for which a wound through skin that has healed by granulation may be pink, or in cold weather blue, is longer than in the case of wounds that have healed by first intention, but gradually, as the cell population decreases, the vessels disappear in the way that we have already discussed, so that an old wound is much paler than the surrounding skin. At this stage a section discloses thick bundles of fibrous tissue with a few compressed nuclei of the original fibroblasts, now mature and known as fibrocytes, retained alive between them. Sometimes the collagen may undergo a further change to form a structureless mass, a process known as hyalinisation.

Infected Wounds

Granulation tissue is in some ways an excellent protection against infection, for it has a good blood supply, there is a continuous exudation of plasma from the new vessels, and large numbers of leucocytes and other cells are present. However, on many occasions, for instance in war, in industrial life and in street accidents, wounds are made that become infected soon after their infliction and before the development of granulation tissue by such pyogenic organisms as staphylococci and streptococci, or on occasion with tetanus or gas-gangrene organisms. The pyogenic cocci come in the great majority of cases from the clothes or skin of the wounded, or from the hands and nasopharynx of those who attend to them, but tetanus and gas gangrene organisms usually come from foreign bodies or soil. Contaminated wounds are never sutured while they contain pathogenic bacteria, but the possibility of early suture, and consequently of better restoration of function, has been greatly increased by the advent of antibacterial substances that can eliminate micro-organisms by chemical means.

Whether they are shallow or deep, the healing of unsutured infected wounds depends on the production of granulation tissue. Infected granulation tissue contains many bacteria on its surface and among the cells. They cause a much greater exudation from the blood vessels than occurs in an uninfected wound, and kill some of the leucocytes and newly formed fibroblasts, so that pus containing bacteria and dead cells may constantly well from the wound. Nevertheless, if the infection is not too severe healing proceeds, though it may be much slowed. Not only does the longer period of healing give time for more fibrous tissue to form, but the inflammation stimulates the proliferation of blood vessels and connective tissue cells, so that the scar is much thicker and denser than that of an uninfected wound. This is one reason for taking every precaution to avoid infection of surgical wounds, especially in plastic surgery where a dense and contracted scar can greatly increase disfigurement or disability.

Organisation and Adhesions

We have spoken of healing of wounds, but the same general process, which is sometimes called organisation, occurs in any part of the body where a deposit of clot, exudate or dead tissue occurs. Thus in blood vessels a thrombus or clot can be, and usually is, organised and turned into fibrous tissue. Exudate may be dealt with in the same way. For instance, a fibrinous exudate in the pleural, pericardial, or abdominal cavity may be turned into fibrous tissue which binds the surfaces of the organs concerned together by what are termed fibrous adhesions. Likewise dead areas of organs, for example infarcts, may in course of time be absorbed and entirely replaced by fibrous tissue.

Closure of the Wound

Other factors beside the formation of new tissue affect the rate of closure of a wound. We are familiar with linear skin wounds that tend to gape because of tissue tension; healing is quicker if the edges are kept together. On the other hand if a piece of mucosa is excised from the stomach the bare area is made considerably smaller by spasm of the muscularis mucosæ. Drying and the formation of a scab tend to draw together the edges of shallow lesions in the skin, though the presence of too solid a scab may mechanically embarrass the growth of epithelium. In the late stages of healing contracture of the fibrous tissue reduces the size of a scar, as we have seen.

Another mechanism that can reduce the size of a defect can be demonstrated in the loose skin of small animals. If a rectangle of skin and subcutaneous tissue 2 or 3 cm. square is excised from the back of a guinea-pig or rat the wound closes in, say, 15 days, with the most rapid inward movement of the edges between the fifth and tenth days. This movement, known as "contraction", is of the cut edges of the pre-existing dermis, and is independent of epithelial regrowth, though this goes on at the same time. FIGURE 21 shows how by tattooing the dermis this movement can be demonstrated. It is maximal before much collagen

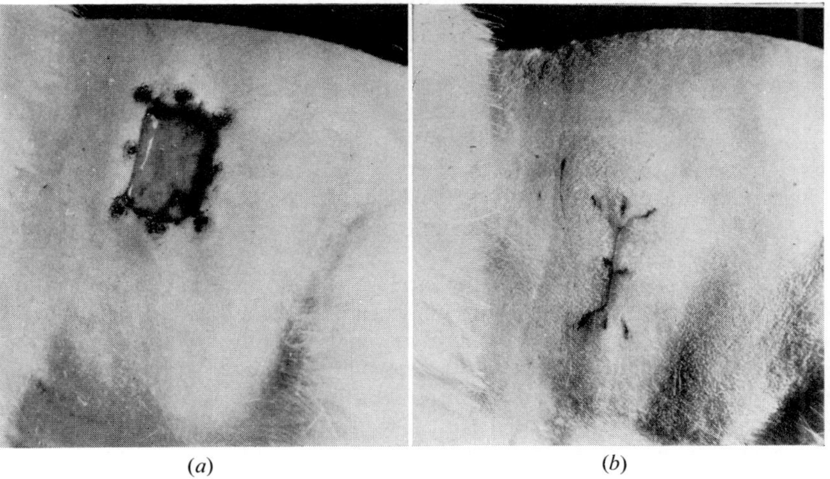

(*a*) (*b*)

17/FIG. 21.—Contraction of a wound in the skin of a guinea-pig. The guinea-pig's head is to the left. A rectangle of skin and panniculus carnosus was excised touching the inner borders of a series of tattoo marks in the dermis (*a*). After 15 days the wound had closed with the tattoo marks at or close to the line of healing (*b*). (From Grillo, Watts and Gross.[11])

has formed and is independent of muscle contraction, and none of the mechanisms mentioned above fully accounts for it. It has been suggested that the connective tissues have, like epithelium, some capacity to remodel themselves to help make good a defect as they do in the regeneration of organs in lower animals, and that this substantially assists closure of the wound quite apart from any new formation of tissue.[12] Others have been inclined to attribute the phenomenon to some unexplained contractile power in the extracellular components of granulation tissue or to contraction of the fibroblasts themselves.[12a]

It is difficult to know how far this mechanism has any importance in healing in man. As far as surface wounds are concerned some degree of useful contraction is said to occur on the back and abdomen but not on the front of the thorax or on the limbs, but on the whole early skin grafting is a more reliable means of obtaining quick healing. It has been suggested that in the loose connective tissues, for instance in the pelvis, this form of contraction may play a significant part in closing defects.[13]

Healing of Epithelium

A gap in epithelium is filled in two ways. Firstly, cells from the lower layers of the remaining skin edge, or corresponding cells in other epithelia, can slide across the bare or fibrin-covered surface. While doing this they spread out, so that in section they appear as flattened squames, and the nucleus and cytoplasm increase in bulk. It has been stated that the epithelial cells move by amœboid motion, but if amœboid motion is taken to mean progression as a result of pseudopod formation and streaming of the cytoplasm into the pseudopod, there is no evidence that this occurs in epithelial cells. In a spreading sheet of epithelium on glass the activity of the free surfaces of the cells is likened rather to a wave-like movement of ruffles.[14] In fixed material viewed by electron microscopy blunt projections of cytoplasm are seen on the free surfaces of epithelial cells at the edge of a wound.[14a] Secondly, after a lag of some hours, mitosis takes place, at first predominantly in the millimetre or so of old skin next to the cut edge and later in the spreading epithelium as well. As the cells divide more are available to move out across the bare surface. If the wound is very small considerable epithelial progression can apparently take place without the production of many new cells; indeed, small wounds in the cornea of the rat were completely covered by epithelium by movement of the cells alone; the bare area was covered by cell movement in 12 hours, though mitoses did not reach their maximum for 5 days.[15]

The forward movement of epithelium stops as soon as the cells meet at the middle of the wound and the whole unites into a single layer. One of the subtle mechanisms of cell recognition is involved in this contact inhibition, for movement and proliferation do not stop if a mechanical barrier is put in the path of the advancing cells, and even two epithelia (for example, those of skin and œsophagus) may be so disparate that if placed so that they meet in this way each piles up against the other because movement and proliferation are not arrested. It is now known that contact inhibition is soon followed by the establishment of normal inter-cell communication (as measured electrically) between the two sides.[16]

After covering is complete, or in larger wounds while it is still in progress, the epithelial cells begin to differentiate starting with the older cells at the periphery of the wound. Multilayered and otherwise specialised epithelia have considerable powers of regeneration and in some restoration may be almost complete.

Healing of the Skin

When an incised wound of the skin heals by first intention the epithelium at the cut edges migrates and proliferates rapidly to bridge the gap. In the early stages the epithelium may grow down into the incision and into the stitch holes, but as healing in the underlying dermis proceeds these hyperplastic downgrowths of epithelium recede and the scar is covered eventually by a more or less normal epithelial layer.[17, 18]

In very small skin wounds, involving only epithelium, migration and proliferation of epithelial cells replace those missing without any other disturbance. This is shown in blisters in which the impermeable horny layer is raised by fluid from the more delicate deeper layers of epithelial cells. When the blister is cut away the latter proliferate and rapidly restore the original structure.

With the loss of more tissue more complex events occur which are well seen when the healing of a clean open skin wound is watched. As we have noted, in such a wound granulation tissue forms quickly. While this is proceeding the epithelium at the cut edges starts to spread out over the wound and if the healing edge is observed microscopically or under low magnification it can be seen to shelve from the normal skin towards the granulations, the growing edge being of a pearly translucency.

As the epithelium gradually closes in over the growing granulations it becomes attached to them in some way not precisely known. The passage of epithelium over the granulations stops their further development.[18a] There is a local increase of collagenolytic activity which may be connected with local remodelling of the tissue. Eventually the wound is completely healed and in time its covering takes on somewhat the appearance of normal skin, but the appendages such as hair follicles and sweat and sebaceous glands are not generally reformed in man, nor are the normal papillæ reconstructed. In animals, however, the skin appendages sometimes reform.[19]

On the other hand remains of skin appendages may be a useful source of new surface epithelium. For example, when considerable areas of skin are burnt, if hair follicles and sebaceous glands are left in the depths of the burnt area skin can be reformed from them and spread as islands over the surrounding granulation tissue (FIG. 22).

To speed up the healing of large areas of granulation tissue, such as appears after burning, use is often made of the procedure of skin grafting. In one of its simplest forms, which is often successful, small snippets of skin that include cells of the Malpighian layer, are taken from an undamaged area and are applied to the granulations with the living cells downwards. Under favourable conditions they survive and adhere to the granulations, on which they spread and form an epithelial covering, at first thin, but gradually increasing in thickness until in many cases satisfactory healing results. Gillman and Penn[17] described at length events following skin grafting and those interested can consult their papers.

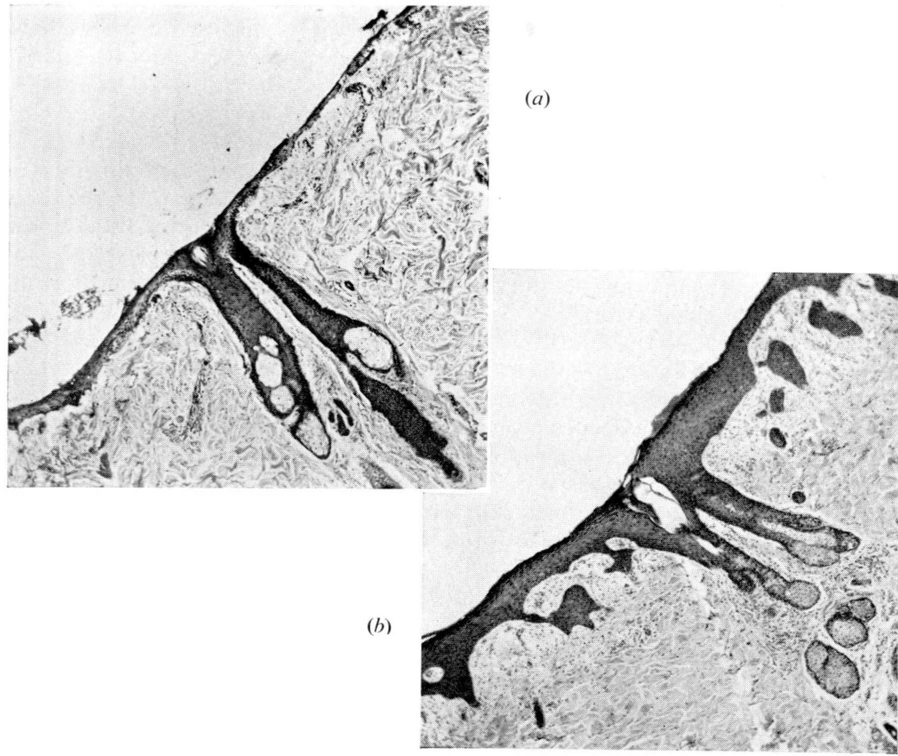

17/FIG. 22.—(*a*) A thin layer of skin, which included all the surface epithelium, was excised from this area for skin-grafting elsewhere. Three days later the bare area was covered by a thin sheet of epithelium which had regenerated from the epithelium of a hair follicle.

(*b*) A similar area nine days after removal of a thin layer of skin. Epithelial regeneration is complete. The epithelium is much thicker than in (*a*), keratinisation is well marked, and newly formed downgrowths can be seen. (From Converse and Robb-Smith.[20])

The Scab

A scab or dry crust forms in wounds that are exposed to the air. It may be supposed to have some function as a cover protecting the tissue from infection, but probably the drying of the superficial layers is the main protection, as bacteria establish themselves less readily on a dry than on a moist surface. On the other hand a scab can delay healing, since the epithelium must circumvent or digest its way through the dense material that it encounters, for it does not attach itself to the surface of the scab.

It has generally been supposed that the scab consists of clotted blood and exudate which has dried, but some anomalies have been noticed. Over 50 years ago Loeb described complicated growth of epithelium in the substance of scabs, and they have been found to contain hydroxyproline. Further, they form apparently unaltered in animals receiving large doses of heparin.

The explanation seems to be that the drying of an exposed wound can involve not only exudate in the surface but some of the superficial tissue as well, so that when the epithelium advances from the edges across the damaged area it finds optimal conditions for growth below the actual surface of the tissue. This has been studied in shallow skin wounds in young pigs, where it was found that in dry wounds the epithelium took a line of growth through the substance of the dermis, so that the more superficial part of the dermis was incorporated into the scab. In moist, occluded wounds, on the other hand, the epithelium "floated" across on the clotted exudate.[21]

Factors Influencing Wound Healing

It has been possible to give a somewhat detailed account of the sequence of morphological events that result in the healing of a wound, but the position is far from satisfactory when consideration is given to analysing the causes of those events.

Control of the Healing Process

It is in line with current thought to suppose that some chemical process is set going by injury which initiates, continues, and finally stops the growth of new tissues. Hypothetical substances supposed to stimulate healing have been called "wound hormones". Attempts have been made to identify such substances by their effect on cells in culture and on the whole animal, but so far without finding anything which is generally agreed to have this kind of activity.

The earlier work stemmed from the discovery of Carrel that the addition of chick embryo extract to tissue cultures promoted their growth. He proposed the name "trephones" for the active components of the extract. It is now known that extracts of many normal tissues, both embryo and adult, and of inflammatory and autolysed tissues, as well as protein degradation products, have a similar effect, and it may well be that proteins and their products liberated at the site of injury are valuable as nutrients in the healing tissue. From time to time effects that are apparently more specific are reported; a recent one is the growth promoting effect on neurons of protein fractions from certain animal tissues.[22, 23] But at present the significance of such observations, and their bearing on the hypothetical *desideratum*, acceleration of healing above the natural rate for well nourished tissues, is not known.

Another school of thought holds that when a tissue is damaged substances that normally keep proliferation in check disappear, and that the proliferation of healing is due to their absence. Abercrombie has discussed the two points of view and has suggested that the terms "promoter" and "depressor" should be used respectively for the two supposed kinds of substance. A stimulant effect might then equally be due to the presence of a promotor or the absence of a depressor.[24]

Another remarkable feature of wound healing is the apparent directional growth of many tissue components. Why do capillary buds growing into a newly established rabbit ear chamber appear only on one side of the existing capillary loops, that is towards the unorganised part of the clot? This directional sprouting cannot be explained in terms of blood pressure within the vessels and would seem to depend on some stimulus external to the vessel wall. What this is is unknown.

Directional growth is seen during the healing of a severed nerve. The proliferating Schwann cells tend to grow across the gap between the peripheral and central parts of the severed nerve. This directional growth appears to depend more on growth along supporting surfaces than on chemotactic influences.[25] The same is true of the growth of axis cylinders from the central stump to the peripheral end by means of which continuity of the nerve is restored. Regenerating axons from the central end which reach the distal end of a cut nerve inhibit the growth of Schwann cells in the distal end by some mechanism that is quite unknown. Other examples of directional growth will be found later in this chapter.

We have at present no knowledge of any substance or conditions that can be used to accelerate healing above the natural rate for the animal and tissue concerned, or will encourage selectively the healing process in any particular tissue. On the other hand a number of factors are known which may retard wound healing.

Local Factors that may influence Healing

Infection.—We have already seen that bacterial infection of a wound modifies the healing process. If the infection is not too severe healing proceeds, but it takes longer and more scar tissue is formed. A severe infection, for instance by a hæmolytic streptococcus, may stop healing altogether and destroy newly formed tissue, so that the wound re-opens.

Before the introduction of antiseptic surgery—still less than a hundred years ago—nearly all operation wounds were infected by the bacteriologically dirty surgeon and his attendants. In fact a wound that produced a nice lot of creamy pus characteristic of staphylococcal infection was considered to be doing well, and such pus was even called "laudable" to contrast it with the more ominous watery exudate seen in some severe infections. Now it is possible to remove infecting bacteria by chemicals from the great majority of wounds of all descriptions, or at least to keep their numbers at such a low level that even heavily contaminated wounds can often be safely sutured after a few days. Even this late, or secondary, suture is of great advantage to the patient, for the apposed granulating surfaces rapidly adhere and unite and by doing so prevent fresh infection of the wound, while the amount of fibrous tissue finally formed is greatly diminished.

Apposition and immobilisation.—It is a familiar fact that a fracture must be "reduced" and the broken bone "immobilised". That is to say the fragments must be brought into correct relation to each other and held in that position while healing takes place. If there is much movement between the broken ends healing occurs by fibrous union instead of by new bone formation.

In the healing of soft tissues conditions are less exacting, as fibrous union is often all that is required. For instance, in abdominal and intestinal wounds no particular care is taken to bring the cut ends of the muscle into exact apposition, though this would be necessary for any substantial regeneration of the muscle fibres to take place. Instead, healing by fibrous tissue is relied on, and in a clean sutured wound this produces a firm narrow junction through the muscle and connective tissue layers which may be difficult to identify in later years. It is only if conditions are unfavourable, especially if there is undue tension for any reason, that the fibrous scar may stretch with the development of what is known as an incisional hernia.

Again, immobilisation is only of limited importance for most soft tissue wounds. The cut surfaces must of course be held together by adequate stitches; but it was shown in dogs that vigorous exercise in no way affected the healing of abdominal wounds while it improved the general condition of the animals,[26] and in a general way this accords with clinical experience.

In some specialised sites good apposition and long immobilisation may be desirable even for soft tissues. These conditions were necessary for the best result in tendons that had been divided and resutured in the legs of dogs, for they resulted in the least ultimate distortion of the tendon and its sheath.[27]

Blood supply.—An adequate blood supply must be present if healing is to proceed normally. Poor circulation in the legs may be the reason for slow healing or lack of healing of leg ulcers in patients with varicose veins; fragments of bone that have had their vessels torn at the time of fracture will undergo necrosis instead of healing; and so on.

Nerves.—Section of the nerves supplying skin, connective tissues and muscle does not alter the rate or quality of healing, as was shown, for instance, in the equal tensile strength of healed symmetrical wounds on denervated and innervated sides of rabbits' backs.[28] Alterations in blood supply due to damage to autonomic nerves could, of course, have an effect.

Size of wound.—As shown in rabbit ear chambers and in various kinds of experimental wounds epithelium, connective tissue and vessels each grow at a uniform rate throughout the period of healing. The initial size of the wound does not affect their rate of growth.[12]

Position of wound in body.—Healing of skin wounds may be slower in one part of the body than another. It is unlikely that this is due to any inherent difference in the tissues. It is probably accounted for by differences in the skin —its thickness, looseness, and so on—between different sites, with consequent differences in contraction, scab formation and other factors.

General Factors that may influence Healing

Presence of another wound.—It has been stated that healing is accelerated if there is another wound already healing somewhere else in the body, with the implication that some growth-stimulating substance is produced by the first wound and circulates in the blood. Such a view should be accepted with great caution. One such result, at least, seems to have been due to the conditions in a particular experiment, for when care was taken that the primary and secondary wounds were made under closely comparable conditions, no difference in the rate of healing could be found.[29, 30] But a concurrent severe injury can delay healing through metabolic processes to be discussed below.

Age.—Wounds in old people heal well, though it should be remembered that in some circumstances the old are more likely than the young to be on a diet deficient in vitamins or other nutrients, and that disease of the blood vessels, which is commoner in later life, may decrease the amount of blood available to a tissue.

In experimental work old animals have not been used, but comparisons have been made between the young and the adult. There is no reason to think that cell proliferation and fibrous tissue formation are any slower or less efficient in the latter. Stomach wounds in adult rats were just as strong after healing as those in young animals, though there was a little more delay before the phase of rapid healing started.[31] This may well have been due to local conditions in the tissue, just as the somewhat longer time taken by skin excisions to heal in adult rats seemed to be due to the fact that the skin was thicker and less mobile than in young animals, so that there was less contraction of the wound.[32]

Nutrition and hormone action.—Any serious deviation from normal metabolism is likely to have some effect on wound healing, but three factors which under experimental conditions can depress or even destroy the capacity of soft tissues to unite have been extensively studied, and a fourth has lately come to attention. This last is *zinc*, which it is now suspected may be widely deficient in agricultural land and in farm animals, at least in parts of the U.S.A. Some evidence has been obtained that it may be concentrated in granulation tissue during the first few days of healing[33] and that its administration to men on a usual diet may speed up healing.[34] The significance of these observations is not altogether clear.

The three better known factors are: deficiency of ascorbic acid, deficiency of sulphur-containing amino-acids, and excess of adrenal cortical steroids, as represented by cortisone. These three conditions all result in impaired collagen formation, but we do not know enough about their point of action to say whether or to what extent they act on healing tissue through a common pathway. There are close metabolic relationships between adrenal cortical steroids, ascorbic acid and proteins, and in severe trauma there are interrelated disturbances of all three (see Chapter 11). Similarly, healing may involve an interaction of these three factors; for example protein-depleted rats show less ascorbic acid in the tissue of a healing wound than normally nourished rats and the administration of methionine to such rats restores the level of ascorbic acid towards, though not fully up to, the normal level.[35]

It has been stated that "the seriously injured patient behaves biochemically like a scorbutic", in that he excretes less ascorbic acid than usual in the urine and shows apparently diminished reserves in the blood and tissues. A severe burn caused the same histological changes in wounds in guinea-pigs as a moderate degree of scurvy, and the administration to the burned animals of extra ascorbic acid (they were already receiving a maintenance dose) prevented these changes from appearing.[36]

(i) *Ascorbic acid deficiency.*—Man is like the guinea-pig in developing scurvy when the diet is deficient in ascorbic acid, though it takes much longer for detectable changes to occur. If guinea-pigs have ascorbic acid removed from their diet on the day of wounding characteristic abnormalities appear during healing of the wound,[36] though the changes are not so extreme as if the animals are already in a state of scurvy when the wound is made.[37] In a man who had been on an ascorbic acid-free diet for three months a wound healed normally, but after six months, when some manifestations of scurvy were present, a wound did not heal and showed the same defect histologically as wounds in scorbutic guinea-pigs.[38] It is possible that some individuals on a poor diet may be in a sub-scorbutic state that could affect healing, especially if substantial trauma were added.

The important aberration of healing which occurs when there is a lack of ascorbic acid is that, according to the degree of the deficiency, collagen fibres are formed little and late or not at all, so that the edges of the wound do not become properly knit together. At first exudate and scab and the growth of epithelium, which is not impaired, may help to conceal this, but in severe deficiency no adequate permanent union occurs, and after a few days the edges separate—the wound is said to "break down". In lesser degrees of deficiency small amounts of collagen are formed though at a slow rate, and the wound is of correspondingly low tensile strength. On the administration of ascorbic acid healing that appears to be normal in all respects immediately gets under way.[39]

Wounds in scorbutic animals contain fibroblasts in considerable numbers, but these do not mature into fibrocytes in the normal way. Macrophages are plentiful, but capillaries are few and sometimes appear ill-formed. Silver-staining fibres of reticulin are laid down, but they are not replaced by van Gieson-staining collagen fibres—some are present, but far fewer than normal. There is a deficiency of hydroxyproline in the wound, and mucopolysaccharides, though normal or increased in amount, are unbalanced, with excess of hyaluronic acid and a marked shortage of sulphated substances such as chondroitin sulphate, one constituent of which, galactosamine, has been shown to be deficient.[40]

Since the mechanisms of normal collagen formation are not well understood the nature of the disturbance brought about by ascorbic acid deficiency is still obscure. There has been conflicting evidence about whether its main action is on synthetic processes inside the fibroblast or on assembly of the collagen fibres in the intercellular space. This has been illuminated by the electron microscopy of wounds from scorbutic animals. The fibroblasts show unusual features, of which the most striking are dilatation of the cisternæ of the endoplasmic reticulum, and redisposition of the ribosomes so that they lose their serried arrangement and are placed singly, as if at random, on the membranes (FIG. 23). The intercellular material contains many fluffy masses of fine filaments though there are generally a few collagen fibres[41] and work with tissue cultures has shown that some collagen is formed.[41a] But evidently the protein synthesising apparatus of the cells is much disturbed, though the nature and results of the disturbance are not yet defined in chemical terms.

It is said that if scurvy develops healed wounds break down.[42] Whether this occurs perhaps depends on the maturity of the healed tissue. The relatively recent "old" lesions of experimental animals are said to show signs of loss of collagen, but it does not follow that old scars in man would do so. It seems certain that collagen of ordinary tissue is turned over more slowly, and is less susceptible to the influence of ascorbic acid, both in formation and in maintenance, than that of healing tissue, but whether this is a difference of kind or only of degree is uncertain.

(ii) *Protein.*—A patient who is severely undernourished often heals his wounds normally; it has been said that "the wound seems to heal at the expense of the patient's tissues".[43] Experimental work lends some support to this suggestion.

It is easier to demonstrate an effect from protein deficiency in animals than in man, and in them the healing process can be totally inhibited if starvation is very prolonged,[44] and delayed in lesser degrees of starvation. The crucial

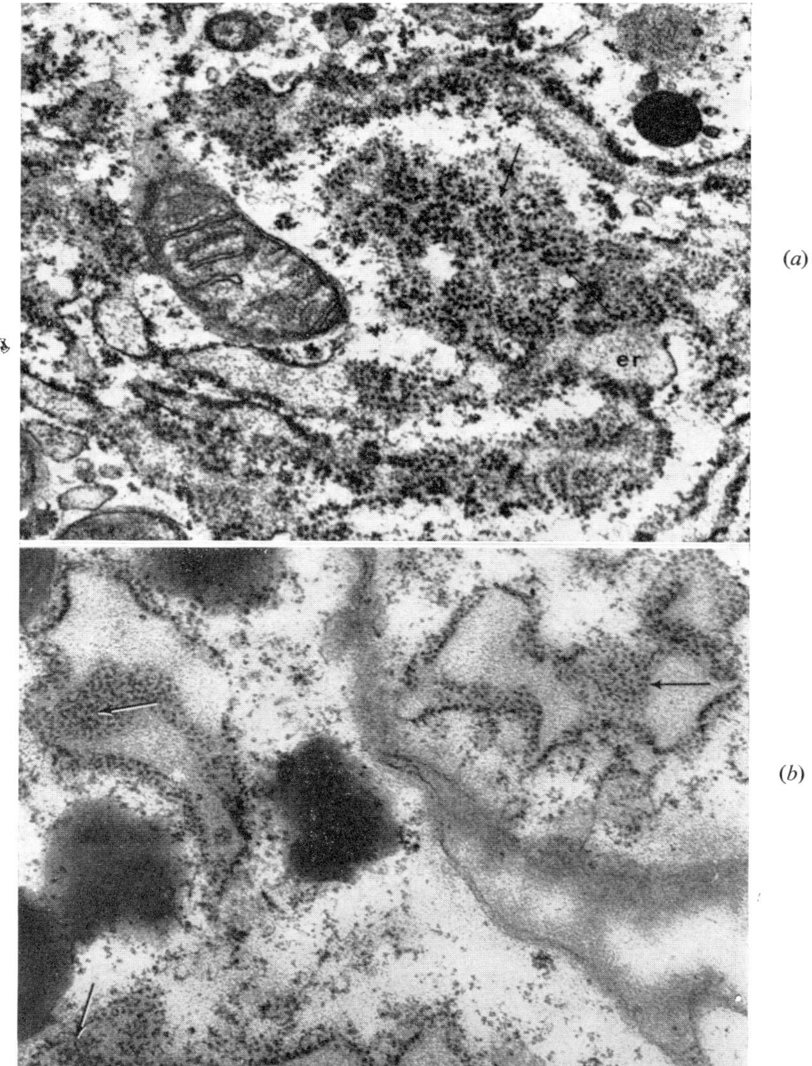

17/Fig. 23.—Parts of Fibroblasts from 7-day-old Wounds in Guinea-pigs

(*a*) From a normal animal. At the centre is an area where the rough endoplasmic reticulum has been grazed tangentially and shows as a relatively electron dense layer (er). On its surface the ribosomes are arranged in curves and spirals, sometimes in double rows and sometimes apparently connected by a fine thread (arrows). (× 39,000).

(*b*) From a scorbutic animal. The endoplasmic reticulum is here again cut tangentially and appears electron dense, but the ribosomes appear to be randomly dispersed, without any special arrangement (arrows). Collections of lipid (the dark areas) and free ribosomes can also be seen in the fibroblasts in this condition. (× 26,000) (From Ross and Benditt.[41])

deficiency is that of the sulphur-containing amino-acids, since they are essential to the synthesis of the new proteins which make up the connective tissues of the wound. If methionine is provided healing proceeds normally even if starvation and weight loss continue.

Histologically the wound in methionine deficiency looks much like that in ascorbic acid deficiency, that is to say the fibroblasts do not mature into fibrocytes or become properly oriented and collagen formation is delayed.[45] There is a corresponding lack of hydroxyproline[46] and of tensile strength in the wound.

By the use of methionine labelled with ^{35}S injected into animals before or after wounding it has been shown that the methionine required by the wound is largely supplied from the proteins of existing tissues. Over a period of many days the radioactivity which at first is incorporated in the liver and other tissues is transferred to the wound. Some of it can be recovered there as ^{35}S-methionine, but as time goes on an increasing amount is found in the form of ^{35}S-cystine and ^{35}S-cysteine.[47] Only traces of the activity appear in the mucopolysaccharides.[48] This transference of amino-acids from the proteins of existing tissues to those of the healing tissue can take place in the presence of a negative nitrogen balance,[49] and to some extent in starvation. This is the basis for saying that a healing wound has a priority claim on the body's proteins.

It might be thought that a general protein deficiency would interfere with healing by upsetting osmotic relationships in the wound but this does not seem to be so. Plasma proteins, like the wound proteins, have a certain metabolic priority and even when their level falls below normal healing is said to proceed in spite of some œdema of the wound.[50]

It seems clear that patients with healing wounds, whether made by accident or by the surgeon, should receive a suitably nourishing and well-balanced diet, but that a high protein diet or a specific protein supplement is not likely to have much effect on the healing process.

(iii) *Adrenal cortical steroids and other hormones.*—It is evident that hormones can influence the growth of connective tissues in the body when we consider the great increase in collagen, as well as muscle, that takes place in the uterus during pregnancy and the regression that follows parturition. The hormone disturbances that cause disease in man do not usually have any obvious effect on wound healing, though probably most of the hormones in the gross excess or deficiency that can be produced under experimental conditions have some effect. In view of the intricate interaction of the endocrine glands the mechanism of any such effect is likely to be complex; for example, wounds made in the abdominal walls of rats healed less strongly in pregnant then in non-pregnant animals, but the workers who showed this suggested as a possible cause a disturbance not of the sex-hormones but of the adrenal cortical hormones, whose output is increased during pregnancy.[51]

In thyroid deficiency in man (cretinism, myxœdema) there are alterations in the mucopolysaccharides of the connective tissues, but in spite of the close relationship between thyroid hormone and connective tissue metabolism healing is generally satisfactory in these conditions, as also in hyperthyroidism (Graves' disease). In animals the administration of thyroxine has been said to impair tensile strength and the uptake of ^{35}S-sulphate in wounds, that is, to affect both collagen and mucopolysaccharide formation in wound tissue.[52] Thyroxine depressed mitosis in the corneal epithelium of rats after burning, and surprisingly, since the animals were stunted, thyroidectomy somewhat increased it.[53]

Pituitary growth hormone when given in large amounts to hypophysectomised rats is said to produce an increase above normal in the number and size of the fibroblasts and in the amount of collagen formed in granulation tissue. An inhibitory effect on healing usually results from the administration of large doses of œstrogens and androgens.[54] Much of the above work, and that on the effects of the adrenal cortical steroids, has been done on the granulation tissue forming around a turpentine abscess, a lesion in which there is inflammation and, usually, necrosis as well as healing. In these circumstances some of the substantial effects which cortisone has on inflammation may well have secondary consequences for the healing process. However, many experiments have shown that the adrenal cortical hormones can influence healing itself.

The introduction of cortisone as a drug for clinical use made this an important question. Some of the first and most elegant work was done on the healing of lesions in the corneas of rabbits, and from this it was clear that the proliferation and migration of fibroblasts and the new formation of blood vessels could be strikingly retarded by cortisone, but that with doses equivalent to those used systemically in man the effect was slight or absent. The healing of epithelium was unaffected except by very large doses, which tended to retard it.[55] The discovery that new vessel formation could be suppressed was of great importance to ophthalmology. By applying appropriate corticosteroids locally to a damaged cornea vascularisation and hence the development of permanent opacities can often be inhibited without preventing satisfactory healing.

Work in other sites and species has confirmed that, according to the dose used and the susceptibility of the animal, cortisone can retard or prevent healing. Less collagen and fewer blood vessels are formed than in control wounds of the same age, and the amorphous matrix has different properties which are probably due to chemical differences in the mucopolysaccharides formed. By light microscopy these effects are very like those due to ascorbic acid or methionine deficiency, though with cortisone there is said to be a dearth of fibroblasts.[56]

There has been difficulty in showing whether the actions of ascorbic acid and cortisone are closely related—for instance whether giving cortisone would exacerbate the effects of scurvy—as the guinea-pig, so suitable for the study of scurvy, has "unorthodox" responses to adrenal cortical hormones.[40]

Dogs were used for trying to assess the possible effect of cortisone on human wounds and it was found that healing was not affected by doses similar to, or larger than, those used for therapeutic purposes in man.[57, 58] Happily in man the dosages of steroids that are generally useful have no deleterious effect on wound healing.

The effects of cortisone apparently represent those of adrenal cortical activity as a whole, for the administration of ACTH[59] and the establishment of a condition of stress (if the adrenals have not been removed)[60] can retard wound healing. But it is stated that the mineralocorticoids when given in large doses have a stimulating effect on the formation of granulation tissue.[54] After adrenalectomy wounds healed with about normal tensile strength.[60]

HEALING OF SOME SPECIAL TISSUES

In all organs the connective tissue and the blood vessels proliferate in response to wounding or loss of tissue and their activities produce the scars which are familiar to us all. But other tissues also react to loss to a greater or less degree, as for instance the epithelium of the skin, which has already been considered. The different organs of the body vary enormously in the extent to which their structure can be restored or their special cells replaced. For example, in the lung there is scarring with no effective restoration of alveoli; in nerve tissue cell processes regenerate but no new neurons arise; in the kidney there is limited proliferation of tubule and glomerular epithelium but no new nephrons are formed; while the liver can proliferate so as to restore its functional capacity completely, and its structure very largely, apparently almost indefinitely.

The rest of this chapter will discuss the healing behaviour of some specialised tissues and organs.

Healing of Mucous Membranes

Epithelial surfaces such as line the trachea, the gastro-intestinal tract, and the bladder may be injured by disease or accident or by the surgeon's knife. The structures beneath such epithelium heal by the formation of fibrous tissue in the way we have considered. Thus, if the surgeon joins the intestine to the stomach, or performs an end-to-end anastomosis between two pieces of intestine, the muscle at the edges of the opening, even if most accurately apposed by the surgeon, does not play any significant part in the repair. Instead, fibrous tissue unites the muscle edges. Serous cells proliferate and cover the peritoneal surface.

We have seen that the skin is able to effect only a relatively simple repair, but the cells of reforming mucosæ are able to differentiate to a remarkable extent. A good idea of their capabilities was obtained by excising a piece of mucosa from the first part of the duodenum of a number of cats, which were then killed at intervals and the events taking place in the defects traced by histological examination. In the area of duodenum that was excised there were not only the common surface structures of the small intestine, with crypts of Lieberkühn and villi, but also Brunner's glands which, by ducts passing through the muscularis mucosæ, open into the crypts of Lieberkühn.

After the excision the area fills with clot, which is then invaded by cells and organised by exactly the same process as elsewhere. Muscle contraction tends to approximate the cut edges, the crypts close in, and from the cut edges a sheet of epithelium begins to grow over the newly forming granulation tissue in the usual way, that is by cell movement followed after a few hours by cell multiplication behind the advancing edge (FIG. 24). By the end of the first day mitoses are present in the acini of the Brunner's glands around the edge of the defect, and on succeeding days mitoses are frequently seen in them and in the neighbouring crypts of Lieberkühn.

From the layer of new epithelium, which is usually only one cell thick, downgrowths occur which in the course of time form crypts of Lieberkühn, while outgrowths form villi (FIG. 25). The epithelium of these newly formed structures soon differentiates to produce the usual intestinal epithelial cells and the goblet cells, and sometimes cells may develop resembling those of the surface of the

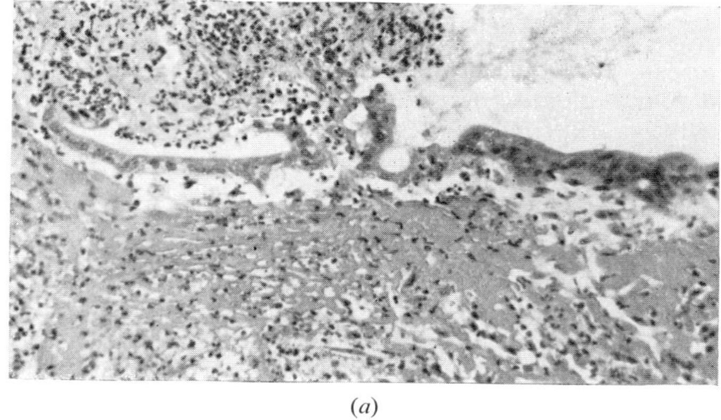

(a)

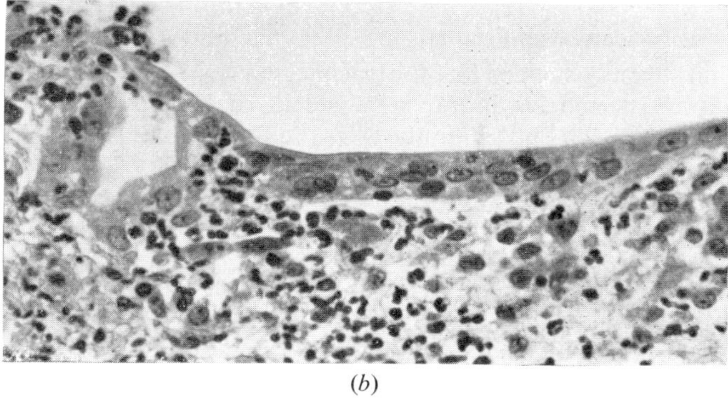

(b)

17/FIG. 24.—HEALING OF EPITHELIUM IN AN ARTIFICIAL DEFECT MADE BY EXCISION OF AN AREA OF THE DUODENAL MUCOSA OF A CAT

(a) Flattened epithelium originating from columnar epithelium of the crypts is passing across newly formed granulation tissue. It is burrowing into clot adherent to this granulation tissue.

(b) Shows a layer of new epithelium several cells deep and the beginning of crypt formation at the left of the picture.

stomach. In the bases of the newly formed crypts of Lieberkühn cells begin to appear with a content of mucus that stains in the same way as that of Brunner's glands, but because the muscularis mucosæ does not reform cells producing mucus typical of Brunner's glands come to form the lower portion of the crypts rather than separate acini. Nevertheless, there is very satisfactory repair.

Repair of gastric mucosa occurs by a similar process, although full restoration of the fundal glands may take many months. Mucous glands are formed at first and then oxyntic and peptic cells appear. After a gastroenterostomy the epithelium of stomach and small intestine heal together but each reforms perfectly, so that a sharp line demarcates the mucosæ of the two organs. The epithelium of other mucous membranes has equally remarkable powers of regeneration and restoration of mucosal structure is often complete.

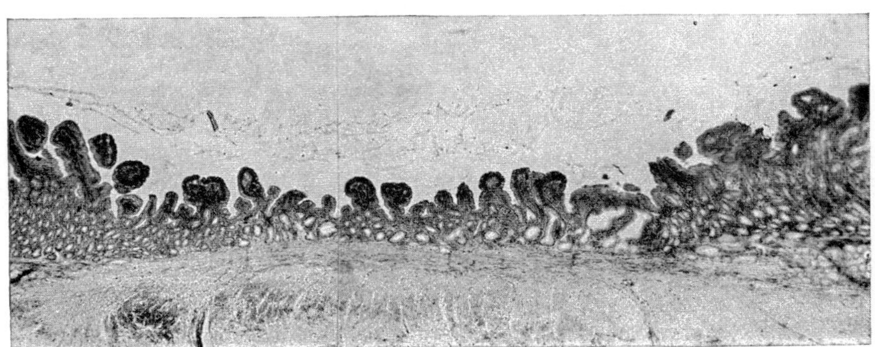

17/FIG. 25.—HEALING OF EPITHELIUM IN AN ARTIFICIAL DEFECT IN THE DUODENAL MUCOSA OF THE CAT

After 31 days the defect is covered with epithelium in which villi and crypts have differentiated, resting on a base which is now well developed fibrous tissue. (From Florey and Harding.[61])

Although healing of the mucosæ of healthy animals and man can be very complete and satisfactory, it should not be supposed that all defects in man heal so readily. A very common lesion of civilised man is peptic ulcer, in which the patient has an area in the stomach or first part of the duodenum that is completely devoid of mucosa with a base of granulation tissue and newly formed fibrous tissue. The cause of the ulceration is not known for certain, nor is it clear why repair of the epithelium is greatly retarded or stopped. The HCl of the gastric juice probably plays some part, but it does not ordinarily prevent healing so other factors must also be operating. Spasm of the blood vessels is one such factor that has been suggested. Ulcers of the intestine also occur, usually in the colon, but these can sometimes be traced to a cause. For example, the colon may become infected by an amœba, *Entamœba histolytica*, and accompanying bacteria, and when the amœbæ are removed healing takes place. The serious disease ulcerative colitis does not seem to be directly due to any infecting organism and its cause is still being elucidated.

Healing of Endothelium in Large Blood Vessels

We have seen how important the sprouting of capillary vessels is in the formation of a fibrous scar during healing. With increasing interest in vascular surgery and the development of ideas on the pathogenesis of atherosclerosis (see Chapter 18), it becomes of more importance to understand the behaviour of the coats of arteries, especially the intima which is presumably of great importance in preserving the normal constitution of the contained blood. It has been supposed that the endothelial cells lining arteries have an unlimited life,[62] but this is certainly untrue. It has also been supposed that endothelial cells divide by amitosis[63] but this is improbable. Mitotic figures are occasionally seen in the endothelium of the normal rat's aorta, and when a normal rat is injected with thymidine labelled with ^3H autoradiographs show labelling of some of the nuclei of its aortic endothelium, indicating that synthesis of desoxyribonucleic acid is taking place and consequently that the cells are multiplying.[64] It has been shown that in man bi- or multi-nucleate endothelial cells increase in number with increasing age.[65, 66] Such cells can be produced in the rabbit's aorta by scraping away the endothelial lining and allowing healing to occur.[67] FIGURES 26 and 27 show some of the stages of endothelial regeneration in these circumstances.

It took many months for the endothelium of the scraped rabbit aorta to regenerate over a length of 1½ to 2 cm. Under some experimental conditions healing is faster than this. This is of considerable importance now that it is surgically possible to replace segments of large vessels such as the aorta or to

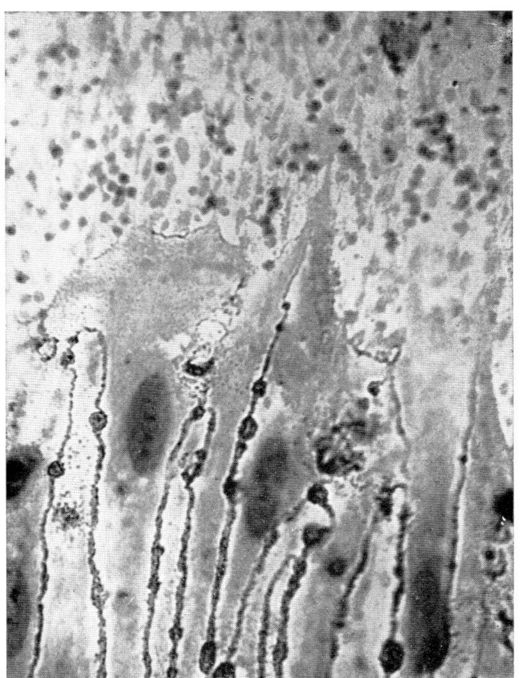

17/FIG. 26.—The edge of growing endothelium 24 hours after scraping away the intima of the abdominal aorta of a rabbit. In the upper half of the picture is the surface from which endothelium was removed. The small round objects may be platelets adhering to the denuded surface. The endothelial cells below are apparently extending a cytoplasmic film over the denuded area. The endothelial cells here and in Figs. 27 and 29 have been outlined by treatment with silver nitrate. (× 800) (From Poole, Sanders and Florey.[67])

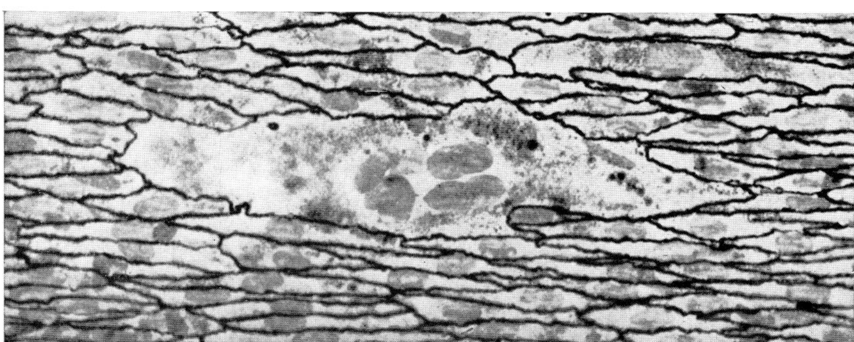

17/FIG. 27.—From a scraped aorta of a rabbit. A giant cell in a healed area is surrounded by endothelial cells with single nuclei of varying size. (× 360.) (From Poole, Sanders and Florey.[67])

make by-pass vessels using as a framework prostheses made of woven or knitted synthetic fibres. Before the tube is sewn into position it is dipped in blood which is allowed to clot, and into this clot granulation tissue grows from the peri-arterial tissues and supports the new endothelium. It has been found that a segment 3 cm. long of knitted Dacron tubing substituted for a segment of the lower abdominal aorta of a baboon is completely lined by new endothelium within ten weeks[68] (FIGS. 28, 29 and 30). Beneath the endothelium the new intima develops a layer of smooth muscle cells mixed with collagen and elastic fibres. The origin of these cells is at present obscure.

It is of great interest that small blood vessels, sometimes not much larger in diameter than capillaries, can be seen opening from the new lumen (FIG. 29) and passing into the depths of the intima, presumably to join with blood vessels in the adventitia. These anastomoses may have started in the granulation tissue as capillary sprouts which reached the lumen of the graft and opened there to form new blood channels. It seems possible also that the tips may have spread out and provided foci of growing endothelium between the two ends of the graft, thus speeding up the process of providing a complete endothelial lining. In the

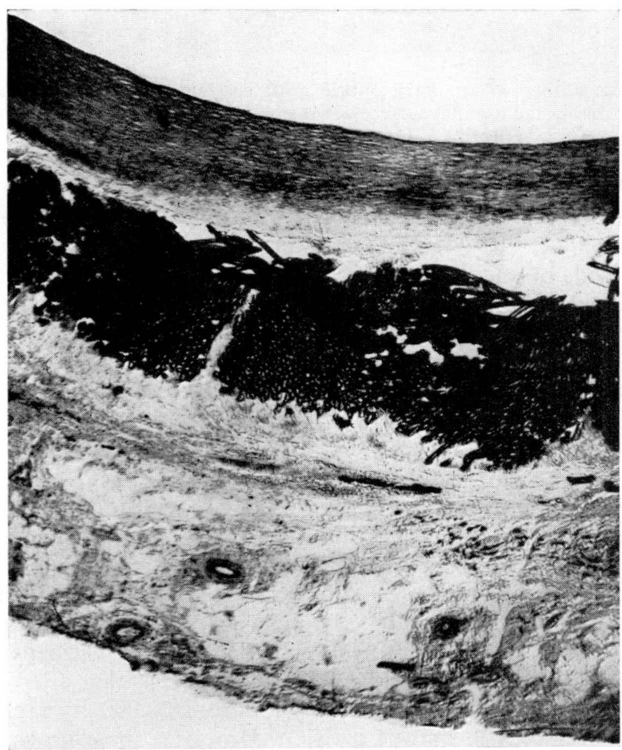

17/FIG. 28.—A section through the wall of a fabric graft in a baboon's aorta. The fibres of the cloth appear black. The new intima is in the upper part of the field. The graft is surrounded by loose connective tissue containing many blood vessels. (× 45) (From Florey, Greer, Poole and Werthessen.[68]

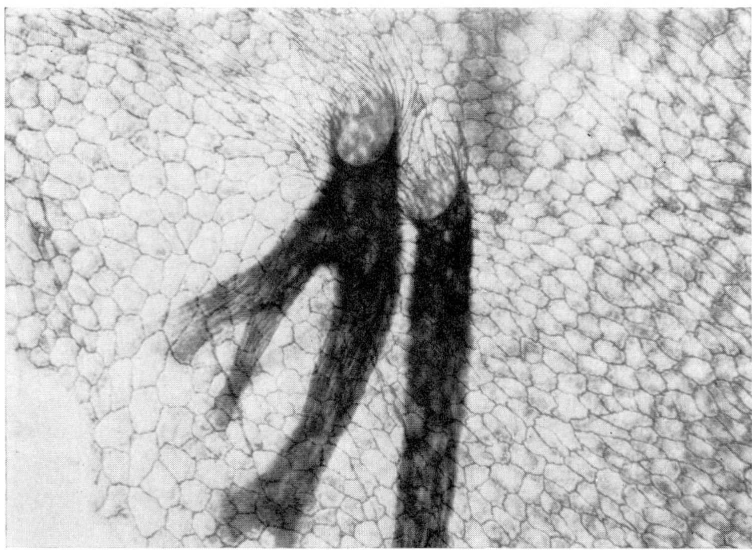

17/FIG. 29.—The surface of an aortic fabric graft showing the outlines of newly formed endothelial cells lining the luminal surface. Two small vessels can be seen to branch from the "aortic" lumen. (× 125) (From Florey, Greer, Poole and Werthessen.[68])

operation of endarterctomy diseased intima is removed from a vessel, and it is possible that the endothelial lining may be reformed in a similar way, by ingrowth not only at the two ends of the bared portion of the artery but also from the cut ends of small vessels in between. These properties of the arterial wall should be kept in mind to give a background to what is theoretically possible in vascular surgery. Grafts and by-passes in man often achieve their purpose very successfuly, though it appears that the organisation of a new intima may be a slower process than in the baboon or dog.

Liver

No organ repays close study as a site of regeneration more than the liver. Such a statement is apt to cause surprise to the student of anatomy and physiology, since the liver, of all organs, seems most fixed in mass and form; nevertheless it is continually changing both in its cellular, vascular and lobular patterns. Liver cells mature, divide to form new individuals in a curious diurnal rhythm, grow old and die off, only to be replaced uniformly by new cells so that for the greater part of life the organ shows little alteration. The expert histologist will find, even without special technical tricks, liver cells that are disintegrating, and by diligent search—he may have to scrutinise 20,000 liver cells first—he will also find liver cells in mitotic division. However, these processes go on so slowly, and ageing and removal of dead cells is compensated so perfectly by replacements, that it is difficult to appreciate that there is any change. But when large masses of liver are killed by disease or removed by the surgeon we soon see signs of more active cell proliferation (FIG. 31).

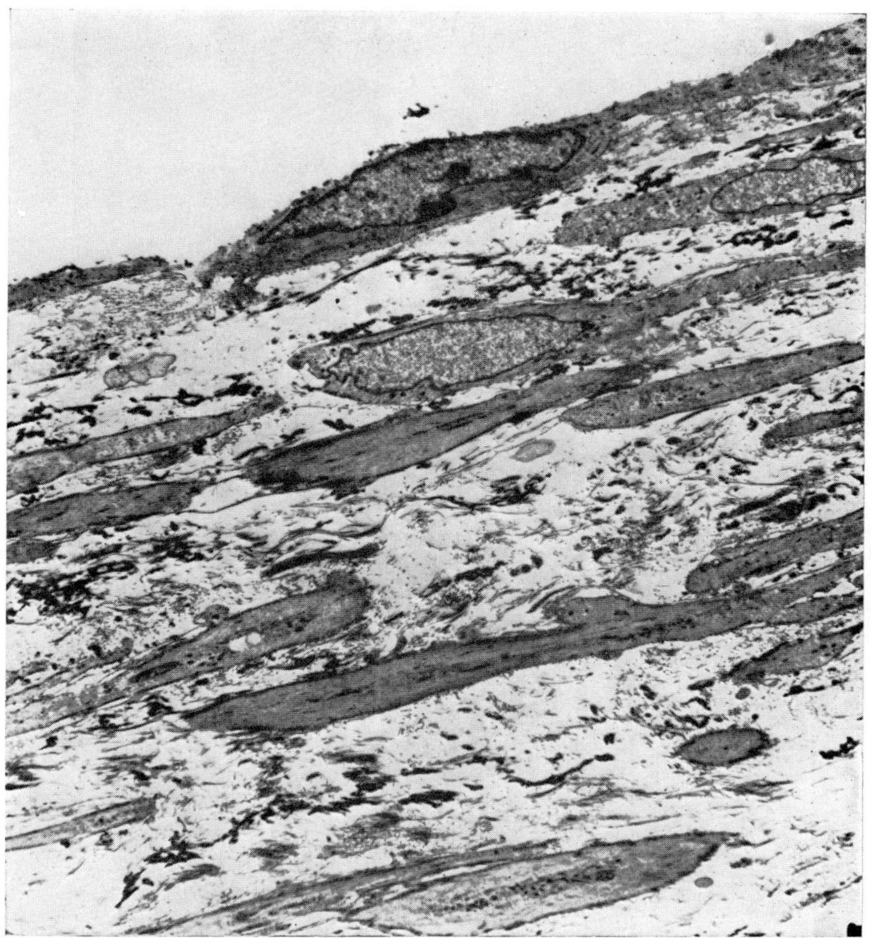

17/FIG. 30.—An electron micrograph through the superficial part of the new intima. Beneath the endothelium the intima consists of elastic tissue which is very electron dense, collagen fibres, and cells which have the appearance of smooth muscle. (× 3,750) (From Florey, Greer, Poole and Werthessen.[68])

The proof of the efficiency of liver regeneration has come from experimental studies on animals (FIG. 32) although, every now and then, the surgeon removes large pieces of liver when cutting out a tumour or a parasite such as a hydatid cyst and proves that the human organ behaves remarkably like that of the experimental animal after partial hepatectomy. A most successful study of liver regeneration after the deliberate removal of different amounts of healthy tissue was one of the earliest to be carried out. Emil Ponfick,[70] a German pathologist who made a number of valuable contributions to pathology though he never attained the fame of some of his contemporaries, opened up the abdominal cavity of a large number of rabbits with careful aseptic technique and cut away

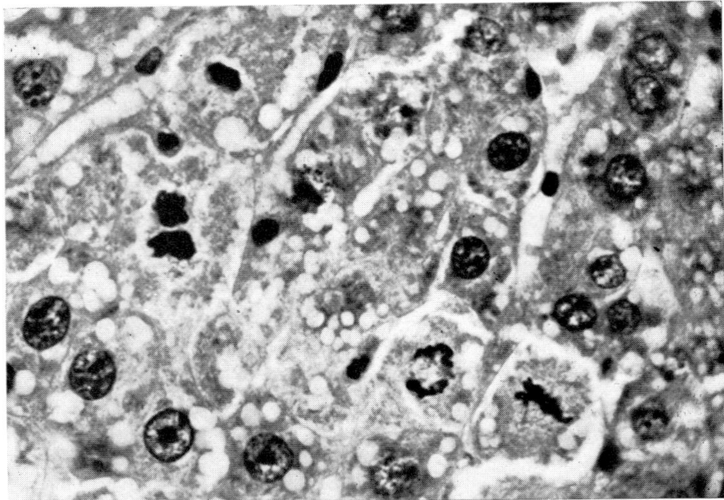

17/FIG. 31.—Mitosis in residual lobe of a rat's liver 43 hours after five-sixths of the organ had been removed. There are four mitoses in the field shown, probably all in parenchymal cells. (×800.)

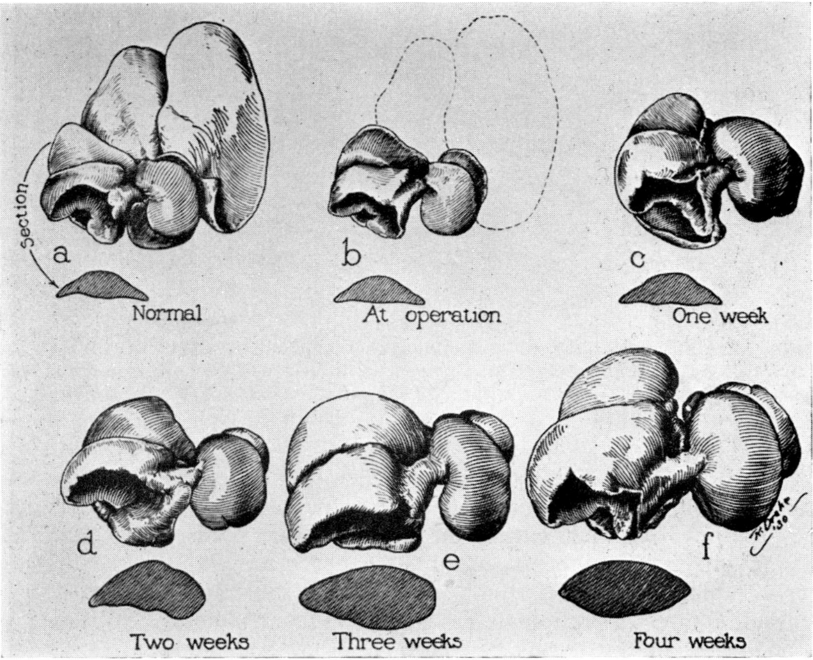

17/FIG. 32.—Regeneration of the rat's liver after partial hepatectomy. The portion removed is indicated by the outline in (*b*). The transverse sections indicate the increase in size of the residual right lobe. (From Higgins and Anderson.[69])

whole lobes of the liver. By determining in a parallel series of animals the ratio of these lobes to the total liver weight, Ponfick could calculate the total liver weight of his operated animals from the weight of the lobe removed. If, then, the rabbits were killed at varying periods after operation and the liver weighed, the amount of new liver tissue added to the remnant calculated as being left behind could be determined, and the percentage regeneration could be estimated. Of course in all such experiments it was important to eliminate any complication which might influence liver growth, such as nutritive disturbance, infection, post-operative hæmorrhage or pregnancy, i.e. the number of variables in the experiment must be reduced to a minimum. Some of Ponfick's figures are given in Table I which shows that regeneration goes on no matter how small or how

17/Table I

Some Data on Liver Regeneration (Ponfick, 1890[70])

Rabbit	*Body weight (grams)*	*Calculated liver weight (grams)*	*Amount of liver removed (grams)*	*Per cent. liver removed*	*Regeneration interval (days)*	*Liver weight at end of experiment (g.)*	*Per cent. liver regeneration*
1	2170	87	17·5	20·1	77	122·0	175
2	2050	82	30·2	36·8	120	136·5	263
3	2600	104	48·5	46·6	450	90·7	164
4	2100	84	53·0	63·1	90	78·0	251
5	2600	104	91·0	87·5	93	91·4	703

large is the amount of liver tissue removed and that considerable amounts may be removed and yet the animal survives. Ponfick gave a brief description of the histology of the regenerating liver tissue and noted that cell division occurred anywhere throughout the active remnant. He deserves most of the credit for establishing the fundamental rule of liver regeneration, viz., that it is chiefly a matter of new formation of liver cells.

Many similar experiments have been done, in a variety of animals, since Ponfick's time and serial operations have been performed whereby liver tissue many times the weight of the original liver has, in total, been removed. They are described in many papers such as those of, Fishback[71], Brues and Marble[72] and Weinbren[73] and in the reviews by Himsworth,[74] Cameron[75] and Harkness.[76] Claims are made, from time to time, that certain zones of the liver lobules are devoted to fat metabolism or to bile salt production, to glycogen storage or to energy concentration. It is true that facts suggestive of some sort of localisation have been brought forward by histologists and physiologists, but it is doubtful whether these indicate anything more than the accentuation of function in some parts more than in others. No matter where the line of transection during partial hepatectomy may be the outcome is the same, for no evidence of disturbed liver function follows upon transection provided a certain minimal amount of healthy tissue is retained. The dog can get along without signs of liver insufficiency with about one-twelfth of his total liver mass; the rat probably needs even less liver. A round figure for all animals is probably 10 per cent of the normal number of liver cells. In some experiments the transections have been multiple but with the same result. So too when a host of tiny areas of the liver are destroyed by a poison such as chloroform, phosphorus or beryllium, no ill effects appear so long as enough healthy tissue, however scattered, is preserved. This is good evidence that each portion of the lobule, as well as of the organ, possesses equivalent functional properties.

In earlier editions of this book G. R. Cameron, who wrote the above historical introduction, propounded three "theorems" of liver regeneration based on his own extensive work on the liver[77], and on other experimental results. These were:

1. "No matter where and how often the liver is transected, regeneration goes on equally well from the surviving fraction, provided that fraction suffice for the maintenance of minimal liver function".

2. "The unit of liver regeneration is something less than the anatomical liver lobule provided an adequate blood supply and excretory system is maintained".

3. "The unit of liver regeneration is independent of a nerve supply". The satisfactory nature of regeneration in the absence of sympathetic stimuli has recently been confirmed[78].

Anatomical pattern of regeneration.—Simpson and Finckh[79] described how they excised about two-thirds of rats' livers on five successive occasions by removing the lobes in turn at intervals of from 5 to 7 weeks. After each interval the original liver weight was almost regained by enlargement of the lobes left behind. Each residual lobe contributed proportionally to the new enlargement (FIG. 33). Their calculation was that one gram of the original liver had given rise

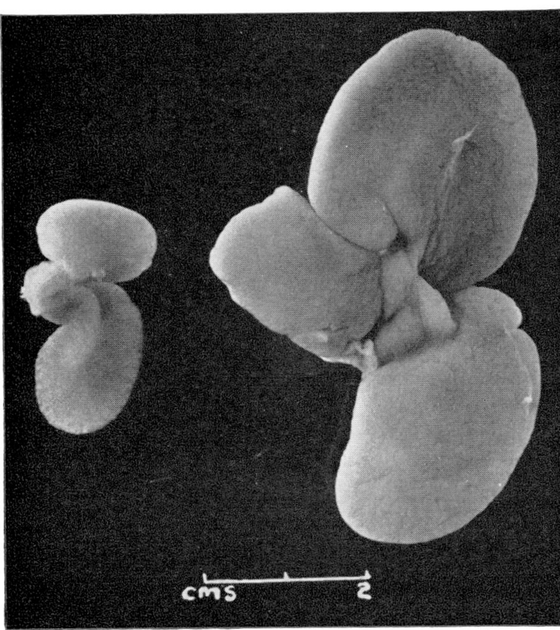

17/FIG. 33.—Regenerated liver of rat after three partial hepatectomies (right). For comparison, the same lobes from a normal rat of the same size are shown (left). There has been diffuse enlargement of all the residual lobes in the operated animal. The two main lobes left at this stage would have been removed at the fourth and fifth operations. (From Simpson and Finckh.[79])

to 18 grams of liver tissue. There was some enlargement of the liver lobules during the early stages of re-growth, the result of the initial burst of mitosis,[80] but the subsequent phase of slow proliferation and remodelling resulted in the formation of new lobules complete with blood vessels and supporting tissue. The picture after the last regeneration was hardly distinguishable from that before the first (FIG. 34). It appeared that while multiplying parenchymal cells

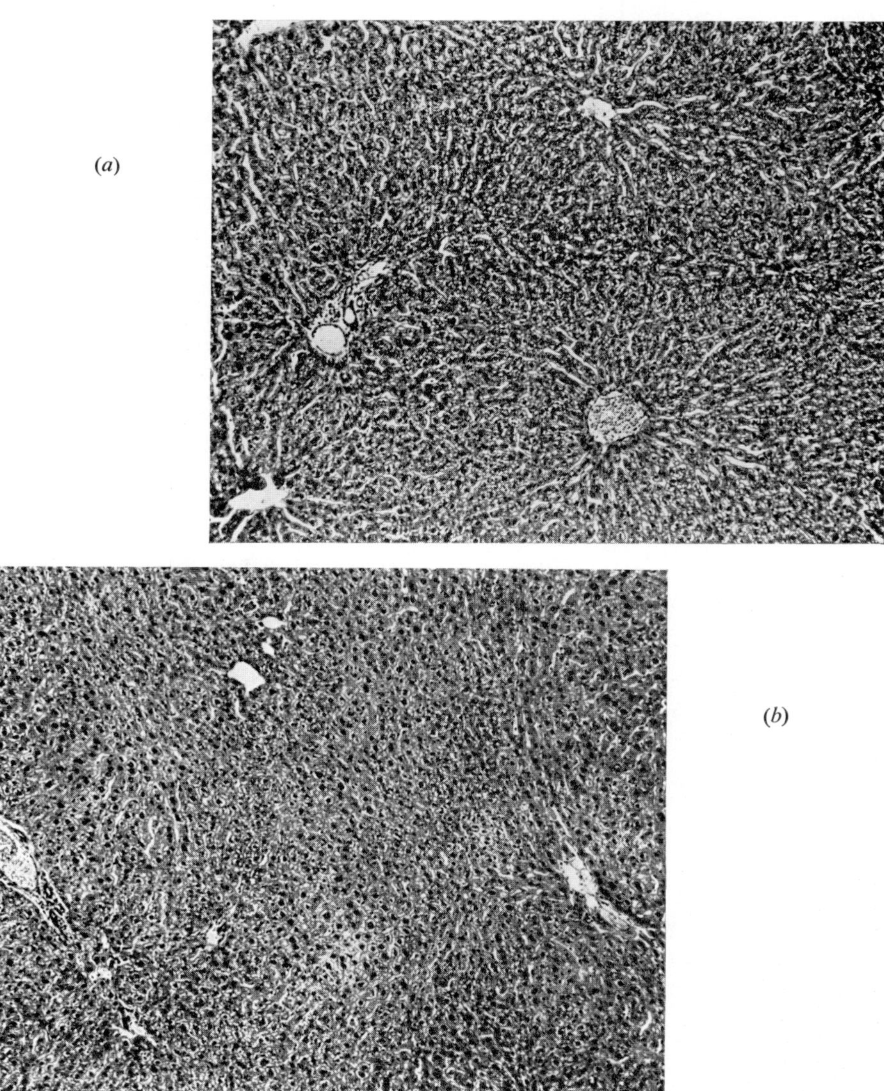

(*a*)

(*b*)

17/FIG. 34.—(*a*) Typical field of normal rat liver. (*b*) Typical field after five successive partial hepatectomies. The pattern of the lobules is normal. Both × 38. (From Simpson and Finckh.[79])

formed new sheets of liver tissue, the sinusoid endothelium proliferated and the portal veins budded off new branches, with enlargement of new or old vessels where necessary, to give a regular blood circulation through the new lobules. Bile ducts and connective tissue similarly proliferated and, presumably, lymphatics and the peritoneal covering of the organ. It is startling to consider the amount of movement and rearrangement of cells that must take place in the organ during such developments.

Cellular basis of regeneration.—Within an hour of a substantial excision from the liver (in practice usually about two-thirds) remaining parenchymal cells begin to swell and to show changes in their organelles which indicate an alteration in their metabolic processes—for example, dispersal of the endoplasmic reticulum and detachment of the ribosomes,[81] which may be connected with a change from synthesis for purposes outside the cell to synthesis for cell needs. They progress through the metabolic and morphological changes leading to mitosis, which reaches its maximum about 26 hours after the excision. Polyploidy becomes commoner after regeneration as many normal liver cells have two nuclei, and these fuse on mitosis. Bile duct epithelium and the endothelium lining the sinusoids are also stimulated to proliferate, but their mitosis reaches its peak about 24 hours later than with the parenchymal cells and the curves are flatter (FIG. 35). The removal of part of the body's reticulo-endothelial

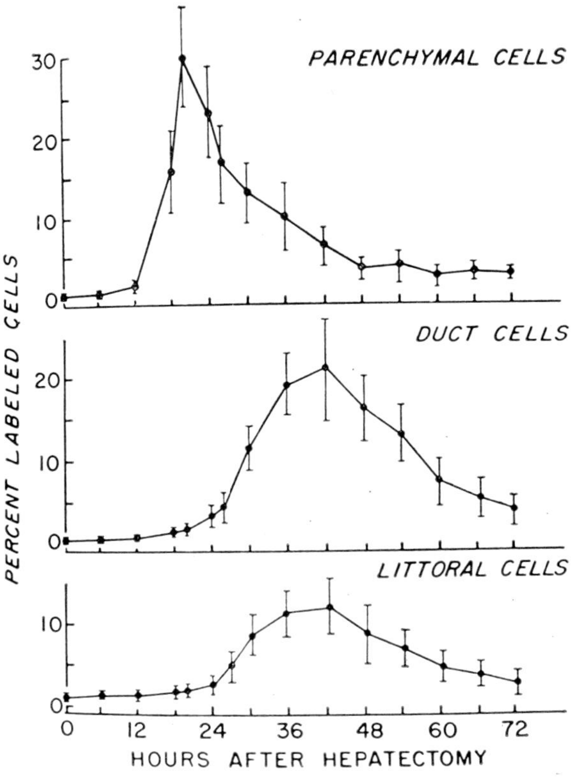

17/FIG. 35.—Curves showing mitotic activity after partial hepatectomy in three kinds of cell in the liver—parenchymal, bile duct epithelium and sinus-lining or littoral cells. Rats were injected with H^3 thymidine at times indicated by points on the curves and were killed 2 hrs. later. The percentage of cells of each type synthesising DNA was determined by counts on autoradiographs of histological sections. Vertical lines show standard deviations. (From Grisham.[80])

system is reflected, too, in the spleen and lymph nodes, where the sinus-lining cells proliferate synchronously with those of the liver[82] (FIG. 36). Other evidence has suggested that the regeneration of the Kupffer cells may be under different control from that of the parenchymal cells[83] and it is now known that under intense stimulation Kupffer cells may be mobilised from outside the liver (see Chapter 4).

After this great burst of activity the increase in number of liver cells goes on more slowly and the original weight of the organ is not restored for some considerable time.[76] There has been much argument over the years as to whether

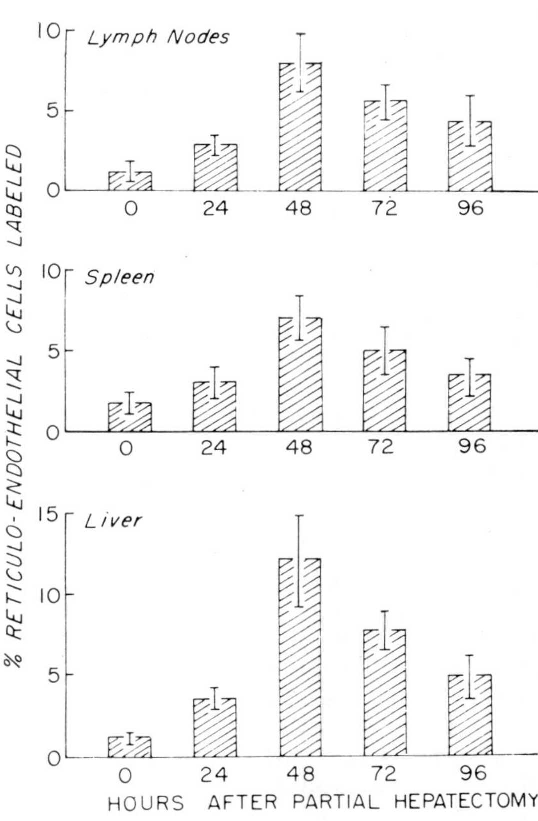

17/FIG. 36.—Curves showing that partial hepatectomy stimulates mitosis in the sinus-lining (reticulo-endothelial) cells of distant organs as well as in those of the residual part of the liver. Conditions similar to those for FIG. 35. (By courtesy of Dr. Grisham.)

the bile duct epithelium is a source of new parenchymal cells but no good evidence has been found for this[84, 85] except in a quite unusual and intense experimental destruction of the parenchyma.[86] If it has this potentiality it is one that seems to be rarely called upon.

In the slow production of liver cells that goes on throughout life mitoses are scattered more or less evenly through the lobule, but when rapid restoration is needed after extensive loss of tissue the replacement mechanism seems to be different. The more peripheral parts of the lobule then become the focus for the

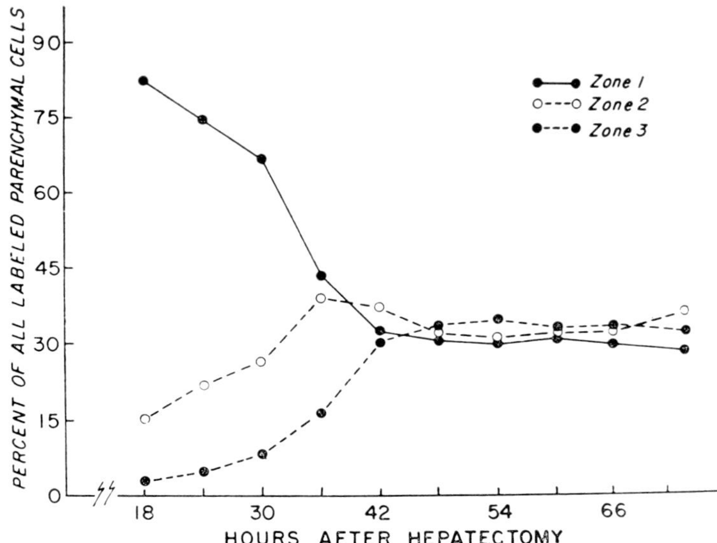

17/FIG. 37.—Curves showing the distribution of mitoses in the conventional liver lobule after partial hepatectomy. The conditions of experiment were similar to those for Fig. 35. Zone 1 is at the periphery of the lobule, zone 3 is at the centre of the lobule, and zone 2 is intermediate. Most of the mitoses are at the periphery. (From Grisham.[80])

production of new liver cells, while the centre remains relatively inactive (FIG. 37). Further, the "wave of mitosis" that passes from the periphery to the centre, as represented by the falling curve for zone 1 and the rising curve for zone 3 in FIG. 37, seems to be due not to enhanced mitotic activity at the centre but to the migration of the new cells from the periphery, possibly because of rising pressure from the increased peripheral cell population, with further division during transit.[80] Here then is some evidence of mobility of the liver cells in an early stage of regeneration, as a first contribution to the extensive remodelling that will be needed as new lobules are formed. It is all too easy, with the liver as with other organs, to think in terms of the usual microscopic picture, and to forget that in life the tissues have not been fixed into immobility as they must be for histological sectioning.

Changes in the blood.—While these changes are going on alterations take place in the composition of the blood. Some of these are due to the trauma of operation and are found equally in sham-operated animals, but some seem to be more specific, in particular a fall in the concentration of some globulins. Considering the increase in the synthesis of nucleic acids and other internal requirements which is going on it is not surprising that the output of substances for use outside the cell is impaired. Nevertheless, the reserve capacity of the liver is such that the animals recover quickly from the operation and the deficiencies are soon made good.

Circumstances influencing regeneration.—The rate and completeness of regeneration may be affected by conditions which have to be taken into account in planning and assessing experiments. Some of these were mentioned earlier and others among the more obvious factors which can have an effect are: species and strain of animal; age of the animals; diet, including vitamins; degree of liver deficiency; conditions affecting the animals in respect of "stress", such as degree of crowding in cages and amount of handling—some investigations with hormones have been made, but no effect of a specific nature has so far been shown. Evidence bearing on these is discussed by Bucher.[87]

Stimuli to regeneration.—It would be satisfactory to conclude the consideration of liver regeneration with an account of the mechanism by which, almost within minutes of the removal of, say, two-thirds of the liver, changes leading to mitosis are initiated in the residual segment. Unfortunately nothing of the kind can be attempted at present, for this has proved a most difficult matter to investigate. There is no evidence that the stimulus is connected with the disturbed bile secretion or the increased portal blood flow that are among the immediate results of the operation. And in the tempting field of chemical stimulation, which has been entered by such experimental methods as establishing parabiosis between two animals and excising the liver of one, the results have been wildly varied and contradictory. Harkness[76] brought together some evidence that lowering of the plasma albumin might be a critical factor (though a measurable fall of albumin in the blood as a whole takes place too late) but Bucher felt that this view could not be sustained as yet. Those who are interested in a discussion of feed-back and other mechanisms that may promote DNA synthesis in the liver when new cells are required are referred to her excellent review.[87]

Regeneration of the liver in pathological states.—In uncomplicated regeneration such as we have been discussing an almost perfect balance is maintained between parenchymal cells and stroma, but in the presence of complications such as sepsis whether in the liver or elsewhere, intoxication, bile duct obstruction, long-continued deficiencies in the diet, or repeated attacks of liver necrosis, stromal proliferation may outweigh liver cell production and result in the condition known as cirrhosis. In this the liver is traversed by sheets of fibrous tissue which has apparently originated from the periportal fibrous tissue but comes to divide up the organ into irregular islands which have little relation to the original lobules. Sometimes it replaces tissue killed by liver poisons such as chloroform or by the virus of infectious hepatitis—this is sometimes called post-necrotic scarring. But it can also develop more insidiously, perhaps replacing cells degenerating slowly in long-continued toxic states or dietary deficiencies; the classical examples of this are chronic alcoholism in man and certain deficiencies of diet in experimental rats. It has been shown that the fibrous tissue can to some extent disappear when the damaging agent is withdrawn[88].

The most notable feature in the cirrhotic liver, and the one that gives it a place in this chapter, is the persistent growth that takes place in the surviving liver tissue, so that functional nodules of liver, always rounded in outline because they are expanding, may be widespread among the fibrous tissue. The condition is sometimes given the name of "multiple nodular hyperplasia" (FIG. 38). As the nodules to be effective have to make or maintain connections with the bile ducts an apparently excessive formation of buds of duct epithelium in the fibrous bands is often a prominent feature (FIG. 39). Sometimes gross distortion of the lobular architecture persists indefinitely, or the liver becomes completely disorganised. The same injurious agent may give different results under different circumstances. Thus in rats and mice long-continued intoxication with carbon tetrachloride may lead, on the one hand, to cirrhosis and nodular hyperplasia associated with numerous attacks of focal liver necrosis; or, on the other hand, by varying the dose, it can give rise predominantly to large regenera-

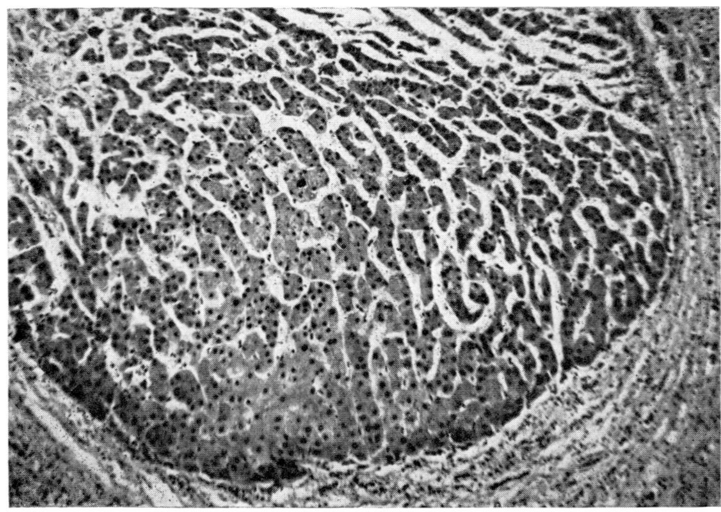

17/FIG. 38.—Regeneration in a human liver that has undergone widespread necrosis. The expanding nodule of liver tissue has taken on a rounded form and is pushing aside the surrounding fibrous tissue of which there was a great excess (cirrhosis). The young liver cells are assuming a columnar arrangement as in the normal lobule. (×95.)

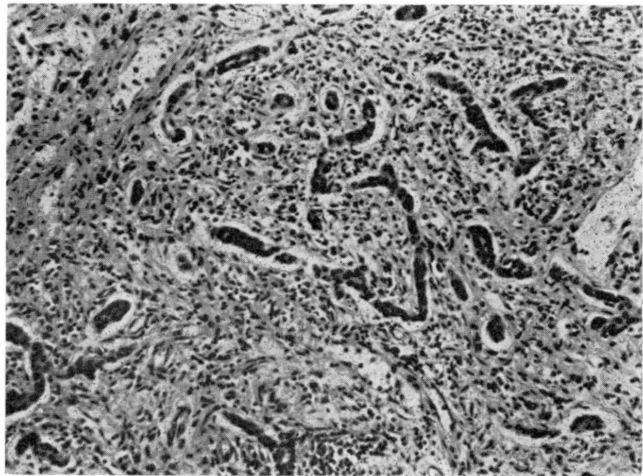

17/FIG. 39.—From the same liver as FIG. 38. In the fibrous tissue that now occupies much of the damaged organ are many newly formed bile ducts, branching in all directions. (×76.)

tion nodules which may develop into tumours (hepatomata). So, too, the dye *p*-dimethylaminoazobenzene ("butter yellow") may lead to cirrhosis of the liver with liver cell and bile duct proliferation and eventually liver carcinoma, or, if the diet is modified, it may produce carcinoma alone without any cirrhosis. The dividing line between benign and malignant tumours of liver cells is not a sharp one, and heptatomata though nominally benign are potentially carcinomata.

Pancreas

There is a good deal of uncertainty about regeneration of the pancreas in man, perhaps because pathologists are not accustomed to routine examination of the organ. As far as the *exocrine gland* composed of the acinar tissue is concerned, there seems to be a considerable reserve capacity, so that function can be satisfactory after loss of part of the organ without necessarily any replacement of acini.[89] Many observations over the years in man and animals have shown that mitotic figures and appearances suggestive of regeneration are quite common when the pancreas is disturbed, particularly in duct epithelium which readily proliferates and which may be a source of acinar and possibly other cells.[75]

In the small laboratory animals acini can be rapidly and fully regenerated after partial excision or toxic damage. It was calculated that rats on a protein-free diet injected with the toxic substance ethionine lost over 90 per cent of their acinar cells in 10 days, but when they were returned to normal conditions the pancreas regained its original weight in about three weeks. A sharp rise in DNA syntheses in the acinar cells with a corresponding wave of mitosis accompanied the regeneration.[90] Electron microscopy showed that most of the mitoses were in damaged but surviving acinar cells, with some also in duct epithelium.[91]

The pancreatic *endocrine gland*, consisting of the islets of Langerhans, is composed mainly of α cells, possibly producing glucagon, and β cells producing insulin. The growth in volume of the islets during life apparently depends on the division of both types of cell, with the β cells becoming proportionally more numerous as the animal (rat) grows older.[92] Mitoses in the β cells have been reported in human subjects dying from various systemic diseases, and they are found in greater numbers than usual in rats and rabbits maintained under conditions that increase the demand for insulin. The dog is reported to be unable to make this response. There is some evidence from the rat and rabbit that, for instance after destruction of part of the pancreas, islets can arise from duct epithelium as well as from residual islet tissue.[93]

It is thought that the β cells of man may be able to respond to increased demand for insulin like those of the rat,[93] but in diabetes any such faculty is lost and such changes as appear in the β cells are those of degranulation and degeneration.[94]

Salivary Glands

Considerable portions of the salivary glands may be removed from animals and, provided infection is prevented, regeneration goes on successfully through mitotic division of secretory cells and ducts. Removal of as much as five-sixths of the total submaxillary tissue of a rabbit or rat can be tolerated, but restoration of lost tissue is never complete.[95]

Milstein[96] found that mitotic division of the cells of pre-existing acini can be demonstrated during the first week of repair, following by proliferation of ducts and formation of new acini in the terminal segments of these ducts. Pathologists every now and then see signs of regeneration in human salivary glands, for instance after removal of a calculus in a salivary duct, but these signs are scattered and rather insignificant.

Kidneys and Urinary Passages

Regeneration in the *kidney* is a very restricted affair, mainly confined to mitotic division of tubule cells in replacement of those dying off from disease or ageing. The book by Oliver[97] is full of interesting information about this and related problems. No complete nephrons are formed, though tubular parts of nephrons can be replaced by new cells. The kidney, of course, possesses an alternative and highly efficient method for increasing the functional activity of its nephrons in the process of hypertrophy. Here enlargement of cells is the chief feature. All surgeons know how efficient the *urinary bladder* is at regeneration. Large portions may be resected from cancer patients and be repaired by overgrowth of new epithelial cells derived from adjacent regions. The entire bladder of dogs has been removed and a regeneration pouch has formed later, with a lining of transitional epithelium, smooth muscle in its wall and capable of functioning normally.[98]

Genital Organs

Endometrial epithelium and the sex cells are the most competent of all cells at cyclical regeneration. Endometrial lining cells spread over the bare connective tissue surface from the mouths of the gland tubules after each menstruation, to cover the defect with a simple layer of columnar cells.[99] Under pathological conditions, the uterus still remains very efficient at repair, but the organs producing sex cells become notoriously incompetent, with the exception of the interstitial cells of Leydig in the testis. These can proliferate in great numbers when given the proper stimulus, which is frequently bound up with atrophy of the seminiferous cells. Regeneration in the prostate and other accessory sex organs is limited so far as division and replacement of specific cells is concerned, but hyperplasia and hypertrophy are common enough and are frequently excessive as the result of hormonal stimulation.

Ductless Glands

The question of regeneration in these glands, as apart from hypertrophy, is still a matter of controversy and investigation.

Thyroid gland.—It is not known for certain how thyroid follicles are formed during development, growth or the hypertrophy that results from iodine deficiency. Some appear to be formed from solid buds, others through constriction of pre-existing follicles, while still others may develop from undifferentiated cells. Mitotic figures are found occasionally in the lining epithelium of follicles which suggests that new follicles or parts of follicles are being manufactured. Apart from the well-established relationship between thyroid size and function and iodine metabolism, we know little about the factors that influence growth of thyroid cells.

We are even more ignorant about the *parathyroids* which may hypertrophy in association with disturbances of calcium metabolism found with some bone diseases and chronic nephritis,[100] but apparently have little power of regeneration.

Suprarenal tissue.—Regeneration goes on actively in the cortex of the infant, especially following the remarkable hæmorrhage and involution that is a constant feature in the cortex during the early weeks after birth.[101] In the adult it seems to be confined to mitotic division of cortical cells around areas of localised injury.[102]

Pituitary gland.—Mitotic figures are found in the anterior lobe of the pituitary after injury of various kinds and, provided that damage of the organ is not too extensive, division may lead to complete replacement of lost cells. There is reason to believe that various hormones control cell division in the organ.[75]

Respiratory Tissue

Surgical wounds of the lung with the sides approximated by suture are repaired in the main by a fibrous scar, though when this was studied experimentally in cats it was seen that there were some attempts at new alveolus formation by the budding of bronchial epithelium into the granulation tissue.[103] Defects in the bronchial lining are rapidly filled in by migrating and dividing epithelium and, judging by events in the trachea,[104] differentiation of the epithelium should follow. The mesothelial cells of the pleura proliferate at the margins of the wound and the pleural surface reforms, with a new layer of serosal cells lying on collagen and elastic tissue.[103]

The question to what extent the lung can replace lost tissue has become of especial interest since improving techniques have enabled surgeons to remove part or the whole of a diseased lung with little risk to life. Does the remaining lung when called on to fill out the vacant space generate new alveoli, or does it remain permanently over-expanded? Present evidence, reviewed by Reid,[105] suggests that a child or young animal can form new alveoli, presumably by an extension of the natural growth process by which, in the human being, the number of alveoli goes on increasing up to the age of about 8 years.[106] On the other hand a fully grown animal or man when deprived of one lung seems to be dependent on a lasting enlargement of the alveoli remaining to him. But even under these circumstances recovery of function is extremely good and it is surmised that the alveolar capillaries enlarge to increase the area for gas exchange; it is not known whether they proliferate as well.

Adipose Tissue

Regeneration in adipose tissue is a controversial subject which has not yet been settled. It is still disputed whether mature fat cells can divide to form daughter cells or whether there is a precursor adipose cell which initially divides and finally settles down to maturity by storing large amounts of lipid. Cameron and Seneviratne[107] found no quantitative evidence of adipose tissue regeneration in the rat but Pochin[108] demonstrated local production of fatty tissue in the rabbit.

Cartilage

Cartilage possesses restricted powers of regeneration, wounds healing by the formation of fibrous scars around which cartilage cells divide and in time replace the scar tissue. Metaplasia also plays a part in repair, and fibro-cartilage precedes the transformation into hyaline cartilage.[109] Regeneration is a slow process lasting over many weeks and apparently varies a great deal in different types of cartilage. Some evidence exists of an endocrine control of cartilage growth in young animals and pressure and attrition help to maintain the integrity of joint cartilage.

Bone

The healing of bone is one of nature's great successes, in that with favourable conditions the highly specialised tissue needed to support weight can be regenerated and remodelled to serve its purpose correctly and completely, provided that osteogenic cells are available.

In spite of increasing knowledge the process of healing in bone persists in seeming a difficult subject, and perhaps a useful approach is to look squarely at the reasons for this. Fundamentally, healing in bone is an example of healing in connective tissues; it depends in the first place on the same tissue reactions as, say, healing of the abdominal wall. But in order to produce the right end-product—a rigid, weight-supporting tissue—some extra steps have to be imposed on the basic process. These are provided by the osteogenic cells, that is, the bone-forming cells of the peri- and endosteum, which in two different phases of healing play a decisive part. Under their influence changes are brought about which terminate in the production of new bone, complete with a Haversian system. Naturally the biological and chemical processes concerned are intricate, and this constitutes the first difficulty. However, the steps seem to be entirely analogous to those by which bone is formed in the embryo and young animal, and knowledge about the one is applicable to the other.

Secondly, bone is a difficult tissue to work with chemically and histologically. No doubt if sections of bone could be prepared as easily as say, sections of a subcutaneous granuloma, many more people would be doing experiments and knowledge would be acquired faster.

Thirdly, the nomenclature of bone healing is complicated by special, traditional terms, in particular the term "callus" or "provisional callus". This simply means the temporary tissue which embeds and encloses the broken ends. It may be likened to granulation tissue in other sites, but it has some special properties and feels firm.

Steps of the healing process.—The commonest bones to break are the long bones of the arms and legs, and healing in these, that is in bones arising in cartilage, is the situation usually described and investigated. Healing in membrane bones is a variant which follows the same principles. This account is based on the former, as to both general description and accounts of experiments.

An admirable short account of bone physiology and healing has been given by Ham,[110] who has worked on the subject for many years, and the student is referred to that or to his earlier article[111] for description and discussion and for related references. Briefly, the steps by which a bone heals are as follows:

1. A bone is a vascular tissue, and as soon as it is broken, with consequent tearing of the vessels in and near it, there is profuse hæmorrhage into the soft tissues round the broken ends, with formation of a clot round and between the ends. As in other situations, if the blood does not clot, healing is delayed.

2. Into the clot, just as we have seen in the rabbit ear chamber and elsewhere, grow capillaries and fibroblasts accompanied by macrophages and other leucocytes. But as the periosteum lining both the outside and the inside of the bone has been torn along with other soft tissues, osteogenic cells also begin to proliferate and these become more numerous and more conspicuous than the fibroblasts. By three days an experimental fracture in a small animal is surrounded by a mass of proliferating periosteal cells, looking like big, plump fibroblasts and showing many mitoses. Parts of the clot between the ends of the bone and not immediately adjacent to the multiplying cells may remain unaltered for some time.

3. These proliferating periosteal cells do not begin to form bone, as might be expected, but secrete the constituents of cartilage—collagen and sulphated mucopolysaccharides—and thus come to lie in holes in a solid matrix with the appearance of cartilage. It is mainly this cartilage-like substance in the tissue round a fracture that gives callus its characteristic firmness and, indeed, its name (Latin: *callum*, hardened thick skin or flesh). However, the formation of this temporary tissue ("provisional callus") does not stop at this stage. The cells begin to secrete phosphatase, with consequent deposition of calcium in the matrix. This calcified cartilage is sometimes referred to as "osteoid tissue". It is thought that the cells, which in cartilage are nourished by diffusion of materials through the matrix, die as soon as calcium is deposited because the necessary diffusion can no longer take place. The fracture is now enveloped by calcified callus which forms a bulging, fusiform collar round it and helps to immobilise and support the broken ends.

4. But the production of cartilage-like material is not the only activity of the disturbed system of osteogenic cells. Firstly, some of these cells begin to lay down bone directly, without any preliminary cartilage stage. These are the cells that are closest to the bone, both on the outside and lining the trabeculæ, and they form bony trabeculæ attached to, and jutting from, the original bone. Similarly, osteoblasts attached to the fibrous periosteum that was raised off the bone by hæmorrhage begin to form trabeculæ on the outside of the callus (Fig. 40). There is some evidence that whether the cells produce bone or cartilage may be determined by the amount of blood available, those with the poorer blood supply being the ones that become cartilage cells. The amount and position of bone which is formed directly probably varies a good deal in different situations.

Secondly, osteoblasts throughout the area proliferate and in an orderly and systematic way invade the calcified cartilage that has been laid down and destroy it and replace it with trabeculæ of bone. This is the last of the rapid tissue transformations in the clot round the fracture.

5. The final process, which may extend over a long period, is the remodelling of the new bone by the activities of osteoclasts and osteoblasts, so that those parts in the lines of stress become stronger and more compact, while unwanted bone at the periphery of the swelling is removed (Figs. 41 and 42).

Mechanisms of bone regeneration.—As was said above, knowledge of the growth, maintenance and remodelling of bone throws light on the processes of bone repair. The reader is referred to specialized accounts (see end of bibliography) for discussion of these intricate subjects, which have been far more

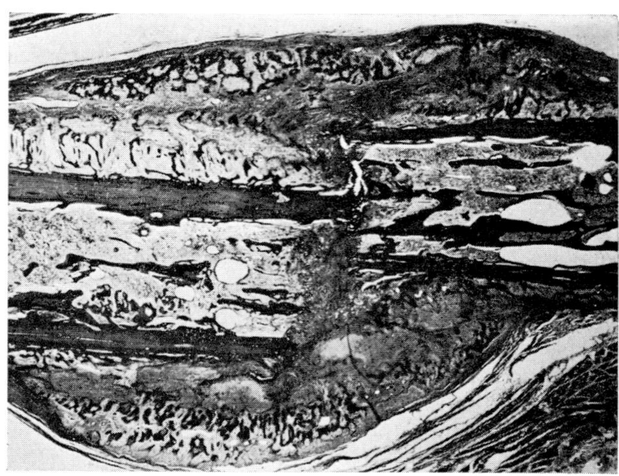

17/FIG. 40.—Healing fracture, early stage. The shaft of the fractured bone shows as dark solid lines, and the callus as a swollen mass around the fracture. The bony fragments are not in good apposition, but the callus is well formed. Trabeculæ of bone are extending into the callus from both outside and inside. (× 3.)

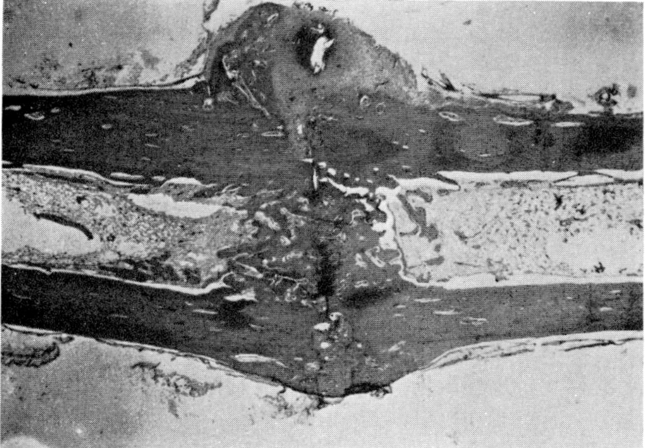

17/FIG. 41.—Healing fracture, beginning of remodelling. In this fracture the fragments are in good apposition. The amount of periosteal callus has been greatly reduced, and there is now a dense mass of cancellous bone in the medullary cavity. (× 3.)

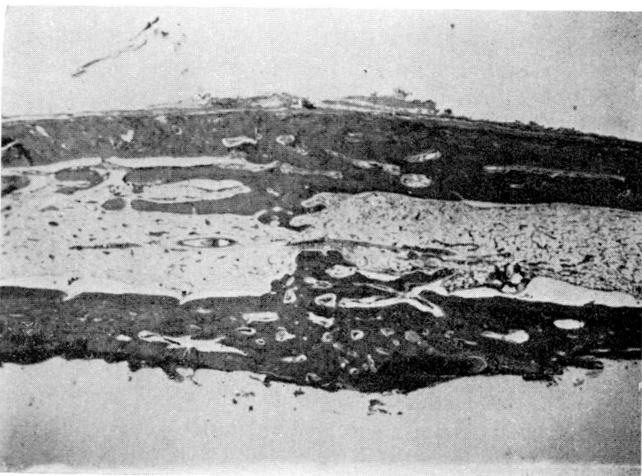

17/FIG. 42.—Healing fracture, remodelling almost complete. There is very little callus still remaining and the cortical bone is in continuity, although the Haversian pattern of the blood vessels at the point of fracture is still irregular. (× 3.)

studied than bone healing itself. A few points that have special relevance to healing may be mentioned here.

Source of new osteogenic cells.—It has often been stated that cells not usually osteogenic, in particular fibroblasts of the neighbouring connective tissue, may under some stimulus provided by the bone cells at a fracture site take over osteogenic functions.

The induction of bone formation in one tissue by another has been described in numerous situations, but the inducing tissue has not generally been an osteogenic one.[112] It is certain that the bone cells themselves are predominant in the formation of new bone when a fracture is repaired, and some recent experiments have provided no evidence of the involvement of fibroblasts. The transplantation of fractured bones to and from irradiated limbs of mice appeared to give clear-cut evidence that cells associated with the bone were needed for repair, and that connective tissue cells could not replace them.[113] The soft tissues naturally suffer considerable injury when a fracture takes place, and by the injection of tritiated thymidine in mice scattered mitosis has been shown to occur initially up to some distance from the site. But by the second day mitosis was markedly concentrated at the fracture and there was no evidence that this concentration was due to anything but the local proliferation of the osteogenic cells of the periosteum.[114]

The suggestion that bone marrow cells may contribute to osteogenesis is not easy to assess as the marrow is so closely associated with bony structures, but there is no firm evidence for it at present.

Conditions determining the formation of bone or cartilage.—As we have seen, some osteoblasts when stimulated by a fracture may begin to form bone directly, while others form cartilage as a stage on the way to final bone formation. Why should there be this difference in their activities? The factors determining it are certainly not simple, as Bassett[115] stressed, but he identified two factors that will induce osteogenic cells in culture to produce the one or the other. These were the oxygen concentration in the surrounding atmosphere and the degree of mechanical stretching of the cells. With cells not subject to stretching the matrix produced was bone when the oxygen tension was high and cartilage when it was low, but if the cell mass was stretched only a tendon-like structure was produced even with high oxygen tension. This effect of oxygen is in harmony with the idea mentioned above that the amount of the blood supply may affect the direction in which the cells differentiate.

The wave of cartilage formation in the fracture site as a whole, shown by the deposition of sulphated mucopolysaccharides, and its overtaking and supersession by the wave of bone formation have been well illustrated histologically by special staining and autoradiography,[116, 117] and chemically.[118]

Healing of bones in vitro.—It has been known for over 30 years that chick embryo long bones when placed in isolated organ culture and deliberately fractured will heal. By a remarkable refinement of technique it has now been shown that they will heal in a synthetic culture medium, that is to say, one containing no complex natural ingredients such as serum or tissue extract.[119] The bones—tibiæ taken from 14-day-old chick embryos—bleed when cut and a small hæmorrhage forms between the ends. Thereafter fibroblasts and osteogenic cells of the periosteum proliferate and cover the area and osteogenic cells fill the gap between the bones, producing collagen and later bony trabeculæ. At the stages so far examined no cartilage was seen. In experiments with this preparation high oxygen tension in the atmosphere was found to improve healing, but a low oxygen concentration did not produce signs of cartilage formation. However, if insulin was added to the medium cartilage sometimes formed, delaying the appearance of trabeculæ of bone. This method seems to be full of promise for the anaylsis of factors that influence healing.

Tendon

When a tendon is severed or partly injured, fibroblasts grow in from the surrounding connective tissue and arrange themselves on strands of fibrin, which form as the outcome of the preliminary aseptic inflammation induced by the injury and extend from one stump to the other. Subsequently these cells become elongated and form collagen fibres which as usual are fine at first and gradually become thicker. They are accompanied by newly formed capillaries which increase in number as the tissue cells proliferate, and run parallel with the long axis of the tendon. Fibrous tissue cells at the divided ends of the tendon play little part in repair, at the most providing fibres which link up with those formed in the gap by migrating fibroblasts from the loose surrounding tissue.

Many interesting experiments have been performed to test the theory that tension playing over the region of regeneration determines the structure of the new tissue. Certainly the parallel alignment of fibres in a tendon and their orientation along the direction of maximum tension exerted by the associated muscle suggests such an idea. Experimentalists have altered the tension vector during repair by ingeniously inserting threads whereby a pull may be exerted transversely to the regeneration field, or by eliminating muscle pull or exaggerating it through division of its nerve supply. Results give much support to a mechanical theory. Weiss[25] has shown how important to alignment are the mechanical conditions provided by structures such as grooves or fibres along which mesenchymal cells tend to grow, and it seems likely that at least in part the effect of tension is to pull the fibrin of the clot into a longitudinal pattern thus initiating the longitudinal development of the fibroblasts. The orientation of the collagen fibres, which roughly follows that of the fibroblasts, does not seem to depend on tension alone.[120]

Muscle

We are familiar with the fact that *skeletal muscle* divided at operation heals in the main by fibrous tissue union, fortunately usually with little impairment of function in the long run. So too we know that part of a muscle mass removed by a missile or in a traffic accident is not replaced by muscle to any useful extent, but that the gap is covered and the sides drawn together by fibrous tissue.

Nevertheless, experiments that extend as far back as the eighteenth century have almost consistently shown that skeletal muscle has some powers of regeneration.[121] It should be remembered that individual fibres are up to 4 cm. in length and have many nuclei, so that a fibre may easily be damaged in one part and survive in another. Nuclei may survive along the sarcolemmal covering and an early sign of regrowth is the appearance of groups of nuclei, apparently proliferating although mitotic figures are rare. At the same time macrophages invade and remove the damaged parts of the fibre and buds of new sarcoplasm grow forward from the surviving end. The buds may be single or multiple, and they advance along the sarcolemmal sheath, or if this has been destroyed along the planes of the endomysium or other connective tissue. It appears that, as with a nerve, regeneration of a muscle fibre depends on the presence of well aligned supporting structures. Good descriptions have been given of these events.[121, 122]

There is less certainty as to whether new fibres can arise after injury. It has been suggested that nuclei which remain on the sarcolemma can form cytoplasm round themselves and develop into new muscle cells. It is also suggested that after injury fibres may develop from unspecified mesenchyme cells in the surrounding tissue. At present much depends on the interpretation of what is seen in histological sections of fixed tissues, and these questions are not settled.

In terms of gross injury such as a surgical wound the regeneration of which muscle is capable is perhaps not of much importance. But there are diseases which can damage individual muscle cells to an extent that may seriously impair the function of the whole muscle. For example, in severe infections or intoxications muscle fibres may be damaged ("Zenker's degeneration"), particularly in sites like the diaphragm, abdominal wall and intercostal muscles which cannot be rested. It is believed that such damaged fibres may regrow inside the sarcolemmal sheaths, which remain intact, and so the function of the muscle may be largely or completely restored. There is, too, a group of diseases whose cause is obscure known under the name of polymyositis. Among other changes there are degeneration and necrosis of voluntary muscle fibres. Histologically there are signs that the fibres attempt to regenerate, and it is believed that if the rate of damage slows down, as for example during the administration of corticosteroids, regrowth of fibres may contribute substantially to recovery of power in the affected muscles.[123]

Less work has been done on *cardiac muscle* than on skeletal muscle, but it seems that similar conditions may apply. That is to say the fibres do not seem to multiply, and if there is general destruction of the tissue, as in an ischæmic infarct, the muscles does not regrow, but it is possible that individual fibres may have some power of regeneration.

Smooth muscle is said to show mitosis after injury and to have some capacity to proliferate. Certainly there are events which involve the appearance of smooth muscle cells in new situations, for example in the wall of a young differentiating arteriole or in an atherosclerotic plaque. But it has not yet been ascertained whether these arise by the migration and division of existing cells or by differentiation *de novo* from mesenchymal precursor cells. It seems clear that the healing of smooth muscle in surgery, as for instance in an anastomosis in the gut, depends in the main on the development of fibrous tissue.

Nervous Tissue

When a *nerve fibre* is divided, the peripheral portion that has been cut off from its nerve cell soon shows irregular fragmentation of its axone, associated with myelin degeneration during the first 24 hours after injury. During the next week the myelin deposits increase in amount and may be converted into isotropic granules of triglyceride through enzyme activity. Macrophages accumulate around the degenerating nerve and remove much of the myelin and other fats.

These changes are essential preliminaries for true nerve regeneration since newly formed fibres prefer to grow along the old pathways, provided these have been cleared of debris. But certain preparations seem to be necessary before the new sprouts from the central part of the divided nerve can take this course. These include the elongation, migration and proliferation of Schwann cells derived from the degenerating stumps into the space between the cut ends. Fibroblasts from supporting connective tissue are also concerned in this union.[124]

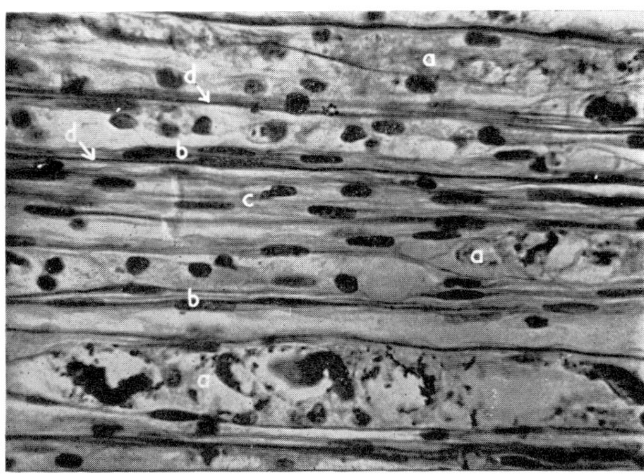

17/FIG. 43.—Early repair of a nerve injury. Longitudinal section of the distal portion. The degenerating myelin (*a*), Schwann cell proliferation (*b*) and collapsed Schwann tubes (*c*) are apparent. In addition new axones (*d*) growing from the proximal stump can be seen to be penetrating the Schwann tubes. (×400.)

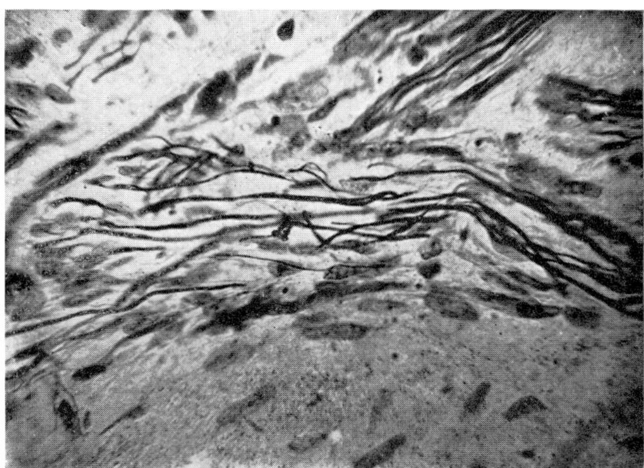

17/FIG. 44.—Early repair of a nerve injury. Longitudinal section of the proximal portion. A leash of axones, showing slight nodularity of the distal tips, can be seen penetrating a Schwann cell syncytium. (×560.)

Meanwhile the axones of the central stump degenerate adjacent to the cut, and its Schwann cells proliferate and migrate to join those emerging from the peripheral stump. As early as the second day after section new axone sprouts grow down among the Schwann cells and within their protoplasm—the details are still disputed—at a rate of 3–4 mm. per day[125] (FIGS. 43 and 44). At first these are naked, but after a week or so they become enclosed in a myelin covering, or medullary sheath, probably through a kind of bandaging action of the

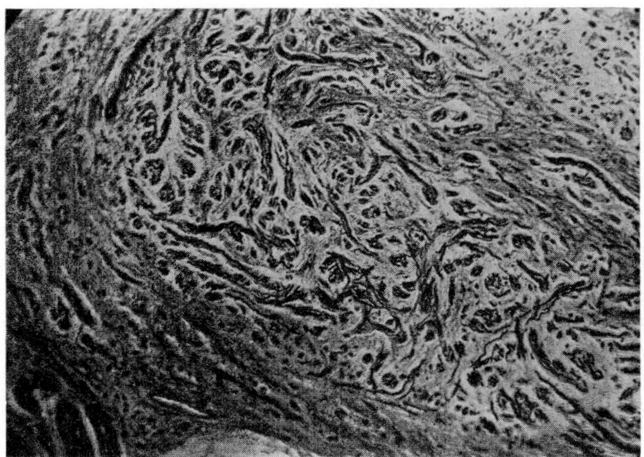

17/FIG. 45.—Late repair of a nerve injury. Transverse section of the point of union between the proximal and distal portions. The leashes of axones can be seen penetrating the collagenised collapsed Schwann tubes of the distal portion. (×160.)

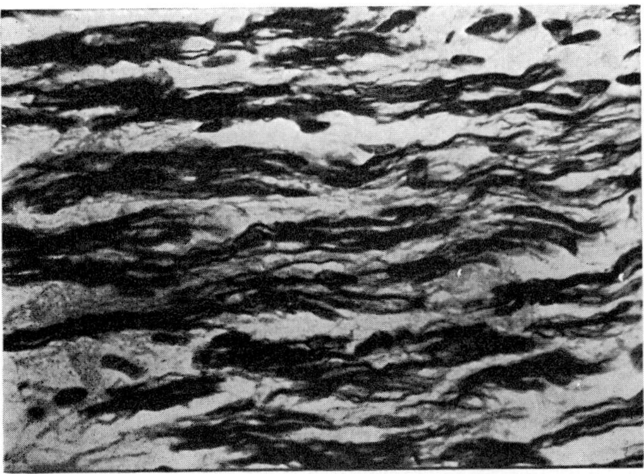

17/FIG. 46.—Late repair of a nerve injury. Longitudinal section of the point of union between the proximal and distal portions. The nerve fibre leashes can be seen spreading into the Schwann cell syncytium. (×400.)

Schwann cells which form successive layers of myelin around the axones[126]; thus they thicken and show evidence of functional regeneration for they now can transmit nerve impulses (FIGS. 45 and 46). The progress of functional regeneration in man may be at the rate of 2·4 mm. per day.[127] Control of regeneration lies in the first instance with the nerve cells belonging to the nerve fibres, but speed and degree of success are largely the outcome of the efficiency with which the phagocytes and Schwann cells perform their duties ahead of the new advancing nerve fibres. The surgeon can facilitate recovery by apposing the divided segments accurately but not too tightly and, if there has been delay in treatment, by removing interposed scar tissue. Weiss[25] has described how the growth of the sprouts may itself put tension on intervening fibrin so that it aligns with the nerve and helps to direct the new fibres from the central to the peripheral stump.

Regeneration in the *central nervous system* is now believed to be in essence the same as in peripheral nerves, that is to say, although the nerve cells do not divide axons and dendrites can regrow if the cell survives; under experimental conditions extensive regrowth has been found.[128] It is suggested that mechanical conditions such as the density of central nervous tissue and the ready formation of scar tissue by the glial cells account for the lack of functional recovery in mammals. The subject of regeneration in the central nervous system has been reviewed by Clemente.[129]

REFERENCES

1. SANDISON, J. C. (1928). *Amer. J. Anat.*, **41,** 475.
2. EBERT, R. H., and FLOREY, H. W. (1939). *Brit. J. exp. Path.*, **20,** 342.
3. PALADE, G. E. (1955). *Anat. Rec.*, **121,** 445.
4. CLIFF, W. J. (1963). *Phil. Trans. B.*, **246,** 305; (1965). *Quart. J. exp. Physiol.*, **50,** 79.
5. CLARK, E. R., HITSCHLER, W. J., KIRBY-SMITH, H. T., REX, R. O., and SMITH, J. H. (1931). *Anat. Rec.*, **50,** 129.
6. CLARK, E. R., and CLARK, E. L. (1932). *Amer. J. Anat.*, **51,** 49.
7. CLARK, E. R. (1936). *Ann. intern. Med.*, **9,** 1043.
8. PULLINGER, B. D., and FLOREY, H. W. (1937). *J. Path. Bact.*, **45,** 157.
9. STEARNS, M. L. (1940). *Amer. J. Anat.*, **66,** 133.
10. ROSS, R., and BENDITT, E. P. (1961). *J. biophys. biochem. Cytol.*, **11,** 677.
11. GRILLO, H. C., WATTS, G. T., and GROSS, J. (1958). *Ann. Surg.*, **148,** 145.
12. VAN DEN BRENK, H. A. S. (1955–56). *Brit. J. Surg.*, **43,** 525.

12a. JAMES, D. W., and TAYLOR, J. F. (1969). *Exp. Cell Res.*, **54,** 107.

13. DUNPHY, J. E. (1960). *Ann. roy. Coll. Surg. Engl.*, **26,** 69.
14. VAUGHAN, R. B., and TRINKAUS, J. P. (1966). *J. Cell Sci.*, **1,** 407.

14a. ODLAND, G., and ROSS, R. (1968). *J. Cell Biol.*, **39,** 135.

15. AREY, L. B., and COVODE, W. M. (1943). *Anat. Rec.*, **86,** 75.
16. LOEWENSTEIN, W. R., and PENN, R. D. (1967). *J. Cell Biol.*, **33,** 235.
17. GILLMAN, T., PENN, J., BRONKS, D., and ROUX, M. (1955–1956). *Brit. J. Surg.*, **43,** 141.
18. GILLMAN, T., and PENN, J. (1956). *Med. Proc.*, **2,** 121.

18a. GRILLO, H. C., and GROSS, J. (1967). *Develop. Biol.*, **15,** 300.

19. BREEDIS, C. (1954). *Cancer Res.*, **14,** 575.
20. CONVERSE, J. M., and ROBB-SMITH, A. H. T. (1944). *Ann. Surg.*, **120,** 873.

21. WINTER, G. D. (1964). *Advances in Biology of Skin, Vol. 5. Wound Healing*, p. 113. Eds. MONTAGNA, W., and BILLINGHAM, R. E. Oxford: Pergamon Press.
22. LEVI-MONTALCINI, R., and ANGELETTI, P. U. (1968). *Physiol. Rev.*, **48,** 534.
23. SCOTT, D., and LIU, C. N. (1964). *Progress in Brain Research*, Vol. 13, p. 127. Eds. SINGER, M., and SCHADE, J. P. Amsterdam: Elsevier Publishing Co.
24. ABERCROMBIE, M. (1964). *Advances in Biology of Skin. Vol. 5. Wound Healing*, p. 95. Eds. MONTAGNA, W., and BILLINGHAM, R. E. Oxford: Pergamon Press.
25. WEISS, P. (1961). *Harvey Lect.*, **55,** 13.
26. ROYSTER, H. P., MCCAIN, L. I., and SLOAN, A. (1948). *Surg. Gynec. Obstet.*, **86,** 565.
27. MASON, M. L., and ALLEN, H. S. (1941). *Ann. Surg.*, **113,** 424.
28. MUREN, A. (1953). *Acta physiol. scand.*, **30,** Suppl. 111, p. 148.
29. SANDBLOM, P., and MUREN, A. (1954). *Ann. Surg.*, **104,** 449.
30. SAVLOV, E. D., and DUNPHY, J. E. (1954). *New Engl. J. Med.*, **250,** 1062.
31. HOWES, E. L., and HARVEY, S. C. (1932). *J. exp. Med.*, **55,** 577.
32. CUTHBERTSON, A. M. (1959). *Surg. Gynec. Obstet.*, **108,** 421.
33. SAVLOV, E. D., STRAIN, W. H., and HUEGIN, F. (1962). *J. Surg. Res.*, **2,** 209.
34. PORIES, W. J., HENZEL, J. H., ROB, C. G., and STRAIN, W. H. (1967). *Lancet*, **1,** 121.
35. EDWARDS, L. C., and DUNPHY, J. E. (1957). *The Healing of Wounds*, p.47. Ed. WILLIAMSON, M. B. New York: McGraw-Hill Book Co.
36. LEVENSON, S. M., UPJOHN, H. L., PRESTON, J. A., and STEER, A. (1957). *Ann. Surg.*, **146,** 357.
37. PENNEY, J. R., and BALFOUR, B. M. (1949). *J. Path. Bact.*, **61,** 171.
38. CRANDON, J. H., LUND, C. C., and DILL, D. B. (1940). *New Engl. J. Med.*, **223,** 353.
39. DUNPHY, J. E., UDUPA, K. N., and EDWARDS, L. C. (1956). *Ann. Surg.*, **144,** 304.
40. ANTONOWICZ, I., and KODICEK, E. (1968). *Biochem. J.*, **110,** 609.
41. ROSS, R., and BENDITT, E. P. (1962). *J. Cell Biol.*, **12,** 533; (1964). *ibid*, **22,** 365.
41a. SCHAFER, I. A., SILVERMAN, L., SULLIVAN, J. C., and ROBERTSON, W. VAN B. (1967). *J. Cell Biol.*, **34,** 83.
42. HUNT, A. H. (1941). *Brit. J. Surg.*, **28,** 436.
43. MOORE, F. D. (1959). *Metabolic Care of the Surgical Patient*, p. 130. Philadelphia: W. B. Saunders.
44. FINDLAY, C. W., Jr., and HOWES, E. L. (1952). *New Engl. J. Med.*, **246,** 597.
45. PEREZ-TAMAYO, R., and IHNEN, M. (1953). *Amer. J. Path.*, **29,** 233.
46. UDUPA, K. N., WOESSNER, J. F., and DUNPHY, J. E. (1956). *Surg. Gynec. Obstet.*, **102,** 639.
47. WILLIAMSON, M. B., and FROMM, H. J. (1955). *J. biol. Chem.*, **212,** 705.
48. NORDLIE, R. C., and FROMM, H. J. (1958). *Proc. Soc. exp. Biol. (N.Y.)*, **97,** 246.
49. WILLIAMSON, M. B., and FROMM, H. J. (1953). *Proc. Soc. exp. Biol. (N.Y.)*, **83,** 329.
50. MOORE, F. D. (1959). *Metabolic Care of the Surgical Patient*, p. 132. Philadelphia: W. B. Saunders.
51. LOCALIO, S. A., and CHASSIN, J. L. (1952). *Surgery*, **32,** 39.
52. MOLTKE, E. (1957). *Acta endocr. (Kbh.)*, **25,** 179.
53. SMELSER, G. K., and OZANICS, V. (1954). *J. cell. comp. Physiol.*, **43,** 107.
54. TAUBENHAUS, M. (1957). *The Healing of Wounds*, p. 113. Ed. WILLIAMSON, M. B. New York: McGraw-Hill Book Co.
55. DUKE-ELDER, S., and ASHTON, N. (1951). *Brit. J. Ophthal.* **35,** 695.
56. RAGAN C., HOWES, E. L., PLOTZ, C. M., MEYER, K., BLUNT, J. W., and LATTES, R. (1950). *Bull. N.Y. Acad. Med.*, **26,** 251.
57. COLE, J. W., ORBISON, J. L., HOLDEN, W. D., HANCOCK, T. J., and LINDSAY, J. F. (1951). *Surg. Gynec. Obstet.*, **93,** 321.

58. Muller, W. H., Spencer, F. C., and Lewis, A. E. (1953). *Surgery*, **33,** 399.
59. Alrich, E. M., Carter, J. P., and Lehman, E. P. (1951). *Ann. Surg.*, **133,** 783.
60. Chassin, J. L., McDougall, H. A., Staal, W., Mackay, M., and Localio, S. A. (1954). *Proc. Soc. exp. Biol. (N.Y.)*, **86,** 446.
61. Florey, H. W., and Harding, H. E. (1935). *J. Path. Bact.*, **40,** 211.
62. Altschul, R. (1954). *Endothelium*, p. 123. New York: Macmillan.
63. Sinapius, D. (1952). *Virchows Arch. path. Anat.*, **322,** 662.
64. Poole, J. C. F. (1964). *Symp. Zool. Soc. Lond.*, **11,** 131.
65. Sinapius, D. (1956). *Z. Zellforsch.*, **44,** 27.
66. Cotton, R. E., and Wartman, W. B. (1961). *Arch. Path.*, **71,** 3.
67. Poole, J. C. F., Sanders, A. G., and Florey, H. W. (1958). *J. Path. Bact.*, **75,** 133; (1959). *ibid.*, **77,** 637.
68. Florey, H. W., Greer, S. J., Poole, J. C. F., and Werthessen, N. T. (1961). *Brit. J. exp. Path.*, **42,** 236; Florey, H. W., Greer, S. J., Kiser, J., Poole, J. C. F., Telander, R., and Werthessen, N. T. (1962). *ibid.*, **43,** 655.
69. Higgins, G. M., and Anderson, R. M. (1931). *Arch. Path.*, **12,** 186.
70. Ponfick, E. (1890). *Verh. dtsch. Ges. Chir.*, **19,** 28; (1895). *Virchows Arch. path. Anat.*, **138,** Suppl. p. 81.
71. Fishback, F. C. (1929). *Arch. Path. Lab. Med.*, **7,** 955.
72. Brues, A. M., and Marble, B. B. (1937). *J. exp. Med.*, **65,** 15.
73. Weinbren, K. (1959). *Gastroenterology*, **37,** 657.
74. Himsworth, H. P. (1949). *The Liver and its Diseases.* Oxford: Blackwell Scientific Publications.
75. Cameron G. R. (1952). *Pathology of the Cell.* Edinburgh: Oliver and Boyd.
76. Harkness, R. D. (1957). *Brit. med. Bull.*, **13,** 87; Abercrombie, M., and Harkness, R. D. (1951). *Proc. roy. Soc. B*, **138,** 544.
77. Cameron, G. R. (1950). *Studies in Pathology*, p. 29. Melbourne Univ. Press.
78. Clerici, E., Mocarelli, P., and Provini, L. (1964). *Exp. molec. Path.*, **3,** 569.
79. Simpson, G. E. C., and Finckh, E. S. (1963). *J. Path. Bact.*, **86,** 361.
80. Grisham, J. W. (1962). *Cancer Res.*, **22,** 842.
81. Jordan, S. W. (1964). *Exp. molec. Path.*, **3,** 183.
82. Grisham, J. W. (1966). *Gastroenterology*, **50,** 417.
83. Leong, G. F., Pessotti, R. L., and Brauer, R. W. (1959). *Amer. J. Physiol.*, **197,** 880.
84. Grisham, J. W., and Porta, E. A. (1964). *Exp. molec. Path.*, **3,** 242.
85. Rubin, E. (1964). *Exp. molec. Path.*, **3,** 279.
86. Wilson, J. W., and Leduc, E. H. (1958). *J. Path. Bact.*, **76,** 441.
87. Bucher, N. L. R. (1963). *Int. Rev. Cytol.*, **15,** 245.
88. Quinn, P. S., and Higginson, J. (1965). *Amer. J. Path.*, **47,** 353.
89. De Reuck, A. V. S., and Cameron, M. P., Eds. (1962). *The Exocrine Pancreas*, p. 358. Ciba Foundation Symposium. London: J. & A. Churchill.
90. Fitzgerald, P. J., Carol, B. M., and Rosenstock, L. (1966). *Nature (Lond.)*, **212,** 594.
91. Herman, L., and Fitzgerald, P. J. (1962). *J. Cell Biol.*, **12,** 297.
92. Hellman, B., Petersson, B., and Hellerström, C. (1964). *The Structure and Metabolism of the Pancreatic Islets*, p. 45. Eds. Brolin, S. E., Hellman, B., and Knutson, H. International Wenner-Gren Symposium. Oxford: Pergamon Press.
93. Lazarus, S. S., and Volk, B. W. (1962). *Clinical Diabetes Mellitus*, p. 107. Eds. Ellenberg, M., and Rifkin, H. New York: Blakiston Division, McGraw-Hill.
94. Berkman, J. I. (1962). *Clinical Diabetes Mellitus*, p. 123. Eds. Ellenberg, M., and Rifkin, H. New York: Blakiston Division, McGraw-Hill.
95. Ribbert, H. (1894). *Arch. EntwMech. Org.*, **1,** 70.
96. Milstein, B. B. (1950). *Brit. J. exp. Path.*, **31,** 664.

97. OLIVER, J. (1939). *Architecture of the Kidney in Chronic Bright's Disease.* New York: Paul. B. Hoeber, Inc.
98. BOHNE, A. W., OSBORN, R. W., and HETTLE, P. J. (1955). *Surg. Gynec. Obstet.*, **100,** 259.
99. NOVAK, E. (1947). *Gynecologic and Obstetric Pathology*, 2nd edit., Chaps. 7, 8, 9. Philadelphia: W. B. Saunders.
100. ALBRIGHT, F. (1933). *New Engl. J. Med.*, **209,** 476.
101. SWINGARD, G. A. (1943). *Anat. Rec.*, **87,** 141.
102. HOERR, N. L. (1931). *Amer. J. Anat.*, **48,** 139.
103. MONTGOMERY, G. L. (1943–44). . *Brit. J. Surg.*, **31,** 292.
104. WILHELM, D. L. (1953). *J. Path. Bact.*, **65,** 543.
105. REID, L. (1967). *The Pathology of Emphysema*, Chaps. 6 and 17. London: Lloyd-Luke.
106. REID, L. (1966). *Development of the Lung*, p. 109. Eds. DE REUCK, A. V. S., and PORTER, R. (Ciba Foundation Symposium.) London: J. & A. Churchill.
107. CAMERON, G. R., and SENEVIRATNE, R. D. (1947). *J. Path. Bact.*, **59,** 665.
108. POCHIN, E. E. (1949). *Clin. Sci.*, **8,** 97.
109. SHANDS, A. R. (1931). *Arch. Surg.*, **22,** 137.
110. HAM, A. W., and LEESON, T. S. (1961). *Histology*, 4th edit. Philadelphia: J. B. Lippincott.
111. HAM, A. W., and HARRIS, W. R. (1956). *The Biochemistry and Physiology of Bone*, p. 475. Ed. BOURNE, G. H. New York: Academic Press.
112. ANDERSON, H. C., and COULTER, P. R. (1967). *J. Cell Biol.*, **33,** 165.
113. COOLEY, L. M., and GOSS, R. J. (1958). *Amer. J. Anat.*, **102,** 167.
114. TONNA, E. A., and CRONKITE, E. P. (1961). *J. Bone Jt. Surg.*, **43A**, 352.
115. BASSETT, C. A. (1964). *Bone Biodynamics*, p. 233. Ed. FROST, H. M. (Henry Ford Hospital Symposium.) London: J. & A. Churchill.
116. DUTHIE, R. B., and BARKER, A. N. (1955). *J. Bone Jt. Surg.*, **37B**, 691.
117. UDUPA, K. N., and PRASAD, G. C. (1963). *J. Bone Jt. Surg.*, **45B**, 770.
118. MACDONALD, N. S., LORICK, P. C., and PETRIELLO, L. I. (1957). *Amer. J. Physiol.*, **191,** 185.
119. PRASAD, G. C., and REYNOLDS, J. J. (1968). *J. Bone Jt. Surg.*, **50B**, 401.
120. BUCK, R. C. (1953). *J. Path. Bact.*, **66**, 1.
121. FIELD, E. J. (1960). *The Structure and Function of Muscle*, Vol. 3, p. 139. Ed. BOURNE, G. H. New York: Academic Press.
122. ADAMS, R. D., DENNY-BROWN, D., and PEARSON, C. M. (1962). *Diseases of Muscle: A Study in Pathology*, 2nd edit, p. 193. London: Henry Kimpton.
123. PEARSON, C. M. (1965). *Muscle:* Proceedings of a Symposium at the University of Alberta, p. 423. Eds. PAUL, W. M., DANIEL, E. E., KAY, C. M., and MONCKTON, G. Oxford: Pergamon Press.
124. ABERCROMBIE, M., and JOHNSON, M. L. (1942). *J. exp. Biol.*, **19**, 226.
125. YOUNG, J. Z. (1942). *Physiol. Rev.*, **22,** 318.
126. PETERSON, E. R., and MURRAY, M. R. (1955). *Amer. J. Anat.*, **96,** 319.
127. TROTTER, W., and DAVIES, H. M. (1909). *J. Physiol.* (*Lond.*), **38,** 135.
128. ROSE, J. E., MALIS, L. I., KRUGER, L., and BAKER, C. P. (1960). *J. comp. Neurol.*, **115,** 243.
129. CLEMENTE, C. D. (1964). *Int. Rev. Neurobiol.*, **6,** 257.

REVIEWS RELATING TO HEALING.

A discussion, with many historical references, of many of the matters dealt with in this chapter can be found in:

CAMERON, G. R. (1952). *Pathology of the Cell.* Edinburgh: Oliver and Boyd.

GENERAL AND WOUND HEALING

EDWARDS, L. C., and DUNPHY, J. E. (1958). Wound Healing. I. Injury and normal repair; II. Injury and abnormal repair. *New Engl. J. Med.*, **259**, 224 and 275.

PATTERSON, W. B., Editor (1959). *Wound Healing and Tissue Repair*. Chicago Univ. Press.

JOHNSON, F. R., and MCMINN, R. M. H. (1960). The cytology of wound healing of body surfaces in mammals. *Biol. Rev.*, **35**, 364. (Includes mucous membranes, lung, etc.).

WEISS, P. (1961). *Harvey Lect.*, **55**, 13.

GOULD, B. S. (1963). *Int. Rev. Cytol.*, **15**, 301. (Collagen formation).

MONTAGNA, W., and BILLINGHAM, R. E., Editors. (1964). *Advances in Biology of Skin. Vol.* 5. *Wound Healing*. Oxford: Pergamon Press.

SCHILLING, J. A. (1968). *Physiol. Rev.*, **48**, 374.

PHYSIOLOGY AND HEALING OF BONE

BOURNE, G. H., Editor (1956). *The Biochemistry and Physiology of Bone*. New York: Academic Press.

MCLEAN, F. C., LACROIX, P., and BUDY, A. M., Editors (1962). *Radioisotopes and Bone*. International Organizations of Medical Sciences Symposium. Oxford: Blackwell Scientific Publications.

FROST, H. M., Editor (1964). *Bone Biodynamics*. (Henry Ford Hospital Symposium.) London: J. & A. Churchill.

BLACKWOOD H. J. J., Editor (1964). *Bone and Tooth*. (First European Symposium.) Oxford: Pergamon Press.

REGENERATION OF LIVER

HARKNESS, R. D. (1957). *Brit. med. Bull.*, **13**, 87.

WEINBREN, K. (1959). *Gastroenterology*, **37**, 657.

BUCHER, N. L. R. (1963). *Int. Rev. Cytol.*, **15**, 245.

FABRIKANT, J. I. (1968). *J. Cell Biol.*, **36**, 551.

Chapter 18

ATHEROSCLEROSIS

By J. E. French

The change in the clinical significance of different diseases which has occurred in recent years is particularly striking in the case of a chronic disorder of the major arteries, known as atherosclerosis. This condition used to be considered a natural consequence of increasing age and appeared to have little effect on the normal life-span. As the life-expectation in the population increases it is obvious that disease of later years will become more prominent, but this is not the only explanation of the present importance of atherosclerosis. There appear to be some other aspects of modern life which are making its clinical effects, particularly as they concern the coronary circulation, much more prevalent than they used to be. When it is pointed out that the effects of atherosclerosis are now at least as important as the tumours or the bacterial infections as a cause of death in this country, it becomes clear that some attempt must be made to understand the pathological basis of the lesions, and if possible to explain them in terms of disordered function.

Definition and Morphology of Atherosclerosis

Atherosclerosis affects the intima of the aorta and the larger distributing arteries. It takes the form of focal thickenings or plaques of fibrous and fatty material, which often encroach on the lumen of the vessel and, particularly when complicated by thrombosis, may lead to impairment of the arterial circulation and ischæmia in the tissues supplied. This descriptive definition serves to distinguish atherosclerosis from the other types of chronic arterial change, which occur in the smaller arteries in hypertension (diffuse hyperplastic sclerosis) or in the media of certain muscular arteries (medial or Mönckeberg's sclerosis). Thus as now used the term *atherosclerosis* is not synonymous with *arteriosclerosis*, which should be used only in a generic sense to include the three types of arterial change. The term *atheroma*, some times used as a synonym for atherosclerosis, is more satisfactorily used as a descriptive term for advanced atherosclerotic lesions in which the fatty element predominates.

The lesions of atherosclerosis are most common in the aorta, where they range from flat, or only slightly elevated, yellow spots or streaks to large raised greyish yellow nodules or plaques. As the lesions advance, they become confluent and may be ulcerated at the surface, partly calcified or complicated by hæmorrhage and thrombosis (Fig. 1). The names fatty streak, fibrous plaque and complicated lesion are given to these various appearances[1]; they may represent successive stages in a single process, but there is some doubt whether the fatty streak is necessarily the precursor of the fibrous plaque. Similar lesions are often widespread in the main branches of the aorta where, on account of the smaller lumen of the vessels, they may appear in cross-section as crescentic or

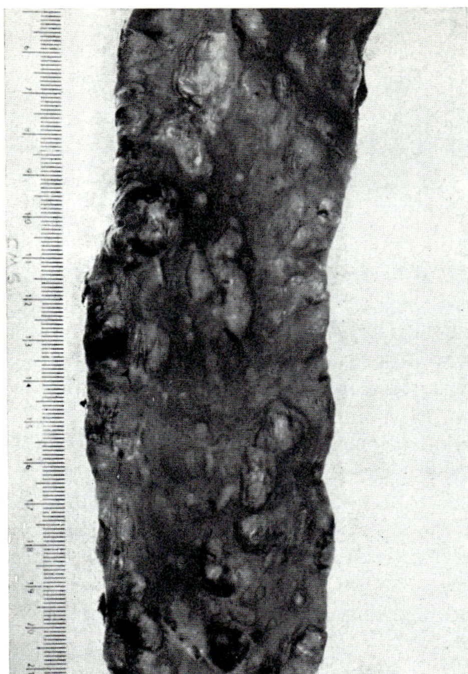

18/Fig. 1.—Advanced atherosclerosis of the human aorta.

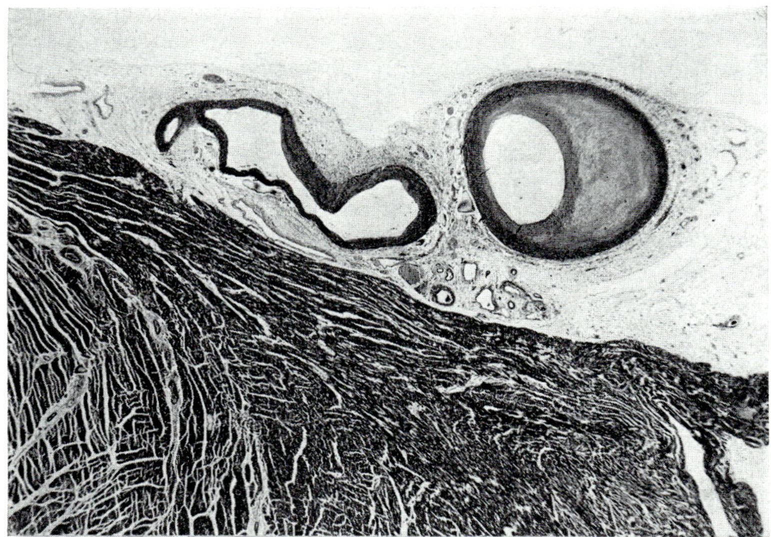

18/Fig. 2.—An atherosclerotic plaque causing narrowing of the lumen in a human coronary artery. ×9.

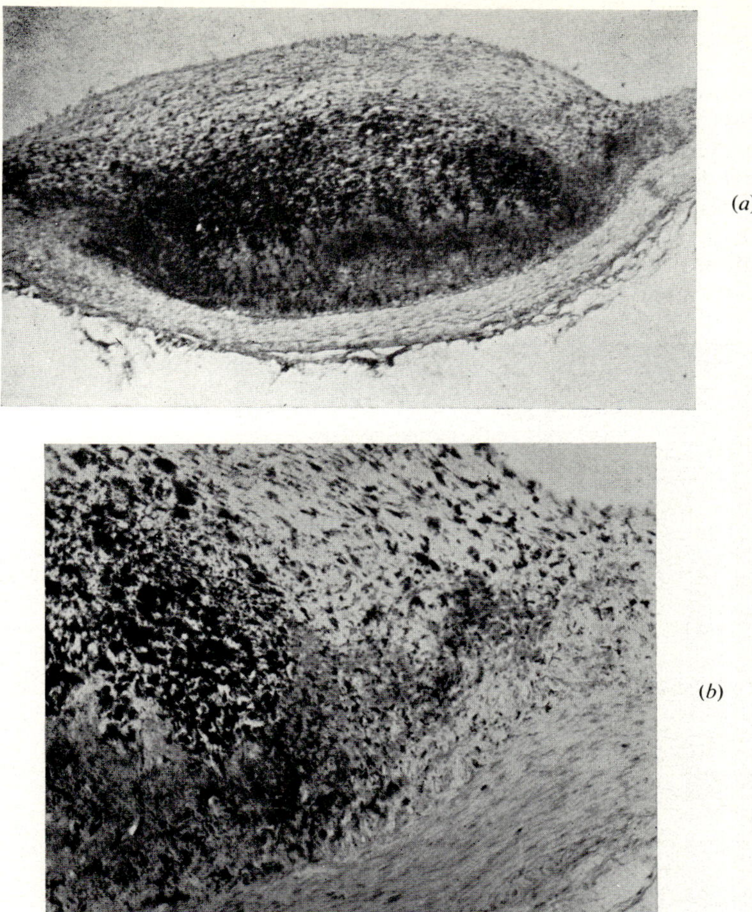

18/FIG. 3.—An atherosclerotic plaque in a coronary artery. The dark areas show the distribution of lipids in discrete macrophages and in amorphous debris at the base of the lesion. The pale zone near the endothelial surface is predominantly fibrous tissue. Hæmatoxylin and Sudan IV. (*a*) ×26. (*b*) ×60.

ring-like thickenings of the intima (FIG. 2). The impairment of the arterial circulation caused by these lesions has important clinical effects at three main sites in the body: the heart, the brain and the lower limbs.

The microscopic appearances of a typical raised plaque are illustrated in FIG. 3. The main features, either of which may predominate, are proliferation of fibro-elastic tissue and accumulation of lipids in the intima. The fibrous tissue is usually most prominent in the superficial layers where it may show extensive hyaline degeneration and sometimes zones of fibrinoid necrosis. The lipid occurs more deeply in the intima, often as a central pultaceous mass of necrotic material and free fat which contains visible cholesterol crystals (*athêrê* = porridge or gruel). The fatty material is mostly cholesterol and its esters, but it also contains some phospholipid and a variable amount of glyceride. Calcification is common in the more advanced lesions. There is usually some fraying and fragmentation of the internal elastic lamina, and when the lesions are advanced there is often thinning and fibrosis of the media and an in-growth of blood vessels from the vasa vasorum into the base of the plaque. The adventitia may also appear fibrotic and show infiltration by small round cells, presumably lymphocytes.

In the fatty streak, the lipid is more superficial and is found mostly in the cytoplasm of macrophages or smooth muscle cells; the tunica media underlying the fatty streak shows very little apparent change.

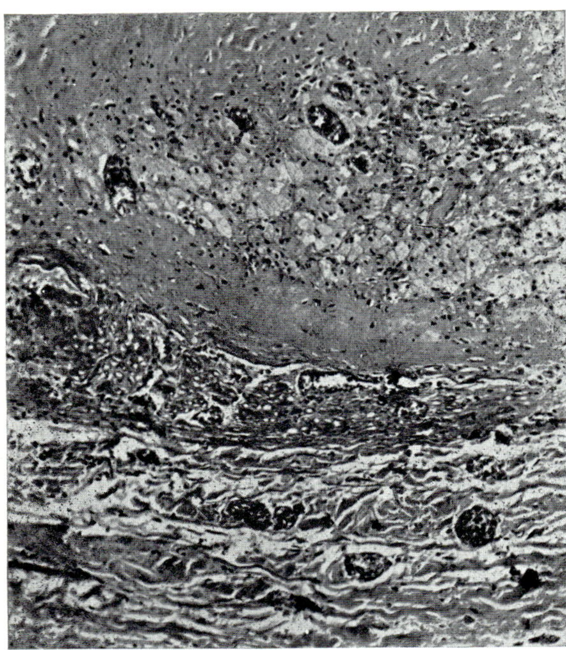

18/FIG. 4.—Blood vessels growing into the base of an atherosclerotic plaque from the vasa vasorum in the media of a coronary artery. ×100. (From Geiringer.[3])

Secondary Changes in Atherosclerosis

When an intimal plaque has become established its subsequent development is influenced by two processes, usually considered to be of a secondary nature. These are hæmorrhage into the intima and thrombosis.

Intimal hæmorrhage.—The vessels which grow into the base of the plaque from the vasa vasorum are often poorly supported by the degenerate intimal connective tissue (FIG. 4), so that injury to them from the functional movements of the arteries may lead to hæmorrhage. The iron pigment, which is frequently found in the plaques, is usually a relic from these episodes. In advanced lesions, capillaries may also be present in the superficial parts of the plaques. Injection studies have shown that some of these vessels are in direct continuity with the arterial lumen, so that they are probably exposed to a high pressure which makes them particularly liable to rupture.[2] Blood may also infiltrate directly from the lumen into the plaque if there is a break in the endothelium covering a necrotic part of the intima. Hæmorrhages occurring in any of these ways will contribute to the accumulation of debris in the intima and, when extensive, may cause occlusion of the lumen or possibly initiate thrombosis.[3]

Thrombosis.—The formation of arterial thrombi in relation to atherosclerotic plaques has been discussed in Chapter 9. If the formation of an occluding thrombus in atherosclerosis is compatible with survival its subsequent organisation or recanalisation brings about a marked change in the character of the lesion. Thus segments of an artery may be found in the heart or lower limbs in which the lumen is completely obliterated by organised thrombus or in which a drastically reduced lumen is the end result of recanalisation. The formation of non-occluding or mural thrombi in atherosclerosis also has very significant effects. Duguid,[4] by examining serial sections of the coronary arteries, has reached the conclusion that mural thrombi form very commonly over the intimal plaques in these vessels. As the thrombi are organised and covered with endothelium they become in effect part of the plaque and may be no longer distinguishable from it. The process can be repeated, so that by successive steps of mural thrombosis and organisation the thickened intima causes extreme narrowing of the lumen (FIG. 5). In these various ways the occurrence of thrombosis has a major role in the development of occlusive and stenotic lesions in the arteries and in determining the effect of the lesions on the circulation; indeed, it has been argued that in the absence of thrombosis, degenerative changes in the wall of an artery are more likely to lead to dilation than to narrowing of the arterial lumen.[5]

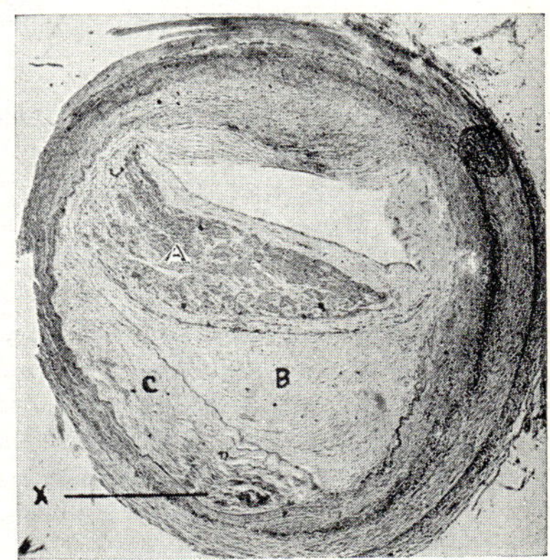

18/FIG. 5.—Atherosclerosis of a coronary artery showing the incorporation of three successive mural thrombi in the thickened intima. ×18. (From Duguid.[4])

Prevalence of Atherosclerosis

Atherosclerosis is not a new disorder. Although there is no clear account of the condition in medical literature before the 17th century, arterial fragments which have survived in Egyptian mummies dating from 1580 B.C. to A.D. 525 show that the condition was apparently prevalent in ancient Egypt. One of the earliest written accounts is a description of the aorta of a famous doctor, J. J. Wepfer, who died in 1695 at the age of 75. His aorta (FIG. 6) contained bone-like plaques throughout and "the internal coat in several places was ruptured, lacerated and rotten". More detailed descriptions appeared in the standard

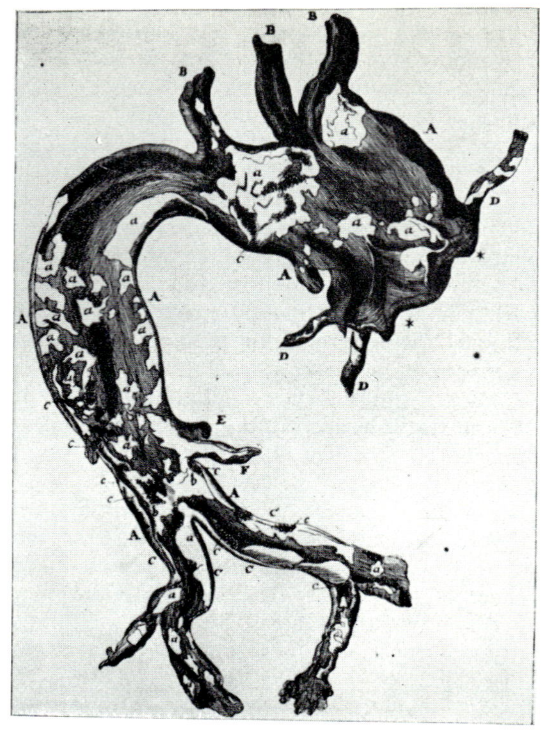

A.A.A.A. *Aortæ inciſæ & apertæ tota interior facies conſpicitur.*
* * *Ejuſdem exortus.*
B.B.B. *Arteriæ caput petentes, ſeu carotidum &c. exortus.*
C.C.C. *Arteriæ iliacæ.*
D.D.D. *Coronariæ arteriæ.*
E. *Arteria cæliaca.*
F. *Arteria renalis ſeu emulgens.*
a.a.a.a.a.a.a.a. *Oſſea ſubſtantia Aortæ per portiones incertæ figuræ & magnitudinis hinc inde conſpicuas.*
b.b.b.b. *Circulus ejuſdem plane oſſeus.*
c.c.c.c. *Tunica interior lacera atque fracida, obſcuri coloris, non citra ruptionis periculum.*

18/FIG. 6.—The aorta of Johann Jakob Wepfer (deceased 1695). This illustration appears in the posthumous edition of his *Observationes Medico-Practicæ de Affectibus Capitis Internis et Externis* (1727).

works on pathological anatomy published in the 18th and 19th centuries. Edward Jenner in the early 1770s first noticed the relationship between coronary sclerosis and the symptoms of angina pectoris, and Cruveilhier in 1850 observed that the lesions could lead to thrombosis and obliteration of the arterial lumen.

Post-mortem data.—At the present time atherosclerosis is particularly common in countries which have a high living standard. Reliable information about the prevalence of the lesions has to be obtained from post-mortem reports rather than from morbidity or mortality statistics since, as will be discussed below, there is no straightforward relationship between the extent or severity of the lesions and their clinical effects. The fatty streaking may be seen frequently in the posterior wall of the aorta in childhood and by the age of 20 some evidence of atherosclerosis can always be found on careful inspection of the aorta. Visible lesions in the coronary arteries may develop later than in the aorta but are also frequently present at an early age. For example, among 300 American soldiers, with an average age of 22 years, who were killed in the Korean War, there was gross evidence of coronary atherosclerosis in 77 per cent.[6] In this country an attempt has been made by Morris and his colleagues[7] to estimate from post-mortem data the extent and severity of coronary atherosclerosis in the population as a whole. The results for men between the ages of 60 and 64 are summarised in Table I. It can be seen that by the early sixties close to 100 per

18/TABLE I

ESTIMATED PREVALENCE OF CORONARY ATHEROSCLEROSIS IN BRITAIN

Males (ages 60–64)

Post-mortem Data	*Rates per cent.*	
Visible atherosclerosis in the coronary arteries		100 (approx.)
Widespread confluent lesions in the coronary arteries	25	
Visible narrowing of a main coronary artery		33
Occlusion of a main coronary artery	15	
Clinical Data		
Deaths from ischaemic heart disease per annum		0·6–0·8
New clinical cases, per annum		1·5
Prevalence of clinical disease		10

(By courtesy of Prof. J. N. Morris)

cent of males in the population have coronary atherosclerosis which is visible to the naked eye. In general, lesions are less extensive in women than in men, particularly in the younger age groups.

It is commonly assumed that the prevalence of the *lesions* has increased since the beginning of the century, but reliable information on this point is extremely difficult to obtain. Even when the most careful post-mortem records have been kept by an unbiased observer it is hazardous to make direct comparisons in the absence of any standardised grading procedure. Nevertheless we can at least be sure that atherosclerosis of the coronary arteries was common fifty years ago. At the London Hospital during the years 1907–14 Turnbull made a special study of arterial disease and kept careful records of the state of the coronary arteries in all patients examined post-mortem. These records have been reviewed by Morris.[8] He came to the conclusion that widespread atherosclerosis of the coronary arteries was at least as common then as it is now. However, during the course of these investigations it was recognised that a distinction could be made between cases in which there was severe narrowing or occlusion of the lumen of the coronary arteries and cases in which there was little effect on the lumen even though lesions in the arterial wall were severe. When this was done a significantly greater prevalence of the occlusive type of lesion was found now than there was in Turnbull's series.[9]

Comparisons of the current prevalence and extent of atherosclerotic lesions in the populations of different countries or racial groups can be made provided that the techniques of post-mortem examination and grading of the lesions are standardised. Several reports of this type have been published and attempts are being made to carry out systematic studies on a world-wide scale.[10] It is already clear that intimal lesions of some kind are always present in the aorta and main arteries, regardless of race or geographical location. Fatty streaking is remarkably constant in younger age groups; however, there are marked quantitative differences in the extent of raised plaques and complicated lesions, particularly as they affect the coronary arteries. Advanced coronary atherosclerosis is, not surprisingly, most widespread in communities which have a high mortality from ischæmic heart disease, but it is noteworthy that raised lesions in the aorta are quite common in communities such as the South African Bantu or Jamaican Negro which have little clinical disease that can be attributed to the effects of atherosclerosis.

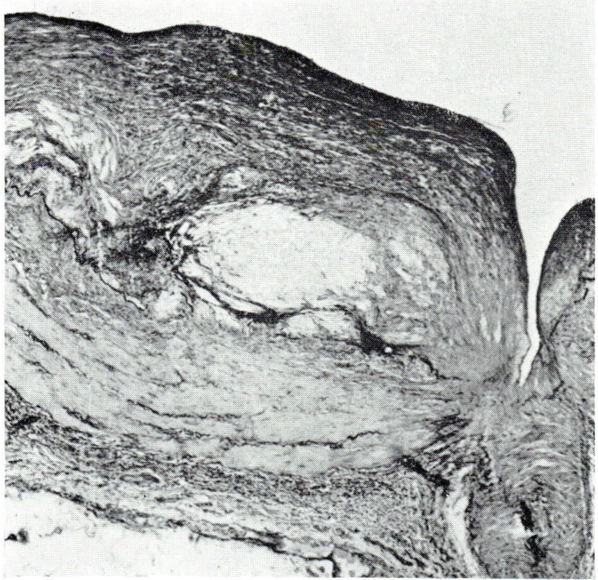

18/Fig. 7.—Intimal lesion near the orifice of a branch in the left coronary artery of a pig aged 8 years. The thickened intima contains much collagen and elastic tissue. The pale areas contain foam cells and crystal clefts possibly indicating the start of atheromatous softening. Weigerts' elastin and van Gieson × 63. (From French *et al.*[12]).

Lesions which resemble *advanced* atherosclerosis in man are very rare or do not occur at all in other mammals. Intimal thickenings which are predominantly fibrous have been described in the arteries of many of the larger mammals and these may be more extensive if the animals survive to old age. Lesions which contain histologically demonstrable fat, and in this respect resemble more closely the uncomplicated lesions in man, occur in non-human primates and have been described in some detail in the baboon and squirrel monkey.[11] Domestic pigs which have been kept to a relatively old age develop lesions of the intima of the aorta and coronary arteries which are very similar to the raised plaques in human arteries[12] (FIG. 7). Fatty plaques are more common in the aortæ of birds; in certain breeds of pigeons such lesions may ulcerate and develop thrombi on their surface so that they bear a very close resemblance to the more advanced lesions in man.[13]

Clinical Data

It has already been mentioned that the clinical effects of atherosclerosis are more prevalent than they used to be. The changes are most striking in the case of ischæmic heart disease. Before the First World War coronary disease was considered a clinical rarity, but since 1917 it has been recognised with increasing frequency. This is shown in the Registrar-General's returns of causes of death, which indicate that in Britain coronary disease as a cause of death has increased by fifteen or more times. The increase is in part explained by the changing age constitution of the population, and by greater accuracy in diagnosis or certification of death; but when all these factors are taken into account the changes still appear highly significant. The figures for recent years, which are shown in Table II, indicate that the increase is still continuing. In the younger age-groups the increase is more marked in males than in females.

18/TABLE II

MORTALITY FROM ISCHAEMIC HEART DISEASE IN ENGLAND AND WALES

Death rate per 100,000

	Males			*Females*		
Age	1941–45	1951–55	1961–65	1941–45	1951–55	1961–65
35–44	14·6	31·6	56·7	2·5	4·5	7·9
45–54	71·0	154·1	225·1	13·6	26·6	36·1
55–64	201·0	463·2	650·2	58·2	131·7	173·8

(Data from the Registrar-General's Reports provided by Prof. J. N. Morris.)

The Relationship of Clinical Disease to Atherosclerotic Lesions

The lesions of atherosclerosis may be well marked without giving rise to any clinical disease. This is illustrated for the coronary arteries in Table I, where it can be seen that a majority of the middle-aged men who have widespread coronary atherosclerosis do not suffer from ischæmic heart disease.

Because it is mainly the occlusive type of lesion which has clinical effects the key factor in the development of clinical disease is often thrombosis. However, the occurrence of thrombosis cannot be related simply to the overall extent of the lesions; it may be absent when lesions are widespread, or present when lesions are relatively few, and it is likely to be influenced by independent factors among which a thrombotic tendency in the blood is considered important. Moreover, when thrombosis does occur the degree of ischæmia may still depend on the exact site and on the availability of a collateral circulation. It can be seen from Table I that even when occlusive lesions are present in the coronary arteries they are not invariably associated with clinical disease.

The relationship between clinical disease and the pathological lesions is therefore much less straightforward than it is in many disease states and it is important to keep this in mind when considering the clinical problem. In this chapter the pathogenesis of the *lesions* will be discussed, but it will be seen that the discussion of arterial thrombosis and its effects in Chapter 9 is equally relevant to an understanding of the clinical effects of atherosclerosis.

THE PATHOGENESIS OF THE LESIONS IN ATHEROSCLEROSIS

Several hypotheses have been put forward which seek to explain in terms of a single pathological process the march of events which transforms the normal arteries of childhood to the diseased arteries of later life. It has been suggested that mechanical wear and tear; infiltration of materials from the lumen; incorporation of surface deposits; or metabolic disturbances in the wall itself may be the cause of atherosclerosis. However, none of these various hypotheses has gained universal acceptance and on closer scrutiny does not appear to include all the known facts. For the present it seems best to consider that all these processes contribute in varying degree to the development of the lesions and to keep an open mind about their order of priority.

These processes will be discussed separately, but in subdividing the subject in this way it must be kept in mind that there are many points at which the different processes interact. It will also be necessary to consider certain special features of the structure of arteries which are relevant to the problems of pathology and to discuss in rather more detail the chemical changes which occur in the arteries as lesions develop.

The Normal Arterial Wall

A diagram illustrating the main structural features of the human aorta is shown in Fig. 8. The intima, comprising about one-sixth of the thickness of the wall, consists of a network of fibro-elastic tissue supported in a mucinous ground substance. On its inner surface it is covered by a single continuous layer of flattened endothelial cells. The elastic fibres are coarser in the deeper parts of the intima where they mingle with some muscle fibres and give a poorly defined inner edge to the internal elastic lamina. This intimal connective tissue develops during infancy and childhood and its growth is probably completed by early adult life. At birth there is only a narrow zone of ground substance between the endothelium and the internal elastic lamina, but thereafter a progressive separation of the two layers occurs by the formation of new collagen and elastic fibres.

Similar changes are observed in the intima of the larger distributing arteries during growth and are particularly marked in the coronary arteries. During

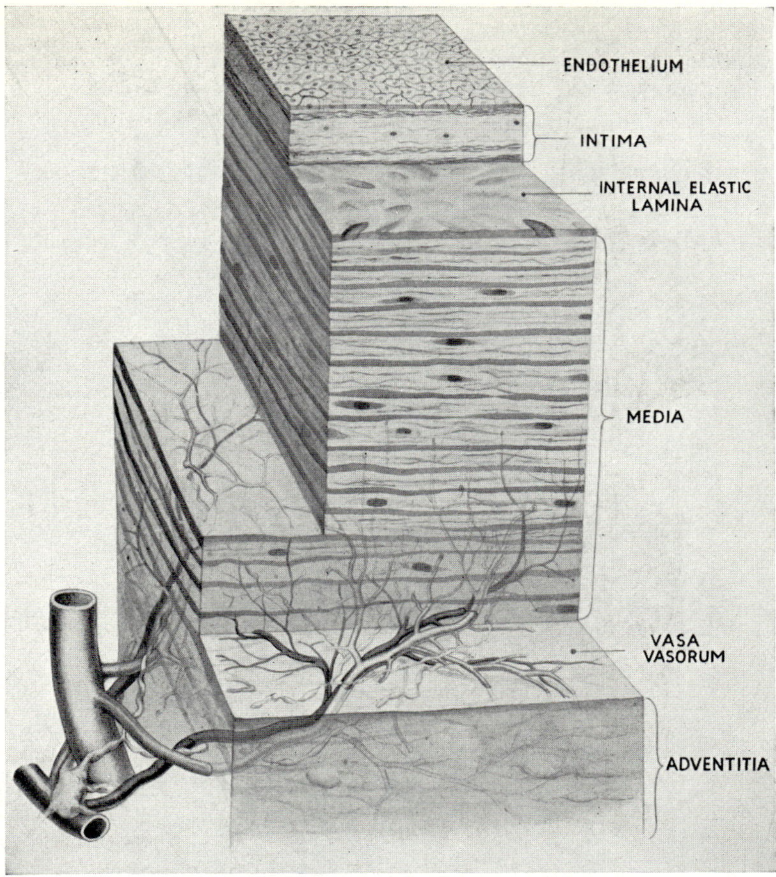

18/FIG. 8.—A diagram of the wall of the human aorta showing the relative thickness of the three coats and the distribution of blood vessels and lymphatics.

childhood there is apparently a penetration by smooth muscle cells of the space between endothelium and internal elastic lamina to form a so-called musculo-elastic layer in the intima. This occurs first in relation to the orifices of proximal branches but later extends widely to form a substantial part of the total thickness of the wall. An elastic hyperplastic layer, composed of circularly directed elastic fibres with relatively few cells among them, then forms on the lumenal side of the musculo-elastic layer. Finally in the third decade an additional connective tissue layer is formed immediately beneath the endothelium.

This thickening of the intima in the larger arteries is usually considered to be a normal growth process, but it is often not possible to distinguish it clearly from early pathological changes. Thus the focal areas of increased thickening seen in the intima of the coronary and cerebral arteries and the aorta even in infancy have a striking similarity in distribution to the atherosclerotic lesions of later life. It can at least be said that the thickening of the intima "sets the scene" for the subsequent development of arterial disease. A distinct sub-endothelial layer also develops in the tunica intima during growth in the arteries of many other large animals but is normally inconspicuous in the smaller laboratory animals. The detailed structure of the intima of the coronary arteries of the pig

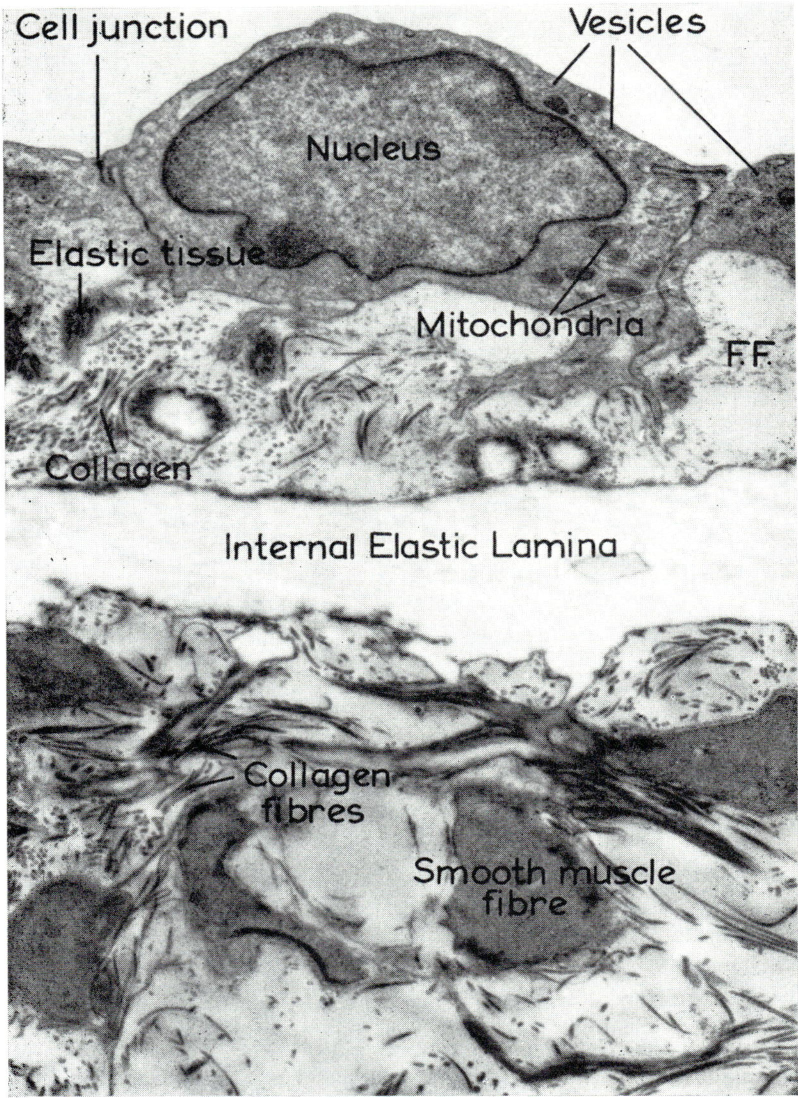

18/Fig. 9.—Coronary artery of a young pig. The endothelial cells are closely apposed at their junctions. The cytoplasm contains mitochondria and the so-called pinocytic vesicles. In the subendothelial space are collagen, elastic and other fine fibres (FF). The inner part of the media is seen below a clearly defined internal elastic lamina. (× 17,500.) (From Florey.[15])

as seen by electron microscopy at different ages is illustrated in FIGS. 9 and 10. (For review on the structure of the intima see French[14]).

There are no capillary vessels in the inner part of the wall of normal arteries. In the relatively thin-walled aortas of small mammals, such as the rat or rabbit, the vasa vasorum are more or less confined to the tunica adventitia, and in larger mammals, including man, the media of the aorta is only partly vascularised. The factors which determine the width of the avascular gap between the endothelium and the vasa vasorum are not fully understood, but it seems probable that the most important factor is the pressure gradient which exists across the arterial wall, and prevents the ingress of vessels beyond a critical depth. In the human aorta, this lies at about the junction of the inner and middle thirds of the media. Lymphatic plexuses occur in the adventitial coat of the arteries and probably penetrate for some distance into the media of the aorta in large mammals, but from consideration of the pressure factors, it seems unlikely that they penetrate as far towards the lumen as do the blood capillaries.

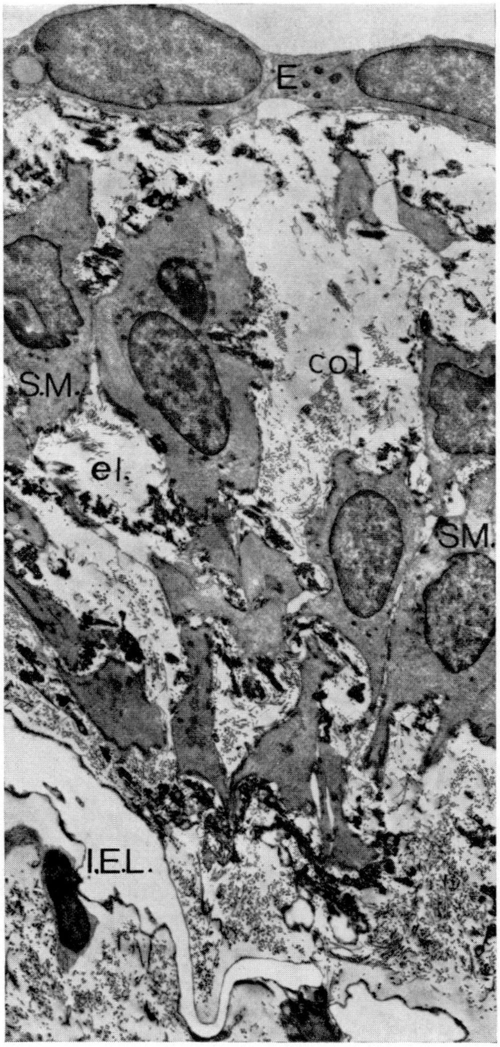

18/FIG. 10.—Coronary artery of an 8-year-old pig showing the full thickness of the intima 2 cm. from the origin of the vessel. The space between endothelium (E) and an interrupted internal elastic lamina (I.E.L.) contains several layers of smooth muscle cells (SM), collagen fibres (col) and densely stained fragments of elastin. Electron micrograph × 5,000. (From French.[14])

The inner part of the wall of large arteries therefore presents a unique situation with regard to nutrition and lymph drainage. Nutrition depends on the blood in the lumen of the artery itself and on the blood in the vasa vasorum, with a somewhat precarious balance between the two sources. Thus diffusion from the lumen appears to be adequate to compensate for the lack of capillaries in the intima and inner media in normal arteries but when the wall becomes thickened with ageing or in disease there is likely to be an intermediate zone of impaired nutrition unless adequate adaptive changes occur in the distribution of the vasa vasorum.[16]

The permeability properties of arterial endothelium appear to be similar to those of capillary endothelium in allowing a slow leakage of large molecules. The staining of the inner part of the arterial wall which occurs when colloidal dyes such as trypan blue are introduced into the blood stream was until recently the main evidence that substances could enter the intima by passing across the endothelium from the lumen, but more precise information on the ability of protein and lipoprotein molecules to enter the intima from the lumen has now been obtained from experiments in which the concentration gradient across the wall can be measured by isotope labelling or immuno-chemical methods.[17,18] Observations by electron microscopy on the distribution of "marker particles" in the arterial wall also confirm that molecules with the dimensions of plasma proteins can enter the sub-endothelial space from the lumen[18a] (FIG. 11).

There is little detailed information about the mechanism of lymph drainage in the arterial wall but it appears that protein molecules, which in other tissues are rapidly returned to the blood via the lymph, must be able to diffuse through

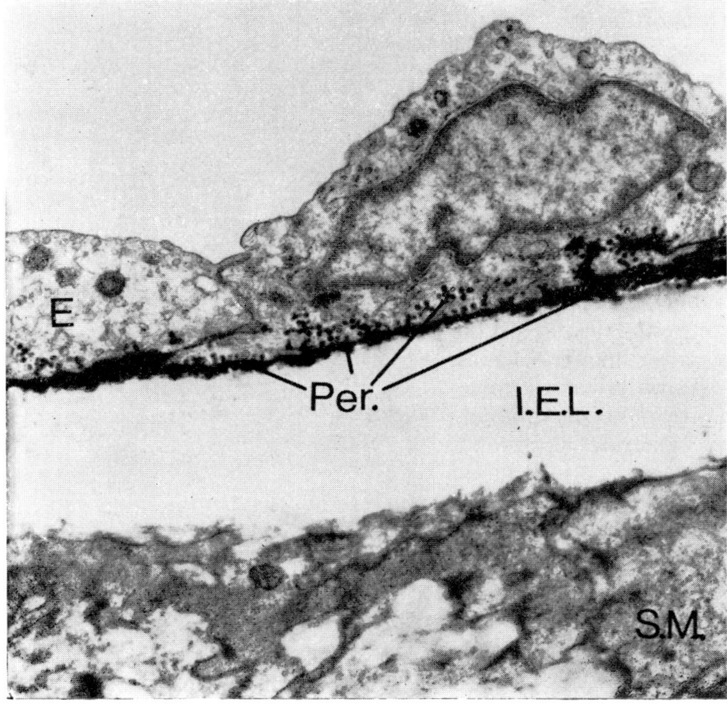

18/FIG. 11.—Aorta of a rat injected intravenously with horseradish peroxidase (M.W. 40,000) 10 minutes previously. The localisation of a dense reaction product shows that the enzyme protein (Per) had entered the space between endothelium (E) and the unstained internal elastic lamina (I.E.L.) from the lumen. Electron micrograph × 16,000.

the ground substance of the relatively broad avascular zone and through several lamellæ of elastic tissue to reach the lymphatics if they are not to be trapped in the wall.

The tunica media of the aorta and distributing arteries, consisting of elastic and collagenous tissue and smooth muscle, maintains a tension which opposes the expansive force of the blood pressure and acts as a shock absorber for the circulation. It is important to realise that the actual stretching force in the wall is proportional to the radius of the artery as well as to the blood pressure, and is therefore much greater in large vessels than in small. It follows that the main arteries of large animals sustain a degree of wall tension which is not normally encountered in small animals; in man, the tangential stretching force in the wall of the aorta is probably a hundred or more times greater than that in the arterioles.[19] In general, arteries are so constructed that these tensile forces are distributed uniformly through the wall and are balanced by structural adaptations which involve principally the tunica media. In the aorta in man, for example, there are 58 medial elastic laminæ compared with only 20 in the much smaller aorta of the rabbit.[20]

In addition to the effect of the blood pressure there are local factors which may influence the tension in an arterial wall. There will be variations in tension at curves, and increases at points where the lumen widens, for example at bifurcations. Longitudinal stretching of the aorta, which may occur with the pulse wave, will impose a strain at the point of attachment of side branches. It is possible also that eddies or turbulent flow at particular points in the circulation or shearing forces may impose a localised strain on the arterial wall.[21]

The resistance of the arteries to the various stretching forces changes with age. This is due in part to an increase in the amount of collagenous tissue in the media, but also to degenerative changes in the elastic tissue. Histological evidence of the ageing of elastic tissue is seen in fragmentation or granulation of the fibres, particularly in the region of the internal elastic lamina. When elastic tissue is extracted from the aorta and examined chemically it is found that its calcium content increases with age and there are changes in its amino-acid composition.[22] The effect of these changes in the artery as a whole is a weakening of the initial resistance to stretch, and a marked reduction in the range of extensibility. In old age the arteries may appear to be fixed in a dilated state and quite rigid from the overgrowth of collagenous tissue.

Chemical Constituents of Normal and Diseased Arteries

The prominence of fatty material in many atherosclerotic arteries, which has long been recognised by histological methods, has led to the view that this material must play a key role in the pathogenesis of the lesions. As a result chemical research into atherosclerosis has been very largely concerned with the study of lipids. This line of investigation has been further stimulated in recent years by the considerable advances in the techniques of lipid analysis. That comparable interest has not been taken in other constituents that may be important in pathogenesis, such as the mucopolysaccharides of the arterial wall, can in part be attributed to this pre-occupation with the lipids; although again it is only recently that precise analytical methods for mucopolysaccharides have become available.

Lipids

The aorta has been used most often for chemical studies because a single specimen provides enough material for analysis and it is possible to separate intima from media or lesions from normal areas and to analyse them separately. With small arteries, bulked material from several specimens may be needed for a complete analysis and, because of the technical problem of separating the intima precisely, it is usually preferable to use a combined sample of intima and media, even though this may obscure changes which are restricted to the intima. Böttcher and his colleagues[23] in Leiden have undertaken an extensive series of investigations in which the overall lipid composition of such combined samples from the coronary arteries, from the circle of Willis, and from intima: media preparations of the aorta, has been determined at different stages in the development of atherosclerotic lesions (Table III). The most striking increase in lipid

18/Table III

Lipids of the Arterial Wall in Atherosclerosis

Site	*Aorta*		*Coronary Arteries*		*Circle of Willis*	
Stage of disease	0–I	II–III	0–I	II–III	0–I	II–III
Weight of lipid analysed (mg.) per preparation	20–60	200–2000	5–20	15–75	10–15	20–60
Lipids as percentage of dry weight (mean):	4	13	15	19	16	20
Percentage composition of lipids (mean):						
Phospholipids	58	33	31	24	58	37
Free fatty acids	8	2	11	3	6	4
Cholesterol	10	19	19	20	9	15
Cholesteryl esters	9	36	15	42	7	28
Glycerides	15	10	27	12	20	16

(By courtesy of Prof. C. J. F. Böttcher)

content with the development of atherosclerosis occurs in the aorta where, in advanced disease, the total lipid content of the intima and media may be increased to ten or more times the normal value. The increase occurs mainly, but not entirely, in the intima and especially in areas with visible lesions; it is responsible for most of the increase in the dry weight of the aorta that occurs as lesions develop. Cholesteryl esters, and to a lesser extent free cholesterol, are the principal components of this added lipid but there is a significant, though relatively smaller, increase in phospholipids and glycerides. It has been found consistently that the increase in phospholipids is accompanied by a change in the proportion of the different phospholipids with a notable increase in the amount of the sphingomyelins. The same general trends are followed in the other arteries that have been examined. In the coronary arteries, the increase in the lipid content as the lesions develop is relatively less than it is in the aorta and it is responsible for a smaller proportion of the increase in the dry weight. The lipid content of normal coronary arteries is relatively high with a particularly large amount of glyceride, though this observation might be misleading because of the difficulty of removing the adventitia completely.

In these analyses of total aortic lipids, particular attention was given to the fatty acids in the cholesteryl esters and phospholipids. A striking increase was observed in the percentage of polyunsaturated acids in the cholesteryl esters as the lesions develop, while changes in the phospholipid fatty acids were in the opposite direction, namely towards a greater degree of saturation. The latter was largely explained by the increase in sphingomyelins, which characteristically contain a high percentage of long chain saturated fatty acids. With the developmet of techniques for the analysis of much smaller samples of tissue it is becoming clear, however, that these overall changes in the lipid content of the aorta represent a combined effect of changes in normal intima with ageing and the more localised changes in the lesions themselves. There are, moreover, quite significant differences in the lipid composition of lesions of different morphological type.[24, 25, 26]

All the lipid components (free and esterified cholesterol, phospholipids and glycerides) of the normal aortic intima increase steadily after the age of ten years. In the young child virtually all the cholesterol is in the unesterified form and there is a relatively high amount of phospholipid which even at this age contains a distinctively high proportion of sphingolipids. With increasing age, cholesteryl esters, which were initially the smallest component, show the greatest rate of increase. Cholesteryl linoleate increases greatly so that the esters come to resemble those of the low density lipoproteins in the plasma.

Fatty lesions, in which the stainable lipid is mainly intracellular, contain at all ages more lipid than the normal parts of the intima and there are notable differences in the detailed composition; there is a much higher proportion of oleic acid in the cholesteryl esters and relatively more lecithin in the phospholipids. In fibrous plaques there is also an increase in lipid content compared with "normal" parts of the intima. The cholesteryl esters predominate; but in contrast to the esters in the fatty streak, they contain a high proportion of linoleic acid and so resemble those in the macroscopically normal parts of the adjoining intima. In an atheroma, i.e. an advanced lesion in which there is a central core of pultaceous lipid, the lipid pattern is broadly similar to that of a fibrous plaque but there is an apparent increase in free cholesterol at the expense of cholesteryl ester, and the sphingolipids may increase to 70 per cent of the total phospholipid present.

It may be premature to draw firm conclusions from these complex lipid analyses but they are at least consistent with certain proposals which have been made concerning the accumulation of lipids in the arteries. Thus the changes which occur in normal intima with ageing and in a more pronounced form in the fibrous plaque could be accounted for by the infiltration and retention of low density plasma lipoproteins. In more advanced lesions the lipid composition may be modified by metabolic changes (for example, hydrolysis of cholesteryl esters) occurring within the plaque. Finally, the lipids of the fatty streak are so different from those in other types of lesion as to suggest that these lesions may develop by a separate mechanism.

Mucopolysaccharide and Glycoproteins

The ground substance, which fills the spaces between the cells and fibres, provides the pathway by which nutrients and the plasma filtrate pass through the arterial wall. This has suggested that the physico-chemical properties of this material and the changes which occur in it with ageing or in disease may have an important bearing on certain features of the atherosclerotic lesion. The main approach to the study of the ground substance has been through the use of histochemical staining methods to detect the presence of acid mucopolysaccharides and glycoproteins; as techniques are developed for the extraction and separation of the various components more attention is being given to quantitative chemical analysis (for review see Muir[27]).

It had been suggested by the histochemical studies that a marked increase in the mucopolysaccharide content of the arteries was associated with atherosclerosis. This has not been confirmed by quantitative chemical analyses and the more significant changes now appear to be in the relative proportions of the different components and in the way in which they are bound to protein rather than in their overall concentration. The main acid mucopolysaccharide (glycosaminoglycan*) components to be characterised in the human arterial wall are: hyaluronic acid; heparitin (heparan) sulphate; chondroitin sulphate B (dermatan sulphate); and chondroitin sulphate C (chondroitin 6-sulphate). The highest total concentration, expressed as a percentage of the dry weight of defatted tissue, is found in the intima and remains fairly constant with increasing age, but in all the main arteries the general trend with age is a fall in the proportion of hyaluronic acid and a rise in the proportion of chondroitin sulphates. These age changes appear to be more advanced in the aorta and coronaries than in the peripheral arteries and to be accelerated in association with hypertension.[28]

The distribution of the individual acid mucopolysaccharides and their relationship to atherosclerosis has been studied in some detail in the aorta where it is possible to excise the different types of lesion and analyse them separately.[29] Compared with surrounding apparently normal intimal tissue the total concentration of acid mucopolysaccharides is slightly raised in fatty streaks, slightly reduced in fibrous plaques and markedly reduced in calcified or ulcerated lesions. The proportion of chondroitin sulphate B remains fairly constant at all stages of the disease, but the ratio of hyaluronic acid to chondroitin sulphate C falls in the different types of lesion (as, indeed, it does in the normal intima with advancing age). Heparitin sulphate reaches its highest relative concentration in the fatty streaks; the value is significantly lower in fibrous plaques and complicated lesions.

This line of investigation is likely to develop further in the future. At present it is possibly only to draw attention to some of the ways in which these changes in the mucopolysaccharide composition could be significant in the processes leading to atherosclerosis. The molecular complexes of which hyaluronic acid and chondroitin sulphate form a part probably have a regulatory function on

* The more recent nomenclature is shown in brackets.

transport of fluid and solutes in the arterial wall, since it is known from *in vitro* studies that these complexes can restrict the passage of water and have a sieving effect through their ability to retard the movement of other large molecules.[30] Chondroitin sulphate C is more effective in restricting transport than is hyaluronic acid so that a change in their relative concentration could be associated with differences in the ease with which metabolites and large molecules pass through the wall. Moreover, as chondroitin sulphates can bind calcium and, under appropriate conditions, can precipitate low-density lipoproteins or fibrinogen from solution, they may well play a role in the retention of such materials.[31] Heparitin sulphate, from its relationship to heparin, may have a protective role in the intima when present in normal concentration by prevention of fibrin formation or by activation of clearing factor lipase.

Reactions of the Intima to Injury

The connective tissue in the intima of arteries may increase in response to a variety of stimuli. This occurs, apparently as a physiological process, during the growth of large arteries and during the obliteration of the ductus arteriosus and umbilical artery at birth. There is an increase also when arteries are deprived of their blood flow by ligation.

The proliferation which occurs in atherosclerosis has usually been interpreted as a reparative process analogous to the proliferation of connective tissue in response to injury at other sites in the body. There are however some unusual features in the proliferation of intimal connective tissue. Typical fibroblasts are inconspicuous, and it appears that the smooth muscle cells, which increase in number in the thickened intima,[32] are capable of elaborating the extracellular ground substance and elastin or collagen. There is an absence of capillary blood vessels, at least in the early stages of intimal proliferation, and a marked tendency for the new tissue to undergo degenerative changes.

The factors which may cause injury and so act as a stimulus to proliferation of intimal tissue are mechanical stresses within the arterial wall—the so-called wear and tear of the arteries—and the accumulation of materials, mostly lipid in nature, which may act as irritants. In this account, the mechanical factors will be discussed first; the effects of irritants, and the changes which occur during the incorporation and organisation of thrombi, will be considered in more detail in later sections.

Mechanical Factors

There is circumstantial evidence that mechanical factors play an important part in determining the localisation and severity of the lesions in atherosclerosis. Lesions occur only in the larger vessels where, as already pointed out, the tangential stretching force is the greatest, and they are often localised at the points of particular mechanical strain. The lesions also tend to be more severe when there is a weakening of the mechanical resistance of the media. This association is seen in its most extreme form in syphilis of the aorta, in which an inflammatory process damages the media, but medial degeneration may also be a factor in determining the increasing severity of atherosclerosis with age. There is also evidence that an increase in the arterial blood pressure predisposes to atherosclerosis. Lesions tend to be more severe in the systemic arteries in generalised hypertension. They occur in the pulmonary arteries, even in early life, in those conditions in which the pulmonary blood pressure is raised, although lesions are otherwise rare at this site.[33]

It can be shown experimentally that a number of injurious stimuli which damage and weaken the walls of arteries lead in the process of repair to a localised thickening of the intima. If the media of the aorta of rabbits is damaged by freezing, for example, there is at first an aneurysmal dilatation at the site of injury. This is followed by proliferation of connective tissue on the inner margin of the injured area with the formation of a greatly thickened intima. This new tissue eventually shows differentiation of muscle and elastic tissue and forms a new vessel wall.[34] If the injury is more or less confined to the region of the internal elastic lamina, healing occurs within the original framework but is associated with penetration of muscle cells into the sub-endothelial space, an increase in the metachromatic staining of the ground substance and the formation of new intimal collagen and elastic fibres.[35]

Features which are consistent with a response to mechanical injury can be seen in many of the intimal thickenings which occur spontaneously at points of mechanical strain in the main arteries. Thus, there is rupture or fragmentation of the internal elastic lamina, penetration of the intima by smooth muscle cells and increased staining of the ground substance with elaboration of new fibres of collagen and elastin.[36] The hæmodynamic factors represent a less intense type of injury than those which have been studied experimentally but it should be borne in mind that they operate throughout life. There may also be circumstances in which their effects are exaggerated; for example, the injurious effects of pulsatile forces and shear will increase when a relatively rigid plaque develops in the intima.[37] In experimental animals it has been shown that dietary measures which impair the normal development of collagen or elastin in the arterial wall may make it more susceptible to injury by hæmodynamic factors. An association of intimal lesions showing the features of the repair reaction with a defect in elastic tissue occurs, for example, in young pigs which have been maintained from birth on a diet deficient in copper.[38] Impaired formation of connective tissue and consequent increased susceptibility to mechanical stress may also be the explanation of the intimal lesions which have been induced by pyridoxine deficiency in rhesus monkeys.[39]

Infiltration of the Intima from the Lumen (The Filtration Hypothesis)

Virchow believed that constituents of the atherosclerotic lesion were derived from the blood in the arterial lumen and had passed *through* the endothelium into the intima. From what has already been said about the nutrition and lymph drainage of the inner part of the wall, it is evident that substances entering the wall from the lumen might be trapped in the sub-endothelial space if they were relatively unstable in solution or did not diffuse readily through the rest of the wall to be removed by the lymphatics.[40] (Fig. 12). This so-called *filtration hypothesis* takes a prominent place in most accounts of the pathogenesis of the lesions; it has mainly been considered in relation to the lipid component, but the same principle might explain the accumulation in the intima of fibrin (derived from infiltrated fibrinogen) and of other plasma proteins.

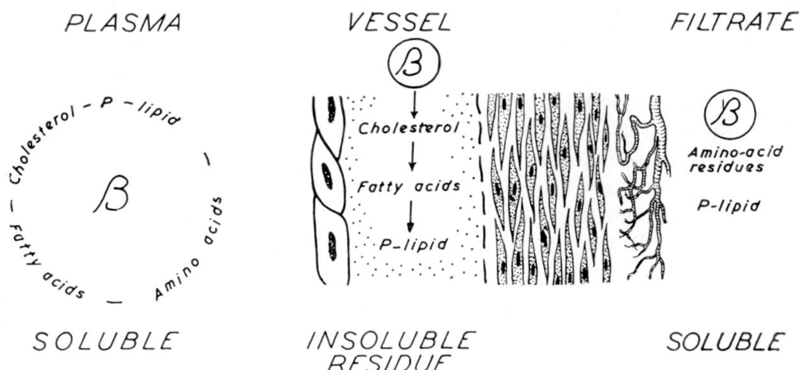

18/FIG. 12.—Diagram illustrating the inherent instability of β lipoproteins which may lead to precipitation of insoluble lipids in the intima of arteries. (Redrawn, by permission, from Page.[40])

Infiltration of Lipids

The lipids which accumulate in normal intima with ageing, and in greater amount in fibrous plaques and advanced lesions, are qualitatively similar to those in the plasma so there is no essential difficulty in the idea that one is derived from the other. Before reaching the intima, however, lipids from the blood must cross the endothelium so that the really significant factor is likely to be the physico-chemical properties of the complex molecules in the plasma filtrate which permeates the sub-endothelial ground substance.

The plasma lipids.—The lipids do not occur in the free state in the body fluids but are conjugated with each other and with carrier proteins to form lipoproteins. About 90 per cent of the cholesterol and phospholipid in plasma is present in one or other of two major classes of lipoproteins, which can be separated by zone electrophoresis, chemical fractionation, or in the ultracentrifuge. On electrophoresis, these two classes migrate with the α and β globulins respectively and are called the α and β lipoproteins. The chemical method of fractionation depends on differences in the solubility of the lipoproteins and isolates two components which have the same electrophoretic properties as the α and β lipoproteins in whole plasma. Separation in the ultracentrifuge depends on differences in density between the major classes, and high density components, corresponding to the α lipoproteins, and low density components, corresponding to the β lipoproteins, can be distinguished. If the density of the solvent is adjusted to 1·063, that is a value between the densities of the α and β lipoproteins, only the low density (β) lipoproteins will float to the surface in the ultracentrifuge; components of different density within this low-density class form a spectrum of molecules which can be distinguished in terms of their flotation rate, usually expressed as Svedberg units of flotation (normal range Sf* 0–20).

When the high and low density lipoproteins are analysed it is found that they each contain protein, phospholipid, cholesterol, cholesteryl esters and triglyceride, but there are significant differences in their relative composition.

* 1 Sf unit = flotation rate of 1×10^{-13} cm./sec./dyne/gm. at 26°C.

When compared with the high density lipoproteins, the low density lipoproteins are larger molecules; they contain a greater proportion of cholesterol to phospholipid and a greater proportion of total lipid to protein. These are all factors which are believed to make the low density lipoprotein molecules relatively unstable in solution.

The concentrations of the α and β lipoproteins remain fairly constant so that they can be considered to form a basic pattern upon which the fluctuations that occur during the transport of glycerides in the plasma are superimposed. This relationship has been described as one of vehicle to cargo with the glycerides associated with the α and β lipoproteins in such a way that they decrease their density still further. There are, however, two fairly distinct forms in which triglycerides are transported. During the ingestion of a fatty meal, dietary fat enters the blood from the thoracic duct in the form of visible particles or chylomicra which have the lowest density of all the plasma lipid components and are made up largely of triglyceride. They contain small amounts of cholesterol phospholipid and protein, contributed in part by α and β lipoprotein molecules. On the other hand, glycerides which are synthesised in the liver by re-esterification of fatty acids released from the fat depots, or from ingested carbohydrate, are transported in a class of very low density lipoproteins and "endogenous particles". The very low density lipoproteins show a range of Sf values from 20–400 depending on the proportion of glyceride in the molecule; they show increased electrophoretic mobility over the β lipoproteins and are therefore sometimes designated pre-β; the protein component is thought to be derived from both the α and β lipoproteins. The endogenous particles contain even more glyceride than the very low density lipoproteins and show Sf values in excess of 400, but though they may be visible in the light microscope they are smaller than the chylomicra and contain relatively more protein and cholesterol.

The main characteristics of these various lipid complexes in human plasma are summarised in Table IV and a detailed account will be found in recent review articles.[41, 42]

18/Table IV

The Major Human Plasma Lipoproteins

Class	*Chylomicra*	*Very low density (pre β)*	*Low density (β)*	*High density (α)*
Density (mean)	0·94	0·98	1·03	1·12
Sf class (approx.)	10,000 ± 5,000	20–400	0–20	—
Molecular diameter (A°)	5,000	700 × 300	350 × 150	300 × 50
Per cent composition				
Protein	2	10	21	50
Phospholipid	7	22	22	26
Cholesterol	2	8	8	3
Cholesteryl ester	8	5	37	15
Glyceride	81	55	11	6
Free fatty acid	—	—	1	—

(Data from Scanu[41] and Fredrickson *et al.*[42])

In other animals the lipoproteins have not been so fully investigated, but it appears that, although the principal classes are present, the distribution of lipids between them shows a considerable species variation. Compared with most other mammalian species man has a relatively high plasma cholesterol concentration, a relatively high proportion of total cholesterol in the low density (β) lipoproteins and a relatively high cholesterol: phospholipid ratio in the plasma as a whole[43] (Table V).

18/TABLE V

COMPARISON OF PLASMA LIPID VALUES IN MAN AND OTHER MAMMALS

	Man	*Baboon*[58]	*Pig*[12]	*Dog*[43]	*Rabbit*[43]
Total cholesterol mg./100 ml.	200	120	90	210	51
Phospholipid mg./100 ml.	250	214	90	430	88
Cholesterol: phospholipid ratio	0·80	0·56	1·0	0·49	0·58
Percentage of total cholesterol in β lipoprotein	70	—	52	17	47

Endothelial permeability to lipids.—In the peripheral vascular bed the basic lipoprotein molecules behave as other plasma proteins with respect to permeability: that is to say, they leak slowly from the bloodstream into the tissue fluid and lymph at a rate which depends on their molecular size. The low density lipoproteins, being the larger molecules, escape less readily than the high density lipoproteins but there is nevertheless an exchange of these large molecules between plasma and lymph. Permeability to lipoproteins is increased by endothelial injury and is also known to be high in the growing vessels of healing tissue where there are intercellular gaps in the endothelium which allow the passage of large molecules.

The permeability of endothelium to glycerides presents a special problem. The chylomicra, endogenous particles and very low density lipoproteins are very much larger than the other protein complexes and do not pass directly from the blood to tissue fluid[44] except at sites of vascular injury; yet, paradoxically, the glyceride component of these giant complexes can leave the bloodstream extremely rapidly. The probable explanation is that a lipolytic enzyme (clearing factor or lipoprotein lipase) is localised at or near the endothelial surface, and that fatty acids released by the activity of this enzyme, rather than the intact chylomicra or macromolecules, are transported across the endothelium.[45]

If it is assumed that the permeability of the arterial endothelium is the same as that of endothelium in small vessels, then proteins and lipoproteins would enter the sub-endothelial ground substance in the proportions observed in peripheral lymph and unhydrolysed triglycerides would be excluded.[14] At present there is no way in which lymph derived exclusively from the inner part of the arterial wall can be obtained but evidence obtained by other techniques indicates that influx of protein and lipoprotein can occur from the lumen in normal arteries and may be exaggerated when atherosclerotic lesions are present (see p. 562). It has also been shown that circulating lipoproteins enter the arterial wall very readily when the endothelial lining is destroyed by injury.

Causes of variation in plasma lipids in man.—The factors which determine the concentration of the plasma lipids in man are numerous and at present not fully understood. The basic pattern of the plasma lipoproteins in an individual depends on genetic factors but can be modified according to his dietary habits and by conditions which interfere with endogenous lipid metabolism.[41, 42, 46]

Differences in the lipoprotein patterns occur that are related to age. The concentration of low-density lipoproteins doubles or trebles within the first week of life; thereafter it increases very slowly into the third decade and then more rapidly. The maximum concentration of cholesterol and of low and very low-density lipoprotein is probably reached during middle age. There are differences in the composition of the plasma lipoproteins between young men and young women and between women before and after the menopause which are probably determined by œstrogenic hormones. When œstrogens are given to women after the menopause, or to male patients with ischæmic heart disease, the plasma cholesterol concentration, the cholesterol: phospholipid ratio and the proportion of cholesterol in the low-density lipoproteins are all decreased. Androgens have the opposite effect.

There are a number of inherited conditions in which the cholesterol or triglyceride values with their respective lipoproteins are grossly elevated. Hypercholesterolæmia with elevation of the low-density lipoproteins (e.g. in familial hypercholesterolæmia xanthomatosis) is the more common type but there are also inherited conditions in which both cholesterol and triglycerides or triglycerides alone are affected. Hypercholesterolæmia as a secondary phenomenon is seen most frequently in thyroid deficiency and when thyroxine is administered either to hypothyroid or euthyroid patients the concentration of cholesterol and of low-density lipoproteins falls.

Extensive studies on the plasma lipid composition in different human populations have shown that differences occur which depend more on the composition of the diet than on genetic or other environmental factors. In less developed communities the low levels of plasma lipids may be determined in part by the low intake of total fat in the diet, but the low intake of protein is recognised as a further significant factor. In other communities, in which dietary fat makes a larger contribution to the total caloric intake, the quality of the fat is probably more important than the total amount in determining the concentration of plasma lipids. It has been established in several studies that the feeding of equivalent amounts of animal fats such as butter, eggs or beef dripping maintain the plasma cholesterol at a higher level than do fish or vegetable oils. This difference can be related to the total mean unsaturation of the fatty acids in the fats used; the addition of unsaturated fat to the diet will reduce the level of plasma cholesterol provided there is a simultaneous reduction of the saturated fat intake. The susceptibility to dietary cholesterol is less in man than in some animal species, e.g. the rabbit, but when cholesterol intake is high, this too has a significant effect on the plasma cholesterol values. Plasma triglycerides are elevated transiently when the diet is changed to contain a high proportion of carbohydrate but it is not clear that an habitual carbohydrate-rich diet will lead to a persistent change. Populations with a high living standard certainly consume a much higher proportion of saturated fats and cholesterol in their diet than poorer communities and this is now thought to be the important factor determining their relatively high concentrations of cholesterol and low-density lipoproteins in the plasma.[47]

Characteristics of plasma lipids in atherosclerosis.—Lipids accumulate in the intima of arteries in man when the plasma values are within the range accepted as normal; but the process is exaggerated in some inherited conditions associated with marked hyperlipidæmia. In most other mammals lipids do not accumulate in appreciable amounts in the intima but the process can be induced by procedures which cause an increase in the concentration and a change in the pattern of distribution of the plasma lipids. These observations suggest that the accumulation of lipids in the arteries is largely determined by the composition of the plasma. Animal experiments have played an important part in developing this point of view.

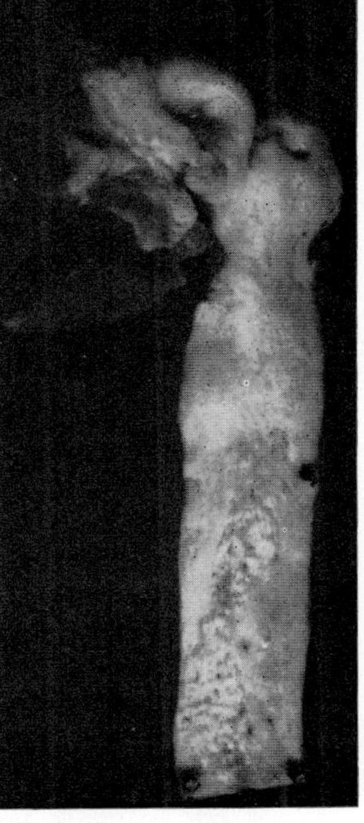

18/FIG. 13.—The aorta of a rabbit which had been fed 0·7 g. of cholesterol daily for 9 months. The plaques on the intimal surface have mostly become confluent. The first part of the pulmonary artery, seen in the foreground at the top, also shows plaques in the intima.

(a) *In experimental animals.*—Until recently the rabbit has been the animal more frequently used in this type of investigation. In 1908 Ignatowski noticed that rabbits given a diet rich in animal proteins developed nodular fatty thickenings of the intima of the aorta. A few years later Anitschkow[48] showed that the significant factor in the diet was cholesterol and produced similar results by feeding pure cholesterol dissolved in olive oil; this type of procedure has been followed in numerous experiments by later investigators.[49]

When the diet of a rabbit is supplemented with $\frac{1}{2}$ to 1 g. of cholesterol daily the lesions appear in about 3 or 4 weeks. They are seen first as raised yellowish-white dots or streaks in the intima and increase progressively in size over a period of six months or more to form confluent plaques of irregular outline (FIG. 13). The lesions are most conspicuous in the aorta but they are also found

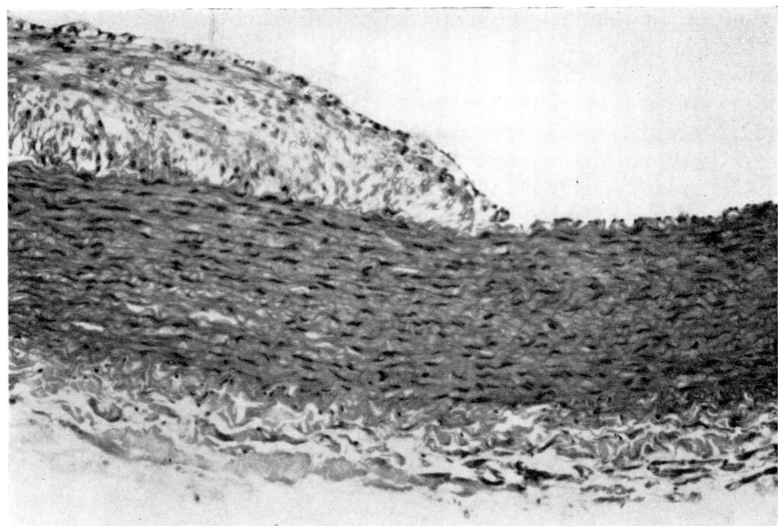

18/FIG. 14.—The edge of an intimal plaque in the aorta of a rabbit which had been fed 0·7 g. of cholesterol daily for 9 months. Hæmatoxylin and eosin. × 175.

in its larger branches, including the coronaries, and in the pulmonary arteries. Microscopically, there is considerable localised thickening of the intima (FIG. 14) with accumulation of lipid, mostly within macrophages or foam cells, in the superficial region, and an overgrowth of collagen and elastic fibres and of

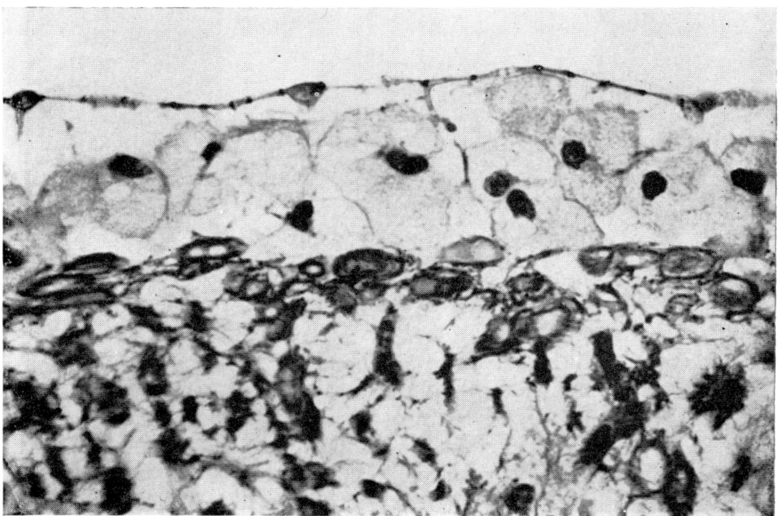

18/FIG. 15.—A collection of foam cells covered by endothelium at the surface of an intimal plaque. The deeper part of the intima shows an overgrowth of cells and fibres. Iron hæmatoxylin. × 960.

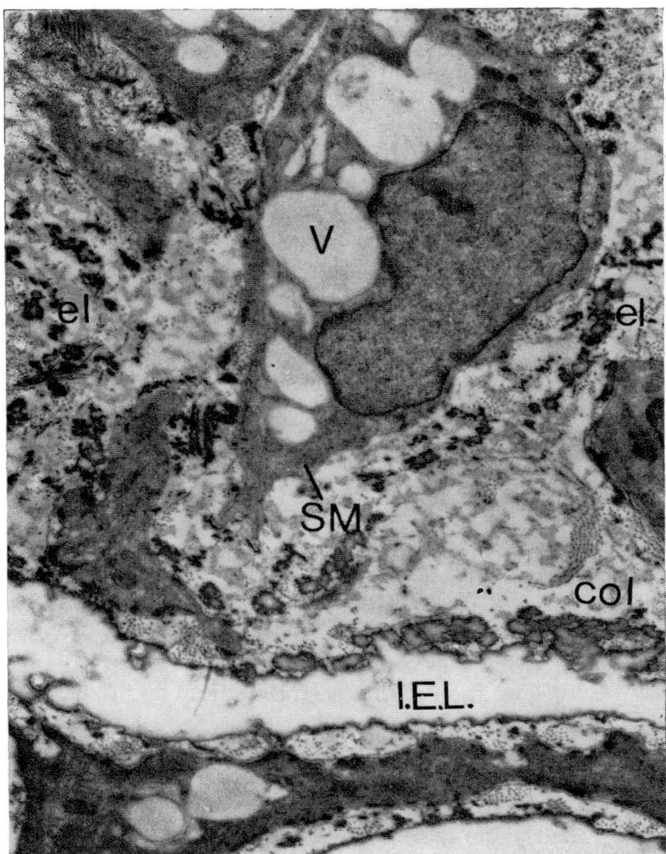

18/Fig. 16.—Smooth muscle cells (SM), at the base of a plaque in the thoracic aorta of a rabbit fed cholesterol, contain cytoplasmic vacuoles (V). Collagen (col) and elastin (el) are seen in the extracellular spaces. The internal elastic lamina (I.E.L.) has an irregular inner surface. Electron micrograph × 10,000.

smooth muscle cells in the deeper parts (Figs. 15 and 16). Chemical analysis of the aorta shows an excess of free cholesterol and cholesteryl esters, as well as a significant increase in phospholipid, including sphingomyelin, and triglyceride.[50]

An alteration in the lipid composition of the blood precedes the changes in the arteries. If one per cent of cholesterol is added to the diet of rabbits there is a sustained elevation of the concentration of cholesterol in the blood, which increases up to 25–30 times the normal values. This is associated with a significant, but smaller, increase in the other lipids. At the height of the lipæmia, which occurs after 2–3 months on the diet, the concentration of phospholipids has increased to about seven times, and triglycerides to about five times the normal values[50]; the cholesterol-phospholipid ratio, which is normally about 0·5, increases to 2·0. Fractionation of the plasma lipoproteins shows that the greater proportion of the total cholesterol now separates with the low-density lipoproteins.[51]

This is a reversal of the distribution found in the normal animal. The changes in the plasma lipids are reflected in the lymph which shows an increase in its cholesterol and lipoprotein content; as a result there is an increase at least fourfold in the total amount of cholesterol which is exchanged between blood and lymph during a 24-hour period.[52]

In general the extent of the arterial lesions can be correlated with the concentration of cholesterol in the blood and with the duration of the hypercholesterolæmia. However, it has been found that some procedures which augment the degree of hypercholesterolæmia which follows cholesterol feeding may actually diminish the severity of the arterial lesions. This effect has been observed in rabbits with alloxan diabetes and following administration of the detergents Tween 80 and Triton A20.[53] It appears that the severity of the lesions in these animals is more closely correlated with the cholesterol: phospholipid ratio and with particular components in the low-density lipoproteins than it is with the absolute concentration of cholesterol in the blood.

Similar lesions to those in the rabbit can be produced in other herbivorous animals and also in fowls by feeding an excess of cholesterol in the diet. In most other animals, cholesterol feeding alone does not have the pronounced effect it does in the rabbit, but marked hypercholesterolæmia and intimal lesions have been obtained when cholesterol feeding was combined with thyroid deficiency in dogs, or with thyroid deficiency and the administration of sodium cholate in rats (see ref. 11).

The experiments discussed so far provide experimental support for the filtration hypothesis by showing that cholesterol can accumulate in the intima of the arteries when the concentration in the plasma is raised and that when it does so it will provoke proliferative changes in the intimal connective tissue. The relevance of these experiments to the situation in man has been questioned on the grounds that the hypercholesterolæmia is of an extreme degree never encountered naturally and that the lesions themselves, with their predominant content of foam cells, may merely be an expression of an overloading of the reticulo-endothelial system with lipids, as can indeed be observed in the liver and spleen of these animals. However, it should be kept in mind that these are acute experiments in which an attempt is made to reproduce rapidly the changes in the arteries which may take many years to develop in man. If the time course of the experiments is prolonged by feeding cholesterol intermittently rather than continuously, the proliferative changes in the intima are more pronounced and the lipid tends to localise more in the centre of the plaque with the formation of an overlying cap of connective tissue.[49] Such lesions correspond more closely to the atherosclerotic lesions in man.

Experiments concerned with the filtration hypothesis are less open to criticism if the animals used resemble man in their arterial structure and in their lipid metabolism; this has led in recent years to the use of non-human primates and pigs in studies on the effects of elevation of plasma lipids in the hope that more informative results may justify the high cost of such experiments.[11] Lesions of the intima containing lipid can be *induced* in the main arteries of some non-human primates by diets which elevate plasma cholesterol to values in a range (250–650 mg./100 ml.) that could be encountered in man. This has been achieved in Cebus monkeys by combining cholesterol feeding with methionine deficiency[5] or by adding cholesterol and large amounts of butter fat or coconut oil to the diet;[55] and in rhesus monkeys by diets containing added cholesterol and butter fat.[56] The latter experiments are of particular interest since the distribution of the lesions and their morphological appearance resemble uncomplicated lesions in man quite closely and continuation of the dietary regime for long periods (40 months) has led to occlusion of the coronary arteries and to fatal myocardial infarction.[57] Another approach has been to determine whether modification of the plasma lipids by diet can affect the development of the spontaneous intimal lesions which occur in the baboon, monkey and pig. The addition of cholesterol and saturated fats to the diet, so that the composition approximates to that in human diets, leads to an accentuation of the lesions and an increase in their lipid content.[11, 58]

(b) *In man.*—The pattern of plasma lipids in man resembles the pattern in the experimental animals in which lesions have been induced by the dietary procedures rather more closely than it does the pattern in the untreated controls. Man has a relatively high plasma cholesterol concentration, a relatively high cholesterol: phospholipid ratio and a relatively high proportion of total cholesterol in the β lipoproteins. If these are important factors in the animal experiments, then man can be said to be naturally predisposed to accumulate lipids in his arteries by infiltration from the blood.

The next question to consider is whether differences in the plasma lipid pattern in different populations or individuals may operate through the filtration process to determine the *severity* of atherosclerotic lesions in man. It has already been mentioned that lesions may be relatively extensive in association with gross hyperlipidæmia and relatively few in undernourished populations which have very low plasma lipid values. The differences in extent of lesions in young men and young women may also be related to the differences in their plasma lipids. Thus, although in young men and women the plasma cholesterol concentration is about the same, women have a lower cholesterol : phospholipid ratio and a smaller proportion of the total cholesterol associated with low-density lipoproteins. Such observations are compatible with the filtration hypothesis but more conclusive evidence would be obtained if it were possible to correlate in individual subjects the plasma lipid pattern during life with the extent and lipid composition of the lesions found *post-mortem*. The one study of this type which has been completed has failed to show any correlation between plasma lipid values and the severity of disease in the coronary arteries or the lipid content of the coronary or cerebral arteries.[59] However, in this study the subjects were all in the age group 60–69 at the time of death and it can be argued that the findings are not representative of what may be happening in the arteries of younger individuals.[60]

Although there are still uncertainties about the significance of lipid infiltration in the pathogenesis of the lesions in man, there is clear evidence that hyperlipidæmia is in some way linked with the *clinical manifestations* of the disease. The mortality rate from ischæmic heart disease, for example, in different racial groups, can be correlated with the mean plasma lipid values in the population as a whole. When the mortality rate is low, so are the mean lipid values; when the mortality rate is high, the mean cholesterol, triglyceride and β-lipoprotein values tend to be high, particularly in middle-aged males in the population.[47] In the populations with a high mortality it is also possible to show a correlation in individuals between the plasma lipid values and the development of ischæmic heart disease. A method commonly adopted is to compare a group of patients who have survived a coronary thrombosis with a healthy group of the same age and sex. When this is done the patients with coronary thrombosis have, on average, a higher concentration of plasma cholesterol, a higher fasting triglyceride level and a higher concentration of the respective low-density lipoproteins. In addition, various prospective studies have demonstrated that presumably healthy men who have high plasma lipid concentrations are especially liable to develop ischæmic heart disease subsequently. Cholesterol, triglyceride and low-density lipoprotein concentrations all have a predictive value in this respect, but it appears that the cholesterol concentration is the most significant.[61] The view that certain components of low-density lipoproteins within the range Sf 0–400 might have a particular significance in the development of coronary disease[60] is not widely accepted at the present time.

It must be emphasised that these clinical data, though in some respects consistent with the filtration hypothesis, do not by themselves provide direct evidence for it. What is really being investigated is not the accumulation of lipids in the arterial wall, but a predisposition to coronary thrombosis. It is therefore possible that the observed changes in the plasma lipids may in part exert their effect through other mechanisms, and in particular through the thrombotic processes which are discussed more fully in a later section. But whatever may be the mechanism, the clinical data provide a clear indication that a reduction in the concentration of plasma lipids could be of value in the prevention or therapy of ischæmic heart disease. Several clinical trials on the effectiveness of particular diets or drugs are now being carried out to this end.[62]

The reactions of the intima to infiltration.—The accumulation of lipid in the intima in experimental animals is accompanied by proliferation of smooth muscle cells, an increase in elastin and collagen fibres, a change in the mucopolysaccharides of the ground substance, and the appearance of foam cells. This is usually interpreted as an irritative response to insoluble components of the lipoproteins though it might also be a response to other residues of the filtration process.

When certain lipids are introduced into connective tissue at other sites in the body they excite a "foreign-body" type of reaction in which there is an accumulation of macrophages and an overgrowth of surrounding fibrous tissue. The most striking irritative effect is shown by cholesterol, either free or esterified with saturated or mono-unsaturated fatty acids; polyunsaturated esters of cholesterol, phospholipids and triglycerides are relatively innocuous and are rapidly resorbed.[63] A similar proliferative reaction occurs when cholesterol, but not intact lipoprotein, is injected into the arterial wall;[64] it appears, however, from other types of experiment, that smooth muscle cells, rather than typical fibroblasts are the cells in the wall responsible for the formation of the new extracellular fibres and ground substance. In addition to their irritative effect in the arterial wall it has been proposed that lipids may damage elastic tissue more directly by forming a solid solution in it.[65]

Foam cells are generally present and often numerous in atherosclerotic lesions both of man and of experimental animals. Various suggestions have been made about their origin but the relative importance of these possibilities is still uncertain (see ref. 14). Many of the cells have the morphological features of lipid-filled macrophages and as with macrophages at other sites in the body they may be derived either from local cells or from cells which migrate into the lesions from the blood; it has been shown in the rabbit that these cells can increase in number in the intima by mitotic division. A potential local source is the few cells in normal intima which appear to be analogous to tissue histiocytes. Other macrophages could be derived from blood monocytes which had migrated into the intima from the lumen of the artery or, in advanced lesions where vascularisation of the intima has occurred, from the vasa vasorum. Occasional monocytes and lymphocytes have been observed in the intima of normal arteries, and they are more frequent at the edges of atherosclerotic lesions, but there is little evidence about the way in which these normal circulating cells are able to pass through the arterial endothelium. There is no doubt, however, that foam cells, already containing lipid, can be seen clinging to the endothelium and occupying gaps between endothelial cells at the surface of the lesions induced by cholesterol feeding in experimental animals and of fatty streaks in man. This does suggest that the cells may be entering the lesions from the blood but there is no conclusive proof that they are not passing in the reverse direction and are in effect being extruded from the lesions.[66] Finally, histological studies, particularly by electron microscopy, have shown that not all the foam cells in experimental and spontaneous lesions are of the macrophage type. Intracellular lipid is frequently observed in the intimal smooth muscle cells which may become highly vacuolated as a result of this intracellular accumulation. Such cells have been designated "myogenic foam cells"[67, 68] to distinguish them from the lipid containing macrophages.

Local factors and the filtration hypothesis.—The evidence from animal experiments and from clinico-pathological observations in man provides considerable support for the view that the concentration of low-density lipoproteins in the plasma is the important factor determining the accumulation of lipids in the arteries in atherosclerosis. This view is consistent with many of the chemical findings and with the demonstration by immuno-chemical methods of the localisation of low-density lipoproteins (but not, apparently, high-density lipoproteins) in the lesions.[31] Although attempts have been made to incriminate particular sub-fractions of the low-density lipoproteins, there is at present no clear evidence to justify this and it appears that an increase in the concentration of any or all of the sub-fractions may be associated with lipid accumulation.

Emphasis has been placed on the role of phospholipids and protein in maintaining the solubility of cholesterol so that a relative instability of the low-density lipoproteins with their high cholesterol : phospholipid and lipid: protein ratios may account for their being selectively retained in the intima. Since the lesions are unevenly distributed in the arteries it is clear, however, that there must be local factors in addition to the general mechanism which make the intima a more effective trap in some regions than in others. A discussion of this localising effect will impinge upon the other processes which are concerned in the pathogenesis of the lesions, but this is not to say that the filtration hypothesis itself is basically unsound.

When an artery is injured in an animal which has been made hypercholesterolæmic, lipid accumulates selectively at the injured site. Lesions can be induced in this way at sites where they would not occur in uninjured vessels; they also develop more rapidly than in undamaged arteries and at lower plasma cholesterol values. For example, while it takes two months and a terminal plasma cholesterol of 800 mg./100 ml. to produce gross lesions in the aorta of a normal rabbit, it takes only three weeks and a cholesterol level of 150 mg./100 ml. to produce comparable lesions in rabbits with injured arteries.[49] This clear association with gross injury has suggested that localisation in vessels which have not been deliberately injured may have a similar basis and be attributable to the mechanical factors which at certain sites in the arterial tree give rise to signs of injury and repair.

The mechanism whereby arterial injury promotes the accumulation of constituents of the plasma filtrate is not fully understood. The local thickenings of the intima which follow injury in animal experiments, or occur spontaneously at certain sites in the arterial tree, particularly in large mammals, might exaggerate the problem of lymph drainage in the arterial wall by increasing the radial diffusion distance between the lumen and the lymphatics. However, it has been found that a healed intimal scar, though it may increase the thickness of the arterial wall by as much as twofold, shows no greater tendency to accumulate lipid when hypercholesterolæmia is induced subsequently.[69] It appears that increased intimal thickness is not by itself an adequate explanation and that the association of lipid accumulation with injury depends in some way on the active stages of injury and repair.

It has been pointed out that an injury which involves the endothelium will allow macromolecules to enter the wall more readily from the plasma and will also permit the entry of the still larger complexes which are normally excluded. This greater influx of lipoprotein and protein, by upsetting the balance between entry and lymph drainage, can be expected to favour accumulation at sites of deliberate injury. In normal animals, regional differences in the permeability of aortic endothelium to labelled protein can be demonstrated at sites where there may be spontaneous injury from mechanical factors[70] and it is probable that such differences in permeability are an important factor in the localisation of lesions. If endothelial permeability were greater over the surface of a developing lesion this would tend still further to accentuate the influx of lipid. The increased permeability of regenerating endothelium to large molecules appears also to be an important factor in the accumulation of lipid which occurs in organising thrombi (p. 582).

Regional differences in the physico-chemical properties of the intimal ground substance, as reflected by increased metachromasia and increased turnover of sulphated mucopolysaccharides at sites of injury or in atherosclerotic lesions, are also thought to have an important effect on the accumulation of large molecules. A change in the relative proportions of the different acid mucopolysaccharides could, by increasing the molecular sieving effect of the intimal gel, lead to a greater accumulation of large molecules in some regions than in others.[29] Moreover the selective retention of low-density lipoproteins, and to a lesser extent of fibrinogen, could depend on a specific interaction between these molecules and components of the ground substance with the formation of insoluble complexes or coacervates, since complexes of this kind have been shown to form *in vitro*.[31] This would have a localising effect if the conditions for this interaction were more favourable in certain regions of the arterial tree. Finally other metabolic processes in the arterial wall, which are discussed in greater detail later, may also be concerned in determining whether, at a particular site, constituents of the plasma filtrate will accumulate in the wall rather than be dispersed.[16]

The Organisation of Surface Deposits

(The Encrustation or Thrombogenic Hypothesis)

In 1842 Rokitansky in his handbook of pathological anatomy put forward the suggestion that thickening of the walls of arteries might be caused by an excessive deposition from the blood of materials which he termed "fibrin". This idea was opposed by Virchow, who pointed out that the lesions were covered by endothelium and therefore concluded that the pathological changes began within the wall and not on its surface. His authoritative view discouraged further investigation of this possible cause of the lesions for many years; nevertheless, a number of observations were later made on the laminated character of certain atherosclerotic lesions and on the presence of blood constituents within them, which would be consistent with thrombosis having occurred during their development. For example, Clark, Graef and Chassis[71] in 1936 described material staining like fibrin in the lesions and concluded that lesions increased in size as a result of repeated deposition of blood elements.

The credit for establishing the hypothesis on a more secure basis may be given to Duguid.[4, 72, 73] Shortly after the Second World War he published a series of papers on the histological appearances of lesions in the coronary arteries and aorta in which he emphasised two points. First, that if a mural thrombus forms on the surface of an artery it will be covered by new endothelium and so become, in effect, a thickened part of the intima of the arterial wall. Second, that having been incorporated in this way, it will with time undergo degenerative changes and organisation that will tend to obscure its thrombotic origin.

These morbid anatomical observations have been repeated and extended by others workers[74, 75] and it is now fairly widely accepted that many atherosclerotic plaques, and particularly those which encroach significantly on the lumen, can be interpreted as the end result of a succession of mural thrombi. In later studies immuno-fluorescent techniques have been used to demonstrate the presence of layers of fibrin or platelet material in plaques when this would otherwise escape notice in sections stained by routine histological methods.[76] The opportunity to examine in the fresh state material from the lining of the aorta or major arteries which has been removed at surgical operation has also provided very clear illustrations of the deposits of platelets and fibrin that may form on the surface of plaques and of the degenerative changes they undergo[77] (Fig. 17).

The first experiments designed to test the hypothesis were based on the assumption that the deposit most likely to form on the surface of arteries would be fibrin. It was shown that when fibrin or whole blood clot was injected intravenously in rabbits the emboli which lodged in the pulmonary arteries were subsequently organised with the formation of localised thickenings of fibro-elastic tissue. It was therefore established that incorporation of fibrin into the arterial wall by growth of endothelium over its surface could indeed give rise to a type of intimal thickening though, under the conditions of these experiments, the lipid component of a typical atherosclerotic lesion was inconspicuous or absent.

It is now more widely appreciated that the deposits likely to form on the surface of arteries are thrombi in the usual sense of the term and consist mainly of blood platelets initially, though they come to contain more fibrin with the passage of time (see Chapter 9). When fragments of a thrombus containing platelets, rather than fibrin clot, are injected intravenously in rabbits it is found that fibro-fatty plaques, resembling atherosclerotic lesions more closely, are formed in the pulmonary arteries.[78] Foam cells similar to those seen in many atherosclerotic lesions appear within the plaques and are probably formed from macrophages which have phagocytosed platelets or platelet material. The organisation of mural thrombi in the aorta of rabbits or in the carotid artery and aorta of pigs gives rise to intimal plaques consisting of smooth muscle cells, collagen and elastin fibres but with less lipid than in the organised emboli.[79] The amount of lipid in the rabbit lesions can, however, be increased if the animal is first made hyperlipæmic.[80] In the pig, the lesions develop a fibromuscular cap overlying a basal pool of thrombotic residue and, even when the blood lipids are within the normal range, stainable fat is present in the cytoplasm of smooth muscle cells and as extracellular droplets in the vicinity of the internal elastic lamina[81] (FIG. 18). It appears from these experiments that intimal lesions which resemble in many ways atherosclerotic lesions in man could develop by the organisation of typical mural thrombi.

As a result of these studies in man and experimental animals it is now established that thrombosis should not be considered only as a late complication in atherosclerosis but that it can play an important part in the progression of at least some of the lesions. However, this should not be taken to imply that the other processes in the pathogenesis of the lesions which have been discussed in this chapter can be ruled out. This will perhaps be made clear by drawing attention to the weak points which emerge when an attempt is made to explain naturally occurring lesions in man entirely in terms of the thrombogenic hypothesis.

The first concerns the amount and chemical composition of the lipid in the lesions. Platelets have a high content of lipids which could contribute to the fatty debris, particularly if the central core of a lesion derived from a mural thrombus were poorly organised. However, platelets contain relatively little esterified cholesterol and much less sphingomyelin in the phospholipid components than is found in the intimal lesions. Considerable metabolic changes would therefore have to occur in the wall for the plaque lipids to be derived entirely from this source. The amount of lipid present in the lesions would also require that a very large mass of platelet material, some twenty times greater than that of the lesion itself, had been deposited.[82] This difficulty could be overcome, however, by invoking the filtration hypothesis. It has been shown by means of the fluorescent antibody technique that there is infiltration of plasma lipoproteins into organising human thrombi.[83] Moreover, experimental thrombi

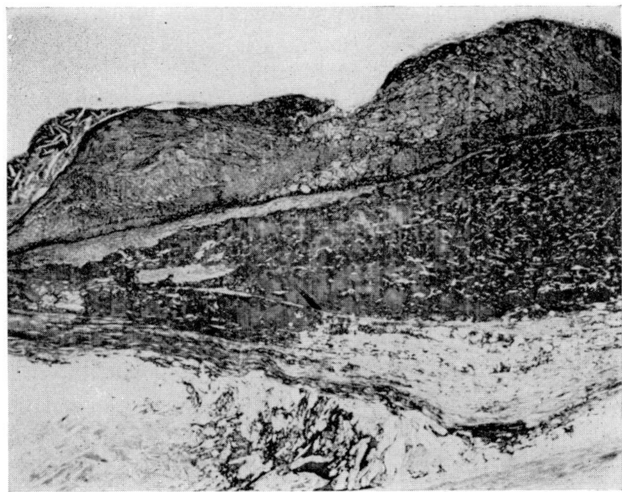

18/Fig. 17.—A mural thrombus, consisting of platelets and fibrin, on the surface of an atherosclerotic plaque in a human iliac artery. Endarterectomy specimen. Mallory's trichrome stain × 22.

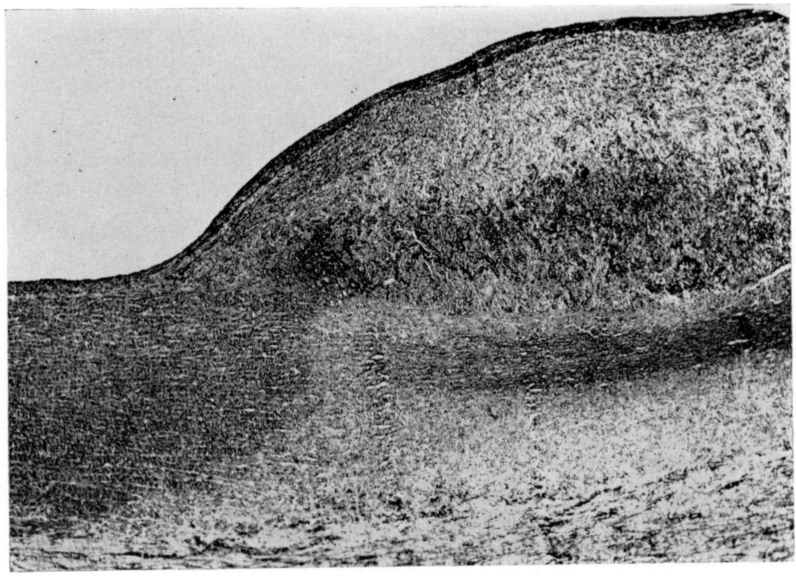

18/Fig. 18.—Organisation of a mural thrombus in the abdominal aorta of a pig has led to the formation of a riased plaque with a fibro-muscular cap and a central core of thrombotic residua. The thrombus had been induced 1 month previously by injuring the intimal surface. Picro-Mallory stain × 40. (By courtesy of Crawford and Woolf.)

become much richer in lipids as they are organised in an animal in which a hyperlipidæmia has been induced.[80]

A more fundamental difficulty in the interpretation of the thrombogenic hypothesis is that it is not known at what stage in the development of natural lesions thrombosis can first begin. The most widely held view is that even though mural thrombi may begin to form very early in the development of some lesions, and account for many of the features of the more advanced plaque, they still represent a *complication*; they thus can only occur when a pre-existing atherosclerotic lesion, due to some other cause, has already impaired the surface properties of the arterial wall. An extension of the thrombogenic hypothesis beyond this, in an attempt to explain the *cause* of atherosclerotic lesions in terms of deposits of fibrin or platelets, is at present much more controversial.

Duguid described fine encrustations of fibrin and like material on the surface of otherwise normal arteries which he thought could be overgrown by endothelium to form the beginning of an intimal plaque. This led to suggestions that deposits might be formed on the walls of arteries if there were an imbalance between a continuing formation of fibrin in the circulation and its removal by fibrinolysis. There is still no convincing proof that such an imbalance can occur. With regard to the platelets, more information is required about their behaviour in the circulation before their possible role in the initiation of intimal lesions can be assessed. Mustard and his colleagues[84] have detected small platelet deposits on apparently normal endothelium of the pig's aorta at points where flow is disturbed. The importance of hydraulic factors in predisposing to platelet deposition at particular sites in the circulation has already been discussed in Chapter 9 but it is not known whether such deposits could persist long enough to be incorporated in the intima if there were no underlying lesion which had already impaired the normal protective mechanisms in the vessel wall. Doubts about this aspect of the hypothesis (i.e. whether some lesions can begin as surface deposits) in no way detract from the convincing evidence that mural thrombosis is important in the later stages of the disease.

Metabolism of the Arterial Wall

Attention has been given to the study of the metabolism of the arterial wall by histochemical and biochemical methods with a view to determining whether the wall has special metabolic properties which can explain its propensity to develop atherosclerotic lesions.[85] It is clear that the arterial wall is not metabolically inert and shares with other tissues the processes of intermediary metabolism which are essential for cell survival. Limitations are imposed by the unique character of its blood supply and by the scarcity of cells in comparison with the abundance of extracellular elements. The changes which occur with ageing and disease are complicated by the fact that there may be alterations not only in the total cell population but also in the proportions of cells with different metabolic properties (e.g. smooth muscle and macrophages).

The arterial wall has a low oxygen consumption and is largely dependent on glycolysis, ærobic or anærobic, for its energy. In consequence there is a high lactic acid production and a low energy reserve. The thickness of the avascular zone between the lumen and vasa vasorum is very close to the maximum diffusion distance for oxygen in the arterial wall so that even in normal large arteries it seems likely that an intermediate region in the inner part of the wall is constantly subjected to hypoxia. If further intimal thickening occurs with disease, and is not accompanied by compensatory changes in the vasa vasorum, it is possible that an intermediate region of ischæmia will develop.[16] Histochemical studies indicate that there is a decline in enzymatic activity in this region which could lead to the accumulation of lipids or other metabolites that would otherwise be removed.[86]

Reference has already been made to the ways in which local metabolic changes in mucopolysaccharides may be important in the permeability of the wall and in the trapping of macromolecules. Other metabolic studies have been concerned primarily with the behaviour of lipids in the wall. It is now generally accepted that the filtration hypothesis can explain the origin of the major part of the lipid which accumulates in atherosclerosis, though in particular lesions at least some may be derived from the degeneration of incorporated thrombi and possibly by the degeneration of elastic tissue. It seems probable that when low-density lipoprotein accumulates in the intima the lipid components are dissociated from the complex and that while the relatively insoluble cholesterol and cholesteryl esters are retained the other lipid components are in part eliminated. At present it is not possible to give a full account of the active processes which may be involved. It is clear, however, that the composition of the lipids deposited in the intima is modified by metabolic processes within the wall itself. Thus, not only does the composition differ quantitatively in many types of lesion from that of the low-density lipoproteins, but the composition alters as the lesions become more advanced. The most striking differences observed are those in the pattern of the fatty acids in the cholesteryl esters of the fatty streak; in the high proportion of sphingomyelin in the phospholipids generally; and in the increasing ratio of free to esterified cholesterol and of total cholesterol to phospholipid as the lesions become more advanced.[87]

There is evidence that some of the lipids in the lesions are formed *in situ*. There has been considerable debate whether a proportion of the cholesterol may actually be synthesised locally but if this does occur at all it is only at a very slow rate which could not apparently account for the bulk of the cholesterol in the lesions. It has been shown, however, that the arterial wall can synthesise fatty acids and that some of these newly formed fatty acids may be incorporated in the cholesteryl esters in the lesions.[88] It is probable that the cholesteryl esters of unusual composition (i.e. high in oleic and low in linoleic acid) which are identified when lipid is predominantly intracellular, as in the fatty streak, have been synthesised *in situ*. Hydrolysis of cholesteryl esters by esterase activity, which has been demonstrated histochemically in the lesions, could account for the increase in the proportion of unesterified cholesterol observed in the more advanced lesions. Fatty acids released in this way may then be rapidly utilised or removed in some other way from the arterial wall. Lipases can also be demonstrated in the arterial wall and are thought to be responsible for removal of the triglyceride component.[86]

Aortic tissue can incorporate inorganic phosphate or acetate into phospholipid and there is evidence that phospholipid synthesis occurs at a high rate in the lesions in experimental animals and in man.[89] It has been suggested that this formation of phospholipid is part of a defence mechanism which may lead to the removal of some cholesterol by the rebuilding of soluble molecular complexes. It is to be noted, however, that sphingomyelin is synthesised less readily than lecithin so that the high proportion of sphingomyelin appears to be accounted for by the selective retention of this component of the phospholipid rather than by an increased local production.[87]

These metabolic processes are an expression of the activities of the cells in the lesions, though it is uncertain what are the relative contributions of the smooth muscle cells and macrophages. Observations on the fine structure of smooth muscle cells in experimental lesions in dogs have suggested that these cells are actively engaged in lipid synthesis.[90] The role of macrophages in lipid metabolism has been investigated more extensively. Cells of the reticulo-endothelial system have the ability to esterify ingested cholesterol, to hydrolyse cholesteryl esters and to oxidise fatty acids and triglycerides. They can also be stimulated by cholesterol uptake to synthesise fatty acids and phopholipids.[91] The foam cells in the lesions from rabbits fed cholesterol have similar properties and it has been suggested that these cells, through their ability to esterify cholesterol with polyunsaturated fatty acids and to synthesise phospholipid, may play an active role in the removal of cholesterol from the lesions.[92] Isotope studies have indicated that some cholesterol can be withdrawn from the atherosclerotic artery, though lipid in the centre of advanced lesions appears to be metabolically inert. These observations suggest that the accumulation of cholesterol in the wall should be considered as an imbalance between the influx of cholesterol on the one hand by the filtration mechanism and on the other an attempt at its removal by local metabolic processes.

Summary and Conclusions

The pathology of atherosclerosis has still to be discussed largely in descriptive terms; many of the changes in function responsible for the alterations in structure and chemical composition of the arterial wall are incompletely understood. The filtration hypothesis has been most investigated, but this should not give undue weight to the role of lipid accumulation, and it is clear that the additional processes concerned in the development of human lesions merit detailed study.

It is possible to observe some general principles about the nature of the process. In the first place, atherosclerosis as a pathological process involves principally the intima of large arteries. This indicates that the characteristic tissue reaction is conditioned by structural and metabolic factors which apply only at this site. Of these the most important appear to be the existence of a higher tension in this tissue than elsewhere, the absence of capillary blood vessels and lymphatics, and the contact on its inner surface with the circulating blood. Thus throughout life the intima is exposed to potentially injurious influences; mechanical forces, accumulation of materials which infiltrate from the blood and formation of surface deposits.

Among the stimuli which initiate the change there are local and general factors. Particular hæmodynamic stresses within the wall appear to be the most important local stimulus causing change in the endothelium and intimal connective tissue and determining the sites at which lesions occur. Of the general factors, the level of blood pressure and the lipid composition of the tissue fluid permeating the wall are clearly important. When lipids accumulate in the thickened intima they delineate and magnify the local tissue response which may then become progressive.

Finally, whether mural deposits are concerned in the initial stages or not, there can be no doubt that thrombosis is the important factor which leads to occlusive lesions and to clinical disease. Whether the formation of thrombi is determined by some particular feature of the lesions or by a change in the blood as a whole is largely unknown. This is the aspect of the problem which appears the most likely to provide the explanation of the high incidence of clinical disease.

REFERENCES

1. World Health Organization (1958). Technical Rep. Series, No. 143.
2. Winternitz, M. C., Thomas, R. M., Le Compte, P. M. (1938). *The Biology of Arteriosclerosis*. Springfield, Ill.: Chas. C. Thomas.
3. Geiringer, E. (1951). *J. Path. Bact.*, **63,** 201.
4. Duguid, J. B. (1946). *J. Path. Bact.*, **58,** 207.
5. Duguid, J. B., and Robertson, W. B. (1955). *Lancet*, **1,** 525.
6. Enos, W. F., Beyer, J. C. and Holmes R. H. (1955). *J. Amer. med. Ass.* **158,** 912.
7. Morris, J. N. (1964). *Uses of Epidemiology*, 2nd edit. Edinburgh: E. & S. Livingstone.
8. Morris, J. N. (1951). *Lancet*, **1,** 1 and 69.
9. Morris, J. N., and Crawford, M. D. (1961). *Lancet*, **1,** 47.
10. Robertson, W. B. (1967). The geographic pathology of atherosclerosis. In *Modern Trends in Pathology*, **2,** p. 176. Ed. Crawford, T. London: Butterworth.
11. Roberts, J. C., and Straus, R. Eds. (1965). *Comparative Atherosclerosis*. New York: Hoeber Harper.
12. French, J. E., Jennings, M. A., Poole, J. C. F., Robinson, D. S., and Florey, H. W. (1963). *Proc. roy. Soc. B*, **158,** 24.
13. Prichard, R. W., Clarkson, T. B., Goodman H., O., and Lofland, H. B. (1964). *Arch. Path.*, **77,** 244.
14. French, J. E. (1966). *Int. Rev. exp. Path.*, **5,** 253.
15. Florey, H. W. (1960). *Brit. med. J.*, **2,** 1329.
16. Adams, C. W. M. (1964). *Biol. Rev.*, **39,** 372.
17. Duncan, L. E. (1963). In *Evolution of the Atherosclerotic Plaque*. Ed. Jones, R. J. Chicago: Chicago Univ Press.
18. Kao, V. C., and Wissler, R. W. (1965). *Exp. molec. Path.*, **4,** 465.

18a. Florey, Lord, and Sheppard, B. L. (1969). *Proc. roy. Soc. B.* In press.

19. Burton, A. C. (1954). *Physiol. Rev.* **34,** 619.
20. Wolinsky, H., and Glagov, S. (1967). *Circulat. Res.*, **20,** 99.
21. Glagov, S. (1965). *Acta cardiol.* (*Brux.*), Suppl. **11,** 311.
22. Shiu Yeh Yuh, and Blumenthal, H. T. (1967). In *The Connective Tissue*. Eds. Wagner, B. M., and Smith, D. E. Baltimore: Williams and Wilkins.
23. Böttcher, C. J. F., and Woodford, F. P. (1962). *Fed. Proc.*, **21,** Suppl. 11, 15.
24. Böttcher, C. J. F. (1963). In *Evolution of the Atherosclerotic Plaque*. Ed. Jones, R. J. Chicago: Chicago Univ. Press.
25. Smith, E. P. (1965). *J. Atheroscler, Res.*, **5,** 224.
26. Smith, E. P., Evans, P. H., and Downham, M. D. (1967). *J. Atheroscler. Res.*, **7,** 171.
27. Muir, H. (1965). In *The Amino Sugars*, **2A,** 311. Eds. Jeanloz, R. W., and Balazs, E. A. New York: Academic Press.
28. Manley, G. (1965). *Brit. J. exp. Path.* **46,** 125.

29. Klynstra, F. B., Böttcher, C. J. F., van Melsen, J. A., and van der Laan, E. J. (1967). *J. Atheroscler. Res.*, **7**, 301.
30. Laurent, T. C., and Persson, H. (1964). *Biochim. Biophys. Acta* (*Amst.*), **83**, 141.
31. Walton, K. W., and Williamson, N. (1968). *J. Atheroscler. Res.*, **8**, 599.
32. Haust, M. D., More, R. H., and Movat, H. Z. (1960). *Amer. J. Path.*, **37**, 377.
33. Heath, D., Wood, E. H., DuShane, J. W., and Edwards, J.E . (1960). *Lab. Invest.*, **9**, 259.
34. Taylor, C. B., Baldwin, D., Hass, G. M. (1950). *Arch. Path.*, **49**, 623.
35. Ssolowjew, A. (1932). *Virchows Arch. path. Anat.*, **283**, 213.
36. Moon, H. D. (1959). *Connective Tissue, Thrombosis and Atherosclerosis*, p. 33. Ed. Page, I. H. New York: Academic Press.
37. Duguid, J. B., and Robertson, W. B. (1957). *Lancet*, **1**, 1205.
38. Coulson, W. F., and Carnes, W. H. (1963). *Amer. J. Path.*, **43**, 945.
39. Rinehart, J. F., and Greenberg, L. D. (1951). *Arch. Path.*, **51**, 12.
40. Page, I. H. (1954). *Circulation*, **10**, 1.
41. Scanu, A. M. (1965). In *Advances in Lipid Research*, 3. Eds. Paoletti, R., and Kritchevsky, D. New York: Academic Press.
42. Fredrickson, D. S., Levy, R. I., and Lees, R. S. (1967). *New Engl. J. Med.*, **276**, 32, 94, 148, 215, 273.
43. Barr, D. P. (1953). *Circulation*, **8**, 641.
44. Schœfl, G. I., and French, J. E. (1968). *Proc. roy. Soc. B*, **169**, 153.
45. Robinson, D. S. (1969). In *Comprehensive Biochemistry*, **18**, 51. Eds. Florkin, M., and Stotz, E. H. Amsterdam: Elsevier Publishing Co.
46. Furman, R. H., Alaupovic, P., and Howard, R. P. (1967). *Progr. biochem. Pharmacol.*, **2**, 215.
47. Stamler, J. (1967). *Lectures on Preventive Cardiology*. New York: Grune and Stratton.
48. Anitschkow, N. (1913). *Beitr. path. Anat.*, **56**, 379.
49. Constantinides, P. (1965). *Experimental Atherosclerosis*. Amsterdam: Elsevier Publishing Co.
50. Weinhouse, S., and Hirsch, E. F. (1940). *Arch. Path.*, **30**, 856.
51. Gofman, J. W., Lindgren, F., Elliott, H., Mantz, W., Hewitt, J., Strisower, B., and Herring, V. (1950). *Science*, **III**, 116.
52. Morris, B., and Courtice, F. C. (1955). *Quart. J. exp. Physiol.*, **40**, 149.
53. Duff, G. L., and McMillan, G. C. (1951). *Amer. J. Med.*, **11**, 92.
54. Mann, G. V., Andrus, S. B., McNally, A., and Stare, F. J. (1953). *J. exp. Med.*, **98**, 195.
55. Wissler, R. W., Frazier, L. E., Hughes R. H., and Rasmussen, R. A. (1962). *Arch. Path.*, **74**, 312.
56. Taylor, C. B., Cox, G. E., Manalo-Estrella, P., and Southworth, J. (1962). *Arch. Path.*, **74**, 16.
57. Taylor, C. B., Patton, D. E., and Cox, G. E. (1963). *Arch. Path.*, **76**, 404.
58. Gresham, G. A., Howard, A. N., McQueen, J., and Bowyer, D. E. (1965). *Brit. J. exp. Path.*, **46**, 94.
59. Paterson, J. C., Armstrong, R., and Armstrong, E. C. (1963). *Circulation*, **27**, 229.
60. Gofman, J. W., Young, W., and Tandy R., (1966). *Circulation*, **34**, 679.
61. Kannel, W. B., Dawber, T. R., Friedman, G. D., Glennon, W. E., and McNamara, P. M. (1964). *Ann. intern. Med.*, **61**, 888.
62. Oliver, M. F. (1967). In *Modern Trends in Pharmacology and Therapeutics*. Ed. Fulton, W. F. M. London: Butterworth.
63. Abdulla, Y. H., Adams, C. W. M., and Morgan, R. S. (1967). *J. Path. Bact.*, **94**, 63.

64. HOLLANDER, W. (1967). *Exp. molec. Path.*, **7**, 248.
65. PARKER, F. (1960). *Amer. J. Path.*, **36**, 19.
66. POOLE, J. C. F., and FLOREY, H. W. (1958). *J. Path. Bact.*, **75**, 245.
67. BALIS, J. U., HAUST, M. D., and MORE, R. H. (1964). *Exp. molec. Path.*, **3**, 511.
68. PARKER, F., and ODLAND, G. F. (1966). *Amer. J. Path.*, **48**, 197.
69. TAYLOR, C. B., TRUEHEART, R. E., and COX, G. E. (1963). *Arch. Path.*, **76**, 14.
70. PACKHAM, M. A., ROWSELL, H. C., JORGENSEN, L., and MUSTARD, J. F. (1967). *Exp. molec. Path.*, **7**, 214.
71. CLARK, E., GRAEF, I., and CHASIS, H. (1936). *Arch. Path.*, **22**, 183.
72. DUGUID, J. B. (1948). *J. Path. Bact.*, **60**, 57.
73. DUGUID, J. B. (1955). *Brit. med. Bull.*, **11**, 36.
74. MORGAN, A. D. (1956). *The Pathogenesis of Coronary Occlusion.* Oxford: Blackwell.
75. MITCHELL, J. R. A., and SCHWARTZ, C. J. (1965). *Arterial Disease.* Oxford: Blackwell.
76. CRAWFORD, T. (1967). In *Modern Trends in Pathology*, 2. London: Butterworth.
77. GUNNING, A. J., HACKETT, M. E. J., MACKENZIE, J. R., OLIVER, D. O., PICKERING, G. W. and TIBBS D. J. (1966). *Quart. J. Med.*, **35**, 475.
78. HAND, R. A., and CHANDLER, A. B. (1962). *Amer. J. Path.*, **40**, 469.
79. JORGENSEN, L., ROWSELL, H. C., HOVIG, T., and MUSTARD, J. F. (1967). *Amer. J. Path.*, **51**, 681.
80. FRIEDMAN, M., and BYERS, S. O. (1965). *Amer. J. Path.*, **46**, 567.
81. WOOLF, N., BRADLEY, J. W. P., CRAWFORD, T., and CARSTAIRS, K. C. (1968). *Brit. J. exp. Path.*, **49**, 257.
82. SMITH, E. B. (1967). *Cardiovasc. Res.*, **1**, 111.
83. WOOLF, N., PILKINGTON, T. R. E., and CARSTAIRS, K. C. (1966). *J. Path. Bact.*, **91**, 383.
84. MUSTARD, J. F., MURPHY, E. A., ROWSELL, H. C., and DOWNIE, H. G. (1964). *J. Atheroscler. Res.*, **4**, 1.
85. KIRK, J. E. (1963). *In Atherosclerosis and its Origin*. Eds. SANDLER, M., and BOURNE, G. H. New York: Academic Press.
86. ADAMS, C. W. M. (1967). *Vascular Histochemistry.* London: Lloyd-Luke.
87. SMITH, E. B., SLATER, R. S., and CHU, P. K. (1968). *J. Atheroscler. Res.*, **8**, 399.
88. LOFLAND, H. B., ST. CLAIR, R. W., CLARKSON, T. B., BULLOCK, B. C., and LEHNER, N. D. M. (1968). *Exp. molec. Path.*, **9**, 57.
89. ZILVERSMIT, D. B., MCCANDLESS, E. L., JORDAN, P. H., HENLEY, W. S., and ACKERMAN, R. F. (1961). *Circulation*, **23**, 370.
90. GEER, J. C. (1965). *Amer. J. Path.*, **47**, 241.
91. DAY, A. J. (1964). *J. Atheroscler. Res.*, **4**, 117.
92. DAY, A. J., and WILKINSON, G. K. (1967). *Circulat. Res.*, **21**, 593.

Chapter 19

PATHOLOGICAL CONSEQUENCES OF CHROMOSOMAL ABNORMALITY

BY C. E. FORD

INTRODUCTION

Historical

The word *chromosome* was introduced by Waldeyer in 1888 shortly after the first investigations of mitosis by Flemming, Strasburger, van Beneden and others. These early investigations demonstrated the normal regularity of the mitotic process and the normal morphological constancy of the chromosome set within the species. The interpretation of the maturation divisions of gametogenesis as *meiotic* or *reduction* divisions followed shortly after: the *diploid* (2n) chromosome set of the germ cell is halved to yield the *haploid* (n) set of the gamete by a process that involves the prior intimate association of the chromosomes in pairs. This complemented Hertwig's discovery of nuclear syngamy as the central event of fertilization and verified Weissman's prediction that there must be a compensatory event at some point in the life cycle.

Shortly after the turn of the century, Sutton and Boveri independently realized that the behaviour of the chromosome pairs in meiosis formed a close parallel to Mendelian segregation, then a newly rediscovered principle. They therefore suggested that the chromosomes were the physical carriers of the Mendelian factors, a postulate that received overwhelming proof during the following half century from correlated chromosome observations and breeding experiments. The chromosome theory of heredity became the cornerstone of genetics and provided the justification for the name "cytogenetics", introduced by Muller for investigations of chromosomes that are relevant to genetic phenomena.

Chromosome Structure and Function

The typical chromosome at mitotic metaphase (FIG. 1) is divided longitudinally into *two chromatids*, the future daughter chromosomes, except for one point, the *centromere*. Division of the centromere initiates the polar movement of the daughter chromosomes at anaphase. In suitable preparations each chromatid can be seen as a closely coiled spiral, the number of gyres can be counted and their pitch measured. Below this level the physical organisation of the chromosome is still controversial, morphologists tending to claim that it has a multistranded structure, geneticists that it must be fundamentally single stranded to satisfy the facts of meiotic recombination and of some experiments on induced mutation.

Chemically, chromosomes are composed largely of desoxyribonucleic acid (DNA), the molecules of which are interlaced twin spirals of great length consisting of a linear sequence of nucleotide pairs of two kinds in which the associa-

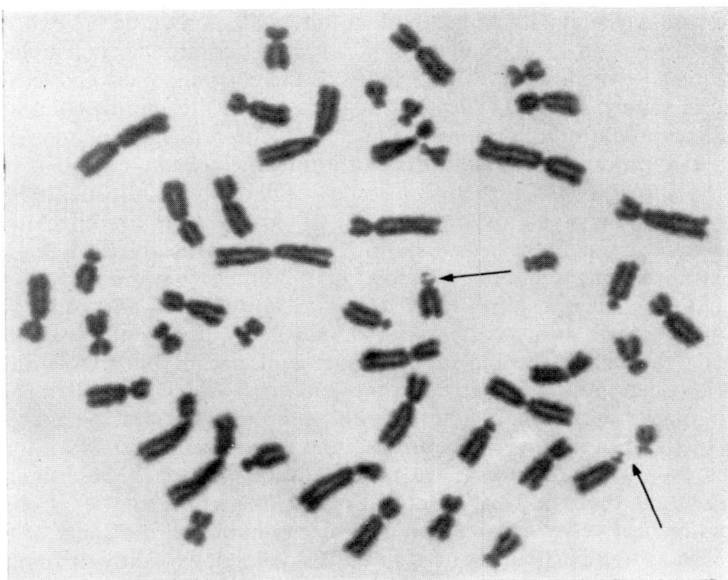

19/Fig. 1.—Cell of a normal human male at mitotic metaphase. Arrows indicate two satellited D group chromosomes one of which is associated with a chromosome of group G. Blood culture. Air dried preparation stained in acetic-orcein.

tion is between the bases adenine and thymine and between guanine and cytosine respectively. Current dogma holds that this sequence constitutes the genetic code, that in the living interphase cell a process of *transcription* occurs in which smaller messenger ribonucleic acid (RNA) molecules are synthesised of nucleotides complementary to those in segments of one strand of the DNA, and that the messenger RNA molecules pass into the cytoplasm where their own base sequences are *translated* into the amino-acid sequences of specific polypeptide chains at special structures usually associated with endoplastic reticulum, the *polyribosomes*. The total DNA of single nuclei of diploid cells is normally constant for the species. Within the class Mammalia it differs little from one species to another, the amount being approximately 6×10^{-12} grams, equivalent to approximately 6×10^{9} nucleotide pairs.

Basic proteins known as histones are the principal constituents of chromosomes additional to DNA. Recent evidence assigns them a role in the regulation of genetic activity.

Human Somatic Chromosomes

Human somatic chromosomes are usually studied in preparations obtained from cells in culture. These may be conventional tissue cultures established from any convenient source (principally dermal fibroblasts), or short-term cultures of peripheral blood in which small lymphocytes are induced to transform into actively dividing large mononuclear cells by the action of phytohæmagglutinin (PHA), a substance present in the seeds of many plant species of the family

Leguminosae. An adequate number of mitotic cells is assured by exposing the culture to the action of a spindle-inhibiting drug (commonly colchicine). This arrests mitosis at metaphase. It also shortens the chromosomes and leaves them dispersed in the cytoplasm, instead of aggregated on the spindle as in a natural mitosis. The preparative method requires first, the replacement of the culture media by a hypotonic fluid, next, the fixation of the cells in a swollen state and finally, the spreading of the chromosomes of individual mitotic cells on the slide, by squashing or air drying (FIG. 1). Fluid transfers are effected by first centrifuging to sediment the cells. Essentially the same procedure can be employed for biopsy specimens (e.g. bone marrow) taken direct from the body.

An array of chromosomes from a single cell like that shown in FIG. 2 is termed a *karyotype* and its obvious purpose is to display the essential morphological features of the chromosome set and permit more accurate comparisons between individual chromosomes or chromosome pairs than is possible in the original photograph. The term is also used in an abstract sense to denote the sum of the morphological features of the chromosome set of an individual or species. Nearly parallel terms are *genotype* and *phenotype*. These signify, for a given individual, the totality of genetic information and the totality of observable characters respectively, or, and perhaps more commonly, that part of the total that is relevant to a particular question that is defined, explicitly or implicitly, in the context.

The 46 chromosomes of a diploid cell from a normal human male (FIGS. 1 and 2) include the *sex chromosomes*, X and Y, and 44 *autosomes*. They normally range from about 1·5μ to about 7μ in length, though the degree of contraction varies considerably from one cell to another. Following the convention agreed upon at Denver in 1960, the pairs are numbered in serial order of length. The letter system for distinguishing the groups of similar pairs was introduced later by Patau and has been widely adopted. The karyotype of a normal female differs from that of a normal male only in the presence of two X chromosomes instead of an X and a Y.

The individual pairs of chromosomes are distinguished primarily by relative length and centromere position though only pairs 1, 2, 3 and 16 can be identified decisively in this way. A chromosome with its centromere located somewhere in the middle, like those of groups A, C and F, is termed *metacentric*; one with its centromere very close to one end, like those of groups D and G, is *acrocentric*. Notwithstanding their lack of exact definition, these terms are useful. The chromosomes of pairs 4, 5, 17 and 18 fall neither into one class nor the other. The terms "sub-metacentric" and "sub-acrocentric" have been employed by some and might be useful here.

The paired X and Y chromosomes of the male are conspicuous at the first meiotic division (FIG. 3), which therefore provides a guide to relative size. At mitotic metaphase the Y can generally be picked out without difficulty. It is commonly about the same length as the chromosomes of group G but has a less prominent short arm and chromatids that may be diffuse terminally and typically lie closely parallel (FIG. 2). The fact that there are 15 members of group C in the male, 16 in the female, immediately places the X in this group. There is little doubt that it is one of the longest of the group, but neither the single X of the normal male nor the paired Xs of the normal female can be identified with certainty.

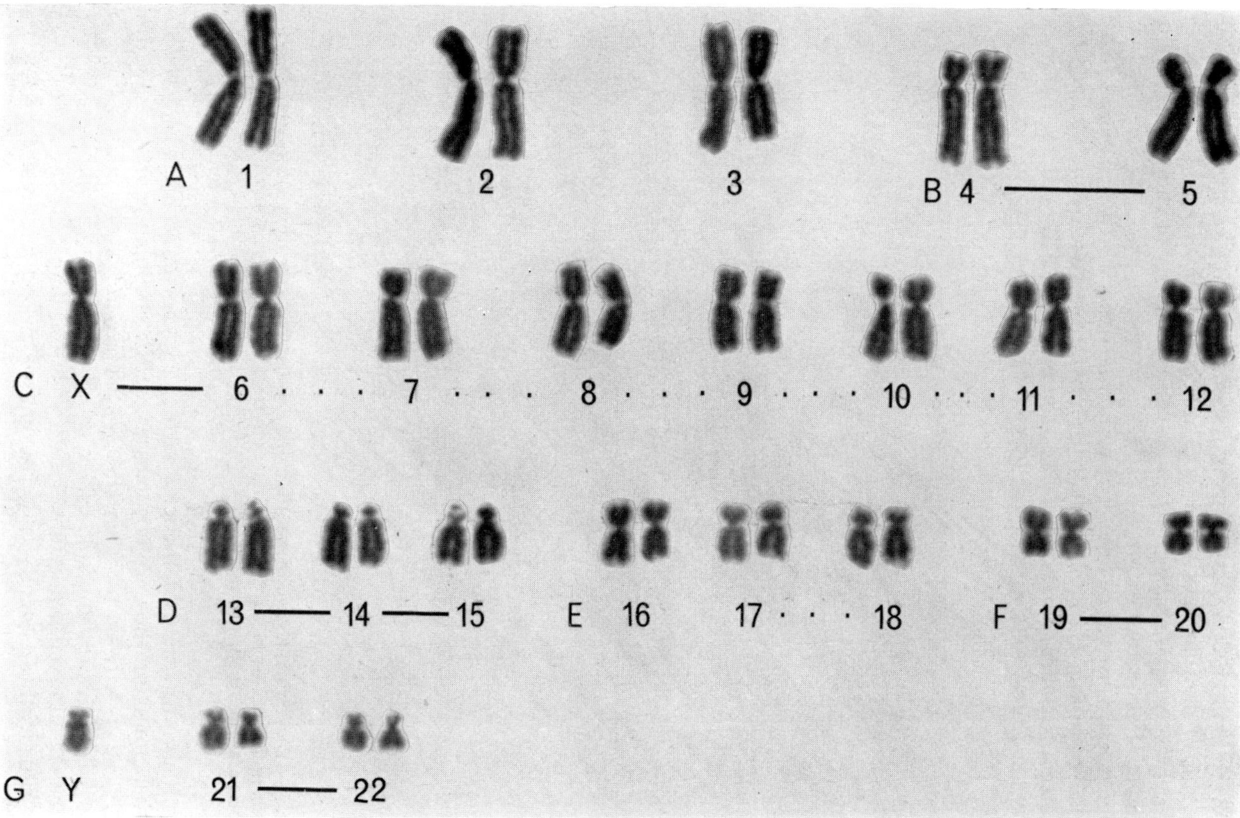

19/Fig. 2.—Karyotype of a normal human male prepared from the cell shown in Fig. 1.

Minor morphological features such as satellites and secondary constrictions may be of value in the identification of particular pairs in other species but they are of very limited usefulness in man. *Satellites* are minute appendages to the chromatids of the short arms of acrocentric chromosomes (FIG. 1). The number of these chromosomes that bear satellites varies from zero to a maximum of ten, but tends to be constant within the cells of a particular subject. Each is attached to its chromatid by a thin thread, the *satellite stalk*, which is believed to be a nucleolar organiser. Human acrocentric chromosomes are frequently seen to be associated proximally in groups of two or more (FIGS. 1 and 4). These may represent relic relationships derived from former attachment to the same nucleolus.

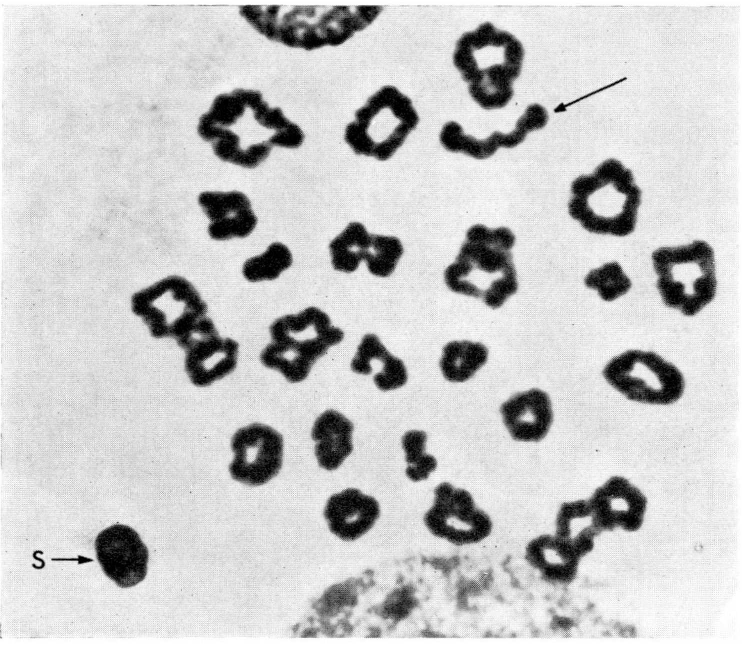

19/FIG. 3.—Diakinesis stage of meiosis in a primary spermatocyte from a normal human male. 22 autosomal bivalents plus the XY bivalent (arrow). The letter S indicates a sperm head. Air dried preparation. Acetic-orcein stain.

Each chromosome is constricted at the centromere. *Secondary constrictions* are other points on the chromosomes where the chromatids are narrowed and (usually) lie close to one another (FIG. 4). Unlike the centric constrictions they are variable in expression from cell to cell even of the same individual, but are nevertheless observed in the same locations in presumptively the same chromosomes sufficiently frequently to be recognised as real features of the chromosome set. The one most frequently seen in human cells lies in the long arm of a medium-length C-group chromosome, close to the centromere.

Autoradiography with tritiated thymidine is at present the most valuable supplement to simple observations of relative length and arm ratio for purposes of chromosome identification. Tritiated thymidine is incorporated into the chromosomes during the period of DNA synthesis (S phase) of the cell cycle, which in cultured cells terminates about five to six hours before metaphase. If tritiated thymidine is given to cells in culture and preparations are made from aliquots taken at intervals thereafter, the first cells in metaphase to show label will have been at the end of S when the istope was administered. In these cells some chromosome segments show a heavy label, others a light label or none, the pattern being a repeatable property of the individual segment. It is supposed that the segments with the heavy label were still actively replicating their DNA close to the end of S and that those with no label had completed it. By this technique it has been found possible to distinguish with a high degree of confidence between some chromosomes otherwise uncertainly distinguishable, if at all.[1] For example, the six very similar long acrocentric chromosomes of group D are divided into three pairs, one of which shows a very weak label, another a heavy label at the tip of the long arm and the third a heavy label over the greater part of the long arm.

Special Properties of the X Chromosome

The most striking result that has emerged from autoradiographic studies however was the discovery that in cells from normal females given tritiated thymidine at the end of S, one of the longest members of the C group shows an exceptionally heavy label (FIGS. 4 and 5). No corresponding heavily labelled chromosome was found in cells from normal males and there is now good evidence that the exceptional chromosome in females is one of the two X chromosomes. It is commonly referred to as the "hot" X. In normal females also, but not in males, one of the longer members of the C group is claimed to contract precociously in prophase, a phenomenon known as *heteropycnosis*. Another important property shown by normal females but not by normal males of many mammalian species, including man, is the presence of a prominent chromocentre that usually lies just within the nuclear membrane in a high proportion of the cells of suitable tissues (FIG. 6). This body, which is most conveniently sought in smears of cells from the buccal mucosa, is generally known as sex chromatin. It has played an important part in the investigation of intersexual states, subjects that possess it being described as "*chromatin-positive*", those that lack it as "*chromatin-negative*". Current hypothesis links the hot X, the heteropycnotic chromosome and the sex chromatin body and supposes them to be different expressions of the same X chromosome. The relationship of this chromosome to the postulated "inactive" X chromosome in normal females is considered later.

Many cases have been reported in which two, three or even four sex chromatin bodies are present. These cases have 17, 18 and 19 chromosomes respectively in the C group. Furthermore, in appropriately timed autoradiographic preparations two, three or four show up as "hot" chromosomes comparable in intensity of labelling to the single "hot X" of normal females. It has become the convention to accept observations of this kind as evidence of the number of X chromosomes present, though they fall short of formal proof.

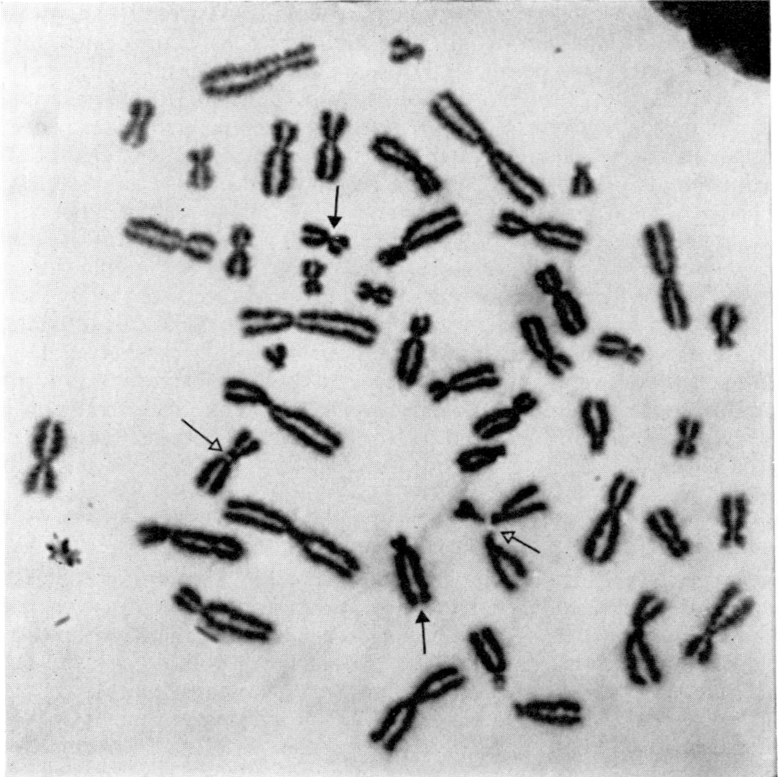

19/FIG. 4.—Aneuploid cell of a human female at mitotic metaphase with 47 chromosomes. Open arrows point to a secondary constriction in a chromosome of group C and to a proximal association of three acrocentric chromosomes. The patient was heterozygous for a presumptive reciprocal translocation between chromosomes of the C and E groups. The rearranged chromosomes, one of which resembles a No. 16, are shown by solid arrows.

Meiosis

Studies of meiotic chromosomes, whether in spermatogenesis or oogenesis, have not yet made much contribution to human cytogenetics. Some knowledge of the meiotic process is nevertheless essential for understanding many of the findings. The broad outlines of meiosis are much the same in the vast majority of higher organisms though there are a great variety of superimposed modifications in individual species or in particular sexes of individual species. The successive phases of normal meiosis are as follows: the chromosomes first appear as long, thin, single strands (*leptotene*); they come to lie side-by-side in homologous pairs or *bivalents* (*zygotene*), the high specificity of pairing being demonstrated by the exactly matching, but irregular linear sequence of variably enlarged, heavily stained regions of the chromosomes, the *chromomeres*; the pairs become shorter and thicker, revealing their specific chromomere patterns more clearly (*pachytene*); the separate chromosomes of each bivalent become visibly double

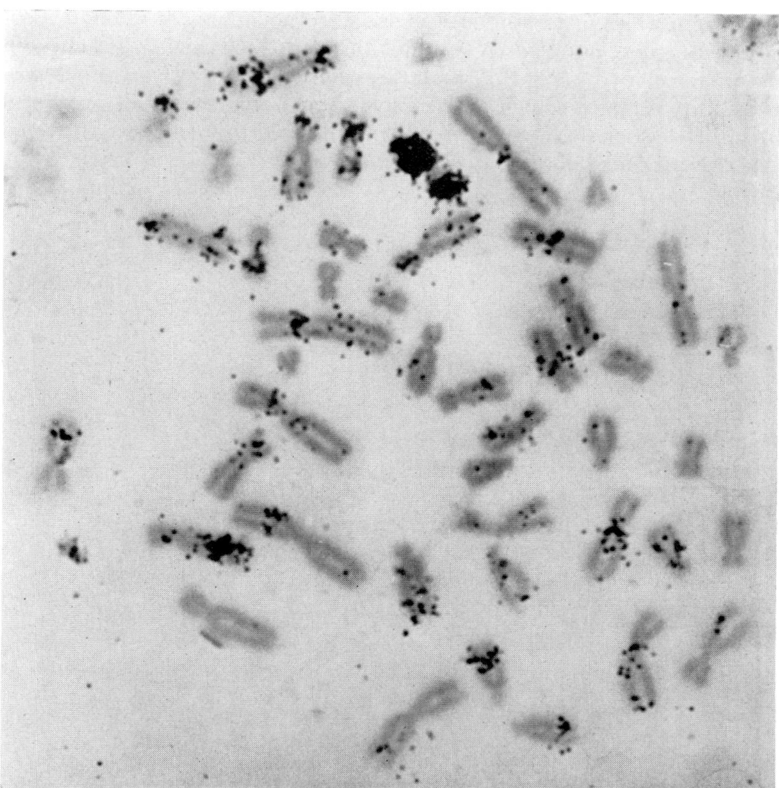

19/FIG. 5.—Tritiated thymidine autoradiograph of the cell shown in Fig. 4. The 'hot' X chromosome is prominent.

and simultaneously move apart from one another, leaving points of apparent attachment (*chiasmata*) where, in favourable preparations, the four constituent strands can be seen to exchange partners (*diplotene*); the bivalents contract still further, during which process some of the chiasmata may move distally and even attain a fully terminal position (*diakinesis*); the bivalents assemble on the spindle (*metaphase 1*) and disjoin into half-bivalents (*anaphase 1*); the half-bivalents pass on to newly formed spindles (*metaphase 11*) and disjoin into single chromatids (*anaphase 11*); finally, daughter nuclei are organised from the resultant polar groups (*telophase 11*). The net result of the whole process is the division of one diploid nucleus into four haploid nuclei, which, since each chiasma involves exchange between only two of the four strands, have different, but complementary combinations of the parental chromosomes, taken segment by segment. The fact that in oocyte meiosis the first polar body may not divide again does not affect the principles involved. A human spermatocyte in diakinesis is shown in FIG. 3.

In the human male and the males of many other mammalian species the detail of the pairing of X and Y in meiosis has not been resolved. When first clearly recognisable (in diplotene) the sex chromosomes are already associated end-to-end but it is not known whether this represents an earlier chiasma that has terminalised or a non-chiasmate association that was terminal *ab initio*. The possibility remains that X and Y have short homologous terminal segments by which they associate. These have been termed *pairing segments*, the remainder of each chromosome being its *differential segment*.

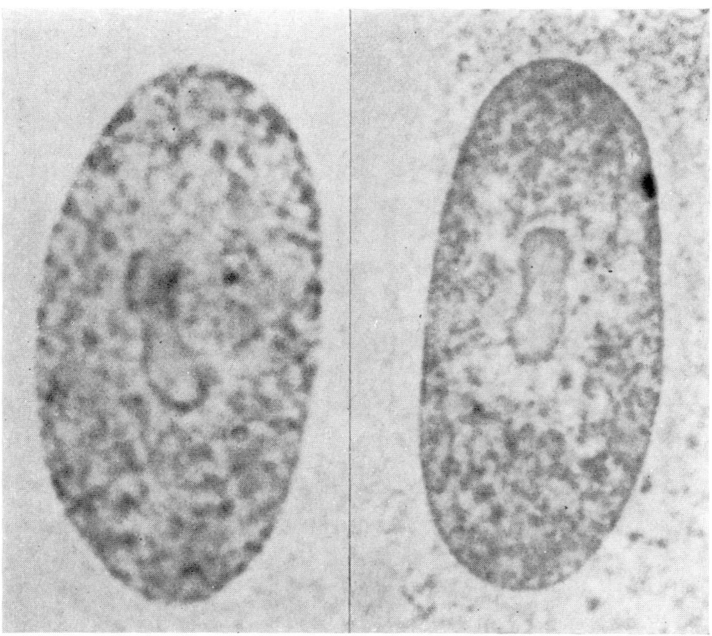

19/FIG. 6.—Nuclei from cells of a normal human male (left) and female (right). The sex chromatin body is prominent in the female nucleus. Fibroblast cultures. Feulgen stain.

Meiosis in female mammals differs in one very important way which interrupts rather than changes the sequence of events. The process is initiated in the primary oocytes of the embryonic ovary and may reach the diplotene stage at or shortly before birth. The bivalents, however, instead of continuing to contract, extend again until a nuclear organisation resembling mitotic interphase results. The oocytes remain in this (*dictyate*) stage until follicular maturation begins. Meiosis is then resumed at the point where it was interrupted. In the human female it is believed that first meiotic anaphase occurs in the oviduct immediately after penetration of the ovum by a sperm.

There is much evidence in favour of the hypothesis that chiasmata are the physical representation of genetic crossovers. Each chiasma would be equivalent to a genetic map length of 50 crossover units, so that in human spermatogenesis, with a mean of about 55 chiasmata per cell, the mean genetic length of the autosomes would be approximately 125 units and the total, 2750 units.

Karyotypic Abnormalities: Numerical Changes

Abnormalities of the karyotype are conveniently considered in two classes, *numerical* changes and *structural* changes. Numerical change may involve the addition (or subtraction) of single chromosomes, or groups of chromosomes, to give a nonintegral multiple of the basic haploid number (*aneuploidy*) or the addition of whole chromosome sets (*polyploidy*). Simplest among the aneuploids are *trisomic* (2n + 1) and *monosomic* (2n — 1) forms.

Numerical changes presumptively arise in consequence of anaphase abnormalities or other errors of mitosis or meiosis that are rarely seen. Anaphase abnormalities include *non-disjunction* (the movement of both daughters of one chromosome or bivalent to the same pole) and *lagging* (the failure of one or both of the disjoining daughter chromosomes to reach the poles, followed by exclussion from the daughter nuclei and eventually the formation of micronuclei that disintegrate in the cytoplasm). Other abnormalities generate *tetraploid* (4n) cells. These include abortive anaphase in which the disjoining chromosomes are not adequately separated and a single nuclear membrane forms round both groups to form a *restitution nucleus*. Tetraploid cells may also result from *endoreduplication*. This is a not very happily chosen term and implies a process whereby the chromosomes are believed to replicate twice in interphase. So much is inferred from the observation at mitotic metaphase of what at first appear to be quadripartite chromosomes but which on closer examination are seen to be closely associated pairs. Fusion of diploid nuclei is also a possible source of tetraploid cells. It has been demonstrated between mammalian cells growing in tissue culture but is not proven for somatic cells *in vivo*. Grossly irregular chromosome numbers may be generated through the appearance of *multipolar spindles* and the partition of the chromosomes of a diploid, or more usually, polyploid cell between three, four or more polar groups. *Chromosome mosaics*, in which cells of two or more different chromosome constitutions are present, are relatively common in human subjects. They presumptively originate very early in development as a result of one or more of the abnormalities just described.

The genetic consequences of aneuploidy are illustrated by the chromosomal mutants of the plant, *Datura stramonium*.[2] Twelve kinds of primary trisomic occur, one corresponding to each chromosome of the haploid set. Each kind has its own distinctive phenotype that deviates from the normal by a whole series of differences, mostly of a minor nature, but which involve almost all the observable plant characters from growth habit to the detailed form of the spines on the fruits. Monosomic plants have not been found in this species and plants with two extra chromosomes, if they are viable at all, are much more severely affected.

These and similar observations on other forms contributed to the development of the important concept of chromosome *balance*. It can be supposed that the proportions of the chromosomes within the normal set of any species are harmoniously adjusted. Should this adjustment be altered by addition or subtraction of a particular chromosome or chromosome segment, the dosage of the corresponding set of genes would be altered. This could be expected to lead to disturbed rates of particular metabolic reaction chains and so to modified developmental pathways. In the extreme, when the degree of unbalance is severe, development may cease at an early stage and death ensue. The precipitating chromosome constitution is then said to be *lethal*.

Karyotypic Abnormalities: Structural Changes

Structural changes arise in consequence of chromosome breakage and the rejoining of the broken ends to give new segmental combinations. In this context therefore, the word "structural" is used to connote linear, segmental constitution, not physical architecture. The processes of breakage and rejoining are largely, if not quite exclusively, confined to interphase. Structural changes are rare in normal tissue whether germinal or somatic, but are greatly increased in frequency by exposure to ionising radiation or certain chemical agents.

A single break that is not healed or rejoined leads to the appearance of a pair of fragments at the ensuing metaphase. The *acentric fragment* is incapable of moving on the spindle and is almost invariably excluded from the daughter nuclei at telophase at the first mitosis after origin. In the rare instances where it is passively included in one telophase nucleus, it reproduces with the other chromosomes in interphase, and is then again exposed to risk of loss at the next anaphase. The complementary *centric fragment* may pass through one or two mitoses but with few possible exceptions it is incapable of indefinite transmission. Muller postulated that without a centromere and two special particles, *telomeres*, one at the end of each arm, a chromosome is not mechanically stable.

Structural changes requiring two breaks and two rejoins include *reciprocal translocations*, in which chromosomes of the segmental constitution AB and CD exchange distal segments to become AD and CB; and *inversions*, in which the two breaks occur in one chromosome and the middle segment is rotated through 180° before rejoining. If the centromere is included within the middle segment the inversion is *pericentric*, if not, it is *paracentric*. An *interstitial deletion* results if the two end segments rejoin; the middle segment is then left as an acentric fragment and lost. A deletion may also arise as the complementary product to a *duplication* by the equivalent of a reciprocal translocation between homologous chromosomes, or between the two chromatids of one chromosome, thus: ABC, ABC → ABBC, AC. A short deletion may be called a *deficiency*.

Three-break changes are less frequently recognised. They include *transpositions*, or *shifts* (ABCDE → ACDBE) and *insertions* (ABC, DE → AC, DBE). Such changes can only be identified if evidence of linear specificity of morphological pattern or of pairing properties can be obtained as in dipteran salivary gland chromosomes or at meiosis. More complex structural changes are also possible.

A special type of rearrangement, widespread throughout the animal kingdom, involves the conversion of two acrocentric chromosomes into one metacentric chromosome. This is often referred to as *centric fusion* although it could represent a special case of reciprocal translocation where both breaks are close to the centromeres and the complementary product (which may be genetically silent) is lost. It is also known as *Robertsonian translocation*.

Misdivision is the name given to errors in the division of the centromere which can give rise to structurally changed chromosomes of a different class. It has been observed in univalents at meiosis in various plant species and though the phenomenon is rare, its consequences have been studied in forms where univalents are regularly present. Transverse division of the centromere takes place rather than the normal longitudinal division and results in two monocentric structures each with two identical chromatids. Should either structure be included within a daughter nucleus it may be perpetuated as a chromosome with two equal and genetically equivalent arms, called an *isochromosome*. Another form of misdivision involves the partition of the four half-chromatids of a metaphase chromosome into a group of three and a single one, each group being attached to one daughter centromere. Should the single half-chromatid be perpetuated, it becomes a *telocentric* chromosome which, by failure of its centromere to divide at a later mitosis, may give rise secondarily to an isochromosome. Misdivision itself has not been demonstrated in mammalian species but the occurrence of presumptive isochromosomes is now well established in man.

In experimental material, duplication and deletion, being unbalanced changes, may have a pronounced phenotypic effect and may mimic dominant gene mutations in their genetic behaviour. Balanced changes, like most reciprocal translocations and inversions, do not usually modify the phenotype: if they do, their interpretation as balanced changes may be questioned since the association of a small duplication or deficiency with the rearrangement is difficult to exclude. Alternatively, *position effect* may be invoked. Structural change without an associated phenotypic effect is often first suspected from the observation of reduced fertility that is transmitted to a portion of the offspring (hereditary semi-sterility). Confirmation may be sought from breeding tests (changed linkage relations) or from cytological examination. In the special case of species of the genus *Drosophila* and related forms the large salivary gland chromosomes can provide detailed information regarding the nature of a change and the exact loci of breakage and reunion.

Examination of somatic chromosomes can only reveal a structural change if it has brought about a decisive alteration of the relative length or arm ratio of at least one chromosome. Paracentric inversions, and reciprocal translocations involving the exchange of approximately equal segments, for example, would not be detectable. Furthermore, even when morphologically abnormal chromosomes are identified, evidence from somatic mitosis alone does not permit the exact nature of the change to be determined. It is therefore the usual practice to accept the simplest explanation that will fit the facts and refer to the interpretation adopted as "presumptive".

The limitation indicated in the last paragraph applies with particular force in human cytogenetics where the greater opportunities for analysis provided by meiotic cells are rarely available. The special value of meiotic cells comes from the very high specificity of chromosome pairing in meiotic prophase, which is retained on a segmental basis whatever the nature of the rearrangement. For example, in an individual heterozygous for (i.e. a carrier of) a reciprocal translocation, the two rearranged chromosomes and their two structurally normal partial homologues are paired segment-by-segment at pachytene in a cross-like pattern (Fig. 7). The number of chiasmata subsequently formed at diplotene and their distribution may vary considerably. Should chiasmata be formed in each arm of the cross, a ring-like association of four (ring *quadrivalent*, ring IV) results (FIG. 7). Failure of chiasma formation in one or more arms leads to the appearance of a linear association of four (chain IV), or a linear association of three and a singleton (*trivalent* plus *univalent*, III + I), or two bivalents, or a bivalent plus two univalents, or in the very rare extreme, four univalents. The complexities are compounded at first anaphase by different modes of congression on the spindle, leading to different types of disjunction. Suffice it to say that 10 different euploid gametic combinations (of chromosome segments) are possible and that if non-disjunction is taken into account, the number is increased to 36, of which only two are balanced.

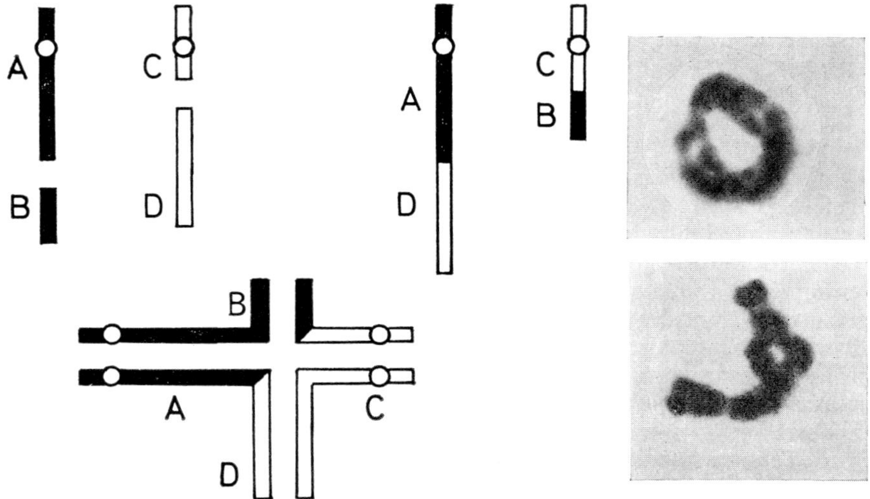

19/FIG. 7.—(*Left*). Diagram indicating the origin of an unequal reciprocal translocation between two D group chromosomes and the cross-like association expected in pachytene. The small circles symbolise the centromeres. The letters A to D indicate the four segments produced by two breaks in two chromosomes. (*Right*). Ring and chain quadricalents from spermatocytes of a mouse heterozygous for a reciprocal translocation similar to that shown in the diagram.

Reciprocal translocations have been well studied in one mammalian species only, the mouse. Despite the number of disjunctional possibilities, in heterozygotes of most translocation lines the output of balanced gametes is not greatly different from 50 per cent. The corresponding figure in human translocations is unknown. The important points are that sperm and ova carrying unbalanced combinations of chromosome segments are fully viable and functional and that an unbalanced *zygotic* combination may lead to death of the resultant embryo *in utero*. In the mouse this is almost invariably so. In man, many of the unbalanced fœtuses have been carried to term and born alive as grossly abnormal children. It remains to add that since chromosome breakage and reunion are essentially random processes, each reciprocal translocation is effectively unique in its detailed cytogenetic properties, including the probability that a given zygote will be unbalanced and the probability that a given unbalanced combination will complete uterine development.

Symbolic Designation of Human Karyotypes

At a conference in Chicago in 1966 a system for the representation of human karyotypes was agreed upon and recommended for general adoption.[1] According to this system, which was designed to be suitable for computer handling, the minimum designation includes the chromosome number and the sex chromosome constitution. To this may be added other numbers, letters, abbreviations or symbols to indicate additional or missing autosomes, the nature of presumed or proven structural changes and other karyotypic features. The principal ones are: 1–22, the autosome numbers (Denver system); A–G, the chromosome groups; p, the short arm of a chromosome; q, the long arm of a chromosome; r, ring chromosome; t, translocation; inv, inversion; i, isochromosome; + or −, extra or missing chromosome *or* longer or shorter structure; ?, interpretation presumptive or uncertain.

Examples, are:

45, X	45 chromosomes, one X chromosome.
47, XXY	47 chromosomes, XXY sex chromosomes.
47, XX, G+	47 chromosomes, XX sex chromosomes, extra chromosome of G group.
46, XY, ?t(Bq − Gq+)	46 chromosomes, XY sex chromosomes, presumptive balanced reciprocal translocation between the long arm of a B group chromosome and the long arm of a G group chromosome.
46, XX/47, XXY	A chromosome mosaic with two cell types, one with 46 chromosomes and XX sex chromosomes, the other with 47 chromosomes and XXY sex chromosomes.
45, X/46, X(Xqi)	A chromosome mosaic with two cell types, one with 45 chromosomes including a single X, the other with 46 chromosomes including one normal X and one X long arm isochromosome.

SEX CHROMOSOME ABNORMALITIES

The discovery of the sex chromatin body gave a great impetus to the investigation of errors of sex development. Attention was given particularly to two conditions, *Klinefelter's syndrome*, with an essentially male phenotype and *Turner's syndrome*, with an essentially female phenotype. It was soon found that, contrary to the rule in normal subjects, the great majority of Klinefelter cases were sex chromatin positive and the great majority of Turner cases were sex chromatin negative. Investigation of the frequency of colour blindness, the sex-linked condition with the highest incidence in the general population, showed that in Klinefelter cases the frequency was similar to that recorded for normal females (0·5 per cent) and that in Turner cases the frequency approached the level in normal males (7 per cent). It was inferred that Klinefelter patients had two X chromosomes, Turner patients only one. When methods for chromosomal examination became available these inferences were verified: typical

Klinefelter cases were found to be 47, XXY and typical Turner cases to be 45, X.

These successes prompted the extension of chromosome investigations to further subjects exhibiting Klinefelter's and Turner's syndromes and to other irregularities of the sex phenotype. Case material has been obtained from sex chromatin surveys of the newborn and of inmates of institutions for mental defectives, among male cases attending infertility clinics, among cases of primary amenorrhœa and among cases of all ages with ambiguous genitalia. Very many types of karyotypic abnormality involving the sex chromosomes have been identified, including a great variety of chromosome mosaics. The occurrence of mosaics raises difficulties of two kinds: first, some of the cases present intermediate phenotypes and second, in no individual case can the possibility of a mosaic constitution be excluded, whatever the number of different anatomical sites from which cells are taken for chromosomal examination.

Phenotypic Males

Klinefelter's Syndrome

Most of the cases of abnormal sex chromosome constitution with a male phenotype[3] exhibit Klinefelter's syndrome,[4] the essential feature of which is the failure of normal testicular development at puberty. In the adult the testes are small, the seminiferous tubules are empty of all but Sertoli cells and the urinary excretion of gonadotrophin is increased. Associated but variable features are gynæcomastia, eunuchoidism, reduced growth of facial hair, osteoporosis, and mental defect. Puberty may be late and ageing premature.

Clinically, the syndrome is probably encountered most frequently at male infertility clinics. It has been stated that in sex chromatin-negative cases, which may amount to 20 per cent of the total, the testes present a quite distinct histological picture, with many tubules of approximately normal size, occasional signs of spermatogenesis and diffusely increased, but cytologically normal Leydig cells. In sex chromatin-positive cases the tubules are smaller, fewer in number and have hyalinised or partly hyalinised membranes, the Leydig cells are aggregated into clumps and have pleomorphic nuclei. It may be that these histological changes are initiated at puberty since in the prepubertal male (who can be recognised by sex chromatin pattern or chromosome constitution) the tubules present a normal appearance except for some reduction of spermatogonia. The sex chromatin-positive form has sometimes been distinguished as "true" Klinefelter's syndrome from the "false" sex chromatin-negative form. Some consider the eponym unsatisfactory and have used alternative names including "seminiferous tubule dysgenesis", "testicular dysgenesis", "medullary gonadal dysgenesis" and "primary micro-orchidism".

Examination of the chromosomes in additional cases of chromatin-positive Klinefelter's syndrome has fully confirmed that the typical constitution is 47,XXY. The same syndrome, or a more extreme form of it, has also been observed in subjects with the following karyotypes: 48,XXYY; 48,XXXY; 49,XXXYY; and 49,XXXXY. Very few examples of the second of these karyotypes have been described and only one of the third. More examples of the first and fourth are on record, but they are infrequent in comparison with the

47,XXY karyotype. As the number of X chromosomes is increased, the reduction in the size of the testes, the histological changes in the seminiferous tubules and the degree of mental retardation become more severe and skeletal defects, of which radioulnar synostosis is the most characteristic, are often present.

Many types of chromosome mosaics also exhibit Klinefelter's syndrome or its variants. All of them include cell lines with one or more of the karyotypes just mentioned. The type most often encountered is 46,XY/47,XXY which seems to occur between five and ten times more frequently than the corresponding 46,XX/47,XXY type. Several of the others include three cell lines, some of which require the assumption of two separate errors to account for their origin. Among the 46,XY/47,XXY mosaics are some that show a less severe expression of the syndrome and some indeed of proven fertility. But as indicated earlier, it is not possible to generalize about the phenotype of mosaics since much presumably depends on the proportion of the different cell types in critical organs, among which the gonads, without doubt, will take first place. It is therefore entirely possible that some 46,XY/47,XXY mosaics are clinically normal individuals whose karyotypic abnormality would only be detected if they chanced to be investigated for some independent reason.

The abnormal karyotype of the typical Klinefelter case presumably originates from a non-disjunctional event. This could be at gametogenesis and result in the fertilization of a normal X ovum by a non-disjunctional XY sperm or of a non-disjunctional XX ovum by a normal Y sperm. Error at an early cleavage division of an XY zygote is also a possibility. Should non-disjunction of the X chromosome occur at the first zygotic division, the complementary products would be cells with the karyotypes 45,Y and 47,XXY, respectively, and since there is reason to believe that the first of these is lethal, the surviving cell might develop into a non-mosaic embryo and a potential Klinefelter subject. Should non-disjunction occur at a later cleavage division, a non-mosaic 47,XXY embryo could still result by chance assortment of cells into the germinal disc from a mosaic blastocyst. The two modes of origin lead to different expected frequencies of expression of recessive sex-linked genes. Evidence from investigations using the sex-linked red cell antigen Xg^a is compatible with a contribution from zygotic non-disjunction. This might account for the greater frequency of 46,XY/47,XXY mosaics compared with 46,XX/47,XXY mosaics, since the latter must originate either by loss of the Y chromosome from 47,XXY zygotes or from 46,XY zygotes through the unlikely occurrence of errors at two separate divisions (XY $\rightarrow$ XXY $\rightarrow$ XX) *and* the effective exclusion of cells carrying the original zygotic combination.

Notwithstanding their apparent unlikelihood, mosaic karyotypes *have* been identified that require errors at two different mitoses for their explanation. An example is the 46,XY/46,XX/47,XXY, combination just considered, found in an elderly Klinefelter subject.

Karyotype 47,XYY

Subjects with the karyotype 47,XYY are rare. The first to be described was a clinically normal male who came to attention as the father of three abnormal children. Very few further examples were recorded until 1965, when it was announced that nine cases had been found among 315 men examined in a survey of men detained in a maximum security hospital.[5] Seven of the nine were mentally subnormal and all had a criminal record, mostly of crimes against property. The mean age at first conviction was low (13·1 years). They came from families with a negligible criminal record or none and from all social classes.[6] A similar high frequency of 47,XYY men has also been recorded among the patients in three similar institutions. The subjects tend to be appreciably taller than the average but apart from this no noteworthy clinical or phenotypic feature has been described. The initial investigation was prompted by the discovery of an unexpectedly high frequency of 48,XXYY subjects in one of these institutions, following a sex chromatin survey of the inmates. These men are also taller on the average than 47,XXY Klinefelters and members of the normal population.

Karyotype 46,XX

Rare chromatin-positive phenotypic males have been recorded with an apparently normal and non-mosaic 46,XX female karyotype, despite the examination of an adequate number of cells from two or more different anatomical sources.[7] Gynæcomastia has been reported, the testes are somewhat reduced in size and histological examination of some of the cases has shown tubules lined by Sertoli cells only. It is not yet clear whether these "XX males" exhibit a characteristic phenotype of their own.

Phenotypic Females

Phenotypic females with abnormalities of the sex chromosomes have been detected by sex chromatin surveys of the newborn and of the inmates of institutions for the mentally retarded, among cases of primary or secondary amenorrhœa and among cases referred in childhood for physical abnormality or retarded growth.

Turner's Syndrome

The patients reported by Turner in 1938 exhibited sexual infantilism, webbing of the neck and cubitus valgus.[8] As now generally understood, sexual infantilism and dwarf stature are cardinal features of a syndrome that also includes any or all of a series of congenital malformations, mostly of a minor nature (Fig. 8) These, which are sometimes referred to collectively as Turner stigmata, include shield chest, multiple pigmented nævi, low hair line, hypoplastic fingernails, short fourth metacarpals and lymphœdema at birth, in addition to neck webbing and cubitus valgus. More serious anatomical abnormalities that may be present include horseshoe kidney and cardiovascular defects, particularly coarctation of the aorta. Laparotomy almost invariably reveals that the ovaries have been replaced by elongated structures composed of connective tissue resembling ovarian stroma but lacking any follicles. They are commonly referred to as "streak" gonads. Menstruation is uncommon and if it occurs at all it is often irregular and secondary amenorrhœa sets in early. Breast development is usually very poor or absent but is often improved by œstrogen treatment. Urinary excretion of gonadotrophins is usually low.

There is difficulty in summarising the information about these cases, partly because of the variety of different karyotypes and the great variability of the phenotype but also because of the considerable number of synonyms and partial synonyms for the condition that have been used in the literature. Principal among these are gonadal dysgenesis, Bonnevie-Ullrich syndrome, ovarian agenesis and ovarian dysgenesis. There is something to be said for the last of these, particularly now that it has been shown that normal or nearly normal ovaries with germ cells may be present in 45,X fœtuses and even newborn infants.[9] However, the name "ovarian dysgenesis" suggests that ovarian defect is the primary lesion and that the associated dwarf stature and congenital defects are secondary. There are no grounds for supposing that this is so.

Ferguson-Smith has clarified the problem by showing that almost all subjects with Turner's syndrome are deficient for at least part of the short arm of one of the X chromosomes in at least some of their cells, and that the remainder are sufficiently few in number to make the assumption of cryptic mosaicism reasonable.[10] The basic karyotypes in which there is such a deficiency are: 45,X; 46,X(Xqi); 46,X(Xp—) and 46,X(Xr), the first being much the most frequent. The bracketed symbols indicate X long arm isochromosome, X short arm deficiency and X ring chromosome respectively. The really significant comparisons are between the 46,X(Xqi) and 46,X(Xp—) types on the one hand and the rare 46,X(Xpi) and 46,X(Xq—) types on the other. The former have the long arm of the X represented two or three times and part or all of the short arm represented once only; they exhibit Turner's syndrome. The latter have the short arm of the X represented two or three times and the long arm represented once only; they do not exhibit Turner's syndrome as here understood, though they may have streak gonads, infantile genitalia and poorly developed secondary sexual characters and fail to menstruate. This condition, known as "pure gonadal dysgenesis", is distinct from Turner's syndrome and is considered later,

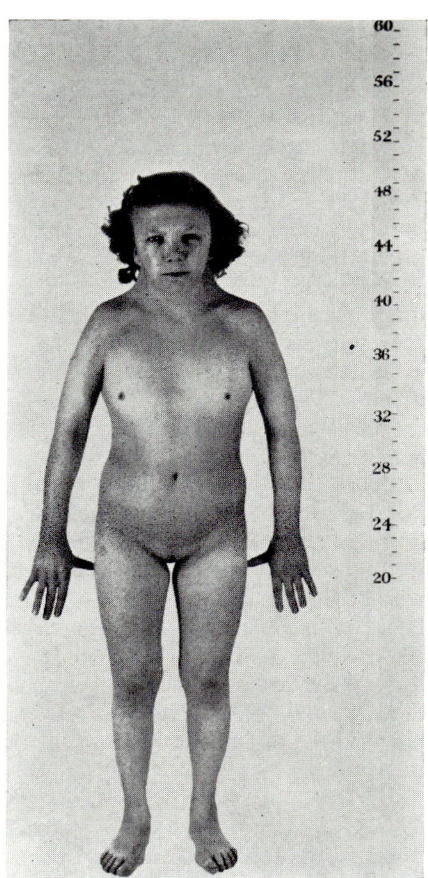

19/FIG. 8.—Turner's syndrome. Age 21. Primary amenorrhoea. Dwarfed. Neck webbing, cubitus valgus, widely spaced nipples, multiple nævi. Patient had horseshoe kidney, coarctation of the aorta and was red/green colour blind. Sex chromatin negative.

The basic karyotypes associated with Turner's syndrome may be compounded with 46,XX; 46,XY; 47,XXX and other karyotypes to form an enormous range of mosaic combinations. They may exhibit typical Turner's syndrome, an intermediate condition or a normal female *or male* phenotype. Apart from adding that those with a male phenotype have at least one cell line carrying a Y chromosome, nothing more can usefully be said about them at present.

In the light of the facts just given it seems reasonable to adopt a working hypothesis of two parts: first, that Turner's syndrome is a genetic deficiency syndrome attributable to the absence of part of the short arm of one X chromosome; and second, that in mosaic subjects the cellular constitution during embryogenesis of the gonadal primordia is critical.

Karyotypes 47,XXX; 48,XXXX; and 49,XXXXX

Many females with a 47,XXX karyotype have been described. They appear to have an essentially normal phenotype with no distinctive clinical picture.[11] However they are liable to menstrual disorders and to an early onset of secondary amenorrhœa or premature menopause. A deficiency of follicles in the ovaries has been reported. Nevertheless many are fertile. Most of the cases reported were identified as a result of sex chromatin surveys of institutional populations and it has been estimated that they constitute approximately five per 1000 female mental defectives, a frequency that is significantly greater than the one estimate among the newborn (1·2 per 1000). If these figures can be taken as representative they imply that the proportion of 47,XXX females who are eventually committed to an institution is appreciably greater than among normal women. They also imply that unless 47,XXX subjects have a particularly high mortality in childhood, a majority of the adults must be living unsuspected in the general population.

Theoretically it could be expected that 47,XXX women would produce normal 23,X ova and abnormal 24,XX ova in equal numbers and would be the mothers of 47,XXY Klinefelter sons and 47,XXX daughters like themselves, as well as equivalent numbers of normal sons and daughters. Yet all the children who have been examined so far have been chromosomally normal, the numbers being sufficient for the difference from expectation to be very highly significant. A possible explanation is loss of one of the three X chromosomes from oogonia by non-disjunction or lagging so that most of the oocytes that mature are, in fact, normal 46,XX. Alternatively, an asymmetrical first meiotic division could result in the inclusion of two of the three X chromosomes in the first polar body nucleus.

A few examples of females with a 48,XXXX karyotype and one with a 49,XXXXX karyotype are known, the latter a child. They are mentally subnormal but present no noteworthy clinical features. One of the 48,XXXX women is reported to have had two children, one a daughter with Down's syndrome.

Pure Gonadal Dysgenesis

The condition known as *pure gonadal dysgenesis*[12] shares with typical Turner's syndrome the streak gonads, primary amenorrhœa, failure of secondary sex development and raised excretion of gonadotrophin in the urine. In other respects the subjects differ. Specifically they are of normal or even tall stature and they do not exhibit any Turner stigmata (FIG. 9). Mental development, as in most cases of Turner's syndrome, appears to be unimpaired.

Chromosomally, there are three groups: mosaics that include a 45,X cell line; subjects with 46,X(Xpi) or 46,X(Xq−) karyotypes; and subjects with apparently normal 46,XX *or* 46,XY karyotypes. The latter are of particular theoretical interest because they appear to provide a natural parallel in the human species to the agonadal rabbits obtained by the French endocrinologist, Jost, following surgical removal of the gonads from 19-day embryos. These animals all had female external internal genitalia and sufficient were obtained to make it unlikely that, by chance, only female embryos had been operated on. A series of unilateral ablation experiments put the matter beyond doubt: they showed that in potential male embryos, Mullerian duct derivatives developed on the operated side and normal male structures on the side with the intact testis.

The possibility may therefore be considered that in pure gonadal dysgenesis with a 46,XY karyotype, the condition results from a *primary* failure of gonadal development. No vestiges of male internal genitalia have been reported in the cases that have come to laparotomy. The 46,XX cases could be parallel. It is most unlikely that they, and the 46,XY cases, could all be explained by cryptic mosaicism involving a 45,X cell line, because detected mosaics are few compared with the number of cases recorded with normal karyotypes. Furthermore, the fact that there are several instances on record of affected sisters suggests that a specific genetic factor (or factors) may be involved. Altogether it seems most reasonable to consider that pure gonadal dysgenesis is a condition *sui generis* and that some mosaics containing a 45,X cell line may simulate it, just as others may simulate normal males or females.

The existence of the 46,X(Xpi) and 46,X(Xq−) cases does not necessarily conflict with this view since genetic information necessary in double dose for normal ovarian development could be located on the long arm of the X, and if so, deficiency or mutation could produce the genetic conditions in mind.

The foregoing interpretation is one of gonadal *agenesis* rather than *dysgenesis*.

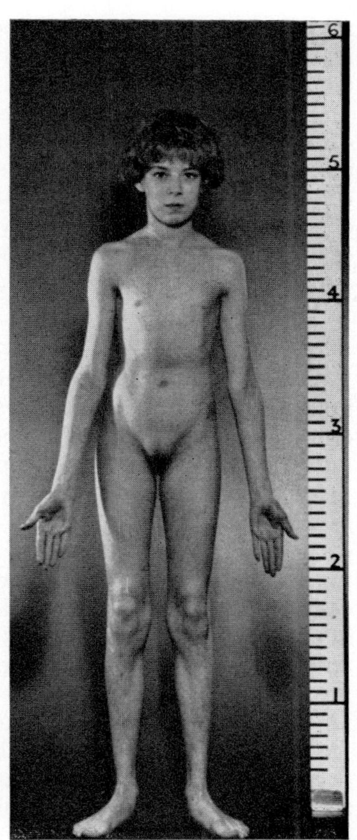

19/FIG. 9.—Pure gonadal dysgenesis. Age 16. Primary amenorrhœa. Eunuchoid habitus. Absence of stigmata of Turner's syndrome. Sex chromatin negative. Karyotype 46,XY.

Nevertheless, the name "pure gonadal dysgenesis" is well established and a change is not advocated. Only if the interpretation should be verified would it be appropriate to think again.

Testicular Feminisation

Mention should be made of another condition, *testicular feminisation*,[14] in which the affected individuals are phenotypic females with a normal 46,XY karyotype.[11] In the typical case the body confirmation is essentially, and often attractively, feminine; pubic and axillary hair is sparse or absent, the external genitalia are feminine, there is a short vagina and occasionally a rudimentary uterus. The most noteworthy feature however, is the presence of testes and associated ducts. The testes are often located in bilateral inguinal hernias but may alternatively be found within the abdomen or in the labia majora. Cases may be recognised in childhood when advice is sought in connection with the inguinal swellings or later, for primary amenorrhœa. There is also a risk of malignant change in the gonads.

The condition is familial, the evidence being consistent with the segregation of normal females, carrier females, affected females and normal males in equal numbers. This suggests that it is determined by either a sex-linked recessive gene or a sex-limited autosomal dominant gene. A satisfactory explanation in developmental terms has not yet been found, however. No evidence has been obtained of abnormal steroid metabolism and the level of androgens in the blood appears to be within normal male limits.

True Hermaphroditism

True hermaphrodites are defined as subjects who have gonadal tissue of both kinds. This tissue may be represented by one ovary and one testis. Alternatively either or both gonads may contain ovarian and testicular tissue variously combined into an *ovotestis.* Exceptionally, ovarian and testicular tissue may be present in distinct structures lying closely adjacent to one another. Testes and ovaries are usually located in their normal scrotal and abdominal positions; ovotestes are found to lie in scrotal, inguinal or abdominal positions with roughly equal frequency. Ovarian tissue may be apparently normal histologically even into adult life. Testicular tissue may approximate to normal during infancy, but germ cells disappear after puberty and the tubules become hyalinised and sclerosed. Strictly, therefore, the term "true hermaphrodite" is a biological misnomer. It ought to be reserved for individuals with *functional* gonads of both kinds. Widespread use is the justification for its retention here.

The internal genitalia usually correspond with the gonad on the same side, derivatives of the Müllerian duct (fallopian tube, uterus) being associated with an ovary, derivatives of the Wolffian duct (vas deferens, epididymis) with a testis and derivatives of either with an ovotestis. But there are many exceptions to these simple rules.

True hermaphroditism is extremely rare. In most of the cases whose chromosomes have been examined, cells with the normal female complement 46,XX have alone been found.[15] This holds even for cases where several different anatomical sites, including the gonadal structures themselves, have been sampled. A single case has been reported to be 46,XY though this, being so far unique, could represent an instance of unrecognised mosaicism. Chromosome mosaics with cell lines including the Y chromosome have indeed been identified. They include: 45,X/46,XY; 46,XX/47,XXY; 46,XX/47,XXY/49,XXYYY and 46,XX/46,XY. The origin of the last type is discussed in the next section.

The cytogenetic problem presented by true hermaphroditism is a matter of great theoretical interest. Its discussion is deferred to a later section.

Mosaics and Chimæras

Chromosome mosaics have been a recurrent theme of the foregoing presentation. The associated phenotypic diversity, the possibility of undetected cell lines and the importance of critical organs are given a remarkable demonstration by cases of monozygotic mosaic twins with discordant phenotypes. Three pairs have been recorded in which the sex chromosomes are involved. The absolute concordance observed in the investigation of polymorphic genetic systems (red cell antigens, serum proteins, enzyme variants) in each case makes the formal probability of origin from two independent zygotes low or negligible; and when this evidence is supplemented by the observation of closely similar dermal ridge patterns (two pairs), by obstetrical evidence of a synchorial placenta (two pairs) and by evidence of remarkably close physical similarity, no remaining doubt can be left that the twins were truly the products of single zygotes.

The first pair reported were a phenotypically normal 46,XY brother and his 45,X Turner sister.[16] The chromosomes were examined in cultures established solely from fascia lata and no evidence of mosaicism was obtained in either twin. Concordance in respect of seventeen different genetic polymorphic systems was recorded and the combined probability of origin from independent zygotes was calculated to be 0·00074. Reciprocal skin grafts were exchanged and accepted like autografts.

The second pair were also a phenotypically normal, though rather short brother and a Turner sister.[17] Cultures of blood and skin fibroblasts from the sister revealed that she was a 45,X/46,XY mosaic, though with a great excess of 45,X cells. Surprisingly, only 45,X mitoses were identified in similar cultures from the brother, although in his case skin fibroblasts from two different sites were cultured and a total of 181 cells was examined. In view of this result it is particularly significant that his external genitalia were of normal appearance and that his testes were "of normal size and consistency". There is therefore a very high probability that normal 46,XY cells contributed to the development of the testis, although none was detected in blood or skin.

The third pair were infant sisters who were found to be 45,X/46,XX mosaics.[18] The one twin was clinically normal. The other was mentally subnormal and showed a considerable number of Turner stigmata. Necropsy after she died aged $3\frac{10}{12}$ years revealed a minor cardiac defect and horseshoe kidney but histologically normal ovaries. Notwithstanding the striking clinical difference between the twins, approximately equal numbers of cells of each type were identified in blood and skin cultures of both.

Exchange of blood-borne cells between fœtuses as a result of placental vascular anastomosis is a regular phenomenon in dizygotic twin cattle and marmoset monkeys. A circulatory exchange between dizygotic fœtuses might therefore be suggested to explain the identity of serotype and the acceptance of recriprocal skin grafts in the twin pairs just described. However, in cattle, two distinct red cell types can be demonstrated in each twin and in the very few human (unquestioned) dizygotic twin pairs reported to have identical serotypes the same is true.[19] No mixing of red cell types was found in the twins under discussion and the weight of evidence in favour of monozygotic origin remains overwhelming.

The observations on discordant monozygotic twins therefore suggest that when a blastocyst that is already mosaic cleaves into two separate embryonic masses, the cell types may be partitioned unequally between the products; and that in the development of a mosaic embryo the cell types may similarly be partitioned unequally between different anatomical sites or organ rudiments, even to the extent of total exclusion of the one type.

Evidence from red cell antigens and serum proteins shows that in the 46,XX/46,XY true hermaphrodites, two serologically distinct cell types may be present in the circulation, as in the cattle twins.[20] However, they differ from the cattle twins in that the chromosomal mosaicism extends to cultures from fixed tissues, implying that the mosaic constitution was established early in embryogenesis. One possible explanation is fusion of two independent zygotes or early embryos. An alternative possibility is retention of a polar body nucleus within the ovum followed by double fertilization.

It is now usual to refer to individuals containing mixtures of cells derived from different zygotes, like the twin cattle, as *chimæras* and to reserve the term *mosaic* for individuals with cell mixtures arising from a single zygote. By this definition the 46,XX/46,XY cases just discussed are chimæras.

The Inactive X Chromosome Hypothesis

Classical sex-linked inheritance is due to the presence of two sets of the genetic loci concerned in the female, one set only in the male. Muller pointed out that a mechanism of *dosage compensation* must exist to adjust for the resultant sex difference in the dosage of sex-linked genes relative to the dosage of autosomal genes.

A hypothesis has been advanced by Lyon which provides a possible mechanism for dosage compensation in mammals and at the same time accounts for a number of hitherto unexplained mosaic phenotypes in female mice heterozygous for sex-linked genes affecting coat character.[21] The essential postulate is that at an early stage in the development of normal female embryos a process of random determination occurs, separately in each cell, whereby one of the two X chromosomes becomes genetically inactivated, the inactive state thereafter being maintained at each cell division. By hypothesis the body then becomes a mixture of cell lines or clones, some with an inactive paternal X chromosome, some with an inactive maternal X chromosome, each clone being derived from a single ancesteral cell at the time of inactivation. If the cellular progenitors of the hair follicles, or of the melanocytes in the dermis, should tend to remain associated after they have divided it is easy to appreciate how a macroscopically recognisable pattern of the coat could result.

An example in man is the rare sex-linked condition *anhidrotic ectodermal dysplasia*.[22] The affected male is unable to sweat and histologically there is a gross deficiency of sweat glands. Heterozygous (carrier) females have localised patches of skin from which sweating is absent, distributed in an erratic pattern over the whole body. Sex-linked glucose-6-phosphate dehydrogenase deficiency is one of several examples that have been described at the biochemical and cellular level. Cloning experiments with cells in tissue culture have shown that female heterozygotes contain cells of two kinds, those that show enzyme deficiency and those that do not. Normal females have only normally active cells; affected males have only inactive cells.[23]

The hypothesis offers an explanation of the sex chromatin body and the late-labelling chromosome: both could be different morphological expressions of the inactive chromosome. This extension has neither been proved nor refuted but meanwhile it offers a highly plausible integration of otherwise unexplained cytological observations with correlated genetic phenomena.

It may be thought that the existence of an inactive X chromosome is disproved by the dissimilarity of the 45,X (Turner) female and the normal 46,XX female since, by hypothesis, the two types should be genetically equivalent, with a single active X chromosome in all their cells. However, the hypothesis has explained so much that it is reasonable to consider subsidiary assumptions and to suppose than genetic information might be supplied by both X chromosomes of the normal 46,XX embryo before the stage at which inactivity is determined, or alternatively that inactivation does not extend over the whole chromosome. (The explanation of dosage compensation would still be valid if activity were retained by a terminal pairing segment, postulated to be homologous with a corresponding segment on the Y (see p. 598)).

The Function of the Y Chromosome

The central role of the sex chromosomes in sex determination has been understood in general terms for over half a century. Some of the information presented in the foregoing sections enables the action of the human Y chromosome to be examined further. The principal facts to be considered are that in the presence of a Y chromosome, testes are almost invariably formed, and a masculine phenotype developed, whatever the number of associated X chromosomes (e.g. subjects with the karyotype 49,XXXXY); and that in the absence of testes, otherwise presumptively normal 46,XY embryos develop into agonadal females (pure gonadal dysgenesis). The working hypothesis can therefore be adopted that the primary action of the masculinising locus (or loci) on the normal Y chromosome is to ensure that the gonadal primordia shall develop into testes. The development of masculine internal and external genitalia and later, secondary sex characters, would then follow as normal consequences of the primary event. Doubtless much genetic information is concerned in the regulation of the development and function of the whole genital system. In testicular feminisation, though the karyotype is 46,XY and testes are present, a single mutant gene results in the development of a female external phenotype. In pure gonadal dysgenesis, factors unknown, but probably at least partly genetic, are presumed to lead to failure of development of the gonadal primordia, so that the phenotype becomes that of an agonadal female whether the karyotype is 46,XX or 46,XY. Neither of these conditions therefore conflict with the basic hypothesis.

Mosaic subjects in whom some cells contain a Y chromosome but who nevertheless exhibit a female phenotype also do not conflict with the hypothesis because, by chance, the Y-bearing cells may have been excluded from the gonadal primordia, or not have been included in sufficient proportion to ensure testicular development. Support for the idea that the developmental information provided by the Y chromosome may be expressed on a quantitative cellular basis is provided by observations of human 45,X/46,XY mosaic subjects who bear an abnormal testis on one side and a streak gonad on the other. The sexual development of XX/XY chimæras of the mouse produced experimentally by fusion of early embryos also suggests that the direction of gonadal development may depend on the proportions of XY to XX cells in the gonadal promordia and that XY cells are dominant.[24]

Karyotypes that include structurally modified Y chromosomes (or presumed Y chromosomes) are on record and the associated phenotypes provide several features of considerable interest.[25, 26] Two types are of particular importance. In the one a presumptive long arm of Y isochromosome takes the place of the normal Y. The two subjects who have been recorded with this abnormality are phenotypic *females*. In the other type, the normal Y chromosome is replaced by a dicentric chromosome which appears to represent a symmetrical doubling of the Y about a break point in the short arm. Again, two subjects are known, who are phenotypic *males*. If the interpretations of these abnormal chromosomes are correct, the inference can be drawn that the genetic information concerned with the primary action of the Y chromosome, namely the induction of testicular development, is located in the short arm.

A further series of observations would seem to run counter to this interpretation. A small number of phenotypic females is on record who have an enlarged phallus and show other signs of masculinisation and whose karyotype includes an abnormal small chromosome believed to be a centric fragment of the Y. If this structure is correctly intepreted, the short arm is intact; it is the long arm which is reduced in length. Reconciliation with the inference drawn in the last paragraph, which is based on more secure interpretations of structure, would then require the assumption of a further locus or loci concerned with masculinisation located on the long arm of the Y chromosome.

The presence of testicular tissue in the apparent absence of the Y chromosome in most true hermaphrodites and in XX males is not contrary to hypothesis, which provides for the possibility that the potentiality of developing testicular architecture is inherent in the primordial gonads of all individuals. The two conditions may represent different facets of a single one, since if embryonic XX gonadal tissue, normally destined to become ovarian, can variably develop into testicular tissue, the intermediate stage is the true hermaphrodite and the extreme, where all the gonadal tissue has become testicular, could be the XX male. In any case the problem of explanation is formally the same in both.

Two types of developmental hypothesis are possible. The one is genetic and postulates that testicular tissue and ovarian tissue develop differently because they are genetically distinct. This embraces the gross chromosomal mosaics known to be represented among true hermaphrodites and also the possibility of mosaicism of a more subtle kind. The alternative type of hypothesis supposes that the gonadal primordia are genetically identical, in which case differential development could only be attributed to the effect of indeterminate fluctuation of inductive processes operating on a labile system.

One form of the mosaic hypothesis invokes two assumptions: first, translocation of a segment of the Y chromosome bearing the masculinising locus or loci on to an X chromosome; second, genetic inactivation of this segment when the attached X chromosome segment is inactivated.[27] By hypothesis the subject would be a mosaic of two kinds of cells, those with the normal X active and those with the X plus attached Y segment active. Random distribution of the two types of cells to and within the gonadal primordia could then theoretically result in the development of two testes, two ovaries, or any combination of testicular and ovarian tissue.

AUTOSOMAL ABNORMALITIES

It is now widely known that Down's syndrome (mongolism) is caused by an autosomal trisomy. Apart from this condition, numerical abnormalities of the autosomes are much less frequent among the live born than sex chromosome abnormalities and much more severe in their effects. In addition to Down's syndrome, two other trisomic syndromes and one deletion syndrome are now well recognised. Autosomal mosaics are relatively infrequent but structural changes involving the autosomes are relatively much more common. In the following account the sex chromosomes will be excluded from the symbolised karyotypes.

Down's Syndrome

This syndrome,[28] described and given the name mongolian idiocy by Langdon Down in 1866 has an incidence at birth of approximately 1 in 700 in white populations. The cases are therefore sufficiently numerous to constitute an important social problem and in consequence it has become by far the most extensively studied of all the syndromes attributable to chromosomal abnormality. It is characterised by severe mental retardation and an enormous array of minor anatomical abnormalities, no one of which is invariably present. In a typical case the aggregate impression given by the abnormal features of the face and head alone is highly characteristic. The principal stigmata are: oblique palpebral fissures, epicanthic folds and speckled irides (Brushfield spots); a flat nasal bridge; an open mouth with a furrowed, protruding tongue and small, malformed teeth; prominent malformed ears with absent lobes; a flat occiput with a short, broad neck; loose skin at the back of the neck and over the shoulders (in early infancy); short, broad hands; short, curved little fingers with dysplastic middle phalanx; and specific features of the dermal ridge pattern, of which a transverse palmar crease is the most typical. Visceral abnormalities, principally cardiovascular defects, are frequent and anomalous hæmatological and biochemical traits have been described. There is perhaps no organ or system in the body that is not affected in some way. Though in the typical case a sufficient number of the external stigmata will be present to permit an unambiguous diagnosis, examples of partial or incomplete expression do occur and may present diagnostic difficulties.

Many Down's syndrome (DS) children die during infancy or childhood. The expectancy of life at birth has nevertheless risen considerably over the past

30 years, a recent estimate derived from an extensive survey in Victoria, Australia being 18 years. Respiratory disease and cardiac defects have been reported as the principal causes of death. Malignancy may be increased compared with the general population and it is established that the incidence of leukæmia during childhood is appreciably greater than in control children.

The incidence of Down's syndrome in relation to maternal age increases slowly until the early thirties but much more rapidly thereafter so that at ages of 45 and over it reaches the high figure of approximately 1 in 50. The changes are independent of paternal age and parity. The curve is not a simple one and Penrose has shown that it can be analysed into a major and a minor component, the minor component being independent of maternal age. This indicated that the causative factors are separable into two groups.

Before the introduction of modern cytogenetic methods, four types of observation provided evidence that a genetic factor is implicated. First, there is the widespread and sporadic distribution of DS births, apparently not influenced by environmental variables such as season, climate and epidemic infection (though in Australia recent evidence points to a possible second order effect of the infectious hepatitis virus). Second, sibship and familial concentrations of DS cases are well known. Third, monozygotic twin partners of DS cases are (almost) invariably affected whereas dizygotic twin partners are rarely affected. Fourth, both affected and unaffected children have been born to DS mothers and though the numbers are small they do not exclude a 1:1ratio. (There is no proven case of a child having been fathered by a DS male.)

Waardenberg in 1932 was the first to suggest that DS might be the consequence of a chromosomal anomaly, but it was not until 1959 that Lejeune, Gautier and Turpin provided the first direct evidence of the presence of an extra small chromosome in cultured cells from three cases.[29] This observation was quickly confirmed and the basic event in the ætiology of the condition at last shown (by inference) to be non-disjunction during meiosis in the ovum in the mother. The maternal age effect can therefore be attributed to an increasing risk of oocyte non-disjunction as the mother gets older. Several possible explanations for this have been put forward but it still remains a matter for conjecture.

The additional chromosome is one of the short acrocentric (G group) chromosomes. The two pairs of this group are very similar morphologically and cannot be distinguished with confidence. The formal possibility that the extra chromosome is sometimes of the one type, sometimes the other, is therefore not yet excluded. Nevertheless it is unlikely and it has become the convention to refer to the extra as a No. 21. The karyotype is written as 47,G+, or 47, 21+.

Trisomy also accounts satisfactorily for the enormous range of minor stigmata, the high frequency of the condition, its sporadic distribution, the difference between monozygotic and dizygotic twins and transmission from affected mother to about half her children.

Familial transmission by unaffected carriers received an explanation when it was discovered that in some DS cases the extra chromosomal material was, in effect, attached to another chromosome of the normal set. There are two types, both involving apparent "centric fusions" (see p. 600). In one, a D chromosome and a G chromosome are attached; in the other, two G chromosomes. It is usual to refer to them as DG and GG translocations respectively, though on the evidence of chromosome morphology alone the latter could equally be G long arm isochromosomes. The karyotypes of the unaffected carriers are written 45,D-,t(DqGq)+ and 45,G-,t(GqGq)+.

About five per cent of DS cases have translocation chromosomes. Their parents may have normal karyotypes or one may carry the translocation chromosome of their child. In the first instance the translocation chromosome must have originated as a chromosomal mutation either during early embryogenesis of the child itself or as a late event in one of the parents, perhaps in a spermatocyte or oocyte. The mutation rate has been estimated to be approximately one per 40,000 gametes,[30] which is an order of magnitude greater than that of the most mutable of human gene loci. Carrier parents appear to be phenotypically unaffected and may themselves have inherited the translocation chromosome from a parent or even a more remote ancestor.

When a mother is a DG translocation carrier the risk of a DS child is high. The limited information available suggests that normal children, carrier children, DS children and abortions plus stillbirths are about equally likely. When the father is the carrier, DS children, abortions and stillbirths are infrequent and the live born children are divided approximately equally between carriers and normals. The origin of a DS karyotype would require the union of a normal gamete with a gamete carrying the DS translocation chromosome plus an extra G chromosome. It is to be expected that in meiosis the D chromosome would form a trivalent by pairing with the single homologous D and G chromosomes. This has been verified for spermatogenesis. Non-disjunctional separation of the DG and G chromosomes from the single D would lead to the formation of the unbalanced gametes implicated. The difference between male and female carriers in respect of the chance of having a DS child may then be due to differences in the fre quency of non-disjunction of the trivalent between spermatogenesis and oogenesis.

Familial examples of GG translocations are less frequent. In contrast with DG translocations the abnormal chromosome appears to be transmitted more often by male carriers than females. Several DS cases are on record with unbalanced karyotypes derived from presumptive reciprocal translocations involving autosomes of other groups. These exceptional karyotypes are nevertheless consistent with effective duplication of a chromosome 21.

Mosaic karyotypes probably account for most instances of partial or incomplete expression of the syndrome. They have been identified in about three per cent of cases. Most of them are 46/47,G+ or, less frequently, 46/47,G+/48,2G+. The proportion of aneuploid cells varies greatly from case to case and is almost invariably considerably lower in blood cultures than in cultures of dermal fibroblasts. Mosaicism has been found in a small number of young mothers of DS children and may be more widespread than is realised. It could explain some of the instances of sibship concentration and would augment the maternal-age-independent group. A pair of monozygotic twins, one normal and one with DS is on record.[31] As discussed earlier (p. 611), this is understandable in terms of unequal partition of cells at the cleavage of a mosaic embryo.

A question of considerable importance is the risk faced by young parents whose first child had DS and who wish to add to their family. If the parental karyotypes are both normal it has sometimes been said that the risk is the same as the general risk-for-age in the population at large. However, this does not take account of the possibility of hidden mosaicism (which can never be wholly excluded) nor of the possibility of a genetic or adventitious factor that increases the chance of oocyte non-disjunction.

Trisomy D and Trisomy E

These conditions, first associated with autosomal trisomy in 1960, are now well known to pædiatricians. Like Down's syndrome, each presents a specific array of congenital anatomical abnormalities and other features none of which is invariably expressed. The affected children have a low birth weight and few survive for more than a few months. In both types there is apparently severe

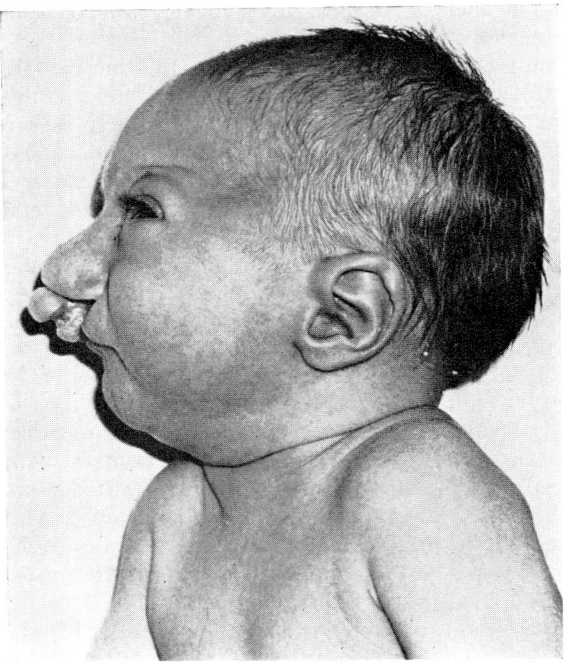

19/FIG. 10.—Trisomy D. Severe bilateral harelip with cleft palate, bulging pre-maxilla, low set and malformed ears, sloping forehead. Eye defects not recorded in this case. Karyotype 47, XY, D+.

mental retardation, though this is difficult to evaluate objectively. Pregnancies that result in the birth of a trisomy E child are often complicated by hydramnios and the placenta is usually small.

The principal external stigmata of trisomy D (FIG. 10) include: micropthalmia or anopthalmia; colobomata of the irides; corneal or lens opacities; low set and malformed ears; harelip or cleft palate or both; sloping forehead; facial angiomata; cryptorchidism; narrow, hyperconvex finger nails; fingers flexed or overlapping or both; polydactyly of hands or feet or both; posterior prominence of the heels ("rocker bottom feet"); and characteristic features of the dermal ridge pattern, including transverse palmar creases. Common internal abnormalities include cardiac and renal malformations, absence or hypoplasia of the olfactory lobes, and bicornuate uterus in females. To these can be added apnœic spells, apparent deafness, minor motor seizures and hypotonia.

In trisomy E (FIG. 11), affected females greatly outnumber affected males. The principal external stigmata include: low set, malformed and rotated ears; micrognathia; narrow palatal arch; head with prominent occiput, relatively flattened laterally; short sternum; narrow pelvis, often with luxation of the hips; fingers flexed, with the index overlapping third and/or fifth overlapping fourth; hallux short, dorsiflexed; and characteristic features of the dermal ridge pattern including an exceptionally high number of arches. Frequent internal abnormalities include cardiac and renal malformations, Meckel's diverticulum and heterotopic pancreatic tissue. Other general features are severe debility and moderate hypertonicity.

The identity of the extra chromosome is not yet established in either syndrome. In trisomy D the extra could be any one of the three D group chromosomes; in trisomy E, No. 16 is excluded but the extra could be either a No.17 or a No. 18. Some cases are on record in which the syndromes, sometimes fully and sometimes only partly expressed, are associated with structural changes or mosaicism. They are still too few to justify detailed consideration and no point of special interest has emerged from them.

The frequency of occurrence of the trisomy D[32] and trisomy E[33] syndromes has not yet been ascertained accurately but appears to be about 1 to 2 per 10,000 live births. The age of a mother at the birth of her D trisomy child is not obviously greater than the general population mean. In E trisomy, on the other hand, there is clear evidence of increasing risk with increasing maternal age, though present evidence makes it unlikely that the rate of increase is so steep as it is in Down's syndrome.

A Deletion Syndrome—"Cri du chat"

A specific syndrome of congenital abnormalities that has recently come to light is associated with apparent absence of about two-thirds of the short arm of a B group chromosome, arbitrarily designated No. 5. The principal clinical signs include severe mental retardation, microcephaly, hypertelorism, epicanthic folds, microganthia and low set ears. The outstanding and unique feature is, however, the characteristic cry, which is said to resemble the miaowing of a cat, hence the name (given in Paris) "cri du chat". Several independent examples of at least two other types of specific presumptive deletion are known but in neither has an associated phenotype yet been clearly defined. These and the cri du chat cases suggest that there are some loci in the human chromosome set that are particularly liable to breakage. The most economical hypothesis would be to suppose that the apparent losses represent simple terminal deletions and are therefore exceptions to the general rule of conservation of telomeres given earlier. However, interstitial deletion cannot be excluded, nor even reciprocal translocation, on the present evidence of mitotic chromosome morphology alone.

Reciprocal Translocation

Most of the examples of reciprocal translocation so far recorded in man have been identified through child propositi with multiple congenital abnormalities.[35, 36] These have often presented a phenotype that is unique to the individual propositus (FIG. 12), except, occasionally, for a similarly affected sib. Their karyotypes have almost invariably proved to be unbalanced with a single abnormal chromosome, usually longer than the one it replaces, included in a normal diploid number of 46. Frequently one parent has been found to have an abnormal karyotype also, but an apparently balanced one that includes the child's abnormal chromosome and a second, complementary, abnormal chromosome (FIG. 4). In some families there is evidence that such a balanced rearrangement has been transmitted through several generations, in one instance from an ancestor born in the late eighteenth century.

The four chromosomes, two original, two rearranged, of any reciprocal translocation heterozygote can be written AB, CD, AD, CB, where B and D represent the segments exchanged (FIG. 7). Such an individual can be expected

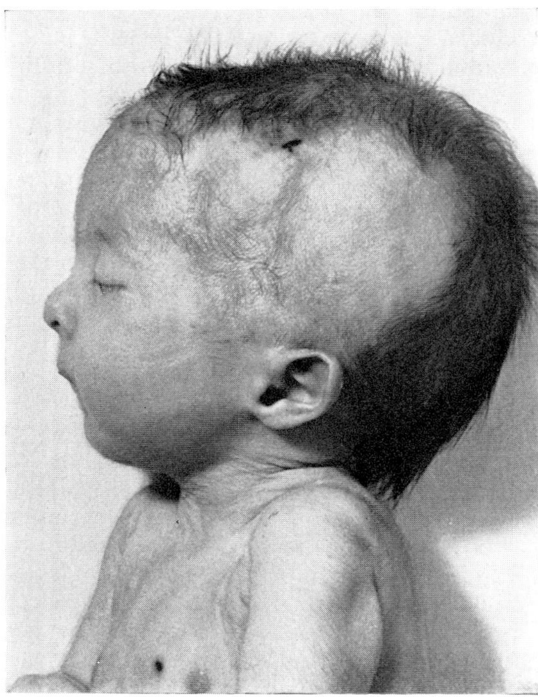

19/FIG. 11.—Trisomy E. Low set, malformed and rotated ears, micrognathia, prominent occiput, wizened skin. Karyotype 47,XX, E+.

to produce unbalanced gametes AB, BD and AD, DC regularly and other unbalanced gametic types less regularly. Participation in fertilization would lead to the production of two principal types of unbalanced zygote, one or both of which may be inviable and lead to death *in utero*. A record of spontaneous abortion is frequent in matings between partners one of whom is a translocation heterozygote.

Relatively little is yet known of reciprocal translocations in man but if they follow the pattern observed in other species the break points will be nearly randomly distributed over the whole chromosome set, so that each is effectively unique in respect of the specific chromosomes concerned and the length of the segments exchanged. These differences of structure would then be reflected by differences in the frequencies of different disjunctional arrangements at first meiotic anaphase and consequently of frequency of output of gametes of dif-

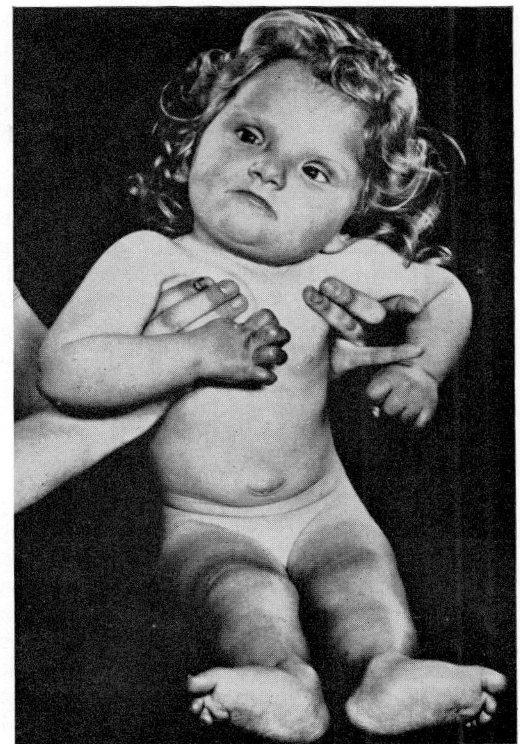

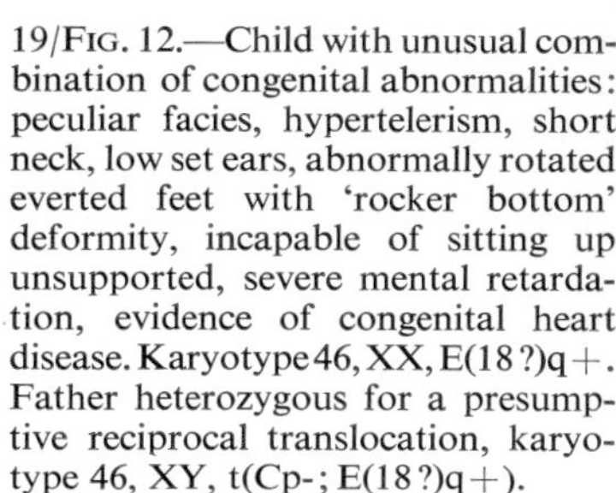

19/Fig. 12.—Child with unusual combination of congenital abnormalities: peculiar facies, hypertelerism, short neck, low set ears, abnormally rotated everted feet with 'rocker bottom' deformity, incapable of sitting up unsupported, severe mental retardation, evidence of congenital heart disease. Karyotype 46, XX, E(18 ?)q+. Father heterozygous for a presumptive reciprocal translocation, karyotype 46, XY, t(Cp-; E(18 ?)q+).

ferent segmental constitution. The known human reciprocal translocation heterozygotes represent a group selected largely because one of the potential unbalanced zygotic combinations happened to be born alive. If therefore, a heterozygote should be identified other than through an abnormal propositus, the risk of abortion or of a malformed child, should he or she wish to have children, could not be stated with any precision. It might be negligible: it might be greater than 1 in 2. The foregoing remarks do not apply to the centric fusion type of translocation, discussed under Down's syndrome, which presents a special situation.

A small number of cases are on record where an apparently balanced reciprocal translocation has been identified in a malformed child itself. In some instances the association of chromosome change and malformations might be coincidental. An alternative formal explanation is associated small deletion or duplication, too small to be detectable.

Inversion

A very few instances of presumptive pericentric inversion have also been recorded in children with congenital malformations. The remarks of the last paragraph apply to them also. Paracentric inversions could not even be suspected from observations of mitotic chromosomes. Prophase pairing at meiosis in an inversion heterozygote, whether peri- or paracentric, can give a loop structure where the direction of homology changes. If crossing over occurs within this loop a proportion of severely unbalanced gametes will be produced, and could be expected to lead to the formation of corresponding severely unbalanced, inviable zygotes. Inversion heterozygosis in a parent is therefore unlikely to be identified through a malformed infant propositus and is correspondingly of much less clinical significance than heterozygosity for a reciprocal translocation.

As yet little direct information about the meiotic behaviour of structural changes in man has been obtained, and all cases have been identified, at least initially, from mitotic chromosomes. It has already been pointed out that the inferences regarding the nature of structural changes that can be made from observation of mitotic karyotypes, though useful, are limited, and that it is appropriate to refer to all such inferences as *presumptive*. However it is right to add that they are only presumptive in the sense that more complex changes are not ruled out.

POPULATION CYTOGENETICS

Normal Variation of the Chromosomes

It is now well recognised that the normal human chromosome set is not absolutely constant but that some true variation in length occurs in at least four of the chromosomes.[37] Each variant type is a constant and characteristic feature of an individual's karyotype and is inherited in a simple Mendelian manner. The variants therefore serve as useful marker chromosomes. No phenotypic consequences of these variations have been recognised.

The Y chromosome varies in length in different normal males from clearly shorter than the G group autosomes to longer than the F group metacentrics. At least one member of the D group and at least one member of the G group may have an exceptionally prominent short arm. The long arm of one or both members of pair 16 may be exceptionally long. Individual satellites also vary in size from one subject to another and occasionally one of them (i.e. that attached to a specific D or G group chromosome) may be very prominent. All these features appear to vary continuously between one person and another so that an objective distinction between standard and variant may be impossible.

Frequency at Birth of gross Chromosome Abnormalities

An estimate of the frequency of sex chromosome abnormalities at birth can be obtained from systematic sex chromatin surveys of the newborn.[11] The best current estimate for chromatin-positive males is 10 per 10,000 births of both sexes, for chromatin double-positive females, 6 per 10,000 and for chromatin-negative females, 2 per 10,000, giving a total of 18 per 10,000 for sex chromosome anomalies of all types. This is a minimum estimate since 47,XYY subjects, some 45,XO/46,XX mosaics and female carriers of structurally altered X chromosomes would be undetected.

The frequency of autosomal abnormalities has to be estimated directly and is well established only for Down's syndrome (15 per 10,000 births),[28] All the remainder are very uncertainly determined. For trisomy D the figure may be 2 per 10,000 and for trisomy E much the same.[32, 33] The frequency of the "cri du chat" condition and of unbalanced structural change may each be approximately 1 per 10,000 so that the overall estimate for sex chromosome and autosomal abnormalities combined becomes 39 per 10,000, or approximately 1 in 250 live births. Although this figure seems high it may well underestimate the numbers of individuals who are more or less severely malformed or otherwise incapacitated in consequence of their chromosomal abnormality. Even so, it does not include a contribution from balanced rearrangement. One systematic survey of samples from an adult population has provided an estimate of 5 balanced rearrangements per 1000.[37] This figure seems high but if it should be confirmed it would mean that very nearly 1 in every 100 newborn babies would be karyotypically abnormal and potentially of clinical interest.

Spontaneous Abortion

Karyotypic abnormality is a common observation in tissue cultures established from spontaneously aborted embryos. The specificity of the observations upon individual cultures enables the abnormalities to be referred to the embryos themselves. Estimates of the frequency of abnormality have ranged from two per cent to 64 per cent of successful cultures, with a mean of approximately 20 per cent.[38] Over twenty different groups of investigators have contributed information from North America, Japan and Europe. The reasons for the wide range of the estimated frequency are not known but could include differences due to method of selection of material, to technical factors and perhaps to differences in the sociological background of the mothers.

Autosomal trisomy is the most frequent of all the individual types of abnormality recorded and accounts for about 40 per cent of the total. All chromosome groups are represented, though group E and particularly group G are dominant. Monosomy of a C group chromosome accounts for a further 20 per cent. Since monosomy of other groups has not been found and trisomy of C group chromosomes (which could be expected to cause a lesser degree of unbalance) is, jointly with group F, the least common of all the trisomies, it seems safe to assume that these cases have the 45,X karyotype characteristic of the major group of Turner subjects. If so, only a small proportion of 45,X embryos can survive to be born alive and the problem is therefore raised of reconciling an exceptionally high pre-natal mortality with a reasonably good expectation of life for those that survive to birth. Another 20 per cent of the abnormal karyotypes is taken up by triploid embryos with 69 chromosomes and tetraploid embryos with 92 chromosomes, the triploids being the more numerous. About 10 per cent are mosaics of various kinds and the remainder include several presumptive translocations and a minor group of unspecified abnormalities.

An estimate of the overall contribution to human infertility from karyotypic abnormality requires knowledge of four things. First, the frequency of clinically recognised pregnancies that terminate in spontaneous abortion. Second, the frequency of karyotypic abnormality in spontaneously aborted embryos. Third, the frequency of conceptions that fail to lead to clinical signs of pregnancy. Fourth, the frequency of karyotypic abnormality in conceptuses of the latter group. The last two are totally unknown, but are likely to be real by analogy with other species and also on the specific grounds that autosomal monosomic zygotes should be approximately as frequent as autosomal trisomic zygotes, yet unequivocal autosomal monosomy has not been recorded. The first two frequencies may be tentatively set at 15 per cent and 20 per cent respectively. The product is 3 per cent, which may be taken as a first, and probably low, estimate of zygotic loss due to chromosomal abnormality. A useful comparison is provided by studies of tissue cultures established from embryos after induced abortion, two per cent of which were found to be karyotypically abnormal in a total of over 450.[38]

EFFECTS OF IONIZING RADIATION ON CHROMOSOMES

It has already been stated that structural changes of the chromosomes arise spontaneously at very low frequency in normal tissues and that the rate of occurrence can be greatly enhanced by exposure to ionizing radiation. At the first metaphase following irradiation an enormous variety of abnormal configurations (chromosome abberations) can be observed, all of which can be explained in terms of breakage either of whole chromosomes or of single chromatids followed by rejoining of some of the broken ends to give new segmental combinations.[39] *Chromosome* breakage and reunion occurs when the cell is irradiated early in the mitotic cycle; *chromatid* breakage and reunion when it is irradiated late in the mitotic cycle.

Radiation-induced breakage and subsequent reunion at both chromosome and chromatid levels are essentially random processes. Where two chromosomes are broken, therefore, the four broken ends may rejoin to form a dicentric chromosome and an acentric chromosome, or two monocentric chromosomes, with approximately equal frequency. New monocentric chromosomes are mechanically stable and capable of indefinite transmission at mitosis but dicentric and acentric chromosomes lead directly to abnormalities at anaphase. The dicentric is almost certain sooner or later to result in a chromosome bridge between the two disjoining anaphase groups. (The rare exception is when the two centromeres are so close together that the disjunction of the daughter centromeres is co-ordinated.) Acentric chromosomes and fragments are almost invariably excluded from both daughter nuclei and form micronuclei in the cytoplasm. Rarely they are included passively in one daughter nucleus, but when this happens they are subject to the same risk of loss at the next anaphase.

In consequence of irregularities at anaphase a restitution nucleus may be formed incorporating both disjoining groups of chromosomes and most or all of the acentric fragments as well. If such a nucleus comes into mitosis again, each of the abnormal structures originally produced is seen to be represented twice in consequence of the intervening replication (FIG. 13).

It is more usual, however, for the daughter groups to separate completely and for the bridges to break. The result of broken dicentric chromosomes and excluded acentric structures is a pair of daughter nuclei which are deficient, or at least unbalanced. Such nuclei have only exceptionally been seen to re-enter mitosis in mammalian tissues. The great majority must die, or alternatively lose the capacity for further proliferation. By this chain of events chromosome breakage can contribute in an important way to the biological effects of irradiation. Regeneration of depleted tissue must come from the surviving cells that by chance escaped chromosome change or in which the chromosome changes were of a balanced kind. In the latter case one or more of the changed chromosomes may be morphologically distinct, *marker* chromosomes. Continued proliferation of the descendants of such a cell can result in the appearance of a distinct clone of cells in the regenerated tissue. In the mouse that has recovered from heavy irradiation, though not yet in man, it has been found that the members of a single clone may become widely distributed throughout the various organs of the lympho-myloid complex.[40]

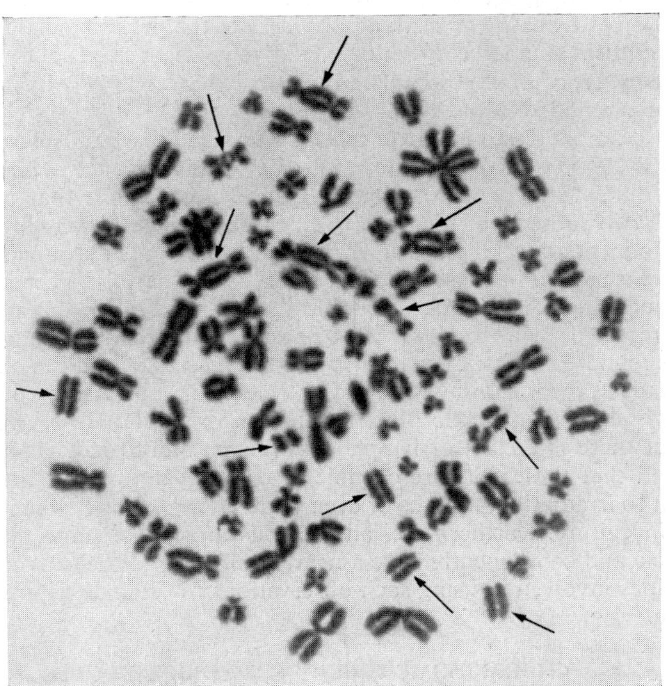

19/FIG. 13.—Tetraploid cell from an irradiated subject presumptively the product of a restitution nucleus. Matching pairs of dicentric and acentric chromosomes (arrows). Blood culture. Air dried preparation. Acetic orcein stain.

Similar clones have been identified in cultures of irradiated human skin but in this situation the possibility that clonal expansion was confined to growth in culture cannot be excluded. It has been shown that different clones within the lympho-myloid complex of the same mouse have different proliferative capacities; more strictly, that one can outgrow another.[40] A plausible but unproved explanation is that a different array of gene mutations was induced in each clone founder cell, rendering each clone physiologically distinct. It is reasonable to suppose that such differential clonal proliferation would occur in all tissues that are depleted by irradiation and retain the capacity for regeneration. If so the animal or man exposed to whole-body irradiation would become in part a patchwork quilt of cell colonies and clones of varying size, but blurred to the extent that cell migration can occur from one site to another.

A parallel may be drawn between different clones in the bone marrow of an irradiated mouse and different cell lines in a human mosaic subject. The latter are chromosomally distinct and presumptively genetically distinct. It is logical therefore to look for evidence of differential proliferation between the different cell lines. In view of the dosage compensation system it is not surprising that no clear evidence of such an effect is evident in the data on sex chromosome mosaics. Nor is the evidence very much stronger in Down's syndrome mosaics with normal and trisomy-21 cell lines. However, some cases of mosaicism involving other autosomes have shown striking increases in the proportions of normal to aneuploid mitoses in blood cultures over relatively short periods of time.[41] It may be that many types of autosomal mosaicism, where one cell line is normal, rapidly become undetectable by blood culture.

Where it is possible to irradiate cells at a specific phase of the mitotic cycle and examine them at the first ensuing metaphase, the frequency of simple breaks has been found to increase linearly with dose. Aberrations that require two breaks and two subsequent reunions, such as dicentric and ring chromosomes, increase exponentially as the dose is increased, the exponent approaching closer to 2 as the dose rate is increased.[39] Consideration has therefore been given to the possibility of using counts of chromosome aberrations as a means for estimating the dose received by human subjects accidently exposed to radiation. The problem is rendered difficult by the fact that to be useful at all, the observations must be made at the first mitosis following irradiation, and also by the variation in sensitivity according to the phase of the mitotic cycle. However, it is now known that there is a class of lymphocytes in the blood that has a very long half-life and that these cells are capable of entering mitosis for the first time subsequent to irradiation, months or even years after exposure, when stimulated by PHA in culture. Furthermore, all the cells are in the same phase of the mitotic cycle and consequently have a nearly uniform radiosensitivity. Even so, the difficulties involved in using such observations to estimate exposure remain formidable.

CHROMOSOME CHANGES IN NEOPLASIA

It has been known for a long time that abnormal chromosome numbers are very common in dividing neoplastic cells. Structural changes are now also recognised to be frequent. In most human carcinomas and sarcomas, the recorded chromosome counts vary considerably from one cell to another, the modes for individual cases usually lying in the sixties or seventies, not far removed from the triploid level. This gross disorder of chromosome number (and often, structure) stands in striking contrast to the great constancy of the karyotype in normal tissues.

More recent and much more significant are the examples, few as yet in man, of repetition of the same (or a closely similar) abnormal and often unique karyotype in all the cells sampled from the same individual neoplasm. The inference is that these cells are the product of the proliferation of a single original cell and constitute a clone. The phenomenon is formally related to the clonal proliferation seen in irradiated tissues discussed above, though the frequent identification of karyotypic variants of neoplastic clones contrasts with the karyotypic constancy of radiation-induced clones, which appear to be as stable as the cells of normal tissue. It may be surmised that the variants of a main neoplastic clone, being karyotypically distinct, could also be genotypically distinct and physiologically distinct, and consequently show different capacities for survival and proliferation. In at least one case a "take over" of an original clone by a related, derivative clone has been demonstrated by serial examination during the course of the disaese.[42]

Bone marrow cells and cells in blood cultures from cases of acute leukæmia not infrequently have the sharply defined, clonal karyotypes just mentioned. The chromosome counts lie at or close to the diploid level and show little numerical variation, or none at all, in the samples of cells examined. Structurally abnormal marker chromosomes are frequent and, of course, provide the only means of identifying an abnormality when the count is 46.

Other evidence and arguments can be advanced to support the proposition that the cell populations of many malignant neoplasms are in a state of active evolution in which variant cell types arise continuously at a high rate and are subject to the operation of selective forces. This may be true not only of the more readily analysed quasi-diploid neoplasms, but also of the karyotypically highly variable carcinomas and sarcomas first mentioned, since karyotypic evidence of earlier clonal proliferation could have been obscured by extensive later numerical and structural variation. This view of the neoplastic process could account for two of the outstanding biological features of neoplasms, namely the changes in cellular properties that may occur during the course of the disease (neoplastic progression) and the specificity, even uniqueness, of individual malignant neoplasms of the same general type when their cytological, biochemical and immunological properties are compared in detail.[42]

Mention must finally be made of a specific marker chromosome that is almost invariably present in the affected cells of patients suffering from chronic granulocytic leukæmia. This is a minute acrocentric chromosome that takes the place of a normal G group chromosome and is presumptively derived from it by deletion of about half its long arm. This chromosome is known as the Philadelphia chromosome (Ph 1) after the city of its discovery. It is rarely absent from mitotic cells in bone marrow biopsy specimens taken from clinically recognisable cases of the disease and may or may not also be identifiable in blood cultures. Chronic granulocytic leukæmia frequently terminates in an acute phase, in which case additional chromosome abnormalities may be superimposed, but during the chronic phase the karyotype of the cells that carry the Ph 1 chromosome shows very little variability.

As the Ph 1 chromosome has been shown to be present in cells of the erythrocytic series[44] it is reasonable to suppose that whatever physiological change is associated with the deletion, it operates at the level of the stem cell, before the differentiation of specific granulocytic and erythrocytic precursors.

REFERENCES

1. Chicago Conference: Standardisation in Human Cytogenetics (1966). Birth Defects (Original Article Series) **2,** 1–21. New York: National Foundation—March of Dimes.
2. Avery, A. G., Satina, S., and J. Rietsema (1959). *Blakeslee: The Genus Datura.* New York: Ronald Press.
3. Hambert, G. (1966). *Males with Positive Sex Chromatin.* Göteborg: Elanders Boktryckeri Aktiebolag.

4. Klinefelter, H. F., Reifenstein, E. C., and Albright, F. (1942). *J. clin. Endocr.* **2,** 615.
5. Jacobs, P. A., Brunton, M., Melville, M. M., Brittain, R. P., and McClement, W. F. (1965). *Nature* (*Lond.*), **208,** 1351.
6. Price, W. H., and Whatmore, P. B. (1967). *Brit. med. J.*, **1,** 533.
7. Therkelsen, A. J. (1964). *Cytogenetics*, **3,** 207–218.
8. Turner, H. H. (1938). *Endocrinology* **23,** 566.
9. Singh, R. S., and Carr, D. H. (1966). *Anat. Rec.*, **155,** 369.
10. Ferguson-Smith, M. A. (1965). *J. med. Genet.*, **2,** 93.
11. Court-Brown, W. M., Harnden, D. G., Jacobs, P. A., Maclean, N., and Mantle, D. J. (1964). Abnormalities of the Sex Chromosome Complement in Man. *Spec. Rep. Ser. med. Res. Coun.* (*Lond.*), No. 305.
12. Boczkowski, K., and Teter, J. (1966). *Acta endocr.* (*Kbh.*), **51,** 497.
13. Jost, A. (1958). In *Hermaphroditism Genital Anomalies and Related Endocrine Disorders*. Eds. Jones, H. W., Jr., and Scott, W. W. Baltimore: Williams & Wilkins.
14. Morris, J. McL., and Mahesh, V. B. (1963). *Amer. J. Obstet. Gynec.*, **90,** 1078.
15. Jones, H. W., Jr., Ferguson-Smith, M. A., and Heller, R. H. (1965). *Obstet. and Gynec.*, **25,** 435.
16. Turpin, R., Lejeune, J., Lafourcade, J., Chigot, P. L., and Salmon, C. (1961). *C.R. Acad. Sci.* (*Paris*), **252,** 2945.
17. Edwards, J. H., Dent, T., and Kahn, J. (1966). *J. med. Genet.*, **3,** 117.
18. Mikklesen, M., Froland, A., and Ellebjerg, J. (1963). *Cytogenetics*, **2,** 86.
19. Uchida, I., Wang, H. C., and Ray, M. (1964). *Nature* (*Lond.*), **204,** 191.
20. Race, R. R., and Sanger, R. (1968). *Blood Groups in Man*, 5th edit. Oxford: Blackwell Scientific Publications.
21. Lyon, M. F. (1961). *Nature* (*Lond.*), **190,** 372.
22. Kerr, C. B., Wells, R. S., and Cooper, K. E. (1966). *J. med. Genet.*, **3,** 169.
23. Davidson, R. G., Nitowski, H. M., and Childs, B. (1963). *Proc. nat. Acad. Sci.* (*Wash.*), **50,** 481.
24. Tarkowski, A. K. (1964). *J. Embryol. exp. Morph.*, **12,** 735.
25. Jacobs, P. A., and Ross, A. (1966). *Nature* (*Lond.*), **210,** 302.
26. McIlree, M. E., Price, W. H., Court-Brown, W. M., Tullock, W. S., Newsams, J. E., and Maclean, N. (1966). *Lancet*, **2,** 69.
27. Ferguson-Smith, M. A. (1966). *Lancet*, **2,** 475.
28. Penrose, L. S., and Smith, G. F. (1966). *Down's Anomaly*. London: J. & A. Churchill.
29. Lejeune, J., Gautier, M., and Turpin, R. (1959). *C.R. Acad. Sci.* (*Paris*), **248,** 602.
30. Polani, P. E., Hamerton, J. L., Gianelli, F., and Carter, C. O. (1965). *Cytogenetics*, **4,** 193.
31. Lejeune, J., Lafourcade, J., Scharer, K., de Wolfe, E., Salmon, C., Haines, M., and Turpin, R. (1962). *C.R. Acad. Sci.* (*Paris*), **254,** 4404.
32. Conen, P. E., and Erkman, B. (1966). *Amer. J. hum. Genet.*, **18,** 374.
33. Conen, P. E., and Erkman, B. (1966). *Amer. J. hum. Genet.*, **18,** 387.
34. Miller, O. J., Breg, W. R., Warburton, D., Miller, D. A., Firschein, I. L., and Hirschhorn, K. (1966). *Cytogenetics*, **5,** 137.
35. Edwards, J. H., Fraccaro, M., Davies, P., and Young, R. B. (1962). *Ann. hum. Genet.*, **26,** 163.
36. Brøgger, A. (1967). *Translocation in Human Chromosomes*. Oslo: Universitatsforlaget.
37. Court-Brown, W. M., Buckton, K. E., Jacobs, P. A,. Tough, I. M., Kuenssberg, E. V., and Knox, J. D. E. (1966). *Chromosome Studies on Adults*. Eugenics Laboratory Memoirs XLII. London: Cambridge Univ. Press.

38. Geneva Conference: Standardisation of Procedures for Chromosomal Studies in Abortion. (1966). *Cytogenetics*, **5**, 361.
39. LEA, D. E. (1946). *Actions of Radiations on Living Cells*, London: Cambridge Univ. Press
40. FORD, C. E. (1964). In *Cytogenetics of Cells in Culture*. Ed. HARRIS, R. J. C. New York: Academic Press.
41. LA MARCHE, P. H., HEISLER, A. B., and KRONEMER, N. S. (1967). *R.I. med. J.*, **20,** 184
42. FORD, C. E., and CLARKE, C. M. (1963). In *Canadian Cancer Conference*, 5. New York: Academic Press.
43. TOUGH, I. M., JACOBS, P. A., COURT-BROWN, W. M., BAIKIE, A. G., and WILLIAMSON, E. R. D. (1963). *Lancet*, **1,** 844.
44. RASTRICK, J. M., FITZGERALD, P. H., and GUNZ, F. W. (1968). *Brit. med. J.*, **1,** 96.

The following general references may be useful:

COURT-BROWN, W. M. (1968). Males with XYY sex chromosome complement. *J. med. Genet.*, **5,** 341–359.

DARLINGTON, C. D. (1965). *Cytology*. London: J. & A. Churchill. (A reprint of the classic second edition of *Recent Advances in Cytology* (Cytogenetics) with a summary of the main developments 1937–1964.)

EVANS, H. J., COURT-BROWN, W. M., and MCLEAN, A. S., Eds. (1967). *Human Radiation Cytogenetics*. Amsterdam: North Holland. (Proceedings of an International Symposium).

FORD, C. E., and HARRIS, H., Eds. (1969). New Aspects of Human Genetics. *Brit. med. Bull.*, **25,** 1. (A series of reviews).

MITTWOCH, U. (1967). *Sex Chromosomes*. New York: Academic Press.

MOORE, K. L., Ed. (1966). *The Sex Chromatin*. (A series of reviews).

OVERZIER, C., Ed. (1963). *Intersexuality*. New York: Academic Press. (A series of reviews).

TAYLOR, A. I. (1968). Autosomal Trisomy Syndromes: A detailed study of 27 cases of Edward's syndrome and 27 cases of Patau's syndrome. *J. med. Genet.*, **5,** 227–352.

TURPIN, R., and LEJEUNE, J. (1965). *Les Chromosomes Humains*. Paris: Gautier-Villars.

WATSON, J. D. (1965). *Molecular Biology of the Gene*. New York: Benjamin. (A clearly written account for the general reader).

WHITE, M. J. D. (1961). *The Chromosomes*, 5th edit. London: Methuen. (An excellent brief introduction to general cytogenetics).

Chapter 20

CELL GROWTH AND MULTIPLICATION

BY H. HARRIS

THE tissues of the body normally grow by a process of cell multiplication. Each cell, between one mitosis and the next, roughly doubles its mass and divides into two daughter cells each having about half the mass of the parent cell. The course of events taking place within the cell between two mitoses is commonly called the *cell cycle*. During this cycle the genetic material in the cell nucleus is replicated, so that after mitosis each daughter cell has the diploid amount of DNA, and before mitosis the tetraploid amount. Mistakes in the replication of the DNA are rare and, in general, the two daughter cells receive identical sets of genetic material at mitosis. The rest of the cell substance is not partitioned so accurately between the two daughter cells, but in the somatic cells of vertebrates cell cleavage does not usually produce great deviations from an approximate halving of the cytoplasmic contents.

Synthesis of Macromolecules during the Cell Cycle

In most higher cells the replication of the DNA occurs at one particular stage of the cell cycle. This has been established by a number of different methods, of which perhaps the most versatile is the technique of autoradiography. For autoradiography cells must be exposed to a radioactive precursor of some cellular constituent which remains *in situ* when the cell is fixed. For example, radioactive nucleosides are incorporated into nucleic acids and radioactive amino-acids into proteins; these substances are not, on the whole, extracted when the cell is fixed by the usual methods. The fixed cells, attached to a glass slide, are then covered with a layer of a specially prepared photographic emulsion of high resolution, and are left in contact with this emulsion for some days. The radioactivity emanating from the fixed cell passes into the overlying emulsion and sensitizes the silver halide crystals. When the emulsion is developed the tracks produced by the passage of the radioactivity appear as black silver grains. The energy of the particles released by the radioactive disintegration depends on the nature of the isotope used and it is this which determines the length of the tracks in the photographic emulsion. With some isotopes, for example tritium, the energy of the particles is very low, and the tracks consequently very short. With istopes of this sort autoradiographs can be produced in which the presence of radioactivity can be accurately localized in quite small parts of the cell. By special techniques autoradiographs can also be made of water-soluble radioactive compounds in the cell; but these techniques have not yet attained the precision which is now routine for water-insoluble compounds.

In studying the cell cycle tritiated precursors of DNA, RNA and protein are of special importance. For DNA we have a highly specific precursor in the nucleoside, thymidine. In animal cells this is incorporated almost exclusively into DNA, and, except in special circumstances, it is only incorporated into the

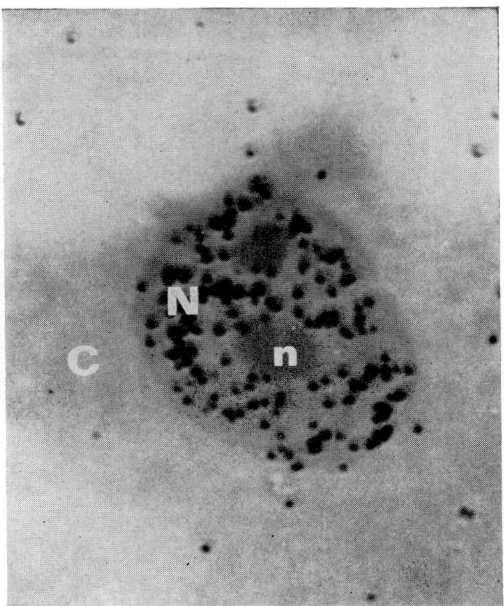

20/FIG. 1.—Autoradiograph of a connective tissue cell exposed to tritiated thymidine during the phase of DNA synthesis. The nucleus (N), but not the nucleolus (n), is labelled. The cytoplasm (C) is not labelled. (From Harris.[1])

DNA in appreciable amounts when this is being replicated. Tritiated thymidine has therefore been extensively used in the study of DNA synthesis. FIGURE 1 shows an autoradiograph of a connective tissue cell which was exposed to tritiated thymidine at a time when the cell was replicating its DNA. The incor-

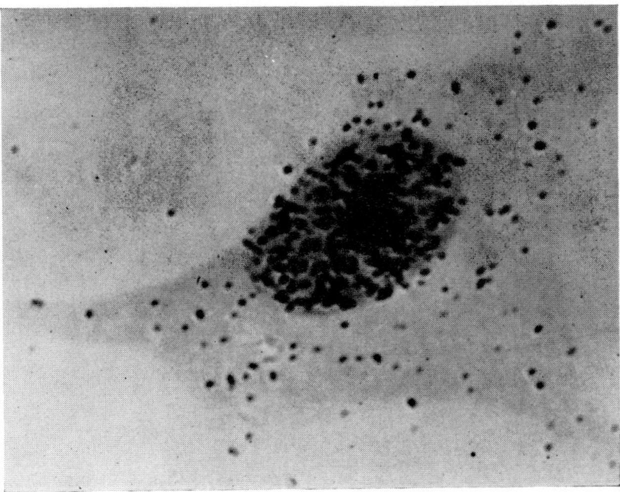

20/FIG. 2.—Autoradiograph of a connective tissue cell exposed for 20 minutes to tritiated adenosine. The RNA in the nucleus is more heavily labelled than the RNA in the cytoplasm. (From Harris.[2])

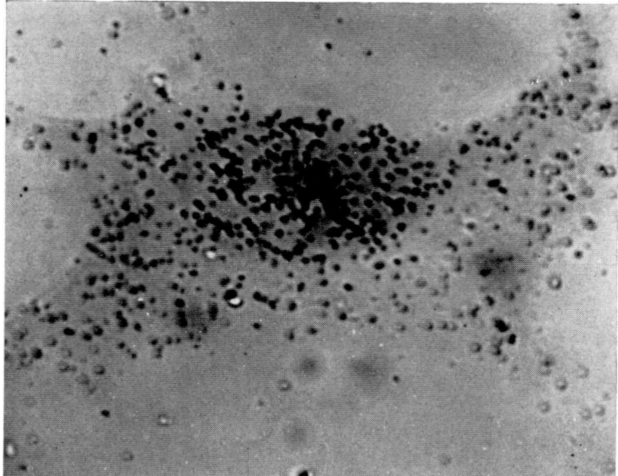

20/Fig. 3.—Autoradiograph of a connective tissue cell exposed for a longer period to tritiated adenosine. There is increased labelling of the cytoplasmic RNA. (From Harris.[2])

poration of the tritiated precursor into the DNA is revealed by the black silver grains over the cell nucleus. We do not have any precursor which is incorporated only into RNA, but tritiated ribonucleosides such as adenosine, uridine and cytidine, are incorporated into RNA much more rapidly than into DNA; and they can be used as specific precursors for RNA, if the DNA of the fixed cells is digested away before the cells are exposed to autoradiography. When the incor-

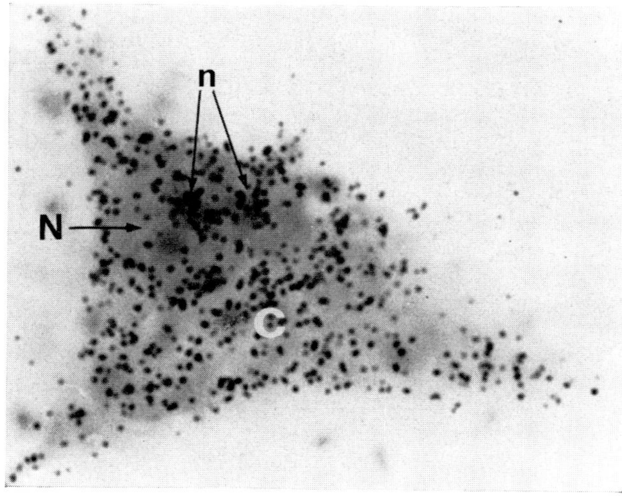

20/Fig. 4.—Autoradiograph of a connective tissue cell exposed for one hour to tritiated valine. Labelling of protein is more marked over the cytoplasm (C) than over the nucleus (N). However, the nucleoli (n) are heavily labelled. (From Harris.[3])

poration of tritiated ribonucleosides into RNA is studied it is found that the RNA in the cell nucleus becomes labelled much more rapidly than the RNA in the cytoplasm. FIGURE 2 is an autoradiograph showing the predominantly nuclear labelling which occurs when a cell is incubated with a tritiated RNA precursor for a few minutes. FIGURE 3 shows the increase in the amount of radioactivity in the cell cytoplasm on more prolonged incubation with the precursor. This pattern of RNA labelling is found in almost all vertebrate cells. If the cell is suitably fixed, tritiated amino-acids may be used as specific precursors for the cell proteins, and autoradiography of cells which have been exposed to tritiated amino-acids therefore reveals information about the synthesis of protein. FIGURE 4 shows an autoradiograph of a connective tissue cell exposed for an hour to tritiated valine. There is generalized labelling over the cytoplasm of the cell and rather less labelling over the nucleus. The nucleolus is more heavily labelled than the rest of the nucleus. This is a common pattern for the synthesis of protein in animal cells.

When a population of animal cells growing exponentially in culture is exposed for one hour to tritiated thymidine, autoradiographs show that not all the cells have labelled nuclei. This indicates at once that DNA is not synthesized throughout the whole cell cycle, because, if it were, all the cells, whatever stage of the cell cycle they were in, would be labelled. It is possible to determine, by autoradiographic means, where in the cell cycle the period of DNA synthesis falls. One way of doing this is to use the time of mitosis as the reference point. The cells are exposed for about an hour to tritiated thymidine and then transferred to non-radioactive medium. Samples are fixed after various periods of growth in this medium. In the autoradiographs made from such preparations mitotic figures are examined to see whether or not they are labelled. If a mitotic figure is labelled, this indicates that the cell must have been in the phase of DNA synthesis at the time of exposure to the tritiated thymidine; and as the cells were fixed at various times after their exposure to the radioactive precursor, a graph of the phase of DNA synthesis can be plotted with the time of mitosis as the reference point. FIGURE 5 shows a graph derived from an experiment of this sort carried out on rat connective tissue cells growing in artificial culture. It will be seen that the phase of DNA synthesis falls largely in the second half of the cell cycle. Both preceding and succeeding the phase of DNA synthesis there are periods in which DNA synthesis does not occur. The two non-synthetic periods are usually referred to as G_1 and G_2, and the phase of DNA synthesis as S. This pattern is quite general in somatic cells and has been confirmed by other types of autoradiographic experiment involving double labelling of the cells with two different types of isotope, and also by direct measurement of the amount of DNA in individual cells by the technique of Feulgen microspectrophotometry. In this technique the cells are stained by the Feulgen reaction, which is specific for DNA, and the amount of red coloration produced in the cell nucleus by this reaction (a value determined by the amount of DNA present) is measured with a microspectrophotometer. In synchronized cell populations it can be shown that the doubling of the DNA takes place in the period delineated by autoradiography as the S period. Extensive studies on a wide variety of somatic cells have shown that there is little variation in the duration of the S period, which usually lasts from 6 to 8 hours. The G_2 period may extend from about

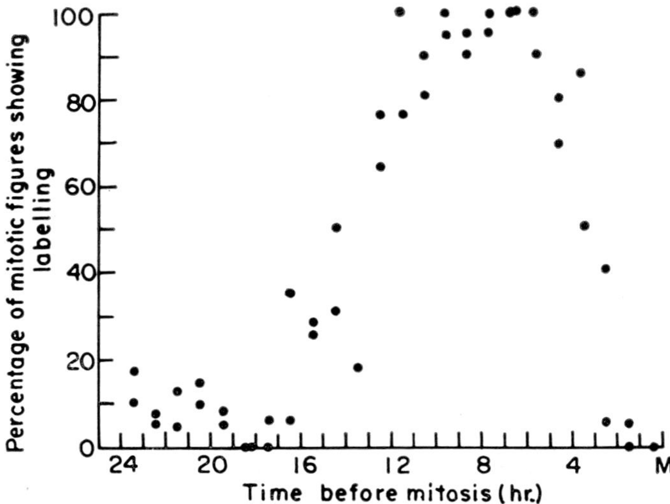

20/FIG. 5.—A graph delineating the phase of DNA synthesis relative to mitosis (M). The experiment was carried out by scoring labelled mitotic figures in autoradiographs of cells exposed to tritiated thymidine at various times prior to mitosis. (From Harris[1].)

$1\frac{1}{2}$ to 4 hours, or occasionally even longer; and the period of mitosis from half an hour to one hour. But the great range of variation in the rate of multiplication of the cells in the body appears to be determined larged by differences in the length of the G_1 period. A diagrammatic representation of a typical cell cycle is shown in FIG. 6. Cells in the body which do not normally multiply, or which have

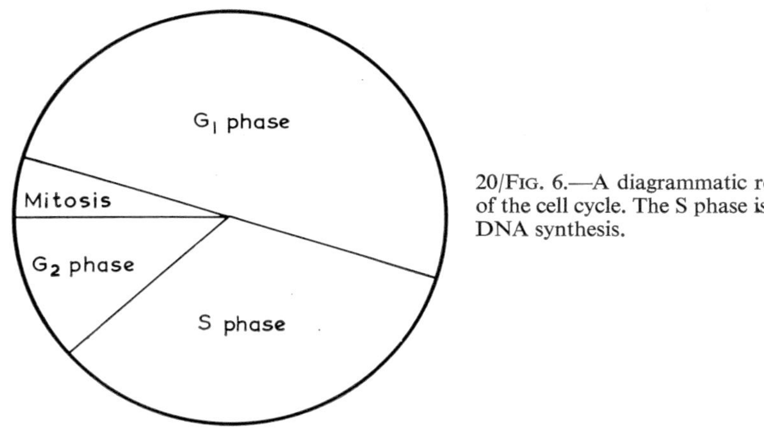

20/FIG. 6.—A diagrammatic representation of the cell cycle. The S phase is the phase of DNA synthesis.

lost the capacity to multiply altogether, usually have the diploid, not the tetraploid, amount of DNA and may thus be regarded as arrested in the G_1 period.

Unlike DNA, the synthesis of both RNA and protein takes place throughout the intermitotic period. This is revealed by the fact that all interphase cells in a growing population are labelled by a short period of exposure to a radioactive

RNA or protein precursor. During the act of mitosis most, if not all, of the RNA synthesis in the cell nucleus is closed off by the condensation of the chromosomes, but synthesis of protein may continue throughout mitosis. Several studies have been made in a variety of cell types on the rate of RNA and protein synthesis throughout the cell cycle and on the rate of DNA synthesis during the S phase. In mammalian cells DNA appears to be synthesized at an approximately constant rate throughout the S phase, but the rates of synthesis of RNA and protein increase during the cell cycle; these rates are about twice as high at the end of interphase as at the beginning.[5] The increase in the rate of RNA synthesis seems to occur predominantly during the second half of interphase at the same time as the doubling of the amount of DNA. However, the rate of protein synthesis appears to increase over the whole of the interphase period in proportion to the amount of RNA present. A simplified statement of these relationships might be that for cells in exponential growth, the rate of RNA synthesis during the cell cycle is determined by the amount of DNA present and the rate of protein synthesis by the amount of RNA present. This direct relationship between the RNA content of the cell (essentially a measure of the number of ribosomes which it contains) and the rate at which it synthesizes protein appears to hold true for both micro-organisms and animal cells over a wide range of physiological conditions.[6] In animal cells in exponential growth there is a close relationship between the mass of the cell and the beginning of the S phase, the point at which the synthesis of DNA is initiated. It appears as if a critical mass must be reached by the cell before it begins to replicate its DNA; and cells in a population which have low initial masses must synthesize more protein before the synthesis of DNA is initiated, than cells with higher initial masses.[7]

Interference with Synthetic Processes at various stages of the Cell Cycle

Because, in general, the cell must attain a certain critical mass before DNA synthesis is initiated, it is not surprising to find that substances which interfere with the synthesis of RNA or protein in the G_1 phase prevent the onset of the S phase. If, for example, cells in culture are exposed during the G_1 phase to an amino-acid analogue or a nucleoside analogue which inhibits either protein or RNA synthesis, or causes the production of spurious protein or RNA, these cells do not, on the whole, reach the S stage in which they will incorporate thymidine into DNA[1]. If, however, these analogues are given when the cells are already in the S phase, DNA reduplication will continue and may go to completion, although usually the rate of DNA synthesis gradually falls. Cells arrested by inhibition of protein or RNA synthesis in the G_1 phase thus have the diploid amount of DNA; those in which these processes are arrested during the S phase will have varying amounts of DNA up to the full tetraploid amount.

It is possible to inhibit the reduplication of DNA specifically, without impairing the synthesis of other cellular constituents including RNA and protein. When this is done the cell may continue to increase in mass, so that the ratio of DNA to RNA and protein progressively falls. Cells blocked in this way do not undergo mitosis. In bacteria this type of metabolic block may produce enormous enlargement of the cells, but each of these huge cells only contains a normal DNA complement. A very dramatic demonstration of this effect is seen in a strain of *Thermobacterium acidophilus* which requires preformed deoxyribosides for DNA synthesis. If these organisms are grown in medium lacking deoxyribosides, synthesis of protein and RNA continues and the bacterial bodies become enormously elongated, but, since DNA synthesis is blocked, formation of new bacterial nuclei is inhibited[8] (FIG. 7). This type of effect can also be produced in bacteria by certain antibiotics which inhibit DNA synthesis. The resulting elongated forms of the organisms are sometimes referred to as "spaghetti" forms. A similar, although less clear-cut dissociation of growth from DNA sysnthesis can be produced also in animal cells. Connective tissue cells cultivated in a medium which supports only a limited degree of multiplication may undergo progressive enlargement as the reduplication of their DNA is suppressed. Eventually such cells become several times as large as they were originally, but they do not undergo mitosis[9] (FIGS. 8 and 9). Synthetic processes

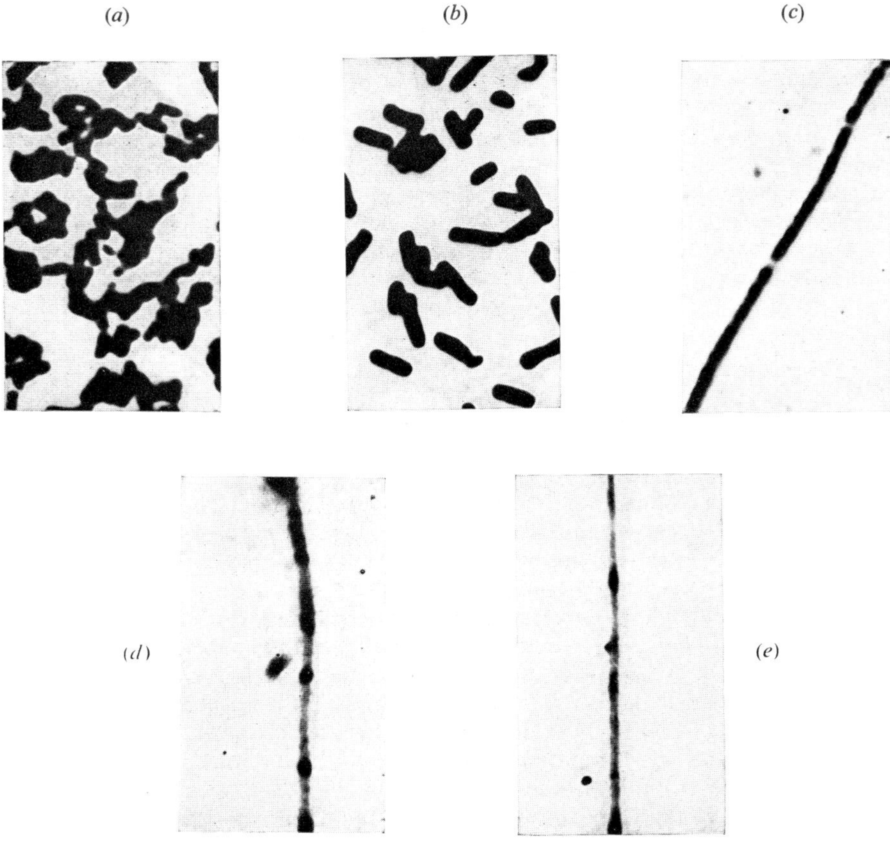

20/FIG. 7.—The morphology of a deoxyriboside-requiring strain of *Thermobacterium acidophilus* grown in a medium deficient in deoxyribosides. (*a*) The normal appearance of the organism. (*b*) and (*c*) Gradual elongation of the bacterial bodies. (*d*) and (*e*) The bacterial bodies are greatly elongated and have formed long chains; the nuclei are seen as dense swellings at intervals along these chains. (From Jeener and Jeener.[8])

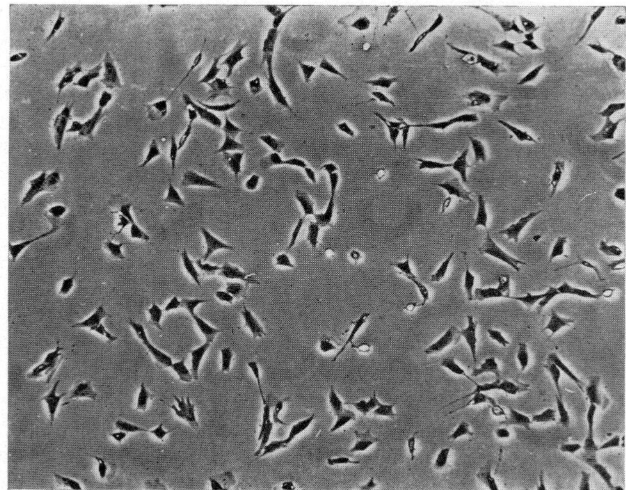

20/FIG. 8.—Dissociated connective tissue cells multiplying *in vitro* 40 hours after they have been isolated from the heart of a 5-day-old rat. (From Harris.[9])

may also be blocked in the G_2 phase, or the act of mitosis itself may be suppressed. If all the synthetic processes in the cell are unimpaired, but the cell cannot undergo mitosis, it may continue to grow until its mass is two or three orders of magnitude greater than normal. Such giant cells can readily be produced by appropriate doses of X-irradiation. Their growth is characterized not

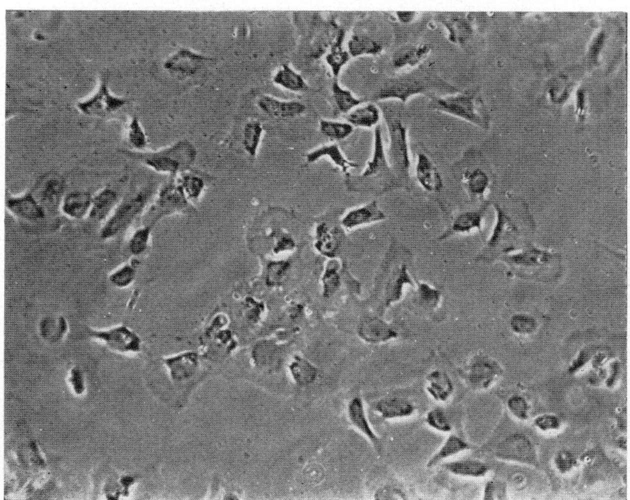

20/FIG. 9.—The same cells after 208 hours in a medium which supports only limited growth. Note the marked increase in the size of the cells, and their abnormal morphology. (From Harris.[9])

only by continuing synthesis of RNA and protein, but also by continuing synthesis of DNA, so that the cells contain huge nuclei having many times the normal amount of DNA. These giant cells eventually die.

Certain pathological conditions involving abnormalities in the growth or multiplication of cells in the body may now be discussed. Enlargement of an organ due to an increase in the size of the cells composing it is known as *hypertrophy*. Enlargement due to an increase in the number of cells present is known as *hyperplasia*. Hypertrophy or hyperplasia may occur singly or together in the one tissue.

Hypertrophy

Pure hypertrophy occurs in organs composed of cells which have lost the capacity to undergo mitosis. In such organs a demand for an increase in the amount of functional tissue is met by the synthesis of more cytoplasm. An increase occurs in the amount of protein and RNA per cell and in the number of specialised cytoplasmic inclusions such as mitochondria. But although this progressive increase in the mass of functional cytoplasm may continue until the cell is many times larger than normal, reduplication of DNA and mitosis do not occur. Hypertrophy is thus, in principle, analogous to the enlargement of bacteria or animal cells which takes place when the synthesis of DNA is blocked without impairment of the synthesis of RNA and protein.

Stimuli to Hypertrophy

Hypertrophy is conventionally divided into two types: compensatory and hormonal. Hypertrophy of an organ is said to be compensatory when it occurs in response to an increase in the amount of work thrown on that organ. For example, removal of one kidney may result in an enlargement of the other; cardiac hypertrophy may result from vascular lesions which cause an increase in the work of the heart; groups of skeletal muscles may hypertrophy as a result of intensive exercise. Hypertrophy which has been shown to be associated with the action of some hormone is known as hormonal. However, the distinction between these two types of hypertrophy may not be as fundamental as it sounds. It has been shown, for example, that hypertrophy of the remaining kidney after unilateral nephrectomy does not occur in hypophysectomized dogs and rats.[10, 11] This sort of experiment would seem to imply that increase in the amount of work thrown on the remaining kidney cannot produce hypertrophy unless certain conditions provided by the secretions of the pituitary gland are also present. Even in the case of cardiac muscle, where the relationship between increased load and hypertrophy seems to be incontrovertible, there are experiments suggesting that this relationship is more complex than would at first appear. For example, Eyster[12] has claimed that if acute dilatation is produced for a short period in the hearts of dogs by constricting the ascending thoracic aorta with a rubber band, hypertrophy occurs *after* the rubber band has been removed; and this hypertrophy is of the same extent and takes place over the same period of time as the hypertrophy in animals where the rubber band remains *in situ*. Eyster found histological evidence of acute injury in the muscle fibres subjected to the stretching and considered that it was this injury rather than the increase in work which was the stimulus to the hypertrophy. It should be mentioned, however, that Herrmann and Decherd[13] failed to confirm this work in rats and rabbits.

It does not really advance matters much to say that increased work or increased hormonal activity is the cause of hypertrophy. In neither case do we have any information about the cellular mechanisms responsible for the hypertrophy, and it is not impossible that the same sort of mechanisms may be at work under both sets of conditions. It has been shown that injections of the growth hormone of the anterior pituitary gland, which produce hypertrophy and hyperplasia of the liver and hyperplasia of the thymus in rats, increase the RNA content of the liver and the rate of RNA turnover in the thymus.[14] While these findings may mean that the hormone exerts its influence through some effect on nucleic acid metabolism, they possibly mean no more than that an increase in the amount or turnover of nucleic acids is a part of the process of hypertrophy or hyperplasia. One of the great difficulties in the way of an experimental approach to this problem at the cellular level is the time scale over which hypertrophy occurs. For example, in dogs in which the ascending thoracic aorta is constricted by means of a rubber band, hypertrophy is said not to begin before the period of acute dilatation has subsided, a period of 3 to 6 days, and it reaches its maximum at about the 80th day after the initial injury. It is difficult to think in conventional biochemical terms about processes occurring over such a length of time, and ordinary biochemical techniques do not lend themselves to the investigation of processes on this time-scale.

A few words should be added about the suggestion which was first made in the very early days of cellular pathology, that hypertrophy is due to an increased "nutrition" of the tissue or, more specifically, to an increased blood flow. A distinction should be made between increased "nutrition" and increased blood flow. The amount of material which passes across the cell membrane and the amount of substrate which is consumed by the cell are determined by a great many factors other than the amount of material brought to the cell by the blood. It seems a little naïve to think that an increase in blood flow would necessarily be followed by an increase in substrate consumption or "nutrition". What evidence there is does not support the view that hypertrophy is caused by increased blood flow. On the contrary, the studies of Wearn *et al.*[15] have shown that, at least in cardiac muscle, the hypertrophy of the muscle fibres precedes and may outstrip the development of an increased capillary blood supply. Wearn contends that it is the failure of the capillary blood supply to keep pace with the hypertrophy of the muscle fibres which eventually causes the hypertrophied heart to fail. On the other hand, increased work on the part of an organ, whatever the state of the blood supply, must presumably entail an increased consumption of substrate by the cells. It has been shown that the concentration of certain enzymes in animal tissues is increased when the substrates of these enzymes are administered in excess.[16] This process in animal tissues has been studied most carefully in certain enzyme systems in the liver and shows some resemblance to the phenomenon of "induced enzyme synthesis" in bacteria.[17] It is tempting to suppose that a general increase in the turnover of substrate might induce increased synthesis of a large number of enzymes, and thus form the basis of hypertrophy. However, at the moment, this possibility is little more than speculation.

Hyperplasia

The conditions which produce "compensatory" hypertrophy in tissues composed of non-multiplying cells may produce hyperplasia in tissues composed of cells which have retained their capacity to multiply. For example, removal of one kidney produces essentially a hypertrophy of the cells of the remaining kidney, but removal of some of the lobes of the liver produces not only hypertrophy but also hyperplasia in the residual lobes. The increased load thrown on the cells of the residual lobes produces first an increase in the size of the cells. In the liver cell, however, these circumstances induce not only the formation of more cytoplasm, but also reduplication of DNA, so that a wave of increased mitosis occurs. The increased mitotic rate continues until the mass of functioning liver tissue is restored to normal. The hypertrophy of the cells, which is a marked feature in the early stages of the regenerative process, becomes increasingly less marked as more and more cells are produced. When the regeneration is complete the cells are again of normal size. Different organs show varying degrees of hypertrophy, hyperplasia, or both, depending in the first place on whether the cells are capable of multiplication, and in the second on whether the multiplication is adequate to meet the demand for more functional tissue.

In the case of "hormonal" hyperplasia, the tissue response is again more or less characteristic for each target organ. Thus the growth hormone of the anterior pituitary produces an apparently pure hyperplasia of the thymus gland in rats, but mixed hypertrophy and hyperplasia of the liver. Œstrogens induce mainly hypertrophy of the uterine muscle—although it has been shown that some multiplication of the smooth muscle cells also occurs—but they induce mainly hyperplasia, and under special circumstances even neoplasia, of the endometrium.

Other Stimuli to Cell Multiplication

Apart from "compensatory" or "hormonal" hyperplasia there are three other principal circumstances which provoke mitotic activity in excess of that normally occurring in the tissue concerned.

(1) Repair of a wound.
(2) Infection with certain viruses.
(3) Neoplasia.

1. Repair of a Wound

The mechanisms of repair have been discussed in Chapter 17. Conditions in a healing wound provide the necessary stimuli for increased mitotic activity in a number of different cell types. What these stimuli are has exercised the speculation of pathologists for more than half a century. One of the most favoured hypotheses is that certain substances released by the injured cells act as mitotic stimuli, and thus initiate the healing process. In 1892, Wiesner,[18] discussing repair in plants, wrote: "If an incision is made in an organ which is capable of producing new adventitious tissue in response to the wound, it will be seen that the injured cells disappear even before the formation of new cells has begun, or at least simultaneously with the latter. Resorption of the damaged cells takes place, and there is no doubt that the products of these cells enter into the metabolism of the surviving tissues. . . . This fact leads one to think that the substances which are released by the damaged cell and which pass into the adjacent tissues, are the cause of the transformation of resting cells into adventitious meristematic cells." Essentially similar theories were put forward about wound healing in man. Bier[19] discussed the possible role of "wound hormones" in the healing of human wounds: "The hormones to be considered are, in my opinion, produced at the site of injury and exert their effect in part locally by diffusion into the surrounding tissues, and in part on other organs in the body, which they reach by the blood stream. As a result of the stimulus provided by these substances, these organs produce building materials for the regenerative process, which again reach the site of regeneration by the blood stream. To make matters clear I should like to mention that not only secretions of glands, tissues and cells are to be regarded as hormones in this context, but also tissue decomposition products."

In animals no "wound hormones" have yet been identified; in fact, there is no convincing evidence that such compounds really exist. There have been a great many experiments showing that tissue extracts of various sorts and certain protein digests increase the rate of multiplication of some tissue cells *in vitro*. But this type of experiment does not necessarily mean much more than that the multiplication of these cells *in vitro* is limited by the absence or low concentration of certain substances which are present in the extracts. None of these extracts initiates cell multiplication in intact tissues. *In vivo*, an essential part of the stimulus to cell multiplication appears to be the actual disorganisation of the architecture of the tissue, that is to say, a disruption of the normal relationship which the cells have to one another. There has been some experimental analysis of the possible role of this relationship in cell multiplication. Wigglesworth[20] has shown that in the bug *Rhodnius prolixus*, which has only a single layer of cells beneath its cuticle, removal of a small area of epithelium provokes multiplication not of the cells immediately adjacent to the bare area, which might have been expected if stimulatory substances were produced by the injured tissue, but of cells somewhat further removed from the edge. The adjacent cells at first move out over the bare area and re-epithelialise it. This movement of cells results in a "loosening up" of the surrounding epithelium, so that the number of cells per unit area is diminished. It is this fall in the cell density which, according to Wigglesworth, stimulates cell multiplication. When enough cells have been produced to restore the cell density to normal, multiplication ceases. In the case of connective tissue cells, Abercrombie and Heaysman[21] have shown that the amœboid movements which these cells exhibit when they are dissociated ceases once the cells make contact with each other, and it has been shown that the multiplication of many types of tissue cell in culture ceases when a sheet of continguous cells is formed. While it is plausible that dissociation of cells which are normally contiguous, as tissue cells are in the body, may stimulate cell multiplication, this sort of explanation is not very satisfying. We still have no idea of *how* dissociation stimulates multiplication, or, conversely, how contiguity suppresses it, and it is precisely this that we want to know.

2. Infection with Viruses

Many of the local lesions produced by animal viruses show some degree of cellular proliferation. Some virus lesions, such as infectious warts in man, the

Shope papilloma, myxoma and fibroma of the rabbit, or the Rous sarcoma of birds, are almost entirely proliferative lesions, and can justifiably be regarded as neoplasms. But apart from these extreme cases, a large number of viruses initiate multiplication in the cells which they infect, and this proliferation, subsequently accompanied by various degrees of necrosis, is the essential basis of the lesion produced. How virus particles initiate proliferation in resting cells is one of the most interesting problems in cell physiology. The cells infected with virus are stimulated to proliferate while they still have the normal relationship to each other; the architecture of the tissue is only subsequently destroyed. Proliferation usually begins before necrosis occurs, and in some conditions there may be no necrosis. It is thus difficult to implicate tissue breakdown products or local "wound hormones" in the proliferation caused by viruses. The current view is that the virus takes over some of the synthetic mechanisms of the cell, or releases these mechanisms from their normal system of controls; the cell is induced to increase its rate of autosynthesis and cell multiplication occurs. We are still very far from understanding how this modification of the synthetic mechanisms of the cell is brought about, or, for that matter, what, in biochemical terms, the modification is.

3. **Neoplasia**

Since the problem of neoplasia is the subject of the following four chapters, only a few comments will be made here. In normal cells, as has been described, multiplication occurs only in response to specific external stimuli and ceases when these stimuli are no longer present. In neoplastic cells progressive multiplication occurs irrespective of external stimuli; the only limiting factors are space and the availability of the necessary substrates, that is to say, an adequate blood supply. The rate of cell multiplication in neoplastic cells may vary widely, just as the generation time of bacteria varies widely, and there is no reason to assume that the neoplastic cell is necessarily less exacting in its growth requirements than the normal cell. Some neoplasms grow very slowly, for example, the "rodent ulcer" of the skin, and some have quite specialized growth requirements, for example, some cancers of the breast or prostate, in which cell multiplication is to a large extent dependent on the presence in the blood of certain hormones. "Autonomy" is thus not an essential feature of the neoplastic cell, if "autonomy" is taken to mean complete independence of the factors which normally control the multiplication of that cell type. What is characteristic of the neoplastic cell, as opposed to its normal homologue, is the fact that multiplication occurs in the absence of any discernible stimulus, and continues under conditions in which the multiplication of normal cells ceases.

The Control of Cell Multiplication

It would be satisfying to suppose that the actions of many of the stimuli to cell multiplication discussed in this chapter will eventually be brought together in terms of some general biochemical mechanism controlling cell division. Any such mechanism would have to account for at least the following facts:

1. Some cells, for example, connective tissue cells or epithelial cells, are stimulated to multiply when the normal spatial relationship between them is

disturbed; multiplication ceases when the normal relationship is restored. This phenomenon is illustrated by the observation that many dissociated tissue cells, cultivated *in vitro*, cease to multiply once a sheet of contiguous cells has been formed, even though there is ample nutrient to support further multiplication.

2. Viruses may initiate multiplication in cells which have a normal spatial relationship to each other.

3. The multiplication of neoplastic cells is not inhibited by contiguity with other cells, or by the normal architecture of the tissues.

A natural tendency is to imagine that cells stay in the intermitotic or "resting" state until something stimulates them to divide. It becomes easier to construct a hypothesis that fits the facts if one assumes the opposite—that cells capable of division would go on dividing except when restrained. It seems reasonable to suppose that if multiplication is inhibited as a result of contiguity between cells something more than mere contact is involved. It has been suggested that this inhibition is brought about by substances which pass from one cell to another across the area of contact. If this is so, certain guesses can be made about the nature of these substances. They must be substances which do not ordinarily exist in adequate concentrations in the extracellular environment. If this were not the case, inhibition would be produced without contiguity of the cells. This requirement probably rules out most of the common metabolites and suggests the possibility of macromolecules, such as nucleic acids or proteins, or even organized cytoplasmic particles. It has recently been shown that the cells of some tissues, notably epithelia, are linked by specialized junctions which permit the free flow from cell to cell of both electrolytes and proteins [22, 23]; and there is evidence that cytoplasmic particles, and presumably other cytoplasmic constituents, do pass across the intercellular bridges which link connective tissue cells cultivated *in vitro*.

A general statement of this theory would be that cells in contact with each other in the tissues are restrained from multiplying by a constant interchange through specialized areas of contact of certain specific substances. When the tissue architecture is disturbed and the flow of these substances is interrupted, the restraint is removed and cell multiplication takes place. When contact is re-established by the restoration of the normal tissue architecture, the flow of these substances is also re-established and multiplication is again inhibited. The ability of certain viruses to initiate multiplication in the cells of intact tissues might be explained if the virus material combined with the specific receptor groups for these inhibitory substances and thus rendered the cell refractory to their action. The interference of the virus with the action of the inhibitory substances could be envisaged as similar in nature to the various "interference" phenomena which occur between different strains of virus or between killed and living virus. The multiplication of neoplastic cells could be explained either by the inability of the inhibitory macromolecules to penetrate the membrane of neoplastic cells, or, more plausibly, by the permanent loss or alteration of the necessary specific receptors in the cells.

No one who reads this should carry away the idea that the theory propounded is more than a speculation. At best, it provides a way of thinking in general terms about some apparently unrelated phenomena, and it does appear to lend itself to experimental investigation.

REFERENCES

1. HARRIS, H. (1959). *Biochem. J.*, **72,** 54.
2. HARRIS, H. (1959). *Biochem. J.*, **73,** 362.
3. HARRIS, H. (1960). *Biochem. J.*, **74,** 276.
4. PILGRIM, C., and MAURER, W. (1965). *Exp. Cell Res.*, **37,** 183.
5. ZETTERBERG, A., and KILLANDER, D. (1965). *Exp. Cell Res.*, **39,** 22.
6. MAALØE, O., and KJELDGAARD, N. O. (1966). *Control of Macromolecular Synthesis.* New York: W. A. Benjamin, Inc.
7. KILLANDER, D., and ZETTERBERG, A. (1965). *Exp. Cell Res.*, **40,** 12.
8. JEENER, H., and JEENER, R. (1952). *Exp. Cell Res.*, **3,** 675.
9. HARRIS, H. (1955). *Brit. J. exp. Path.*, **36,** 115.
10. WINTERNITZ, M. C., and WATERS, L. L. (1940). *Yale J. Biol. Med.*, **12,** 705.
11. MCQUEEN-WILLIAMS, M., and THOMPSON, K. W. (1940). *Yale J. Biol. Med.*, **12,** 531
12. EYSTER, J. A. E. (1927). *Trans. Ass. Amer. Phycns.*, **42,** 15; (1928). *J. Amer. med. Ass.*, **91,** 1881.
13. HERRMANN, G., and DECHERD, G. M. (1939). *Ann. intern. Med.*, **13,** 794.
14. LI, C. H. (1952). *Harvey Lect.*, **1950–51,** 195.
15. WEARN, J. T., SHIPLEY, R. A., and SHIPLEY, L. J. (1937). *J. exp. Med.*, **65,** 29.
16. KNOX, W. E., AUERBACH, V. H., and LIN, E. C. C. (1956). *Physiol. Rev.*, **36,** 164.
17. MONOD, J., and COHN, M. (1952). *Advanc. Enzymol.*, **13,** 67.
18. WIESNER, J. (1892). *Elementarstruktur und das Wachstum der lebenden Substanz.* Vienna: A. Holder.
19. BIER, A. (1917). *Dtsch. med. Wschr.*, Nos. 27–30.
20. WIGGLESWORTH, V. B. (1937). *J. exp. Biol.*, **14,** 364.
21. ABERCROMBIE, M., and HEAYSMAN, J. E. M. (1953). *Exp. Cell Res.*, **5,** 111.
22. LOEWENSTEIN, W. R., SOCOLAR, S. J., HIGASHINO, S., KANNO, Y., and DAVIDSON, N. (1965). *Science*, **149,** 295.
23. KANNO, Y., and LOEWENSTEIN, W. R. (1966). *Nature* (*Lond.*), **212,** 629.

Chapter 21

THE NATURE OF TUMOUR GROWTH

By I. Berenblum

THOUGH it is customary, in a course on tumour pathology, to start with a definition, little is really gained by it, since the student, coming new to the problem, can hardly benefit from a highly condensed précis of something he does not yet know. In the case of tumours, there is the added difficulty that most of the recognisable features are inconstant, being peculiar to some tumours but not to all, and cannot, therefore, be included in a definition. And yet, when these are excluded, what is left is almost meaningless.

The purpose of a definition is, by sifting the available knowledge, to bring into relief the essentials of the subject under discussion; and since the reasoning that leads to the construction of a definition can be more revealing than the formula itself, the conventional procedure will be reversed here, with the definition being built up step by step as the subject unfolds. The end result may still fall short of an ideal definition, but one will, at least, become aware of its limitations and thereby acquire a truer understanding of the problem.

The Tumour Cell

The first, rather obvious but nonetheless important, fact about a tumour, or "neoplasm", is that it is composed of living cells, generally but not invariably supplied with a supporting stroma and blood vessels. *The living cell is the essential unit of a tumour, as it is of any normal tissue of the body.*

The second important fact about a tumour is that the component cells are not alien to the body but are actually descendants of normal cells. *A tumour cell is a modified normal cell.*

From these two basic axioms one can already draw a number of far-reaching conclusions, at least in circumscribing the problem of neoplasia. For instance, the distinction between neoplasia and inflammation becomes more understandable, once it is realised that the essential unit, in the one case, is derived from the body, and in the other case, is an extraneous micro-organism. In inflammation the leucocytes, macrophages and other cellular elements represent a *reaction* against the disease; in neoplasia the cellular elements of the lesion *themselves* represent the disease. The distinction is also apparent in the therapeutic approach which, in the case of inflammation, is designed to destroy the micro-organisms but not the leucocytes, while in the case of neoplasia it is directed towards the eradication of the very cells that comprise the lesion.

Though the tumour resembles normal tissue in being composed of living cells, important differences naturally exist between the two. Structurally, a tumour manifests some degree of exaggerated variability and of abnormalities in the size, shape and staining properties of the cells and their nuclei, and more especially of derangements in the spatial relationship of the cells to one another.

The functional peculiarities are more fundamental, and refer to (*a*) a diminution, and sometimes even a total loss, of the more specialised functions; (*b*) an accentuation of the more vegetative functions, e.g. those concerned with proliferative vigour; and (*c*) the acquisition in the case of *malignant* tumours of certain new functions, such as the ability to invade the surrounding tissues and to continue to grow in distant parts of the body after transportation of fragments of the tumour tissue through the blood or lymph stream.

A further deduction that can be made from the two basic axioms is that insofar as tumour cells are originally derived from normal cells, there should be different kinds of tumours according to the different normal cell types that exist in the body. This is, in fact, the case; indeed, the variety of types of tumours is one of the most striking features of the disease.

We have now to consider to what extent a tumour *resembles* the normal tissue from which it is derived.

Potentially, every cell type in the body can give rise to a tumour, and in each case the specific functional propensities (e.g. the ability to produce keratin, fat, cartilage, bone, or specific enzymes and hormones) are handed on to the tumour cells. Thus, a tumour derived from squamous epithelium has potentially the capacity to produce keratin; that of bone-forming cells, the capacity to produce bone tissue, and so on. But with rapidly growing tumours, these propensities are not fully realised, and the more rapid the growth rate of the tumour, the more "primitive" it appears both with respect to structure and specialised function.

The situation is actually more complicated, because not only is there an inverse relationship between rate of growth and specialisation, but also an interplay between the normal characteristics and those derived from the neoplastic transformation. One may thus speak of tumours having a double heritage—normal and neoplastic; and much of the complexity of tumour growth stems from the varying ratio of these two heritages, each modified by the growth rate of the tumour.

Tumour cells may be considered as *changed* fibroblasts, *changed* osteoblasts, *changed* liver cells, as the case may be; but while the change is, in some cases, so slight that the tumour cells appear little different from the parent cell type ("minimal deviation" tumours), in other cases their resemblance to the parent cell type may be entirely obliterated.

There is, of course, nothing unusual in a normal cell changing its appearance and behaviour in response to an altered environment. This is often reversible, persisting as long as the modifying influence acts, and known as metaplasia. But the change involved in the transformation of a normal into a tumour cell is irreversible, the newly-acquired properties being handed on to the daughter-cells at each division. When, for instance, through the action of a carcinogenic agent on a normal tissue, a tumour is induced, the latter thereafter continues to grow without the necessity of further action by the inciting agent. The evolution of a tumour thus represents *the development of a colony of permanently altered cells*. Since irreversible changes may also occur in the normal development of tissues—I refer particularly to the series of irreversible differentiations in morphogenesis in the embryo—we may provisionally describe a tumour as representing *an abnormal type of irreversible differentiation.*

From what has so far been discussed, the inception of a tumour may be visualised as follows: As a result of some peculiar stimulus, a normal cell undergoes an irreversible change, becoming endowed with certain new functional properties; this cell divides into two, and these divide again, until a large colony is formed, each component cell possessing these newly-acquired properties superimposed upon the pattern inherited from the normal, parent cell. Though ultimately the tumour mass may assume enormous proportions, exceeding in size the organ or tissue within which it had arisen, all the component cells are, according to this "focal origin" concept, descendants of the one that originally underwent the irreversible transformation from the non-neoplastic cell.

Though this picture seems to arise logically from the two basic axioms described at the outset, we already find ourselves in conflict with views held by many pathologists. The "focal origin" concept, just described, implies that once the initial transformation has taken place, the subsequent development and growth proceed exclusively by the division of the existing tumour cells, as opposed to the idea of a contiguous conversion of the surrounding normal cells. Also implicit in the idea of the focal origin is that the initial change occurred in a single cell, in contrast to the "field effect" hypothesis of Willis.[1]

Those who maintain that a tumour arises diffusely base their belief largely on histological appearances of human tumours, in which it is often impossible to draw the exact demarcation line between the tumour cells proper and the surrounding non-neoplastic cells that happen to have undergone hyperplasia. They also point to the fact that where the neoplastic lesion is still very small, the histological appearances are suggestive of multiple foci of origin. But this is not necessarily in conflict with the "focal origin" of a tumour, because multiple tumours commonly occur in the same tissue, *each tumour having originated independently*. Confusion arises from the failure to distinguish between the concept of *multiple tumours each of focal origin, fused into one mass*, and that of *a tumour supposedly originating through a "field effect" on the whole area of tissue*.

The distinction between these two hypotheses is more than academic, in view of the bearing it has on the interpretation of "precancerous" lesions.

The Role of Proliferation in Tumours

In a sense, cellular proliferation is the *sine qua non* of neoplasia, for without it the most conspicuous feature of the disease—growth—would be lacking. And yet, a tumour cell may, for many years, remain in a dormant state without apparently undergoing division. We are, therefore, faced with a curious paradox: if we accept the dormant tumour cell as neoplastic, then the factor of *growth* cannot be an essential part of the definition of a tumour. If, on the other hand, we choose to ignore the dormant tumour cell, then the irreversible nature of neoplastic transformation, at the inception of the tumour, would have to be excluded. In the one case, the clinical picture of the disease would be distorted out of all recognition; in the other, the theoretical concept of neoplasia, tenuous enough as it is, would become meaningless.

The difficulty arises from the fact that we are trying to define two things at the same time: tumour tissue and the tumour cell. This is a common conflict in pathology. There are, for instance, many examples of *hypertrophy* of an organ involving *atrophy* of its component cells, also of hypersecretion of an endocrine gland in which each individual cell secretes *less* than the normal. Logically, one should aim at two independent definitions—one for the tumour cell and the other for the tumour as a tissue. The former is concerned with the mechanism of carcinogenesis (tumour induction). Here we are dealing with the tumour as a tissue in which cellular proliferation is undoubtedly a constant feature.

This brings us to one of the crucial problems in tumour pathology: what is the essential difference between the proliferation of a tumour and that of a non-neoplastic tissue?

Normal Cell Division, Hyperplasia and Neoplasia

Hyperplasia is cellular proliferation in excess of the normal. But excessive cellular proliferation is also a feature of neoplasia; and though the degree of proliferation in the latter is usually much greater, this is not invariably the case; from which we must deduce that the essential difference is a qualitative one.

The relation between normal proliferation in an adult tissue and hyperplasia is well illustrated in skin epithelium, in which the cells in the deeper layers (which I shall refer to as "stem cells") proliferate, while those at the surface die, to be converted into keratin, and eventually shed. The fact that the thickness of the skin epithelium remains more or less constant throughout life indicates that an equilibrium normally exists between division at the base and death at the surface. A pathological stimulus (non-specific irritation) speeds up the process, until a new equilibrium is reached between the increased proliferation at the base and the increased death rate at the surface. This is hyperplasia, which may persist for a long time, but which is never progressive, irrespective of the intensity of action of the inciting stimulus. The net effect of hyperplasia is essentially the same as that of normal cell division: the reaching of an equilibrium.

Neoplasia differs from both normal cell division and hyperplasia in that its growth never attains an equilibrium. Irrespective of whether the growth of a tumour is rapid or slow, *it is progressive*, i.e. without limit, other than that imposed by the death of the host. Under certain experimental conditions in animals, when there is absence of ulceration, secondary infection, hæmorrhage, invasion of important organs, or the development of secondary deposits in other parts of the body—i.e. of factors which might otherwise shorten the life of the host—the size of the tumour may eventually exceed that of the animal.

When the stem cells, in the deeper layers of the skin epithelium, divide, one must suppose, if a growth equilibrium is to be maintained, that 50 per cent of the daughter-cells remain as stem cells and 50 per cent move upward and die. Conversely, in the case of a *tumour* of the skin epithelium, where growth is progressive, one must assume that there is a persistent excess of division rate over death rate. Since, under normal conditions, this excess is automatically compensated, after a relatively short period, by a commensurate increase in death rate, brought about by the maturing of 50 per cent of the daughter-cells, it must be concluded that *the absence of an equilibrium in neoplasia of skin epithelium results from a delay in maturation of the* (*neoplastic*) *stem cells.*[2] The same principle presumably operates in other tissues or organs in which a similar steady state of cell division is attended by an equilibrium, e.g. in hæmopoiesis, spermatogenesis, and in such organs as the intestinal mucosa, lymph follicles, etc. The mechanism is not so readily demonstrable in the brain, where cell division does not normally occur, nor at the other extreme, in the case of fibroblasts, where the contrast between the quiescent state and hyperplasia is very pronounced. But the principle may still apply, once the cells begin to divide.

Delay in maturation at the stem-cell stage also accounts for the tendency of a tumour to display deficiency in specialisation. There are, in fact, three aspects of maturation: *functionally*, it represents an expression of the degree of specialisation of the particular cell type; *developmentally*, it represents the passing beyond the stem-cell stage; and *in terms of the ultimate fate of the cell*, it represents the onset of ageing of the cell, which, in most tissues, eventually leads to its death. Stem cells, on the other hand, do not, strictly speaking, have a definable life span, as only 50 per cent of their progeny, not they themselves, mature and die.

It is necessary, at this point, to clear up certain ambiguities in terminology. In modern biology the term "differentiation" is used to describe an irreversible change in cell morphology and function in contrast to "modulation", which refers to a reversible change.[3] In pathology, the term "differentiation" has a wider and looser meaning, with emphasis on the change from a lower to a higher state of specialisation, but without insisting on the irreversible nature of the change. An "undifferentiated" cell, in pathology, is one that has not yet reached a high degree of specialisation (e.g. an embryonal cell, or a "stem cell" in the adult); while a "dedifferentiated" cell is one that has supposedly reverted from a highly differentiated to a relatively undifferentiated level. Since tumours usually display less specialisation than their tissue of origin, they are generally considered to have undergone "*de*differentiation". But since the specialised cells of a tissue, either normal or neoplastic, arise from undifferentiated stem cells, the relative deficiency of specialisation in a tumour is an expression of *inadequate maturation* rather than of *dedifferentiation*. For this reason, the term "dedifferentiation" should be avoided, except possibly for very special cases, e.g. in tissue culture.

A fact sometimes forgotten is that tumour cells do mature to some degree, and that these maturing neoplastic cells, which probably form the bulk of the tumour mass, are presumably no longer viable. If they do undergo a few more divisions, they probably give rise to the bizarre tumour giant cells and other monstrosities so frequently seen in rapidly growing tumours. The fact that a high proportion of the cell population in a tumour consists of neoplastic maturing cells has important implications in tumour chemotherapy studies. An agent that causes dramatic shrinking of the tumour mass may possibly achieve its effect by speeding up the death of the *maturing* cells, and thus have no relation to true therapy, which demands the destruction of the neoplastic *stem* cells. (This may explain why chemotherapeutic drugs against cancer are so often transitory in their action.)

Tumour Autonomy

The most concise definition of a tumour and the one most widely quoted is that of Ewing,[4] which states that "a tumour is an autonomous new growth of tissue". This definition is inadequate and confusing, since it begs the question of what we mean by "autonomy". This term, with its vitalistic connotation, only obscures the issue of what really constitutes a tumour.

Superficially the meaning is clear enough: a tumour seems autonomous in that it appears to be less under the controlling influence of the body than normal tissues. But two questions immediately present themselves: (1) in what precise manner does a tumour defy the normal homeostatic laws that govern a multicellular organism? and (2) what is responsible for this apparent anarchy?

One aspect of this problem has already been discussed: while normal and hyperplastic growth reach an equilibrium, that of a tumour does not. Instead of labelling it as "autonomy", this property of progressive growth has been shown to result from a delay in maturation at the stem cell stage. The cause of this delayed maturation is not yet clear; but one can hazard the guess that while the effect on the organism may appear "uncontrolled" the mechanism involved is simply an imbalance of *normal* processes.

Another example of apparent autonomy is the ability of a tumour to divert towards itself a disproportionate allocation of the available foodstuffs in the body. The harmful effects of this are most evident in the case of malignant tumours: the body wasting away while the malignant tumour flourishes. The phenomenon can even be recognised in very slowly growing benign tumours, e.g. in the case of a lipoma (a benign tumour of adipose tissue), which may continue to accumulate fat in an emaciated person in whom no trace of fat is detectable elsewhere. Here, then, is an illustration of the "uselessness" of a tumour in the body economy.

The problem of fat deposition in a lipoma is a very special case, and only of academic interest. Of far greater importance is the extent and manner of protein synthesis in the course of the growth of a tumour, especially under conditions of partial starvation of the body—i.e. when there is a negative nitrogen balance. One should point out, in passing, that nutritional studies in animals, in relation to tumour growth, involve other complicating factors, such as the increased energy requirements of the animal bearing the tumour, loss of appetite after the tumour has reached a certain size, and the possibility of special nutritional requirements of the tumour, in comparison with those of normal tissues.[5] The fact that a growing tumour may disturb the endocrine balance of the body, which may affect enzymic and metabolic processes, further complicates the issue.[6] There are, in addition, such obvious complications as secondary infection of the tumour and anæmia.

The fact remains that a tumour can continue to increase in size while the host is suffering from starvation, and that this increase in size involves synthesis of new proteins out of building blocks which, if not provided by the food intake, will be derived from the breakdown of proteins of the normal tissues of the body.[7] But the same is true for the growth of a fœtus *in utero*,[8] and probably for many normal organs of the body, yet no one speaks of these as "autonomous".

The allocation of foodstuffs in the body is by no means egalitarian; and loss of weight during extreme starvation is also very unequal among the different organs and tissues of the body. What actually determines the priorities for the amino-acids, etc., among the various tissues in the body, is not known; but it is a fact that each tissue somehow transmits to the body its minimal requirements, and that during nutritional stress "urgent" demands by some tissues are satisfied at the expense of other tissues.

If this is a biological law in multicellular organisms one must not be surprised that tumour cells can also exert a claim, and as it happens a very pressing claim, for "urgent" food allocation. A tumour probably does disturb the homeostatic metabolic mechanism more markedly than a fœtus, or any other growing tissue; but this is merely an exaggeration of a normal process, not a defiance of the laws governing *in vivo* metabolism.

Then there is the concept of tumour autonomy in the more general sense, referring to what is generally alluded to as the "uselessness" of the lesion in the body economy. Even this—for which the term "autonomy" would seem more justified—also requires looking into.

The keratin produced by a tumour of squamous epithelium does not perform its normal function of surface protection; a tumour of muscle tissue rarely exhibits contractile properties, and when it does the contractions are dissipated in an ineffectual manner; the fat stored by a lipoma is, as already pointed out, not usually available for the rest of the body; and the hormones secreted by a tumour of an endocrine organ, though usually normal in function, are produced in amounts unrelated to the needs of the body. Other examples could be quoted.

But here too the "autonomous" nature of the process is deceptive. If the keratin of an epithelial tumour displays no effectual function, this is because of its erratic distribution in the tumour. The same applies to the contractility of neoplastic muscle fibres. Potentially, the specialised products of tumours, be they keratin, fat, bone, or specific hormones, would function normally, but for their situation and the disproportion of the amount produced in relation to the needs of the body. We must also remember that there are many non-neoplastic diseases of endocrine glands that cause a hormonal imbalance. We do not call these examples of autonomy because in such cases the physiological cause and effect relationship is assumed to be still operative, though set at an abnormal level.

There is, however, an important difference between disturbances in homeostasis in non-neoplastic diseases and in malignant tumours. In the former, the defect is in the homeostatic mechanisms; in the latter, in the response of the tumour cells to the homeostatic mechanisms *which may themselves be functioning normally*.

We might digress here for a moment to consider the validity of such terms as "purpose", "usefulness", "orderliness", etc., as applied to cells or tissues. Such anthropomorphic and teleological phraseology only tends to confuse the issue. Can one say, for instance, that fibrosis of the heart valves is useful? As a stage in the healing of a rheumatic lesion it is useful and apparently purposeful; yet with respect to the subsequent functioning of the heart it leads to chronic valvular disease which is eventually fatal. (For a masterly treatment of this problem in relation to tumour growth see Nicholson.[9])

We must, for the time being, pass over those aspects of "autonomy" which are peculiar to malignancy, and therefore irrelevant to a discussion of neoplasia in general, which comprises benign as well as malignant tumours. I refer not only to the two outstanding properties of malignancy—invasion and secondary growth (metastases)—and to the morphological expression of malignancy—"anaplasia"—but also to certain other unusual properties which a tumour may develop in the course of its growth, such as the tendency of a tumour (e.g. of the breast) to lose its dependence on hormonal influences,[10, 11] or the property of certain tumours to become transplantable into foreign species.[12, 13]

The Chemistry of Tumour Tissue

It is natural to assume that the differences in biological behaviour between a tumour and a normal tissue must ultimately depend on chemical differences, either in a qualitative sense—the tumour lacking some essential constituent or, conversely, possessing something which is absent in normal tissue—or in a quantitative sense—measurable by the amounts of certain key constituents per cell or in terms of intensity of metabolic activity.

Much of the early work on the subject was vitiated by failure to take into account the dissimilarities of different tumours according to their cell types of origin, and the range of variability among those within any one group. The more constant chemical characteristics, noted in these early studies, included a high water content, an increased potassium : calcium ratio, and a relatively high glycogen content, in comparison to normal tissues.[14] Since similar trends were also found in embryonic and hyperplastic tissues, they probably represented an expression of high growth rate and deficiency in differentiation of the tumours tested, rather than a specific property of neoplasia.

The comparative study of the metabolic activity of tumour and normal tissues *in vitro*[15] provided a new approach to the problem. The method involved the use of slices of living tissue, in a fluid medium to which glucose or some other substrate was added, placed in a vessel attached to a microrespirometer, whereby the uptake of oxygen and the liberation of carbon dioxide, lactic acid, etc., could be measured per unit volume of tissue over a given period.

The living cell acquires most of its energy by fermentation (the splitting of the sugar molecule) and by respiration (its further breakdown into carbon dioxide and water, involving the utilisation of oxygen). In animals, fermentation leads to the formation of lactic acid, the process being called *anærobic glycolysis* when occurring in the absence of oxygen, and *ærobic glycolysis* in its presence. A number of normal tissues, tested by Warburg, exhibited a high respiration with some anærobic glycolysis, but a low ærobic glycolysis. In embryonic tissue, respiration was found to be low; ærobic glycolysis also low; while anærobic glycolysis was high. Tumours, on the other hand, were found to have a low or normal respiration, but a *high glycolysis both in the presence and in the absence of oxygen.* Warburg concluded that the high glycolysis was a consequence of a damaged respiration, and that this was the underlying defect of neoplasia, accounting not only for the behaviour of tumour growth, but also, through a process of selection of the cells during carcinogenesis, for its mode of origin.

Many normal tissues (retina, kidney medulla, cartilage, placenta, fibroblasts, intestinal mucosa, skin epithelium) were later shown to possess this "tumour type" of ærobic glycolysis; while a few tumours, on the contrary, exhibited the "normal" pattern of carbohydrate metabolism. Though attempts have been made to account for these discrepancies by modifying the original theory in various ways, the validity of Warburg's theory is now seriously questioned.[16]

The more recent advances in the field of intermediary metabolism, involving phosphorylation mechanisms, specific coenzymes of known constitution, and the elucidation of the Krebs citric acid cycle, permitted a more detailed analysis of the role of carbohydrate metabolism in tumours[16, 17] without, however, bringing to light any fundamental deviation from the normal pattern.

For a broader study of tumour enzymology, concerned with biosynthetic processes as well as energy metabolism, it was necessary to explore in a systematic fashion the existence and extent of activity, in tumours, of all enzyme systems known to occur in normal tissues. Greenstein[18] and his associates, who were largely responsible for this enzymological survey, paid particular attention to comparisons of enzyme patterns between a tumour and its parent tissue of origin; and in analysing their results they drew attention to the importance of distinguishing between basic enzyme systems, common to most tissues, and those concerned with the specific functions of the specialised cells of parenchymatous tissues. Only by such means was it possible to discern a coherent picture of what appeared at first to be a collection of contradictory results.

On the whole, the enzyme patterns of tumours tend to resemble more closely those of their parent normal tissues than those of other normal tissues. Where differences between the tumour and the parent tissue are observed, these are, in most cases, associated with enzymes involved in specialised activities, though including a few enzymes of a more general kind, such as catalase and succinoxidase, which are depressed in tumours. Since "specialised" enzyme systems determine the features that distinguish one normal tissue type from another, their deficiencies in tumours would tend to iron out these distinguishing features.

This tendency for a common enzyme pattern in tumours is the biochemical counterpart of the biological findings, that tumour tissue is usually less differentiated than its parent normal tissue. No basic enzymic defect has so far been demonstrated in neoplasia, though the concept of a deletion of some unknown enzyme has been postulated as an essential feature of neoplasia (see p. 773).

A different approach to the problem of tumour chemistry, concerned with metabolic processes *in the intact animal*, was made possible with the introduction of the use of isotopically-labelled amino-acids and other building blocks for biosyntheses, and the use of "antimetabolites", which compete metabolically with normal essential chemical units. These methods have been largely directed to protein synthesis in tumours and to the biosynthesis of nucleic acids[19]—both important in so actively growing a tissue as tumours. Though the impetus has been mainly from the angle of chemotherapy, i.e. with the object of discovering specific means of interfering metabolically with the growth of the tumour,[20] the work has nevertheless helped to lay the groundwork for the study *in vivo* of the chemical nature of neoplasia. Current studies in this field are in line with recent advances in molecular biology—e.g. with the transfer of genetic information from nucleus to cytoplasm, specific control of protein synthesis in the ribosomes, viral replication in the cell (see below), etc. Essential differences should eventually be detected by these means.

A final word, before leaving the subject of the chemistry of tumours, about the histochemical approach to the problem. Recent advances in the subject[21] have opened up new possibilities of qualitative and quantitative analyses of tissues at the microscopic level, in contrast to the empirical staining methods of conventional histology.

The Role of Viruses in Neoplasia

While tumour viruses are generally considered from the ætiological angle (see Chapter 24), they also have a bearing on the nature of tumour growth. A viral agent capable of transmitting neoplastic properties could also be responsible for the specific behaviour pattern of the affected cell. Tumour viruses thus differ from carcinogens, which only participate in the neoplastic transformation but play no part in the ensuing development and growth of the tumour.

Some tumours are readily transmitted by cell-free, virus-containing extracts; but they are the exception rather than the rule. The crucial question, then, is whether the non-filtrability of the majority of tumours is due to the absence of virus in such cases or whether it is attributable to technical difficulties in demonstrating its presence.

The theory postulating *an obligatory virus in every tumour* is still far from established; but with so many examples of viral participation in tumours, the theory can no longer be lightly dismissed. Assuming, then, a hypothetical, obligatory virus, or group of viruses, how might they account for the characteristic behaviour pattern of neoplasia?

Recent studies have thrown some light on the subject, at least on the more general problem of necrotising versus growth-promoting viruses. This distinction is no longer believed to be as rigid as was previously supposed. The outcome seems rather to be determined by the relative multiplication rates of the virus and the cell that harbours it: a balanced virus-cell relationship is conducive to cell proliferation; excessive virus multiplication causes the cell to burst. By varying the experimental conditions, the cell can be made to change from one extreme type of reaction to the other in response to the same virus.

But why a *stable* virus-cell relationship should stimulate cell division is still not properly understood. One can only draw general inferences from the fact that viruses are chemically related to those cellular components responsible for the genetically-determined control of the living cell—both being essentially composed of nucleoproteins. New or altered genic material would naturally cause the cell to acquire new characteristics; and the more these particles multiplied within the cell, the more pronounced their influence would presumably be, up to the point where, by their numbers, they began to interfere with the viability of the cell. Assuming that the "altered gene" type of virus were concerned with the growth-controlling mechanism of the cell, the scheme would begin to make sense. The issue is not so simple, however, as there are both DNA and RNA tumour viruses; and while the DNA viruses may become incorporated in the nuclear genome, thus losing their viral identity, RNA tumour viruses generally continue to multiply *as such* in the cytoplasm.

How to Define a Tumour

We have now reached the stage where an attempt must be made to define what we mean by a "tumour".

We have seen that a tumour is composed of living cells, forming a growing colony; that these cells are derived from a normal cell that has undergone an abnormal type of irreversible differentiation; that cellular proliferation is a characteristic feature of tumour tissue, though not necessarily an essential attribute of the individual tumour cell; that the growth of a tumour differs from both normal proliferation and hyperplasia in that it is progressive—i.e. that it fails to reach an equilibrium—this phenomenon being due to a delay in maturation of the neoplastic stem cells; that the avidity of a tumour for the limited food supply in the circulation, and the "uselessness" of a tumour in the body economy, are probably secondary to exaggerations of normal processes, rather than primary defections of the principle of homeostasis; that the dramatic features of "autonomy"—invasion, metastases, etc.—are peculiar to malignant tumours, and do not, therefore, form part of a definition of a tumour proper; and that no fundamental characteristics of a tumour, in chemical terms, have yet been discovered, while the essential participation of specific viruses in neoplasia, though gaining support, still remains unproved.

This summary may be further condensed into the following statement:

> *A tumour is an actively-growing tissue, composed of cells derived from one that has undergone an abnormal type of irreversible differentiation; its growth is progressive, due to a persistent delay in maturation of its stem cells. The essential nature of the irreversible differentiation, whether in biological or chemical terms, and whether necessarily determined by a virus, is still unknown.*

The nearest we can get to a definition, on the basis of this analysis, is that *a tumour is a cellular tissue in which the normal growth-controlling mechanism is permanently impaired, permitting progressive growth.* The fault lies in the tumour cell, not in the controlling mechanisms of the body. The individual tumour cell, while possessing this potential impairment, need not necessarily manifest its effects (*cf.* "dormant tumour cell").

The Distinction between Benign and Malignant Tumours

All that has been said so far applies equally to a benign and a malignant tumour. But the latter has three additional qualities—two functional and one morphological. The two functional qualities of a malignant tumour are *invasion* (the ability to infiltrate and actively destroy the surrounding tissues) and *metastasis formation* (the development of secondary centres of tumour growth at a distance from the primary focus); the morphological quality of a malignant tumour, known as *anaplasia*, consists of certain structural derangements of the component cells, and serves as a histological means of detecting malignancy even when the clinical manifestations are not sufficiently well established. (How far these three qualities of malignancy are inter-related is a matter of considerable importance, and will be discussed later in more detail.)

A benign tumour is often surrounded by a fibrous-tissue capsule. This is not, as some believe, responsible for preventing the benign tumour from doing harm to the host; nor does its absence round a malignant tumour enable the latter to invade the surrounding tissues and eventually kill the host.

To understand the origin of a capsule and its limited function, one must remember that any tissue which expands generally displaces normal tissue that was there before, and that the latter will, in time, undergo pressure atrophy, leaving behind its connective tissue stroma in a condensed form. This constitutes the essential origin of a capsule, not only round a benign tumour, but potentially also round a malignant growth, and even round a non-neoplastic cyst or other progressively expanding mass. There may be the additional factor of new fibrous tissue being laid down as a mild inflammatory reaction, but this too is an indirect effect and not the result of any specific action by the tumour. The absence of a visible capsule round a *malignant* tumour is no doubt due to the fact that it is destroyed as rapidly as it is formed, through the invasive action of the malignant cells. The fact that a benign tumour growing outwardly at the surface of the body, or within the lumen of a hollow organ, has no capsule is therefore not surprising, as in such cases pressure atrophy of pre-existing normal tissue is not involved.

Nevertheless, the encapsulation of a benign tumour has clinical significance, in that the lesion can be shelled out surgically, with the reasonable assurance that the growth will not recur; while in the case of a malignant tumour that has no capsule, and where actively growing tumour cells permeate well beyond the apparent margin of the mass, a wide zone of surrounding normal tissue has to be removed (e.g. the whole breast, and usually the whole contents of the axilla, in the case of cancer of the breast), if recurrence is to be avoided. Even by such radical treatment recurrence may yet occur if the tumour is at all far advanced. Knowledge of the likely paths of invasion is an important consideration for the surgeon in planning the extent of excision necessary in each particular organ affected. The importance of knowing whether a tumour is benign or malignant thus influences the scale of surgical treatment; and when there is an element of doubt the lesion is usually treated as malignant.

Properties of Invasion

Before discussing the mechanism of invasion some consideration must be given to the anatomical patterns of invasion in different tissues.

A malignant tumour growing in a cellular organ of fairly uniform consistency (e.g. in the liver or brain) tends to invade equally in all directions, though microscopically the growing edge is far from regular. Under these conditions even the thin outer capsule of the organ acts temporarily as a barrier, the tumour finding it easier to invade the cellular parenchymatous tissue than the capsule. Another example of this principle of invasion along the lines of least resistance is that of "lymphatic permeation" within the lumen of a lymphatic channel, after the tumour cells have gained entrance through the wall of the vessel. In such a case the growth may extend rapidly and reach very far from the primary site of entry. The actual penetration through the lymphatic wall or, for that matter, through walls of arterioles and venules, and even large arteries and veins, represents a more active process than that described as "invasion along the lines of least resistance". Yet another common pattern of invasion is along tissue spaces between planes of fascia, though it is often difficult to judge whether the spread is not actually within thin-walled lymphatics lying in these spaces. Invasion through the serous membrane lining the peritoneum or other cavity has special significance because of the ease with which the growth can then extend as a continuous sheet of tumour tissue covering the mesothelial lining of the cavity, and also permit trans-cœlomic dissemination. Finally, there is the unusual intra-epithelial invasion, as exemplified in the condition known as "Paget's disease of the nipple", the tumour originating probably in mammary duct tissue and extending *within the epithelium* to the nipple and the skin beyond it.

Examples of the histological appearances of tumour tissue invading surrounding tissues are illustrated in FIGS. 1–3.

There is one type of invasion—of a malignant tumour derived from acinous glands—which manifests itself histologically as breaking through the basement membrane of the acini. The bursting of the membrane, due to the expansive growth of the multi-layered tumour acini (unlike the single-layered pattern of normal acini or of most benign tumours), no doubt contributes to the "invasion" across the membrane. In fact, all anatomical forms of invasion probably involve complex features.

This brings us to the actual mechanism of invasion by malignant tumour cells,

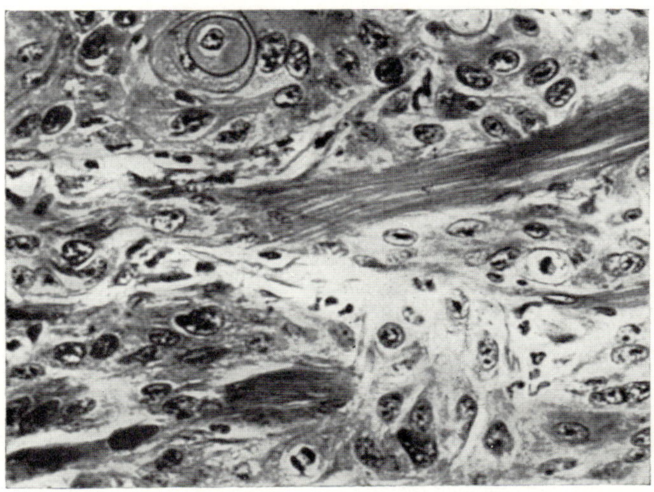

21/FIG. 1.—Squamous carcinoma of the skin invading muscle. The section shows epithelial cell nests, cells in mitosis, and many features of anaplasia.

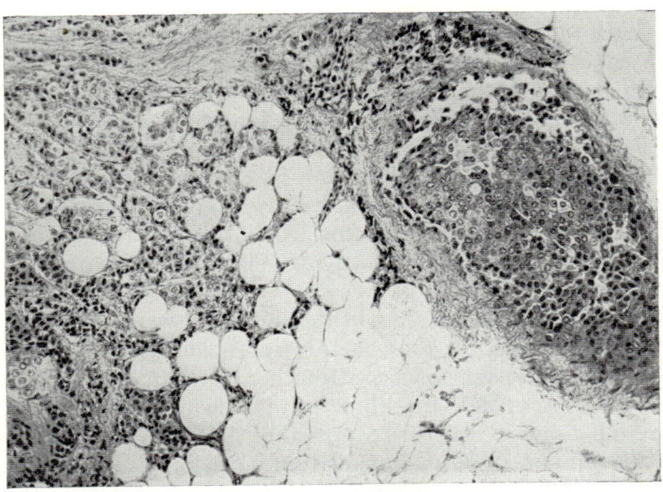

21/FIG. 2.—Carcinoma of the breast invading adipose tissue and a large blood vessel.

about which there has been much speculation, largely based on inferences derived from histology.[22, 1]

(1) *Rapidity of Growth:* The high division rate among the outgrowing cells at the margin of an invading malignant tumour, and the histological evidence of "invasion along the lines of least resistance", provide the popular analogy between the pattern of invasive tumour growth and that of "extending rootlets of a plant thrusting their way through the soil". But analogies rarely offer a clue to mechanisms of action, and only too often serve as lazy substitutes for thinking.

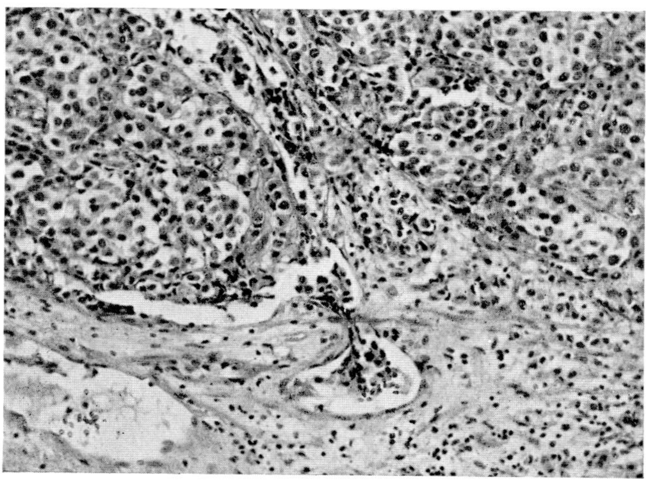

21/Fig. 3.—Carcinoma of the breast in a lymph node, showing actual penetration into a peri-capsular vein.

The evidence for attributing invasion to rapidity of growth is far from convincing. Rapid division leads to expansive growth, pressure atrophy of the surrounding tissues, and the formation of a capsule, *but not to invasion.* Malignant tumours, on the other hand, invade even when they grow very slowly. Non-neoplastic invasion by leucocytes or free macrophages is not accompanied by cellular division *in situ*, while invasion by normal chorionic tissue, though proliferative in character, is self-limiting.

Even as a mere contributing factor, rapidity of growth only affords the *scope* for invasion, by providing new tissue. The *mechanism* obviously involves other factors.

(2) *Motility:* If the older claims in the literature were true, that malignant tumour cells are more motile than their normal counterparts, a case might be made out for motility serving as a contributing factor in invasion. Actually, the claims themselves are open to question, as it is now believed that the previously observed motile tumour cells were probably non-neoplastic wandering cells present in the tumour. That malignant tumour cells often display motility in tissue culture is not a valid argument, as most cells tend to migrate more actively *in vitro*, but see below under (5).

Another weakness of the motility hypothesis of invasion is that truly motile cells migrate singly, while tumour invasion is by finger-like extensions from the main tumour mass. However, Coman[23] has demonstrated that malignant cells have a lowered adhesiveness of their cell surface, presumably owing to a low calcium content, enabling the cells to detach themselves from one another. Such a property might conceivably further the scope for invasion, but could hardly be responsible for the process of invasion itself.

(3) *Phagocytosis:* The alleged phagocytic properties of malignant tumour cells have been considered to be partly responsible for invasion. Here too there is some doubt about the accuracy of the observation. The postulated association also seems dubious on *a priori* grounds.

Many of the examples of malignant tumour cells exhibiting phagocytosis were probably ordinary macrophages, or alternatively, tumour cells with *inclusion bodies* in the cytoplasm, rather than with phagocytosed particles. Normal tissues known to possess phagocytic properties (e.g. the fixed cells of the reticulo-endothelial system) do not invade surrounding tissues, even when stimulated to activity.

(4) *Loss of Growth Restraint of the Surrounding Tissues:* This old hypothesis of Ribbert, repeated faithfully and reverently from one textbook to another, is based on a misconception.

The idea behind it is that the potential growth capacity of each tissue in the body is normally restrained by that of its neighbouring tissues; and when this balance is disturbed the growth of one of the tissues can proceed unimpeded and over-run the surrounding tissues. But this would mean that the neoplastic defect resides in the surrounding tissues and not in the actual tumour. If so, a metastatic deposit, or an experimental transplant of the tumour, finding itself in a normal milieu, should become "restrained" back to normal. The whole concept is obviously fallacious.

(5) *Loss of Contact Inhibition: Normal* cells, grown in tissue culture, wander out on the surface of the solid medium as a monolayer until the whole area is covered, after which growth and spread virtually cease. This self-limiting process is known as "contact inhibition".[24] It does not occur when *malignant tumour cells* are grown in tissue culture, the cells stepping over each other in a somewhat chaotic fashion. Assuming that loss of contact inhibition also applies to tumour growth in the body, this might constitute an essential factor in the invasive process, without however accounting for the destruction of the tissue prior to its invasion.

(6) *The Elaboration of Lytic Products:* The most plausible way to account for the actual destruction of surrounding tissue, as a prerequisite to active invasion, is to postulate the elaboration of lytic products by the malignant cells at the growing margin.

Here is a rich field for future research, once the appropriate histochemical or other micro techniques, required for the solution of the problem, have been worked out. In this connection, Burstone[24] reported that aminopeptidase activity is histochemically demonstrable in the stroma adjacent to invading tumour tissue, but not in that of normal or inflammatory tissues.

Some indication of the nature of the postulated lytic products may be gathered from the relative differences in susceptibility to invasion by various tissues. Thus, cartilage is impervious to tumour invasion, and elastic and dense fibrous tissues (e.g. tendons, ligaments, sclera, etc.) also present serious obstacles; on the other hand, bone and muscle are invaded with ease. Arteries are much less readily invaded than veins, presumably because of the presence of elastic tissue in the former. The exceptional vulnerability of lymphatics to invasion has already been mentioned. While malignant tumour tissue grows extensively in the brain the myelinated peripheral nerves seem to resist direct invasion, though they may suffer from pressure effects by the tumour mass. The extension of tumour growth round nerves occurs in the peri-neural lymphatics (FIG. 4), and not along the nerves themselves.

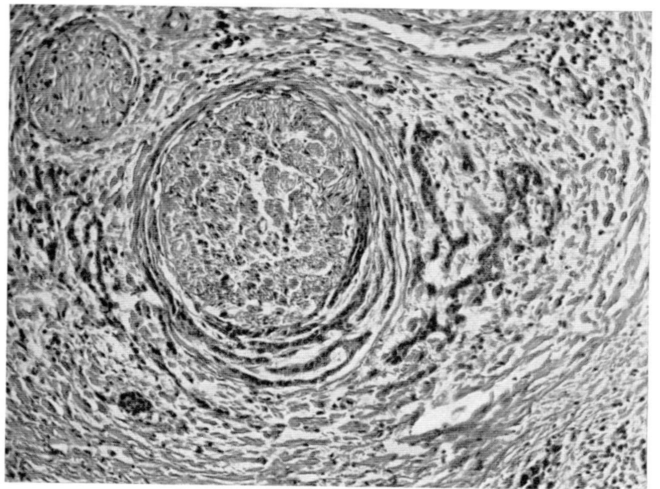

21/FIG. 4.—Carcinoma of the prostate invading peri-neural lymphatics.

With the discovery of antibody production against one's own proteins (auto-immunity),[26] and of the part played by lymphocytes, or more specifically of plasma cells in antibody formation,[27] the long-forgotten theory of Murphy[28]—that the accumulation of lymphocytes (and plasma cells) round a malignant tumour might represent an abortive defence mechanism—deserves re-examination.

The prevalent view that lactic acid, liberated by malignant tumour cells, might help to destroy fibrous tissue at the invading edge and thus be responsible for invasion by the tumour tissue can be ruled out, since the product does not appear *in situ* as the free acid but as the neutral salt, through the buffering of the tissue fluids. Moreover, as already mentioned, there are many normal tissues which glycolyse as much as tumours; yet they show no evidence of invasion.

Anaplasia

Anaplasia is difficult to define or describe because (*a*) it comprises a number of different qualities that do not necessarily appear together in every case, and (*b*) it represents an attempt to depict histologically what is, in fact, a clinical or functional concept—malignancy. The fact that the term has undergone frequent changes in meaning since it was first introduced by Hansemann is irrelevant, since its value is essentially utilitarian: it represents those features by which the histopathologist is able to diagnose malignancy under the microscope.

Some of the histological features of malignancy are merely an exaggeration of those discernible in a benign tumour; and it is sometimes difficult to tell whether they are basic to neoplasia or merely the result of rapid growth rate.

Adult tissue normally displays a remarkably constant architectural pattern. The orientation of the cells in relation to one another or to their connective tissue stroma and vascular supply represents the "organisation" of the tissue in question; and the orientation of the structures within the cells, with respect to the tissue as a whole, is referred to as their "polarity". Disturbance of the polarity of the cells, already detectable to some extent in a benign tumour but much more pronounced in a malignant growth, is an important, though subtle, feature of neoplasia, and of malignancy in particular. The spatial relationship of the various layers of normal skin epithelium, the orientation of the component cells of the gastric or intestinal mucosa, the architectural pattern of the liver lobule, of the kidney nephron or, in a more intricate fashion, of the various parts of the central nervous system, are all examples of the organisation of adult tissues; and evidence of disturbance of these normal patterns is a characteristic feature of malignancy. Naturally, much experience is required to recognise finer shades of such disturbance and to distinguish these from structural abnormalities that may arise from inflammatory or other pathological processes. Attention has already been drawn to the tendency of a tumour—particularly of a malignant tumour—to display morphological evidence of deficiency in differentiation (specialisation); and this feature usually goes hand in hand with the disturbance in orientation. Variability in structure, not only as between one tumour and another derived from the same cell type of origin, but also in different parts of the same tumour, constitutes yet another architectural derangement in malignancy. The more malignant the tumour, the more marked are the variations.

As for the intracellular changes in malignant cells,[29] many peculiarities have been described, some relatively common to most malignant tumours and of diagnostic value, others encountered only in extreme forms of anaplasia. Malignant cells tend to vary in size, and in the shape and size of their nuclei. The latter tend to stain hyperchromatically, though this is not the rule, and the nucleoli are often very prominent. Mitoses are seen in large numbers and are often irregular in form, with distorted spindles, tripolar mitoses and other abnormalities in the more anaplastic forms. Similarly, giant cells with multiple nuclei or enormous single nuclei are occasionally seen, and these are probably degenerated cells in the process of abnormal maturation and death.

The study of cells by electron microscopy has brought to light a wealth of detail not visible by the light microscope, e.g. the precise structure of the nuclear membrane, the double membrane of mitochondria, the fine structure of the endoplasmic reticulum, with the RNA-containing ribosomes aligned along its surface, and the occasional presence of viral particles. Similar studies of tumour cells (see Bernhard[30]) have confirmed the presence of these entities, often showing simplication of detailed structure of blurring of membranous outlines. Though bodies resembling virus particles are also seen in tumour cells, often in greater numbers than in comparable normal cells, they are not invariably seen in tumour cells. Nothing specifically characteristic of neoplasia has thus been demonstrated by electron microscopy; but the field has not yet been adequately explored.

The connective tissue stroma of a malignant tumour may be deficient, as though the growth of the tumour is too rapid for the stroma reaction to keep pace with it. The accompanying deficiency in the blood supply may lead to (*a*) central necrosis of the tumour (commonly occurring in carcinomas), or (*b*) the formation of immature blood vessels, which may appear as mere vascular clefts among the tumour cells, with hardly any endothelial lining (occurring in rapidly growing sarcomas). On the other hand, certain slowly growing but highly invasive carcinomas may have a super-abundance of connective tissue stroma (described as "scirrhous" tumours), in contrast to "encephaloid" tumours (which describes the brain-like consistency of those which are highly cellular and poor in stroma).

It might be imagined that with such a galaxy of histological peculiarities the diagnosis of malignancy should be easy. In most cases this is so. But when the tumour is atypical and the tissue of origin obscure, and more particularly when it is an early or borderline lesion, diagnosis may be very difficult. In the last resort it is based on an assessment of slight inferences, with many of the characteristic features absent. Is the epithelial tumour benign or malignant? Is the peculiar connective tissue lesion a sarcoma or an extremely reactive type of post-inflammatory repair? Is the undoubtedly malignant tumour of strange structure a primary growth in the organ in which it is found, or is it a metastasis from some unrecognised primary lesion elsewhere? These are frequent questions that confront the histopathologist, which cannot be answered by rule-of-thumb methods but depend on keen observation of minute details found here and there in the section.

Attempts have been made to mechanise or quantitate histological diagnosis of malignancy, as by Broders' method[31] of grading malignancy into four or five categories according to the proportion of anaplastic cells in the tumour. This has serious technical limitations, since different fields of the same tumour may display different grades, and since the application of the method has to be arbitrarily modified for each tumour type. It also has objections in principle, in that the numerical values give a spurious impression to the clinician of an accuracy which the method, in fact, does not possess. More useful systems of grading are those based on clinical, as distinct from fine histological, criteria—e.g. according to the extent of local invasion, involvement of regional lymph nodes, of distant lymph nodes, of other organs, etc.

The histological criteria of malignancy on which most reliance is normally placed are (*a*) evidence of invasion, and (*b*) disturbance in the organisation of the tissue. Both of these are architectural derangements, as distinct from cellular abnormalities. Yet modern pathology is beginning to accept more and more the diagnosis of malignancy on the basis of the morphology of individual tumour cells, as evidenced by the recognition of "carcinoma *in situ*", in which no invasion of the underlying tissues has yet appeared,[32] and by the use of the Papanicolaou test,[33] whereby malignancy is diagnosed by examination of specially stained smears from body secretions in which isolated tumour cells are present. The latter, which requires considerable skill for correct interpretation,

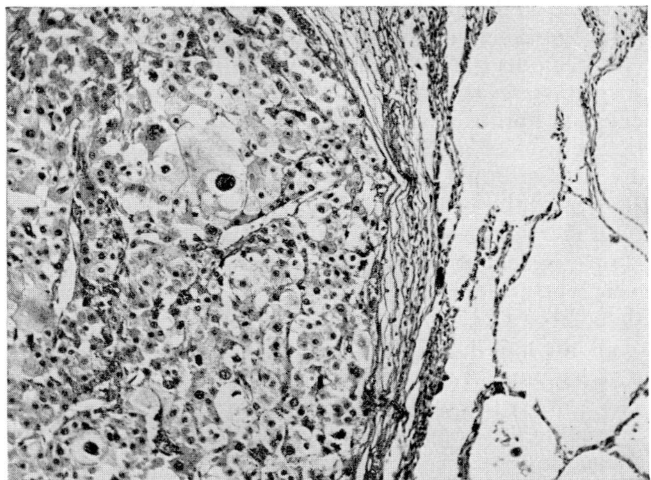

21/FIG. 5.—Carcinoma of the adrenal gland—metastasis in the lung. The characteristic morphology of an adrenal carcinoma is preserved in the metastasis.

should be considered as an additional tool, rather than a substitute for histological examination of biopsy material.

Metastases

A "metastasis" is a secondary centre of tumour growth at a distance from the primary focus (FIGS. 5 and 6). It is derived from transported live cells of the primary mass, which it resembles both in histological structure and in functional behaviour. Thus, in a tumour which is sufficiently differentiated, one can usually recognise from a histological study of the metastases the cell type of origin of the

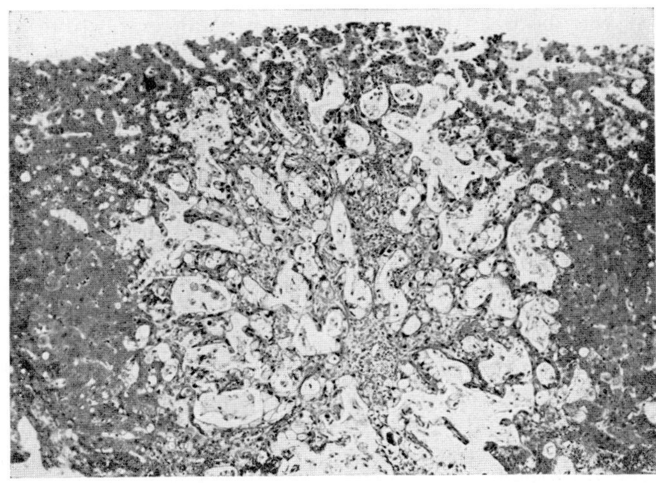

21/FIG. 6.—Carcinoma of the pancreas; metastasis in the liver (from a needle biopsy specimen).

primary growth (e.g. by the presence of keratin whorls in a squamous carcinoma, distorted but recognisable acini in a tumour of glandular origin, and colloid formation in a carcinoma of the thyroid). Minor differences between the primary tumour and its metastases may result from local modifying factors, such as differences in vascularity, fibrous tissue framework, etc., in the new surroundings.

Metastases are usually multiple, and in terminal cases these may be found in their hundreds, distributed all over the body. Their number and size bear no relation to the size of the primary tumour except, of course, that in each particular case both increase progressively with the passage of time. There are, for instance, certain pigmented tumours (malignant melanomas) which tend to metastasise very early indeed, sometimes even when the primary growth is clinically undetectable. Occasionally a spontaneous fracture of the femur in an elderly woman is the first indication of a bone metastasis, secondary to a small unrecognised carcinoma of the breast. But more often metastases begin to appear after the primary tumour has reached a fair size. The importance of early treatment is to enable the tumour to be removed or destroyed before metastases have had a chance to develop.

Regarding the way metastases are formed, the simplest and most plausible concept first to be considered was that they arose by embolic dissemination of detached tumour fragments, set free in the blood stream either directly, by penetration of blood vessels, or indirectly, through the thoracic duct. As for metastases in the regional lymph nodes, a similar *lymphatic* form of embolic dissemination was postulated. Since capillaries and venules are more easily invaded by tumour cells than arterioles, it was to be expected that dissemination peripheral to the local arteries would be rare. Dissemination through the venous route would lead to tumour emboli being trapped in the lungs (from tumours located in the body as a whole) and in the liver (from tumours located in organs that drain into the portal circulation). In fact, the regional lymph nodes, the liver and the lungs are the three most common sites for metastasis formation. As for the occurrence of metastases in other organs supplied by the systemic circulation, it was assumed that these developed after the tumour cells had "somehow slipped through the lung capillaries".

A closer examination of the distribution of metastases in the body did not, however, provide the kind of pattern one might have expected from the probable distribution through embolic dissemination. Why should some tissues (e.g. bone) be so common a site for metastases, and others (e.g. skeletal muscle) be so rare? And why should the distribution in certain organs (e.g. in liver, bone, brain, lungs, adrenal) vary according to the nature of the primary tumour? (For a detailed analysis of the distribution of metastases see Willis.[34])

Those who first recognised this "illogical" distribution[35] attributed it to a specific predilection of certain tissues, realising that only a small proportion of tumour emboli actually developed into metastases. Many explanations have been postulated for this failure of so many tumour emboli to take root. In the case of skeletal and heart muscle, it was attributed to the powerful contractions disturbing or even destroying the tumour cells. Yet, in the fowl, heart muscle is the commonest site for metastases. Others have postulated specific toxic products secreted by certain organs, which were supposed to be antagonistic to tumour cells; and unsuccessful methods of therapy have even been devised on the basis of this (e.g. using spleen extracts for the treatment of malignant disease). The true explanation is probably more straightforward—the tissues receiving the emboli must be capable of speedily providing an adequate blood supply for the new tumour tissue, and the emboli must be able to survive the period before the vascularisation. Furthermore, only tumour emboli which are at the stem-cell stage of development would be capable of giving rise to metastases, since maturing tumour cells would die. This could account for the infrequency of metastases, but would not, of course, explain the peculiar organ distribution pattern.

So far we have assumed that metastases arise only from tumour emboli. A very different mechanism was postulated by Handley,[36] who stressed the role of lymphatic permeation for long distances from the primary focus, *with the obliteration (through fibrosis resulting from an inflammatory reaction round the occluded vessels) of the intervening strands of tumour tissue, originally connecting the growing tip to the primary mass.* Not only could this account for "metastases" in the subcutaneous tissues round the primary growth, but supposedly also in such distant organs as bone, liver, etc. While Handley probably over-stressed the extent to which this process is responsible for metastasis formation, there is no doubt that it does play a significant role.

Another way in which metastases may develop is by trans-cœlomic dissemination, of which the best known example is the development of bilateral metastases in the ovaries, secondary to a carcinoma of the stomach. Among the rarer forms of metastasis formation are (*a*) the transfer, by contact, of an ulcerating tumour from one lip of a mucous surface to another, and (*b*) accidental implantation of tumour cells to a new site by means of a contaminated scalpel or needle. (Experimental tumour transplantation represents, in a sense, an artificial metastasis in another animal.)

That tumour emboli may take root, yet not develop into metastases till years later, is a phenomenon occasionally observed in man, and in keeping with the concept of "dormant tumour cells" which can be shown experimentally to require "promoting action" to stimulate them to progressive growth (see p. 770).

The Inter-relationship between the Different Properties of Malignancy

Not every malignant tumour possesses all the functional and structural features characteristic of malignancy, nor is it possible to define malignancy on the basis of certain minimal requirements; though invasion comes nearest to it, since without it metastasis formation could hardly occur. It might perhaps be correct to say that *the potential capacity for invasion* is the basis of malignancy; and in this way "carcinoma *in situ*" is the histological expression of a condition which, if left to progress, would eventually exhibit manifestation of invasion.

Metastasis formation is the most important clinical feature of malignancy, since its presence or absence virtually determines whether the disease is curable or not. Regional metastases in lymph nodes can often be successfully removed together with the primary growth; but the presence of metastases in other organs usually denotes that the process has gone too far for it to be cured by the conventional methods of surgery or radiotherapy.

The fact that in borderline cases histology may fail as a diagnostic technique is not surprising. It is not necessarily due to the fallibility of the observer but may represent the region in which the inter-relationship between structure and function breaks down. Nevertheless, histological diagnosis remains the most precise method of recognising malignancy.

Histological examination of a suspected neoplastic lesion tells more than whether it is benign or malignant. Such questions as the probable tissue of origin of the tumour, its vascularity and *degree* of anaplasia, and the extent of invasion of surrounding lymphatics, the amount and pattern of stroma and the maturity of the new blood vessels are all important to the clinician in determining the form of treatment best suited for the case, as well as to the diagnostician in appraising the prognosis of the condition.

Systemic Aspects of Neoplasia

Attention has already been drawn to the high metabolic requirements of a rapidly growing tumour, and the tendency of the tumour to grow even when the rest of the body suffers from relative starvation. Loss of weight is an important clinical symptom of malignant disease; and both the loss of weight and anæmia, associated with a peculiar sallowness, represent the condition known as "cachexia".

Though there is little to support the belief in a specific tumour toxin responsible for cachexia, a substance called "toxohormone"[37] has been detected in tumours, and in the urine of tumour-bearing patients, which, when injected into animals, causes a lowering of liver catalase activity. (It will be recalled that low catalase activity is characteristic of most tumour-bearing animals.)

Systemic effects resulting from secretory activity of specific tumour cell types, as distinct from their neoplastic properties, may be observed in cases of tumours of endocrine organs. While the amount of hormone secreted per cell is usually lower in neoplastic than in normal cells of an endocrine organ, the total amount secreted by the tumour mass may be appreciable, giving rise to symptoms of hypersecretion—e.g. masculinisation in cases of arrhenoblastoma of the ovary, secondary sexual changes in cases of tumours of the adrenal gland, alterations in bone (von Recklinghausen's disease) in connection with tumours of the parathyroid, and hypoglycæmia in cases of tumours of the pancreatic islets. Strangely enough, thyrotoxicosis is not a common accompaniment in tumours of the thyroid gland. The excessive secretion of specific hormones may, with some types of tumour, serve as a diagnostic aid—e.g. the exceptionally high levels of gonadotrophic hormone in the urine of patients with chorion carcinoma, or the increase in acid phosphatase in the blood of patients with prostatic carcinoma. (The opposite effect—a hormonal deficiency—may, of course, arise from the destruction of an endocrine gland through invasion by a neighbouring tumour or by a metastasis from a distant site.)

Some malignant tumours kill the host before metastases have had time to appear, and where other complicating factors, such as severe hæmorrhage, secondary infection, or serious interference with the function of the organ primarily affected, do not necessarily operate. Some types of tumours rarely if ever metastasise (e.g. "basal cell carcinoma" of the skin, and most types of brain tumour), and yet eventually kill the host if left untreated. On the other hand, the body may be riddled with metastases, and certain vital organs in the body (e.g. the liver) may be almost entirely destroyed by the metastatic deposits, yet life may continue for weeks or months.

Experimental studies of tumour-host relationships[5, 6] have not, so far, provided a satisfactory explanation of the many anomalies concerning the overall effects of tumour growth on the body.

REFERENCES

1. WILLIS, R. A. (1960). *Pathology of Tumours*, 3rd edit. London: Butterworth & Co.
2. BERENBLUM, I. (1954). *Cancer Res.*, **14,** 471.
3. WEISS, P. (1939). *Principles of Development*. New York: Henry Holt & Co.
4. EWING, J. (1940). *Neoplastic Diseases*, 4th edit. Philadelphia: W. B. Saunders Co.
5. FENNINGER, L. D., and MIDER, G. B. (1954). *Advanc. Cancer Res.*, **2,** 229.
6. BEGG, R. W. (1958). *Advanc. Cancer Res.*, **5,** 1.
7. WHITE, F. R. (1945). *J. nat. Cancer Inst.*, **5,** 265.
8. SEEGERS, W. H. (1937). *Amer. J. Physiol.*, **119,** 474.
9. NICHOLSON, G. W. DE P. (1950). *Studies on Tumour Formation*, Chapters 11–13. London: Butterworth & Co.
10. FOULDS, L. (1954). *Cancer Res.*, **14,** 327.
11. FURTH, J. (1953). *Cancer Res.*, **13,** 477.
12. GREENE, H. S. N. (1951). *Cancer Res.*, **11,** 899.
13. SNELL, G. D. (1959). *The Physiopathology of Cancer*, 2nd edit., Chapter 8. New York: Paul B. Hoeber Inc.
14. STERN, K., and WILLHEIM, R. (1943). *The Biochemistry of Malignant Tumours*. Brooklyn: Chemical Pub. Co.
15. WARBURG, O. (1930). *The Metabolism of Tumours*. London: Constable & Co.
16. WEINHOUSE, S. (1955). *Advanc. Cancer Res.*, **3,** 269.
17. POTTER, V. R. (1951). *Cancer Res.*, **11,** 565.
18. GREENSTEIN, J. P. (1954). *Biochemistry of Cancer*, 2nd edit. New York: Academic Press Inc.
19. GREENBERG, D. M. (1955). *Cancer Res.*, **15,** 421.
20. SKIPPER, H. E. (1953). *Cancer Res.*, **13,** 545.
21. PEARSE, A. G. E. (1960). *Histochemistry. Theoretical and Applied*, 2nd edit. London: J. & A. Churchill Ltd.
22. COWDRY, E. V. (1940). *Arch. Path.* (*Chicago*), **30,** 1245.
23. COMAN, D. R. (1944). *Cancer Res.*, **4,** 625.
24. ABERCROMBIE, M. (1961). *Proc. Fourth Canadian Cancer Conf.*, 101.
25. BURSTONE, M. S. (1956). *J. nat. Cancer Inst.*, **16,** 1149.
26. VARIOUS AUTHORS (1965). *Ann. N.Y. Acad. Sci.*, **114,** 413.
27. NOSSAL, G. J. V. (1962). *Int. Rev. exp. Path.*, **1,** 1.
28. MURPHY, J. B. (1926). *Monograph, Rockefeller Inst. for Med. Research*, No. **21.**
29. COWDRY, E. V. (1955). *Cancer Cell*. Philadelphia: W. B. Saunders Co.
30. BERNHARD, W. (1958). *Cancer Res.*, **18,** 491.
31. BRODERS, A. C. (1926). *Arch. Path.* (*Chicago*), **2,** 376.
32. FOOTE, F. W., and STEWART, F. W. (1941). *Amer. J. Path.*, **17,** 491.
33. GRAHAM, R. M. (1963). *The Cytologic Diagnosis of Cancer*. Philadelphia: W. B. Saunders Co.
34. WILLIS, R. A. (1952). *The Spread of Tumours in the Human Body*. London: Butterworth & Co.
35. PAGET, S. (1889). *Lancet*, **1,** 571.
36. HANDLEY, W. S. (1922). *Cancer of the Breast*. London: John Murray.
37. NAKAHARA, W., and FUKUOKA, F. (1958). *Advanc. Cancer Res.*, **5,** 157.

Chapter 22

THE CLASSIFICATION, MORPHOLOGY, AND BEHAVIOUR OF TUMOURS

By A. C. Ritchie

CLASSIFICATION

The classification of tumours usually used today has been evolved over the centuries to describe the tumours physicians have observed in their patients. It is thus essentially a clinical classification, describing the appearance and behaviour of human tumours. It can be adapted for statistical studies, elaborated for special investigations of a particular type of tumour, or, often rather unsatisfactorily, applied to animal tumours, but it remains in essence a description of human tumours. As would be expected, a classification which has been developed over so long a time is often inconsistent, and bears many traces of theories and forms of nomenclature which are no longer current.

In its main features, the classification is clearly derived from those in use 2,000 or 3,000 years ago. Then, as now, tumours were divided into groups according to their appearance, their behaviour, and their site. Though the ancient Egyptians 1,500 years before Christ had no clear idea of the nature of tumours, and certainly had no formal classification of the type we now employ, they did realise that tumours arising in different sites were different, distinguishing between tumours of the breast, tumours of the uterus, tumours of the soft parts, and so on, and did realise that tumours which differed in appearance were different, remarking that hard tumours were dangerous, and should be treated surgically, an observation still of considerable practical use today. A more formal classification was given by Hippocrates (460–375 B.C.), who divided tumours according to their behaviour into two large groups, the relatively innocuous "carcinos", a mixed group of lumps of various kinds which included hæmorrhoids and other non-neoplastic swellings as well as many benign tumours, and the dangerous "carcinoma" which killed the patient. Galen (A.D. 131–203) lessened the confusion between the true neoplasms and non-neoplastic lumps with his famous division of lumps into those according to nature, such as physiological swelling of the uterus in pregnancy; those exceeding nature, reparative or inflammatory masses, such as the callus around a fracture; and those contrary to nature, a group which included the true neoplasms. But the main bases of the classification of tumours remained their appearance, their behaviour, and their site.

There has been only one major extension of this system. With the advent of the microscope, it became possible to divide tumours according to their tissue of origin. Last century, when tumours were first studied microscopically, it was found that some resembled epithelium, and were in continuity with non-neoplastic epithelium; others resembled connective tissue, and were in continuity with non-neoplastic connective tissue; and yet others resembled and were in continuity with other tissues. After some debate, it was accepted that the tumours which resembled epithelium arose from epithelium, that those which resembled connective tissue arose from connective tissue, and that those which resembled other tissues aroses from those tissues. This division of tumours according to the tissue of origin rapidly became the principal basis of classification, and about 100 years ago the type of classification usual today became well established. In it tumours are classified according to four criteria; their tissue of origin, their behaviour, their site, and their appearance.

Before coming to the classification itself, it will be useful to discuss at greater length these bases of classification, and to consider two other bases which have been suggested as being more logical, but which have been found unsatisfactory.

The Bases of Classification

1. Histogenetic Classification

As has been mentioned, this is now the principal basis of classification. Tumours are divided into groups according to the type of tissue from which they arise. Usually, six such groups are distinguished, tumours of epithelium, tumours of connective tissue, tumours of hæmopoietic tissue, tumours of nervous tissue, tumours containing more than one kind of tissue, and a miscellaneous group of tumours which do not fit easily into one of the other groups. This classification has proved most valuable, for not only do the tumours of each group tend to resemble one another grossly and microscopically, but they tend to behave alike, while tumours of different groups tend to look different, and to behave differently. For example, all epithelial tumours tend to look alike, and to behave alike, and all connective tissue tumours tend to look alike, and to behave alike, but a typical epithelial tumour neither looks nor behaves like a connective tissue tumour.

There are, however, some minor difficulties. The tissue of origin of a tumour can only be determined by deduction, from its gross and microscopical appearance. This is usually easy, but there are tumours in which the histogenesis remains obscure. Fortunately such tumours are uncommon. In some, the tissue of origin is altogether unknown; in others, different tissues of origin have been suggested by different authorities. To mention only one example, Ewing's sarcoma of bone (James Ewing, 1866–1943) is considered by some writers to be a tumour of connective tissue, by others a tumour of hæmopoietic tissue. Another difficulty is that while it is usually obvious what is epithelium, and what is connective tissue, and what is hæmopoietic tissue, it is not always so. In general, the tissues are divided empirically so that like tumours will be grouped together, but there are exceptions. For example, while the adrenal cortex is considered epithelial, the adrenal medulla is classed as nervous. This is in spite of the fact that tumours of the adrenal cortex may so closely resemble those of the medulla that it may be difficult to distinguish them grossly or microscopically. But while it is important to note these and other difficulties and inconsistencies, they are not so numerous or important as seriously to lessen the value of this basis of classification.

2. Behaviouristic Classification

The second major basis of classification is the division of tumours into benign and malignant forms. The practical value of this subdivision is obvious.

A malignant tumour may invade or metastasise, severely injuring the patient, but a benign tumour remains localised, and so is much less dangerous. But it is most important to realise that the division between benign and malignant is not absolute, as is the division between black and white, but is rather as the division between hills and mountains. In most cases the distinction is clear, but there are intermediate forms. Some kinds of malignant tumour invade so little, or so slowly, and metastasise so rarely, that they are almost benign.

To emphasise these intermediate forms, Morehead has proposed a modification of the behaviouristic classification. He suggests that tumours be divided into three groups, benign, intermediate, and malignant. In the benign group, he places those types of tumour which are unequivocally benign, which grow only by expansion, which never invade or metastasise, and which do not endanger the life of the patient unless by ill chance they press upon some vital structure or suffer some complication. In the malignant group, he places the types of tumour which are unequivocally malignant, which invade locally, metastasise widely, and which will kill the patient unless eradicated. In the intermediate group are placed the rest, the kinds of tumour which invade locally but metastasise rarely, the kinds which metastasise only slowly and to a limited degree, and those which are multifocal though otherwise benign. The principle behind this suggestion is excellent, though it is doubtful if it justifies further complication of the terminology.

Rather it should be realised that each type of tumour has it own pattern of behaviour. Each kind of tumour must be studied individually. Its habit of growth must be learnt, the rate and extent of its invasion determined, and the pattern of its metastases established. All variations exist. At one extreme, it is sometimes difficult to distinguish between a benign neoplasm, in which the tumour cells are abnormal, and a focal hyperplasia, in which normal cells are reacting to a stimulus. For example, it is difficult to distinguish between a true benign tumour of the thyroid and a reactive nodule. It may also be difficult to distinguish between a benign tumour and a congenital malformation. The hæmangiomata of the skin are usually listed among the neoplasms, but in most cases they are in truth malformations. The common port-wine mark is a good example. Similarly, all gradations exist between the clearly benign tumours and the malignant. The common type of tumour of the islets of Langerhans is considered benign, though tumours of this kind often invade just a little. The tumours of the skin called basal cell carcinomata are more aggressive. They take origin in the epidermis, and grow slowly, invading the dermis, but do not metastasise once in a million cases. The anaplastic carcinomata of the pharynx sometimes show an opposite pattern of behaviour. The primary tumour remains very small, and invades so little that it may be extremely hard to find, and yet metastases in the neck grow rapidly and to large size. Some malignant tumours, such as the osteogenic sarcoma, metastasise in almost every case. In others, such as carcinoma of the breast, metastases are found at the time of operation in only about 50 per cent of cases. In yet others, they occur even more rarely. The adenomata of the bronchus metastasise in only about 10 per cent of cases. Each kind of tumour must be studied individually. The devision into benign and malignant forms is only a very rough guide.

The terms "benign" and "malignant" are usually used statistically. When we say that a tumour is malignant, we mean that if we study a large number of tumours of that kind, many or most will be found to invade, and a certain proportion will be found to metastasise. When we see an individual patient with one of these tumours, we do not know how that individual tumour will behave. Even within a group of similar tumours, there is still room for individuality. Some progress more rapidly, some more slowly. Some metastasise sooner, some later. We can only draw on our experience of the group as a whole to determine the probability that the patient will develop metastases, and to determine the probable habit of growth of his tumour.

3. Regional Classification

It is clearly important to know where the tumour is. However, alone, a regional classification is inadequate, for different kinds of tumour may arise in the same part of the body. For example, a tumour of the stomach could be a benign epithelial tumour, a benign connective tissue tumour, a benign nervous tumour, a primary or secondary malignant epithelial tumour, a primary or secondary malignant connective tissue tumour, a primary or secondary tumour of hæmopoietic tissue, and so on. One needs to know not only where the tumour is, but from what tissue it takes origin, whether it is benign or malignant, and whether it is primary or secondary.

Secondary tumours are sometimes described as being secondary tumours of the organ affected, being called, for instance, secondary tumours of the lung, or secondary tumours of the liver, but more often they retain the regional name of their primary, and are designated as, for example, secondary carcinoma of the breast in the lung, or carcinoma of the colon secondary in the liver.

4. Descriptive Classification

To the names describing the histogenesis, behaviour, and site of tumours are often added terms describing their gross or microscopical appearance. Sometimes these descriptive terms are added merely because it is customary to do so. One often speaks of a clear cell carcinoma of the kidney, because the cells of the common form of renal carcinoma have a clear cytoplasm in the usual microscopical preparations, even though this descriptive term adds little or nothing to the designation carcinoma of the kidney.

In other cases, descriptive terms are added to subdivide tumours of some particular type into smaller groups, perhaps in the hope that in this way more information will be gained about the prognosis of the individual tumours. Carcinoma of the thyroid, for example, is very often subdivided into papillary carcinoma, in which the tumour forms papillary structures which project into cystic spaces; follicular carcinoma, in which the tumour forms acini more or less like those of normal thyroid; and anaplastic carcinoma, in which the tumour tends to form solid masses of tumour cells. This subdivision is important clinically, because these different types of carcinoma behave differently, the papillary carcinoma growing more slowly, and metastasising much more slowly than does the anaplastic carcinoma. The follicular carcinoma behaves in an intermediate fashion.

In yet other cases, different kinds of benign or malignant tumour may arise from the same tissue, in the same region. Descriptive terms are added to distinguish between these different kinds of tumour which would otherwise have the same name. For example, two kinds of malignant tumour arise from the epidermis, the basal cell carcinoma and the squamous cell carcinoma. These behave so differently that it is important to give them different names. The basal cell carcinoma has already been mentioned. If often arises on the face, and grows slowly to form a small ulcer. At this stage it is easily cured by excision or radiotherapy. However, if it is left alone it will continue to grow, and continue to invade, until half the head is eaten away. Nevertheless, it almost never metastasises. The squamous cell carcinoma tends to grow more rapidly, and to form a somewhat different kind of ulcer, but more importantly it often metastasises to the regional lymph nodes, and so is much more dangerous. It too can be cured if treated early, but the treatment needed may be more extensive. The descriptive terms "basal cell" and "squamous cell" are used to distinguish between the two kinds of tumour. The names are derived from the microscopic appearance of the tumours. The basal cell carcinoma is made in large part of cells which resemble the basal cells of the epidermis, while in the squamous cell carcinoma the tumour cells tend to become flattened and to develop intercellular bridges as do the squamous cells of the epidermis.

Other tumours have what are really nick-names. Some are called after men who described them, as, for example, the carcinoma of the kidney is sometimes called a Grawitz tumour (Paul Grawitz, 1850–1932). Others are named after some striking feature. The basal cell carcinoma of the skin, for example, is sometimes called a rodent ulcer, because of the way in which it may erode away the face if left untreated. Yet others have names derived from mistaken theories as to their nature, or because no more simple term was available. The carcinoma of the kidney is still often called a hypernephroma, a name given under the mistaken belief that the tumour arose from adrenal tissue, and many of the tumours in the sixth histogenetic group, those which do not fit easily into one of the other groups, have strange names devised to indicate their supposed nature. It is, however, most desirable that terminology be kept as simple as possible, and where a satisfactory orthodox term is available it should be used. One should, for instance, speak of a carcinoma of the kidney, not a Grawitz tumour or a hypernephroma. Nevertheless, the nick-names are sometimes very useful. As has been mentioned, there is no agreement as to the histogenesis of Ewing's tumour of bone, and so it is very convenient to retain this name which does not imply any theory of histogenesis. Or again, the term Hodgkin's disease (Thomas Hodgkin, 1798–1866) is more desirable than the terms that have been devised to replace it, for it too provides a non-committal name for a curious tumour, the nature of which is not clear.

5. Embryological Classification

Coming now to the two bases of classification which have been proposed as more logical than the system which has been described, but which have been abandoned as unsatisfactory, the most famous is that based on embryology. With the growth of knowledge of embryology, the many similarities between tumours, especially malignant tumours, and embryonic tissues, were noted, and it became customary to think of neoplasia as being a return towards the embryonic state, or a failure to evolve from it, as is implied by the terms "dedifferentiated" or "undifferentiated". These theories have now become untenable. Tumours do have some similarity to embryonic tissues, but the differences are very great. Most now believe that, with the exception of the few tumours that arise from embryonic tissue, usually during fœtal life or soon after birth, tumours are derived from adult cells, and that in becoming neoplastic they develop qualities which are quite different from those of embryonic tissue. However, while the theories that all tumours were derived from embryonic cells, or had returned towards the embryonic state, were in vogue, attempts were made to devise a classification in which tumours were classified as were embryonic tissues, according to the germ layer theory.

Perhaps the most famous of these attempts is that of Adami (1861–1926). He divided tumours into three great groups, those arising from ectoderm, those arising from endoderm, and those arising from mesoderm. Each group was subdivided further into tumours arising from cells lining surfaces, and those arising from pulp cells; and again into benign and malignant forms. Though logical on paper, this classification is most unsatisfactory in practice. A good classification groups like things together, and separates unlike things into different groups. In the embryological classification similar tumours are placed in different groups, and unlike tumours are grouped together. For example, squamous cell carcinoma of the mucosa of the lip is ectodermal, squamous cell carcinoma of the œsophagus is endodermal, and squamous cell carcinoma of the cervix uteri is mesodermal. These tumours are very similar morphologically and behave similarly, but under an embryological classification such as Adami's, they would be placed in different groups. Or conversely, carcinoma of the endometrium, osteogenic sarcoma, and myelogenous leukæmia are all malignant mesodermal tumours, and so would be grouped together in Adami's classification, but they are as different one from another as any three malignant tumours that might be chosen.

This method of classification is now of historical interest only. It is unsatisfactory in practice, and no longer has any theoretical justification.

6. Ætiological Classification.

The second of the bases of classification which have proved unsatisfactory was supported by MacCallum (1874–1944), who claimed in his textbook of pathology that the only satisfactory classification of tumours would be one based on ætiological considerations. He regretted that our knowledge of the ætiology of tumours was too little to permit such a classification. Though this view seems at first sight to be reasonable, an ætiological classification of tumours would not be satisfactory either. Once again, like tumours would be placed in different groups, and unlike tumours would be grouped together. This is because different ætiological agents can cause the same kind of tumour, and the same agent can cause different kinds of tumour. For example, in animals squamous cell carcinoma of the skin can be induced by chemical carcinogens, ionising radiation, and viruses, and so in an ætiological classification would have to be classified in at least these three different groups. Or again, in man ionising radiation can produce, or contribute to the production of squamous cell carcinoma of the skin, carcinoma of the thyroid, myelogenous leukæmia, osteogenic sarcoma, and other types of tumour. In an ætiological classification these diverse types of tumour would have to be grouped together.

But if ætiological considerations cannot provide a good basis for the classification of tumours, the importance of discovering more of the ætiology of tumours can scarcely be overstated. Further knowledge of their ætiology would not only add to our understanding of neoplasia, but would be of great value in the prevention of tumours, and might be of use in their treatment.

The Classification

Table I shows a simple classification of the usual type. As can be seen, the classification divides the tumours according to their tissue of origin into the six groups already listed. Each group is then subdivided into benign and malignant forms. To these names, one must add terms indicating the site of the particular tumour under consideration, and usually descriptive terms which make clearer its nature.

Such a classification is, of course, only a skeleton. A large number of different tumours have been isolated, each with its own morphological features, and its own peculiarities of behaviour. The study of these various tumours forms part of special pathology, but it will be easy to fit them into the simple classification given, complicating and enriching it as seems necessary.

Terminology

As it appears in the classification given in Table I, the terminology is relatively simple and consistent. Most of the names end in "-oma", an ending that usually, but not always, implies a neoplasm. There are a few names ending in "-oma" still in use to designate non-neoplastic lesions which in some way resemble neoplasms. For example, a tumour-like tuberculous abscess is often called a tuberculoma. Such terms arose before the distinction between neoplastic and non-neoplastic lesions was drawn as clearly as it is today. It is perhaps interesting to note in this context that as late as 1860 Virchow (1821–1902) in his book *Cellular Pathology* still discussed tuberculous lesions together with what we now consider true neoplasms.

A benign tumour of epithelial tissue is called a papilloma or an adenoma, a malignant one is called a carcinoma. Benign tumours of connective tissue have names made by joining the Greek term designating the type of connective tissue involved to the ending "-oma", and malignant tumours of connective tissue have names made by joining the appropriate Greek term to the ending "-sarcoma". For example, the Greek for cartilage is chondros, and so a benign tumour of cartilage is called a chondroma, and a malignant one is called a chondrosarcoma. The term sarcoma can also be used alone to designate a malignant tumour of connective tissue without specifying the particular type. The terminology of the other groups of tumour is less logical, but it will be noted that in them there is a tendency to use names ending in "-sarcoma" to designate malignant tumours.

A few malignant tumours have names ending in "-blastoma". This implies that they have arisen from embryonic tissue or are made up of embryonic cells. Such names can be used properly to designate tumours which arise in the embryo, and so do really take origin from embryonic or "blast" cells. The neuroblastoma,

22/Table I

A Simple Classification of Tumours

Tissue of Origin	*Benign*	*Malignant*
Group 1. Epithelial tumours		
Surface epithelium	papilloma	carcinoma
Glandular epithelium	adenoma	carcinoma
Group 2. Connective tissue tumours		
Fibrous tissue	fibroma	fibrosarcoma
Cartilage	chondroma	chondrosarcoma
Bone	osteoma	osteogenic sarcoma
Fat	lipoma	liposarcoma
Blood vessels	hæmangioma	hæmangiosarcoma
Lymph vessels	lymphangioma	lymphangiosarcoma
Smooth muscle	leiomyoma	leiomyosarcoma
Striped muscle	rhabdomyoma	rhabdomyosarcoma
Group 3. Hæmopoietic tumours		
Lympho-recticular tissues		Malignant lymphoma
		follicular lymphoma
		lymphosarcoma
		reticulum cell sarcoma
		Hodgkin's disease
		Lymphatic leukæmia
		Monocytic leukæmia
		Histocytosis "X"
		Reticulosis
Bone marrow		Myeloid leukæmia
		Polycythæmia vera
Plasma cells		Multiple myeloma
Group 4. Nervous tumours		
Glial tissue		glioma
Meninges	meningioma	meningeal sarcoma
Peripheral nerve cells	ganglioneuroma	neuroblastoma
Retina		retinoblastoma
Adrenal medulla	phæochromocytoma	
Schwann cells	Schwannoma	malignant Schwannoma
Group 5. Tumours of more than one tissue		
Breast	fibroadenoma	cystosarcoma phylodes
Embryonic kidney		Wilms' tumour
Multipotent cells	teratoma	teratoma
Group 6. Tumours which do not fit easily into one of the other groups		
Melanoblasts	pigmented nævus	malignant melanoma
Placenta	hydatidaform mole	chorionepithelioma
Ovary	cystadenoma	cystadenocarcinoma
	granulosa cell tumour	granulosa cell tumour
	fibroma	
	Brenner tumour	
		carcinoma
		arrhenoblastoma
Testis	interstitial cell tumour	
		seminoma
		embryonic carcinoma
Thymus	thymoma	thymoma

for example, usually arises from embryonic neuroblasts before or very soon after birth. Unfortunately, however, certain tumours which arise in the adult also have names ending in "-blastoma". These names were introduced when it was believed that all tumours arose from embryonic cells or from cells which had reverted towards the embryonic state. The ending "-blastoma" was reserved for malignant tumours because it was thought that they were nearer to the embryonal state than were benign tumours. With the abandonment of this theory, names ending in "-blastoma" are no longer appropriate for tumours which arise in the adult, and should be reserved for those which arise during embryonic life.

As more knowledge of tumours is gained, and as the simple classification given is enriched and complicated, a great many tumours will be found to have illogical, and even misleading names. Also, it will be found that different authorities sometimes use different names to designate the same tumour, and, what is even worse, make up new names that are more congruent with some favourite theory. However, if the simple classification given here is understood clearly, there need be no confusion.

The terminology will be considered in more detail as the morphology and behaviour of the various groups of tumours are discussed.

THE STRUCTURE OF TUMOURS

The Stroma

As seen grossly, tumours form a lump. This lump is made up of tumour cells, together with the material, if any, that they produce, and the stroma which supports and nourishes them. One can think of a tumour as being something like a sponge. The solid parts of the sponge represent the stroma, while the holes should be thought of as filled with the tumour cells and the material that they produce.

The stroma is not neoplastic, but is provided by the normal tissues of the host. As the tumour cells multiply they stimulate the connective tissue of the host to proliferate, so that the connective tissue of the host forms new vessels and new collagenous tissue around and between clumps of tumour cells. As the tumour grows, more connective tissue is produced by the host, so that the stroma grows with the tumour. In some tumours the stroma makes up a large part of the tumour mass, in others, it is sparse. But even when it makes up the greater part of the tumour mass, the stroma is not neoplastic. It is a reaction to the tumour, and not truly part of it.

The stroma consists of vascular connective tissue. If extensive, it may be made of coarse, or even sclerotic collagenous tissue, with few vessels. If delicate, it may consist of little but blood vessels supported by a minimal quantity of collagenous tissue. Often, it is something in between. It may contain elastic fibres or mast cells. It may even develop islands of bone or cartilage, presumably by metaplasia. Occasionally it may incorporate pre-existing nerves, but it has not been established that new nerve fibres grow into the tumour mass. It very rarely, if ever, contains lymphatics.

Sometimes the stroma is acutely or chronically inflamed. Usually the cause of the inflammation is obvious. If the tumour is ulcerated, it may be infected and the infection may give rise to inflammation. If the tumour is partially necrotic, the necrosis may cause an inflammatory response, though in many cases necrosis within a tumour causes no reaction whatsoever. Of more current interest is a different kind or reaction to tumours. Occasionally, lymphocytes accumulate at the margin of a tumour, as if in reaction to its growing edge. This kind of reaction is usual with primary malignant melanomata of the skin, but is uncommon with other tumours. Its significance is unknown. Because of the association between lymphocytes and the immunological defences of the body, some have thought it evidence of an attempt by the body to defend itself against the tumour by immunological means. Some tumours do contain abnormal antigens which might make such a defence possible, and it is interesting to note that the rare encephaloid carcinomata of the breast which are associated with a pronounced lymphocytic reaction do have a better prognosis than other carcinomata of the breast. On the other hand, the highly malignant anaplastic carinomata of the pharynx are also often associated with a marked lymphocytic reaction. Yet another type of association between lymphocytes and tumours is sometimes seen. In a few types of tumour, the whole of the stroma is filled with lymphocytes. Again, the explanation is unknown. The benign cystadenoma lymphomatosum papilliferum of the parotid gland is an example.

In some malignant tumours the invading tumour cells extend beyond the limits of the stroma, so that at the periphery of the tumour mass, columns of tumour cells lie among the pre-existing tissue elements, without stroma around them. In such cases, as the tumour enlarges, more stroma is formed, but always a little behind the growing edge of the tumour. In other malignant tumours, the stroma surrounds even the most peripheral tumour cells.

One of the principal functions of the stroma is to provide a blood supply within the tumour mass. Tumour cells, like the other cells of the body, need oxygen and the nutrient substances derived from the blood, and need some means by which their excretory products may be carried away. These needs are met by the stroma. As the blood vessels of the stroma course through the tumour mass, they carry oxygen and nutrition to the tumour cells, and carry away their waste products. If it were not for the stromal vessels which penetrate into the tumour mass, the tumour could not form a large lump. The tumour cells in the centre of the lump would become so far removed from the nearest blood vessels that they would die from lack of oxygen and nutrition, or from poisoning by their own metabolites. Occasionally one does see a tumour which fails to induce the host tissues to form a suitable stroma for it, and does find that it tends to form large masses of tumour cells which become necrotic in the centre, even though they continue to grow at the periphery. Sometimes a tumour will supplement or replace the stroma by making use of pre-existing structures. For example, occasional tumours in the lung grow round the alveoli, using the alveolar walls in place of stroma.

In those tumours which have a considerable quantity of stroma, the stroma serves also to give the tumour mass mechanical strength and rigidity. It serves as a framework, or skeleton, for the tumour. This function of the stroma is best seen in epithelial tumours, particularly malignant ones, which often have a massive stroma. In such cases, it is the stroma which determines the texture of the tumour. A carcinoma is classically described as being stony hard, and this hardness is due to the stroma. A tumour which is made up mainly of tumour cells is soft, with a texture not unlike that of normal brain.

Material Produced by the Tumour Cells

In some kinds of tumour, the tumour cells secrete or induce the formation of extracellular material. For example, in tumours of cartilage the tumour cells lay down an extracellular cartilagenous matrix. This is well formed in the benign chondromata, so that the tumour is histologically similar to normal cartilage, but usually ill-formed and myxomatous in the malignant chondrosarcomata. Some kinds of tumour produce considerable quantities of extracellular material of this kind, others little or none. In general, benign connective tissue tumours produce the kind and quantity of extracellular tissue that would be expected. Chondromata lay down cartilage; fibromata form collagen fibres and the intercellular material associated with them; osteomata make bone. Connective tissue tumours material also have little extracellular material. There is little between the muscle cells in normal smooth muscle, and little between the neoplastic muscle cells in a leiomyoma. In malignant connective tissue tumours, the extracellular material produced by the tumour cells is usually abnormal. It may be excessive in quantity or scant, and tends to be ill-formed and often myxoid. Epithelial tumours also may produce extracellular material. Adenomata of the thyroid, for instance, often secrete colloid into their acini. Occasionally, a carcinoma which secretes mucus releases the mucoid material into its stroma, giving the tumour a curious, slimy, myxoid appearance. Such tumours are sometimes called "colloid carcinomata". Other epithelial tumours form keratin. The keratin tends to appear in the middle of a clump of tumour cells, and to form a small whorled nodule called a "keratin pearl". Hæmatopoietic tumours rarely produce extracellular material, though some reticulum cell sarcomata do lay down reticulum fibres between the tumour cells, and fibrosis is often a striking feature of Hodgkin's disease.

This extracellular material produced by the tumour cells should not be confused with the stroma of the tumour. The extracellular material produced by the tumour cells is a product of the neoplasm; the stroma is produced by the normal tissues of the host in response to the neoplasm.

The Arrangement of the Tumour Cells

The tumour cells tend to be arranged differently in different kinds of tumour. In epithelial tumours they are usually arranged in one way, in connective tissue tumours in another, and in hæmopoietic tumours in a third.

In epithelial tumours, the tumour cells tend to form sheets or clumps. If the neoplastic epithelium covers a surface, it forms sheets or fronds which are supported by an underlying stroma. If it is within a tumour mass, it forms clumps, columns or acini which are surrounded by the stroma. But whatever the arrangement of the neoplastic epithelium, each epithelial tumour cell is fastened directly to the next, just as each normal epithelial cell is fastened directly to the next. The stroma between the groups of neoplastic cells may be small in quantity, but often is of considerable bulk, making up much of the tumour mass.

In connective tissue tumours it is different. Instead of being grouped into clumps in which each tumour cell is in contact with the next, the tumour cells lie singly, each separated from the next by the intercellular substance they themselves have produced. In a fibroma, for example, each tumour cell is separated from the next by the bands of collagen which the tumour cells have produced. In connective tissue tumours the stroma is sparse, consisting of little but blood vessels and a little fibrous tissue around them. The intercellular substance produced by the tumour cells serves to give the tumour the mechanical strength which is provided by the stroma in epithelial tumours.

In hæmopoietic tumours it is different again. The tumour cells form groups, but instead of being fastened together, as are the cells of epithelial tumours, or separated by the intercellular substance they produce, as are the cells of connective tissue tumours, the cells of hæmopoietic tumours are closely packed, but remain discrete. They are clumped together, but not joined together. The stroma is again sparse, consisting of little but blood vessels which run through the masses of hæmopoietic cells. As would be expected, such cellular tumours which have neither an extensive stroma nor produce large quantities of intercellular substance form a soft, homogeneous tissue.

The other major groups of tumours listed in the classification have no such typical patterns. Some of the tumours more or less resemble epithelial tumours; some are like connective tissue tumours; a few are similar to hæmopoietic tumours; and occasionally one has some other structure.

The Effect of Anaplasia on Structure

Anaplasia may be defined as a variation from normal structure or behaviour. The term is usually restricted to the kind of abnormality seen in neoplasms, but is occasionally used to describe other kinds of variation from normal. The more anaplastic a tumour, the more it varies from the normal, and from what are considered well-differentiated examples of that particular kind of tumour. Tumours show all degrees of anaplasia. Benign tumours usually resemble closely the tissue from which they arise. Malignant tumours are more bizarre, and much more variable, but in most cases still bear sufficient resemblance to their parent tissue to permit their identification. Only in the rare highly anaplastic tumours is this resemblance lost completely.

Tumours which show little anaplasia are often described as "well differentiated" or "highly differentiated", and anaplastic tumours are commonly called "poorly differentiated" or "ill differentiated", and sometimes "undifferentiated" or "dedifferentiated". These terms are too firmly embedded in usage to be avoided, but unfortunately imply a theory of neoplasia which is unlikely to be true. Differentiation is a term used to describe the changes which occur as primitive cells develop into more specialized forms, gaining new structure and new functions, but losing some of the potential they once had. To call an anaplastic tumour cell undifferentiated, or dedifferentiated, is to suggest that it is similar to the primitive precursors of that type of cell, either because it arose from a primitive cell and failed to differentiate or because it arose from an adult cell and regressed towards a more primitive form. Neither suggestion is justified. In all probability, the great majority of neoplasms arise from normal, fully differentiated adult cells. When such normal cells become neoplastic, they do not revert towards the primitive precursors from which they arose, though they may regain some of the characters of primitive cells. Instead, they develop new and different properties, new and different functions, new and different characters. To take only a gross example, the ability to invade and metastasise which is so prominent a property of the cells of a bronchogenic carcinoma is a new character, not shared by the cells of normal bronchial epithelium at any time during their differentiation. Tumour cells are not less differentiated than normal cells. They have suffered a further and aberrant differentiation. They are not poorly differentiated, they are wrongly differentiated.

Anaplasia is of different types. Most tumours show a marked degree of what may be called organ anaplasia. The tumour cells are not arranged so as to form an organ of the type formed by the normal cells of the tissue from which the tumour arises. Instead, they usually form an abnormal structure which is usually useless functionally. For instance, a tumour of the smooth muscle of the stomach does not form sheets of muscle which surround the viscus as does the normal smooth muscle of the stomach, but instead makes a more or less spherical mass in which the muscle fibres form intertwining bundles, to give an "organ" which is abnormal structurally and useless functionally. Similarly, a carcinoma of the colon does not form an epithelial layer to line a portion of gut, but grows as a mass in which the neoplastic epithelium lines glandular spaces within the mass, again giving an abnormal "organ". This crude kind of anaplasia is present in the great majority of tumours, benign or malignant.

A more subtle form of anaplasia is also seen. Not only does the tumour form an abnormal "organ", but the relationship of the tumour cells one to another may be abnormal. For example, in a basal cell carcinoma of the skin, the orderly sequence from basal cell to prickle cell and keratinized cell seen in normal epidermis is lost. Instead, the clumps of tumour cells show a peripheral palisade of basal cells enclosing a disorderly confusion of similar cells, arranged at random without the relationship to the basement membrane seen in normal epithelium. Keratinization is usually absent, or if it does occur is seen only in occasional foci, where sudden keratinization occurs to give small keratin pearls. A similar kind of structural anaplasia may be seen in connective tissue tumours, where again the tumour may not only form an abnormal "organ", but may show gross or slight abnormalities in the relationship between the tumour cells. They may be separated by too little or too much extracellular material, and particularly in malignant tumours may be separated by abnormal extracellular material.

Anaplasia may also be evident in the tumour cells themselves. They may differ from the cells of their tissue of origin in many ways. They may be too big or too small. They may have an abnormal shape. The ratio between the volume of the nucleus and the volume of the cytoplasm is often increased. Their cytoplasm may not show features present in the cytoplasm of normal cells of the same type, or may show features that the normal cells do not. Similarly, the nuclei of tumour cells are often abnormal. They are commonly bigger than those of the normal cells of the same type, and often contain abnormal quantities of chromatin, abnormal numbers of chromosomes, irregularly disposed chromatin, prominent nucleoli, or any of a great many other abnormalities. In general, benign tumours show little cellular anaplasia. Indeed, the individual tumour cells are often indistinguishable from normal, and the diagnosis depends on the "organ" anaplasia. The naked eye may be of more help in diagnosis than is the microscope. In malignant tumours, the more marked the cellular anaplasia the more likely the tumour is to invade extensively and quickly, and the more likely it is to metastasise widely and rapidly. The degree of cellular anaplasia is thus a good guide to the future behaviour of the tumour. It should, of course, be considered together with all other information that can be obtained, and in particular with our experience with other tumours of the same type.

Tumours also show functional anaplasia. In most cases, the deviation from normal is manifested by a failure to function. For instance, tumours of muscle do not contract, and most carcinomata of the thyroid do not secrete hormone. Rarely the opposite occurs. A tumour functions excessively and without regard to the needs of the body. Overaction of this kind is particularly important in some of the benign tumours of the endocrine glands. The oversecretion may be far more important and far more dangerous than the tumour itself. For example, some phæochromocytomata of the adrenal medulla secrete excessive quantities of catecholamines, continuously or intermittently, causing serious systemic hypertension. Some adenomata of the parathyroid gland secrete excessively causing a complicated syndrome classically including hypercalcæmia, hypophosphatæmia, lytic lesions in the bone, calcification of the kidneys, and many other lesions. Even less commonly a tumour may produce an abnormal secretion. A few carinomata of the lung have given rise to a syndrome similar to that of hyperparathyroidism, perhaps by secreting an agent similar to parathormone. Rare tumours of the retroperitoneum or mediastinum which seem to be well differentiated fibrosarcomata have caused a syndrome similar to hyperinsulinism, presumably by secreting some agent. Less clear is the relationship between certain tumours, particularly carcinoma of the lung, and a peripheral neuropathy which develops in a small proportion of cases. These overactions are important and dangerous, but should not obscure the fact that the vast majority of tumours do not secrete hormones or any other substance which acts at a distance. Most damage the body only by growing and taking up space.

Pleomorphism is closely related to anaplasia. It is defined as a variation in structure from one part of a tumour to another. Like anaplasia, pleomorphism may be divided into various types. Sometimes pleomorphism can be appreciated with the naked eye, one part of a tumour having one appearance, another a different appearance. For example, carcinoma of the kidney is usually markedly pleomorphic to the naked eye, a section of the tumour showing one part to be firm and white, another bright yellow, and a third soft, red, and hæmorrhagic. In other cases, a tumour may show itself pleomorphic when viewed with a low power of the microscope. In one part there may be much stroma, in another little; or in one part the tumour cells may be arranged in one manner, and another part in some different manner. In some carcinomata, for example, one finds that in some areas the tumour cells form glandular spaces, while in other areas they make solid masses of tumour cells. Or again, pleomorphism may be evident in the tumour cells themselves, one being different to the next. One cell may be big, the next small; one may have one huge nucleus, the next two small ones; almost any sort of variation is possible. In general, the degree of pleomorphism correlates well with the degree of anaplasia, and, indeed, pleomorphism can be considered a form of anaplasia.

The more anaplastic a tumour, the more difficult it will be to determine its origin histologically. The features which distinguish between epithelial tumours, connective tissue tumours and hæmopoietic tumours are lost. All highly anaplastic tumours look alike histologically and macroscopically. They form soft, ill-defined masses which are highly cellular, with bizarre, pleomorphic cells, little stroma, and no evidence of an attempt to produce a recognisable product. Necrosis and hæmorrhage are common. Such highly anaplastic tumours are rare. Usually an area which permits diagnosis can be found. In most cases, however, the identification of the origin of such a tumour is only of academic interest. The tumour will kill the patient within a few months. Of course, all intermediate forms exist between the most anaplastic tumour and the most high differentiated.

The Shape of Tumours

Tumours may be of many shapes. Those arising from a surface epithelium or from the connective tissue close beneath it may form plaques or nodules and show themselves as a thickening in the surface or be felt as an induration beneath it. Other tumours arising from a surface project above it. If such a tumour forms a bulbous mass which is joined to the surface by a relatively narrow stalk, it is sometimes called a polyp, or is said to be polypoid. Not all polyps are neoplastic. Sometimes inflamed or œdematous mucosa will give rise to a polypoid excrescence. The common polyps which occur in the nose are an example in point. Other tumours arising from a surface form fronds which stand above the surface. Such tumours are often called papillary. Similarly, tumours in which fronds project into glandular spaces may be called papillary. If a tumour forms a large mass which stands above a surface, it is said to be fungating. Yet other tumours of a surface form ulcers, and not uncommonly a papillary or a fungating tumour becomes secondarily ulcerated.

Tumours which grow in a solid organ or tissue tend to be spherical, though often distorted by the pressure of fascial planes or other structures which are not easily deformed. Such tumours may be completely separated from the surrounding tissue by a collagenous capsule, in which case they are said to encapsulated, or may appear well demarcated or delimited, distinct from the surrounding tissue even though they do not have a capsule. Other tumours are poorly defined, extending vaguely out into the surrounding tissue, so that with the naked eye it is impossible to be sure just where the tumour ends. Sometimes a tumour which seems well demarcated to the naked eye, proves on microscopical examination to have long projections, which run through the surrounding tissue beyond the apparent limit of the tumour, but which are not large enough or numerous enough to alter the gross appearance of the involved tissue.

If a tumour of a surface extends into the underlying tissue, as they often do, its appearance in the deeper tissues is similar to that of the tumours arising within a solid organ or tissue. A surface tumour invading deeper structures will rarely appear encapsulated, but it may be well defined, or may merge vaguely with the surrounding structures.

THE MORPHOLOGY AND BEHAVIOUR OF THE VARIOUS TYPES OF TUMOUR

In a short chapter such as this, it is not possible to consider even in outline the morphology and behaviour of even the more important and common tumours. Large books have been filled with descriptions of the morphology and behaviour of tumours. Among the more important of these works in English are the *Pathology of Tumours* by Willis, and the profusely illustrated Fascicles on tumour pathology being issued by the Armed Forces Institute of Pathology of the United States of America. In this chapter, a few examples will be chosen to show the usual structure and behaviour of the various types of tumour. This will serve as a basis which can be elaborated and modified by subsequent study.

It should be emphasised that the behaviour of the various kinds of tumour should be studied. Their habit of local growth, and their manner and rate of metastasis, are at least as important as their morphology. It is little use recognising a tumour, if you do not know what it is likely to do.

1. Tumours of Epithelial Tissue

Benign

Benign tumours of epithelium are common. Those arising from the epidermis or the epithelium of the body's tubes are called papillomata; those arising from endocrine or exocrine glands are called adenomata.

Papilloma

Papillomata may form a focal thickening in the epithelium which stands above the surface as a well-defined plaque, or may form a structure sometimes called a true papilloma, in which fronds of neoplastic epithelium supported by a connective tissue stroma project above the surface somewhat after the manner of a fern, or the head of a palm tree.

Two of the more common types of benign epithelial tumour arise in the skin, often the skin of the face, and usually in older people, though they may occur at any age. Both form plaque-like lesions. Both have special names which have become established by long usage. One, usually called a seborrhœic keratosis, is made of a proliferation of the basal cells of the epidermis, and is often markedly pigmented and markedly hyperkeratotic, so that it appears as a black, greasy lesion. This type of tumour is quite benign, and can be thought of as a benign relative of the basal cell carcinoma, indeed being occasionally

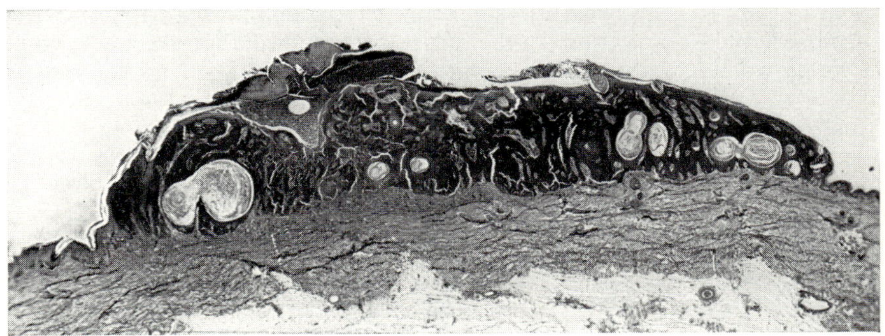

22/Fig. 1.—Seborrhœic keratosis of the skin. The plaque-like tumour stands above the surface of the skin.

called a basal cell papilloma (FIG. 1). The other is usually called a senile keratosis, though it often occurs on patients who are by no means senile. It, too, forms a local lesion, but tends to appear more warty, and when examined microscopically is seen to be made up of a proliferation of epidermal cells which show a relatively normal pattern of differentiation, with basal cells giving way to prickle cells and to keratinised cells as in normal epidermis. In this type of lesion, however, there is often some disorder and atypicality of the basal cells, and though the lesion is benign, it sometimes gives rise to a squamous cell carcinoma. It is, therefore, more dangerous than the seborrhoeic keratosis.

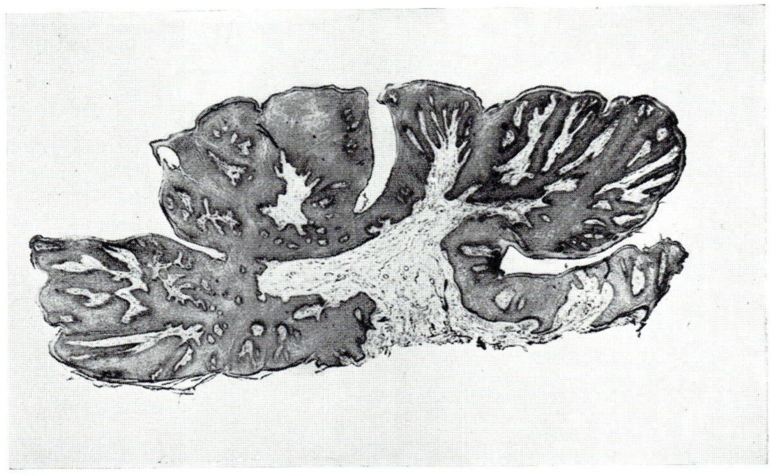

22/FIG. 2.—Squamous cell papilloma of the skin. The short fronds are covered by neoplastic squamous epithelium.

True papillomata may be simple, with a few, short, thick fronds, or complicated with many delicate branches (FIG. 2). Simple papillomata with stratified squamous epithelium may arise in the mouth, larynx, or elsewhere, but only rarely do they give rise to malignancy. More complicated papillomata may arise in the breast or rectum. In the breast, for instance, they are most common in young women, and often occur in the large ducts near the nipple. They may have a simple structure, but more often appear cribriform on section, with fronds which branch and rejoin. These soft lesions can rarely be felt, but often give rise to bleeding from the nipple. It is easy to understand how the delicate fronds of such a papilloma might be damaged and cause bleeding.

Adenoma

Adenomata are common in the endocrine glands, where, unless distorted by some external pressure, they tend to be spherical, and are often encapsulated. They are made up of well differentiated glandular tissue, usually with a scanty stroma. The glandular tissue nearly always forms structures reminiscent of the tissue of origin. Adenomata of the thyroid, for instance, form acini which may contain colloid (FIG. 3); and adenomata of the islets of Langerhans form cords and clumps of cells which may contain the granules typical of the islets. Adenomata of endocrine glands are often multiple. There may be more than one in the same gland, or adenomata in more than one gland. They may or may not secrete hormone. If they do, they may do so in physiological quantities, or may secrete excessively. An adenoma of the beta cells of the islets of Langerhans, for example, may secrete excessive quantities of insulin, giving rise to hypoglycæmia,

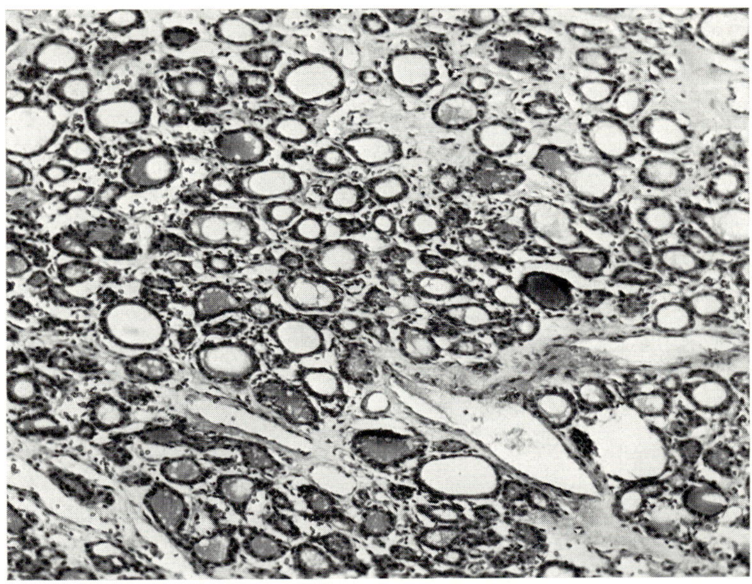

22/FIG. 3.—Adenoma of the thyroid. The tumour is made of well-formed acini, some of which contain colloid.

or an adenoma of the pituitary gland secrete excessive quantities of growth hormone, giving rise to gigantism or acromegaly. The adenomata of endocrine glands have not been shown clearly to become malignant in man, but some of them do show evidence of limited invasion. The islet cell adenomata are a case in point.

Adenomata may also arise from exocrine glands. Many different kinds occur in the skin, and have been given long and curious names. They are also common in the salivary glands, both major and minor. Again, there are many different kinds. The most common is the mixed tumour, so called because it contains a curious mixture of epithelial and stromal elements, and because it was once thought that both its epithelium and stroma were neoplastic. It is now accepted that only the epithelium is neoplastic, the changes in the stroma being secondary. Histologically the epithelium and stroma are sometimes hard to distinguish, the epithelium fraying into the stroma in a confusing manner. Another characteristic feature is the presence in the stroma of deposits that closely resemble cartilage. Many mixed tumours behave as benign tumours should, growing slowly, remaining well differentiated, and being curable by excision. Many are rather more active. They grow slowly and remain well differentiated, but recur if not widely removed. A few are even more active. They grow more rapidly, become more anaplastic, and may metastasise. This serves to emphasise again that there is no clear distinction between benign and malignant tumours. All forms occur, from the most benign to the most malignant. The mixed tumours of the salivary glands are usually considered benign tumours which occasionally become malignant. It would be equally logical to consider them malignant tumours which by good fortune are often removed before they have metastasised or invaded beyond the line of resection.

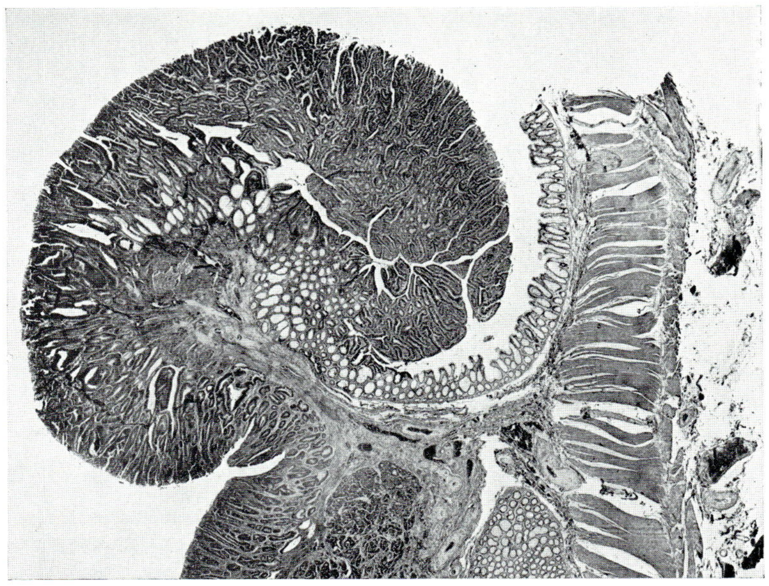

22/FIG. 4.—Adenomatous polyp of the colon. One frond of the polyp is shown. A second passes out at the lower edge of the picture. Normal mucosa can be seen lining the upper side of the stalk.

One other type of benign epithelial tumour must be mentioned. Polypoid tumours of the colon and rectum are common. They are usually found in patients of 50 or more years of age, and become increasingly common with increasing years. Very often they are multiple, and even if only one or two are present when a patient is first examined, others may appear subsequently. These tumours are usually called adenomatous polyps. They have something of the structure of a papilloma, something of the structure of an adenoma. The tumour itself typically forms a small ball which hangs from the wall of the bowel by a stalk covered by normal epithelium (FIG. 4). Less commonly it forms a sessile plaque in the mucosa. The tumour is made of one or more broad fronds covered by neoplastic epithelium, and set closely together so that the surface of the tumour appears evenly granular. Within these broad fronds one finds acinar spaces also lined by neoplastic epithelium. The importance of these common tumours is that most believe that they may turn malignant, giving rise to a carcinoma of the colon or rectum. This view has been challenged recently, and it is certain that not more than a small proportion of polyps become malignant, but many think the risk sufficient to justify the removal of adenomatous polyps of the large intestine whenever practicable.

Malignant

Malignant tumours of the epithelial tissues are called carcinomata. They make up the great bulk of the malignant tumours seen in practice. Most patients dying of cancer, die of carcinoma. Any epithelium can give rise to a carcinoma. They are common in the skin, the oral cavity and pharynx, and in the œsophagus and stomach. They are rare in the small bowel, but very common in the colon and rectum. They are also common in the larynx and bronchi, particularly in men, and may arise in the kidney, renal pelvis or bladder. If one excludes the ovary and testis, which will be considered among the special tumours of Group 6, they are not common in endocrine glands, except the thyroid, but often occur in the exocrine pancreas and in the prostate. Carcinoma of the endometrium and cervix uteri are both common, and, in women, carcinoma of the breast is one of the most common of all carcinomata. The morphology and behaviour of these important tumours cannot be discussed in detail here, but some generalisations are possible.

Gross Appearance

As seen by the surgeon or pathologist, the gross appearance of the various types of carcinoma varies widely. Carcinomata of the skin usually form shallow ulcers, with raised, indurated edges. They are usually a centimetre or so across when the patient seeks medical advice. Similar ulcers may be formed by other carcinomata arising from a surface epithelium, particularly those of the alimentary tract. In the gut, the ulcers are often larger (FIG. 5). By the time the patient comes to surgery or to autopsy, they are often several centimetres across, and in the smaller tubes such as the œsophagus tend to become elongated in the long axis of the tube. Because of the scarring associated with the invasion and destruction of the wall of the tube, a stricture is likely to develop at the site of the carcinomatous ulcer, and together with the protrusion of the raised edges of the ulcer into the lumen, is likely to cause complete or partial obstruction. Cases of carcinoma of the œsophagus or colon, for example, often present with signs and symptoms of obstruction.

In other cases, the carcinomata arising from a lining epithelium project into the lumen, giving rise to a large polypoid tumour in which there may be little or no ulceration. Such tumours are seen in the large, easily distended cæcum. Another common site for papillary carcinomata is the urinary bladder, where the tumours have many very fine fronds. It is easy to understand how such ulcerated or fungating tumours could give rise to the small hæmorrhages often associated with carcinomata, and which explain at least in part the anæmia often found in patients with carcinoma.

Less commonly, a carcinoma of a surface epithelium causes little or no ulceration, and does not project above the surface, but instead infiltrates the

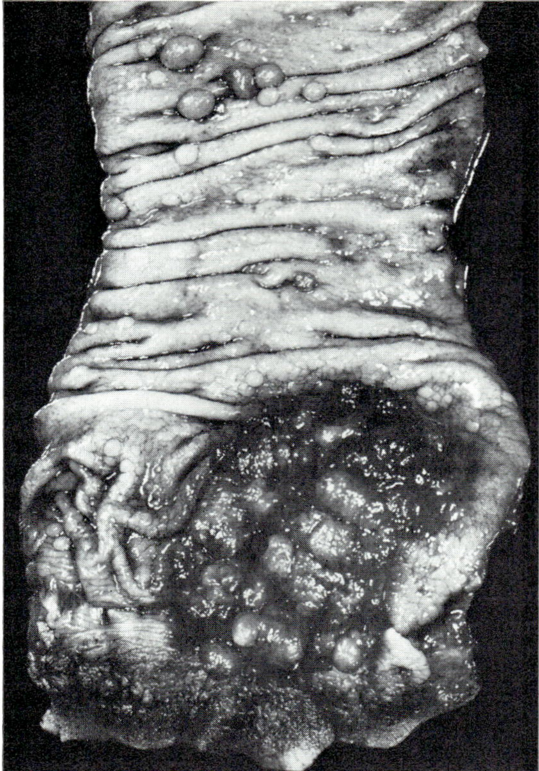

22/Fig. 5.—Adenocarcinoma of the rectum. The anal margin can be seen at lower edge of the specimen, with the partially polypoid, partially ulcerated carcinoma adjacent to it. Several adenomatous polyps can be seen in the upper part of the picture.

wall of the affected organ, thickening and replacing it by a hard mass of tumour. Such carcinomata are sometimes seen in the stomach, and are one of the commoner types of carcinoma of the bronchus.

Carcinomata arising within solid organs, from glandular cells or ducts, usually form an ill-defined mass. Carcinoma of the breast is the classical example. Here, in a typical case, the carcinoma forms an irregular mass some 2 or 3 centimetres across, which replaces the normal breast tissue (Fig. 6). The mass is hard and white, because of the dense fibrous stroma associated with the carcinoma, and extends into the surrounding tissue, giving off the processes which have been compared with the legs of a crab, a comparison that is more satisfactory in theory than when one examines an actual lesion. Because of this extension, the surrounding tissues are often puckered in towards the carcinoma. Other carcinomata occurring within organs are similar, being usually white and hard, though occasionally soft, and brown or reddish, the texture and colour depending mainly on the nature and quantity of the stroma. In some carcinomata, carcinoma of the kidney being the usual example, necrosis and hæmorrhage are common within the tumour. In such a case, the whitish viable tumour tissue will be intermixed with necrotic zones which are often yellow, and with dark red zones of hæmorrhage. Occasionally a carcinoma may appear to be well demarcated or even encapsulated. Carcinoma of the kidney is again the usual example.

If a carcinoma arising from a surface epithelium is sectioned, the cut surface will show the same features as do the carcinomata arising within organs, hard white tissue replacing and infiltrating the wall of the affected organ.

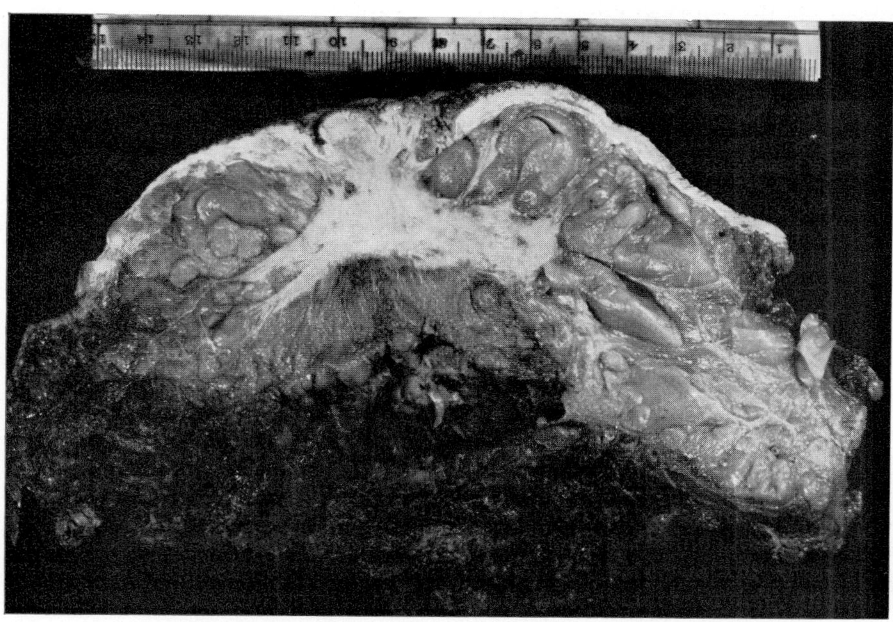

22/FIG. 6.—Carcinoma of the breast. The nipple is in the centre of the skin surface. Immediately below it is the carcinoma, which extends irregularly into the surrounding breast and has caused retraction of the nipple. The pectoral muscles can be seen in the lower part of the picture.

Microscopical Appearance

Microscopically, carcinomata may show many different kinds of structure, though within any single carcinoma the structure is usually similar throughout. However, as has been mentioned earlier, they do share with the benign tumours of epithelium one common feature which distinguishes them sharply from the tumours of connective tissue and of hæmopoietic tissue. In a carcinoma, the tumour cells form sheets or clumps in which the carcinoma cells are fastened one to the next. Neither the connective tissue tumours nor the hæmopoietic tumours form clumps of this sort. Carcinomata may be divided into types according to the microscopical appearance of the tumour cells and their arrangement.

One of the more common kinds of carcinoma is the squamous cell carcinoma, which may arise from any squamous epithelium, or by metaplasia as in the bronchus. In a well-differentiated example, the clumps of tumour cells seen microscopically show a differentiation which is distorted and atypical, but which preserves some similarity to the normal differentiation of squamous epithelium (FIG. 7). At the periphery of the clumps of carcinoma cells are basal cells, and as one moves towards the centre of the clump these tend to differentiate into prickle cells, and to show evidence of the formation of keratin, even, in well-differentiated tumours, giving rise to keratin "pearls", little balls of laminated keratin in the centre of a mass of tumour cells.

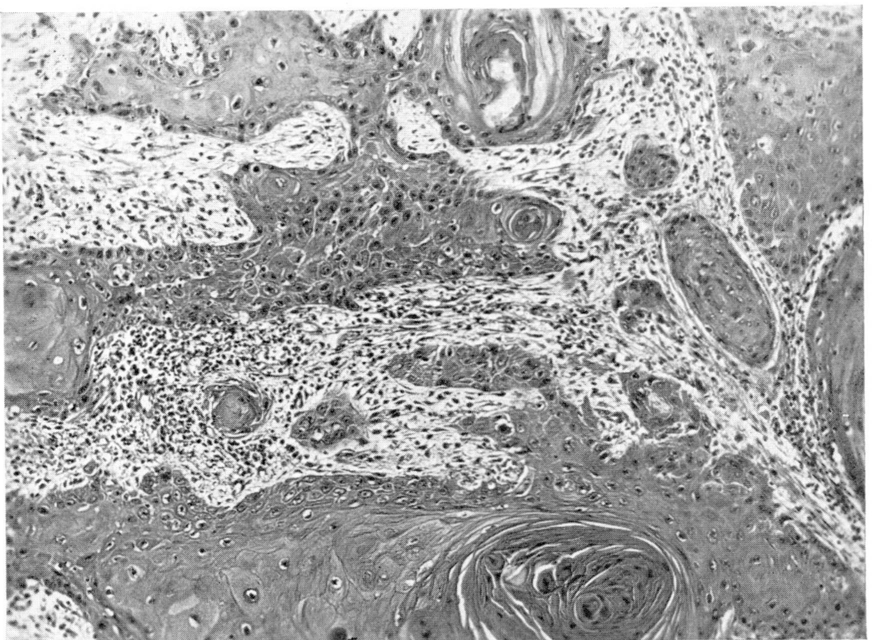

22/FIG. 7.—Squamous cell carcinoma. The clumps of carcinoma cells lie in a slightly inflamed stroma. Within each clump, the tumour cells are applied directly one to another. The carcinoma cells show differentiation into prickle cells, and the formation of keratin at the centre of some of the tumour masses.

In contrast, the basal cell carcinomata of the skin form clumps of tumour cells in which basal cells form a palisade around the periphery, but inside, instead of the differentiation seen in the squamous cell carcinomata, is a disorderly mass of basal cells showing no evidence of differentiation, though occasionally in these tumours, too, keratin pearls may be found.

The carcinomata arising from the transitional epithelium of the urinary system may form clumps in which the cells preserve their transitional features, or may give rise to papillary carcinomata such as those of the bladder, where the delicate fronds are covered by a typical transitional epithelium. Not uncommonly, carinomata of the bronchus form masses in which the tumour cells closely resemble those of the transitional cell carcinomata of the urinary bladder.

Carcinomata arising from glands, whether glands such as the pancreas or glands such as those of the stomach and colon, give rise to tumours in which the clumps of invading tumour cells usually form acini (FIG. 8). These acini do not reproduce the structure of their tissue of origin very well. The glands of the tumour often differ from those of their tissue of origin in size and arrangement, and are usually lined by cells which do not well reproduce the features of their cell of origin. In the prostate, for example, a common type of carcinoma is made of very small glands, which are closely packed, lined by pale cells, and which give no sign of the lobular arrangement of the normal prostate.

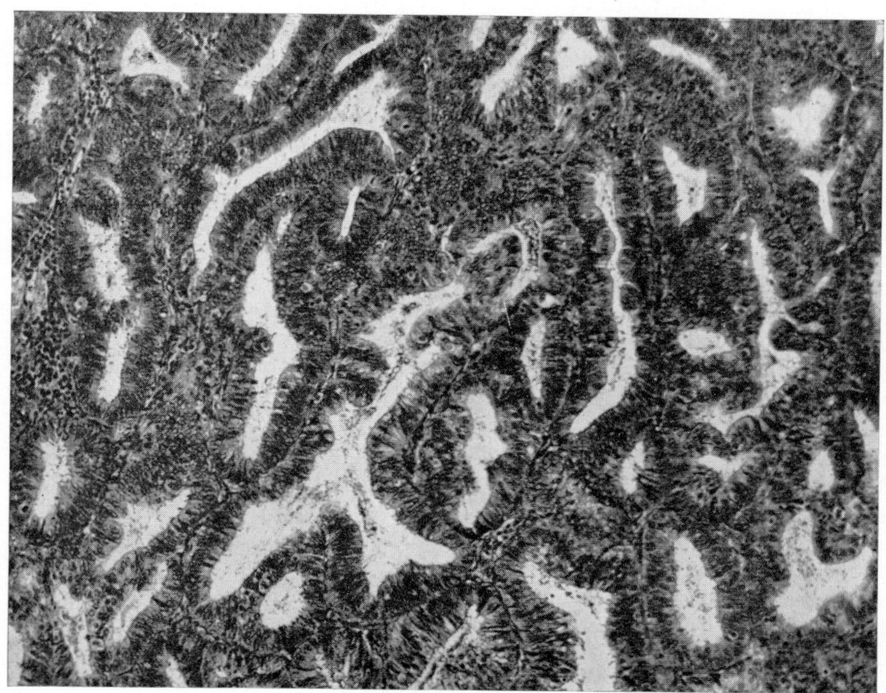

22/FIG. 8.—Adenocarcinoma of the endometrium. Irregular neoplastic glands are closely packed with little stroma.

Yet another arrangement of carcinoma cells is common in the breast. Here the clumps of carcinoma cells show little evidence of differentiation, forming clumps of fairly uniform cells which are all much alike. These clumps may be large or small. They may be any shape.

The microscopical appearance of a carcinoma is also affected by the quantity and texture of the stroma. Whatever may be the appearance and arrangement of the carcinoma cells themselves, the stroma may be so extensive that it makes up most of the tumour mass, or it may be scant, or may be anything between. It may be of coarse hyaline collagen, or fine and vascular, or anything between.

Finally, with all these types of carcinoma, in the more anaplastic examples, the clumps of tumour cells tend to become less and less clearly defined, and the tumour cells less and less obviously epithelial, until in a highly anaplastic carcinoma the microscopical appearance may become indistinguishable from that of any other highly anaplastic tumour. Masses of pleomorphic, highly atypical cells lie jumbled together with little attempt to form any recognisable structure.

Behaviour

Though there are considerable differences in the behaviour of different types of carcinomata, and in the behaviour of carcinomata arising at different sites, they all tend to show more or less the same pattern of invasion and metastasis. Some will invade quicker than others, some will extend further by local extension than others, some will metastasise earlier than others, some prefer one site for their metastases, some another. But, in general, all carcinomata grow first by local extension, invading the surrounding tissues and producing a local mass. In very many cases, fortunately, the tumour can be detected at this stage, while it is still readily curable by surgery. Sooner or later, however, the carcinoma cells will enter the lymphatics, and in nearly all cases the first metastases are to the regional lymph nodes, the lymph nodes which receive the lymph draining the tumour site. Here again, in many cases, there seems to be a delay. The regional nodes are involved, but further spread does not occur for some time. A surgical cure may be still possible, but a more radical operation will be needed. However, sooner or later, if the carcinoma has not been eradicated, further lymphatic spread will occur, and more distant nodes will be involved. The blockage of lymphatics may set up abnormal patterns of lymph flow, so that, for example, carcinoma cells may be carried in the lymph from the hilus of the lung out into its substance, giving rise to lymphogenous metastases throughout the lung. Moreover, sooner or later, blood-borne metastases will occur. In most carcinomata they occur late, but occasionally may occur early, as in some cases of carcinoma of the lung with cerebral metastases. As would be expected, hæmatogenous metastases are most common in the liver and lung, but may occur anywhere, the organs most commonly involved by secondaries being different for different kinds of carcinoma.

Carcinoma of the female breast can serve as an example of the way in which carcinomata behave. This tumour is often found quite early, the patient noticing a lump in her breast, though sometimes the mass is allowed to grow large before the patient seeks advice. On examination, a hard mass is felt in the breast. It may be fixed to the overlying skin or to the underlying muscle, if the extending carcinoma has invaded these structures. It may be associated with local lymphœdema, if the carcinoma has obstructed the lymphatics. The nipple may be retracted if one or more of the major ducts has been involved, the retraction of the collagenous tissue of the tumour's stroma pulling the ducts into the breast, and dragging the nipple after them. But more important than these local signs is the possibility of metastasis. In all probability, the first metastases will be to the regional lymph nodes. It is therefore most important to examine the axillary nodes carefully. Any enlarged nodes, and particularly any nodes which are enlarged and hard, would be most suspicious. If no evidence of more distant metastases can be found, most patients come to operation. Unfortunately, some will be found to have already metastases in the bone or lung, and so are inoperable. A common operation is radical mastectomy, in which the whole breast, the pectoral muscles and the content of the axilla are removed in one mass. In this way it is hoped that the carcinoma can be eradicated, the primary being removed together with the structures it may have invaded, and together with the lymphatics it may have permeated, and the nodes to which it may have metastasised. Unfortunately, this operation does not always succeed. Sometimes the carcinoma is already beyond the limits of the resection. It may recur locally, forming subcutaneous masses in the scar of the operation, or may extend from the site of operation subcutaneously, to form a progressive induration of the skin of the chest. Or it may show evidence of further lymphatic extension, involving nodes in the base of the neck or in the mediastinum, or appearing as a mass in the other breast. It may involve the lung by lymphatic permeation, or may cause a malignant pleural effusion. It may pass by the blood stream to set up metastases in the bones, in the liver, in the lung, in the brain, or elsewhere. And this whole process of extension and metastasis may occur rapidly, killing the patient in a few months, or may progress very slowly, taking many years. Some patients show one form of extension, others another. In some, evidence of recurrence appears soon after mastectomy; others may remain well for many years after operation, only to develop metastases in the bone, or elsewhere. But this gloomy list of possible means of extension should not obscure the fact that of patients who come to operation before the axillary nodes are involved and who are treated by radical mastectomy, 75 per cent survive more than 5 years, and even of those in which the nodes were involved at the time of operation, 45 per cent are still well after 5 years.

Terminology

The terminology of the tumours of epithelial tissues gives rise to few difficulties. When speaking of carcinomata, some sort of descriptive term is usually added to qualify or further describe the tumour. For example, one speaks of squamous cell carcinoma of the cervix uteri, or papillary transitional cell carcinoma of the urinary bladder, or follicular carcinoma of the thyroid. In the case of those carcinomata which form glands, the descriptive term is usually combined with the word carcinoma, and these tumours are called adenocarcinomata, as for example, adenocarcinoma of the stomach, or adenocarcinoma of the endometrium. If in an adenocarcinoma or an adenoma the glandular spaces formed by the tumour are very large, the tumour is sometimes called a cystadenocarcinoma, or a cystadenoma.

A few carcinomata have special names. A carcinoma of the liver is often called a hepatoma, and one form of carcinoma of the pharynx is sometimes called a lymphoepithelioma, but such special names are not common. The term epithelioma is sometimes used to describe epithelial tumours. In English this term is little used, and implies an epithelial tumour, without any clear indication whether it is benign or malignant. One sometimes hears, for example, of a basal cell epithelioma, when the speaker means basal cell carcinoma. Others use the term as synonymous with squamous cell carcinoma. It is perhaps worth noting that the word "épitheliome" in French, and the word "epitheliom" in German, should usually be translated into English as "carcinoma", not "epithelioma".

Special Cases

A few malignant epithelial tumours deserve special mention. In some organs, more than one kind of primary malignant epithelial tumour may arise. In the lung, for example, there are three fairly common kinds of primary epithelial tumour. The most common is the highly malignant bronchogenic carcinoma. This may occur in any part of the lung, is much more common in men than in women, is usually found in patients over 50, and is likely to metastasise early to the hilar lymph nodes or by the blood stream, often, unfortunately, before the tumour is discovered. To be contrasted with this is the adenoma of the bronchus, also a malignant tumour, but a much less dangerous one. The adenomata usually arise in the large bronchi, are equally common in men and women, are usually found in patients between 20 and 40, and grow slowly and metastasise slowly. At the time that these tumours come to surgery, only about 10 per cent have metastases, and these are usually confined to the hilar nodes. Even in cases with involved nodes, cure is likely, because the extension of this type of tumour is so slow that complete extirpation is still possible. It should be particularly noted that this malignant tumour is called an adenoma. This is because when first described it was thought to be benign. Further experience has shown that it is not so, and it would be logical to call the tumour an adenocarcinoma, if it were not that this term is already in use to describe one of the forms of the much more highly malignant bronchogenic carcinoma. The misleading name adenoma has, therefore, been retained. The third kind of primary epithelial malignancy arising in the lung is the tumour sometimes called an alveolar cell carcinoma, sometimes a bronchiolar carcinoma. This has patterns of growth which are different again, and gives rise to tumours which may differ greatly from the other two types both grossly and microscopically. It is of a degree of malignancy intermediate between the bronchogenic carcinoma and the bronchial adenoma. Other examples of organs in which more than one type of primary epithelial malignancy occur will be encountered. Fortunately, in most cases, descriptive terms of the usual type serve to distinguish the different forms of carcinoma.

Finally, there is a lesion which occurs in epithelium, usually in stratified epithelium, which is called carcinoma-in-situ, or intra-epidermoid carcinoma. It is common in the cervix uteri, and may occur elsewhere. In this lesion the normal stratified epithelium is replaced by a disorderly sheet of anaplastic epithelial cells. The lesion shows all the histological signs of malignancy, except that there is no invasion, the abnormality being confined to the epithelium. It can be seen that this lesion is not malignant in the usual sense of the word. There is no invasion, and so can be no metastases. However, it is usually considered an early form of carcinoma because it so closely resembles carcinoma microscopically, and because in some cases carcinoma-in-situ is known to have developed into an invasive carcinoma. It is interesting to note that often a primary invasive carcinoma is surrounded by an irregular zone in which the epithelium has been replaced by carcinoma cells, giving an appearance identical with that of carcinoma-in-situ. Whether this means that the carcinoma arose in an area of carcinoma-in-situ, or whether it means that the carcinoma invading outwards from its site of origin has replaced the pre-existing epithelium to imitate carcinoma-in-situ, or whether it means that a wide area of epithelium was undergoing a gradual change into carcinoma, is not known.

2. Tumours of Connective Tissue

Benign

Benign tumours of connective tissue are common, but are usually small, and are often overlooked. Leiomyomata, for example, are rarely found in the stomach either at operation or at autopsy, but in one series in which the stomach was examined particularly carefully small leiomyomata were demonstrated in 23 of 50 stomachs. Other types of benign tumour may be equally common. The benign tumours of connective tissue usually form well-defined masses, which tend to be spherical, unless distorted by some extrinsic pressure. They are made up of well-differentiated connective tissue cells of the appropriate type, separated by the intercellular structures the cells form. Their stroma usually consists of nothing but blood vessels, and a little perivascular fibrous tissue. They arise in the areas where they would be expected, leiomyomata arising from smooth muscle; lipomata arising from adipose tissue; chondromata in or near bones formed in cartilage; and so on. Not uncommonly, they are multiple. Particular attention has been paid to multiple hæmangiomata, and a number of syndromes have been given special names. The benign tumours of connective tissue are unlikely to harm the patient unless they are unusually large, or occur in some critical spot where the tumour compresses some important structure.

Of the benign connective tissue tumours of clinical importance, two of the more common are the leiomyomata of the uterus, and the benign connective tissue tumours of the skin. The uterine leiomyomata, often called "fibroids", are common after the age of 40. They are often multiple, and may grow to a large size, sometimes necessitating hysterectomy because of their size and weight, or because they cause irregularities in the cyclic changes of the endometrium (Fig. 9). The connective tissue tumours of the skin can be found by the patient, and so often come to be removed. Unlike the typical benign connective tissue tumour, they are not well delimited, but mix intimately with the surrounding dermis, often having processes which extend well beyond the apparent edge of the tumour. Histologically, they are usually dermatofibromata, made of plump fibrocytes separated by bundles of collagen, or hæmangiomata with large or small blood vessels admixed with a variable quantity of collagenous tissue.

Just as there is no sharp division between benign and malignant tumours, so there is no sharp division between true benign tumours and congenital malformations. It is usual to consider hæmangiomata, for example, as neoplasms, but there can be little doubt that in most cases they are really malformations. This is obvious enough if one considers the form of hæmangioma called a port-wine mark. This is present at birth, grows with the part on which it is, and stops growing when that part stops growing. This is the behaviour of a malformation, not of a true tumour. On the other hand, there is no doubt that some benign tumours, as, for example, the leiomyomata of the uterus, are true neoplasms.

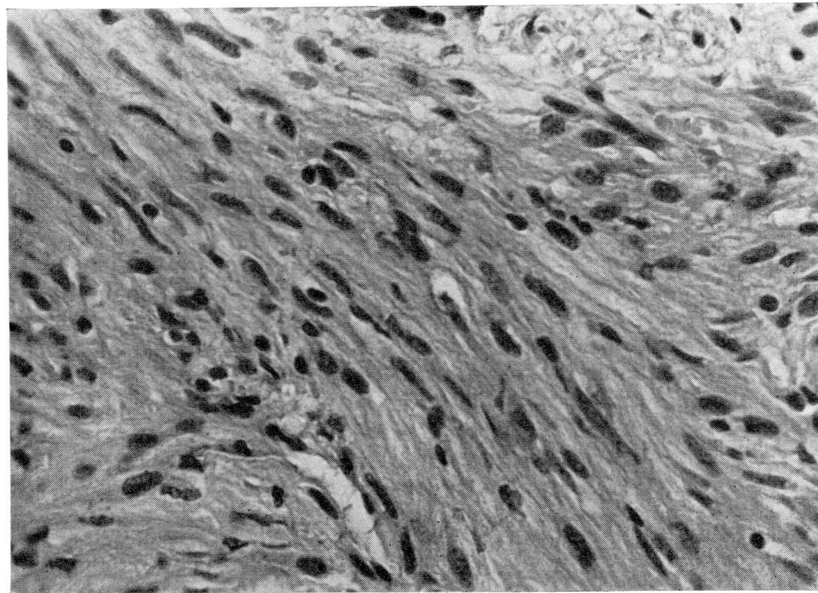

22/FIG. 9.—Leiomyoma of the uterus. The individual tumour cells are well differentiated myocytes, but are separated one from another by intercellular substance.

Malignant

Malignant tumours of connective tissue are relatively uncommon, the fibrosarcoma being probably the most common. They may arise from almost any of the connective tissue structures. Usually, each kind of connective tissue gives rise to the type that would be expected of it, liposarcomata arising from fatty tissue, rhabdomyosarcomata from the skeletal muscles, and so on. Occasionally, a malignant connective tissue tumour may be found in a place where a sarcoma of that type would not be expected. Synovial sarcomata, for example, often arise at some distance from a joint, and some types of rhabdomyosarcoma may be found in unlikely places, such as the bile duct.

It is usually assumed that sarcomata are highly malignant tumours, which kill quickly. This is not necessarily true. Some sarcomata, such as the osteogenic sarcomata, do grow fast, metastasise early, and kill quickly, usually in under two years. But other forms of sarcoma may grow very slowly, infiltrating locally, but metastasising only after a long delay, if at all. In recent years, more attention has been paid to these slow-growing tumours of low or border-line malignancy. It is, indeed, not always easy to distinguish between a slow-growing fibrosarcoma and a fibrosing lesion which is benign, or even not neoplastic at all. But bearing in mind this wide divergency in growth rate, and in the likelihood and speed of metastasis, some generalisations can be made about the way sarcomata grow. The malignant tumours of connective tissue all tend to infiltrate locally, very often penetrating for considerable distances, far beyond the apparent limits of the tumour. For this reason they often recur after attempted removal, and can only be cured by an extensive operation. They may metastasise to lymph nodes, but blood-borne metastases are usually more prominent, and, as would be expected, occur first and most prominently in the lung.

Most malignant tumours of connective tissue form moderately large masses, which destroy and replace their tissue of origin, and extend out into the surrounding tissues. In some cases, however, they seem well delimited, or even encapsulated. Oddly, it is often the more malignant sarcomata which show the most clear delimitation. The malignant synovioma, which grows rapidly and metastasises early, is often sharply demarcated, and the more malignant types of fibrosarcoma may appear well delimited, although the more slow growing

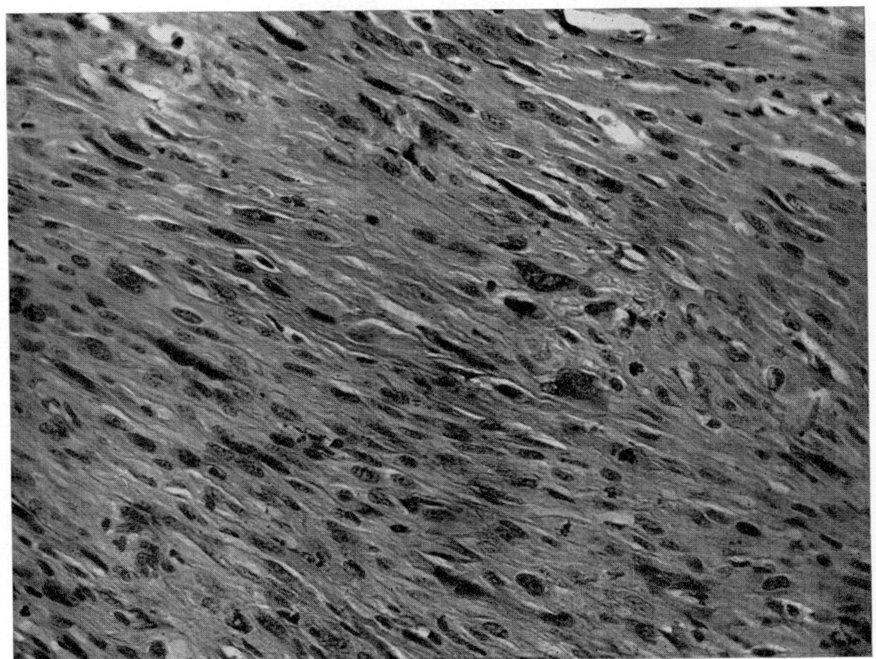

22/FIG. 10.—Fibrosarcoma of the thigh. Spindle cells lie separated one from another by intercellular substance. The cells are anaplastic, with abnormal mitoses, and occasional giant forms.

forms clearly infiltrate the surrounding tissues. The more anaplastic sarcomata may show areas of hæmorrhage and necrosis on section, but in the less anaplastic tumours and in the better preserved parts of anaplastic ones, the tumour tissue is often homogeneous, firm and white in fibrosarcomata, fatty or myxoid in liposarcomata, chondroid in chondrosarcomata, and so on.

Microscopically, the sarcomata vary greatly. In general, fibrosarcomata are made of more or less atypical fibrocytes separated by the collagen they produce. In well differentiated tumours, the cells and their collagen may closely resemble normal fibrocytes and normal collagen, but as one examines more and more anaplastic fibrosarcomata, the cells become more and more bizarre, often becoming large, very pleomorphic, with giant forms, and numerous atypical mitoses (FIG. 10). The intercellular substance tends to become less as the tumour becomes more anaplastic. Instead of well-formed collagen, there are only a few strands of collagen in a mucoid intercellular substance, or no collagen at all. Similarly, in the other forms of connective tissue sarcoma the tumour cells are relatively like those of their tissue of origin in well-differentiated cases, and the appropriate intercellular substance is well formed, but in the more anaplastic tumours, the tumour cells become bizarre, and the intercellular substance is scanty and ill-formed, tending to be mucoid.

Terminology

The terminology used to designate the tumours of connective tissue has been described above. As more is learnt of these tumours, many exceptions to the rules will be found. Some tumours have names which should designate a benign tumour, but which is usually applied to a malignant one. The term synovioma, for example, is used by many writers to mean malignant synovioma, or synovial sarcoma, although its form suggests a benign tumour. Again, many connective tissue tumours, especially the more malignant ones, show more than one kind of neoplastic connective tissue. At one time it was usual to give these tumours compound names, such as leiomyofibroma, a name used to designate the fibroid of the uterus, which may contain collagen and fibrocytes as well as smooth muscle cells, or fibrolipomyxosarcoma, to describe a liposarcoma in which some areas were fibrous, others myxoid. These complicated names are not often used now. Instead, such tumours are called by the name suitable to their principal component. Occasionally, when a tumour contains several kinds of neoplastic connective tissue, and none of the usual names seem suitable, the term mesenchymoma, or malignant mesenchymoma, is used.

In recent years a number of new types of connective tissue tumour have been described, and many of these have been given special names; for example, alveolar soft part sarcoma, chondromyxoid fibroma, hæmangiopericytoma, and so on. The nature of these relatively rare tumours, and their behaviour, cannot be described here.

3. Tumours of Hæmopoietic Tissue

The usual division into benign and malignant forms has not proved useful in classifying the tumours of hæmopoietic tissue. Almost all hæmopoietic tumours invade or are multifocal, and so are considered malignant. This is not to say that forms equivalent to the benign tumours of other tissues do not exist. They may occur, but we cannot recognise them. This is because benign tumours are distinguished from malignant by two principal criteria, invasion and metastasis. These criteria are not useful in the classification of hæmopoietic tumours, and cannot be used to distinguish between benign and malignant tumours, because even normal hæmopoietic cells invade and metastasise. Neutrophils invade the damaged tissues in every acute inflammatory reaction, and every abscess is in a sense a metastasis of hæmopoietic cells. As invasion and metastasis are properties of normal hæmopoietic tissue, benign hæmopoietic tumours would also be expected to invade and metastasise. Rather than belabour the question of benignancy and malignancy, it is easier to assume that the hæmopoietic tumours are all malignant, and to classify them differently.

Hæmopoietic tumours occur in two forms. In one, the principal feature is the presence of focal tumour masses; in the other, the predominant feature is the presence of large numbers of circulating tumour cells in the blood. Some kinds of hæmopoietic tumour occur almost always in the form with local tumour masses, others almost always in the form with many circulating tumour cells. Yet others may occur in either form, or show both features. At one time it was suggested that these two forms of hæmopoietic tumour were different. Some thought the form with local masses was truly neoplastic while the form with many tumour cells in the blood was not. This controversy has been largely abandoned, and almost everyone agrees that the two forms of disease are only different methods of presentation of a single kind of neoplasm.

Terminology.—Many terms are in use to describe the hæmopoietic tumours. Some centres prefer one set of terms, others another. Moreover, many writers continue to make up new names to designate conditions which differ in some minor fashion from one of the more usual kinds of hæmopoietic tumour. Only a few of the more common terms can be mentioned here. The many synonyms and alternatives can be added later.

Table II shows a simple scheme of nomenclature for the tumours of the hæmopoietic tissues. It can be seen that some tumours have two names, one for the form in which local masses are the most striking feature, the other for the form in which circulating tumour cells are predominant. If a patient shows both local masses and many tumour cells in the blood, either name can be used. It can also be seen that "leukæmia" is a general term which can be used to describe any kind of hæmopoietic tumour in which many tumour cells circulate in the blood. Adjectives are added to indicate the nature of the tumour.

22/Table II

A Form of Nomenclature for Tumours of Hæmopoietic Tissue

Tissue of Origin	*Form with Local Masses*	*Form with Circulating Tumour Cells*
Lympho-reticular tissues	Malignant lymphoma	
	Follicular lymphoma	
	Lymphosarcoma	Lymphatic leukæmia
	Reticulum cell sarcoma	Monocytic leukæmia
	Hodgkin's disease	
	Histiocytosis "X"	
	Reticulosis	
Bone Marrow		Myeloid leukæmia
		Polycythæmia vera
Plasma cells	Multiple myeloma	(Plasma cell leukæmia)

Tumours of the Lympho-reticular Tissues

The malignant lymphomata are by far the most common of the lympho-reticular tumours which present with local masses. Patients suffering from this kind of disease usually seek medical advice because of enlargement of one or more groups of lymph nodes. At that time the patient may be otherwise well. As times passes, the disease extends. More nodes become enlarged, and there may be involvement of the spleen, liver, gut, or other organs. The patients grow weaker. Infections become common. Death often comes gradually and quietly. The rate of extension varies a good deal from case to case. In general, the follicular form tends to progress slowly, 60 per cent of the patients being alive 5 years after the diagnosis was established. The other lymphomata have a much worse prognosis. Only about 25 per cent of the patients with lymphosarcoma or Hodgkin's disease survive 5 years, and only about 12 per cent of those with reticulum cell sarcoma. Unfortunately most patients with malignant lymphoma have either lymphosarcoma or Hodgkin's disease, each making up about 45 per cent of all lymphomata. Recently it has been realised that a malignant lymphoma can be diagnosed before it becomes widespread, and that with proper therapy the prognosis is much better in such cases. Cases of Hodgkin's disease or lymphosarcoma in which the disease was limited to a single group of lymph nodes and which have been treated by radiotherapy have shown a 50 per cent five-year survival. About half the cases of lymphosarcoma have many tumour cells circulating in the blood at some time, and such cases may show the lesions of lymphatic leukæmia as well as those of lymphosarcoma. Leukæmia is rare in the other forms of lymphoma, though it may complicate reticulum cell sarcoma.

The lymph nodes affected by a lymphoma are enlarged. Usually they remain discrete, though in Hodgkin's disease they tend to become matted together. On section, the node is usually completely replaced by the lymphoma. The cut surface has a characteristic smooth, damp, uniform surface, usually described as reminiscent of fish flesh (FIG. 11). Foci of hæmorrhage or necrosis may occur in the more anaplastic tumours. If the liver or spleen is involved, it may show diffuse enlargement or, less commonly, discrete tumours similar to the metastases of other neoplasms.

Microscopically, lymph nodes involved by follicular lymphoma show a proliferation of neoplastic follicles throughout the cortex and medulla. The follicles retain some resemblance to normal germinal follicles, and should not be confused with focal deposits of some other kind of lymphoma.

In lymphosarcoma and reticulum cell sarcoma, the affected lymph nodes are partially or completely replaced by lymphomatous tissue. The normal structure of the node is lost, and replaced by masses of closely packed tumour cells. There is little or no stroma. In lymphosarcomata, the tumour cells are lymphocytes. They may be well differentiated and closely resemble normal lymphocytes (FIG. 12), but are often more anaplastic and tend to resemble lymphoblasts. In well differentiated tumours, the cells are monotonously uniform, but in more anaplastic examples they become more variable and more irregular in shape, until it seems better to call the tumour a reticulum cell sarcoma rather than a lymphosarcoma. Histologically, there is no sharp distinction between these two forms of lymphoma. The better differentiated examples are called lymphosarcoma,

22/FIG. 11 (*see opposite*).—Lymphosarcoma in para-aortic lymph nodes. The enlarged nodes are discrete. They have been sectioned to show the homogeneous, white lymphosarcoma tissue.

22/FIG. 12 (*see opposite*).—Lymphosarcoma in a lymph node. The node is replaced by small cells resembling lymphocytes. The cells are closely packed, but each is separate from the next. A blood vessel can be seen in the left upper corner.

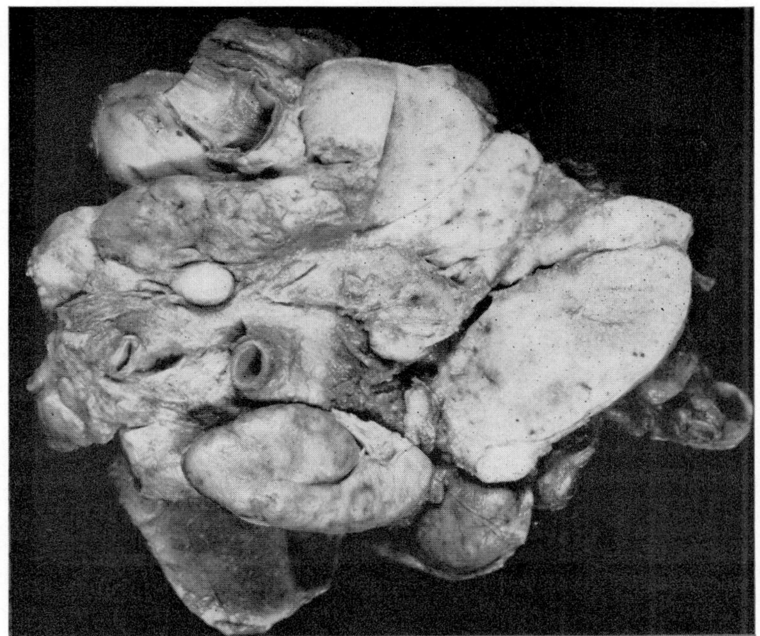

22/FIG. 11

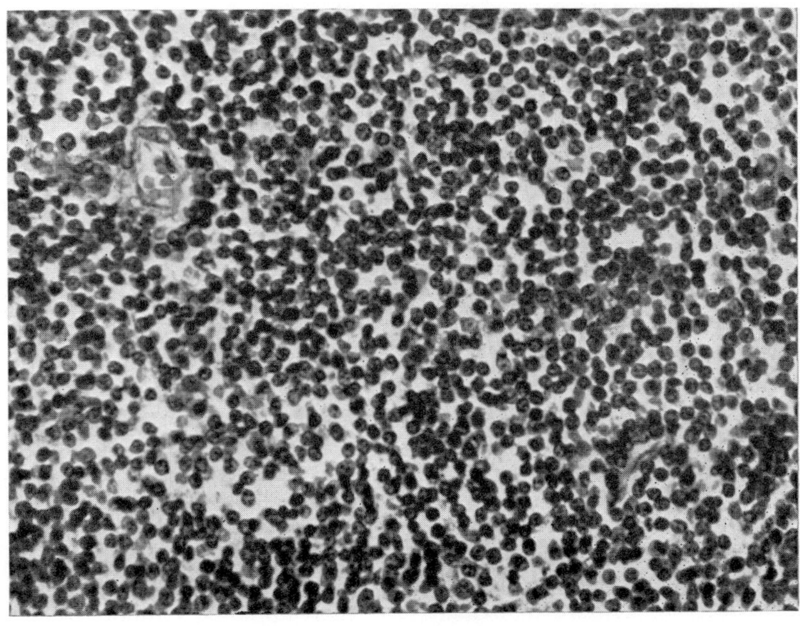

22/FIG. 12

the more anaplastic ones reticulum cell sarcoma. If other tissues are involved, they may be replaced completely by malignant tissue similar to that seen in the lymph nodes, or the lymphoma cells may infiltrate between pre-existing elements.

Hodgkin's disease is different. The affected lymph nodes are replaced completely or partially by the lymphoma, but instead of the uniformity of lymphosarcoma and reticulum cell sarcoma the microscopical appearance is varied and often bizarre. One case varies greatly from the next, and in a single case one lesion may vary from another. The Hodgkin's tissue is a mixture of many elements. Normal lymphocytes and abnormal reticulum cells are always present, and there may be as well normal reticulum cells, normal neutrophils, normal eosinophils, normal plasma cells, areas of fibrosis, or foci of necrosis. The proportions of these various elements varies enormously. Lymphocytes may make up 95 per cent of the cells, or may be rare. Abnormal reticulum cells may be so abundant that it is hard to distinguish the tumour from a reticulum cell sarcoma, or may be hard to find. Any of the other elements may be abundant, or may be absent. In some cases the tumour is almost destroyed by scarring; in others there is no fibrosis at all. Sometimes eosinophils are numerous; sometimes they do not occur. Particular importance is given to the form of abnormal reticulum cell which has two nuclei, each with a large nucleolus, and which has eosinophilic, well-defined cytoplasm. Such cells are called Dorothy Reed cells, or Reed-Sternberg cells. They are not diagnostic of Hodgkin's disease as they occur also in reticulum cell sarcoma, and similar cells may occur in certain viral infections, but they always occur in Hodgkin's disease and most authorities require them in order to establish the diagnosis. For the last 20 years, it has been usual to divide Hodgkin's disease on histological criteria into three forms, Hodgkin's paragranuloma, Hodgkin's granuloma, and Hodgkin's sarcoma. In Hodgkin's paragranuloma, the prognosis is much better. Some 80 per cent of cases survive five years. In Hodgkin's sarcoma, the prognosis is very bad. The value of this division is limited by the rarity of both the paragranuloma and sarcoma. Most cases fall in the intermediate category. Recently a new subdivision has become more popular. Cases are divided into those with many lymphocytes, those with few lymphocytes, mixed forms and those with a curious form of nodular fibrosis. The cases with many lymphocytes do well, some 73 per cent surviving 5 years, and those with few lymphocytes do badly, only 13 per cent surviving five years. The mixed cases fall between. About 30 per cent survive five years. The cases with nodular fibrosis also do reasonably well, about 44 per cent surviving five years, but this form of the disease is usually confined to the mediastinum and adjacent lymph nodes. In view of the relationship between lymphocytes and immune reactions, it is interesting that the forms of Hodgkin's disease in which lymphocytes are few are often associated with a failure of the body's immune defences. When Hodgkin's disease involves other tissues, it usually forms well-defined tumours in which the pre-existing tissue is replaced by Hodgkin's tissue.

The malignant lymphomata all have a tendency to change to a more malignant form. Patients with follicular lymphoma, for example, are likely to change sooner or later to a more malignant type of lymphoma, lymphosarcoma or Hodgkin's disease. Or patients with one of the more favourable lymphocytic forms of Hodgkin's disease are likely to change sooner or later to one of the more malignant lymphopenic forms.

Patients who present with lymphatic leukæmia have symptoms similar to those of patients with myeloid leukæmia. The disease may be chronic, or acute. As would be expected, enlargement of lymph nodes soon becomes evident, and the nodes show the changes seen in lymphosarcoma. In addition, there is usually massive replacement of the bone marrow by leukæmic cells, and diffuse infiltration of the spleen and liver is very common. Infiltration of any organ may occur. There are large numbers of malignant cells circulating in the blood, and they may escape anywhere. In chronic lymphatic leukæmia, the leukæmic cells can be recognized as lymphocytes or lymphoblasts, but in the acute form of the disease they are more anaplastic and resemble stem cells. Rarely, the leukæmic cells resemble monocytes.

Histiocytosis "X" is a term coined in 1953 to include three conditions which are now thought to be different forms of a single disease. Not all agree that they should be grouped together, though intermediate forms are common, and not all agree that they are neoplastic. Letterer-Siwe disease is the most malignant of the group. It usually occurs in young children, and is characterized by lesions in the skin, bone, and many other organs. The lesions are made up of accumulations of anaplastic reticulo-endothelial cells. The outcome is usually fatal. Hand-Schüller-Christian disease is more benign. It affects children and young adults. There are again multiple lesions in bone and other organs, but they are made up of well differentiated reticulo-endothelial cells which characteristically contain large quantities of cholesterol. The lesions tend to become fibrotic and to heal. Most cases recover. Eosinophilic granuloma is the most benign of the group. It usually occurs in young adults. There may be one or a few lesions in bone, or the disease may involve the lung or other organs. Again, reticulo-endothelial cells are predominant in the lesions, though eosinophils are often also present. The bony lesions are readily cured by curetting, and probably tend to heal by fibrosis.

The reticuloses are a rare and ill-understood group of neoplastic and hyperplastic conditions affecting the reticulo-endothelial system. A few forms of reticulosis have been well described and clearly defined, but most await clarification. The group includes clearly reactive and non-neoplastic lesions such as the lipo-melanotic reticulosis which affects lymph nodes draining skin lesions, clearly malignant lesions such as the medullary histiocytic reticulosis which is a highly malignant tumour of lymph nodes, and a great many intermediate conditions whose nature and behaviour are ill understood.

Tumours of the Bone Marrow

The tumours of the bone marrow have excited a good deal of discussion in recent years. It has become clear that it is very difficult to distinguish sharply between reactive, non-neoplastic hyperplasia and true neoplasms. In both, any or all of the bone marrow cells may be involved, granulocytes, erythrocytes, megakaryocytes, reticulo-endothelial cells, or fibrocytes. There may be proliferation of one, some, or all of these types of cell, or proliferation of some and hypoplasia of others. Marrow cells may appear in the spleen and other organs in both neoplastic and non-neoplastic conditions. If the marrow cells in other organs seem normal, the condition is often called "myeloid metaplasia", though it is not clear that the extra-osseous deposits of marrow cells arise by metaplasia rather than by colonization. In both neoplastic and non-neoplastic disease, abnormal cells may appear in the circulating blood, and again it is sometimes difficult to distinguish between neoplasia and reaction. Because of these difficulties, many now group together all the proliferative lesions of the bone marrow, neoplastic and non-neoplastic, and call the whole group the "myeloproliferative disorders". There is not space here to discuss even briefly all of these interesting conditions, and we must confine ourselves to those which are clearly neoplastic, the various forms of myeloid leukæmia.

Patients with myeloid leukæmia often seek medical advice because of vague complaints of weakness or tiredness. A moderately severe anæmia is common and on examination the tumour cells are found in the blood. In the majority of patients, the spleen is enlarged, sometimes so greatly that it extends into the pelvis. The liver tends to enlarge later. Enlargement of lymph nodes is less marked than in lymphatic leukæmia. As time passes other organs and tissues may be infiltrated by the tumour cells, the anæmia grows more severe, the patient grows weaker, infection becomes more and more likely, and death follows. Sometimes the disease is acute, killing the patient in a few months, but often it is chronic, going on for years with remissions and exacerbations, but leading at last to death.

In chronic myeloid leukæmia, the bone marrow is usually extensively replaced by leukæmic cells, explaining at least in part the anæmia and osteoporosis often seen in these patients. The spleen is usually infiltrated by huge numbers of leukæmic cells, but its normal sinusoidal architecture is preserved in most cases. The liver and other organs tend to show patchy involvement, with leukæmic cells escaping from the vessels to infiltrate the tissues in a manner reminiscent of an inflammatory reaction, the leukæmic cells spreading through the tissues as do their cousins in acute inflammation. In severely involved foci, the pre-existing tissue may be destroyed and replaced by leukæmic cells. Any or all of the various types of marrow cell may proliferate in the bone marrow. The disease is not a neoplasm of one particular kind of marrow cell, but a condition which affects them all. However, as the disease progresses one kind of marrow cell tends to become predominant. Usually, the neutrophilic granulocytes establish dominance, and the term chronic myeloid leukæmia is usually reserved for this form of the disease. In the rare cases in which some other kind of marrow cell becomes dominant, other terms are used, as for example eosinophilic leukæmia, megakaryocytic leukæmia, and so on. If the erythrocytes become dominant, the condition is called polycythæmia vera. The cells which proliferate in the bone marrow are not normal. There is an excess of the more primitive forms, and there may be other abnormalities. The extra-osseous lesions of chronic myeloid leukæmia also show several kinds of marrow cell. Usually the various granulocytic series, the erythrocytic series, and megakaryocytes can all be recognized. Again, there tends to be an excess of primitive forms.

In acute myeloid leukæmia, the findings are simpler. There is extensive replacement of the bone marrow, but other lesions are usually less marked. The leukæmic cells are anaplastic, resembling the blast cells of the marrow. They give rise to an infiltrate which is uniform, more like the uniform infiltrate of a poorly differentiated lymphosarcoma or a reticulum cell sarcoma than the polymorphous proliferation characteristic of chronic myeloid leukæmia.

In chronic myeloid leukæmia, very large numbers of tumour cells may circulate in the blood. There may be tens of thousands or even hundreds of thousands per cubic millimetre. As might be expected, various kinds of abnormal cell can be found but usually the neutrophilic series predominates. In acute myeloid leukæmia, the number of circulating tumour cells is usually much less, not more than ten or twenty thousand per cubic millimetre, and the cells are anaplastic, resembling the blast cells of the marrow. In practice, it is very difficult to distinguish between acute myeloid leukæmia and acute lymphatic leukæmia. In both conditions the leukæmic cells resemble the stem cells of the bone marrow, and the course of the two diseases is very similar. Many authorities therefore group these two conditions together, and divide the leukæmias into three main groups, chronic myeloid leukæmia, chronic lymphatic leukæmia, and acute or stem cell leukæmia. This is not to deny that both acute myeloid leukæmia and acute lymphatic leukæmia exist, but only to admit our inability to distinguish between them.

Like the lymphomata, the myeloid leukæmias tend to change to the worse. Patients who have suffered for years with chronic myeloid leukæmia or polycythæmia vera may develop acute myeloid leukæmia, and die of it in a few months.

Tumours of Plasma Cells

Although rare benign tumours of plasma cells may occur, plasma cells usually give rise to the malignant tumour called multiple myeloma. The tumour cells infiltrate the bone marrow diffusely. They may cause general osteoporosis which can be detected radiographically, or may cause a focal destruction of bone which appears as a punched-out hole radiographically. Extra-osseous infiltrations or deposits may also occur. The tumour cells resemble normal plasma cells, but are often bigger, pleomorphic, multinucleate, or show other evidence of anaplasia. It has long been known that patients with multiple myeloma often have abnormal proteins in the blood or urine, and in view of the relationship between plasma cells and the production of antibodies it is not surprising that some of these proteins have been found to be similar to immunoglobulins. This is not the place to discuss these findings at length, though it is interesting to note that the Bence-Jones protein found in the urine of some patients with multiple myeloma has been shown to be made of isolated "L" chains from the globulin molecule. Amyloidosis is very common in multiple myeloma, presumably because of the dysproteinæmia. As with the other forms of hæmopoietic tumour, the distinction between true neoplasms or plasma cells and non-neoplastic proliferations is not always clear. Not all cases of dysproteinæmia associated with a proliferation of plasma cells seem to be neoplastic. In view of the theory that plasma cells are derived from lymphocytes, perhaps through an intermediate form resembling a reticulo-endothelial cell, it is interesting that tumours intermediate between lymphosarcoma and multiple myeloma and intermediate between reticulum cell sarcoma and myeloma occur.

4. Tumours of Nervous Tissues

The tumours of the nervous tissues form a heterogeneous group, the various types of tumour having little in common with one another. That this should be is not surprising when one remembers that the nervous system is made of many different kinds of tissue, neurones, neuroglia, microglia, blood vessels and their supporting stroma, meninges, Schwann sheaths, and so on. Each of these different kinds of tissue gives rise to its own sort of neoplasm.

Glioma

The tumours of the neuroglia are called gliomata. With rare exceptions, they occur only in the brain and spinal cord. For many years, it was customary to divide the gliomata into many subgroups according to their microscopical appearance, and, in particular, according to the resemblance of their cells to one or other of the forms of neuroglial cell seen in the developing embryo. More recently, a simpler classification has become common. It has been realised that in all probability gliomata arise from adult neuroglial cells, just as other types of tumour probably arise from adult cells. The gliomata are therefore divided into three groups. The astrocytes give rise to the astrocytoma, the ependyma to the ependymoma, and the oligodendroglia to oligodendroglioma.

The astrocytoma is the most common of the gliomata. Indeed, it is the most common primary intracranial neoplasm. It may occur at any age, and is more common in the brain than in the cord. The better differentiated astrocytomata form ill-defined masses of greyish white, firm tissue which merges gradually into the surrounding brain. Often, the tumours are several centimetres in greatest dimension. They may be cystic. The more anaplastic astrocytomata look better defined, but are softer, often with areas of necrosis or hæmorrhage. Microscopically, the well differentiated tumours are made of cells easily recognisable as astrocytes, but in the more poorly differentiated forms the cells are bizarre and pleomorphic cells. In many hospitals, the term astrocytoma is reserved for the better differentiated tumours, and the name gliobastoma multiforme is used for the more anaplastic forms (Fig. 13). This name is a remnant of the more complicated classifications used in the past.

The other types of glioma are relatively uncommon. The ependymomata and oligodendrogliomata both tend to form relatively large, often quite well-defined tumours. The ependymomata are relatively frequent in the cord, where they are one of the more common gliomata. Microscopically, they tend to form spaces lined by ependyma, while the oligodendrogliomata usually form uniform masses of small oligodendrocytes.

The medulloblastoma is a tumour of unknown origin which is in many ways similar to a glioma. It occurs in infants and children and runs a rapid course. Some have thought that it arises from primitive cells able to differentiate either into glial cells or into neurones. Others think it arises from neurones. The tumour nearly always takes origin in the cerebellum, usually near the midline, and grows rapidly to form a soft, well-defined mass. Microscopically, it is made of small, pear-shaped cells which may be arranged around small spaces filled with fibrillary material.

The more rapidly growing gliomata and the medulloblastoma may metastasise by the cerebrospinal fluid, forming plaques or nodules of tumour in the meninges. They may also grow into the scalp through a craniotomy defect. Metastases outside the central nervous system are, however, extremely rare. Because of this failure to form metastases outside the central nervous system, some have thought that the gliomata should be considered benign. Indeed, the better differentiated examples invade little, if at all, and do not metastasise, and so could well be classed as benign. However, the invasive growth of the more anaplastic forms, and their ability to metastasise within the central nervous

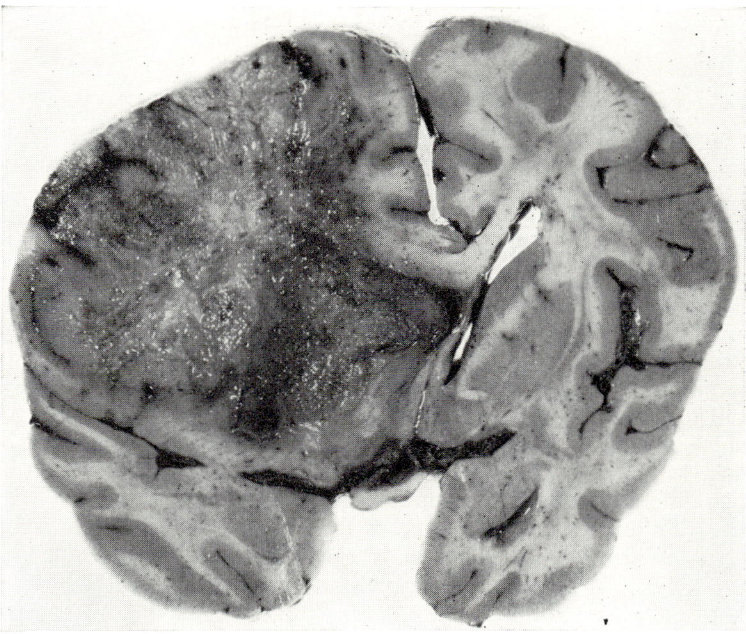

22/Fig. 13.—Glioblastoma multiforme. The tumour shows areas of hæmorrhage and necrosis, but is fairly well defined. It has caused considerable distortion of the brain.

system make their classification as malignant more logical, and it is not useful to attempt an arbitrary division into benign and malignant types. The gliomata are, of course, very dangerous. Unless they can be completely removed without damaging some important structure in the brain or cord, they will increase in size inexorably, killing the patient either by damaging some structure in the vicinity of the tumour, or by serving as a space occupying lesion, expanding within the non-expansible confines of the skull or vertebral canal, and depriving the brain or cord of the space it must have.

Meningioma

Meningiomata are the second most frequent primary intracranial tumour. They commonly take origin in the meninges of the parasagittal region, but are often found along the sphenoid ridge or at other sites within the skull or spinal canal. They usually form a well-defined, firm nodule. They may be small, or may weigh as much as 200 gm. They do not usually invade the brain, but push into it, displacing it and causing pressure atrophy. They may invade the adjacent bone, causing a reactive overgrowth. Microscopically, some meningiomata are made of sheets and clumps of large, flattened cells; others contain many psammoma bodies, small calcified balls which develop in hyalinised tissue in the centre of masses of meningioma cells arranged in whorls; yet others resemble fibromata. Meningiomata are usually benign, causing symptoms because they are space-occupying lesions, or because they press on important structures. Unfortunately, their anatomical relationships sometimes make resection difficult.

Tumours of Neurones

Tumours of the neurones of the central nervous system are very rare, but tumours of peripheral neurones are not unusual. Two types are usually distinguished, though intermediate forms exist. The neuroblastoma is a highly malignant tumour of infants and children. It usually takes origin in or near an adrenal, grows rapidly and metastasises extensively. Microscopically, it is made of masses of small cells which somewhat resemble lymphocytes. These cells may be arranged around a space containing fibrillary material, an arrangement somewhat similar to that seen in the medulloblastomata. The ganglioneuroma, in contrast, is a tumour of children or adults. It may occur near the adrenal or in the sympathetic ganglia. It is benign and forms a well-defined mass. Ganglion cells and their axons are readily identified microscopically, together with supporting cells and fibres. The relationship of these two types of tumour has been demonstrated elegantly in the rare cases in which a neuroblastoma has been shown to differentiate, changing at last into a ganglioneuroma.

The retinoblastoma is a tumour of the retina which arises in infants and children. It is in many ways similar to the neuroblastoma, though metastases are less frequent, so that it can be cured in a proportion of cases by excision of the eye. In some cases the liability to this tumour is clearly inherited, though the exact Mendelian mechanism is not clear. Its microscopical appearance is similar in the main to that of a neuroblastoma or a medulloblastoma, with small, closely packed cells, which may sometimes be arranged around small spaces.

Other Nervous Tumours

The phæochromocytoma is a tumour of the adrenal medulla. Though it is usually classed as a tumour of the nervous system because the adrenal medulla is derived from the nervous system, it might more logically be considered an adenoma, a benign epithelial tumour. As has been mentioned, it looks grossly and microscopically like an adenoma, being very similar to the adenomata of the adrenal cortex. It also behaves like an adenoma. Some phæochromocytomata secrete noradrenalin and adrenalin, giving rise to paroxysmal or constant hypertension. Malignant forms are very rare.

Similarly, the Schwannoma might be considered a tumour of connective tissue rather than a tumour of nervous tissue, though as it takes origin from Schwann cells it, too, is usually classified with the nervous tumours. As would be expected, the tumour takes origin from a nerve, usually a peripheral nerve, though Schwannomata also arise from the nerves within the skull and spinal canal. Grossly and microscopically, the Schwannoma has the characteristics of a benign, connective tissue tumour. Indeed, it closely resembles a fibroma, though the tendency to have its nuclei arranged in rows, and certain other features, serve to distinguish it. The uncommon malignant Schwannomata look and behave much like fibrosarcomata.

Mention should also be made of neurofibromatosis. In this condition there are multiple tumours and enlargements of the peripheral nerves, together with pigmentation of the skin and other changes. The nerve tumours may be neurolemmomata, or, more commonly, are fibromata of a type sometimes called neurofibromata because nerve fibrils run through them. Not uncommonly, one or more of the tumours becomes malignant.

5. Tumours of more than One Tissue

In the tumours we have considered so far, only one kind of cell has been neoplastic, and the neoplastic cells have been supported and nourished by a non-neoplastic stroma. Now come a few exceptional tumours in which more than one kind of tissue is neoplastic. These tumours still have a stroma, which is provided by the host, and is still non-neoplastic, but the stroma is usually scant. It is, of course, important not to confuse the stromal cells with the true neoplastic cells.

Teratoma

The teratomata are the best example of a tumour of more than one kind of neoplastic tissue, for in a teratoma one may have any kind of neoplastic tissue whatsoever, and any combination of types. Teratomata are most common in the ovary and the testis, though they may occur anywhere along the mid-line of the body, the sacrum, posterior mediastinum and base of the skull being among the more common extra-genital sites. In the testis, they are usually malignant. In the ovary and elsewhere, they are usually benign. They may occur in children, but are more common in adults.

A typical benign, ovarian teratoma gives rise to a cystic tumour. The cyst is usually about 10 cm. in diameter when it is found, though it may be much larger or very small. The wall of the cyst is thin, except at one or more points where there is a thickening of the wall giving rise to a little mound which projects into the cyst. The cyst is usually full of sebaceous matter, and often contains hair, which grows from the stratified squamous epithelium, or skin, which lines most or all of the cyst. The skin is usually well formed, and complete with hair follicles and sebaceous glands, though the arrangement and number of these appendages is usually abnormal. In the mounds which project into the cyst, an extraordinary profusion of tissues may occur. Many different kinds of tissue can be identified. All are reasonably well formed, and often are easily recognised as adult or fœtal tissues, but they are arranged without apparent logic. Spaces are lined with various kinds of epithelium, bronchial epithelium, intestinal epithelium, squamous epithelium, any kind at all (Fig. 14). A single space may be lined with more than one kind of epithelium, perhaps in part with, say, bronchial epithelium, in part by intestinal epithelium, in part by stratified squamous epithelium. In relation to these spaces there may or may not be the appropriate connective tissue structures. For example, a space lined in whole or part with bronchial epithelium may have around it cartilage bars, or muscle, or may have no particular wall at all. Islands of glandular tissue, thyroid, pancreas, and others may occur, and are sometimes the predominant feature, but are again arranged without apparent logic or reason. Nervous

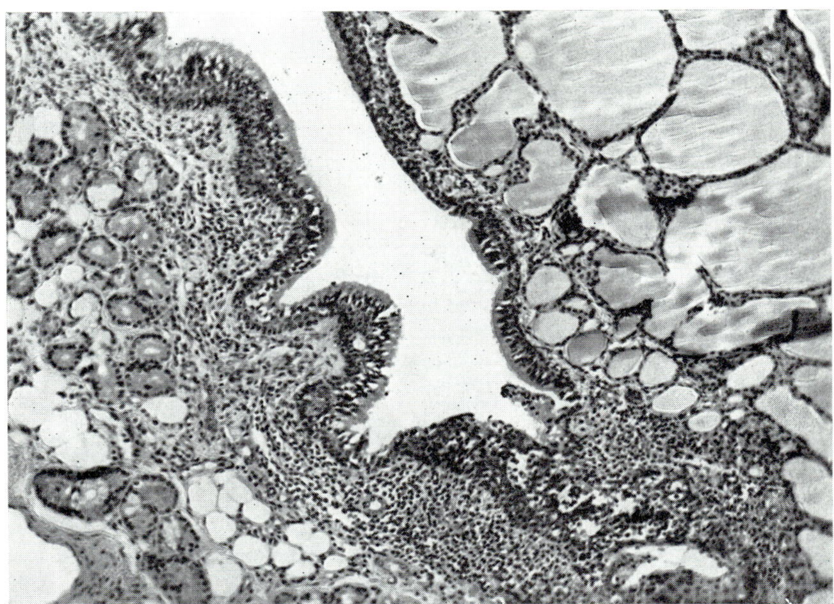

22/FIG. 14.—Teratoma of ovary. A portion of the tumour showing well differentiated thyroid, a tube lined by ciliated epithelium, salivary or pancreatic glands, fat and lymphocytes. This tumour also contained brain, nerves, cartilage, muscle, and other tissues.

structures, particularly structures reminiscent of the embryonic central nervous system, are common, but occur mixed in with the epithelial structures in any sort of relationship whatsoever. Cartilage, bone or joints may be found. Sometimes relatively well-formed organs occur. Teeth not uncommonly project into the cyst of an ovarian teratoma, and rarely fingers may be found. But the predominant feature in a benign teratoma is not organoid structures such as teeth or fingers, but the extraordinary muddle of reasonably well-formed tissues. It is as if one took at random samples of some or all the tissues of the body, put them in a pot, and stirred it all up with a big spoon. The benign teratomata grow slowly, and are not usually dangerous.

The malignant ones tend to grow quicker, and are likely to metastasise to the lymph nodes or by the blood stream. Malignant teratomata may be entirely malignant, or may have only one malignant element. For example, a squamous cell carcinoma can develop from the squamous epithelium of an otherwise benign teratoma, and will behave like a squamous cell carcinoma elsewhere. The entirely malignant teratomata are usually poorly differentiated lesions, in which various kinds of tissue can be found, though their exact nature remains obscure. Such anaplastic teratomata are usually solid, usually small, grow fairly rapidly, and may show in their metastases any or all of the tissues of the primary. Occasionally, there may even be found in the metastases tissues which do not seem to be present in the primary.

The origin of these curious tumours is not known, and, indeed, they may not all be produced in the same way. It has been suggested that they may be parasitic twins, brothers or sisters of the host. This may occasionally be true, for distorted twins may be found attached to the head, sacrum or some other part of otherwise normal infants, but does not seem an adequate theory to explain the teratomata appearing in the adult. One would not expect abortive twins to manifest themselves so late or to show a predilection for the ovary or testis. Nor does the theory explain why in females the "sex" of teratomata is always female when it is determined by the configuration of the nucleus, though in males it may be male, female, or even male in parts, female in others. Another theory suggests that teratomata take origin in the adult, resulting from the parthenogenetic proliferation of one or more gametes, with a reversion to a more or less diploid, or even a polypoid state. A similar theory suggests that the teratomata may arise from the combination of two of the host's own gametes. These theories explain better the observations on the nuclear 'sex' of teratomata. In the female, each gamete has one X chromosome; and so the nuclei of all tumours derived from the proliferation or combination of gametes would have two or more X chromosomes, and so would appear female so far as nuclear sexing is concerned. In the male, the gametes may contain either an X or a Y chromosome, and so the nuclei of the resultant teratomata could be XX, XY, or YY, or some polypoid state such as XXY or XYY, and so could appear as either male or female to nuclear sexing. Teratomata in which part of the tumour is male to nuclear sexing, and part is female, could be explained by assuming that the tumour took origin from two or more gametes or combinations of gametes, or by assuming that different parts of the tumour have acquired different kinds of polypoidy or different abnormalities in their chromosomal content. These theories do not, of course, explain the occurrence of teratomata in the mediastinum and other points in the mid-line. There are many other theories, but this is not the place to go further into the argument.

Wilms' Tumour

Wilms' tumour is much less common than are teratomata. It is a tumour of infancy and early childhood. A large mass develops in close relation to a kidney, grows rapidly, and soon metastasises. The mass is often well defined, and on section is grey, sometimes with cysts, or areas of hæmorrhage or necrosis. Microscopically, the tumour is a combination of malignant connective tissue and malignant epithelium. The malignant connective tissue resembles embryonic connective tissue, but often contains areas of cartilage, and smooth or striped muscle. The malignant epithelium tends to form tubules or solid cords. Occasionally, structures like glomeruli are found. It is believed that the tumour takes origin from the cells of the embryonic kidney. These cells have the power to form almost any kind of connective tissue, but can make only the epithelial structures of the kidney, and so, though any kind of connective tissue may be seen, the epithelial part of the tumour is limited to anaplastic derivatives of fœtal kidney epithelium.

Mixed Mesodermal Tumour

In the adult, a tumour now usually called a mixed mesodermal tumour may arise in the uterus. It shows the same kind of mixture of neoplastic connective tissue and neoplastic epithelium as does Wilms' tumour. The neoplastic connective tissue is of more adult type, but often contains cartilage, smooth muscle, or striped muscle in addition to the anaplastic cells which make up the greater part of its volume. The neoplastic epithelium forms glands not unlike those of an adenocarcinoma of the endometrium. It is believed that the mixed mesodermal tumour of the uterus takes origin from Müllerian remnants which retain their primitive ability to form both connective tissue and endometrial epithelium. Once again, any kind of connective tissue may be formed, but only the epithelium proper to the part.

Fibroadenoma of the Breast

The last of the tumours listed in the classification of this section is the fibroadenoma of the breast. This is a very common tumour, often occurring in young women between 20 and 30, and giving rise to a smooth mass which is freely movable in the breast. On section, it is a well-delimited tumour which on microscopical examination shows a proliferation of both ducts and the loose connective tissue which surrounds them.

It is usual to consider both the proliferation of the epithelium and the proliferation of the connective tissue neoplastic. However, though this is the classical theory, and is accepted by most authorities, it is possible to take a simpler view, and consider the tumour an adenoma which stimulates the formation of a non-neoplastic stroma in the usual way. There seems little reason to continue to hold the classical theory. If it is true, the fibroadenoma is an almost unique type of mixed tumour. If the simpler view is taken, the fibroadenoma is a commonplace adenoma of an exocrine gland.

It may even be that in some cases at least the masses called fibroadenomata are not neoplasms at all, but a local hyperplasia of the ducts and periductal connective tissue of the breast. Such proliferations are common in the female breast, and often involve only a small segment of it.

6. Tumours which do not Fit Easily into One of the Other Groups

In this section are collected a number of types of tumour which, for one reason or another, do not fit easily into one of the other groups. In some instances, the origin of the tumour is curious; in some, the behaviour of the tumour separates it from those which might otherwise be considered similar; and in some instances, the tumour is placed here because there is no agreement as to its nature.

Tumours of Melanoblasts

The tumours of the melanin-producing cells of the skin are a case in which there is dispute about the cell of origin. All agree that these tumours arise from the melanoblasts of the epidermis, but there is no agreement as to the origin of the melanoblasts. On the whole, the evidence seems to support the theory that they are derived from the neural crest, migrating out from the crest during embryonic life together with the developing peripheral nerves, and coming to lie at last in the basal layer of the epidermis, a theory which owes much to the work of Masson (1882–1959). The alternative view is that the melanoblasts of the skin are a special differentiation of the epidermal cells themselves. Unfortunately, this difference of opinion as to the origin of the melanoblasts has been allowed to influence the terminology. Instead of the satisfactory, noncommittal term malignant melanoma, the term melanocarcinoma has been favoured by those taking the second view, and the old term melanosarcoma is sometimes preferred by those accepting Masson's theory. It should be emphasised that it is undesirable to modify a satisfactory, established terminology to make it fit a theory which is at the best controversial.

Before coming to the malignant melanoma of the skin, it is necessary to say a little about a lesion which often, though not always, precedes it. This is a pigmented nævus, or common mole. The common mole is a very common lesion indeed. It has been said that the average person has some 50 of them. They are probably malformations rather than true tumours, but their pathogenesis is of considerable relevance to the understanding of the malignant melanoma. The pigmented nævi begin in childhood as a focal proliferation of the melanoblasts in the basal layers of the epidermis. As time passes, the melanoblasts, or nævus cells, move down into the dermis, where they become quiescent, forming columns and clumps of regular cells. Often the nævus cells shed melanim into the dermis, where it is taken up by macrophages which are called melanophores. The proliferation of melanoblasts in the epidermis continues, and more nævus cells move down into the dermis. At puberty, the proliferation of the melanoblasts in the epidermis ceases, but the nævus cells in the dermis remain, forming the common pigmented mole of the skin. Only in the palms, soles and the genitalia does the formation of new nævus cells persist throughout adult life.

If a pigmented nævus becomes malignant, the proliferation of new, and now malignant, melanoblasts begins again in the basal layers of the epidermis. The new, malignant melanoma cells move down into the dermis as did the nævus cells, but unlike the nævus cells, the melanoma cells continue to proliferate in the dermis. They also invade the overlying epidermis. Clinically, this alteration is shown by an increase in the size or pigmentation of the nævus. Microscopically, instead of the regular, quiescent nævus cells lying in the dermis, there is a marked proliferation of melanoblasts in the epidermis, with the production of the anaplastic melanoma cells which invade the epidermis, and proliferate in the dermis (FIG. 15). The extent of pigment formation is of no prognostic importance in malignant melanomata of the skin. Some produce much melanin, some little or none. In most cases, there is a marked lymphocytic reaction at the deep margin of the tumour.

The malignant melanoma of the skin has a very bad reputation. It often extends very early, before the local mass has become large enough to attract the patient's attention, metastasising to the regional lymph nodes or by the blood stream. It may occur in young adults, and may kill quickly. It is therefore of considerable interest that recent reports have suggested that though the malig-

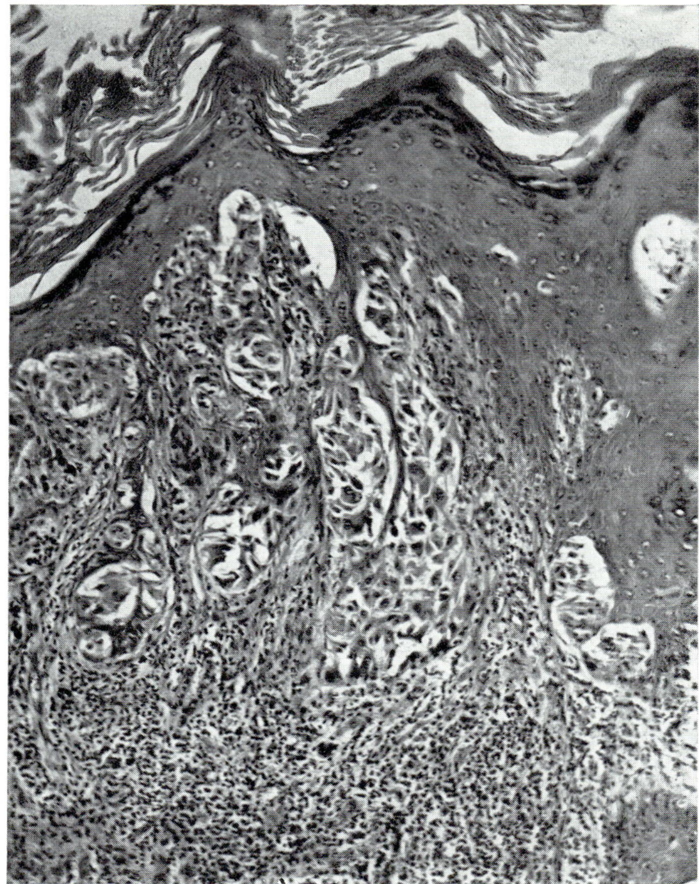

22/FIG. 15.—Malignant melanoma of the skin. Anaplastic melanoma cells are extending down from the epidermis into the dermis. As is usual with malignant melanomata of the skin, a large number of lymphocytes have accumulated in the dermis in the region of the tumour.

nant melanoma of the skin does kill many people, the prognosis is not as bad as had been thought. Some half of the patients can be cured by an adequate, local excision of the primary tumour. This makes it the more imperative that whenever a pigmented lesion of the skin is removed, it be subjected to histological examination, so that, in the remote chance it may be a malignant melanoma, the patient may be given the benefit of an early, wide local excision. There is no way of being sure on clinical grounds alone that a pigmented lesion is not malignant.

Tumours of melanoblasts may also occur in other parts of the body. The blue nævus, for example, is a benign melanin-producing tumour or malformation which occurs in the deep parts of the skin, appearing blue when seen through the overlying tissue. It presumably takes origin from melanoblasts which failed to migrate all the way to the epidermis. Malignant melanomata may also arise in parts of the body other than the skin, but are rare except in the eye, where they are one of the most important primary malignant tumours. Here, too, the cure rate after enucleation of the eye is fairly good, about 50 per cent, though it is hard to be confident of this figure, for the malignant melanoma of the eye is notorious for its tendency to manifest metastases only many years after the removal of the primary. The glass eye and large liver is the classical syndrome of recurrent ocular melanoma.

Tumours of the Placenta

The tumours of the placenta are odd in that, though they grow and metastasise in the mother, they are not tumours of the mother at all, but tumours of the fœtus. They may occur in a benign form, the hydatidiform mole, in which there is a proliferation of the placental tissues so that the enlarged uterus becomes filled with a mass of grape-like œdematous vesicles. They also occur in a more invasive form, called a chorioadenoma destruens; and as the highly malignant chorionepithelioma. In the chorionepithelioma, the uterine wall is invaded by the malignant derivatives of the trophoblast, which easily gain access to the dilated blood vessels, and metastasise widely, giving rise to hæmorrhagic tumours. The diagnosis can often be established by the demonstration in the urine of the gonadotropins produced by the trophoblast of the tumour. Although chorionepitheliomata are rapidly fatal in most cases, their metastases occasionally regress after the removal of the primary tumour.

Tumours of the Ovary

The tumours of the ovary have also been segregated in this section. This is because, though some of the more common ovarian tumours look and behave like carcinomata, other common forms resemble rather connective tissue tumours, and yet other forms have a structure which is suggestive neither of carcinoma nor of a connective tissue tumour. Moreover, the classification of the rarer ovarian tumours is very confused. A great many sub-types have been described and named, the names often reflecting the sometimes fanciful theories of histogenesis proposed. The matter is further complicated because some of the ovarian tumours have hormonal activity, not necessarily œstrogenic, and the sub-types have been further divided according to the degree and type of hormonal activity. And yet again, tumours of remnants of testicular structures, or their ducts, may occur in the ovary. This is not the place to discuss all these varieties of tumour, and not even the more important of them can all be mentioned here.

To take just a few, relatively typical, examples, one of the commoner ovarian tumours is the cystadenoma, and its malignant counterpart, the cystadenocarcinoma. These tumours form cysts which may be unilocular or multilocular, and may be of any size. Indeed, cases have been recorded in which a cystadenoma was so large that after its removal from the abdomen with the help of a crane, the patient remaining weighed less than the tumour. Fortunately, such dramatic cases are very rare, and most cystadenomata are only a few centimetres in greatest diameter when they are found at operation or at autopsy. They may be bilateral. The tumours have a thin wall, and are, if benign, usually lined by a single layer of cuboidal epithelium. They may contain serous or mucinous fluid.

Sometimes there are papillary projections into or outside the cyst. If these are outside, there is considerable danger of metastasis by the breaking off of these projections and their reimplantation into the peritoneum. The cystadenocarcinomata may also metastasise to the regional lymph nodes. Such tumours have no endocrine activity.

Another group of ovarian tumours has several forms. There may be a well-defined nodule usually only a few centimetres across, which is well described by its usual name, fibroma. Intermediate forms exist between this ovarian fibroma and the thecoma, a benign tumour made up of cells resembling those of the ovarian cortex. Sometimes thecomata contain much fat, and may be termed luteomata. They may be associated with another type of tumour, the granulosa cell tumour, in which there are sheets and clumps of rather uniform cells somewhat resembling epithelium, and often containing small spaces reminiscent of ovarian follicles. All these tumours may be œstrogenic. They are benign, except for the granulosa cell tumours, which may spread to the peritoneum and regional nodes. Any of these tumours may be associated with carcinoma of the endometrium if they secrete œstrogens, the endometrial carcinoma being secondary to the continued œstrogenic stimulation.

These two groups of tumours must serve as the inadequate representatives of the great range of benign and malignant ovarian tumours.

Tumours of the Testis

For much the same reasons, the testicular tumours have also been segregated in this section. Benign tumours of the testis are rare. The interstitial cell adenoma can serve as an example. Malignant tumours are more frequent, though not common. With a few exceptions, they are believed to arise from the germ cells, and have been divided into three main groups. The seminoma has a relatively good prognosis, some 85 per cent of the patients living more than 5 years and being probably cured. It forms a well-defined homogeneous, white tumour, which is usually a few centimetres across when detected. Microscopically, it is made of sheets and clumps of moderately large cells, with pale, well-defined cytoplasm, and typically has a fine stroma infiltrated with lymphocytes. It tends to metastasize to the regional lymph nodes. A much more malignant testicular tumour is the embryonal carcinoma. This poorly differentiated tumour forms a soft, hæmorrhagic or partially necrotic mass. It is made of large, anaplastic cells, often resembling epithelium. It metastasises in most cases to the regional nodes, and often also by the blood stream. Only 15 per cent of patients survive 5 years. Of intermediate malignancy is the teratoma, which in the testis is almost always malignant. Mixed forms also occur. For example, a testicular tumour may be part seminoma, part teratoma, or part teratoma part embryonal carcinoma.

The rare benign tumours of the testis may secrete androgens or œstrogens, or may show no hormonal activity. The majority of malignant testicular tumours do not secrete hormones. Occasionally gonadotropins similar to those found in women with a chorionepithelioma of the placenta may be found in the urine of a patient with a seminoma, and they are found more commonly in cases of embryonic carcinoma. Indeed, there is a form of testicular tumour which not only secretes gonadotropins as do the chorionepitheliomata of the placenta, but looks grossly and microscopically like a chorionepithelioma, and behaves like one. Such tumours are sometimes called chorionepitheliomata of the testis. They may be a form of anaplastic embryonal carcinoma, or of anaplastic teratoma.

Other Tumours

Finally, mention might be made of rare tumours of curious structure and behaviour, such as the thymoma which arises from the thymus and may be associated with myasthenia gravis or other systemic effects. This tumour shows a proliferation of both the lymphoid and epithelioid cells of the thymus. Other odd tumours exist, but are of no great theoretical or practical importance.

Relationship between Anaplasia, Extension and Behaviour

As must be now clear, different kinds of tumour behave in very different ways. This raises a clinical problem of some importance. Merely to name a tumour is of little practical use. We need to know how it is likely to behave in the future, so that we can plan appropriate therapy and advise the patient suitably.

Benign tumours offer little difficulty. In most cases, the patient can be reassured, and the tumour removed without difficulty.

With malignant tumours it is different. Their behaviour varies very widely, and generalizations are not of much help clinically. In order to advise the patient, we must decide how the individual tumour that he has is likely to behave in the future. The first thing is to determine the nature of the tumour. To mention extreme cases, we know that basal cell carcinomata of the skin invade but metastasise most rarely, while osteogenic sarcomata metastasise early and widely in almost every case. The majority of types of tumour are less predictable. We know that a certain proportion will metastasise, and that most tumours of the type in question will grow at a certain rate and in a certain manner, but we do not know whether the individual tumour before us will follow the general rule. The patient may be lucky, and his tumour will grow more slowly and metastasise later than is usual for tumours of that type, or he may be unlucky and his tumour may extend more rapidly than is usual in that kind of neoplasm. Two means of predicting the future behaviour of individual tumours have proved of some value. As has been mentioned before, anaplastic tumours tend to grow more rapidly and to spread sooner and more widely than do well-differentiated examples of the same kind of tumour. Various systems of estimating the degree of anaplasia have been proposed and are of some help in predicting the future behaviour of individual tumours. The second method of prediction depends on the past behaviour of the individual tumour. We try to determine what it has done in the past, to discover how far and how quickly it has extended, and to use this information to predict the future.

One of the more famous methods of judging the degree of anaplasia of a malignant tumour is that devised by Broders, who divided squamous cell carcinomata into four grades. In grade 1, more than three-fourths of the tumour cells were well differentiated; in grade 2, about half the cells were differentiated; in grade 3, some three-quarters were undifferentiated; and in grade 4, the cells showed no tendency to differentiate. It is obvious that this is not a very precise method. There is no way of determining with certainty whether a given cell in a carcinoma is or is not well differentiated. Others have attempted to devise more objective ways of grading the anaplasia of various types of tumour, but with little success. It has therefore become usual to grade malignant tumours into four groups, by comparing the example under consideration with other tumours of the same type. If the example is unusually well differentiated, it is called grade 1; if it is in the usual range, but better differentiated than some, it is called grade 2; if it is in the usual range, but relatively anaplastic, it is called grade 3; and if it is unusually anaplastic, it is called grade 4. Thus the anaplasia of malignant tumours is graded not by comparing them with their tissue of origin, but by comparing them with other tumours of the same type. This system is of limited value. Certainly, tumours of grade 1 have a good prognosis, and tumours of grade 4 have a very bad one, but such tumours are rare. The great majority of tumours fall in grades 2 and 3, that is to say, in the usual range, and so may be expected to behave in the usual way. Grading according to the degree of anaplasia does little to indicate whether any individual patient with a tumour of grade 2 or grade 3 will do well or badly.

The division of tumours into grades according to the degree of anaplasia should not be confused with their division into stages according to the extent of their invasion and metastasis. Many schemes to record the extension of various kinds of tumours have been devised, and different methods are used in different centres. Recently, the Unio Internationalis Contra Cancrum has introduced a new system which it hopes will be widely adopted. In this system, the size, and local extension of the primary, the possible involvement of lymph nodes and the presence or absence of distant metastases are all considered. However, one of the best-known methods of recording the extension of a tumour is that introduced by Dukes for carcinoma of the rectum. Carcinomata which have not penetrated through the whole thickness of the rectal muscle are classed as stage A; those which have extended through the muscle into the perirectal fat but which have no metastases are called stage B; and those which have metastases in nodes or elsewhere are called stage C. The value of this method of staging is shown by the observation that some 90 per cent of the cases in which carcinoma of the rectum is found to be of stage A at operation survive 5 years, and more than 60 per cent of the cases in which the carcinoma is found to be of stage B, but less than 20 per cent of the cases in which it is found to be of stage C. Other kinds of tumour may be divided into stages in a similar manner, and often useful information is so gained. Less often, attention is paid to the rate of growth, but again useful information may be obtained. The use of staging as a guide to prognosis is based on the assumption that the individual tumour will continue to behave as it has done in the past, that a tumour which has invaded little will continue to invade little, or that one which has given rise to many metastases will continue to give rise to many metastases. This assumption is usually justified.

REFERENCES

The literature on the morphology and behaviour of tumours is immense. The following books have recently been published on the subject:

1. Ackerman, L. V., and del Regato, J. A. (1964). *Cancer: Diagnosis, Treatment and Prognosis*, 3rd edit. St. Louis: C. V. Mosby Co.

2. American Registry of Pathology (1951–67). *Atlas of Tumor Pathology* (12 sections). Washington, D.C.: Armed Forces Institute of Pathology. (Fascicles in course of publication.)
3. Evans, R. W. (1966). *Histological Appearances of Tumours*, 2nd edit. Edinburgh: E. & S. Livingstone.
4. Masson, P. (1956). *Tumeurs Humaines: Histologie, Diagnostics et Techniques*, 2-éme edit. Paris: Libraire Maloine.
5. Raven, R. W., Editor (1957–60). *Cancer* (7 volumes). London: Butterworth & Co.
6. Willis, R. A. (1960). *Pathology of Tumours*, 3rd edit. London: Butterworth & Co.

Chapter 23

THE EPIDEMIOLOGY OF CANCER

By I. Berenblum

Under the general title of "The Epidemiology of Cancer", the following topics will be discussed: some basic principles of tumour statistics; occupational and other forms of environmental tumours; the incidence and organ distribution of cancer according to geographical location; the interplay between race and environment; and the role of heredity in "spontaneous" cancer in man. Related information from animal experiments will be discussed in the next chapter.

Tumour Statistics in Man

Vital statistics, so boring a subject to the medical student, acquires a strange fascination to the medical graduate reporting on "Five New Cases of X Disease, with a Survey of the Literature". The "statistical" treatment in such a publication may consist of little more than the conversion of scanty data into percentages; from which far-reaching conclusions are then drawn about the incidence of the disease, its relationship to previous illnesses, diet, social habits, etc., with a blissful unawareness of the many pitfalls that may beset such analyses.

To avoid these pitfalls calls for knowledge of the mathematical principles of statistical methods (see Yule and Kendall[1]) and also an understanding of certain special factors peculiar to vital statistics (see Hill[2]). While the mathematical aspects lie outside the scope of this chapter, the special aspects must be examined here, to give meaning and significance to the discussion that follows.

Apart from problems of statistical computations, such as errors of sampling, there are five major sources of error in tumour statistics: (1) the age distribution of the population; (2) the accuracy of diagnosis; (3) the methods of collecting the data; (4) the degree of subdivision of the various tumour types; and (5) the degree of subdivision according to sex, marital status, and other biological factors. How seriously these five potential sources of error can influence the interpretation of statistical analyses will become apparent from the following illustrations.

(1) Age Distribution of the Population

While some diseases may affect all age groups fairly evenly, others are restricted to certain periods of life or are very much more prevalent at some ages than at others. To choose a rather grotesque example, the incidence of infantile diarrhœa in an Old Age Home would hardly provide a clue as to the prevalence of this disease in the country at large. Even when dealing with the incidence of this disease per *total* population, comparisons between two countries or between two different periods in the same country would still have doubtful meaning, unless one were sure that the proportion of infants to the rest of the population were the same in the groups being compared; or failing this, unless one could apply some correction factor to allow for the dissimilarities in the age distributions. Alternatively, one could calculate the incidence of the disease on the basis of the total number of infants under the age of one, irrespective of their proportion in the general population. This would, in fact, be the logical approach *for the particular example chosen here*, since infantile diarrhœa is, by definition, restricted to the first year of life, and the number of adults in the population is really irrelevant in such a case.

The situation about malignant tumours is more complicated, in that cancer is predominantly, though not exclusively, a disease of old age. Not only does the frequency of the disease increase with age, but the curve begins to rise steeply after middle life. This explains why about 50 per cent of all recorded cases of cancer in Western countries occur over the age of 65, *although this old-age group constitutes only about 8 per cent of the total population*. A slight increase in the average age of the population will, therefore, result in a strikingly large increase in the over-all incidence of cancer.

The average expectation of life has been rising steadily for a century or more, and so has the cancer incidence. We are thus faced with an important question: Can this increase in cancer incidence be entirely attributed to the ageing of the population or only partly so? Expressed in more practical terms, is it possible, by statistical manipulations, to "correct" for the increased ageing of the population, and thus detect any *residual* increase attributable to other factors?

This can be done in one of two ways.

By one method, the comparisons are confined to very narrow age groups. Thus, from each of the populations under study, the cancer incidence is determined within, say, 5-year age groups, each group being considered separately. The method has the added advantage of bringing to light any tendency for a shift in the age at which the incidence curve begins to rise sharply, as distinct from any change in total incidence. The method has, however, a serious limitation in that, with the division of each population into small groups, the number of cases per group may become so small as to introduce appreciable errors due to chance; moreover, a large number of separate figures are difficult to take in, and it is useful to have them summarized in the form of a single index.

This is nowadays achieved by the use of a correction factor—the "Standardized Mortality Ratio" (S.M.R.)—which shows the number of deaths registered in a particular year *as a percentage of those which would have been expected had the sex/age mortality of a standard period* (e.g. 1950–52) *operated then*[3]. It permits comparisons to be made, for instance, between recorded incidences from different sources, despite differences in age distribution.

In order to compare cancer incidences at different periods, *as a measure of the true increase in incidence of the disease*, an earlier standard period than 1950–52 would have to be chosen (e.g. 1900–1910). By such means, it is possible to show that part, at least, of the recorded increase in crude incidence of cancer during the past half-century is attributable to the ageing of the population.

Before accepting the "residual" increase, not accounted for by the ageing of the population, as due to a genuine rise in incidence (either through increased carcinogenic hazards in man's environment or because of a higher susceptibility of the population), the possibility of other factors must first be examined.

(2) Accuracy of Diagnosis

The extent to which cancer in man is accurately diagnosed has been variously estimated as ranging, in Western countries, from 60 to 90 per cent, depending not only on the competence of the clinical investigation, but also on the technical facilities available such as X-rays, biopsies, and histological confirmation at autopsy. The accuracy has undoubtedly improved during the past 50 years, partly through the introduction of new diagnostic methods, but more especially as the result of the extension of medical services which has accompanied the rise in living standards and education. With improved diagnosis more cases of cancer have been recognised, and the recorded total incidence has consequently risen. How important is this complicating factor?

When comparisons are attempted between countries in which standards of medical service are very dissimilar, the situation is so complex that often no valid conclusions are possible. For instance, the recorded cancer death rate per 100,000 of population is about 170 for England and Wales, and only about 10–20 for countries like Peru, Mexico, and Ceylon. In more under-developed countries, the figures are still lower, because the average life expectancy there is little more than 30 years, with a consequently low true cancer incidence, and because the few cases that do arise are mostly not diagnosed at all. This should warn one against accepting the common allegation that natives of certain countries are "immune" to cancer.

When comparisons are made between different periods in the same country, the problem is narrowed down somewhat, though the exact influence of improvement in diagnosis is still difficult to assess. Attempts have been made in this direction by comparing the discrepancies between clinical and post-mortem diagnoses at various periods; but such information deals only with hospitalised patients, not with the population at large. One can, however, apply certain indirect methods of gauging the extent to which this factor of improved diagnosis may have operated in accounting for the "residual" rise in recorded incidence: The scope for improvement in diagnosis is naturally greater in cases of tumours remotely situated in the body (where diagnosis is difficult) than in cases of tumours at more accessible sites (where diagnosis is easy). Thus, if after classifying malignant tumours into two categories—those at accessible sites (e.g. of skin, tongue, breast, and uterus) and those at remote sites (e.g. of brain, stomach, lung, and certain other internal organs)—it were found that the increase in recorded incidence affected both categories, one would be tempted to conclude that the increase was a genuine one; if, on the other hand, it were confined to tumours of remote sites, one might deduce that it was due to improved diagnosis.

When the "residual" increases, as defined above, were examined in this light, they were found to be largely confined to tumours at remote sites, thus suggesting that improvements in diagnosis were largely responsible for the recorded increases. In fact, the incidence of cancer at accessible sites seems to be decreasing.

(3) Methods of Collecting Data

There are two major types of vital statistics: *mortality rates*, which refer to the incidence of *deaths* from the disease per 1,000 of the living population, and *morbidity rates*, which refer to the incidence (usually expressed per 100,000 or

1,000,000 of the population), *as diagnosed in the living patient*. Each has its advantages and disadvantages from the point of view of the statistician.

The apparent conflict between the slogan "cancer strikes one in six" and the statement that "about one per 600 of the population develops cancer" is resolved when one remembers that the "one in six" refers to the ratio of cancer deaths to total deaths—the latter, in any one year, being a small fraction of the living population. The fact that a substantial, and growing, proportion of cancer cases is cured, must also be taken into account in attempting to convert mortality into morbidity figures, or *vice versa*. But the problem does not end there, for morbidity and mortality rates are derived from independent sources, and different errors are introduced accordingly.

The usual sources for mortality rates are (*a*) from the Registrar-General's figures (or comparable governmental figures in other countries), compiled from the recorded death certificates; (*b*) from the medical records of Insurance Companies; and (*c*) from autopsy records of hospitals. The first has the merit of comprehensiveness, since all deaths are reported by law; but it suffers from inaccuracy, the diagnosis in the death certificate being generally accepted without check. The second is subject to selection, as it only includes holders of insurance policies. Autopsy records have the highest degree of accuracy of diagnosis, but suffer from a double system of selection—one at admission to the hospital, and the other, with respect to the proportion of dead patients submitted to autopsy.

The usual sources of morbidity rates, in most countries, are from individual hospital records. In some countries, they are also available from lists compiled by Insurance Companies. Selection enters into both these sets of data. A more valuable source, however, is from National Cancer Registries[3]. These are compiled from fairly complete notifications of hospitalised cancer patients in the country, and the filed data include clinical and histological diagnosis, the kind of operation performed, and other useful information.

A few examples will indicate how such factors as selection, differences in accuracy of diagnosis, and changes in treatment can affect the results of statistical analyses: (*a*) a change in the policy for admission to a general hospital (e.g. by diverting patients with chronic lung diseases to tuberculosis sanatoria) will cause a change in the proportion of lung cancer wrongly diagnosed before admission; (*b*) a hospital famous for its brain surgery unit will attract many cases of brain tumours from distant regions, and both the morbidity and autopsy records for this type of tumour will show incidences out of proportion to those truly reflecting the region which the hospital normally serves; (*c*) increase in the staff of the pathology department of a hospital may lead to a rise in the proportion of autopsies performed, thereby minimising the factor of selection and raising the accuracy of recorded causes of death; (*d*) the more widespread use of X-ray equipment and other diagnostic facilities will raise the recorded morbidity rates; and (*e*) new discoveries for curing certain types of cancer will result in a fall in the mortality rates but not in the morbidity rates.

(4) Inclusion of Heterogeneous Types of Tumours in Single Categories

This factor operates in a different manner from those so far discussed, by tending to mask true differences in incidence. To take the extreme example where all forms of cancer are, for statistical purposes, grouped together as a single disease, a true increase in incidence of one type of tumour may be cancelled by a true fall in incidence of another. Even the general practice of listing tumours according to the organs affected is undesirable, since each organ may harbour different types of unrelated tumours. An interesting example of this is seen in the recent studies on the increase of lung-cancer incidence and its possible relation to smoking. The statistical correlation was found to hold for epidermoid cancer of the lung but not for adenocarcinoma of that organ; yet the two are usually classified together for statistical purposes. Other examples where independent ætiological factors are probably implicated in the same organ are (*a*) malignant melanoma of the skin versus other skin tumours, (*b*) carcinoma of the uterine cervix versus that of the uterine corpus, (*c*) osteogenic sarcoma versus other tumours of bone, and (*d*) lymphatic versus myelogenous leukæmia.

Failure to distinguish between metastases and primary tumours, especially in organs such as the liver, lung, and bone, in which metastases from other parts of the body are exceptionally common, may also lead to a serious distortion of the differential tumour incidence.

(5) **Other Factors**

In sorting statistical material according to tumour types, the factor of age distribution can play a complicated role.

The general statement that the frequency of cancer increases with age and that the curve rises steeply after middle life is true for total cancer but not necessarily for each individual type of tumour. The rise in the incidence is, for instance, very steep for carcinomas but only slight for sarcomas. The death-rate per million *for carcinomas* is about 10 for people under the age of 25, and about 12,500 for those over that age; the corresponding figures *for sarcomas* are 25 and 250, respectively. When the sarcomas are further sub-divided, it is found that only some of those affecting "soft tissues" increase gradually with age, while that of bone has a peak incidence in the second and third decades of life. The incidence of leukæmia is actually highest in infancy and early childhood, with a secondary peak in later life.

The other, unconnected, factors that have to be taken into consideration by the statistician in evaluating tumour incidences include sex, marital status, diet, occupation, social status, customs, etc. We shall refer here briefly only to the first two, as the others will be more fully discussed later.

Tumours of reproductive organs in women (i.e. of the breast, uterus, ovary) constitute, in Western countries, well over 30 per cent of all forms of tumours in that sex; those in men (i.e. of the prostate, testis, breast) constitute less than 10 per cent of all forms. Yet the total cancer incidence in the two sexes is about equal. This is not so in all countries, and even where the situation does arise, the incidence for women is higher when calculated for the child-bearing period of life. While some authors[4] still believe that this apparent equalisation between the sexes is an indication of a single, over-all susceptibility to cancer, this is not generally accepted. There is, in fact, a wealth of experimental evidence to show that separate genetic (and environmental) factors operate independently for the different types of tumours in the different organs (see Chapter 24).

Marital status can also affect cancer incidence, and should therefore be taken into account in statistical studies. For instance, cancer of the breast is more common in unmarried than in married women—a difference presumably connected with variations in hormone balance. Another example is that of cancer of the uterine cervix, the incidence of which is higher in married than in unmarried women, and rises with the number of pregnancies, while cancer of the uterine corpus is higher in unmarried women.

Types of Comparisons

In addition to direct comparisons of mortality or morbidity rates, comparisons are often made in the form of percentages of *specific* tumour types to *total* tumours. Cancer of the digestive tract may, for instance, constitute 50 per cent of all tumours in one country, but only 5 per cent in another. By this method, however, errors due to varying age distribution and to differences in accuracy of diagnosis operate at their maximum; furthermore, errors due to small numbers cannot be checked when the results are presented in this form. Consequently, the alleged differences in incidence, judged by this method, are often spurious, and should be interpreted with caution. On the whole, less reliance should be placed on unusually *low* incidences, in comparison with average figures from most other countries, than on exceptionally *high* incidences for certain specific types of tumours, sometimes encountered in particular localities.

There is a useful modification of the method just described, whereby the *ratio between two chosen types of tumour* is taken for comparison. Such values may reveal true differences, even when the age distribution of the populations and the accuracy of diagnosis are dissimilar, provided (*a*) that the pairs of tumour types chosen for comparison do not tend to arise at very different age periods as would be the case, for instance, if carcinomas were compared with sarcomas, or cancer of the lung with that of the prostate; and (*b*) that the ease of diagnosis in the two cases is not too dissimilar as would be the case, for instance, if comparisons were made between skin tumours and those of the brain or lung. Satisfactory examples of such paired comparisons are: tumours of the breast and uterus, uterine cervix and corpus, scrotum and penis, stomach and œsophagus, stomach and large intestine, lung and larynx.

Occupational Tumours

The first authenticated report of an occupational tumour—that of "scrotal cancer in chimney-sweeps"—appeared in 1775. This was long before the establishment of modern pathology and bacteriology, at a time when the very concept of extrinsic causes of disease was still in its infancy. Little progress was made until a century later, when new types of occupational tumours, many resulting from new industrial processes, were discovered. Since then, the field has expanded greatly, and the literature on the subject is now very extensive.[5, 6]

Radiation Effects

One example of tumour development related to occupation, which must have existed for thousands of years, though the association was recognised only towards the end of last century, is that of skin cancer among farmers and fishermen. The condition arises late in life, and is often preceded by the familiar "weather-beaten complexion", technically known as "solar dermatitis", which comprises a wrinkled dry skin and excessive pigmentation, with scaly thickening (keratosis), telangiectases, and later, focal areas of atrophy and depigmentation. The tumours that eventually develop include papillomas which may ultimately become malignant, or initial squamous carcinomas, or basal-cell carcinomas, and are mainly located on the face. Dark-coloured people are practically immune to this form of occupational tumour though not to skin melanomas, which have a different ætiology; and among whites, blondes are the most susceptible. Thus, deficiency of skin pigment is a decisive factor.

The disease is particularly prevalent in Australia, and in other regions in the world where fair-skinned people work long hours out-of-doors in sunny climates. The relation between sunlight and skin tumour induction has been experimentally confirmed in animals, and the carcinogenic effect narrowed down to a range of the U.V. spectrum below 3,200 Å.[7] The significant clinical aspects to be noted are: (*a*) the strict limitation of the condition to the exposed parts of the skin; (*b*) the long latent period, measurable in decades, during which solar dermatitis is a prominent feature; and (*c*) the frequency of multiple tumours.

A more dramatic development of tumours attributable to radiation occurred among the pioneers of the use of X-rays several years after the invention of the X-ray tube. Through ignorance of the harmful effects of these rays and through failure to take adequate precautions, these early workers began to suffer from varying degrees of "radiodermatitis" of the exposed skin of the hands, arms, and face—a condition not unlike the more extreme forms of solar dermatitis. In a high proportion of cases carcinomas and less often sarcomas eventually arose in the affected skin, with a latent period decidedly shorter than that following solar or ultraviolet radiation. The tumours were often multiple, in one case numbering ten independent malignancies in the same person.

Since the low-voltage machines then in use emitted very "soft" rays that had little penetrating power, the harmful effects were largely confined to the skin, and even thin articles of clothing served as a fairly effective protection. With the introduction of machines emitting "harder" rays, which readily penetrated clothing and the various tissues of the body, delayed effects on internal organs became a serious potential hazard. In such cases, however, the association of a tumour developing in later life with any former radiation was often overlooked. Experimental demonstration in animals of the carcinogenic action of X-rays on the ovaries, and on lymphoid and myeloid tissues,[8] confirmed the early impressions of the hazard in man, and subsequent statistical studies established the association, demonstrating, for instance, a raised incidence of leukæmia among the survivors of the Hiroshima atomic explosion.[9]

Several other examples of occupational tumours attributable to radiation call for special comment.

For many centuries the miners of Schneeberg (Saxony) and Jàchimov (Bohemia) were known to suffer from a strange chronic pulmonary disease. A high proportion of the men were affected, and the ultimate outcome was always fatal, the disease being eventually identified as a malignant tumour of the lung. The mines in question are rich in many minerals, including radium, and different components of the inhaled dust (arsenic, cobalt, etc.) have, from time to time, been suspected as the causative agent. While proof is yet lacking, it is generally agreed that the radioactivity of the inhaled dust is responsible for the disease.

Another unusual type of occupational tumour due to radiation was discovered some 40 years ago, in a factory in the United States, where the hands and dials of watches and clocks were painted with a luminous paint containing zinc sulphide with traces of radioactive material. Minute amounts of the paint, swallowed by the working girls while pointing the brushes between their lips, led to the absorption of the radioactive material, its uptake by the reticulo-endothelial cells of the bone marrow, and its ultimate incorporation in the bone. The emitted radiation led to bone resorption, anæmia associated with leucopænia, and several years later, to the development of multiple osteogenic sarcomas of bone.

A further example of a carcinogenic hazard associated with radioactivity—belonging to a category of therapeutic rather than occupational use—is associated with injections of colloidal thorium dioxide (thorotrast) as a contrast medium in diagnostic radiology.This weakly-radioactive substance has been shown to be carcinogenic in animals; while cases of human tumours attributable to it have also been reported in the literature.

A possible danger of some magnitude, which must be faced in the future, is concerned with the use of atomic energy for the generation of domestic power, and more generally, with the use of radioactive materials for industrial application. Though the necessary precautions to be taken are by now well understood and the regulations are no doubt enforced at present, their relaxation will become probable with the more widespread use of these materials throughout the world.

Chemical Agents

As already mentioned, the first recognised cases of extraneously induced cancer were those connected with the occupation of chimney-sweeping. The men in question who, two centuries ago, tended to start work as "climbing boys" in early childhood, began to develop their tumours 20 years or more after entering the hazardous occupation, and sometimes not until several years after relinquishing it. The resulting tumours were usually confined to the scrotal skin (in which the soot persisted longest when personal cleanliness was inadequate). It was clear from the start that the soot was responsible for the disease.

This material, which accumulates in chimneys when coal is burnt in open fire-places, characteristic of English homes, is a by-product of the incomplete combustion of the coal, the products of carbonisation condensing in the colder parts of the chimney. It is noteworthy that England is the only country in which chimney-sweep cancer has ever been described.

High-temperature destructive distillation of coal in the virtual absence of air, as in the manufacture of coal-gas, produces a somewhat similar by-product in much larger quantities, namely *coal-tar*. This material, originally an undesirable by-product in the manufacture of coal-gas, has since acquired wide use in industry, in the form of solvents and lubricants, as the source for the refined aromatic hydrocarbon chemicals, and also in the crude form, or as pitch, for the manufacture of fuels, for roofing, road-surfacing, and other uses. It soon became apparent that coal-tar was even more potently carcinogenic for the skin than soot, and was responsible for many cases of occupational skin cancer, not only among workers engaged in the manufacture of coal-tar itself, but also of the unrefined high-boiling fractions such as crude creosote, anthracene oil and pitch. Unlike chimney-sweep cancer, which accounts for only a few cases annually and is confined to England, tar cancer occurs in larger numbers (over 100 cases per year) in the industrialised countries of the world. Tumours begin to develop only after many years of daily exposure, and the skin of the head and neck, arms and hands are affected as well as that of the scrotum.

Coal itself, from which the tar is obtained, is not carcinogenic; nor are the majority of *purified* end-products derived from the tar, such as benzene, naphthalene, anthracene, and most of their derivatives.

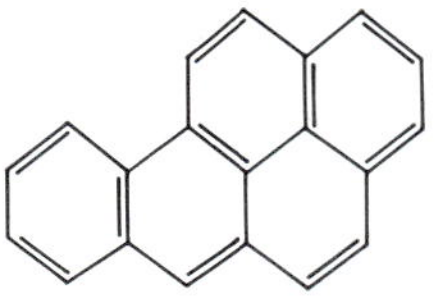

(I) 3:4-*benzpyrene*, potent carcinogen.

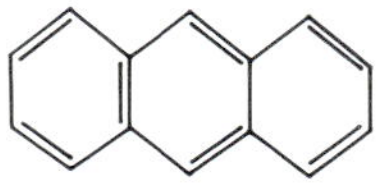

(II) *Anthracene*, non-carcinogenic.

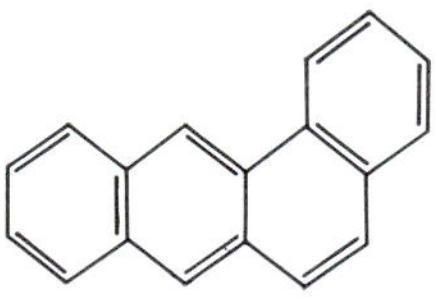

(III) 1:2-*benzanthracene*, possessing borderline carcinogenicity.

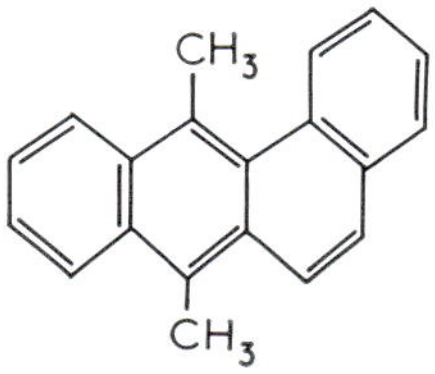

CH_3

CH_3

(IV) 9:10-*dimethyl*-1:2-*benzanthracene*, a very potent carcinogen.

While the chemistry of carcinogenic tars will be discussed in some detail in the next chapter, a few of the essential facts may be mentioned here, because of the bearing they have on the occupational hazard in man: (*a*) the potent carcinogen isolated from coal-tar—3:4-benzpyrene (I)—is a polycyclic aromatic hydrocarbon comprising 5 fused benzene rings; (*b*) tar also contains other carcinogens belonging to the same class of compound; (*c*) experimental studies have shown that carcinogenic activity (for mouse skin) is restricted, among the polycyclic hydrocarbons, to a few of the more complex members (5–6 fused benzene rings), with hardly any activity among the lower members (II and III); yet considerable activity is found among some of the *alkyl derivatives* of 4-benzene ring derivatives (IV), depending on the positions of substitution, and slight activity even among derivatives of 3-benzene ring compounds.[10]

Another important group of occupational skin cancers is that associated with the crude distillation products of mineral oils, including oils derived from shale and asphalt deposits. Here also, the natural products (natural oil from the wells or solid shale) are not carcinogenic; yet the crude products obtained from them by high-temperature distillation are a source of serious carcinogenic hazard. The most active fractions are among the lubricating oils and heavy fuel oils, while the lighter fuels and solvents, the pure long-chained aliphatic hydrocarbons, and the semi-refined waxes are entirely non-carcinogenic. Chemically, the products of mineral oils are olefinic rather than aromatic, though, through the industrial process of "cracking", oils rich in aromatic compounds can be obtained. However, since some oils which contain only traces of 3:4-benzpyrene and related compounds are highly carcinogenic, and since their carcinogenic properties are somewhat different from those of coal-tar, it must be concluded that their carcinogenic constituents belong to a different class of compounds from the aromatic carcinogens of coal-tar.

Knowledge of the carcinogenic hazards of mineral oils came from two different sources: (1) the discovery of skin cancer of the hands and arms of the paraffin workers in the Scottish shale-oil industry,[11] and (2) the observations, in the Lancashire cotton-spinning industry, of similar tumours affecting the scrotum, thighs, abdomen, penis, and other parts of the skin acted upon by the lubricating oils which soaked through clothing.[12] The latter form of occupational cancer, known as "mule-spinner's cancer", began to appear a few decades after the change-over from vegetable to mineral lubricating oils in this industry. Comparative studies of mineral oils from different geographical locations have demonstrated significant differences in potencies, Russian and Pennsylvanian oils having relatively low carcinogenic potencies, while Venezuelan and Scottish (shale) oils have high potencies, though the conditions of refining are probably more important factors than location of origin of the oil.

A very different kind of occupational cancer, this time affecting the urinary bladder, was discovered in Germany in 1895 among men engaged in the manufacture of synthetic dyestuffs. As the industry expanded, cases began to appear in other countries with alarming frequency. Hueper estimates that there were close on 1,500 cases by 1952.

The possibility that the finished dyes were responsible for the disease was soon ruled out although, as will be shown later, some dyes are carcinogenic for some organs other than the bladder. Attention was then directed towards the "intermediate products"—phenolic, quinone, and amino derivatives of benzene, naphthalene, and anthracene from which the dyes are manufactured. At least two of the intermediate products—β-naphthylamine (V) and benzidine (VI)—are now known to be implicated as causative agents of the disease in man.

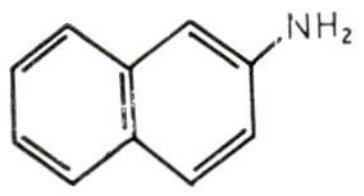

(V) *β-Naphthylamine.*

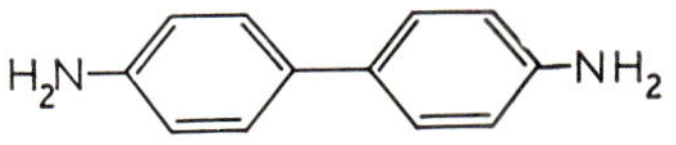

(VI) *Benzidine.*

The tumours—transitional-cell papillomas and carcinomas of the bladder epithelium—usually make their appearance after a latent period of 5–30 years of occupation, during which time intermittent hæmaturia is sometimes observed. The important feature of this type of occupational cancer is that the organ affected is remote from any primary site of action (skin, lung, or gastro-intestinal tract), the causative agent, or more probably its metabolite, reaching the bladder through the urine, after being excreted by the kidneys.

The examples so far discussed illustrate the diversity of occupational tumours, but by no means exhaust the list. Among the more important other forms associated with industrial processes are the following[5,6]: Cancer of the lung associated with hot tar fumes from gas-generator retorts, also with the manufacture of chromates, with exposure to asbestos, and with nickel refining; cancer of the nasal cavity and sinuses in association with nickel refining and with the manufacture of *iso*propyl alcohol (probably due to impurities rather than to the alcohol); and leukæmia connected with long-term inhalation of benzene. Though doubts have been expressed about the older reports that trivalent arsenic is a cause of occupational skin cancer, recent observations seem to substantiate the view that it has a mild carcinogenic action on human skin. The action as systemic, and the tumour distribution unusual, the arms and *especially the palms of the hands and soles of the feet* being mainly affected.

Some mention should also be made of "potential" occupational cancers. This refers to substances whose carcinogenic properties have been demonstrated experimentally in animals, though no cancers have so far been reported in man. The list includes (i) 2-acetylaminofluorene, originally intended as an insecticide, whose carcinogenic properties, on a variety of tissues in animals, were fortunately discovered through chronic toxicity tests before the substance was marketed; (ii) chloroform, carbon tetrachloride, and probably other chlorinated aliphatic hydrocarbons, which are not only highly toxic for the liver, but eventually produce tumours in that organ; (iii) tannic acid, also hepatotoxic, and carcinogenic for the liver; (iv) beryllium, carcinogenic for bone; (v) selenium, carcinogenic for the liver; (vi) thiourea, carcinogenic for the liver and thyroid gland; and (vii) *p*-dimethylaminoazobenzene (butter yellow), once used in traces for colouring butter, which in large doses is a potent carcinogen for the rat's liver. Certain other dyes, used for colouring foods, are suspected of being carcinogenic, though the ones which experimentally produce local sarcomas at the site of subcutaneous injection in animals are innocuous when given by mouth. (For other potential carcinogens in man's environment, not associated with specific occupations, see below.)

Physical Injuries

There is finally the question whether mechanical and thermal injuries are carcinogenic in man. The problem is a difficult one, because unlike occupational tumours restricted to specific industries, where the noxious stimulus is fairly specific, and where the tumour incidence among the men at risk can be compared with that of the general population, in the case of mechanical and thermal injuries the stimulus is non-specific, and the general population itself comprises the men at risk.

Let us first consider trauma, in the restricted sense of *mechanical* injury—single or multiple. Claims in the literature have ranged from the statement that "44·7 per cent of all malignant tumours in man are caused by trauma" to the other extreme that "there is no proof that a single tumour has ever been caused by trauma". This diversity of opinion is partly the result of the lax use of the term "trauma", and partly arises from a number of inherent difficulties of the problem.[13] For instance, (*a*) the tumour, in a reported case, may have been genuine but the injury may have been imagined by the patient later on, as an unconscious process of rationalisation; (*b*) both the injury and the tumour may have been genuine, but the association fortuitous, especially when occurring at accessible sites (breast, bone, etc.) where both injuries and tumours are not uncommon; (*c*) the injury may merely have drawn the patient's attention to a pre-existing tumour; and (*d*) the injury may have served as a precipitating factor in a tissue already rendered preneoplastic.

It is now generally recognised that certain postulates must be satisfied before an alleged association between an injury and a tumour can be accepted: There must be demonstrable evidence of the injury (e.g. a wound, scar, hæmatoma, or fracture) at the site where the tumour later appears; there must be evidence that no tumour was present prior to the injury; there must be histological proof of the neoplastic nature of the alleged tumour; the tumour must be compatible with the local tissue, to exclude a metastasis from elsewhere, localised by the injury; there must be a reasonable time relationship (not too short) between the injury and the appearance of the tumour; and the possibility of other carcinogenic factors operating at the site must be excluded.

The vast majority of reported cases in the literature, in which a tumour was reputed to have been brought on by a *single* trauma, fail to obey these postulates; while the rare examples that appear to conform could readily be attributed to chance association. Thus, the "irritation theory of cancer", in the strict sense of the term, is unacceptable.

The same is probably true of *repeated* mild mechanical injuries, though the problem there is more complicated, because of the length of time of action, allowing for other factors to operate at the same time. For instance, rare cases of carcinoma of the bridge of the nose, attributed to irritation from ill-fitting spectacles, are probably due to sunlight; skin cancers in engineering trades, attributed to mechanical injuries, may owe their origin to carcinogenic lubricating oils; carcinoma of the tongue, attributed to irritation from jagged teeth or an ill-fitting denture, may owe its origin to a variety of factors such as excessive smoking, burns from hot food and syphilitic infection. There is also the added complicating possibility of mechanical irritation merely acting as a contributory (promoting) factor, precipitating a tumour which owes its origin (initiating action) to a true carcinogenic stimulus.[13]

The case for *thermal* injuries being responsible for tumour induction is more definite, though some features of the association are not clear. A number of authenticated cases have been described in which a skin carcinoma resulted from a local burn or scalding, either arising within a year of the injury before it had properly healed, or, in the "latent" form, developing in a scar from a burn 20 years or more after the initial injury. The ease with which a severe burn is characterised and remembered, and the unusual situations in the body in which the burn and the resulting tumour often occur (e.g. on the upper surface of the foot, or at the elbow, where skin cancers are normally almost unknown), substantiate the validity of the alleged association. Moreover, skin tumours have been successfully induced, in small numbers, in mice following single or multiple burns. The unusual feature of the association is that, though burns of various degrees are so common in man, tumours due to burns are extremely rare. It suggests that other factors ("precancerous" conditions, other carcinogens operating at the same site, or an exceptional susceptibility to carcinogenesis of the person's skin) must be required as well. The same applies to frost-bites as a very rare cause of skin tumour induction, substantiated both clinically and experimentally.

Medico-legal Aspects

Before leaving the subject of occupational tumours, a few words should be said about public health and medico-legal aspects of the problem, the former dealing with preventive measures, and the latter with questions of compensation. Public health authorities in the more advanced countries are becoming aware of their responsibility to investigate cases of occupational tumours, to formulate suitable preventive or protective measures for the workers exposed to the hazards, and, more hesitantly, to impose restrictive legislation. The issue has recently been taken up by international bodies such as the International Union Against Cancer, and the International Agency for Research on Cancer (Lyons), who are conducting world-wide surveys of existing, and suspected, types of occupational cancer, and advising governments of the dangers involved and of the steps to be taken to reduce the risks.

The legal aspects, concerned with compensation, are unsatisfactory in most countries, and judgements in law courts sometimes err towards undue generosity when, for instance, claims are allowed for a dubious association between a physical injury and cancer. They often err the other way, by dismissing claims for genuine occupational tumours. In the absence of a clear directive through appropriate legislation, the members of a jury are naturally bewildered by conflicting opinions of "expert" witnesses.

Conclusions

The long latent period (usually 5–25 years) from the commencement of exposure to the appearance of the tumour, is one of the most characteristic features of occupational cancer. In cases where exposure normally starts at a relatively early age, the average age distribution of the resulting tumour tends to be lower than that of the same type of tumour arising "spontaneously" in the general population. From these two facts it is possible to deduce that the length of exposure, and not the age of the individual, is the determining factor in tumour formation. Once this is recognised as a general principle of carcinogenesis, the tendency for the disease to occur late in life becomes understandable. By implication, this helps to disprove the old idea that neoplasia is a consequence of the ageing of the tissues.

The fact that occupational tumours may arise several years after relinquishing the hazardous occupation indicates that the carcinogenic process can become irreversible before the visible appearance of the tumour.

Occupational tumours are histologically indistinguishable from those arising in the same tissue "spontaneously". The pathological changes in the tissue during the latent period have always been considered to represent a "precancerous state"; yet, according to recent experimental evidence, they may, after all, constitute a side reaction unconnected with the neoplastic process. Most carcinogens are toxic, apart from being carcinogenic.

Recognition of a carcinogenic risk, especially in an industrial plant in which the specific tumour incidence is high, provides the opportunity to prevent the disease from arising in the first place, either through avoidance of the use of the incriminating substance, or through adequate protective precautions. Close co-operation between public health authorities and factory managements is necessary for this to be effective.

Non-occupational Environmental Tumours

To divide environmental tumours into *occupational* and *non-occupational* categories may at first seem artificial, especially where the same carcinogenic factor is involved and where the resulting tumour is also the same. Skin carcinogenesis from exposure to sunlight does not differ whether it arises in a farmer, in pursuance of his occupation, or in any other individual who exposes himself unduly to sunlight all his life. The problem becomes more complicated, and the methods of study involved more diverse, when the *occupational* hazard belongs to a restricted industry while the *non-occupational* one is distributed throughout the population. Thus, contact with tar in industry, and the possible role of tarry products dispersed in the atmosphere of a smoky city, are methodologically very different problems.[14] Similarly, X-ray cancer of the skin, first noted as an occupational disease among the pioneers of radiology, has not infrequently been observed among patients receiving excessive X-ray therapy often for a trivial skin disease, while the association of leukæmia with repeated mild doses of radiation, originally recognised among radiologists, is now known also to arise, in rare cases, from repeated therapeutic or diagnostic radiation. To what extent "spontaneous" leukæmia in adults, or other tumours arising in the general population, may be the result of previous, forgotten, exposures to radiation, is a difficult, but important problem to solve. Even a single, massive, dose as suffered by the inhabitants of Hiroshima at the time of the atomic explosion, has been found to be responsible for an increased incidence of leukæmia in later years.[9] At the other extreme, there is the possibility of tumours arising from the cumulative effects of minute amounts of radiation (the background and "fall-out" radiations). Finally, there are the environmental tumours associated with habits and customs, including diets and dietary additives, medicines, and infections. These, too, involve techniques of study and carry implications that are very different from those connected with occupational cancer.

It is becoming more and more apparent that papillomas, squamous carcinomas, and basal-cell carcinomas of the face in old men, even where no marked "precancerous" solar dermatitis is evident, are generally attributable to sunlight except, of course, for those cases which are associated with occupations involving such substances as tar. The same probably holds for cancer of the lip, previously attributed to pipe smoking. The fact that only the lower lip, which is more exposed than the upper lip to actinic rays, is involved, and that the incidence of cancer of the lip and of cancer of the face run more or less parallel on a geographical basis, supports this interpretation. The modern fashion of excessive sun-bathing, or daily exposures to radiation from a U.V. lamp, may involve an element of carcinogenic risk.

There is a rare congenital disease, known as *Xeroderma pigmentosum*, which is characterised by an extreme hypersusceptibility to light, so that the typical "solar dermatitis" develops on the hands and face in early childhood, even when exposure is only to diffuse light. A high proportion of cases develop skin cancer, frequently multiple, by the age of twenty.

Regarding tumour development through thermal injury, some unusual examples have been described, such as the high incidence of cancer of the roof of the mouth in certain regions of South America, India, and Sardinia, among men who practise the strange custom of cigar smoking with the lighted end inside the mouth. That carcinogenic tars from the ash might be a contributory factor is a possibility to be taken into account. Such a double carcinogenic action is more likely still in "Kangri cancer" in Kashmir, which arises as the result of the burning of charcoal in special Kangri baskets worn close to the skin under the clothing, for warmth. Such factors are probably also operative in the reported cases of skin cancer of the legs among stokers and firemen.

The high incidence of œsophageal cancer among Chinese males has also been attributed to thermal injury—from the swallowing of very hot rice. However, the association, in this case, has not been proved.

Another example of cancer of the mouth arising through a strange custom is that occurring among the poorer inhabitants of Travancore (India) and of Ceylon, addicted to "betel nut" chewing. The quid, held in the cheek all day long, and sometimes even during sleep, is composed of a mixture of betel nut, tobacco, and lime. There is evidence to suggest that the carcinogenic action is attributable to the tobacco and lime rather than to the betel nut, despite the name "betel nut cancer".

An important example of tumour formation related to a custom, where the association is, as it were, in reverse, is that of cancer of the penis—a not uncommon type of tumour among uncircumcised people, but never found in Jews, who perform circumcision in infants a week after birth. Among Mohammedans, who perform the operation between the 3rd and 14th year, the condition does occur, though less frequently than among the uncircumcised.[15] The retained smegma is generally credited with carcinogenic or cocarcinogenic properties. It is possible that it merely serves as a vehicle for carcinogenic tarry materials from the environment.

Primary cancer of the lung, which was a rare disease in man 50 years ago, has increased in frequency to a phenomenal degree (up to 50-fold, according to some figures). This increase, which cannot be explained entirely by improvements in diagnosis, has been attributed to cigarette smoking.[16, 17] The fact that for the past 30 years or so, the incidence of lung cancer appears to have followed the consumption of tobacco, is in itself not very convincing evidence. Statistical correlations can serve as pointers but not as proof of a true association: a similar correlation might well exist between the incidence of lung cancer and the sales of refrigerators. More telling evidence is the fact that the incidence is highest among heavy cigarette smokers, less so among moderate cigarette smokers, and lowest among non-smokers and cigar or pipe smokers. (See also recent prospective studies.[3])

Experimental studies in animals were inconclusive, for although tarry extracts of tobacco smoke proved to be mildy carcinogenic when painted on skin, attempts to induce lung tumours by subjecting mice daily to an atmosphere of tobacco smoke proved unsuccessful. The slight rise in the incidence of adenomas of the lung, reported by some investigators, is probably unrelated to the problem of bronchiogenic carcinoma in man. Certain discrepancies, difficult to explain, have also been encountered in the statistical correlations in man, e.g. with respect to (*a*) the incidence of the disease in different countries in relation to their smoking habits; (*b*) the variations in the relative frequencies in the two sexes; and (*c*) the fact that a genuine correlation should have involved a 20–30-year lag period, to allow for the latent period of carcinogenesis.

There is evidence[14,18] that atmospheric pollution is partially responsible for the rise in the incidence of cancer of the lung in some urban districts. It has been suggested that some cancers of the lung may owe their origin to the exhaust fumes from petrol or diesel engines, or from dust of asphalted roads, especially since such fumes and dusts are known to contain carcinogenic constituents. However, no clinical evidence for such an association is yet available, and the products in question must, for the time being, be placed in the category of "potential" carcinogenic hazards only.

One might have supposed that the gastro-intestinal tract should have been the area *par excellence* to be implicated in environmental cancer; for the stomach and large intestine, which account for almost 50 per cent of human cancers in Western countries, though anatomically internal organs, are functionally external in the sense that they are continually under dietary, i.e. environmental, influence. In animals, spontaneous tumours of the gastro-intestinal tract are extremely rare, which would suggest that the complexity of the human diet, and perhaps the factor of cooking, are responsible for the difference. Yet, domesticated animals, which share man's food, fail to reflect the human cancer pattern. The idea that highly spiced food may be a causative factor in gastric cancer, is improbable, since the incidence of this disease is rare in India and South East Asia in general, where such flavouring is most common.

The experimental approach in animals has also proved disappointing[19, 20] for, while the forestomach of mice and rats, *which is covered by squamous epithelium*, responds readily to a variety of carcinogenic agents administered by mouth, the glandular portion of the stomach does not. This applies not only to polycyclic aromatic hydrocarbons, but also to heated fats, heated cholesterol, and a number of other products associated with human cooked foods.

It is important to note, in this connection, that the liver is exceptionally susceptible to neoplastic change through dietary factors, as evidenced by both clinical observations and experimental studies.

In the previous section, a distinction was made between types of occupational cancer where the carcinogenicity of the causative agent is established for man and those, designated "potential" occupational cancers, where the agent is known to be carcinogenic for animals but not proven for man. The same could be applied to non-occupational, environmental cancer—i.e. for substances which find their way into man's normal environment. In this connection, the growing use of synthetic products as food additives, colorants, anti-oxidants and emulsifiers, and as pesticides, cosmetics, pharmaceutical products, etc., raises the problem that some of these might indeed be carcinogenic for man. (Most of them have never been tested for carcinogenicity in animals.) The fact, for instance, that some dyes are carcinogenic for the liver, or subcutaneously, is a warning signal. Attention should also be drawn to recent findings that many simple alkylating agents are carcinogenic.[21] Of particular importance are the recent findings that certain natural products—notably some alkaloids of the *Senecio* groups of plants[22] and of aflatoxin (a product of the common mould *Aspergillus flavus*)[21]—are carcinogenic for the liver in animals.

Finally, while tumours of endocrine and reproductive organs are essentially endogenous in origin, extrinsic factors can play a decisive role in the production of thyroid tumours through iodine deficiency, and in breast cancer through excessive œstrone action, although this latter fact has so far been established only in animals. Note should be taken of the increasing use of synthetic œstrogens in cosmetics, and as implanted pellets in fowl used for human consumption.

The Geographical Pathology of Cancer

The systematic study of cancer according to geographical location, which has received much attention in recent years, is known under the name of "geographical pathology" of cancer. Such comparative studies might appear, at first sight, to contradict the principles laid down in the opening section of this chapter, that marked differences in age distribution of populations, and wide variations in accuracy of diagnosis and reporting of cancer cases, tend to vitiate statistical comparisons among countries of very different levels of civilisation. It was, however, pointed out that allowances could be made for these disturbing factors, and that even where direct comparisons of incidences were not valid, the demonstration of pronounced differences in organ distribution of the disease could, under certain prescribed conditions, be significant. A concise description, in non-mathematical terms, of the techniques employed in studies of the geographical pathology of cancer is given by Dunham and Dorn.[23]

Table I presents schematically the relative frequencies of six important types of cancer in different countries in the world. While minor variations in the Table may be ignored, some of the major ones are so striking as to constitute, without a doubt, true differences in incidence, portraying local conditions—racial or environmental—which profoundly influence the genesis of the disease.

Particularly noteworthy features in Table I are: (*a*) the higher frequency of breast than of uterine cancer in Europe and the United States, the reverse being true in Eastern countries, where cancer of the cervix is particularly common; (*b*) the exceptionally low incidence of breast cancer in Japan (a country where the statistical data are fairly reliable); (*c*) the high incidence of stomach cancer in Northern parts of Europe, Iceland, the United States, and Japan, with a variable low frequency in other countries (though, in some of the latter, poor diagnosis must be taken into account); (*d*) the high frequency of œsophageal cancer in China; (*e*) the very high incidence of primary liver cancer among the Bantu of Portuguese West Africa, and South Africa, and in Eastern countries; and (*f*) the high frequency of cancer of the oral cavity in most Eastern countries which is attributable, at least in part, to the environmental factors already discussed.

Other unusual distribution patterns that have been reported [24, 25] include *high frequencies*: of skin cancer in Australia, of thyroid cancer in Switzerland, of skin melanoma among Negroid people, of angiosarcoma of the skin (Kaposi's sarcoma) in Algeria and Uganda, of urinary bladder cancer in Egypt and Iraq (attributed to Bilharzia infection), of penile cancer and chorioncarcinoma in Viet-Nam, of chorioncarcinoma and malignant lymphoma in the Philippines; of uterine cancer in Latin American countries; of œsophageal cancer in South

Africa, Jamaica and Puerto Rico; and *unusually low frequencies*: of breast cancer in Egypt, of cancer of the colon and rectum in Iceland where gastric cancer is unusually common, and of lung cancer in Japan.

Perhaps the most important of all these unusual tumours is primary cancer of the liver, which is so rare a tumour in European and American countries, and so common in Central and South Africa and the Far East. The subject has been most exhaustively studied among the Bantu in South Africa.[24, 26]

23/TABLE I

SCHEMATIC TABULATION OF THE RELATIVE FREQUENCIES OF SIX TYPES OF CANCER IN VARIOUS COUNTRIES

	Breast	*Cervix*	*Œsophagus*	*Stomach*	*Liver*	*Oral Cavity*
Britain, Northern and Central Europe, and United States .	+++++	+++	++	(+++)[1] +++++	±	+
Japan . .	+	++++	++	+++++	+++	++
China . .	++	+++	++++	+++	(+)[2] ++++	++
Philippines .	+++	++	+	++	+++	++++
Sumatra:						
(*a*) Chinese .	+	+	++	+++	++++	+
(*b*) Malayan .	+	+++	±	+	+++++	+++
India . .	++[3]	+++++[3]	++	+	++	++++
South Africa (Bantu) .	++	++++[4]	±	++	+++++	(+++)[5] +

[1] Lower incidence in Britain than in the rest of Europe or U.S.A.; highest in Sweden, Finland and Iceland.

[2] The high incidence refers to Southern China; the incidence is low in Northern China.

[3] Proportion of breast to uterine cancer in India varies according to communities (e.g. breast cancer is high among Parsees).

[4] Also unusually high incidence of cancer of uterine corpus.

[5] Relatively high incidence if carcinoma of maxillary antrum and of salivary glands is included.

Not only is its incidence very high among these people, but its onset is usually in young adult life, and not infrequently in children. It affects males much more than females, and is invariably fatal.

A racial (hereditary) basis for this disease can be easily ruled out. The extreme rarity of primary liver cancer among the not-too-distantly related American Negro, and its wide geographical distribution in many other parts of the world not only argue against racial influence and in favour of an environmental one, but also suggest that the extrinsic factor involved must be of a very general kind, yet one which is absent in the West. There is finally the significant fact that the age of onset of the disease is very low indeed among the Bantu, and that its pathology is associated with a multilobular cirrhosis, a condition denoting long-term liver damage. All these observations indicate that *the extrinsic ætiological factor probably begins to operate in infancy or early childhood.* This points to diet as the most likely factor.

The diet of the Bantu generally consists of "mealie pap" (maize porridge) and sour milk, supplemented by fruit, and only rarely by meat. Though such a diet has been shown to induce degenerative changes in the liver of rats, leading to cirrhotic changes, there is as yet no evidence that the deficient diet *alone* is responsible for the high incidence of cancer of the liver in man or experimental animal. Carcinoma of the liver can readily be induced experimentally in animals, however, not only with certain azo dyes, *but also by prolonged choline deficiency.*[27] Infection has also been considered as a possible causative factor, but bilharzial infection can readily be ruled out in view of the rarity of cancer of the liver in Egypt. The evidence for other types of infection is also very scanty. Herbal plants containing *Senecio* alkaloids, and mouldy food containing aflatoxin, have been suggested as possible causative agents; but there is, as yet, no proof of this. The absolute morbidity or mortality rates for gastric cancer are notoriously unreliable for underdeveloped countries. Nevertheless, true variations in incidence of this disease do occur according to country, as demonstrated by comparative data from those in which the age distributions and statistical reliability are fairly uniform (e.g. England and Wales, U.S.A., Holland, Bavaria, Scandinavian countries, and Japan). Among these, the proportion of gastric to total cancer ranges from 22·3 per cent in England and Wales to 60·5 per cent in Sweden. The incidence of the disease appears now to be on the decline in the United States[28] and other countries.

A unique example of geographical localisation is the "Burkitt tumour"—a malignant lymphoma of the jaw and other sites, affecting children in restricted areas in Central Africa, especially in Uganda.[29] Circumstantial evidence suggests that a virus may be involved in the transmission of the disease.

Finally, in addition to simple comparisons of data according to countries, useful information can also be derived from (*a*) comparisons of the *same* racial groups in *different* countries (e.g. of whites in Europe, America, and South Africa, or of Negroes in Africa and America, or of Chinese in China, Indonesia, and America), and (*b*) comparisons of *different* racial groups living in the *same* country (e.g. of whites and Negroes in the United States, or of Chinese and Malayans in South East Asian countries).

A good example of the latter type of survey is that of Steiner,[30] in which the cancer records of the Los Angeles County Hospital were analysed according to the six racial groups of the patients—Caucasoid (Whites), Mexican, Negroid, Japanese, Chinese, and Filipino—with added comparisons between these data and those of the countries from which the racial groups had originally migrated.

The Relationship Between Heredity and Environment in Human Cancer

The role of heredity in disease is not always a simple one. Some diseases are truly hereditary in the Mendelian sense, the disease process being itself a consequence of an altered gene. With others, the relationship is only apparent, as when an extrinsic causative agent is transferred from mother to child *in utero* (transplacental infection) or in early post-natal life (through the mother's milk or by contact infection). Others again are under genetic influence *indirectly*, the susceptibility or resistance being genetically controlled but the causative agent being extrinsic in origin. Lastly, a kinship between heredity and disease may be simulated in cases where a non-hereditary disease happens *by chance* to develop in several members of the same family.

From the preceding discussion, it is clear that many types of human tumours (e.g. those of the skin, mouth, respiratory system, gastro-intestinal system, liver, urinary bladder, bone, and hæmopoietic and lymphoid tissues) are often induced by outside stimuli. These cannot, therefore, be attributed to heredity in the strict sense of the term. There are other types of tumours in man, notably of the reproductive and endocrine systems, in which the inducing process seems to be dependent on a hormonal imbalance, usually of endogenous origin though able to be induced by extrinsic influence. These, too, cannot be attributed to heredity in the strict sense, though heredity may play an important and even decisive role, not only in determining the responsiveness of the tissue to the hormonal imbalance but also in effecting the imbalance itself. Since all these examples comprise the majority of tumours in man, it is evident that the role of heredity in human cancer is, at most, of an indirect kind.

On the other hand, there are certain human tumours for which no evidence exists of a carcinogenic environment being implicated, for example those of the nervous system, many types of sarcoma, and most of the rarer types of tumours in children. Furthermore, the development of spontaneous tumours is decidedly under genetic influence in animals. One is thus faced with the situation that a tumour can be hereditary or environmental in origin, according to the tissue affected, and that in the latter case, the responsiveness may itself be determined by genetic factors.

From the point of view of human cancer, the problem resolves itself into the practical question: In the interaction between environment and heredity in tumour development, how important a role does heredity play?

The study of the geographical pathology of cancer is particularly revealing in this connection: While the relative frequencies of the different tumour types are so strikingly different from one country or region to another,[24, 25] the reason for the differences appears to be largely environmental rather than racial.

In some of the cases, the environmental carcinogenic factors are already known, as with cancer of the skin (exposure to sunlight, tar), mouth ("betel-nut" chewing, reversed cigar smoking), urinary bladder (Bilharzia infection), thyroid (iodine deficiency). In others, while the carcinogenic factors themselves are unknown, the environmental circumstances are evident, as with cancer of the penis (phimosis among the uncircumcised), the lung (smoking, atmospheric pollution, etc.), and the breast and uterus (influenced by marital status and numbers of pregnancies). In others still, the indication that environmental factors are involved is derived from circumstantial evidence, as in the case of cancer of the stomach and possibly of the large intestine. On the other hand, the exceptionally low incidence of breast cancer among the Japanese is not entirely attributable to extrinsic factors (e.g. marital status) and seems, therefore, to be dependent on racial characteristics, though probably mediated by specific patterns of hormonal secretion of the body.

Useful information has also been derived from the study of different racial groups living under similar environment in the same country. Emphasis is placed on *similarity* in environment, for it would obviously be fallacious, in studying racial differences, to compare, say, the White and Bantu populations of South Africa, exhibiting such different standards of living. Similarly, where several racial groups in the same country continue to maintain their respective customs and habits (e.g. the Chinese, Malayans, and other racial groups in South East Asia). comparisons on the basis of racial differences would also be deceptive. On the other hand, in a more integrated society, as exists in the United States, where different customs, habits, and standards of living are rapidly being levelled out, such comparisons are more valid.

It is interesting to note, therefore, how closely parallel the cancer organ-distribution patterns are among the white and coloured populations in the United States. Another interesting example is that of the Jews, dispersed throughout the world, whose cancer pattern tends to approximate to that of the majority population among whom they live, except for two specific types of tumour—penile cancer, which is non-existent, and cancer of the uterine cervix, which is relatively infrequent among Jews wherever they live.

One is thus led to the conclusion that, at least when an extrinsic carcinogenic stimulus is involved, the influence of race is of minor importance. Two facts should, however, be kept in mind: (1) the term "race", as applied to man, is a very loose one, and bears little relation to the genetic homogeneity of an inbred strain of animal, *where hereditary influence plays a far more decisive role*; and (2) even though a carcinogenic stimulus, if powerful enough, may override a low genetic responsiveness of the tissue acted upon, there may still be *individual* differences in response, attributable to genetic factors.

Another approach to the problem of the relative importance of heredity and environment is by analysis of the statistical data according to social and occupational standing, the whole population being divided into five categories, with skilled artisans and those in the higher professions (Group I) at one extreme, and unskilled labourers (Group V) at the other.[31] The idea behind the method is as follows: diseases (or in this case, tumour types) which arise through factors determined by genetic constitution should theoretically operate uniformly throughout the population irrespective of social standing, etc.; those that are dependent on, or strongly influenced by, environmental factors would be expected to vary from one class to another. Here are some of the results obtained from such a survey: (A) Tumours of the following organs showed an upward trend in incidence when passing from Group I to Group V: tongue, mouth, tonsil, jaw, pharynx, œsophagus, stomach, larynx, skin, scrotum, penis, and uterus. (B) Tumours of the following showed an opposite correlation: breast, ovary, testis, mediastinum, thyroid, bone, and kidney. (C) Tumours of the following failed to show any difference among the groups: gall bladder, pancreas, bladder, prostate, and lung. While some of the differences may not be statistically significant, the general trend is no doubt significant, supporting once again the view that more types of human tumours are of extrinsic origin than is generally supposed.

The Role of Heredity in Spontaneous Tumours in Man

Apart from the theoretical basis of tumour genetics (to be discussed in the next chapter in connection with tumour development in inbred strains of animals), there is the practical, and essentially statistical, problem of whether such a thing exists as a "family history" of cancer. The term "family history" implies a frequency of the disease significantly higher than that found in the general population. The question of significance is one that can be computed mathematically by calculating what the probability would be for a particular number of cancers arising in the same family *according to the laws of chance*—i.e. without assuming a hereditary predisposition.

Here are the calculated values for cancer (of all types) for a family of ten members, based on a frequency of one cancer death per seven total deaths in the community as a whole. The probability that:

none	will	develop	cancer	is about	1 chance in 5;
one	,,	,,	,,	,,	1 chance in 3;
two	,,	,,	,,	,,	1 chance in 4;
three	,,	,,	,,	,,	1 chance in 8;
four	,,	,,	,,	,,	1 chance in 30;
five	,,	,,	,,	,,	1 chance in 140;
six	,,	,,	,,	,,	1 chance in 1,000;
seven	,,	,,	,,	,,	1 chance in 11,000;
eight	,,	,,	,,	,,	1 chance in 175,000;
nine	,,	,,	,,	,,	1 chance in 4,700,000;
all ten	,,	,,	,,	,,	1 chance in 280,000,000.

In other words, when dealing with a disease with an average frequency of 1 in 7, the chances of 0, 1, 2, or 3 members of a family of 10 acquiring it are almost the same; and even for 4 cases per family, the chances are no more than 1 in 30. The situation is altogether different when dealing with a rare disease. For instance, one having an average frequency of 1 in 1,000 instead of 1 in 7, the probability of 4 members of a family of 10 acquiring it would be, not 1 in 30 but 1 in 5,000,000,000.

For this reason, the finding of multiple cases of cancer in the same family is not significant, whereas such findings with regard to a specific type, especially one of the rarer kinds (e.g. retinoblastoma), becomes very much more significant.

Yet another approach to the problem of the role of heredity in spontaneous tumours is to determine whether tumours appearing in both members of homozygous twins do so more commonly than among heterozygous twins, or among brothers and sisters of different ages, or among unrelated people. Though several cases are on record in which both members of homozygous twins develop cancer, sometimes involving even the same type of tumour (e.g. breast cancer), the question of chance association cannot be ruled out, as the number of cases is too small for application of statistical methods.[4]

To overcome the variability of individual family histories, a method has been devised whereby the incidence of tumours among brothers and sisters of patients suffering from this disease is compared with that of the general population. This can be undertaken on a sufficiently large scale to enable the significance of any difference to be evaluated.

When such analyses were carried out at first with respect to all forms of cancer, no significant differences were observed. When each distinctive tumour type was treated separately the incidence among brothers and sisters of patients bearing that type of tumour tended to be slightly, but significantly, higher than among the rest of the population. The most convincing results so far obtained have been with cancer of the breast.

From these somewhat tentative results in man, and from far more convincing evidence derived from animal experiments (see Chapter 24), it is possible to arrive at certain general conclusions on the subject of the role of heredity in spontaneous cancer in man:

1. Hereditary influences towards cancer manifest themselves only to a slight degree in man.
2. Such hereditary influences operate independently for different tumour types.
3. There is, therefore, probably no such thing as a general over-all hereditary predisposition to cancer.

Conclusions Derived from the Study of Environmental Cancer in Man

With the growing knowledge about human cancer of environmental origin, the concept of cancer prevention has undergone a revolutionary change (see[32]). While tumours of occupational and industrial origin still constitute a relatively small proportion of all human cancers, those of environmental origin in general (including those which, though essentially intrinsic in origin, can be influenced, during their latent periods, by extrinsic factors) now appear to account for more than half, and possibly three-quarters, of all human cancers. The problem is, therefore, no longer one of academic interest only (i.e. as a lead for the scientific study of experimental carcinogenesis), or of limited value in industrial medicine, but also a potential guide for the future, large-scale prevention of cancer in the population as a whole.

REFERENCES

1. Yule, G. U., and Kendall, M. G. (1953). *An Introduction to the Theory of Statistics*, 14th edit. London: Charles Griffin & Co.
2. Hill, A. Bradford (1961). *Principles of Medical Statistics*, 7th edit. London: The Lancet, Ltd.
3. Doll, R., Payne, P., and Waterhouse, J. A. H. (1967). *Cancer Incidence in Five Continents*, UICC Publ.
4. Peller, S. (1952). *Cancer in Man*. New York: International Universities Press.
5. Hueper, W. C. (1942). *Occupational Tumors and Allied Diseases*. Springfield, Ill.: Charles C. Thomas.
6. Hueper, W. C. (1954). *Arch. Path. (Chicago)*, **56,** 360, 475, & 645.
7. Blum, H. F. (1948). *J. nat. Cancer Inst.*, **9,** 245.
8. Furth, J., and Furth, O. B. (1936). *Amer. J. Cancer*, **28,** 54.
9. United Nations Scientific Committee. (1964). Report *The Effects of Atomic Radiation*. U.N. Official Records, 19th Session, Suppl. 14 (A/5814).
10. Clayson, D. B. (1962). *Chemical Carcinogenesis*. London: J. & A. Churchill.

11. Scott, A. (1923). *Eighth Scient. Rep., Imperial Cancer Res. Fund*, 85.
12. Southam, A. H., and Wilson, S. R. (1922). *Brit. med. J.*, **2,** 971.
13. Berenblum, I. (1944). *Arch. Path. (Chicago)*, **38,** 337.
14. Various Authors (1962). *Symposium: Analysis of Carcinogenic Air Pollutants.* Nat. Cancer Inst. Monogr. No. 9, Bethesda, Md.: U.S. Dept. of Health, Education & Welfare.
15. Kennaway, E. L. (1947). *Brit. J. Cancer*, **1,** 335.
16. Royal College of Physicians, London (1962). Report *In Relation to Cancer of the Lung and other Diseases.* London: Pitman Med. Publ. Co.
17. Advisory Committee to the Surgeon General (1964). Report *Smoking and Health.* U.S. Publ. Health Service Publ. No. 1103.
18. Stocks, P. (1952). *Brit. J. Cancer*, **6,** 99.
19. Klein, A. J., and Palmer, W. L. (1940). *Arch. Path. (Chicago)*, **29,** 814.
20. Barrett, M. K. (1946). *J. nat. Cancer Inst.*, **7,** 127.
21. Various Authors (1964). Mechanisms of Carcinogenesis: Chemical, Physical and Viral. *Brit. med. Bull.*, **20,** No. 2.
22. Schoental, R. (1963). *Bull. Wld. Hlth. Org.*, **29,** 823.
23. Dunham, L. J., and Dorn, H. F. (1955). *Schweiz. Z. allg. Path. Bakt.*, **18,** 472 (in English).
24. Higginson, J. (1963). In *Cancer Progress* (Ed. R. W. Raven), Extra vol. p. 77.
25. Various Authors (1964). *Epidemiologic Approaches to Cancer Etiology*, **25**.
26. Berman, C. (1951). *Primary Carcinoma of the Liver.* London: H. K. Lewis & Co.
27. Badger, G. M., and Lewis, G. E. (1952). *Brit. J. Cancer*, **6,** 270.
28. Terris, M., and Hall, C. E. (1963). *J. nat. Cancer Inst.*, **31,** 155.
29. Burkitt, D. (1963). In *Viruses, Nucleic Acids, and Cancer*, p. 615. Baltimore: Williams & Wilkins.
30. Steiner, P. E. (1954). *Cancer: Race and Geography.* Baltimore: Williams & Wilkins Co.
31. *The Registrar-General's Decennial Supplement, England and Wales*, 1951. Part I: Occupational Mortality. London: H.M. Stationery Office.
32. WHO Expert Committee (1964). Report *Prevention of Cancer.* (Wld. Hlth. Techn. Rep. Ser. 276). Geneva: W.H.O.

Chapter 24

THE STUDY OF TUMOURS IN ANIMALS*

BY I. BERENBLUM

CANCER was already a recognised disease a thousand years before Hippocrates (460–375 B.C.) first described some of its diverse clinical manifestations; yet its basic character remained a mystery for more than 2,000 years. The establishment of cellular pathology, a century ago, provided the first indication of the nature of neoplasia *in morphological terms*; and with the development of histopathology, led to the identification of separate structural tumour types, correlated with their behaviour, as an aid to diagnosis. By the end of the last century the principles of tumour morphology were fairly well established.

In contrast to the accumulated knowledge of the structural basis of neoplasia, there was at that time little known about the functional properties of tumours or about their mode of origin. The considerable progress made since then can be traced to the introduction of animal experimentation, belatedly accepted as an essential technique for the study of pathological processes.

Apart from the change in technical approach (from observational, for the study of morphology, to experimental, for the study of functional properties and ætiology), the new interest in animal tumours was itself an important advance in drawing attention to the fact that the disease was not restricted to man. A survey of tumours throughout the animal kingdom was but the logical extension of the study of human tumours beyond the confines of one's own country—as safeguards against false conclusions drawn from limited experience.

The Zoological Distribution of Tumours (see Various Authors[1])

At the end of last century any animal tumour encountered by chance was generally dismissed as a lesion unrelated to the human disease, even when its histological character and clinical course were patently akin to the corresponding tumour in man. The compilation of data by Sticker (1902), Bashford and Murray (1904), Tyzzer (1907), Murray (1908), and others (see also Feldman[2]), reporting on tumours in domestic, captive, and wild animals, including birds, reptiles, and fish, finally overcame this scepticism. Incidentally, it also disproved another erroneous belief—that only animals living in close proximity to man could acquire the disease.

All vertebrates, probably without exception, are liable to develop spontaneous tumours. Whether the tumour-like lesions in insects[3] and in plants[4] are also to be considered neoplastic, is debatable, because of the difficulty in distinguishing true neoplasia from developmental growth aberrations, in the case of insects, and from infective or traumatic hyperplasia, in the case of plants. No such doubts now exist, however, about tumours in higher animals. Indeed, the

* Many names, with dates, appear in the text without being listed among the references at the end, which are restricted to books, reviews, and only a few original papers published too recently to be covered by such reviews.

pendulum has swung from one extreme to another—from doubts as to whether animals can develop tumours at all, to the idea that the disease is as common throughout the animal kingdom as it is in man.

From fairly reliable statistical reports on dogs, involving many thousands of autopsies, the mortality rate for tumours ranges from about 3 to 9 per cent, with an average age of 10 years. Since some of the surveys deal only with carcinomas, the true incidence, i.e. for all malignant tumours, is probably closer to the higher than the lower figure; which suggests that the disease is almost as common in the dog as in man. Comparable, though less extensive, analyses of data for the cat indicate a lower frequency of tumours for that species, ranging from about 0·5 to 6 per cent with the likelihood that the lower figure is closer to the true incidence. In the horse, for which adequate data are also available, the incidence (for carcinoma only) is low, ranging from 0·1 to 1·2 per cent, with a somewhat higher, but still relatively low, figure for total malignancies. The recorded tumour incidence for cattle is lower still (0·1 to 0·5 per cent), and very low incidences have been reported for the pig, goat, and sheep. The fowl, on the contrary, has a high tumour incidence, especially if leukæmias are included. As for random-bred laboratory animals, spontaneous tumours are very common in the mouse, less so in the rat, and rather infrequent in the guinea-pig and rabbit, even when these are allowed to live their full life-span. No reliable quantitative data are available for wild animals, though good descriptions exist of the different tumours observed in them.

When we try to evaluate these results in a comparative fashion, we are faced with rather serious difficulties. The question is, how far one is justified in making quantitative comparisons between tumour incidences of such diverse categories as (i) *animals kept as livestock*, which are usually slaughtered at a very early age; (ii) *animals kept as pets*, which generally live to old age, but which are not regularly submitted to autopsy examination when they die; (iii) *wild animals in their natural habitat*, those captured not necessarily being representative as regards age distribution; (iv) *wild animals kept in captivity*, living under abnormal climatic conditions and in confined spaces; and (v) *laboratory animals*, which are maintained under good living conditions, and which are carefully examined at death, but which may, through inbreeding, exhibit artificial patterns of tumour incidence in comparison with human or other heterogeneous populations. There is, furthermore, the problem of relative versus absolute old age, in animal species having different "natural" life-spans. Does a mouse aged 2½ years really correspond to a dog aged 18 years, from the viewpoint of relative speed of carcinogenesis, and, if so, should they be related to man in Western society—having an average life expectancy of about 70, or to man living in primitive surroundings—having a life expectancy as low as 30? Attempts have been made to allow for these unknown variables, e.g. by comparing the carcinoma : sarcoma ratio in different species, on the assumption that similar ratios necessarily denote comparable age distributions (Dobberstein, 1953). But such an assumption may not be justified in comparing different species.

In fact, there is at present no real solution to the problem raised here, and one can do no more than generalise—that the total tumour incidences in the different species do vary strikingly, even when the animals in question live to old age, and that in most species the disease seems less common than in man.

Turning to the varieties of tumours, every histological type occurring in man has been encountered in one or other of the animal species studied; but their relative frequencies in the different species vary enormously, as indicated in Table I. (Since quantitative comparisons are impossible, the data are presented schematically by plus and minus signs, the latter denoting rarity rather than total absence of the particular type of tumour.)

Since in man, many types of "spontaneous" tumours are attributable to environmental influences (see Chapter 23), it is interesting to note what

24/Table I

Schematic Tabulation of the Relative Frequencies of Tumours in Various Species of Animals

Tumours of	*Dog*	*Horse*	*Cattle*	*Mouse*	*Rabbit*	*Fowl*
Skin papill. + carc.[1]	++++	+++	++	–	(++++)[2]	–
,, melanoma	++	++++[3]	–	–	–	–
Penis	(+++)[4]	+++	–	–	–	–
Breast	+++	+	–	+++++	–	–
Uterus	–	–	+	–	+++	–
Ovary	++	–	+	–	–	++++
Testis	+++	++	–	–	–	+
Forestomach (squamous)	+	++	+++	–	–	–
Stomach (glandular)	–	+	–	–	–	–
Intestine	+	–	+	–	–	++
Liver	+	+	++	++	–	–
Lung	++	+	++	+++	–	–
Thyroid	+++	–	+	+	–	–
Kidney	–	++	–	–	++	+++[5]
Connective tissues:						
(*a*) Benign (fibroma, lipoma, myxoma)	+++	++++	++	–	(+++)[6]	+
(*b*) Malignant	++	++	+	+	+	++
Leukæmia	+	–	++	++	–	++++
Lymphoma	+++	–	+++	+	–	+

[1] Including eye and appendages.
[2] Infectious (viral) "Shope papilloma".
[3] In old grey and white horses, less often in black, never in brown horses—affecting anal region and tail, mouth, etc.
[4] "Transmissible lymphosarcoma"—also in vagina of female, transmitted by coitus from the male.
[5] Embryonal nephroma.
[6] "Infectious fibromas".

the situation is with regard to some of the commoner tumours in animals. These may be classified as follows from the point of view of ætiology:

A. *Definite environmental influences:* "Shope papillomatosis" in wild (cottontail) rabbits, and "infectious fibromas", in rabbits—both viral in origin; "transmissible lymphosarcoma" of the penis and vagina in dogs—transmitted by an uncharacterised agent; some of the leukæmias in mouse and fowl—also viral in origin; and sarcoma of the liver in rats (not listed in Table I), associated with cysticercus infection.

B. *Probable environmental influences:* Skin tumours in the dog, horse, and cattle (? due to actinic radiation); tumours of the forestomach in cattle (? dietetic in origin); tumours of the liver in cattle and the dog (? dietetic in origin); and tumour of the penis in the horse (exact cause unknown).

C. *Probable intrinsic environmental influences* (*hormonal imbalance*): Tumours of the breast, uterus, ovary, testis, and thyroid, in the various species.

D. *No evidence for environmental influence:* This group includes most of the benign and malignant tumours of connective tissues, and the rarer tumours not included in categories A–C. Some sarcomas may, however, be related to the leukæmias, and be viral in origin. See also p. 776 for tumours transmitted by the polyoma virus.

Experimental Approach

The limitations inherent in simple comparative studies of spontaneous tumour incidences among different species of animals prompted investigators (*a*) to explore the role of heredity in tumour development within single species, (*b*) to narrow the range of variability by genetic inbreeding, (*c*) to define the role of hormonal imbalance in relation to tumour development in tissues known to be under hormonal influence, (*d*) to look for other non-genetic factors influencing "spontaneous" tumour development, and (*e*) to establish means of artificially inducing tumours in animals *de novo.*

Thus began the divergence, during the first two decades of this century, into independent experimental disciplines for the study of tumour genesis. It was important, for this kind of work, to choose an animal with the following characteristics: (1) small size, to permit the use of large numbers essential for controlled experiments; (2) rapid breeding cycle, to facilitate the follow-up of as many generations as possible in a short period; and (3) a pronounced tendency for tumours to develop. The mouse, satisfying these requirements, has been the animal of choice, the rat being used far less. Where inbreeding was not essential, e.g. in certain studies on carcinogenesis, mice, rats, and rabbits of random-bred stock were much used, and fowls, guinea-pigs, and hamsters, less frequently so. A few observations on dogs and monkeys are also reported.

The Genetics of Spontaneous Tumours in the Mouse

The possibility that the total tumour incidence of random-bred mice might be higher in families derived from tumour-bearing than in those derived from non-tumour-bearing ancestry, was suggested by the early observations of Tyzzer (1907) and Slye (1913, etc.), though the results of Murray (1911) and others (see Little[5]) pointed to the likelihood that different types of tumours were inherited separately. More exact methods, involving the use of "inbred" strains of mice, were clearly needed for a proper genetic analysis of the tumour problem.

Inbred strains are obtained by successive brother-to-sister matings for about 30 generations. The genetic uniformity, obtained by such a procedure, results from the fact that with each brother-to-sister mating genes from the two parents that happen to be dissimilar have an even chance of being eliminated, while those that are identical continue to be transmitted, with no new types of genes added—thus approximating to a "homozygous" state, in which the corresponding genes in each pair of chromosomes—or "alleles"—are identical.

Such inbred strains do not always remain constant, because of the likelihood of mutations arising during subsequent inbreeding; thus accounting for the different "sub-lines" of the established strains in the various breeding centres in the world. But this does not diminish the value of inbred strains in experimental studies, offering (*a*) decreased variations in the colony, (*b*) a more accurate knowledge of pedigree, and (*c*) the ability to compare the effects of hybrid crosses, with theoretically predicted results based on Mendelian principles (see Russell[5]). These conditions enable one, for instance, to distinguish between dominant and recessive traits, to determine the number of genes involved in a particular effect, and to detect extrachromosomal types of inheritance (see below).

The total tumour incidence was found to vary greatly among the 30 or more inbred strains of mice that were specially developed for the study of tumour genetics (Strong, 1935; Little, 1937, etc., see Heston[6, 7]), ranging from less than 5 per cent in the *C57 leaden strain* to close on 100 per cent in the *C3H strain.* Equally striking were the differences in the relative and absolute frequencies of the individual tumour types among the different strains (see Table II).

Thus, with the use of inbred strains, two important principles were established: (1) that genetic factors can play a decisive role in the development of spontaneous tumours; and (2) that not all tumours are controlled by the same set of genes. The fact that the manifested hereditary expression is so striking in the case of inbred strains, in contrast to the slight evidence of a hereditary influence on tumour development in random-bred man or animal, is a consequence of the development of homozygosity. This artificial exaggeration of a normal trend, though unrealistic for comparative purposes with respect to heterozygous populations, has obvious advantages for purposes of genetic analysis.

Regarding the manner of tumour inheritance, the older belief in a single *recessive* factor for all tumours (Slye, 1926) has given place to the view (Little, 1928) that multiple factors are involved, mostly *dominant*. However, less emphasis is placed nowadays on the distinction between dominant and recessive characters than formerly (*a*) because these qualities refer to the gene characters (or "genotype") rather than to the ultimate expression of their influence (or "phenotype"), the latter being modified by environmental influences, (*b*) because the effects of dominant and recessive influences are often relative rather than absolute, and (*c*) because several genes may be implicated in effecting a single change such as tumour development.

Mammary tumours.—The most detailed and extensive studies on the problem of the genetics of spontaneous tumours in animals are those concerned with mammary carcinoma in the mouse. This tumour was singled out partly because it was the commonest malignant neoplasm arising spontaneously in random-bred mice, and partly because in inbred animals its incidence differed to an exceptional degree between one strain and another (see Table II), indicating a striking dependence on genetic control.

The fact that mouse mammary cancer normally occurs only in the female and develops only after sexual maturity, that its incidence, in certain strains, is higher in breeders than in virgins, increasing with the number of pregnancies,

24/TABLE II

TUMOUR INCIDENCES (PER CENT) IN INBRED STRAINS OF MICE

Strain	*Mammary carcinoma*		*Lung adenoma and carcinoma*	*Leukæmia*	*Remarks*
	Breeders	*Virgins*			
C3H	75–100	95	5–10	<1	also 10 per cent hepatomas in males and 27 per cent in females.
A	70–85	5	80–90	low	
dba	55–75	10–70*	<1	10–40*	*according to sub-line.
CBA	3–20	<1	low	<1	also some hepatomas.
BALB/c	<5	very low	20–30	70	
Ak	low	low	low	60–80	
I	<1	<1	10–20	very low	but tumours of glandular mucosa of stomach very common.
C57 black	<1	0	<1	5	also about 15 per cent other non-epithelial tumours, notably reticulum-cell sarcoma in old age.
C57 leaden	<1	0	<1	3–9	

and that the tissue of origin (the mammary gland) is hormonally dependent, suggested that in the ætiology of the tumour hormonal action might also be implicated (see Shimkin[6]; Gardner[8]; Burrows and Horning[9]). This was supported by the following observations.

Ovariectomy *at a very early age* prevented the subsequent appearance of mammary tumours (Lathrop and Loeb, 1916); conversely, injections of large doses of the ovarian hormone, œstrone, into mice of a strain in which mammary cancer normally develops in a high proportion of the females, caused a rise in the tumour incidence in *females* and the development of such tumours *even in males* (Lacassagne, 1932). The development of mammary tumours in castrated males bearing ovarian grafts (Murray, 1928) should also be mentioned in this connection. (These results demonstrate, incidentally, that the normal absence of mammary cancer in the male of a high mammary cancer strain is due to the fact that male mammary tissue, though potentially responsive, is in a rudimentary state.) In low mammary cancer strains, œstrone injections raised the tumour incidence less effectively, and in very low tumour strains not at all. The carcinogenic effect was also produced with synthetic œstrogens—e.g. diethylstilbœstrol (Lacassagne, 1938), and triphenylene (Bonser and Robson, 1940), their carcinogenic effectiveness being proportional to their physiological activity—thus proving that *œstrogenic action*, rather than anything connected with the chemical configuration of the œstrone molecule, was responsible for the effect. Simultaneous androgen treatment reduced the tumour incidence.

In experiments involving reciprocal crosses between females of a high and males of a low mammary tumour strain, and vice versa, the tumour incidence in the hybrid young was found always to resemble that of the mother's strain (Little *et al.*, 1933; Korteweg, 1934). These results could not be explained on principles of Mendelian inheritance, and pointed to some extra-chromosomal influence at work. The critical experiment to explain this phenomenon was performed by Bittner (1935), who removed the babies from mothers of a high mammary tumour strain *immediately after birth*, and allowed them to be foster-nursed by mothers of a low tumour strain: *these young failed to develop mammary tumours.* The extra-chromosomal factor was evidently something transmitted from mother to young through the milk!

For information concerning the genetic factor, the mammary tumour incidence was analysed further, using different strains, and also crosses between them, *under conditions in which both the hormonal factor and the "milk factor" operated effectively.* One might have expected, under these conditions, that the different strains would exhibit an all-or-none effect, yielding either 0 per cent or 100 per cent mammary tumour incidence; but this was not found to be the case (Bittner, 1940, etc.). The results could be explained by (*a*) involvement of multiple genetic factors in the over-all genetic influence, (*b*) differences in relative effectiveness of the genetic influence, resulting in a lengthening of the latent period beyond the life expectancy of the animal, or (*c*) the overriding effects of (uncontrolled) non-genetic influences.

Regarding the hormonal component, an important question to be answered was whether œstrogens acted as true carcinogens, or whether they merely stimulated the mammary tissue to full physiological activity *as a prerequisite for the action of the "milk agent".* Œstrogens do not, in fact, act directly on the mammary tissue, but indirectly through the pituitary gland, and are ineffective in providing the hormonal requirements for mammary tumour development without the additional participation of progesterone, mammatrophic hormone, growth hormone and corticosterone (DeOme *et al.*[10]).

The agent, swallowed at birth with the mother's milk, appears to have no demonstrable effects until 6 to 20 months later, when the tumour arises. Other tissues in the body also contain the agent, extracts of which are capable, on injection, of causing mammary tumours to appear in later life. The agent was eventually characterised as an RNA virus (see Dmochowski[11]), and is now called the "Bittner virus".

The postulated triple mechanism of mammary tumour development in mice —comprising a genetic, a hormonal, and a viral factor—is, however, an over-simplification of the case.

1. The genetic "factor" involves more than one single gene (Heston[5]), and controls not only the susceptibility of the mammary tissue but also the production of hormone and the multiplication and transmissibility of the virus.

2. Mammary cancers may develop, admittedly in small numbers, in mice of strains apparently lacking the Bittner virus, or in those in which the virus has been eliminated, e.g. by transferring blastocysts (early embryos prior to placenta formation) from the uterus of an agent-containing to that of an agent-free mouse, and breeding therefrom an "agent-free" sub-line (Mühlbock[12]). There are many possible explanations for such tumours developing in "agent-free" mice: (*a*) different types of mammary tumours may exist, some dependent on the virus and others not; (*b*) the virus may be present in undected amounts in the "agent-free" strains; (*c*) the virus may not be an absolutely essential requirement; or (*d*) the virus may possibly arise in the animal *de novo*. In support of (*a*) is the fact that tumours in "agent-free" strains arise only in very old mice, and appear to have a somewhat different morphology (Dunn[13]); in support of (*b*), that electron microscopy studies of mammary tumours have demonstrated virus-like bodies not only in the case of agent-containing strains, but also, in smaller amounts, in "agent-free" strains (Bernhard *et al.*[14]); and in support of (*c*) an (*d*) that injections of carcinogenic hydrocarbons raise the mammary tumour incidence not only in agent-containing (Mider and Morton, 1939) but also in "agent-free" female mice (Strong and Williams, 1941) and rats (Shay *et al.*, 1949; Huggins *et al.*, 1959).

3. Other extrinsic factors, notably caloric restriction of the diet, can reduce the incidence of mammary tumours in mice (see Tannenbaum and Silverstone[15]).

The significance of these experimental results in animals, in relation to the human disease, is not easy to interpret: (1) As mentioned in the previous chapter, cancer of the breast in women appears also to be influenced by heredity, though the manifested influence is slight. (2) There is, as yet, no convincing evidence that prolonged œtrogen administration is carcinogenic for the breast *in humans*; but neither has the possibility been excluded. The fact that in mice mammary tumours develop more frequently in breeders than in virgins, while in women the opposite seems to be the case, has been attributed to the fact that in the mouse the corpus luteum does not produce progesterone *in the virgin* while in women it does (Mühlbock[12]). (3) No evidence has so far been adduced for a "milk agent" virus operating in human breast cancer. (4) Finally, in trying to correlate animal data on mammary cancer with those observed in man, the possibility that the different types of human breast cancer—ductal, canalicular, and acinous (Foot, 1942)—might have different ætiologies should be kept in mind.

Lung tumours.—The discrete pearly nodules on the surface of the lungs of mice in certain strains, known as lung "adenomas" because of the acinar cell arrangement, are derived from lung alveoli (Stewart[13]); they may eventually become carcinomatous. While probably having no relation to lung cancer in man, which is mostly bronchiogenic in origin, these lung tumours in mice serve, nevertheless, as good material for genetic analysis.

From studies of the incidence of the condition in different inbred strains, and from cross-breeding experiments, the genetic factor seems to be dominant (Lynch, 1926), and probably involves more than one gene (Heston, 1942). No hormonal factor is involved, nor has any extra-chromosomal factor been detected. On the other hand, the tumour incidence in susceptible strains may be greatly augmented by injections of carcinogenic hydrocarbons (Andervont, 1940) or urethane (Nettleship and Henshaw, 1943).

Leukæmias.—A more complicated problem is involved in the study of the genetics of leukæmia in mice, partly because of the multiplicity of morphological types (see Dunn[16]), and partly because of non-genetic factors involved in its development.

That a genetic factor is implicated in spontaneous leukæmia in mice is evidenced by the striking differences in incidence in various strains (see Table II). From cross-breeding experiments, it seems that several genes are involved (Cole and Furth, 1941). Most of the mouse leukæmias are lymphocytic in type, judged on the basis of morphological criteria, and also of the organ distribution of the localised lesions, with early involvement of the thymus (Kaplan, 1948). However, myelogenous (Graffi, 1957) and stem-cell types also exist.

With regard to non-genetic factors in its ætiology, the following observations are relevant:

1. In strains of mice exhibiting a low spontaneous leukæmia incidence, significantly high incidences can be produced artificially by injecting large doses of œstrogens (Lacassagne, 1937), or carcinogenic hydrocarbons (Morton and Mider, 1938), or by radiation (Kaplan, 1952).

2. From reciprocal cross-breeding experiments, an extra-chromosomal factor appears to be implicated (MacDowell and Richter, 1935), though *not connected with the milk*.

3. A viral factor has been demonstrated in spontaneous leukæmia of mice (Gross, 1951), transmissible by injection of material from high leukæmia strains into very young mice of low leukæmia strains (see p. 776). A similar virus has also been found in radiation-induced leukæmia (Lieberman and Kaplan, 1959).

Other tumours.—Among the other types of tumours in mice, studied from the genetic angle, the adenomatous and (?) adenocarcinomatous lesions of the glandular mucosa of the stomach in *I strain* mice (Strong, 1944), and some of the sub-lines derived from it, are of special interest, in view of the rarity of such tumours in animals in general. Another unusual tumour is carcinoma of the adrenal cortex in *CE strain* mice that have been gonadectomised at an early age (Woolley and Little, 1945).

Experimental Carcinogenesis

An astonishingly long interval of 140 years elapsed between the first clinical observation of occupational skin cancer in chimney-sweeps (Pott, 1775) and the first production of skin tumours in animals by tar applications (Yamagiwa and Itchikawa, 1915). The field of experimental carcinogenesis expanded rapidly after 1920, and, considering the time-consuming nature of the experimental procedures involved, made remarkable progress.

In little more than a decade, the chemical structure of a potent carcinogenic constituent of the complex coal-tar was identified (Cook, Hewett, and Hieger,

1933), and tar carcinogenesis was thereafter replaced by more refined methods involving the use of pure chemical compounds. By 1951 (see 2nd edit. of Hartwell's *Survey*[17]), about 1,300 compounds, including several hundred newly synthesised ones, had been tested for carcinogenesis, of which more than 350 were found to be active; and the list has increased considerably since then. During this period, important advances were also made on (i) the structural diversity and possible inter-relationship of the various carcinogens; (ii) the metabolism of carcinogens in the body; (iii) the responsiveness of different tissues to local carcinogenic action; (iv) systemic carcinogenic action; (v) carcinogenesis through hormonal imbalance; (vi) similarities and differences between physical, chemical, and viral carcinogenesis; (vii) the influence of genetics on responsiveness to chemical carcinogenesis; and (viii) possible mechanisms of carcinogenic action.

For a general review of chemical carcinogenesis, see Clayson[18]; Various Authors[19]. More detailed reviews of separate aspects of carcinogenesis will be referred to in the appropriate sections.

Tar carcinogenesis (see Woglom[20]).—The first experimental induction of skin tumours with coal-tar was on the ears of rabbits, but the skin of the mouse's back was later found to be equally responsive, and thereafter served as the test object of choice. Repeated applications, at weekly or half-weekly intervals for many weeks or months, eventually led to the appearance of discrete papillomas on the treated skin, though early diffuse changes—epidermal hyperplasia, hyperkeratosis, and mild inflammatory reactions in the corium—were evident throughout the "latent period". While the papillomas induced in the rabbit had a tendency to regress when the tarring was discontinued, and became malignant only when the treatment was very prolonged, the papillomas in the mouse usually became established after their first appearance, and many of them progressed to malignancy even after cessation of tarring.

The skin of many other species was less responsive. Thus, in the rat, treatment for more than a year was necessary for tumours to develop; in the guinea-pig or fowl, tumours rarely appeared even after such long treatment; in the dog, the required latent period of action was about 8 years. When tar treatment, in a responsive species, was tested at different ages, the length of treatment rather than the age of the animal proved to be the decisive factor. This provided proof in support of indications from occupational tumours in man that *the tendency for tumours to develop late in life is due to the long latent period of carcinogenesis and not, as previously supposed, to ageing of the tissues.*

Other general conclusions from these early studies were (*a*) that extrinsic chemical action is capable of inducing tumours *in a previously normal tissue of a healthy animal*, (*b*) that the resulting tumours are often multiple, and (*c*) that each tumour arises from a single minute focus, and not as a diffuse cancerisation of the whole area of treated skin.

The diffuse epidermal hyperplasia, observed before the appearance of the discrete papillomas, and certain degenerative changes in internal organs of tar-painted mice, were more difficult to interpret. Coal-tar is a complex mixture of hundreds of compounds, many possessing toxic properties unrelated to the process of tumour induction. The isolation of a carcinogenic constituent *in pure form* was, therefore, as important from the viewpoint of pathogenesis as the identification of its chemical structure was from the viewpoint of ætiology.

Coal-tar is not a simple distillate of coal—itself non-carcinogenic—but a product of pryolysis at high temperatures, the operative conditions (temperature range and exclusion of air) determining not only the chemical composition of the resulting tar, but also its carcinogenic potency (Kennaway, 1924). Qualitive analyses by Block and Dreifuss (1921), established the fact that carcinogenic constituents of potent crude fractions were neither acid nor base, and contained no sulphur, nitrogen, oxygen, or arsenic, suggesting that the active components were hydrocarbons; and this was supported by the experimental production of a carcinogenic tar *from simple organic compounds consisting only of carbon and hydrogen* (Kennaway, 1925). However, the hydrocarbons known at the time to be present in coal-tar were inactive (Kennaway, 1930).

The isolation and identification of 3:4-benzpyrene (I) from tar (Cook, Hewett, and Hieger, 1933) was hastened by Mayneord's suggestion (Hieger, 1930) that the characteristic fluorescence spectrum of active crude tar fractions might be a measure of their carcinogenic activity, and that the rapid fluorescence

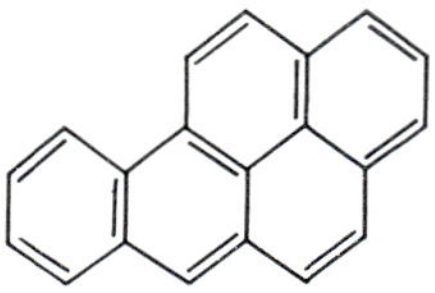

(I) 3:4-benzpyrene

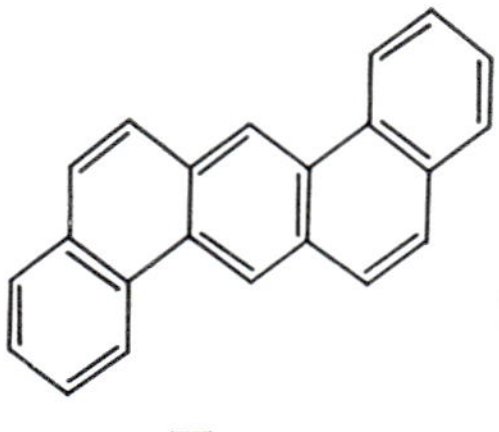

(II) 1:2:5:6-dibenzanthracene

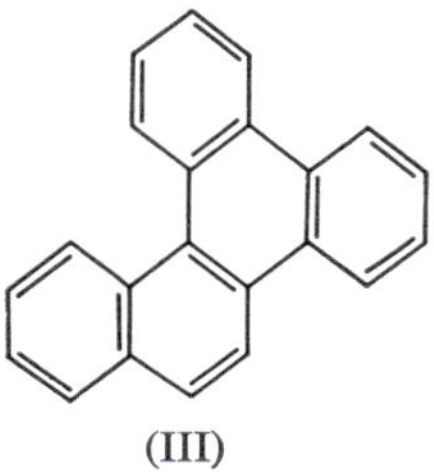

(III) 1:2:3:4-dibenzphenanthrene

spectrographic analysis of the hundreds of separated fractions, instead of the laborious biological testing, might thus save years of work. The validity of this association was supported by the observation that synthetic 1:2:5:6-dibenzanthracene (II)—not present in tar, but possessing a somewhat similar fluorescence spectrum—was carcinogenic (Kennaway, 1930).

Later, it was shown (Berenblum and Schoental, 1943, 1947) that carcinogenic oils and tars contain other carcinogenic constituents as well, which in the case of shale oil may even belong to a different class of compound from the polycyclic aromatic hydrocarbons. All the same, with the isolation and identification of 3:4-benzpyrene, the confirmation of its structure by synthesis, and the demonstration of its high carcinogenic activity, a new phase of carcinogenesis was inaugurated, which provided the biologist with better tools, and the organic chemist with the means of exploring the relationship between chemical structure and carcinogenic activity.

Polycyclic aromatic hydrocarbons (see Clayson[18]).—As is apparent from structural formulas of 3:4-benzpyrene (I) and 1:2:5:6-dibenzanthracene (II), both are composed of 5 fused benzene rings. Of the 15 theoretically possible 5-ring polycyclic aromatic hydrocarbons, all of which were synthesised and tested for carcinogenic activity, only 3:4-benzpyrene (I), 1:2:5:6-dibenzanthracene (II), and 1:2:3:4-dibenzphenanthrene (III) were definitely carcinogenic, the remaining 12 being inactive or displaying, at most, only borderline activity.[16] Structurally, compounds (I) and (II) may be considered derivatives of 1:2-benzanthracene (IV); compound (III), a derivative of 3:4-benzphenanthrene (V); but compounds (I) and (III) also derivatives of chrysene (VI). Of these 4-ring key compounds, 3:4-benzphenanthrene (V) was found to be mildly carcinogenic, 1:2-benzanthracene (IV) to have borderline activity, and chrysene (VI) to be non-carcinogenic.

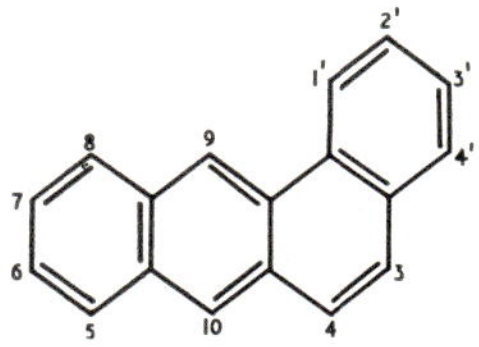

(IV)
1:2-benzanthracene

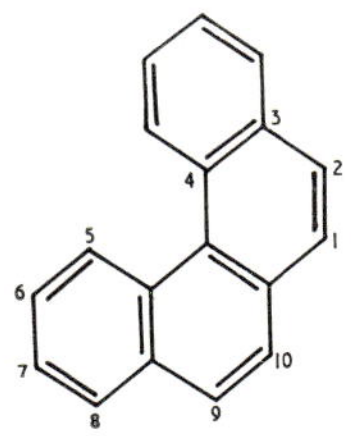

(V)
3:4-benz-
phenanthrene

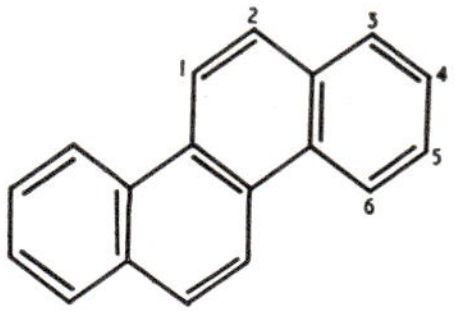

(VI)
chrysene

An extensive study was then undertaken, both in London (by Cook, Kennaway, and others) and in Boston, U.S.A. (by Fieser, Shear, and others), involving the synthesis and biological testing of a large number of related compounds, with particular emphasis on derivatives of the 4-ring hydrocarbons (IV, V, and VI).

Many alkyl derivatives of the 4-ring hydrocarbons were found to be more active than the parent hydrocarbons, *depending on the positions of substitution.* Thus, of the 12 possible methyl-1:2-benzanthracenes, the 9- and 10- derivatives were highly active; the 3-, 4-, 5-, and 6-, moderately so; the 7- and 8-, weakly so; while the 1′-, 2′-, 3′-, and 4′-methyl derivatives had borderline or no activity.

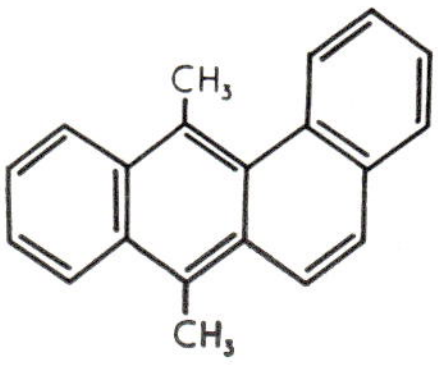

(VII)
9:10-dimethyl-
1:2-benzanthracene

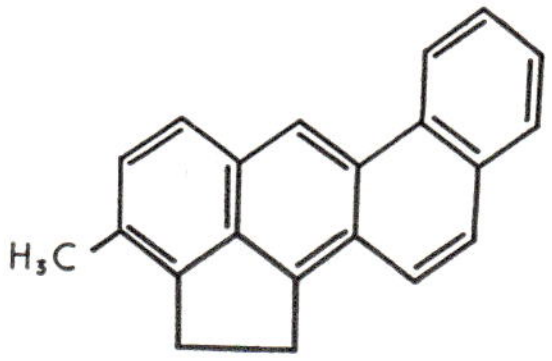

(VIII)
20-methylcholanthrene

In the case of methyl-3:4-benzphenanthrenes, highest activity was with the methyl group in the 2- position; lower activity, in the 1- position; and weak activity in the 6-, 7-, and 8- positions. With chrysene, which was itself inactive, methyl- substitution in the 1- position imparted moderate activity, and in the 2- position, weak activity. Finally, when several "active" positions of the molecule were substituted, carcinogenesis was summated. Indeed, 9:10-dimethyl-1:2-benzanthracene (VII) is the most potent carcinogen known.

Some reference should be made to 20-methylcholanthracene (VIII)—also known as 3-methylcholanthrene by a different system of numbering—one of the most commonly used carcinogens. It was first synthesised from bile acids by cyclisation of the side-chain, followed by dehydrogenation. The hypothesis which prompted the synthesis—that normal steroids in the body might conceivably be converted into carcinogenic hydrocarbons *in vivo* (Kennaway and Cook, 1932), is, however, no longer considered valid.

A common factor in all the carcinogenic compounds so far discussed is the

(X)

(XIII)

(XI)

(IX)
Phenanthrene

(XIV)

(XII)

(XV)

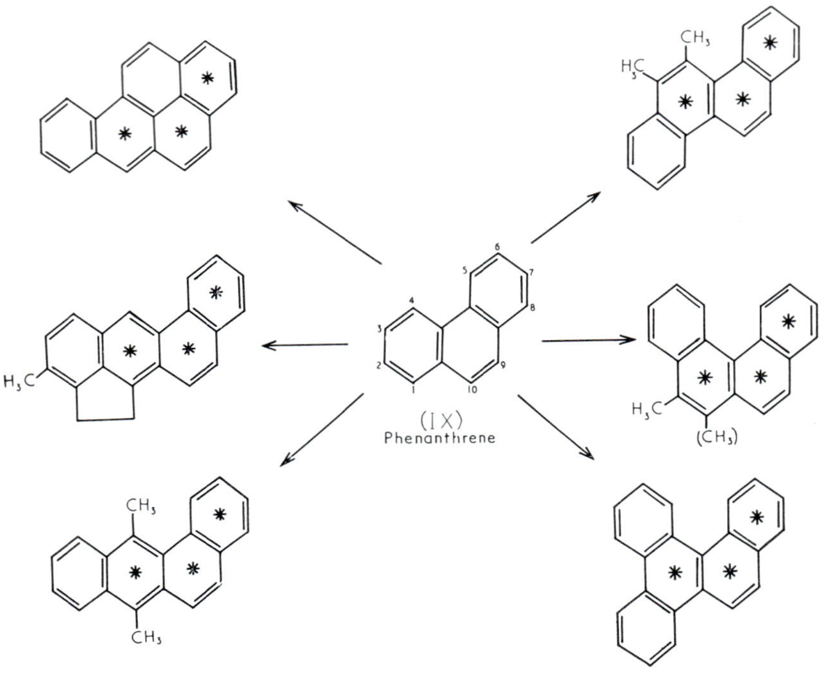

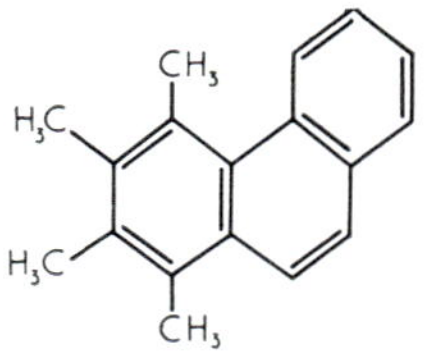

(XVI)
1:2:3:4-tetramethyl-
phenanthrene

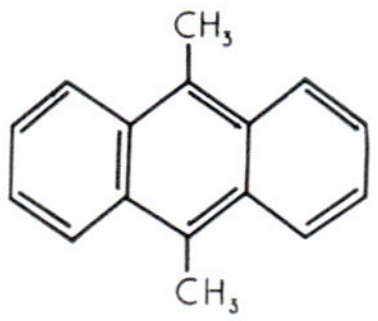

(XVII)
9:10-dimethyl-
anthracene

3-ring hydrocarbon—phenanthrene (IX), substituted in at least three of the four positions: 1-, 2-, 3-, and 4-, either by two additional benzene rings or by one benzene ring and one or two methyl groups (compare formulas IX–XV). One might, therefore, have anticipated that the compound 1:2:3:4-tetramethylphenanthrene (XVI) should also exhibit some carcinogenic activity; and this was indeed found to be the case. But 9:10-dimethylanthracene (XVII), which has no phenanthrene component, was found to have about the same (weak) activity (Kennaway, Kennaway, and Warren, 1942). This was a disappointment with regard to the correlation sought for.

As for other types of substitution in "active" positions, ethyl and propyl groups were also effective, but activity rapidly fell off with further lengthening of the side chain. The influence of other substituents was unpredictable. On the whole, polar groups and halogen substituents, in the case of polycyclic aromatic hydrocarbons, seem unfavourable for carcinogenesis.

These results should, however, be interpreted with caution (*a*) because lack of activity might, in some cases, have been due to the imparting of water-soluble properties to the compound, facilitating its rapid diffusion from the site of action, and thus requiring larger doses than those actually used, and (*b*) because carcinogenic activity might, in some cases, have been due to *in vivo* conversion of essentially inactive into active compounds.

Regarding the ring structure itself, partial or total hydrogenation led to loss of carcinogenic activity. Substitution of a thiophene (sulphur-containing), a pyridene (nitrogen-containing), or a 5-membered carbon ring, for one of the benzene rings, did not significantly interfere with carcinogenic activity, though this depended, to some extent, on the ring involved.

As these pure compounds could be injected into the body without causing appreciable toxic side effects, it now became possible to investigate carcinogenic action on tissues other than the skin. Indeed, the comparative data for different compounds, discussed above, were based both on papilloma and carcinoma production, by skin applications, and on sarcoma production, by subcutaneous injection. For the skin, a benzene or acetone solution of the hydrocarbon was applied once or twice weekly *for 6 months or more*; for the subcutaneous tissues, a *single* injection was usually given of an oily solution, or sometimes of crystals moistened with glycerol. The latter two methods also served for carcinogenicity tests on the various parenchymatous organs in the body.

In skin, multiple papillomas appeared in the painted area after 6 weeks to a year or more, depending on the potency of the compound, its concentration and the frequency of application, the strain of mouse used, and also on individual variations in response within the strain. These papillomas usually grew progressively, and many eventually developed into squamous carcinomas, while some appeared malignant from the start. In mice, basal-cell carcinoma and malignant melanoma of the skin were only rarely encountered. (In guinea-pigs and hamsters, skin painting with potent carcinogenic hydrocarbons leads more often to melanoma formation.)

After subcutaneous injection in mice and rats, the resulting lesions, appearing after 3-18 months, were sarcomas, again arising at or close to the site of administration of the compound. When the injection was made into a parenchymatous tissue, tumours of the specialised cell type, characteristic of the tissue, developed in many cases, e.g. tumours of smooth and striated muscle, uterus, prostate, bone, brain, kidney, breast, testis, thymus (accompanied sometimes by leukæmia), lung, and urinary bladder.

When these compounds were given by mouth, tumours tended to develop in the gastro-intestinal tract, in the form of squamous carcinoma of the cardiac (squamous-lined) portion of the stomach and adenocarcinoma of the small intestine. Adenocarcinoma of the *glandular* portion of the stomach, which did not develop by feeding these carcinogens, readily developed when such substances were injected into the wall of the organ (Stewart and Lorenz, 1942).

Most tissues in the body are thus potentially capable of responding to the local carcinogenic action of polycyclic aromatic hydrocarbons, some being more responsive than others. In the less responsive organs, fibrosarcomas tend to develop from the connective-tissue stroma before the parenchymatous cells have a chance of reacting.

These differences in tissue response are determined by the animal species and strain, and to a much lesser extent by the particular hydrocarbon used. For instance, in the mouse, the skin and subcutaneous tissue are about equally responsive to most carcinogenic hydrocarbons; in the rat, the skin is refractory while the subcutaneous tissue is extremely responsive to them all; in the rabbit, the situation is reversed, the skin being responsive and the subcutaneous tissue not at all. Different inbred strains of mice exhibit considerable variation in skin response and somewhat less pronounced variation in subcutaneous tissue response. The two trends—skin and subcutaneous tissue response—do not run parallel in the different strains (see Woolley[13]).

Localised action of carcinogenic hydrocarbons on specific tissues is also possible by incorporating a few crystals of the carcinogen in a slice or mince of tissue, and injecting the material subcutaneously. Tumours have thus been induced with embryonic tissues (Greene, 1945; Smith and Rous, 1945), including intestinal mucosa, lung, muscle, cartilage, and skin; and with adult tissues (Horning, 1946, 1947) such as prostate and lung. The latent period of carcinogenesis, by this procedure, is very short.

Other locally-acting chemical carcinogens (see Clayson[18]; Various Authors[19]). —The carcinogenic polycyclic aromatic hydrocarbons, discussed above, are characterised by local action at the site of administration, most tissues of the body being responsive and the tumour yield being usually high. But there are also other classes of locally-acting carcinogens, chemically unrelated one to another, which are, on the whole, weakly acting, and effective only on one type of tissue, and in some cases confined to one species. Care must be taken to distinguish between examples of partial carcinogenesis (i.e. "precipitation" of a tumour at a "preneoplastic" site), and those which are truly carcinogenic (see Berenblum[21]).

Among the doubtful, borderline, or extremely weak carcinogens, are the following: *for skin*: arsenite, conc. HCl, conc. NaOH, oleic acid; *for subcutaneous* tissues: conc. solutions of glucose and other sugars, dil. HCl in phthalate buffer, deoxycholic acid, nickel, and other metals, cholesterol-rich fractions of human tissues, and (in rats only) olive oil and lard; *for oral and rectal mucosa*: alcohol; *for bone*: chromium, cobalt, and arsenic.

The more significant examples of locally-acting carcinogens, among this heterogeneous series, include (*a*) zinc chloride, which produces tumours in the fowl testis (Michalowsky, 1928); (*b*) shale oil, and other mineral oils, carcinogenic for mouse skin (Twort *et al.*, 1928, etc.), which, though including traces of 3:4-benzpyrene and other polycyclic aromatic hydrocarbons, probably owe their carcinogenic action to other (unidentified) classes of compounds (Berenblum and Schoental, 1943); and (*c*) a number of substances that produce sarcomas in mice and rats at the site of subcutaneous injection, such as the dye Styryl 430 (Browning *et al.*, 1936), cellophane and many other insoluble polymers in sheet or membrane form (Oppenheimer *et al.*, 1950), and an interesting group of alkylating agents of which "nitrogen mustard" (XVIII) and its sulphur analogue "mustard gas" (Boyland and Horning, 1949), di-epoxides (XIX) (Hendrey *et al.*, 1951) and β-propriolactone (XX) (Walpole *et al.*, 1954) are important examples.

Physical agents.—The knowledge of occupational cancer in man, which led to the development of chemical carcinogenesis in animals, also stimulated the experimental study of carcinogenesis in animals by *physical* means. In fact, the production of sarcoma of the skin in the rat by X-radiation (Marie, Clunet, and Raulot-Lapointe, 1910) preceded tar carcinogenesis in the rabbit; but the method proved less reliable and convenient for the detailed study of carcinogenesis.

Skin tumours—papillomas, carcinomas, and sarcomas—have also been produced experimentally by long-continued ultraviolet radiation (Findlay, 1928; and others; see Blum[22]), and by burns, caused by heat (Bang, 1925) or freezing (Berenblum, 1929). Yet, the numerous attempts to induce skin tumours in animals by single or repeated *mechanical* injuries were without success—thus finally disproving the old idea of "irritation" as a cause of cancer.

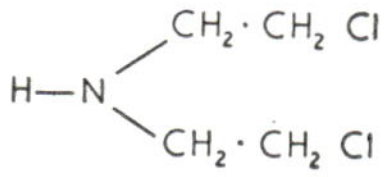

$H{-}N(CH_2 \cdot CH_2Cl)_2$

(XVIII)

di-2-chloroethylamine ("nitrogen mustard")

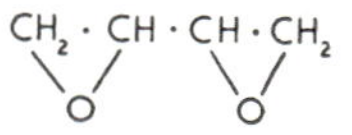

$CH_2 \cdot CH \cdot CH \cdot CH_2$ (two epoxide rings, O bridging each pair)

(XIX)

1:2:3:4-diepoxybutane

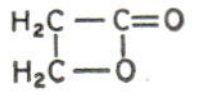

$H_2C{-}C{=}O$ / $H_2C{-}O$ (four-membered ring)

(XX)

β-propriolactone

Subcutaneous implantation of small glass tubes containing radium, produced local sarcomas (Daels, 1926); while insertion of radium into bones produced osteogenic sarcomas (Schinz and Uehlinger, 1931). Administration of radioactive compounds by feeding, or by intravenous or intraperitoneal injection, has also led to the development of tumours in bone and other internal organs (see Martinelli and Brues[13]). Special mention should be made, in this connection, of the results of feeding or injecting into mice, rats, and rabbits various radioactive fission products and plutonium (Lisco *et al.*, 1947). Most of the resulting tumours were in bone, especially with the radium family of elements in the periodic table (e.g. with radio-strontium). With radio-yttrium, given by mouth, adenocarcinomas of the large intestine were produced, as well as other tumours.

Carcinogenesis *in vitro*. —It has recently been demonstrated that normal cells can be transformed into malignant cells in tissue culture through local action of carcinogenic hydrocarbons (Berwald and Sachs[23]). Since systemic influences are eliminated by this procedure, the process of carcinogenesis is thus narrowed down to the cellular level, providing a simplified model for the study of the mechanism of action of carcinogens.

Remotely-acting carcinogenesis—(1) **General**. Many locally-acting carcinogens also have a tendency to influence carcinogenesis at a distance from the site of administration. Thus 1:2:5:6-dibenzanthracene, and certain other hydrocarbons, when injected subcutaneously or applied to the skin, sometimes raise the spontaneous tumour incidence in remotely situated organs—e.g. of lung adenomas, leukæmia, and mammary carcinoma. Another early example of systemic carcinogenesis, already quoted, is that of œstrone in relation to mammary tumours in mice. A more important example of systemic action, which opened up a new field of carcinogenesis, was the discovery by Yoshida (1933) that continued feeding of certain azo dyes led to the development of primary tumours in the liver.

Remotely-acting carcinogenesis—(2) **Azo dyes** (see Miller and Miller[24]). It had been shown long ago that the dye—scarlet red (XXI)—injected under the skin of the rabbit's ear, produced pronounced local epithelial proliferation (Fischer, 1906)—an action subsequently traced to that portion of the scarlet red molecule represented by 2′:3-dimethyl-4-aminoazobenzene (XXII). Though these local skin changes were not truly neoplastic, it was later demonstrated by Yoshida (1933) that in rats, continuous feeding of 2′:3-dimethyl-4-aminoazobenzene led to the development of liver tumours. Kinosita (1935) then showed that 4-dimethylaminoazobenzene (XXIII) was even more effective.

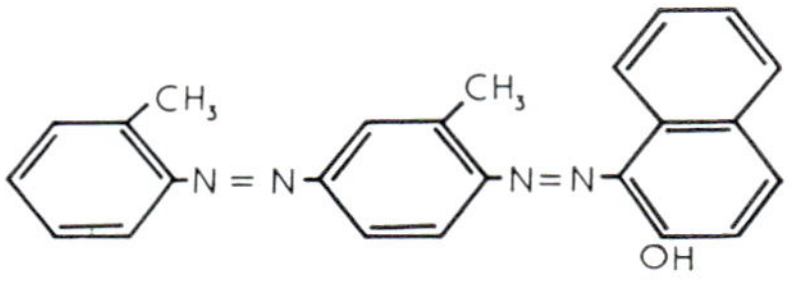

(XXI)
scarlet red

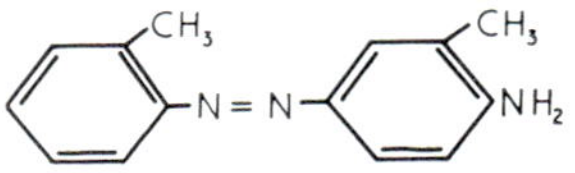

(XXII)
2′:3-dimethyl-
4-aminoazobenzene
(*o*-aminoazotoluene)

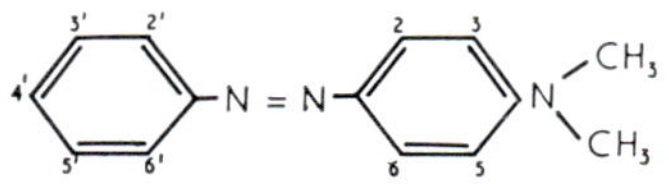

(XXIII)
4-dimethylamino-
azobenzene
("butter yellow")

The carcinogenic action on the liver is a slow process, preceded for many months by hyperplasia of the liver parenchyma, followed by adenoma formation, though usually without cirrhotic changes; and the development of malignant tumours—hepatomas, cholangiomas, and mixed varieties—becomes established in about 8 months, provided the treatment is continuous and the dose is large (e.g. 1 mg. per gm. of food). With lower doses or interrupted treatment the tumour yield is lower and the latent period much longer.

Mice were also found to be susceptible to the action of 2′:3-dimethyl-4-aminoazobenzene (XXII), the tumour yield varying according to strain (Andervont *et al.*, 1942), and the animals responding also to subcutaneous injections of the compound (Shear, 1937). On the other hand, 4-dimethylaminoazobenzene (XXIII)—the more potent of the two compounds for the rat—was only feebly active in the mouse (Andervont *et al.*, 1944).

With regard to the relation between chemical structure and carcinogenicity, once again the position of substitution, as well as the nature of the substituent, was found to be important, though the relation could not always be predicted according to any simple rule. Among the isomers of 2′:3-dimethyl-4-aminoazobenzene (XXII), the 2′:5-dimethyl- and the 2:4′-dimethyl- compounds were carcinogenic for the liver, while little or no activity occurred with other configurations. A more extensive study was made on derivatives of 4-dimethylaminoazobenzene (XXIII): Carcinogenic activity in the liver was maintained when one of the methyl groups was removed (i.e. with 4-monomethylaminoazobenzene) but not when both were removed (i.e. with 4-aminoazobenzene). Additional substituents—especially of another methyl group—led to *augmented* activity when in the 3′- position, but to diminution or even loss of activity when in certain other positions. Fluoro- derivatives were particularly active, even in positions other than 3′-; other halogens less so; while hydroxy-(phenolic) derivatives were inactive. When the —N=N— linkage in (XXIII) was replaced by —C=N— or —N=C—, activity was lost; yet when replaced by —C=C— (producing 4-dimethylaminostilbene), there was marked activity (Elson, 1952).

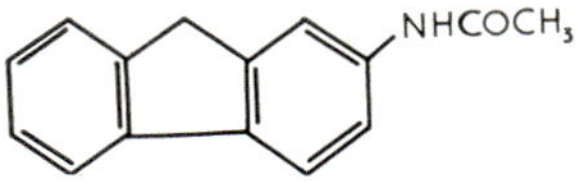

$NHCOCH_3$

(XXIV)
2-acetylamino-fluorene

NH_2

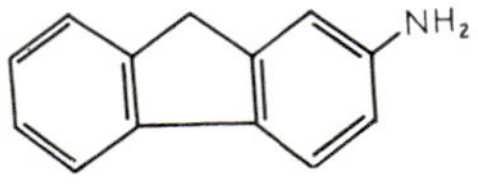

(XXV)
2-aminofluorene

Azo-dye carcinogenesis in the liver is more strongly influenced by diet than any other form of carcinogenesis (see Tannenbaum[13]). The ease with which such tumours were first produced in rats maintained on polished rice (Yoshida, 1933), and the difficulties, by other investigators, using rats maintained on more balanced diets, led to the discovery of "protective factors", especially in yeast and liver. Eventually it was shown that riboflavin prevented liver carcinogenesis by azo dyes (Kenzler *et al.*, 1941); and that the effect was antagonised by biotin (du Vigneaud *et al.*, 1942). The protective action of riboflavin (not effective with other liver carcinogens) is probably connected with the participation of a flavin-adenine-dinucleotide in the enzymatic cleavage of the azo linkage (Kenzler, 1949; Mueller and Miller, 1950), thereby destroying the carcinogen before it can act.

Remotely-acting carcinogenesis—(3) **Other carcinogenic amines** (Various Authors[19]). Unlike the azo carcinogens, which have a restricted systemic action directed mainly to a single target organ—the liver, 2-acetylaminofluorene (XXIV), and its free amine—2-aminofluorene (XXV), when administered by mouth or injection, cause tumours to appear in many different organs. The discovery, made by chance in routine toxicity tests (Wilson, DeEds, and Cox, 1941) before marketing the substance as an insecticide, provided yet another unique type of carcinogen. As an amino- derivative, and by virtue of its systemic or "remote" action, acetylaminofluorene may be classed with the azo compounds; from the viewpoint of general chemical structure, it belongs rather to the polycyclic aromatic hydrocarbons; while biologically it combines some of the properties of each of these classes of compounds.

Carcinogenic action occurs in rats, mice, rabbits, and dogs, with the production of tumours in the liver, external acoustic duct, breast, lung, urinary bladder, intestine, and other organs, and also of leukæmia. The relative frequencies of the different kinds of tumours vary greatly according to species and strain of animal. Thus, liver tumour incidence ranged from 0 to 100 per cent in different rat strains (Wilson *et al.*, 1941) and from 5 to 73 per cent in different mouse strains (Armstrong and Bonser, 1947); and was generally much higher in males than females. Similar, though not parallel, differences were observed with the other kinds of tumours.

Chemical analogues, with the amino- or the acetylamino- group in other positions in the molecule, have been found to be generally non-carcinogenic; but mono- or di-methylation of the amine in the 2- position provided active compounds (Miller and Miller, 1952).

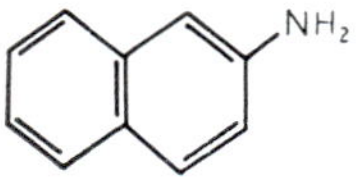

(XXVI)
2-naphthylamine

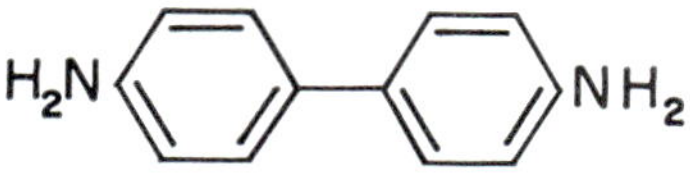

(XXVII)
benzidene

Two important carcinogenic amines, responsible for occupational urinary bladder cancer in man (see Chapter 23), are 2-naphthylamine (XXVI) and benzidine (XXVII). The carcinogenic action of 2-naphthylamine has been confirmed experimentally in dogs (Hueper *et al.*, 1938) and with a weaker action, in rats and rabbits (Bonser *et al.*, 1951).

Another interesting compound, belonging to the series of carcinogenic amines, is dimethylnitrosamine (XXVIII), carcinogenic for the liver and kidneys (Magee and Barnes, 1956). Some analogues of this compound, with replacement of the methyl groups by other substituents, are carcinogenic for the œsophagus, brain and other organs (Druckrey *et al.*, 1961). Dimethylnitrosamine presumably acts as an alkylating agent in the body. Using istopoically-labelled dimethylnitrosamine, Magee and Farber (1962) found evidence of *in vivo* methylation of nucleic acids at the 7-position of the guanine moiety, and of proteins, in liver and kidney cells.

Remotely-acting carcinogenesis—(4) **Natural products** (see Various Authors[19]). The discovery that certain pyrrolizidine alkaloids, derived from wild plants (*Senecio jacobœa*), can produce liver tumours in animals (Barnes and Schoental, 1958) was the first indication that naturally-occurring substances could play an important role in carcinogenesis. The fact that these plants are often used as herbal medicines for man, gave rise to speculations about human liver cancer in Africa being possibly attributable to their use.

The next example was discovered indirectly, following a serious outbreak of a fatal "Turkey X" disease in 1960, with hepatotoxic signs in the dying birds. This was traced to contamination of the groundnut feed with a fungus, *Aspergillus flavus*, which produced a number of related compounds, of which the most active one was subsequently identified as aflatoxin B (XXIX). This proved to be a potent liver carcinogen when tested in different species of animals (Lancaster *et al.*, 1961).

An important feature both of the pyrrolizidine compounds and of aflatoxin B is that even a single dose, administered orally to young animals, is able, after a considerable latent period, to cause liver tumours to develop. The current belief is that aflatoxin, rather than the pyrrolizidine alkaloids, plays a major role in primary liver cancer development in man.

Among the other, recently identified, naturally-occurring liver carcinogens are (*a*) several compounds (a chlorine-containing cyclic peptide and some anthraquinone derivatives), produced by the fungus *Penicillium islandicum*—contaminant of rice in Japan (Miyaki *et al.*, (1959); (*b*) safrole (4-allyl-1:2-methylene dioxy-benzene)—a flavouring agent in root beer (Homburger *et al.*, 1961); and (*c*) cycasin (methylazoxymethanol) present in cycad nuts—sometimes used in the diet in Guam (Laqueur *et al.*, 1963).

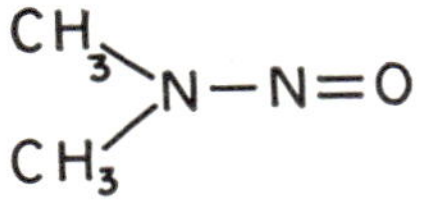

$(CH_3)_2N{-}N{=}O$

(XXVIII)

dimethylnitrosamine

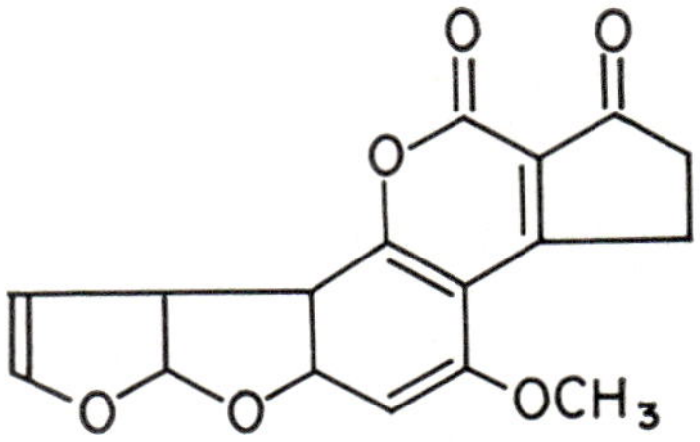

OCH_3

(XXIX)

aflatoxin B

$C_2H_5OCONH_2$

(XXX)
urethane
(ethyl carbamate)

Remotely-acting carcinogenesis—(5) **Miscellaneous compounds** (see Haddow[13]). These include ethyl carbamate or "urethane" (XXVI), carcinogenic for the lung in the mouse (Nettleship and Henshaw, 1943), and weakly so for the liver in the rat (Jaffe, 1947), also weakly carcinogenic for other organs (Tannenbaum, 1960), and an "initiating agent" for skin carcinogenesis (see p. 772; "nitrogen mustard" (XVIII) (Boyland and Horning, 1949) and "mustard gas" or "sulphur mustard" (Heston, 1950), both carcinogenic for the lung in the mouse; also carbon tetrachloride, selenium compounds and tannic acid—all carcinogenic for the liver; thiourea, carcinogenic for the liver and thyroid; benzidene, weakly carcinogenic for the liver, sebaceous glands, and intestinal mucosa; and trypan blue, which produces sarcomas and lymphomas in rats.

With regard to the systemic action of urethane on the lung, mono- and dialkyl substitution of the nitrogen atom leads to diminution of activity (Larsen, 1948) and replacement of the ethyl- by other alkyl groups results in almost complete loss of activity (Larsen, 1947). Response to urethane action on the lung is strongly influenced by the strain of animals used, being related to the tendency to spontaneous lung tumour development (Cowen, 1950).

Remotely-acting carcinogenesis—(6) **Hormonal imbalance** (see Burrows and Horning[9]; Gardner *et al.*,[13]). This section deals with the broader field of hormonal imbalance, rather than with the more limited one of hormonal action, since a sustained disturbance in the hormonal equilibrium of the body is an essential feature of this form of carcinogenesis, which could be brought about by methods other than repeated injections of hormones.

In discussing the part played by œstrogens in the development of mammary tumours in mice (see p. 749), attention was drawn to (*a*) the inhibiting effect of ovariectomy at an early age, and (*b*) the powerfully stimulating effect of repeated œstrogen administration. It is interesting to note here that *in strains of mice in which the adrenal glands are able effectively to take over the function of œstrogen production*, ovariectomy fails to inhibit mammary tumour development (Woolley *et al.*, 1939). (In some of these strains, gonadectomy at an early age not only produces hyperplasia of the adrenal cortex, but later, also, adrenal cortical tumours.) Androgens inhibit mammary carcinogenesis by œstrogens, and this is confirmed by the observation that the grafting of ovaries into males causes mammary tumours to develop later, *but only when the testes had been removed* (Murray, 1928). As already mentioned, the carcinogenic action of œstrogens on mammary tissue operates indirectly via the pituitary gland.

Other tumours which develop, though in smaller numbers, after œstrogen administration include: carcinoma of the uterus, adenoma of the pituitary, interstitial cell tumours of the testis, and lymphoma of the thymus—all in mice; also mammary and pituitary tumours in the rat; fibromatous tumours of the uterus and other organs in the peritoneal cavity in the guinea-pig (Lipschutz[25]), and malignant tumours of the kidney in the hamster (see Kirkman[26]).

There is suprisingly little evidence of carcinogenic activity by any of the other known hormones, with the exception of the growth hormone of the pituitary, which has been reported to produce lymphosarcoma of the lungs, and tumours of the adrenal cortex and ovaries, in rats (Moon *et al.*, 1950).

An interesting case of carcinogenesis by hormonal imbalance is the neoplastic change which ovarian tissue may undergo when grafted into the spleen of gonadectomised rats (Biskind and Biskind, 1944). Since the œstrogenic hormone, produced by the grafted ovarian tissue, now has to pass by way of the portal circulation to the liver, where it is destroyed, it no longer reaches the pituitary gland. The resulting over-production of gonadotrophic hormone by the pituitary causes persistent over-stimulation of the grafted ovarian tissue, and this is presumably responsible for its eventual transformation into a neoplasm.

Remotely-acting carcinogenesis—(7) **by Ionising radiations** (see Kaplan[27]). Malignant lymphomas and leukæmias in mice, which occur spontaneously in certain strains, and which can be artificially induced by systemic action of carcinogenic hydrocarbons or by œstrogens, can also be made to develop by total body irradiation. The subject has become particularly important in view of the significant increase in incidence of leukæmia in man, with the recognition of ionising radiation as a possible cause.

The leukæmogenic action of total body irradiation was first demonstrated by Furth and Furth in 1936. Subsequent studies have shown that multiple small doses are more effective than a single large one; that radiation and chemical leukæmogenic agents can act synergistically; that young females are most susceptible; and that there are marked strain differences in response. However, unlike mammary or lung carcinogenesis, in which the induced effects operate best in strains subject to the respective spontaneous tumours, no such parallel exists between spontaneous and induced leukæmias—indicating that in this case independent genetic factors are involved (Kirschbaum and Mixer, 1947).

A striking feature of the common (lymphatic) type of leukæmia in mice is its early manifestation as a *local* tumour of the thymus, its subsequent dissemination to lymph nodes, spleen, liver and kidneys, but with the leukæmic blood picture only appearing as a terminal complication. Early thymectomy prevents the development of the spontaneous disease in AKR mice (McEndrey *et al.*, 1944) or of that induced by x-irradiation in C57BL mice (Kaplan, 1950). This can be partly reversed, both in the spontaneously-occurring (Law, 1952) and in the induced form (Kaplan *et al.*, 1956) by reimplantation of syngeneic (isologous) thymic tissue.

Gross, in 1951 (see[28]), succeeded in demonstrating the involvement of a virus in spontaneous thymic leukæmia in AKR mice, transmitting the disease by injecting cell-free extracts of the lesions into newborn mice of another strain (C3H) in which leukæmia did not normally occur. Later, Lieberman and Kaplan (1959) found the virus also to be present in *irradiated* C57BL mice, prior to the appearance of the induced disease, but not in *unirradiated* C57BL mice (in which the incidence of the spontaneous disease is less than 1 per cent).

The unique feature of the reversal effect of thymic implantation in irradiated, thymectomised C57BL mice, was that the implanted thymic tissue had never been subjected to the x-irradiation. Three explanations could be postulated *a priori*: (i) that the irradiation produced carcinogenic substances elsewhere in the body, and that these acted on the thymic graft; (ii) that the irradiation induced the leukæmic disease elsewhere in the body, and that leukæmic cells eventually invaded the thymic graft; and (iii) that the irradiation liberated an existing leukæmia virus, lying latent elsewhere in the body, and that this virus then infected the thymic graft. The third (viral-release) hypothesis is by far the most likely explanation.

In fact, the leukæmogenic action of x-irradiation would seem to be more complicated, involving (*a*) release of an existing virus (probably from the megakaryocytes of the bone marrow), (*b*) transient depression of the immune response of the animal (permitting the virus to pass to the intact thymus, or to the thymic graft, without being destroyed in transit), and (*c*) stimulation of the thymic tissue, as an after-effect of initial thymic damage by the radiation (to facilitate its acceptance of the leukæmia virus). Whether the first effect mentioned constitutes a mere release of the virus from the cells in which it exists, or whether it also involves an activation of the virus from a precursor to an active state, is not yet established.

There is still a fourth factor in radiation leukæmogenesis in mice. For leukæmia to develop, the irradiation must be applied to the whole body, lead shielding of one limb, or of the exteriorised spleen, causing a marked depression of the leukæmia incidence. After whole-body irradiation, the incidence can still be depressed by subsequent injection of syngeneic bone marrow or spleen cells (Kaplan *et al.*, 1953). The inhibitory effect can also be obtained by a protein factor extracted from the spleen (Berenblum *et al.*[29]).

Factors Influencing Carcinogenesis

Biological variables.—Carcinogenesis, whether locally-acting or remotely-acting, is not significantly influenced by the age or sex of the animal, or by pregnancy, lactation, or other biological variables. The interesting exceptions are (i) the insensitiveness of newborn skin to *locally-acting* carcinogenesis and the greater sensitiveness of newborn to certain *remotely-acting* forms of carcinogenesis, notably to the leukæmogenic action of urethane; (ii) the influence of sex on mammary carcinogenesis with œstrogens (already discussed); and (iii) the greater sensitivity of the male to both liver and bladder carcinogenesis with 2-acetylaminofluorene, though mammary carcinogenesis with this agent is restricted to the female. There are also minor sex differences with regard to liver carcinogenesis by azo dyes.

Dosage and solvent.—A single injection of about 0·06 mg. is generally adequate for locally-acting *subcutaneous* carcinogenesis with hydrocarbons; while frequently repeated applications, with a cumulative dose of about 3 mg., are generally required for *skin* carcinogenesis with these compounds. This 50-fold difference is presumably due to losses of carcinogenic material from the surface, in the case of skin paintings (see[21]). The requirements for remotely-acting carcinogenesis are very much more variable, ranging from 0·0015 mg. of 1:2:5:6-dibenzanthracene, for systemic lung tumour production, to about 250 mg. of 2-acetylaminofluorene, for effective multiple carcinogenic action. The rate of metabolic destruction and excretion of the carcinogen is no doubt an important factor in determining effective dosage; and in this connection the solvent used as carrier—whether lipoid- or water-soluble, or both, and also whether possessing anti-oxidant properties, etc.—may play an important role.

Diet. The influence of diet may be considered under three headings: (1) the specific role of riboflavin on liver carcinogenesis with azo dyes; (2) the possible effects of vitamins and specific dietary constituents on other forms of carcinogenesis; and (3) the influence of non-specific caloric restriction on carcinogenesis.

The influence of riboflavin on liver carcinogenesis with azo dyes has already been discussed, and shown to be concerned with the metabolic inactivation of the carcinogen rather than with any effect on the responsiveness of the liver cells. Other specific influences of various vitamins and dietary components of the diet have been reported in relation to various types of carcinogenesis (see[15]), but the effects appear to be slight or variable.

The inhibition by caloric restriction operates for both spontaneous and induced tumour genesis. Among the spontaneous mouse tumours affected are mammary carcinoma, lung adenoma, and spontaneous hepatoma (Tannenbaum, 1940, etc.), and leukæmia (Saxton *et al.*, 1944); among the experimentally induced tumours are those of the skin, either by skin painting (Tannenbaum, 1940) or ultraviolet irradiation (Rusch *et al.*, 1945), induced sarcoma (Tannenbaum, 1942), and leukæmia production by carcinogenic skin painting (White *et al.*, 1944).

The inhibitory effects are produced by a caloric restriction corresponding to 50–70 per cent of the control, unrestricted, food intake, involving a balanced diet in which all the components are equally reduced, or in which the essential components are maintained but the caloric restriction is brought about by reduction of carbohydrates alone. Such underfed mice, though remaining smaller than the controls, appear normal and healthy, and actually have a longer average life-span. The resulting decrease in tumour incidence is never complete; the lower tumour yield is associated with a delay in the average latent period.

Several tentative explanations have been put forward to explain the mode of inhibitory action of caloric restriction, such as an influence through the development of anœstrus—in the case of mammary carcinogenesis (White *et al.*, 1944), or through depression of mitotic activity—with respect to skin carcinogenesis (Bullough, 1949). In fact, no satisfactory explanation is yet available.

Local factors.—Histological studies of early tissue changes during experimental carcinogenesis have not added materially to our knowledge of the histogenesis or pathogenesis of "pre-neoplasia".

Pullinger (1940) described certain distinctive appearances in mouse skin after brief treatment with carcinogenic substances, from which the respective potencies of these substances could be evaluated; but in view of the limited range of carcinogens tested, and in the light of subsequent studies, it is doubtful if the observed correlation reflects any basic association. The role of subepithelial tissues in skin carcinogenesis has been extensively studied by Orr (1934, etc.), with special reference to focal ischæmia as a factor favouring the localisation of tumour induction.

The Mechanism of Carcinogenic Action

This can be approached: (1) from the viewpoint of the carcinogens—by correlating their chemical structure with their carcinogenic potencies; (2) from the biochemical angle—by studying the metabolites of carcinogens and determining their role in the carcinogenic process; and (3) from the biological angle —by analysing the carcinogenic effect in terms of cell and tissue response.

Relation between chemical structure and carcinogenic action (Pullman and Pullman[30]).—The early studies with polycyclic aromatic hydrocarbons encouraged the belief that carcinogenic activity was dependent on a characteristic chemical configuration. The discovery of "active" positions for substitution in otherwise non-carcinogenic compounds, the cumulative effects of double or triple substitutions in such "active" positions, and the considerable success in predicting carcinogenic activity for derivatives of simple model compounds, gave support to such an idea. However, several exceptions were noted to any postulated rigid systems of correlation; moreover, the grading of compounds according to their carcinogenicity *when tested on skin* broke down in some cases *when tested by the subcutaneous route*. With the discovery of other carcinogens, e.g. of azo compounds, urethane, carbon tetrachloride, etc., which could in no sense be considered chemically related to the polycyclic aromatic hydrocarbons, the idea of a close parallel between chemical structure and carcinogenic activity became impossible.

Another approach to the problem (see[30]) was based on the following considerations: (*a*) that separate correlations might exist for each class of carcinogenic compounds (e.g. one for hydrocarbons, one for azo compounds, etc.), even though no single over-all correlation was possible; and (*b*) that common factors might be found in physico-chemical rather than structural analogies, as expressed by the electron characteristics of the compounds.

A fair correlation was found to exist between the calculated "electron densities" at the "K" region in angular polycyclic aromatic hydrocarbons (XXIX) and their carcinogenic potencies—the values for the electron densities being an expression of the reactivity of the molecule, varying according to the structure of the ring system in question, and according to the nature and positions of any substituents in other parts of the molecule.

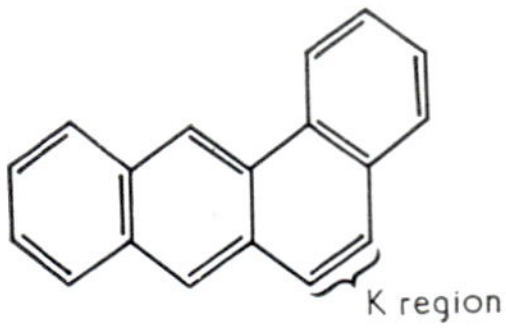

(XXIX)

While this hypothesis enjoys at the moment considerable popularity, it suffers from certain inherent weaknesses, partly in connection with the difficulties in calculating the electron density values (see Coulson[31]), and partly on biological grounds. Though an absolute correlation between electron characteristics and carcinogenic activity is probably illusory, there may be some basis for the association in a limited sense: if the first step in carcinogenic action involves the conversion of a carcinogen into a metabolic intermediary, the electron characteristics of the parent hydrocarbon might indicate the facility with which this specific conversion occurs *in vivo*. This brings us to the problem of the metabolism of carcinogens in the body.

The metabolism of aromatic hydrocarbons (see Peacock[32]; Boyland[19]).—The disappearance of polycyclic aromatic hydrocarbons from the sites of injection (Chalmers, 1934), the absence of their accumulation in other parts of the body or in the excreta (Berenblum and Schoental, 1942), and the detection in the bile of fluorescence differing from that of the injected hydrocarbon (Peacock, 1936,

PHENOLIC METABOLITES OF AROMATIC HYDROCARBONS

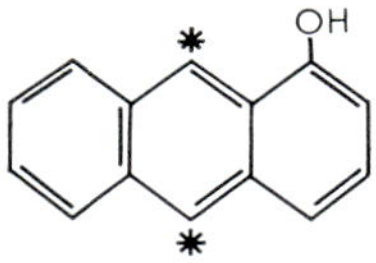

(XXX) 1-anthranol

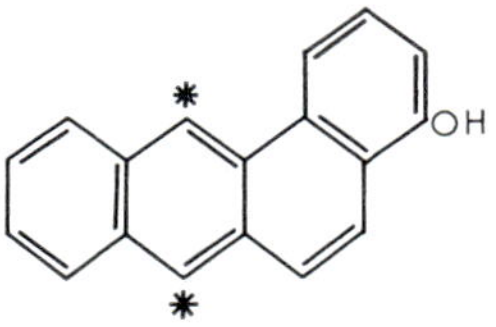

(XXXI) 4′-hydroxy-1:2-benzanthracene

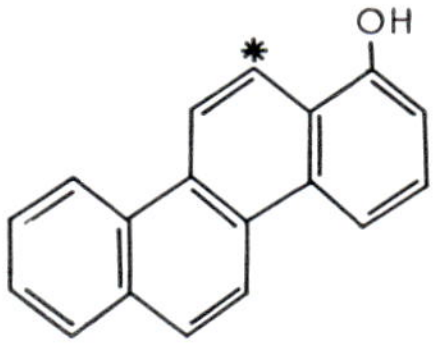

(XXXII) 3-chrysenol

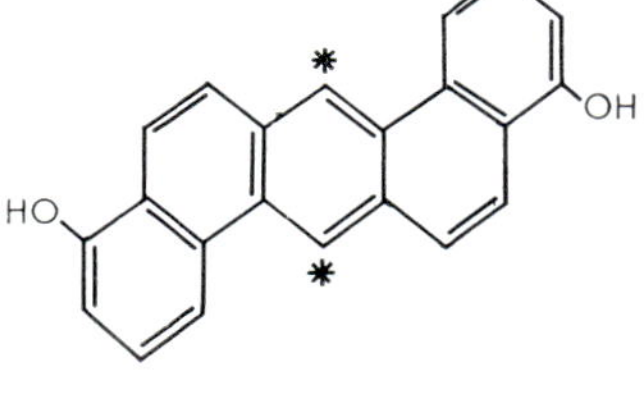

(XXXIII) 4′:8′-dihydroxy-1:2:5:6-dibenzanthracene

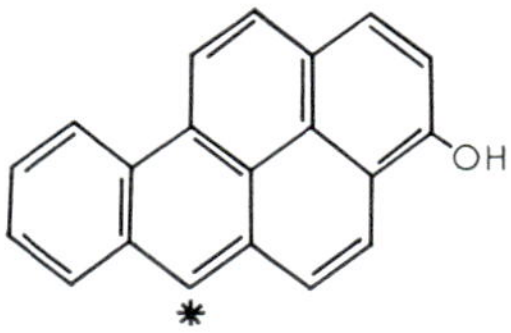

(XXXIV) 8-hydroxy-3:4-benzpyrene

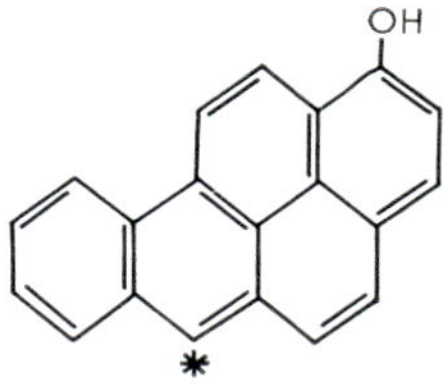

(XXXV) 10-hydroxy-3:4-benzpyrene

Note.—The asterisk in each case denotes the positions of attack by *in vitro* oxidation.

etc.), all pointed to the fact that the body was capable of metabolising these compounds. Subsequent work (Boyland *et al.*, 1938, etc.; Dobriner *et al.*, 1939; Berenblum and Schoental, 1943) led to the identification, in the excreta of animals injected with different hydrocarbons, of a number of phenolic derivatives (XXX–XXXV). The interesting feature about these metabolites is that *the positions in the molecule metabolically attacked are different from those* (*marked by an asterisk*) *obtained by* in vitro *treatment with strong oxidising agents.* (For other sites of metabolic oxidation, see Boyland[19]).

When tested for carcinogenicity, these phenolic metabolites were found to possess, at most, borderline activity, which suggested that they were mere products of detoxication, and that only those molecules which escaped the process were implicated in the carcinogenic action. On the other hand, a synthetically methylated derivative of one of the phenolic metabolites of benzpyrene (8-methoxy-3:4-benzpyrene) proved to be very highly carcinogenic (Cook and Schoental, 1952).

More recent work by Heidelberger and Wiest (1951, etc.) with the use of C^{14}-labelled 1:2:5:6-dibenzanthracene has shown that the body is capable of breaking up these complex molecules with the formation of dicarboxylic acid residues. However, when tested for carcinogenicity, they too were found to be inactive.

The metabolism of azo and amino compounds (see Miller and Miller[24]; Weisburger and Wiesburger[33]).—4-Dimethylaminoazobenzene (XXII), and related azo compounds, tend to lose one or both N-methyl-groups in the process of *in vivo* metabolism, also to be hydroxylated in the para position, and to undergo further degradation by cleavage of the azo linkage. While the monomethyl-derivative is still carcinogenic, no activity is left after the further metabolic changes. These metabolic pathways seem, therefore, to be connected with detoxication and not with carcinogenesis.

From studies with C^{14}-labelled 2-acetylaminofluorene (XXIII), some 12 metabolites were isolated and identified (Weisburger *et al.*, 1954, etc.), involving de-acetylation, and oxidation to hydroxy-derivatives in the 1-, 3-, 7-, and other positions. A different type of metabolite has recently been isolated from rats treated with 2-acetylaminofluorene—namely, the N-hydroxy-derivative (Cramer *et al.*, 1960). This is not only unique as a pattern of metabolic oxidation, but also biologically, since this metabolite proved to be more carcinogenic even than the parent compound. Protein binding *in vivo* has been reported with unidentified derivatives of the parent hydrocarbon (Miller and Miller, 1952).

An interesting aspect of the metabolism of 2-naphthylamine (XXV) is that one of its metabolites—2-amino-1-naphthol—is *locally* carcinogenic for the tissue (urinary bladder epithelium) for which the parent compound is *remotely* carcinogenic (Bonser *et al.*, 1952).

The observation that many carcinogens become bound to proteins *in vivo*, and that in the case of liver carcinogenesis with azo dyes, this binding occurs during the early stages but not in the resulting tumour cells (see Miller and Miller[24]), has given rise to the "deletion" hypothesis of tumours. According to this, tumour cells differ from normal cells in lacking some specific enzyme, which has been permanently destroyed through "protein binding" during the process of carcinogenesis (see p. 773).

Biological mechanism—(1) **Tissue response** (see Berenblum[21]). The "irritation theory of cancer causation"—one of the earliest attempted explanations of carcinogenesis—became untenable when it was shown (*a*) that *mechanical* injury, whether mild or severe, single or frequently repeated, was incapable of producing tumours in animals; and (*b*) that no parallel existed between the carcinogenic potencies of different agents and their "irritating" properties, if by the latter was meant the ability to induce simple reparative hyperplasia (Berenblum, 1944). A necessary implication of the discarded theory was that neoplasia was a kind of extension of hyperplasia; and this also became subject to criticism, since the hyperplasia which precedes neoplasia is a diffuse process, indistinguishable from hyperplasias not connected with carcinogenic action, whereas tumours, in their early stages, are discrete lesions. This raised the more general question: whether the specific tissue changes responsible for the evolution of a tumour could at all be interpreted in terms of morphology.

The alternative approach to the problem was to study neoplastic response in a more functional sense, and under varying experimental conditions, i.e. *when the carcinogenic action is augmented or inhibited by modifying factors.* This represented, in a sense, the biological counterpart to the accepted biochemical techniques of elucidating complicated chain-reactions by adding intermediary substrates, or by blocking metabolic pathways at different points.

Such modifying effects were first observed in experiments designed for other purposes. When tar-painted mouse skin was scarified, the tumours tended to become localised at the wound edges (Deelman, 1923). When application of di-2-chloroethylsulphide ("mustard gas") was added to tar painting, a pronounced *inhibition* of carcinogenesis was observed (Berenblum, 1929); yet, when another skin "irritant"—croton oil—was tested together with a dilute carcinogen, a striking *augmentation* of carcinogenesis resulted (Berenblum, 1941). Many other "anticarcinogens" and "cocarcinogens" have been described (Sall *et al.*, 1940; Crabtree, 1941; Setälä, 1949); however, the majority of substances tested together with carcinogens failed to elicit either effect. Furthermore, though some of the cocarcinogens were themselves mildly carcinogenic, their cocarcinogenic action could not easily be attributed to a simple additive effect.

An important development arose from a study of the regression of tar-induced papillomas in the rabbit's ear (Rous and Kidd, 1941). After marking the site of each papilloma, by injecting India ink at its base, the tumours were allowed to regress by discontinuing the tarring. Later resumption of tarring led again to the appearance of papillomas, *many of which arose at the exact sites where previous ones had disappeared.* Similar effects were obtained with certain non-carcinogenic stimuli for the secondary treatment, e.g. with turpentine, chloroform, and more effectively, by punching holes in the carcinogen-treated ears (Friedewald and Rous, 1947). They concluded (*a*) that "latent tumour cells", irreversibly different from normal cells, could persist for many months, thus constituting "tumours in a sub-threshold state", which required additional aid for progressive neoplasia; and (*b*) that carcinogenesis was therefore made up of at least two independent stages: an *initiating stage*, during which normal cells are irreversibly converted into "latent" (or, to use a preferable term, "dormant") tumour cells, and a *promoting stage*, during which these are made to change from dormancy to progressive growth.

Confirmation of the validity of these conclusions came independently from a detailed study of the cocarcinogenic action of croton oil on mouse skin: When, instead of allowing this substance to act *concurrently* with a carcinogen, it was applied for several months *before starting carcinogen painting*, the tumour yield and average latent period remained unaffected; when the croton oil treatment was begun *after cessation of a brief period of carcinogen painting*, many more tumours developed than in control mice receiving carcinogen alone (Berenblum, 1941). Even a single application of a carcinogen (3:4-benzpyrene), which was insufficient to produce skin tumours by itself, caused many to appear when the action was followed by croton oil treatment (Mottram, 1944). The fact that croton oil could *complete* the process of carcinogenesis but could not *initiate* it, indicated that the two phases of carcinogenesis had different biological mechan-

THE "TWO-STAGE MECHANISM" HYPOTHESIS OF CARCINOGENESIS

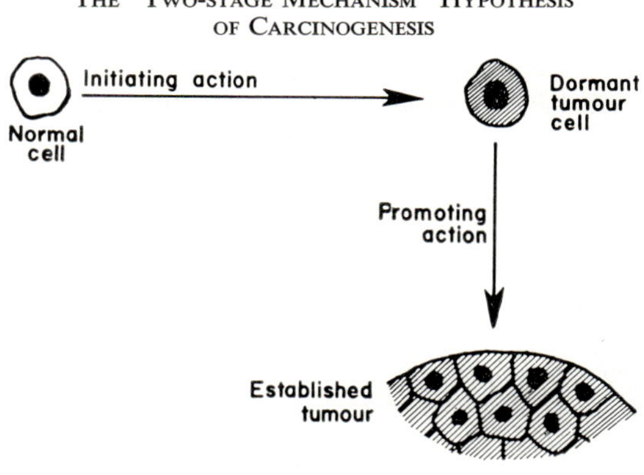

24/FIG. 1

isms (Berenblum, 1941). Tannenbaum (1944) showed that the inhibiting effect of caloric restriction operated on the promoting, but not on the initiating, stage of skin carcinogenesis.

This "two-stage hypothesis" of carcinogenesis lent itself to quantitative analysis: if the specific neoplastic transformation from normal to "dormant" tumour cells occurred at the initiating stage, the subsequent promoting action should theoretically do no more than convert these into visible tumours. In other words, the ultimate *number* of tumours produced should be a function of initiating action, while their *speed of production* should be determined by the promoting action. When this was tested experimentally—by applying different concentrations of carcinogen (once only) as initiating agent, followed by standard croton oil treatment, in one series, and by delaying the croton oil treatment for various intervals, in another series—the theoretical expectations were fully realised (Berenblum and Shubik, 1947).

These experiments were complicated by the fact that (*a*) the agents used for initiating action were actually *complete* carcinogens with the promoting effect suppressed through very short action, and (*b*) the agent used for promoting action also possessed slight carcinogenic activity.

To eliminate completely the possibility that the effects produced by this "two-stage" process were not additive, rather than consecutive actions of different processes, the standard procedure was tested in reverse—i.e. with the croton oil treatment *before* the single carcinogen painting, *under otherwise identical conditions*: virtually no tumours developed under these reverse conditions (Berenblum and Haran, 1955). In order to overcome the other complications, attempts were made in various laboratories to discover "pure" initiating and "pure" promoting agents. So far, one of the two objectives has been realised: *urethane*, carcinogenic for lung, and mildly so for liver, but totally devoid of such action on skin, and failing even to produce demonstrable hyperplastic changes in that tissue, nevertheless proved to be an efficient *initiating* agent for mouse skin—i.e. causing tumours to develop when its application is followed by croton oil treatment (Salaman and Roe, 1953).

There are indications that the "two-stage" mechanism also operates in relation to carcinogenesis in the thyroid (Bielschowsky, 1945) and liver (Glinos *et al.*, 1951); and some investigators have speculated that in mammary gland carcinogenesis, the milk virus agent might be the initiating factor and œstrogens the promoting factor. However, considerable technical difficulties are encountered in testing the two-stage hypothesis for carcinogenesis of internal organs.

Some interesting developments in the field are concerned with the ability of 2-acetylaminofluorene (Ritchie and Saffiotti, 1955), 9:10-dimethyl-1:2-benzanthracene (Graffi *et al.*, 1955), and urethane (Haran and Berenblum, 1956) to act as initiating agents for mouse skin *when administered systemically.*

Biological mechanism—(2) the "Somatic cell mutation" hypothesis (see Bauer[34]; Burdette[35]). This hypothesis, which postulates a gene mutation *in a somatic cell* as the specific cellular change responsible for tumour induction, aims to explain (*a*) the irreversibility of the neoplastic transformation, (*b*) the unlimited variety of types of tumours, and (*c*) the frequency of nuclear abnormalities, at least in the more rapidly growing malignant tumours. Though highly attractive, this hypothesis cannot be convincingly proved or disproved, since the acid test of a mutation—by crossing the alleged mutated cell with a normal cell and analysing the characters of the progeny—is impossible with somatic cells (Haldane, 1934). Indirect evidence in support of the hypothesis is the demonstration that many of the known mutagens for *Drosophila*, *Neurospora*, *E. coli*, etc., are carcinogenic when tested on mice, and that many of the known carcinogens possess mutagenic properties on these organisms (Tatum, 1947; Demerec, 1948). Yet, the correlation is far from close (Latarjet, 1948); and other experimental evidence has been adduced that argues against the alleged association (see Burdette[35]).

The original hypothesis also seemed illogical in one respect: a mutation represents an instantaneous change, whereas carcinogenesis is one of the slowest biological processes. But this difficulty could be overcome on the basis of the "two-stage" mechanism, since only the brief initiating phase of carcinogenesis could possibly be mutational, the promoting phase being concerned with a very different process, namely, a delay in maturation of the dormant tumour cells (see Berenblum[36]). Even this modified "mutation" hypothesis is open to question, since the main characteristic which the hypothesis aims to explain—

irreversibility—could equally well be interpreted on the basis of some abnormal type of differentiation (see Henshaw[37]). Mathematical attempts to support the mutational nature of initiating action seem unconvincing.

Biological mechanism—(3) **Intracellular response.** Apart from the observation that a blue fluorescent material is microscopically demonstrable in the cytoplasm surrounding the nuclei of cells treated with polycyclic aromatic hydrocarbons (Graffi, 1941), there is remarkably little known about the *intracellular* site of action of these, or other types of carcinogens. Unidentified acidic moieties of polycyclic hydrocarbons, bound to proteins, have been demonstrated in treated tissues (Tarbell *et al.*, 1956).

A different aspect of essentially the same problem arose from a study of "radiomimetic" compounds (see Haddow[13]). Attention has already been drawn (see p. 759) to the carcinogenic properties of nitrogen and sulphur mustards, diepoxides, and other "bifunctional" alkylating agents (so called because of double, highly reactive, side chains in the molecule). Originally investigated as potential agents for chemical warfare, these compounds were found to produce cell and nuclear damage of a kind reminiscent of the effects of X-radiation—hence the name "radiomimetic" drugs. Because of this analogy, they were tested both for carcinogenic and tumour-inhibiting properties, and indeed were found to possess both.

In the light of these biological activities, and the knowledge of their chemical properties of combining, at the two reactive ends of the molecule, with cell components, the "cross-linking" hypothesis of carcinogenesis was formulated by Haddow and his associates, which postulated that the carcinogenic action of these compounds might be dependent on cross-linking either within two parts of a protein molecule, thus interfering with its folding properties, or between two adjacent protein molecules, causing, for instance, a disturbance in the separation of the mitotic spindle during nuclear division. The accumulating evidence of dicarboxylic acid residues of hydrocarbon carcinogens may conceivably bring these in line with the compounds discussed here.

In constrast to the theory that irreversible neoplastic transformation of a cell must, of necessity, involve a change in the genome (i.e. in the composition of the DNA of the nucleus, which carries the genetic information of the cell), is that based on the belief that carcinogenic action depends on the combination of the carcinogen, or its metabolite, with a specific *protein* in the cell, which is eventually deleted (Miller and Miller, 1951; Wiest and Heidelberger, 1953). This alternative theory (see Pitot and Heidelberger[38]), by analogy with that of Monod and Jacob (1961) for the control of cellular differentiation, postulates that the protein in question serves as a controller of a repressor gene, which normally regulates the activity of growth-regulating genes, and that the elimination of the protein permits free expression of such growth-regulating genes. (It should be noted, however, that cell division is not the only attribute of neoplasia, or even the most important one—see Chapter 21.)

Tumour Viruses

The "virus theory of tumour causation", originally based on theoretical speculation (Borrel, 1903) and subsequently on experimental findings among restricted groups of tumours (Ellerman and Bang, 1908; Rous, 1911; Shope,

1933; Bittner, 1942), has stimulated a considerable volume of research (see (Oberling and Guerin[39]; Duran-Reynals[13]; Various Authors[19, 40, 41]).

The *aim* of the theory was to account for the progressive growth of tumour cells, and to find a common underlying factor for the diversity of carcinogenic stimuli. The main *support* for the theory was that certain tumours do contain viruses capable of transmitting the disease. The main *controversial issue* was whether this limited verification of the theory for some types of tumours could be taken to mean that a virus mechanism was involved in all tumours.

Those who supported the theory maintained that infectivity was not necessarily an essential condition, since failure to demonstrate a virus might be technical—i.e. that some viruses, like certain enzymes, might be strongly linked to the living cell and, therefore, not extractable. Those who opposed the theory stressed the fact that the recognised virus tumours constituted a very small proportion of all tumours studied, and that they differed in many respects from the "non-virus" tumours. The problem was further complicated by the fact that the older concept of viruses as *living symbionts* later gave place to the idea that viruses might constitute *mutated genic material* which did not really "multiply" itself, but served as a template, enabling the host cells to reproduce its kind. In this sense, the virus theory becomes a problem of innate cell biology.

The first demonstration of a virus being implicated in neoplasia was in connection with fowl leukosis (Ellerman and Bang, 1908)—a very common disease of the fowl, though the importance of the problem of tumour viruses only became apparent after the classic work of Rous (1910, etc.) on "filtrable" fowl sarcomas. Of the many fowl tumours subsequently studied by Rous, Fujinama (1911), Teutchlaender (1921), Begg (1927) and others, several proved to be "filtrable", each possessing distinctive morphological and functional characters faithfully transmitted by their respective "cell-free agents". They were also shown to be immunologically distinguishable (Andrewes, 1933).

The viral nature of these agents was established by evidence of their "multiplication" *in vivo*, and by their passage through bacteria-proof filters but not through collodion membranes. Ultracentrifugation analyses established the size of the virus particle of Rous fowl tumour No. 1 as about 75 mμ, chemical analyses determined its composition as an RNA-protein complex with lipoid and carbohydrate components.

A further impetus to the tumour-virus problem was given by the discovery (Shope, 1933) that spontaneous skin papillomatosis—a common disease of wild cottontail rabbits—was transmissible to domestic rabbits by tattooing cell-free extracts of the lesions into the skin. Here, too, the agent was shown to be viral in nature, though smaller in size than those of fowl sarcomas (Sharp *et al.*, 1946), and of DNA type (Taylor *et al.*, 1942) etc. Virus material, though easily obtained from the lesions of cottontail rabbits, was rarely recoverable from those induced in the domestic rabbit; yet its presence in these animals was demonstrable by immunological means. The virus is strictly specific for the squamous epithelium of the rabbit's skin, the mouth mucosa and other epithelia being unresponsive. In the cottontail rabbit, the papillomas may grow rapidly, but often regress, and rarely become malignant; in the domestic rabbit, growth may be slow, yet malignancy may eventually supervene. When the virus material is injected intravenously into rabbits bearing *tar* papillomas, the latter may rapidly become converted into carcinomas (Rous and Kidd, 1938). Some weeks after local infection of the skin, the rabbits become resistant to further inoculation, when antibodies appear in the blood. The virus already present inside the tumour cells remains protected, however (Kidd, 1938), as is the case with the fowl sarcoma viruses.

The implication of an RNA virus in mammary gland carcinogenesis, transmitted by the mother's milk, has already been discussed. Further examples of viruses involved in animal tumours included a fibroma of the rabbit, serologically related to infectious myxomatosis (Shope, 1932; Ahlström, 1938), and a tumour of the kidney of the frog (Lucké, 1934).

One of the difficulties in accepting the "virus theory" of tumours was the necessity of postulating the existence of thousands of different viruses, to account for the different types and varieties of tumours. Gye and Purdy tried to overcome this difficulty by proposing a single living virus for all neoplasms, and in addition, the requirement of multiple, non-living, protein factors for imparting the specific characters in each case. The evidence in support of this ingenious scheme proved, however, to be based on false premises.

As for the fundamental question, why intracellular viruses should ever cause progressive multiplication of infected cells, Duran-Reynals[12] put forward the view that the two opposite effects—cell stimulation and cytopathic effects—might actually represent different phases of a single basic property, depending on the responsive state of the host. He was able to show that fowl tumour virus, when injected into very young chicks or embryos, did not produce tumours but caused hæmorrhagic lesions. He did not, however, succeed in his attempts to achieve the opposite effect, i.e. so to alter the condition of the host that necrotising viruses should induce tumours. The general principle has, however, received support recently, when it was shown, in *in vitro* studies, that a balanced virus-cell relationship generally leads to cell proliferation, while excessive virus multiplication causes the cell to burst.

Further progress in the study of the tumour virus problem was made possible by recent advances in general virological techniques—e.g. in the purification and chemical characterisation of viruses, the study of their physical properties, determination of their size and morphology by electron microscopy, and analysis of their mechanisms of action (*cf.* phage replication in bacteria, etc.), by studying their behaviour and replication in cells grown in tissue culture.

While some progress has been made in purifying the Rous virus, the "purified" material is still too crude to permit more exact characterisation. Rubin *et al.* (1961) have shown that the Rous sarcoma virus is incapable by itself of causing the neoplastic transformation of normal fibroblasts, but requires the concurrent action of a "helper virus", which appears to be closely related to, or possibly even identical with, the fowl leukosis virus. Since then, examples of "helper viruses", implicated in other systems, have been recognised.

The involvement of a viral factor in *mouse* leukæmia has also been long suspected; yet all earlier attempts to demonstrate its presence (by injecting cell-free extracts of leukæmic tissues into normal adult mice) proved unsuccessful. In 1951, Gross demonstrated that this could, in fact, be achieved by injecting cell-free extracts from Ak mice (high spontaneous leukæmia strain) into *new-born* C3H mice (low leukæmia strain). The resulting leukæmia was lymphocytic in type.

More recently, Graffi[40] was able to induce *myelocytic* leukæmia in mice by means of cell-free extracts obtained from mice bearing a transplantable (Ehrlich) sarcoma.

Even more interesting and significant was the discovery of Stewart, Eddy, and co-workers (see[42]), that when the crude virus material of Gross was cultivated *in vitro* (on monkey kidney tissue or chick chorio-allantoic membrane) and then injected into mice, a great variety of different types of tumours developed, including tumours of the parotid, kidney, mesothelial tissues, connective tissue, mammary gland, etc., *but only rarely did leukæmia appear*. Because of the diversity of tumour types produced, the responsible agent was named "polyoma" virus. This was different from other tumour viruses in several respects: (*a*) as mentioned, it produced a wide spectrum of tumours; (*b*) it proved to be contageous, being transmitted by contact with saliva, urine and fæces; and (*c*) it was found also to be infective when injected into rats, rabbits, guinea-pigs and hamsters.

It was difficult, at first, to decide whether this was a single virus with multiple potentialities or a mixture of independent viruses; and if a single virus, whether it was related to the leukæmia virus, or a mutated form of it developed during the *in vitro* cultivation, or altogether independent from it. Recent work established beyond any doubt that it is a single virus, and independent of the leukæmia virus. The most convincing evidence was obtained by cultivating clones of the polyoma virus from a single virus particle (by the "plaque" technique) and demonstrating that the progeny of such a single virus particle gave rise to the same diversity of tumours (but not including leukæmia) on injection into mice (Winocour and Sachs[43]). The polyoma virus is now known to be DNA in composition.

Among the other recognised tumour viruses in mice are (i) the Graffi chloroleukæmia virus, isolated from a European strain of mice—possibly related to the Gross virus which produces thymic lymphatic leukæmia in AKR mice (Graffi, 1955); (ii) the Moloney virus, obtained from Swiss mice carrying the S37 transplanted sarcoma (Moloney, 1960)—which is distinct from the Gross virus; (iii) the Friend virus, also derived from Swiss mice bearing S37 sarcoma—causing a reticulum-cell type of leukæmia (Friend, 1956); and (iv) the Rauscher virus, similar to, but distinct from, the Friend or Gross virus (Rauscher, 1963).

Two interesting examples of viruses which, while non-oncogenic for their natural hosts, are capable of transforming normal cells of other species into tumour cells, are (i) the SV-40 virus, normally present (as a non-pathogenic carrier virus) in monkey kidney cells in tissue culture, which is oncogenic for *hamster* cells (Eddy *et al.*, 1961) and (ii) certain members of the group of adenoviruses, normally affecting man (in which they cause a variety of inflammatory diseases), which are similarly capable of transforming *hamster* cells into tumour cells (Trentin *et al.*, 1962).

Tumour Transplantation

Early studies (see Woglom[44, 45]).—Many early attempts to transmit cancer from man to animal were motivated by the desire to demonstrate an infective causative agent; *the results were consistently negative*. Transference of the disease was, however, shown to be possible by injecting tumour material from rat to rat (Hanau, 1889) or from mouse to mouse (Morau, 1891); and this species specificity was subsequently confirmed by other investigators. The studies of Loeb (1901), Jensen (1903), and Bashford, Murray, and Cramer (1905), demonstrated how closely the morphology and behaviour of the apparently "induced" tumour always resembled that of the original growth. From these and other results, it became clear that the process was not one of tumour induction at all, but depended on *a transfer of live tumour cells* which continued to multiply in the new host. Only the tumour cells proper were descendants of the original growth, the stroma and blood vessels being provided by the new host. This process of tumour transplantation could be continued successively, apparently for unlimited generations, thus maintaining "standard strains" of tumour material, so valuable for the controlled scientific study of the disease.

The failure of a tumour transplant to take root in a foreign species ("*hetero*-transplant") was at first interpreted as indicative of the development of tumour immunity; and this belief was strengthened by the fact that such failure to "take" also occurred sometimes among animals within the same species ("*homo*transplant"), or could be brought about artificially by surgical removal, or destruction *in situ,* of a previous transplant in a responsive animal. The "failure to take" often took the form of a transitory growth of the graft followed by regression.

Transplantation in inbred strains (see Little[5]; Snell[13]; Law[46]; Gorer[47]).—It was eventually demonstrated (*a*) that tumour transplantation was 100 per cent successful when performed into animals of the strain of origin; (*b*) that transplantation was also 100 per cent successful in F_1 hybrids (first generation hybrids of crosses with animals of a resistant strain), but far less so in F_2 hybrids—thus proving that the factors involved were Mendelian; and (*c*) that *within inbred strains,* a previous transplant of the same tumour did *not* interfere with the taking of the subsequent one.

Rare examples of immunity to *iso*transplants have been reported, but these are attributable either to somatic mutations in the tumour, in the course of successive transplantations, or to germinal mutations in the strains of mice used as recipients (see Snell[13]).

It may be wondered why a tumour transplant ever took at all in the early studies with heterozygous animals. The explanation rests on the following facts: (1) though several "histocompatibility" genes, numbering up to 14 or more, may be involved in tumour transplantability, the number is sometimes very small, in which case the chances of the alleles in the donor (tumour) tissue and the recipient animal being identical may not be so remote; and (2) with successive transplantations of a tumour, several of the dissimilar alleles may, by mutations followed by selection, become eliminated, until the tumour loses altogether its "strain specificity". [The number of histocompatibility genes involved in a particular tumour is determined by the percentage of takes in the F_2 hybrids (see above), based on Mendelian principles affecting multiple dominant genes (see Little[5]). The determination of their precise *loci* in the chromosomes (Gorer *et al.*, 1948; Snell, 1951) demands more intricate genetic analyses, which cannot conveniently be discussed here. For cytological changes during tumour regression, see Gorer.[47]]

Recent Studies in Tumour Immunity[47]

The following refinements in technique have facilitated the re-investigation of the problem of tumour immunity in more precise terms.

1. The availability of tumour strains possessing very few histocompatibility genes.

2. The development of sub-lines of *susceptible* strains of mice, differing from the latter only by a single gene that renders them *resistant* to a particular tumour —called "isogenic resistant sub-lines".

3. The discovery of specific hæmagglutinogens in mice, which appear to be determined by the genes responsible for the histocompatibility factors (Gorer, 1937, etc.).

4. The demonstration of complement-fixing antibodies in rabbits, in response to certain transplantable tumours in that species—probably associated with a tumour virus (Kidd, 1942).

5. The development of "ascitis tumours" (see Hauschka[48])—through adaptation of transplantable tumours to grow *as free tumour cells* in the peritoneal cavity.

6. The important discovery that the body is capable of developing antibodies against its own normal cells, sometimes giving rise to pathological lesions in certain organs (kidney, thyroid, etc.), known as "auto-immune diseases"[50] raised the question whether it could also develop specific antibodies against its own tumours, whether spontaneously arising or artificially induced. This proved, in fact, to be the case for many types of tumours in animals (see[51]).

An interesting outcome of these studies was the difference in specificity observed between tumour antigens of virus-induced tumours and those of chemically-induced tumours. In the former case, all the induced tumours seemed to share a common antigen (for any particular virus system)[52]; in the latter case, each tumour had its own specific antigen.[51] An extreme example of this was seen when the same carcinogen (e.g. methylcholanthrene) was injected at several sites in the same animal. The tumour antigen of each tumour was distinct. (At first sight, this could seem to argue against the notion that all tumours were viral in origin—see p. 774).

Progression of Tumour Growth

If the term "carcinogenesis" is confined, as it should be, to the biological processes leading to the establishment of a neoplasm, all subsequent evolutionary changes in the tumour must be considered independently. That such "post-carcinogenic" changes do occur is shown, for instance, by the tendency of certain benign tumours to acquire malignant properties in the course of their development. The following is a brief summary of other types of irreversible "progressions" in the evolution of a tumour.

1. **Tumour "autonomy" as judged by loss of dependence on hormonal control** (Furth[53]).—Many tumours which are at first dependent for their growth on a hormonal balance in the body—called "conditioned" neoplasms—may lose their dependence as a sudden, apparently mutational, change. Particularly interesting examples of hormonally dependent tumours are some of the X-ray induced pituitary tumours in mice (see Furth *et al.*[54]).

2. **Tumour "progression"** (Foulds[55]).—This is an extension of the concept by Furth, including not only loss of dependence on hormonal control, but also the development of drug resistance, sarcomatous change during serial transplantation of a carcinoma, and other irreversible changes.

3. **Loss of resistance to homotransplantability, associated with polyploidy** (Hauschka and Levan, 1953).—This has already been discussed in the previous section.

4. **Heterotransplantability as a clinical measure of prognosis** (Greene[56]). The successful growth of certain human tumours in the anterior chamber of the guinea-pig eye has been correlated with the poor prognosis of the tumour in the original host, as manifested by its tendency to metastasise or to recur after radical treatment. The validity of the alleged correlation has, however, not yet been established.

REFERENCES

1. Various Authors (1963). *Epizoologic Approaches to Cancer Etiology.* New York: Ann. N.Y. Acad. Sci., Art. 3.
2. FELDMAN, W. H. (1932). *Neoplasms of Domesticated Animals* (Mayo Clinic Monogr.). Philadelphia: W. B. Saunders Co.
3. BURDETTE, W. J. (1950). *Texas Rep. Biol. Med.,* **8,** 123.
4. BRAUN, A. C., and WOOD, H. N. (1961). *Advanc. Cancer Res.,* **6,** 81.
5. Various Authors (1941). *Biology of the Laboratory Mouse.* (Ed.: G. D. SNELL). Philadelphia: The Blakiston Co.
6. Various Authors (1945). *A Symposium of Mammary Tumors in Mice.* (Ed.: F. R. Moulton). Washington: Amer. Assn. Advanc. Sci.
7. HESTON, W. E. (1948). *Advanc. Genet.,* **2,** 99.
8. Various Authors (1947). *Endocrinology of Neoplastic Diseases.* New York: Oxford Univ. Press.
9. BURROWS, H., and HORNING, E. S. (1952). *Oestrogens and Neoplasia.* Oxford: Blackwell Sci. Publns.
10. DEOME, K. B. (1965). *Cancer Res.,* **25,** 1348.
11. DMOCHOWSKI, L. (1957). In *Cancer* (Ed.: H. W. RAVEN). Vol. **1,** 214. London: Butterworth & Co.
12. MÜHLBOCK, O. (1956). *Advanc. Cancer Res.,* **4,** 371.
13. Various Authors (1959). *The Physiopathology of Cancer,* 2nd edit. (Ed.: F. HOMBURGER). New York: Paul B. Hoeber Inc.
14. BERNHARD, W., GUÉRIN, M., and OBERLING, CH. (1956). *Acta Unio int. Cancrum,* **12,** 544.
15. TANNENBAUM, A., and SILVERSTONE, H. (1953). *Advanc. Cancer Res.,* **1,** 451.
16. DUNN, T. B. (1954). *J. nat. Cancer Inst.,* **14,** 1281.
17. HARTWELL, J. L., and SHUBIK, P. (1957). *Survey of Compounds which have been Tested for Carcinogenic Activity.* (Publ. Hlth. Service Publn. No. 149); Suppl. to 2nd edit. (Hartwell, 1951). Washington: U.S. Govt. Printing Office.
18. CLAYSON, D. B. (1962). *Chemical Carcinogenesis.* London: J. & A. Churchill.
19. Various Authors (1964). Mechanisms of Carcinogenesis: Chemical, Physical and Viral. *Brit. med. Bull.,* **20,** No. 2.
20. WOGLOM, W. H. (1926). *Arch. Path. (Chic.),* **2,** 533 and 709.
21. BERENBLUM, I. (1954). *Advanc. Cancer Res.,* **2,** 129.
22. BLUM, H. F. (1950). *J. nat. Cancer Inst.,* 11, 463.
23. BERWALD, Y., and SACHS, L. (1965). *J. nat. Cancer Inst.,* **35,** 641.
24. MILLER, J. A., and MILLER, E. C. (1953). *Advanc. Cancer Res.,* **1,** 339.

25. Lipschutz, A. (1950). *Steroid Hormones and Tumors.* Baltimore: Williams & Wilkins.
26. Kirkman, H. (1959). *J. nat. Cancer Inst.*, Monogr. No. 1.
27. Kaplan, H. S. (1954). *Cancer Res.*, **14,** 535.
28. Gross, L. (1961). *Oncogenic Viruses.* Oxford: Pergamon Press.
29. Berenblum, I., Cividalli, G., Trainin, N., and Hodes, M. E. (1965). *Blood*, **26,** 8.
30. Pullman, A., and Pullman, B. (1955). *Advanc. Cancer Res.*, **3,** 117.
31. Coulson, C. A. (1953). *Advanc. Cancer Res.*, **3,** 1.
32. Peacock, P. R. (1940). *Amer. J. Cancer*, **40,** 251.
33. Weisburger, E. K., and Weisburger, J. H. (1958). *Advanc. Cancer Res.,* **5,** 331.
34. Bauer, K. H. (1954). *Acta Unio int. Cancrum*, **10,** No. 3, 91.
35. Burdette, J. W. (1954). *Acta Unio int. Cancrum*, **10,** No. 3, 97.
36. Berenblum, I. (1954). *Cancer Res.*, **14,** 471.
37. Henshaw, P. S. (1945). *J. nat. Cancer Inst.*, **5,** 419.
38. Pitot, H. C., and Heidelberger, C. (1963). *Cancer Res.*, **23,** 1694.
39. Oberling, C., and Guérin, M. (1954). *Advanc. Cancer Res.*, **2,** 353.
40. Various Authors (1958). Subcellular Particles in the Neoplastic Process, *Ann. N. Y. Acad. Sci.*, **68,** 245.
41. Various Authors (1964). *Viruses of Vertebrates* (Ed.: Sir Christopher Andrewes), London: Baillière, Tindall and Cox.
42. Stewart, S. E., Eddy, B. E., and Stanton, M. F. (1958). 3rd *Canadian Cancer Conf.,* p. 287. New York: Academic Press.
43. Winocour, E., and Sachs, L. (1959). *Virology*, **8,** 397.
44. Woglom, W. H. (1913). *Studies in Cancer and Allied Subjects.* New York: Columbia Univ. Press.
45. Woglom, W. H. (1929). *Cancer Rev.*, **4,** 129.
46. Law, L. W. (1954). *Advanc. Cancer Res.*, **2,** 281.
47. Gorer, P. A. (1956). *Advanc. Cancer Res.*, **4,** 149.
48. Hauschka, T. S. (1957). *2nd Canadian Cancer Conf.*, p. 305. New York: Academic Press.
49. Oudin, J. (1952). *Meth. Med. Res.*, **5,** 335.
50. Various Authors (1965). *Ann. N.Y. Acad. Sci.*, **124,** 413.
51. Old, L. J., Boyse, E. A., Clarke, D. A., and Carswell, E. A. (1962). *Ann. N.Y. Acad. Sci.*, **101,** 80.
52. Sjögren, H. O., Helström, I., and Klein, G. (1961). *Cancer Res.*, **21,** 329.
53. Furth, J. (1953). *Cancer Res.*, **13,** 477.
54. Furth, J., Buffett, R. F., and Haran-Ghera, N. (1960). *Acta Unio int. Cancrum,* **16,** 138.
55. Foulds, L. (1965). *Cancer Res.*, **25,** 1339.
56. Greene, H. S. N. (1951). *Cancer Res.*, **11,** 899.

Chapter 25

SOME BIOLOGICAL EFFECTS OF RADIANT ENERGY

By E. P. Abraham and R. J. Berry

The danger of exposing the human body to excessive amounts of radiation became apparent from the experiences of some of the early workers with X-rays, who were afflicted by serious lesions which tended to become the seat of malignant tumours. This danger is now of more than academic interest to us all. A considerable number of nuclear weapons have already been exploded and many more explosions may yet be made; large groups of people are concerned with the processing of intensely radioactive materials; instruments for the production of subatomic particles with high energy are increasing in size and number; and the use of X-rays and radioactive elements for diagnostic, therapeutic, scientific and industrial purposes is becoming widespread.

These chapters will attempt to provide a general account of the biological effects of radiation and some idea of how far they are understood. It seems worth while to set those aspects of the subject that are of immediate interest to the pathologist against a wider background, by dealing with the action of radiation not only on higher animals but also on other complex organisms, on living cells and on subcellular units, including enzymes and enzyme systems. While experimental work with mammals is essential for estimating the hazards of radiation to man, studies with simpler systems are important if the effects of radiation on the living cell are eventually to be interpreted in biochemical terms.

Origin and Some Physical Properties of Different Radiations

An appreciation of the biological effects of radiant energy requires some knowledge of the nature and energy of the radiations themselves. Radiation consists of electromagnetic waves, or of atomic nuclei or subatomic particles moving at a high velocity. The rays with which we shall be concerned originate from changes within the atom.

Atomic structure.—The atom contains a positively charged nucleus surrounded by negatively charged electrons. Some of these electrons are involved in the formation of bonds between one atom and another, and therefore determine chemical properties.

The mass of an atom, which is due largely to the nucleus, is referred to the mass of the oxygen atom of weight 16. The mass number of a nucleus (A) is the integral number nearest the actual mass.

According to a greatly simplified picture of modern views, atomic nuclei are built up from protons and neutrons. The neutron (n) has a mass number of 1 and is uncharged. The proton (p) has the same mass number but a single positive charge equivalent to the negative charge of an electron. Consequently the mass number of an atom is equal to the total number of particles in the nucleus. The atom is electrically neutral, so that the number of protons in the nucleus equals the number of extranuclear electrons. This is known as the atomic number, Z. It follows that A-Z = number of neutrons.

The neutrons in a nucleus will contribute towards its mass but not towards its charge, and will thus not normally influence the chemical behaviour of the atom. Nuclei which differ in mass but not in charge belong to atoms that are called *isotopes*. In describing isotopes the atomic number is sometimes written as a left subscript to the chemical symbol and the mass number as a superscript. Thus ordinary hydrogen is ${}^{1}_{1}H$ and heavy hydrogen (deuterium, D,) is ${}^{2}_{1}H$.

Origin and Nature of Radiations

Radiation may be a consequence of energy changes in either the extranuclear electrons or in the nucleus, and these changes may occur because the atom is naturally unstable or because it has been purposely transformed into an unstable state.

When an extranuclear electron which has been excited by heat or an extraneous beam of electrons reverts to a lower orbit, energy (E) is emitted in the form of electromagnetic radiation. The frequency, ν, of this radiation is given by the expression $E = h\nu$, where h is Planck's constant. The greater the difference in energy between the electronic levels, the higher the frequency and thus the shorter the wavelength, λ, of the radiation. Large changes in energy, involving electrons of the inner shells of atoms, yield X-rays (λ = 0·05–10Å; 1Å = 10^{-8} cm.), whereas smaller changes yield ultraviolet light (λ = 2000–3000Å). In recent years methods have been evolved for stimulating the emission, from certain materials, of very narrow beams of almost monochromatic light in the ultraviolet, visible or near infra-red range. This is known as Laser radiation, the name being an acronym derived from the first letters of the words of "light amplification by stimulated emission of radiation".

Only certain combinations of neutrons and protons, in which the ratio of the two particles is not far from unity, result in stable nuclei. If the nucleus contains an excess of either neutrons or protons a redistribution occurs, accompanied by the emission of one or several kinds of radiation. Atoms containing such nuclei are said to be radioactive. The discovery of the natural radioactivity of uranium ore by Becquerel in 1896 led to the isolation of radium by the Curies in 1899. In 1934 Curie and Joliot found that certain atoms showed artificial radioactivity after bombardment with α-particles (helium nuclei) emitted by polonium, and following this discovery a wide range of new radioactive isotopes has been obtained by bombarding stable nuclei with certain fundamental particles, particularly deuterons and neutrons. These particles can be produced by high-energy accelerators, such as the cyclotron, or by the uranium pile.

Radioactive atoms emit three kinds of radiation, known as α- or β-particles and γ-rays.

α-particles are double-charged helium nuclei (${}^{4}_{2}He$) with velocities of $1 - 2 \times 10^{9}$ cm./sec. They are emitted by many heavy radioactive elements such as radium, uranium and plutonium.

β-particles are either positive or negative electrons with velocities that may approach the speed of light (3×10^{10} cm./sec.). They are produced by a large variety of radioactive elements; for example, unstable $^{14}_{6}C$ changes to stable $^{14}_{7}N$ by the process $n \longrightarrow p + \beta-$, while unstable $^{11}_{6}C$ changes to $^{11}_{5}B$ by the process $p \longrightarrow n + \beta+$. Positive electrons (or positrons) have only a transitory existence, combining with negative electrons to produce "annihilation" electromagnetic radiation.

γ-rays are electromagnetic radiation and may be considered as X-rays of short wavelength ($\lambda = 0{\cdot}001$–$0{\cdot}1$Å). The emission of γ-rays is often consequent on the emission of α- or β-particles, since the residual nucleus may be left in an excited state.

The Energy of Radiations

The unit commonly used for measuring the energy involved in radiation is the electron volt (EV), that is the kinetic energy acquired by one unit of electric charge moving through a potential of one volt. In terms of heat energy 1 EV per mole equals 23,000 g. cal. per mole.

The energies involved in nuclear transmutations are vastly greater than those of chemical reactions. This is to be expected from the fact that in nuclear transformations there are appreciable changes in total mass, for according to the theory of special relativity energy and mass (M) are related by the expression Energy $= Mc^2$, where c is the velocity of light. The energies of chemical reactions come within the range of 0–10 EV, whereas α- and β-particles emitted from radioactive nuclei may have energies of several million electron volts (MEV). For example, the α-rays from RaC′ have an energy of 7·68 MEV, and ^{32}P emits β-particles with an upper energy limit of 1·69 MEV; γ-rays, which may be described in terms of both wave and particle properties, are encountered with quantum energies varying from 0·1 to 17 MEV. The quantum energies of X-rays depend on the type of generator which produces them and range from about 1000 EV to several MEV and the quantum energies of ultraviolet light are of the order of only 5 EV. However, although the quantum energies of non-ionizing ultraviolet and visible light are relatively very small, Laser beams of light with these wavelengths can produce extremely high energy fluxes at a small focal spot.

The activity of radioactive substances.—The unit of radioactivity is based on the number of disintegrations occurring in unit time. A substance has an activity of one *curie* if it emits the same number of particles per second as one gram of pure radium ($3{\cdot}7 \times 10^{10}$). Millicuries (mCi $= 10^{-3}$ curies) and microcuries (μCi $= 10^{-6}$ curies) are units in common use. One mCi corresponds to $2{\cdot}2 \times 10^9$ particles per minute.

Rutherford discovered that the activity of a radioactive element decays exponentially with time. The period in which half the atoms have undergone disintegration, which is known as the *half-life*, varies enormously from one element to another. For example, the half-life of ^{14}C is about 5,000 years, that of ^{90}Sr nearly 20 years, and that of ^{32}P about 14 days.

Radiation dosage.—The *exposure dose* for X-rays or γ-rays is measured in terms of the *Rœntgen* (R). The Rœntgen is that quantity of radiation which produces ions containing one electrostatic unit of electricity of either sign in one ml. of air at standard temperature and pressure. It corresponds to $1{\cdot}62 \times 10^{12}$

ion pairs per gram of air. The energy absorbed in one gram of air exposed to one Rœntgen is 83 ergs, or $1{\cdot}98 \times 10^{-6}$ calories. The *absorbed dose* in biological tissues is measured in units of *rads*; one rad represents the absorption of 100 ergs per gram of tissue.

The dosage for α- and β-radiations in tissues is also given in rads. For the calculation of the relative biological effectiveness of different radiations, the rœntgen-equivalent (man) (*rem*) unit is used. This unit merely implies that the same biological damage would be inflicted by exposing a man to a dose of so-many Rœntgens, and has limited applications outside the field of radiation protection, where it is used to specify maximum permissible doses.

If the activity of a radioactive substance and the energy of its radiation are both known, it is clearly possible to calculate the dose of radiation obtained from the substance in unit time.

The Dissipation of Energy by Radiations in Matter

When α-rays, β-rays, neutrons, γ-rays and X-rays pass through matter they dissipate much of their energy by the ejection of extranuclear electrons from atoms. The charged α- and β-particles act directly, whereas X-rays, γ-rays and neutrons act indirectly. X-rays and γ-rays produce their effect through the intermediary of swift secondary electrons. Neutrons passing through tissue project the hydrogen nuclei (protons) with which they come into contact.

An atom that has lost an electron is left as a positively charged *ion*, and such radiations may therefore be grouped together as ionizing radiations. Energy is also dissipated, however, by excitation—that is, by raising an electron in an atom to a state of higher energy. This is the only way in which it is dissipated by ultraviolet light, which can be described as a non-ionizing radiation because it is unable to cause the complete removal of an electron from an atom.

There are other important differences between the dissipation of energy by ultraviolet light and by ionizing radiation such as X-rays. The absorption coefficient for ultraviolet light depends on the molecular structure and may thus vary markedly from one part of a cell to another; it will be very high, for example, in cell structures that are rich in nucleic acid. In contrast, the absorption of X-rays is not affected by the chemical combination of the atoms but depends only on their atomic number. It will thus vary little in different parts of a living organism, except for an increased absorption near bone where there is a concentration of atoms with atomic number higher than those in soft tissue.

The penetrating power of electromagnetic radiations in tissue depends on their wavelength. It is large for γ-rays and X-rays and very small for ultraviolet light. Among other radiations, β-rays have relatively little power of penetration and α-rays less still. For example, the range of an 0·35 MEV β-particle in tissue is about 1 mm. and the range of a 5·0 MEV α-particle is only about 35μ. The α-particle, however, produces a much denser ionisation than the β-particle, X-rays or γ-rays. FIGURE 1 provides an idea of the relative ion density in the path of α-rays and of different types of electromagnetic radiation. A high density of ionisation is associated with a high loss of energy per unit distance. This rate of energy loss is known as the linear energy transfer, or LET.

Almost all the energy dissipated by radiation in living organisms is finally degraded to heat. The general rise in temperature caused by ionizing radiation, which is only about 0·25° C. for a dose of 10^5 rads, is far too small to explain the biological changes that ionising radiations bring about. By contrast beams of Laser radiation can produce local heat effects which may be intense, sometimes causing vaporization in the tissue and an intense pressure wave of short duration which may largely explain their biological effects.[2]

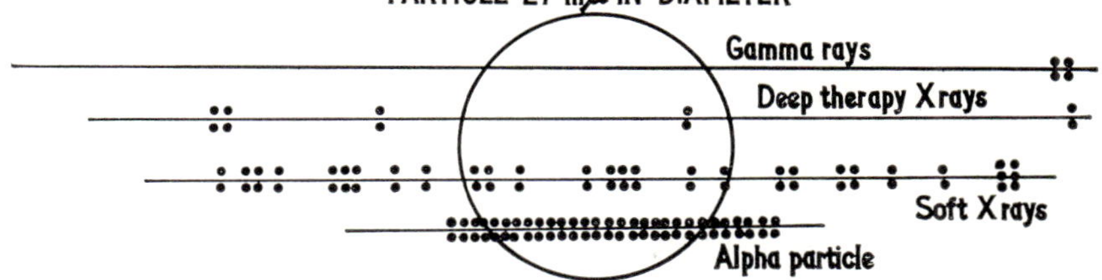

25/FIG. 1. (After Gray.[1])

POSSIBLE MODES OF ACTION OF RADIATIONS ON LIVING ORGANISMS

In some cases marked biological effects have been produced by doses of radiation as low as 5 rads; in other cases doses as high as 5×10^5 rads have been used. Only about 1 in 10^5 of the atoms in tissue are ionized by a dose of 5×10^5 rads, so that in terms of atoms the initial amount of chemical change would be expected to be very small. Such small changes could have important biological consequences, however, if an essential constituent of the cell were destroyed by reaction with ions or radicals formed in the surrounding cellular medium, or if the functioning of an important molecule of high molecular weight was modified by any ionization in a large part of the molecule. These alternatives are assumed in two theories that have been developed to account for the biological actions of radiations—the theory of indirect action and the target theory. It appears that the mechanisms envisaged by both theories can operate, and that sometimes one and sometimes the other is the more important.

Indirect Action

The theory of indirect action may be illustrated by considering the effect of radiation on an organic molecule in dilute aqueous solution. Under these conditions most of the energy will be dissipated in the water, where it will produce free radicals ("activated water") in the following manner:

$$H_2O \rightsquigarrow H_2O^+ + e$$
$$H_2O + H_2O^+ \longrightarrow H_3O^+ + OH$$
$$H_2O + e \longrightarrow H + OH^-$$

In the presence of oxygen the perhydroxyl radical may also be formed:

$$H + O_2 \longrightarrow HO_2$$

Free radicals are highly reactive, and the hydroxyl and perhydroxyl radicals are very strong oxidizing agents. If such radicals were responsible for a chemical change in the molecules of an organic compound in the solution, the amount of the compound changed would be governed by the number of radicals available and would be largely independent of its own concentration. Hence the *proportion* of the compound changed would become smaller as its concentration was increased. This phenomenon is commonly encountered when substances are irradiated in aqueous solution. Moreover, the production of oxidizing agents from water would be expected to be enhanced in the presence of oxygen. We shall see later that the biological injury caused by X- and γ-rays is often reduced under anærobic conditions. With high-LET radiations, such as α-particles and fast neutrons, the effect of oxygen is much less, a fact which has been attributed to the reaction of OH radicals with each other when they are formed close together by a densely ionizing particle, to yield hydrogen peroxide.

$$OH + OH \longrightarrow H_2O_2$$

In the simplest case the amount of solute changed by indirect action will increase linearly with the dose of radiation. If a solution contains two or more solutes, however, the solutes may compete for the free radicals and one may protect the other. In the presence of a protective agent, or if the products of reaction themselves compete for free radicals, the solute under investigation may secure a continually smaller proportion of the radicals available as its concentration diminishes, so that the amount of solute changed will increase less rapidly than the dose of radiation.

Direct Action—the Target Theory

The target theory, which was developed by Lea[3] in England and by Timofeeff-Ressovsky and Zimmer[4] in Germany, has had considerable success in accounting for some of the effects of radiations on viruses, genes and chromosomes. It has attributed these effects to a single ionization, or small number of ionizations, anywhere within a structure of relatively large molecular dimensions. This structure is known as the target.

Suppose that a chemical change occurs in a molecule when an ionization is produced directly within it. A large molecule is more likely to be hit by an ionizing particle than is a small one, and the dose required to change a given proportion of an irradiated substance will therefore be inversely proportional to its molecular weight. This fact has been used for the determination of the approximate molecular size of certain biologically-important proteins which have not yet proved amenable to study by the usual physico-chemical methods.[5]

Assuming that each ionization is effective, we can calculate that a dose of 10^6 rads will produce chemical change in about half the molecules of a substance of molecular weight 10^6. We might thus expect that entities such as genes and the small viruses, which may be considered as molecules of very high molecular weight, would be relatively sensitive to the direct action of radiation.

Certain predictions may be made from the target theory about the shape of the survival curve when the radiation exerts a lethal action, the effect of changing the intensity at which a given dose of radiation is administered, and the relative effectiveness of different types of radiation.

The survival curve.—Suppose that the death of an organism results from an ionizing particle hitting a region of the organism known as the target. The chance of a particle meeting a target will be proportional to the number of living organisms in the space through which it passes. If n_0 is the initial number of organisms and n the number which survive a dose of radiation D, the decrease in the number of viable organisms resulting from an increment dD in the dose will be:

$$-dn = ndD/D_0$$

where D_0 is the dose required to score an average of one hit on the target per organism. By integration

$$n = n_0 e^{-D/D_0} \quad \text{or} \quad ln\, n/n_0 = -D/D_0$$

Hence the survival curve is exponential and a straight line is obtained on plotting the dose against the logarithm of the surviving fraction. D_0 is known as the mean lethal dose, inactivation dose, or 37 per cent dose. It corresponds to 37 per cent survival, since, when $D = D_0$, $ln\, n/n_0 = -1$ and therefore $n/n_0 =$ 0·37.

If the death of an organism were due to the cumulative effect of many ionizations the survival curve would be expected to be sigmoid and not exponential in shape.

Intensity of dosage.—The probability that a given dose of radiation will result in a hit on a target depends on the size of the dose but not on the time in which it is administered. Hence, if the effect of radiation on an organism were due to a single ionization, the chance of the organism being damaged by a given dose would be independent of the intensity of the dose. On the other hand, if the action of radiation were cumulative it would not be surprising to find that a given dose was more effective when administered at a high intensity than at a low one, since the organism might be capable of recovery during the time in which the dose was administered.

Type of radiation.—Ionization is concentrated along the paths of ionizing particles or quanta and it is possible that a densely ionizing particle will produce more than one ionization in traversing the target. If only one ionization were necessary for a biological effect the remaining ionizations would be wasted. A densely ionizing radiation (such as α-rays) would consequently be less effective than a weaker one for a given amount of total ionization. In contrast, if many ionizations were required to produce the biological effect the densely ionizing radiation should be more efficient.

The target size.—If one ionization in a target of given shape and size produces a biological effect it is possible to calculate the 37 per cent dose, because the number of ionizations produced by 1R in a unit volume of tissue is known. Conversely, knowing the 37 per cent dose, it should be possible to calculate the target size.

Direct *versus* Indirect Effects of Radiation

In the following part of this chapter we shall consider some of the experimental relationships between the amount of damage that is caused to molecules or to living organisms by irradiation under various conditions. Some of the simpler entities, such as protein molecules, can be studied in either dilute aqueous solution or the solid state and there may be little difficulty in deciding that a theory of indirect action is valid in the former case and a target theory in the latter. Many living structures, however, can only be studied in a relatively complex environment containing a considerable amount of water. It would be inadvisable to conclude that the action of radiation on these structures was mainly a direct one merely because some of the predictions of the target theory held true.

However, in a number of cases the target theory provides so convenient a method of describing the effect of radiation on living organisms that it is difficult to avoid the impression that the theory must contain a good deal of truth. Nevertheless, the target can scarcely be envisaged as a rigid biological particle within which an ionization produces a stereotyped effect, for the sensitivity of living organisms to radiation varies greatly with certain changes in their environment. A picture of the target as a biological particle together with the layer of fluid immediately surrounding it may be closer to reality. According to this view a hit on the target might be due to an ionization within the particle itself or to a reaction between the particle and an ion or free radical formed in its vicinity.

Some Effects of Radiation on Enzymes and Enzyme Systems

Many attempts have been made to determine whether some of the injurious effects of radiation on the higher animals could be due to damage caused to individual enzymes or to enzyme systems.[6] The results of most of the early work in this field were disappointing, for various degradative enzymes proved to be relatively insensitive to radiation in the kind of environment in which they existed in living cells. Studies of synthetic processes in the cell nucleus promise to be more illuminating. It may be that damage to the organization of certain nuclear enzyme systems represents one of the most important biochemical lesions caused by radiation in the cell, but the most radiosensitive synthetic process is not necessarily the most critical one in relation to the cell's survival, as this will also depend on other factors such as the existence of alternative synthetic pathways.

Degradative Enzymes

Enzymes have been irradiated in the solid state and in aqueous solution. In the solid state very large doses of radiation may be needed to bring about a substantial change. For example, a dry preparation of ribonuclease only lost half its activity when irradiated with about 20×10^6 rads of X-rays[7]. Under these conditions the surviving active fraction decreased exponentially as the dose was increased and the inactivation was probably due to direct action of the radiation (Fig. 2).

A purified enzyme is inactivated much more readily in dilute aqueous solution than in the solid state, but the proportion of the enzyme that is destroyed by a given dose of radiation becomes smaller as the concentration of enzyme is increased. This suggests that the inactivation in aqueous solution is due to a reaction of the enzyme with "activated water". Since the amount of enzyme inactivated increases less rapidly than the dose of radiation when increasing doses are given, it may be assumed that the products of the reaction compete with the unchanged substance for activated water. Many compounds have been shown to exert a protective effect when added to an enzyme solution, particularly compounds such as cysteine and glutathione which react readily with oxidizing radicals.

Enzymes having free SH groups essential for their activity were reported to be particularly sensitive to irradiation in dilute aqueous solution[8], but in tissue homogenates or similar complex biological fluids these enzymes are resistant *in vitro* to doses of radiation that are rapidly lethal to higher animals.[6] Although the SH group itself is radiosensitive, it may be protected in complex media.

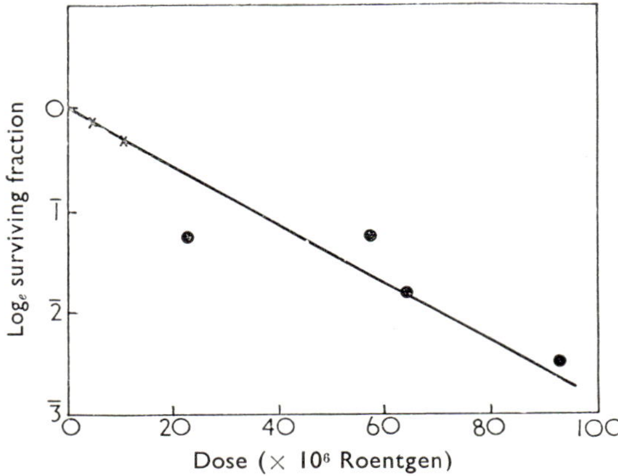

25/FIG. 2.—Inactivation of ribonuclease in the solid state by X-rays. The points and crosses represent results obtained by running the X-ray tube under different conditions. (After Lea, Smith, Holmes and Markham.[7])

Enzyme Systems involved in Oxidative Phosphorylation

Some of the energy released during oxidation in biological systems may be used to generate adenosine triphosphate (ATP) by phosphorylation of adenosine diphosphate (ADP) or monophosphate (AMP), and the ATP so formed provides energy for synthetic processes. When it was discovered that phosphorylation could be easily uncoupled from oxidation by certain chemical reagents, the question arose whether this could also be brought about by radiation.

One of the main sites of ATP generation in the cell is in the mitochondria. Irradiation of mitochondria *in vitro* produced little change in their phosphorylating ability, at least until the doses used were as high as 10,000 rads. But mitochondria isolated from the spleen or thymus of rats which had received doses of 700 rads showed less capacity for generating ATP than mitochondria from normal animals, and the change became apparent two hours after exposure.

Osawa, Allfrey and Mirsky[9] showed that oxidative phosphorylation occurred *in vitro* in isolated calf thymus nuclei, and it has subsequently been shown to occur in nuclei from spleen, lymph node, intestinal mucosa and bone marrow. This nuclear phosphorylation was found by Creasey and Stocken[10] to be exceptionally sensitive to radiation. In cell nuclei from rats irradiated with only 25 rads it was inhibited by from 50 to 80 per cent and the effect could be detected from 3 to 6 minutes after exposure. Subsequently it was shown that phosphorylation of a nuclear histone was depressed by γ-irradiation.

Experiments with bean root tips and bone marrow cultures have indicated that the synthesis of desoxyribonucleic acid (DNA) is depressed after irradiation and that this change occurs most readily when the cells are irradiated prior to mitosis at a stage before DNA synthesis has begun. It has been suggested that one of the reasons for the delay in DNA synthesis, which may be observed with doses of less than 200 rads is a failure, in the nucleus, of the generation of ATP required for the synthesis of DNA precursors.

Some Effects of Radiation on Viruses and Living Cells

A good deal of attention has been given to the ability of radiation to inactivate viruses, which are rich in nucleic acid, and to interfere with cellular division, which is associated with changes in the DNA of the cell nucleus. These studies show that the effect of radiation on the nucleic acid of living organisms is not confined to an inhibition of the preparatory stages for DNA synthesis.

Viruses

The inactivation of purified viruses in dilute aqueous suspension seems to be largely indirect, for the mean lethal dose is increased by increasing the concentration of the virus or by adding a protective agent such as a protein. Figure 3 shows this effect with rabbit papilloma virus. In concentrated solution, or in

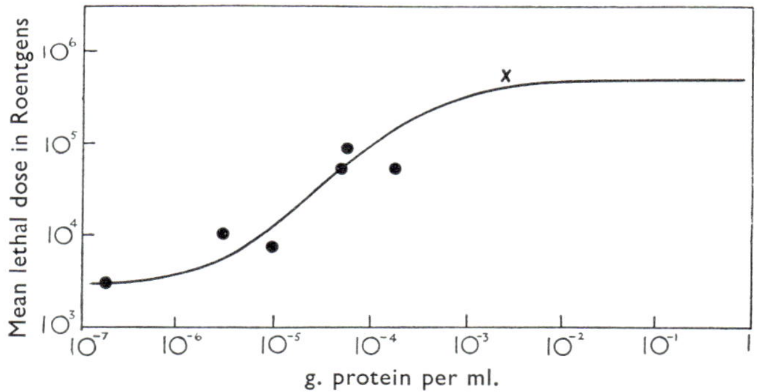

25/Fig. 3.—Dependence on protein concentration of mean lethal dose for rabbit papilloma virus irradiated by X-rays in aqueous solution. ● mainly virus protein; x mainly extraneous protein. (After Lea, Smith, Holmes and Markham.[7])

the presence of a sufficient amount of a protective substance, the mean lethal dose approaches that for the dry virus, and the direct effect of radiation appears to be much more important.

Evidence was collected by Lea[3] for the view that the direct inactivation of viruses by ionizing radiations is caused by a single ionization in each virus particle. Firstly, various plant viruses, animal viruses and bacteriophages show exponential survival curves when irradiated with α-rays, β-rays, γ-rays or X-rays. Secondly, the effect of a given amount of radiation appears to be independent of the intensity at which it is administered. Thirdly, the mean lethal dose increases with the density of ionization produced by the radiation, that is, it increases in the order γ-rays, X-rays and α-rays. Fourthly, with a given type of radiation the mean lethal dose is greater for small viruses than for large ones.

On the assumption that a single ionization within a spherical target is sufficient to cause inactivation, the target volume for a number of viruses has been calculated from the mean lethal dose. With some of the small viruses, as may be seen from FIG. 4, the size of the target is found to be rather similar to

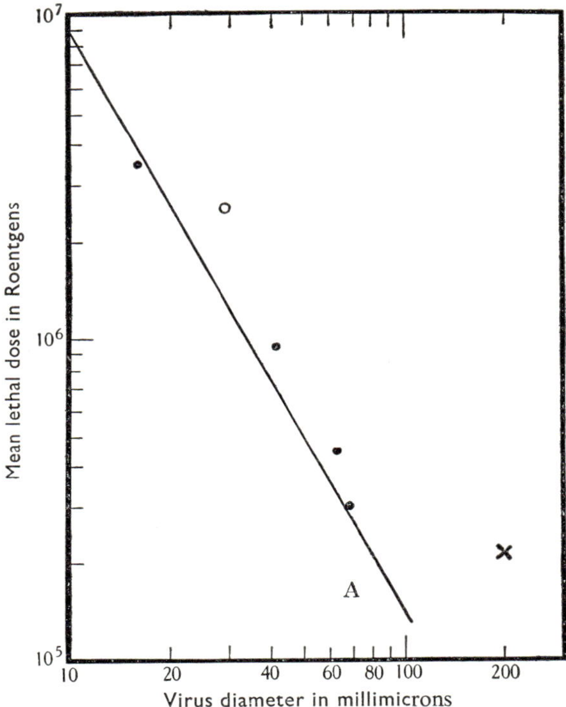

25/FIG. 4.—Relation between virus diameter and mean lethal dose (for α-rays). Curve A is the calculated relation between target diameter and mean lethal dose on the assumption that there is a single spherical target one or more ionizations in which suffice to cause the inactivation of the virus. ● phage; o plant virus; x vaccinia virus. (From Lea.[3])

the size of the virus. With the large vaccinia virus, however, the target appears to be considerably smaller than the virus itself, a result which could be taken to mean that a portion of this relatively complex entity is more radio-sensitive than the remainder.

Bacteria

The survival of bacteria after exposure to ionizing radiations has been studied for organisms irradiated dry, in aqueous suspensions or in suspension in (or on the surface of) complex nutrient media. The criterion of reproductive survival of the bacterial cell is its ability after irradiation to grow into a macroscopically visible colony. The survival curve is often exponential with a mean lethal dose of $10^3 - 10^4$ rads, but in many cases the plot of the logarithm of the number of survivors against dose exhibits a "shoulder" region in which an increasing percentage of the cells is killed for each equal increment of radiation dose, before reaching an exponential part of the curve where each equal increment in radiation dose reduces the fraction of surviving cells by the same factor. In some conditions, bacteria are protected against the effects of radiation by anoxia. The differing degrees of protection afforded by anoxia against radiations of different types and its modification by chemical and physical pre- and post-irradiation treatment have led to the concept of two different types of target site within the bacterial cell, one of which is protected by anoxia, the other which is not [11, 12]. Some protection against radiation damage is also apparent in bacteria irradiated in the presence of cysteine and certain other reducing agents; and this has been attributed to the removal of oxygen-containing radicals by SH containing compounds. Moreover, bacteria are less sensitive when irradiated in the frozen state than at normal temperatures. This may be attributed to a decrease in the rate of diffusion, with freezing, of radicals formed in the track of an ionizing ray.

Cells from Lower Animals

A number of experiments have indicated that a cell is more easily damaged by irradiation of the nucleus than by irradiation of the cytoplasm.[13] Eggs of the wasp *Habrobracon* have an eccentric nucleus which enables either the nucleus or the cytoplasm to be irradiated selectively with α-particles. One α-particle passing through the nucleus prevented hatching, but 10^6 α-particles traversing the cytoplasm were required for the same effect. Other work showed that when an irradiated amœba nucleus was transplanted to an unirradiated amœba the cell was less likely to survive than when a healthy nucleus was transplanted to an irradiated amœba. It has been suggested that the relatively high resistance of the cytoplasm to ionising radiation is due to the fact that many vital cytoplasmic structures are present in multiple form.

Mammalian cells.—Studies of the lethal effects of radiation upon mammalian cells became far more clear-cut in 1956, when Puck[14] succeeded in growing human cancer cells *in vitro* from single cells into macroscopically visible colonies or *clones*. This allowed a direct measurement of the survival of their reproductive capacity after irradiation in a manner similar to that used for bacteria. Doses of X-rays as small as 25 rads produced a measurable decrease in the percentage of cells which were reproductively intact. With this method the radiosensitivity of cultured cells of many types derived from several animal species have now been measured in different laboratories.[15] A further advance was made in 1959, when Hewitt and Wilson made quantitative measurements *in vivo* of the reproductive survival of murine leukæmic cells with a serial dilution-assay technique.[16] Serial dilutions of a suspension of tumour cells were injected into recipient mice of the same inbred strain, and the number of cells necessary to transplant the tumour successfully into 50 per cent of the recipients (the TD-50) was determined statistically. Comparison of the TD-50 values for tumour cells from unirradiated and irradiated donor animals enabled the percentage of tumour cells which remained reproductively intact after a given dose of irradiation to be calculated with precision. This method was applied to other types of murine tumours, including sarcomata, adenocarcinoma and squamous carcinoma. Methods followed for the assessment *in vivo* of the ability of the cell to survive and reproduce after irradiation in skin, cartilage and bone marrow.

The shape of the X- or γ-ray survival curves for most types of cells studied *in vitro* and *in vivo* were consistent with the view that the radiation exerted a *cumulative effect.* When plotted semilogarithmically the curves had a shoulder region followed by a straight-line "exponential" portion. The slope of the latter

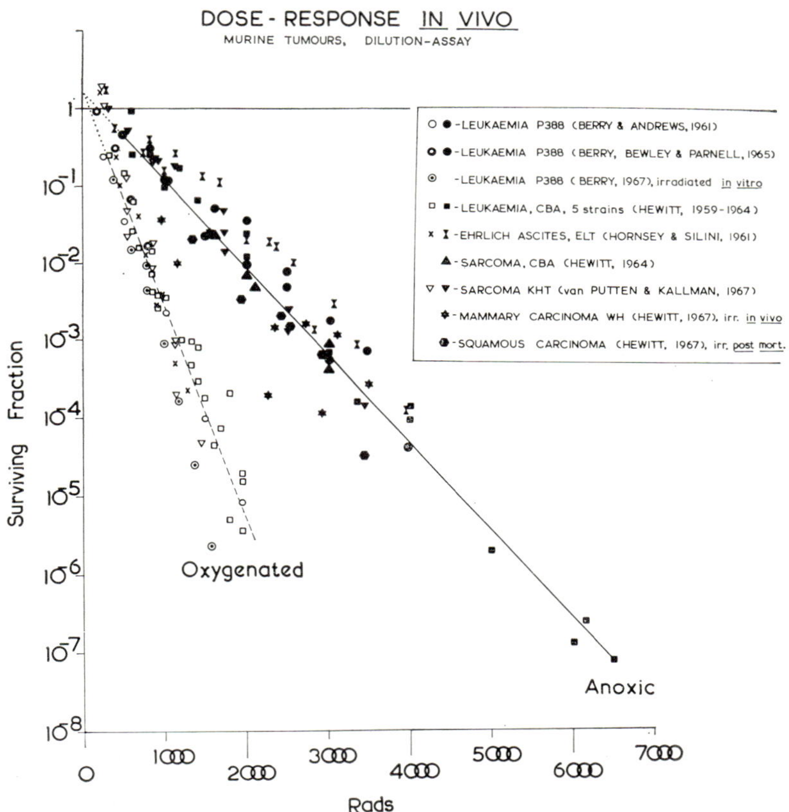

25/FIG. 5.—Survival of cell reproductive capacity after X- or γ-irradiation of several types of murine tumour cells. Assessment of cell survival was made *in vivo* using the technique of serial dilution-assay developed by Hewitt and Wilson.[16]

portion of the survival curve was dependent upon whether irradiation took place under oxygenated or anoxic conditions; with cells which were anoxic at the time of irradiation the dose required to produce a given decrease in reproductive capacity was 2–3 times greater than with ærobic cells. The radiosensitivities of most of the tumour cells studied so far have been very similar (FIG. 5), as have the cells of normal tissue origin studied *in vivo*. For mammalian cells studied in culture *in vitro* differences of a factor of nearly 4 in radiosensitivities have been reported for ærobic cells of different types. This range of radiosensitivities, with cell reproductive death as a criterion is, however, very much smaller than the difference between the mean lethal doses for mammalian cells and the very much larger doses necessary to achieve significant decreases in the survival of bacteria and viruses or in the activity of most biochemical processes. Terzi has concluded that the large and well-developed differences between the radiosensitivity of viruses and bacteria and that of cells of higher animals correspond to discrete levels of structural organisation.[17] According to this view the final sensitivity of the organisms is a function of this complexity of organisation and of the total cell content of nucleic acid.

Elkind and Sutton[18] and many subsequent workers, showed that the shoulder region of the dose-response curve obtained for survival of reproductive capacity of mammalian cells after irradiation with X-rays, reflected a reparable type of

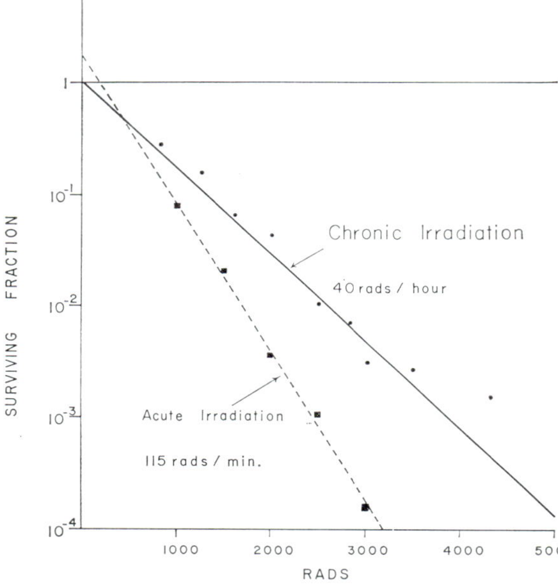

25/Fig. 6.—Survival of cell reproductive capacity after irradiation of murine leukaemia P-388 cells *in vivo* with ^{60}Co gamma rays at high and low dose-rates. The survival after a given radiation dose is increased when the irradiation is delivered over a relatively long time. (Adapted from Berry and Cohen.[19])

injury to the cell; division of a given X-ray dose into two equal doses spaced as little as 30 minutes apart increased the percentage of cells which retained their reproductive capacity. This type of intracellular repair (called *recovery from sublethal damage*) could take place even during irradiation, if radiation was delivered at low dose-rates so that the exposure lasted hours or days (Fig. 6). Thus, a given radiation dose would kill a greater proportion of cells if delivered in a single, short burst, than if given over a prolonged time.[19]

The dose-survival curves for the reproductive capacity of mammalian cells after irradiation with densely-ionizing (high-LET) radiations were shown to be exponential, with no shoulder. Dividing or prolonging the exposure to these radiations did not increase the proportion of cells surviving. In addition, while irradiation under anoxic conditions protected mammalian cells against the lethal effects of sparsely-ionizing (low-LET) radiations such as X- and gamma-rays so that nearly three times the radiation dose was required under anoxic conditions to produce a given degree of depopulation, mammalian cells were protected far less by anoxia against the high-LET radiations (FIG. 7).

The sensitivity of mammalian cells to lethal damage by X- and γ-rays was shown to vary widely, depending upon the position of the cell in the division cycle. For the HeLa cell strain, derived originally from human cancer, Terasima and Tolmach[21] showed that cells in the act of mitosis were radiosensitive. Once having completed mitosis, however, they became extremely resistant for a short while, but then again became extremely radiosensitive until the start of the synthesis of DNA. Having completed DNA synthesis, the cells remained radio-

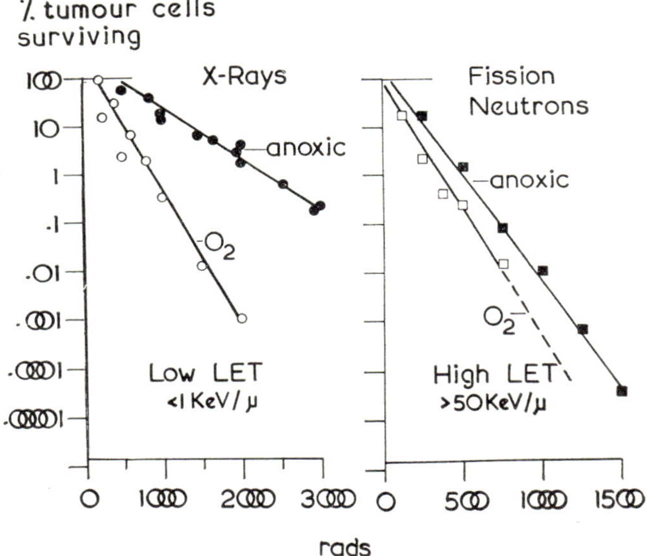

25/FIG. 7.—Survival of cell reproductive capacity after irradiation of murine leukaemia P-388 cells *in vivo* with radiations of high and low ionization density (LET). Note that the degree of protection afforded to the cells by anoxia during irradiation is much reduced for irradiation with high-LET fast neutrons from atomic fission. (Adapted from Berry.[20])

resistant until they again entered mitosis. Other types of cells have shown different cyclic patterns of radiosensitivity through their division cycle, but maximum resistance towards the end of the period of DNA synthesis and sensitivity at the time of mitosis seem to be common to all cells studied so far.

Ionizing radiations can also produce heritable, non-lethal damage to mammalian cells. This was clearly demonstrated by Sinclair's study of the incidence of slow-growing "small clones" among Chinese hamster cells surviving various radiation doses.[22] While capable of unlimited division, cells had a markedly prolonged inter-mitotic interval and a high incidence of "faulty" divisions which resulted in the death of one or both daughters. In addition, these small clones were markedly more radiosensitive than the unirradiated parent population from which they had come.

The importance of the cell nucleus in determining cell survival or cell death at mitosis after irradiation was shown also for mammalian cells by irradiation of portions of cells with microbeams[23], or by irradiation with beta-rays of low energy. When the energy of the beta radiation was too low to allow it to penetrate to the nucleus, large radiation doses (tens of thousands of rads) were necessary to produce cell death. When the nucleus was even partially irradiated death occurred on cell reproduction after radiation doses of less than 100 rads.

All mammalian cells which have been discussed so far die a *reproductive* death after irradiation; i.e. unless called upon to attempt division, they can perform their many biochemical functions after irradiation. Only at the time of cell division is the radiation damage which they carry made manifest. In fact, lethally damaged cells can often complete one or more mitoses. A few cells, however, far more radiosensitive than the majority of those studied, undergo a rapid interphase death which is characterised by nuclear pyknosis and cell lysis within hours after doses as small as 5 rads. This extreme radiosensitivity is observed in small lymphocytes, and in oocytes, but not in other cells derived from all three primordial germ layers.

Radiation and Cell Division

Doses of radiation which are too small to kill cells rapidly may have a marked effect on the ability of the cells to divide.

With bacteria, division may be inhibited without a corresponding change in cell growth, so that there is an increase in the size of the organisms. When a strain of *Bact. coli* was irradiated with γ-rays at 35 rads per minute in a nutrient liquid medium, cell division ceased and the total number of organisms remained constant, while the number of viable organisms decreased since some cells were killed. The rate of increase in length of the cells in the irradiated culture, however, was almost the same as the increase in the length of the cells in the unirradiated culture.[3] Thus the growth rate was similar in both cases.

If division eventually occurs, after a temporary delay, it may precipitate the death of the cell. Direct observation has shown that an irradiated bacterium which cannot give rise to a colony may nevertheless divide once, or even twice.

In mammalian cells as well, radiation can delay division, though not necessarily with consequences lethal to the cell. The advent of the techniques of modern cytology, however, allowed direct observation of the effects of ionizing radiation on the chromosomes of mammalian cells.

Structural Changes in Chromosomes

The production of structural changes in chromosomes by radiation can be observed in the cells of many animal tissues. Irradiation during the later stages of cell division may produce changes which interfere with the separation of the chromatids, so that the process of division breaks down. This is sometimes described as the primary or physiological effect. A secondary or aberration effect may occur when cells are irradiated before division begins or in its very early stages. Abnormal chromosomes may then be observed during division, or in the daughter cells produced after division is complete. These abnormalities are due to chromosome breakage at the time of irradiation.

The parts of a large proportion of the broken chromosomes appear to reunite in the original way, so that no permanent damage is caused to the cell, but there are some parts which either combine in new ways or remain in fragments.[24] Work with the broad bean, *Vicia faba*, has indicated that reunion is inhibited by radiation but accelerated by an increase in the concentration of adenosine triphosphate.[25] If there are breaks in two chromosomes in the same nucleus, reunion may occur symmetrically, giving two new chromosomes each with a centromere; or it may occur asymmetrically to form grossly defective chromosomes, one having two centromeres and the other none. Fragments without a centromere remain inert on the spindle, while fragments with two centromeres may move in an unco-ordinated manner, so that chromosome bridges are formed at anaphase. Changes of this kind, which can be seen in the irradiated carcinoma cell shown in FIG. 8, lead ultimately to cell death. Such cells are said to have unstable chromosome aberrations, whereas cells with abnormal monocentric chromosomes resulting from the reciprocal exchange of material between different chromosomes are said to have stable aberrations.

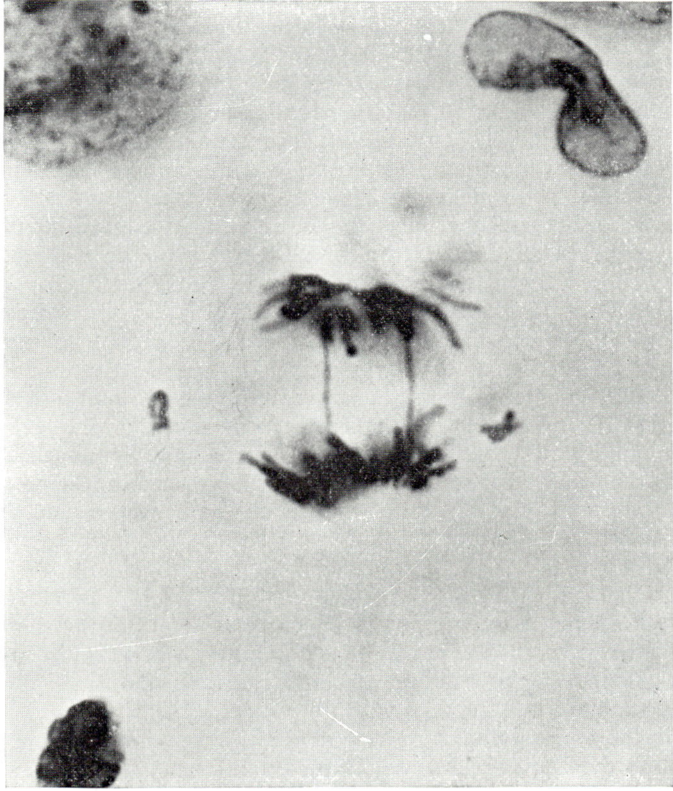

25/FIG. 8.—Dividing cells of Walker carcinoma 24 hours after irradiation with X-rays (300 rads). The two sets of daughter chromosomes show bridges which will prevent separation of the nuclei, and fragments of separated chromosomes. (× 2100.)

The relationship between the number of chromosome structural changes and the kind and dose of radiation varies with the nature of the changes concerned.

The number of persistent simple chromosome and chromatid-breaks produced by X-rays, neutrons and α-rays increases linearly with the dose and is independent of the intensity at which a given dose is administered. Neutrons are more efficient in causing breaks, however, than X-rays, in contrast to their lower efficiency in producing gene mutations. These facts have been thought to indicate that a chromosome may be broken by the passage through it of a single ionizing *particle*, but that the breakage requires several *ionisations*. Radiation which produces ionization of low density, such as X-rays, would often fail to cause the requisite number of ionizations in traversing the chromosome, and would thus have a relatively low efficiency.

The number of structural changes in two chromosomes (interchanges and other two-break aberrations) that are produced by X-rays increases more rapidly than the first power of the dose, and with large amounts of radiation is proportional to the square of the dose. The corresponding changes produced by neutrons and α-particles increase linearly with the dose. It has been suggested that with X-rays a double break involves the action of two separate ionizing particles (electrons), whereas with α-rays and neutrons it is generally caused by a single particle. An electron might only be able to produce a break if it traversed a chromosome at the end of its path, where the ion density is highest, and if this were so it would be unlikely to cause two ruptures.

This view of the process is in agreement with the finding that the number of two-break aberrations produced by a given dose of X-rays decreases as the dose is spread over a longer time, whereas the number produced by neutrons or α-particles is independent of the time within which the dose is given. If two breaks were caused independently, the first might be repaired before the second occurred, but if the breaks were simultaneous this would not be possible. Like other biological particles, however, the chromosome cannot be regarded as a target whose sensitivity to radiation is entirely independent of its environment. Chromosomal aberrations are produced less readily by X- and γ-rays if irradiation is carried out under relatively anærobic conditions.[26]

The possibility of examining chromosome damage produced in man by exposure to radiation arose when a method was developed for the preparation of suitable cultures of white cells of human blood.[27] Some of the changes observed are described in the following chapter.

Genetic Consequences of Irradiation of Cells

Radiation damage which results in the reproductive death of the cell has no genetic consequences, for the cell has lost its ability to hand on its information-carrying capacity. The production of some gross chromosomal abnormalities by ionizing radiation are for this reason of no genetic consequence, as the cells which carry the abnormalities are incapable of further proliferation. Of greater importance to the long-term survival of all species, however, is potentially non-lethal radiation damage to the genetic information of the cell.

In 1927 Muller[28] discovered that X-rays could cause mutations in the fruit fly *Drosophila*, and thereby initiated an extensive series of investigations into the genetic effects of radiation. These investigations have been carried out mainly with organisms such as *Drosophila melanogaster*, the bread mould *Neurospora* or the flowering plant *Tradescantia*, which can be handled in large numbers or contain chromosomes that are relatively easy to study, but the difficult task of extending them to the higher animals has now begun.

Radiation may cause genetic changes in at least two ways. Firstly, it may bring about gene mutations by altering genes without disturbing their position in the chromosome. Secondly, it may break the chromosome threads with the result that there is a rearrangement or loss of genes. Most of the gene mutations produced by radiation in the sperm of male *Drosophila* flies are recessive, so that special methods must be used for detecting them. Among the simplest to detect are the sex-linked recessive lethals, which result from mutations in the X-chromosome.

Each chromosome contributed to the zygote by a male gamete is, in general, homologous with a corresponding chromosome contributed by the female gamete. With many organisms, however, including man and *Drosophila*, the sex chromosomes are exceptional, the female having two X-chromosomes and the male one X- and one Y-chromosome. Thus females will be heterozygous for a mutant gene in a single X-chromosome, whereas males will be hemizygous. The gene may be passed from father to daughter and mother to son, but if it is recessive, only the males, in which it is unmasked, will show it.

Muller made use of these facts in the following manner for detecting mutations in the X-chromosome.[29] Irradiated male flies were mated with a special strain of females known as ClB. These females carry a dominant marker gene, in one of their X-chromosomes (ClB), which confers a characteristic (Bar eye) that can easily be recognised. They also carry a recessive lethal in this chromosome, such that a male zygote containing it will not survive. Each female offspring (F_1) of the mating which has Bar eye will have an irradiated X-chromosome from her father and a ClB chromosome from her mother. All the male offspring of these F_1 females will have only X-chromosomes from their grandfathers, since those receiving a ClB chromosome from their grandmothers will not live. Hence, if there is a recessive mutation due to radiation, all the males of this culture will show it, and if the mutation is a recessive lethal there will be a complete absence of male offspring.

Much laborious work established certain quantitative relationships between the number of sex-linked recessive lethals in *Drosophila* and the dosage and kind of radiation used. Thus, the number of mutations is linearly proportional to the total dose. It is independent of the intensity at which the dose is given and of whether it is administered in fractions or in one exposure (FIG. 9). It is independent of the temperature. Finally, it decreases with an increase in the density of ionization produced by the radiation. Table I shows the number of sex-linked recessive lethals obtained per 1000 rads.

These relationships have been used to support the view that mutations are produced by single ionizations within genes. However, it appears that radicals formed in the presence of oxygen may be important intermediaries. The mutagenic effect of X-radiation on *Drosophila*, like its lethal effect on bacteria, has been found to decrease when the oxygen tension is reduced. In one experiment the number of sex-linked lethals was 12 per cent per 4000 rads when the concen-

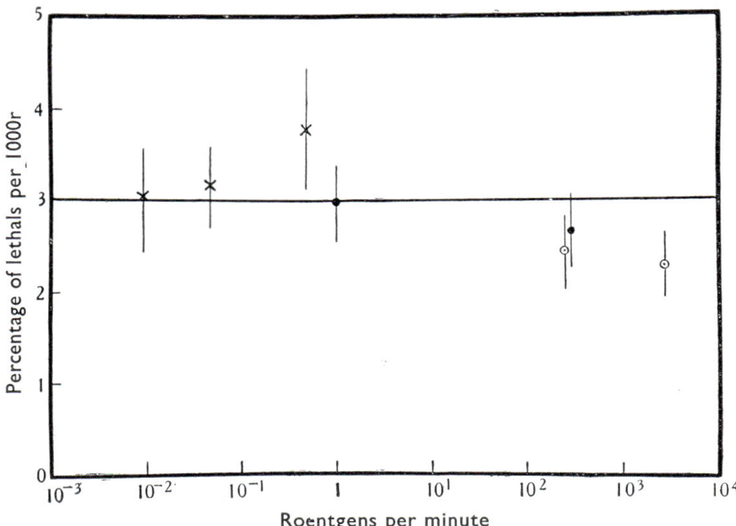

25/Fig. 9.—Yield of sex-linked recessive lethals at different intensities. ● X-rays; ⊙ soft X-rays; x γ-rays. (From Lea.[3])

tration of oxygen was greater than 15 per cent during irradiation, but could be reduced to 8 per cent under relatively anærobic conditions.[26] Moreover, there is evidence that some mutations, at least, result from damage which may be initially repaired.

25/Table I

Radiation	*β-rays, γ-rays or X-rays*	*Soft X-rays*	*Neutrons*	*α-rays*
	per cent	*per cent*	*per cent*	*per cent*
Yield of sex-linked lethals per 1000 rads	2·89	2·23	1·90	0·84

(*After Lea.*[3])

The available evidence suggests that relationships similar to those found for sex-linked recessive lethals hold for other recessive mutations in *Drosophila*, and also that the mutations induced by radiation do not differ in kind from those which occur spontaneously. It appears, however, that genes vary among themselves in stability, for the mutation-rate differs from one locus and one allelomorph to another.

Irradiation of male *Drosophila* flies produces dominant as well as recessive lethals in the sperm[30] and it is thought the dominant lethals are mostly a result of chromosome breakage. Eggs fertilised by such sperm fail to hatch, although they may undergo a number of nuclear divisions before death finally occurs. FIGURE 10 shows the relationship between the dose and the logarithm of the number of eggs hatching. It is of interest that the sex ratio declines as the dose increases, possibly because the X-chromosome is bigger than the male-producing Y-chromosome and thus presents a larger target for irradiation.

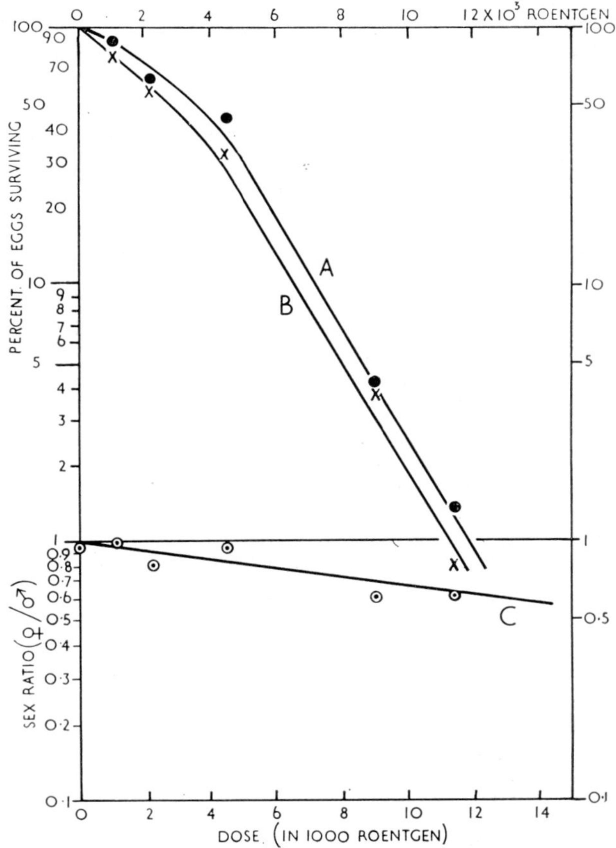

25/Fig. 10—Relation of frequency of dominant lethals produced in sperm to dose of X rays employed. A = percentage of eggs hatching; B = percentage of eggs producing adult flies; C = sex ratio. In each case the logarithm of the frequency is plotted against the dose. (after Catcheside and Lea.[30])

EFFECTS OF NON-IONIZING RADIATIONS

As has been previously noted, irradiation with the highly-collimated beam of coherent light from a laser source probably produces its biological effects by a combination of intense local heating and the pressure wave which is produced at the site. Ultraviolet irradiation, however, owes the majority of its biological effects to the fact that it is selectively absorbed by nucleic acids. Because of this great absorption, the penetration of ultraviolet light into tissue is extremely limited, but within cells exposed to U.V., genetic abnormalities and structural breaks of the chromosomes are produced which are qualitatively similar to those produced by ionizing radiation. In contrast to the effects of ionizing radiation, however, the cell-lethal effect of U.V. light is much greater if the cells are kept in the dark after irradiation than if they are exposed to strong visible light. This ability of visible light to mitigate the damage caused by ultraviolet light is called photoreactivation. It appears to be due to the enzymatic repair of a specific molecular lesion in DNA; the specific light-requiring photoreactivating enzyme splits the dimers of thymine which had been induced by the U.V., so that normal functional lengths of DNA can be resynthesized by the cell.[31] No such specific enzymatic repair system has been demonstrated for the lesions produced by the ionizing radiations.

REFERENCES

1. GRAY, L. H. (1946–47). *Brit. med. Bull.*, **4,** 11.
2. Proceedings of the First Annual Conference on Biologic Effects of Laser Radiation (1965). *Fed. Proc.*, **24,** No. 1, Part III.
3. LEA, D. E. (1955). *Actions of Radiations on Living Cells*, 2nd edit. London: Cambridge Univ. Press.
4. TIMOFEEFF-RESSOVSKY, N. W., and ZIMMER, K. G. (1947). *Biophysik I. Das Trefferprinzip in der Biologie*. Leipzig: S. Hirzel.
5. HUTCHINSON, F. (1961). *Science*, **134,** 533.
6. STOCKEN, L. A., and ORD, M. G. (1961). In *Mechanisms in Radiobiology*. Eds. FORSSBERG, A., and ERRERA, M. New York: Academic Press.
7. LEA, D. E., SMITH, K. M., HOLMES, B., and MARKHAM, R. (1944). *Parasitology*, **36,** 110.
8. BARRON, E. S., DICKMAN, S., MUNTZ, J. A., and SINGER, T. P. (1949). *J. gen. Physiol.*, **32,** 537.
9. OSAWA, S., ALLFREY, V. G., and MIRSKY, A. E. (1957). *J. gen. Physiol.*, **40,** 491.
10. CREASEY, W. A., and STOCKEN, L. A. (1958). *Biochem. J.*, **69,** 17P; ORD, M. G., and STOCKEN, L. A. (1966). *Biochem. J.*, **101,** 34P).
11. ALPER, T. (1963). *Phys. in Med. Biol.*, **8,** 365.
12. POWERS, E. L. (1965). *Radiol. Clin. N. Amer.*, **3,** 197.
13. HOLLAENDER, A., and STAPLETON, G. E. (1959). *Scientific American*, **201,** No. 3, p. 94.
14. PUCK, T. T., MARCUS, P. I., and CIECIURA, S. J. (1956). *J. exp. Med.*, **103,** 273; PUCK, T. T., and MARCUS, P. I. (1956). *J. exp. Med.*, **103,** 653.
15. WHITMORE, G. F., and TILL, J. E. (1964). *Ann. Rev. nuclear. Sci.*, **41,** 347.
16. HEWITT, H. B., and WILSON, C. W. (1959). *Brit. J. Cancer*, **13,** 69.
17. TERZI, M. (1961). *Nature (Lond.)*, **191,** 461.
18. ELKIND, M. M., and SUTTON, H. (1960). *Radiat. Res.*, **13,** 556.
19. BERRY, R. J., and COHEN, A. B. (1962). *Brit. J. Radiol.*, **35,** 489.
20. BERRY, R. J. (1965). *Radiol. Clin. N. Amer.*, **3,** 249.
21. TERASIMA, T., and TOLMACH, L. J. (1963). *Biophys. J.*, **3,** 11.
22. SINCLAIR, W. K. (1964). *Radiat Res.*, **21,** 583.
23. SMITH, C. L., and DENDY, P. P. (1968). *Cell Tiss. Kinet.*, **1,** 225.
24. CATCHESIDE, D. G. (1946–47). *Brit. med. Bull.*, **4,** 18.
25. WOLFF, S., and LUIPPOLD, H. E. (1955). *Science*, **122,** 231.

26. Hollaender, A., Baker, W. Y., and Anderson, E. H. (1951). *Cold Spr. Harb. Symp. quant. Biol.*, **16,** 315.
27. Moorhead, P. S., Nowell, P. C., Mellman, W. J., Battips, D. M., and Hungerford, D. S. (1960). *Exp. Cell. Res.*, **20,** 613.
28. Muller, H. J. (1927). *Science*, **66,** 84.
29. Muller, H. J. (1928). *Genetics*, **13,** 279.
30. Catcheside, D. G., and Lea, D. E. (1945–46). *J. Genet.*, **47,** 1.
31. Kimball, R. F. (1965). In *Advances in Radiology*, **2,** 135. New York: Academic Press.

Chapter 26

SOME EFFECTS OF RADIATION ON THE HIGHER ANIMALS

By E. P. Abraham and R. J. Berry

We shall now discuss, against the background provided by the preceding chapter, the complex effects of radiation on the higher forms of life—effects whose importance to human pathology has been magnified enormously in less than two decades. The development of atomic energy has made it imperative to assess the harm that radiations can cause to man, and to try to find ways of preventing or treating the pathological changes they induce. The wider use of radiation therapy with external beams and radioisotopes in human cancer has increased the need for a better understanding of the action of radiation on normal tissues and on tumours. Extensive investigations are therefore being made of the action of radiation on experimental animals and the data that have so far become available from human patients are being subjected to careful analysis.

A man in contact with highly radioactive material is confronted with two dangers: he may be exposed to excessive amounts of external radiation, and he may absorb radioactive compounds through the mouth, the nose, or the skin. Several factors would influence the consequences of these misfortunes. The damage caused by external radiation depends not only on its amount, but also on its power of penetration. For example, β-rays and X-rays of long wavelength dissipate much of their energy in the outer layers of the body and therefore cause erythema of the skin in smaller doses than the highly penetrating γ-rays, which may cause primary injury, on the other hand, to the deep tissues. The most vulnerable organ to Laser beams appears to be the eye since in this case the energy is focused on the retina. The effect of radioactive compounds which have entered the body depends not only on their initial activity, but on how they are distributed in the body, how long they remain there and how quickly their activity decays. For example, some of the radioactive elements are concentrated in bone and tritiated thymidine is incorporated into the DNA of the cell nucleus. When these factors are allowed for, however, we find that the qualitative effects of different kinds of ionizing radiation on the body tissues are remarkably alike.

We must expect that when the whole body is subjected to large amounts of radiation many pathological changes will occur and that some of them will be secondary changes following primary damage to a vital organ. A great deal of information has been gathered about the sensitivity of the various parts of the body to radiation and about the changes that follow exposure either to massive doses or to quite small doses given repeatedly over a long period of time.

We may say at once that a result of excessive exposure to radiation which seems to be almost invariable is a shortening of life. After very large doses death due to radiation may take place within days or sometimes hours, but after smaller ones it may be delayed for months or years, or may even be reserved for an individual of some future generation.

As the dose of radiation is gradually decreased the gross and obvious injuries that it can bring about merge imperceptibly into the more insidious ones. The immediate cause of death, however, varies with the time at which death occurs and we shall therefore try to distinguish between acute and late effects.

ACUTE EFFECTS OF RADIATION

The effects of massive doses of radiation on man were first seen on a large scale when atomic bombs were dropped on Hiroshima and Nagasaki, and some 25,000 people died. Some of these effects could have been predicted from results obtained in 1935 and 1936 on exposing experimental animals to heavy doses of X-rays, γ-rays or neutrons.

Lawrence and Tennant[1] reported in 1937 that mice exposed to more than 700 rads of X-rays, or an equivalent single dose of neutrons, as whole-body radiation almost invariably died within about ten days. There was a latent period of about two days followed by loss of weight and diarrhœa. Examination of the animals after five days showed complete loss of the epithelium of the intestine, destruction of the lymphoid tissue of the spleen and nearly complete aplasia of the bone marrow. When the amount of radiation was large enough to be fatal within a few days, death was thought to be due to the destructive changes in the viscera and to toxæmia caused by tissue breakdown products. When the animals survived longer the picture was usually complicated by bacterial infection. Bacteria reached the circulation through the damaged intestinal mucosa and met little resistance on account of the effect of radiation on the reticulo-endothelial system.

These findings have been confirmed and elaborated by later work. When exposed to very large doses of radiation indeed, such as 50,000 rads, an animal may die within a few hours in a state of muscular spasm, and the immediate cause of death appears to be damage to the brain, because the neuromuscular symptoms can be reproduced by irradiating the head alone.[2] With doses in the region of the LD_{50} radiation sickness may be observed within an hour and the animal behaves as though in shock, but it does not normally die. After one or two days there is an apparent recovery, but this is soon succeeded by a phase of acute illness and death is then likely to occur, with mice or rats, around the fifth or tenth day after irradiation. In this period the animal shows extreme weakness and loses weight rapidly; towards the end it develops a high fever and rapid heart beat, and finally there is circulatory collapse in a shock-like state.

Some observers have concluded that the early deaths in the acute period are a consequence of damage to the small bowel, because they can be prevented by shielding the abdomen, while the later ones result from damage to the bone marrow. However, the cause of death is not altogether clear. The suggestion that there is a general metabolic disturbance must be given serious consideration, because, for some animals at least, the LD_{50} at thirty days is said to be about the same with β-rays as with γ-rays, although the former only cause primary damage to the superficial parts of the body. The possibility of hæmorrhage must be considered, because petechiæ and hæmatomata appear and there is an increase in the clotting time of the blood, probably due to a fall in the number of platelets; but in some cases the hæmoglobin content of the blood of irradiated animals does not fall greatly below normal and they can hardly be said to die of anæmia.

If death does not occur in the acute period a marked recovery may occur within a month. Nevertheless the animal is liable to be left in a debilitated state, and may never regain entirely the weight that it lost. In this condition it may well succumb to an infection.

The reports of American investigators in Japan[3] have shown that the effects of large doses of whole-body radiation on man are similar to their effects on experimental animals as shown in Table I. The atomic bombs generated vast amounts of heat and ionizing radiations within about one second. People within 500 metres of the explosion appear to have been instantly burned to death. At much greater distances those in the open received severe flash burns, although

26/TABLE I

DOSES OF RADIATION AND THEIR EFFECTS*

Dose (rads)	*Biological Effect*
0·001	Two and one-half days natural background radiation.
0·01	No detectable effect.
1	No detectable somatic effect, minimal genetic effects.
10	Barely detectable qualitative changes in lymphocytes.
10^2	Mild acute radiation sickness in some. Slight diminution in blood cell counts. Possible nausea and vomiting, possible transient reflex changes.
10^3	Depression of blood cell and platelet formation. Damage to gastro-intestinal mucosa. Severe acute radiation sickness. Death within thirty days.
10^4	Immediate disorientation or coma. Death within hours.
10^5	Death of some micro-organisms.
10^6	Death of most bacteria.
10^7	Death of all living organisms, some denaturation of proteins.

* Modified from Warren[4].

quite thin layers of clothing were able to afford considerable protection. People who died from radiation injury were troubled by nausea and vomiting on the day of the bombing. In those who received the largest doses (greater than 600 rads) the initial radiation sickness was rapidly followed by prostration and intractable diarrhœa, and death occurred within ten days. If the dose was somewhat smaller the initial sickness was followed by a period free from clinical symptoms, but after two or three weeks the patients became seriously ill and about half of them subsequently died. Table II summarises some of the changes in people who died within a few months of the bombing. Diarrhœa was one of the earliest symptoms and epilation and purpura, which are illustrated in FIG. 1, preceded death. In those who lived more than two weeks sepsis was a common feature.

26/TABLE II

ONSET OF SYMPTOMS OF RADIATION INJURY

	Most Severe	*Severe*	*Moderately Severe*
Vomiting	Day of bombing	Day of bombing	Day of bombing
Fever	2–7 days	14–28 days	
Diarrhœa	2–7 days	4–21 days	14–35 days
Leucopenia	2–7 days	7–28 days	7–28 days
Purpura	4–7 days	14–28 days	
Epilation		7–28 days	14–35 days
Mucous membrane ulceration		14–28 days	14–28 days
Anaemia		7–28 days	10–35 days
Death	4–10 days	10–42 days	30–90 days

(*From LeRoy*[5])

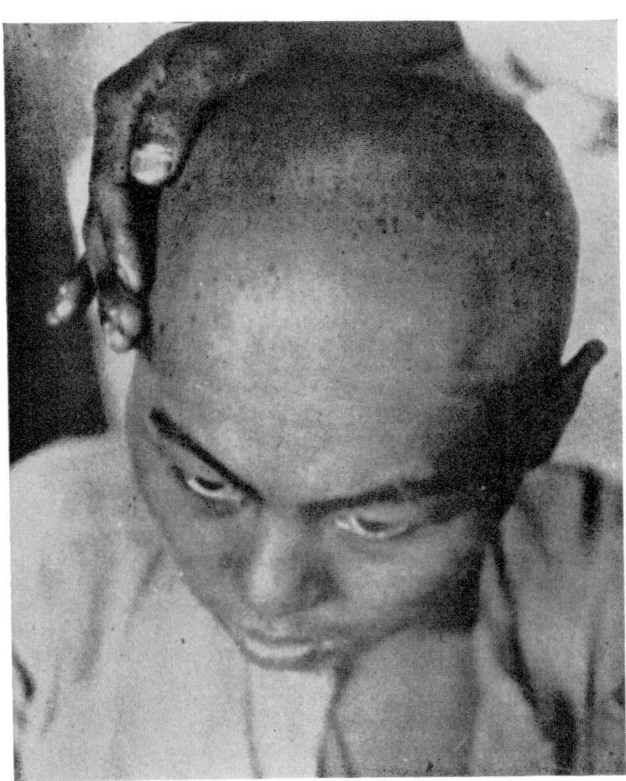

26/FIG. 1.—Epilation and petechiæ following exposure to radiation from atomic bomb. Male, aged 20, 1000 metres from explosion. (From Oughterson *et al.*[3])

Histological Changes

We have already mentioned that large doses of penetrating radiation cause gross damage to the bone marrow, the spleen and the small bowel. The histological changes in these and other tissues of irradiated animals have been studied in considerable detail by Bloom.[6]

Hæmopoietic and lymphoid tissue.—After doses in the region of the LD_{50} to rabbits or mice there is damage to the bone marrow within thirty minutes, mitosis being arrested and the erythroblasts reduced in numbers. Within a few hours many dead cells and a considerable amount of débris can be observed, and after nine or ten days the depleted marrow cavity, which is illustrated together with a normal marrow in FIGS. 2 and 3, is occupied by a gelatinous mass. If the animal survives, regeneration then begins and the erythropoietic elements, although more sensitive to radiation than the myelopoietic, recover more quickly.

In the spleen, mitosis is also inhibited within less than an hour and there is soon evidence of severe damage to the lymphocytes. Once again, regeneration may begin after nine days. In the lymph nodes most of the follicles are completely destroyed and new ones may not begin to form for three weeks.

These injuries to the hæmopoietic and lymphoid tissue will naturally exert an influence on the cell population of the peripheral blood (see Chapter 8). The way in which the damage is reflected in the blood count, however, will depend not only on the radio-sensitivity of the parent cells but on the normal length of life of the cells that circulate in the blood. For example, since many white cells have a rapid turnover, a leucopenia, and in particular a drop in the number

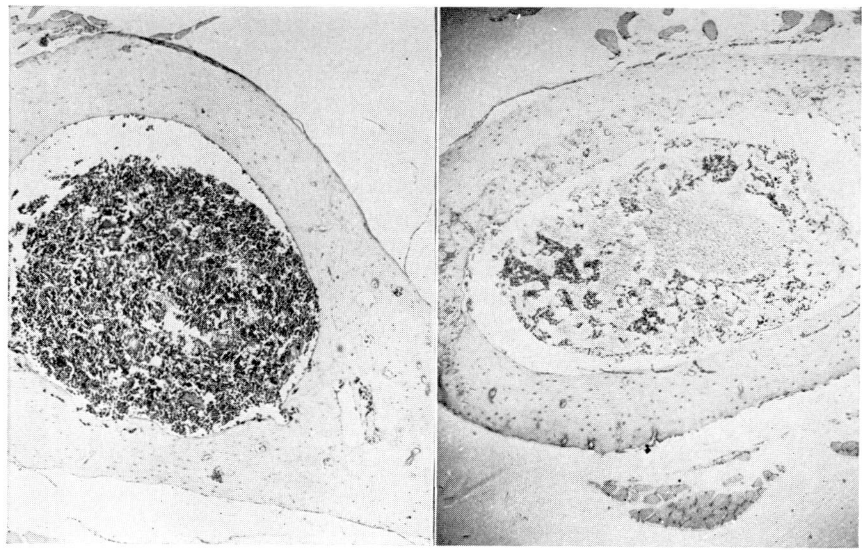

26/FIG. 2.—Shaft of femur of control mouse. (From Mole.[7])

26/FIG. 3.—Shaft of femur of a mouse ten days after irradiation with 600 rads X-rays. (From Mole.[7])

of circulating lymphocytes, is likely to be a fairly sensitive index of radiation injury. On the other hand a change in the number of red cells may be much less obvious, even though the erythroblast is radiosensitive, because it is liable to be obscured by the long life of the red cell and the recovery of the marrow.

The existence of chromosome damage in human lymphocytes has been studied in radiation workers accidentally exposed to doses of radiation between 23 and 365 rads and in patients treated with relatively high doses of X-rays for ankylosing spondylitis. Both stable and unstable aberrations (Chapter 25) have been observed. A typical unstable aberration, with a dicentric chromosome (Di) and an acentric fragment (F) is shown in FIG. 4, and the changes in the proportion

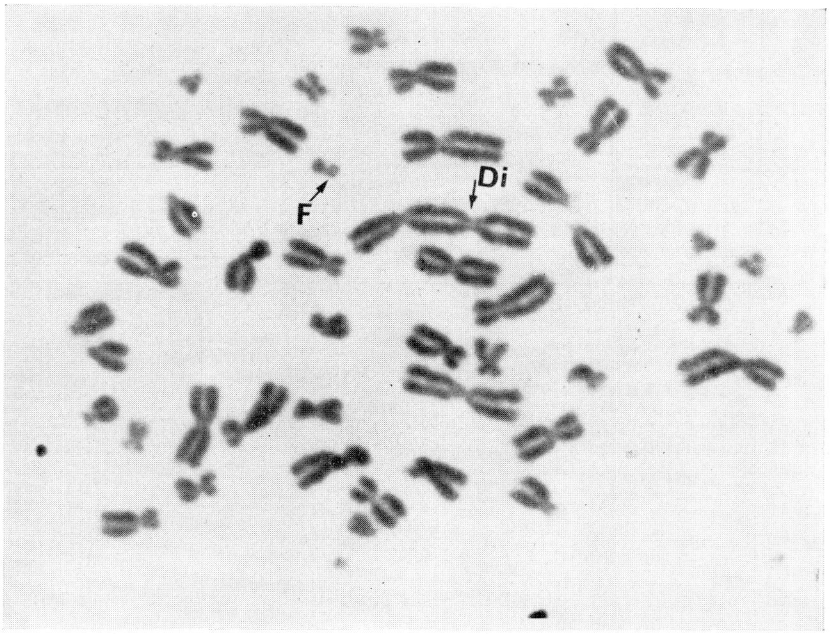

26/FIG. 4.—Cell from a blood culture of patient after treatment with X-rays for ankylosing spondylitis, showing an unstable chromosome aberration composed of a dicentric chromosome (Di) and an acentric fragment (F). (By courtesy of Dr. W. M. Court Brown.)

of normal cells after X-ray treatment is shown in FIG. 5. It is clear from FIG. 5 that detectable chromosome damage may persist for nearly twenty years after exposure. Moreover, despite the fact that work with plant material had indicated that cells with unstable aberrations were unlikely to survive more than three or four divisions, such aberrations can be seen in blood cultures seven or more years after exposure. Many of these cells are probably dividing for the first time when they are recognised, for they contain a dicentric or ring chromosome together with an acentric fragment, which would normally have been lost had a previous division occurred. Their existence thus provides evidence for the

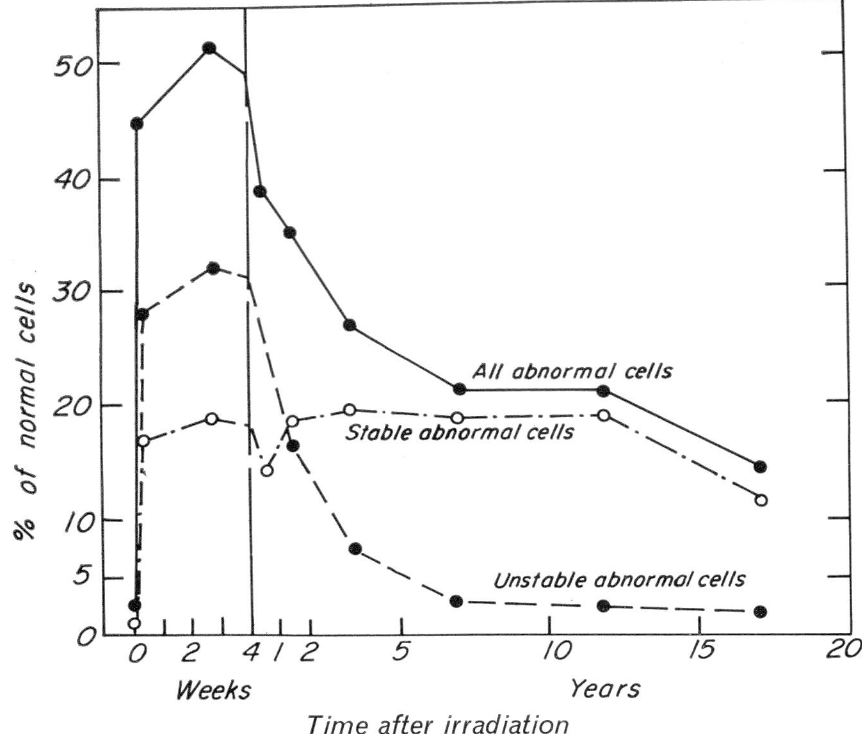

26/Fig. 5.—Changes in the proportion of abnormal cells in relation to normal cells after treatment of 58 men with X-rays for ankylosing spondylitis. (From Buckton, Jacobs, Court Brown and Doll.[8])

survival of a population of lymphocytes in the body for long periods without division.

Gastro-intestinal tract.—Destructive changes in the gastro-intestinal tract are most pronounced in the small bowel. After doses in the region of the LD_{50} mitotic activity ceases within thirty minutes, and nuclear swelling and pyknosis are observed in cells of the epithelium of the crypts, the villi and Brunner's glands. More extensive degenerative changes may proceed for some days, but within a week the process of repair is under way.

The gonads.—In addition to the tissues we have already mentioned the testis or the ovary are severely damaged in animals exposed to large doses of penetrating radiation. This damage may lead to temporary or permanent sterility. In the testis the spermatogonia are the first cells to be affected and some of them may die within a few hours; spermatogenesis is then gradually diminished over a period of one or two weeks, until eventually many tubules contain only the radio-resistant cells of Sertoli; but after a month some of the tubules may begin to recover. In the ovary, pyknosis of the ova is observed within a few days, and not long afterwards the ova begin to disappear and the follicles to degenerate.

Comments on the Mode of Action of Whole-body Radiation

When we consider the results of exposing the whole body to large amounts of radiation it appears that the rapidly proliferating tissues are the most easily damaged. The association of cellular multiplication and apparent radio-sensitivity, which was recognised many years ago by Lacassagne, can scarcely be merely fortuitous. Among the cells that first decrease in number after irradiation, the erythroblasts, myelocytes, spermatogonia and cells of the intestinal epithelium are all actively dividing. In contrast, the cells of highly resistant tissue, such as brain and muscle, seldom undergo mitosis. It is clear that the ability to multiply is not the only factor which determines the sensitivity of a cell to radiation, for the small lymphocyte, which rarely if ever divides, is highly susceptible to radiation injury and may be damaged not only in the lymph nodes but in the peripheral blood.[9] Nevertheless, a cell may be killed by radiation more easily when it is dividing, or preparing to divide, than in the resting state. The apparent radiosensitivity of a tissue will therefore depend on the conditions under which its cells maintain their normal function, as well as on the intrinsic radiosensitivity of the cells themselves. Thus the liver, in which there is normally a low rate of cell turnover, is regarded as a radio-resistant organ because its metabolic functions are not impaired by localised radiation in doses large enough to kill the animal if delivered to the whole body. However, should the irradiated animal be subjected to partial surgical, or chemical, hepatectomy, the latent damage to the liver cells is revealed when the latter are forced to proliferate. The regenerating liver is then a radiosensitive organ, comparable with the hæmopoietic and gastrointestinal tissues.[10]

It seems possible that one of the causes of the acute effects of large doses of radiation is damage to chromosomes. Chromosome breakage, which was discussed in the previous chapter, undoubtedly occurs in animal tissues. Abnormal mitotic figures have been observed, for example, in tumour cells and regenerating liver after irradiation. Work with simpler organisms has indicated that the cell nucleus is more sensitive to radiation than the cytoplasm and it appears certain that one vital target in the cell is its DNA.[11] However, it does not follow that direct chromosome breaks are mainly responsible for the rapid lethal action of radiation.[12]

The acute effects of radiation cannot be well understood until we know not only the ways in which the body cells are first injured, but also the chain of events which link the injury with the final death of the animal. At the present time, the nature of all the links in this chain is little more certain than that of the primary lesions themselves.[13] But it does not seem difficult to understand, in principle, why death is usually delayed. Except in very large doses indeed, radiation does not cause serious damage to tissues whose failure to function would be immediately fatal, such as those of the heart or the brain. Even if cell death were immediate in the radio-sensitive parts of the body, some time might be expected to elapse before its full effects were manifested in other vital organs. Moreover, the cellular changes are seldom completely irreversible, for regeneration is observed even in tissues that have suffered gross destruction if the animal itself can survive. The importance of recovery is implied in the fact that the acute lethal dose varies with the intensity at which it is given. We may conclude that the fate of an animal in the first few weeks after irradiation is decided by the outcome of a race between processes of degeneration and repair.

LATE EFFECTS OF TOTAL IRRADIATION

We have already mentioned that animals which survive the acute period of radiation-injury nevertheless often die earlier than unirradiated controls. Death is sometimes due to infection, and it seems likely that damage to the mechanism for producing antibodies, which will be discussed in Chapter 34, plays a part in this phenomenon. However, mice which appear to have recovered from acute injury, and which do not succumb to infection, may lose weight and die up to nine months after irradiation. Some of these deaths are connected with an ill-defined syndrome which has been called an acceleration of the ageing process.[14] Others are due to the development of malignant tumours. Both kinds of change may follow continued exposure to quite small amounts of radiation as well as a single exposure to a massive dose. In addition to these somatic effects radiation produces genetic effects which are seen in the descendants of the irradiated animal.

Ageing

Animals which die long after a single exposure to radiation, or after they have received daily doses of the order of 8 rads for several months, may appear generally atrophied, with tissues resembling those of very old animals. Daily doses of 1 rad of radiation, and possibly even of 0·11 rad, produce a measurable shortening of the span of life.

Leukæmia

Exposure of animals to radiation is known to induce leukæmia and an analysis of two sets of clinical data has left no doubt that this disease is also induced by radiation in man. The incidence of leukæmia among the Japanese survivors at Nagasaki and Hiroshima has been much greater than that expected in a normal population.[3] An approximately ten-fold increase in the incidence of leukæmia has been noted in England among patients whose spinal marrows had received from 500 to 1,000 rads of X-rays during treatment of ankylosing spondylitis.[15] In both cases the average time between exposure and diagnosis of the disease was about six years. After ten years from the time of exposure the increased risk of leukæmia appears to decline.

Carcinogenic Effects

Many experiments with animals have shown that both external radiation and radioactive substances deposited in the body tend eventually to induce the formation of tumours. Cells of cultures of golden hamster embryos have been transformed into tumour cells *in vitro* by X-irradiation.[16] We have clear evidence that radiation is also carcinogenic in man.

Cases in which skin cancer and other forms of carcinoma developed after exposure to X-rays were described in the first decade of the present century. In 1924 it was suggested that the lung cancer which was common in certain groups of miners was connected with the radioactivity of the ore being worked. At about the same time reports began to appear of people dying with bone tumours who had been employed in the self-luminous dial painting industry. In this industry, which began to develop in 1908 and utilised a preparation containing radium or mesothorium, the girls who did the painting pointed the ends of camel hair brushes in their lips. The subsequent fate of some of these girls, and of other people for whom physicians in the 1920's had prescribed radium water as a medicine, has been described in detail by Martland and his colleagues.[17] In many cases the patients were still excreting radium ten or twenty years after they had ceased to absorb it. Of twenty-six who stored more than 0·7 μg of radium, and received more than about 20 rad/year, twenty-one suffered obvious damage to the bone. Tumours appeared after an average latent period of twenty-three years.

We now know that not only radium and mesothorium, but also a number of other radioactive elements, including uranium, plutonium and an isotope of strontium, are concentrated in the bone if they enter the body. Since some of these elements have extremely long half-lives, and are excreted very slowly, they will irradiate the bone continuously for many years. FIGURE 6 illustrates the distribution of radium in "hot spots" in the femur of a patient who died thirty years after leaving the luminous dial industry. Strontium 90 has become a serious potential hazard, since it is present in relatively large amounts in the fall-out from explosions of nuclear weapons and tends to follow calcium through the human food chain.

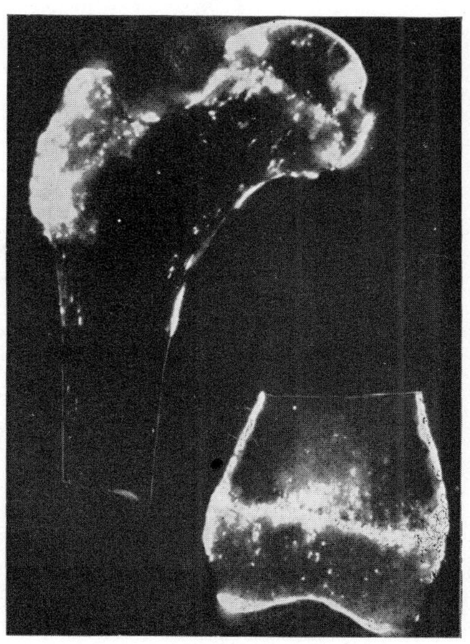

26/FIG. 6.—Autoradiograph of femur showing distribution of radioactivity. The "hot spots" are clearly visible. (From Aub, Evans, Hempelmann and Martland.[17])

The important question arises whether the probability of inducing tumours by radiation is simply proportional to the total dose, or whether tumours cease to develop when either the total dose or the dosage-rate falls below a threshold value. This question may be very difficult to answer, but there is evidence that a threshold for the dosage-rate, if it exists, must be rather low. An increased incidence of tumours of the ovary has been reported in mice irradiated with only 0·11rad of γ-rays daily.

The results of investigations with *Drosophila*, which were discussed in the previous chapter, gave us every reason to expect that irradiation would bring about genetic changes in the higher animals. The number of gene mutations produced by X- or gamma-radiation in the sperm of *Drosophila* is about 3×10^{-8} per gene per rad. If the same number were produced in man, a total dose of about 333 rads per generation would be required to double the spontaneous mutation rate; this figure is probably too high. From the study of conditions such as hæmophilia for which the genetic background has been worked out in detail, the rate of spontaneous mutation is about 10^{-5} per gene per generation. Thus 333 rads ($\times 3 \times 10^{-8}$ gene mutations per rad) would produce an additional 10^{-5} gene mutations per generation. However, results obtained using mice and other higher animals have often been at variance with those obtained in *Drosophila* for reasons which are not yet clear.[18]

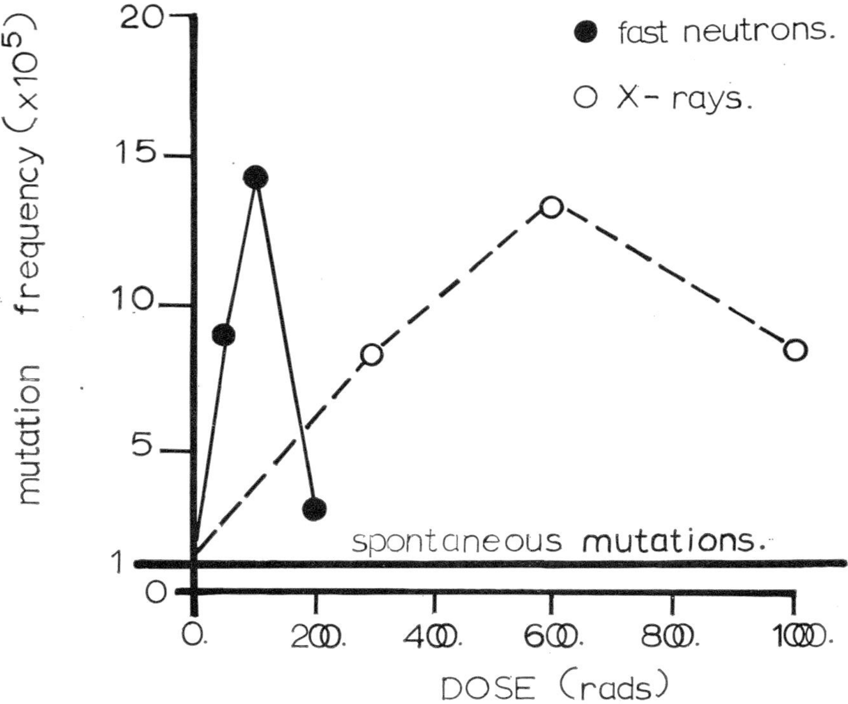

26/Fig. 7.—Specific locus mutation frequencies resulting from acute irradiation of mouse spermatogonia with X-rays or fast neutrons. (Adapted from Searle.[18])

Snell[19] found in 1933 that male mice irradiated with X-rays, before completely losing their fertility, produce offspring containing individuals that are semi-sterile. This semi-sterility, which is inherited, results in small litters, some of the embryos dying in the uterus. It was shown by Koller and Auerbach[20] to be associated with an interchange of chromosome segments. Further work has demonstrated the existence of a number of recessive mutations in irradiated male mice, some of which are lethal, some sublethal and others viable when homozygous.

The calculation of a mutation doubling dose, however, is based on the assumption that the number of mutations produced in human germ cells will be proportional to the dose and independent of its intensity, as is the case in the sperm of *Drosophila*. The assumption may be valid for human spermatozoa but not for immature germ cells. In 1958 Russell, Russell and Kelly[21] obtained evidence that fewer mutations are produced in the spermatogonia and oocytes of mice (though not in the spermatozoa) by a dose of radiation given at a low intensity than by the same dose given at a high intensity. The genetic effects of X and γ radiation at low dose rates on man may therefore be less than some of the earlier data suggested. For densely-ionizing raditions, however, there appears to be a slight *increase* in the mutation frequency at low dose-rates.[18] The problem is further complicated by the fact that increasing radiation doses kill a percentage of the cells which contained radiation-induced mutations, and these mutations are never expressed. This is shown in FIG. 7; for acute exposures to both X-rays and fast neutrons, mouse spermatogonia show a mutation frequency which increases with dose, but then decreases again as the radiation dose is further increased.

It is clear that any assessment of the doubling dose for human genes is attended by great uncertainty. A committee of the Medical Research Council has concluded that a representative value probably lies between 30 rads and 80 rads, but that values lower than 15 rads or higher than 150 rads cannot be definitely excluded. Muller[22] has suggested that a dose of 200 rads, which must have been received by many Hiroshima survivors, would cause each of their offspring to inherit at least one new mutation.

The Permissible Dose

We have seen that relatively small amounts of radiation can cause serious pathological changes in the human body. These changes may remain hidden for months, years, or even generations, but when manifested they are difficult or impossible to reverse. It is therefore of great importance to avoid the primary lesion. The existence of cosmic rays and naturally occurring radioactive elements makes it impossible for us to escape a background radiation of about 3 rads per generation, but we can try to limit our additional exposure to doses which are unlikely to cause widespread harm or to involve a risk that will be unacceptable to the individual and the community. How small should such doses be?

In 1937 it was considered that the maximum permissible exposure should be 0·2 rad per day for continual irradiation of the whole body with X-rays. Later, a dose of 0·1 rad per day was accepted in the U.S.A. for X-rays, γ-rays and β-rays. In 1950 the International Commission on Radiological Protection recommended a reduction of the maximum dose that could be sanctioned to 0·3 rad per week. Subsequently, a British committee added the suggestion that no individual should accumulate more than 200 rads of whole-body radiation during his lifetime, or more than 50 rads from conception to the age of 30 years; and that this allowance should not apply to more than one-fiftieth of the total population. In 1959 and 1965 the International Commission suggested that, for the whole population, the dose to the gonads up to the age of 30 years should not exceed 5 rads plus the natural background and the lowest possible contribution from medical exposure.[23] Doses about ten times as large were regarded as permissible for groups of people subject to controlled occupational exposure.

In the present state of our knowledge any value that is fixed for the permissible dose can only be regarded as provisional.[24] We do not know that even very small amounts of ionising radiation are entirely devoid of carcinogenic action. We have reason to believe that small doses of radiation may be mutagenic, but we cannot predict in detail what the effects of a given dose will be. However, it should be remembered that a dose of 0·3 rads per week will accumulate to 150 rads in ten years, and that this may be more than the amount of radiation which is required to double the spontaneous rate of mutation. Most of the additional mutants will be recessive, and their lethal or detrimental character will sometimes not be expressed until they are paired with others of the same kind. But in the long run each mutation is liable to contribute to the death of one individual and, before being extinguished, to impair the lives of many others.[25] It follows that the total number of individuals that are eventually damaged by a given dose of radiation may be very large, although the proportion of a single generation that is affected is too small to be detectable. A significant number of these individuals is likely to suffer from mental disease.

The total genetic damage to a large population will be related to the sum of the doses of radiation received by the gonads of its individual members. It is therefore important to assess the over-all amount of radiation that various populations are receiving from external sources. From a survey in England some years ago the interesting fact emerged that by far the largest contribution, amounting to about 20 per cent of the natural background, came from diagnostic radiology. The corresponding figure from the Atomic Energy Authority was only about 0·1 per cent. The average contribution from nuclear explosions up to the end of 1958 was about 1 per cent. The testing of these nuclear weapons subsequently declined, but the contribution from this source would eventually rise to a much higher value if testing were resumed on its former scale.

The many benefits to be derived from an increasing use of sources of ionizing radiation clearly need to be weighed against the biological injury with which they may eventually be accompanied. Although the Atomic Energy Establishments have set a high standard of care, a substantial increase in the number of thermonuclear explosions can scarcely be envisaged without anxiety and, until recently, the potential dangers of medical radiology do not seem to have been generally appreciated. For example, fluoroscopic examinations have delivered from 15 to 20 rads to the ovaries of a woman. The abandonment of radiation as an aid to diagnosis cannot be contemplated, but the physician may fairly be asked to exercise all possible care in its use, to avoid large doses if smaller ones will do, and to shield, whenever practicable, the reproductive organs. The young should be treated with special care, for they are most likely to experience the long-delayed carcinogenic effects of radiation, and to hand down genetic defects to future generations which, as Muller has said, lie helpless in our custody.[26] Improvements in techniques should enable the average dose from radiology to be reduced even further without impairment of the radiological services.[27]

OTHER ASPECTS OF RADIATION DAMAGE

Radiation Treatment of Tumours

Within a year of the discovery of X-rays, the damaging effects of these rays on tissues had been turned to the useful purpose of treating surgically inaccessible human cancer. As techniques and equipment have improved over the past 60 years, radiation therapy has become the treatment of choice for many tumours, even those which allowed surgical extirpation, or has become a useful adjunct to surgery as pre-operative irradiation to reduce tumour mass or as post-operative irradiation to ablate local or metastatic tumour discovered at the time of surgery. However, this use of ionizing radiation represents a "blunt knife" with little, if any, greater effect upon tumour than upon normal tissues included in the radiation field. The limitation upon the radiation dose which can be given is not the dose necessary to kill all tumour cells, but the highest dose which will be tolerated by the normal tissues and allow them to heal the tissue defect. For this reason, ways have been sought since the beginning of radiotherapy to maximise the radiation effect upon tumour cells while minimising effects on normal tissues by the use of fractionated courses of X-rays which would allow recovery in normal tissues between the individual radiation doses. Different patterns of dose-fractionation evolved with the empirical clinical experience of several radiotherapy centres, but it is only in recent years that radiobiologists have been able to compare the several commonly-used clinical techniques by the use of experimental tumour systems which resemble human cancer and isotopic methods of analysis of cell population kinetics. Using the response of pig skin as a biological end-point, Fowler and his colleagues have shown that the number of fractions into which a given radiation dose is divided is more important than the total time over which those doses are given; the larger the number of fractions, the smaller the tissue damage produced. Total time also exerts a lesser effect, however; a given radiation dose delivered in five fractions over five days produced a more intense skin response than the same dose given in five fractions over 29 days—but this in turn was much more intense than the response produced by giving the same total dose in 21 fractions over a period of 29 days.[28]

The work of Gray and his co-workers called attention to one area in which the effect of radiation upon tumour cells might be enhanced, while little or no additional damage was done to normal tissues. We have seen in the previous chapter that mammalian cells which were anoxic (or severely hypoxic) at the time of irradiation with X- or gamma-rays were protected so that nearly three times the radiation dose was necessary to achieve depopulation comparable with that from radiation delivered to well-oxygenated cells. Thomlinson and Gray showed that the incidence of necrotic zones in human tumours was clearly related to the distance from the nearest capillary blood supply. Necrosis regularly occurred beyond the maximum calculated diffusion distance for oxygen from the capillary through respiring tissue. Tumour cells on the brink of the necrotic region which were severely hypoxic, although still viable, would be protected from effects of irradiation and could serve as the nidus for the regrowth of the "radioresistant" or "radio-incurable" tumours. As normal tissues were presumed to be well-oxygenated, their cells would not be similarly protected.[29, 30] These studies led to clinical trials of the combination of radiotherapy with hyperbaric oxygen, since the well-oxygenated normal tissues were presumably near their maximum radiosensitivity and the oxygen tension within the tumour could be dramatically raised. This method has shown initially promising results.[31] An alternative approach has been the use of radiations of higher ionization density, for which the protection afforded by anoxia is much reduced (*cf.* previous chapter.

The clinical 'radiosensitivity' of a tumour, i.e. the rate at which the mass shrinks during and after radiotherapy, has been shown to be poorly correlated with the radiocurability of tumours. Hewitt has pointed out that many tumours are "cured" by radiotherapy not because the radiation has destroyed the reproductive capacity of every tumour cell, but because the natural growth-rate of the surviving tumour cells is so slow that the patient dies of other causes before the tumour again presents itself as a clinical problem. One other matter currently exciting interest is the possibility of a weak host-tumour immune interaction so that the use of a dose of radiation sufficient to decrease the surviving tumour cell population below a critical size could allow the immune response to delay or destroy the survivors; this is an area in which a large amount of experimental effort is now going on.

The use of radioisotopes which selectively localize in tumours to deliver a radiation dose only to the tumour and not to the remainder of the body has been relatively unrewarding up to the present time. ^{131}I has been used in this way to treat functional thyroid carcinoma, but few isotopes show sufficiently higher differential uptake in tumour than in a critical normal tissue to allow adequate irradiation of the tumour without an excessive dose being delivered either to the kidney and the excretory pathway or to some other critical organ.

Protection from Radiation Injury

We have previously seen that cells become less sensitive to X-rays and γ-rays when the oxygen tension is lowered, or when they are in contact with certain protective substances. This is true also for the whole animal.[33]

The effect of anoxia is particularly striking. Lacassagne and Latarjet, making use of the remarkable fact that newborn mice are able to survive complete

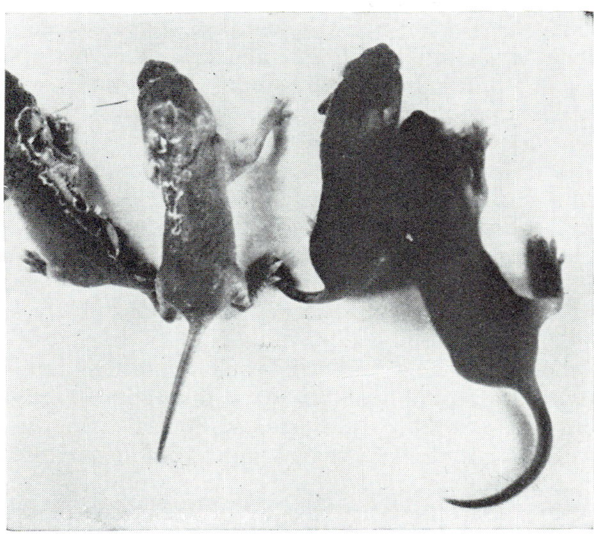

26/Fig. 8.—Effects of anoxic irradiation on newborn mice. *Right to left.* (1) Non-irradiated control; (2) Irradiated in anoxia; (3) and (4) Irradiated under normal conditions. (From R. Latarjet.[11])

asphyxia for as long as twenty minutes, have irradiated these animals under normal and anærobic conditions with 1500rads of soft X-rays. The results of one experiment are shown in FIG. 8. Normal mice generally die within twelve days, showing severe cutaneous lesions and distortion due to deep œdema, whereas mice asphyxiated with nitrogen or carbon dioxide appear to be undamaged, and grow like the unirradiated controls.

A considerable number of relatively simple chemical substances, including cysteine, β-mercaptoethylamine, thiourea, an S-β-aminoethyl*iso*thiuronium salt (AET), histamine, epinephrine and serotonin, afford definite protection to mice if injected intraperitoneally just before irradiation[34, 35, 36]. Such substances appear to have in common an ability to react readily with oxidising radicals or, in the case of the pharmacologically active amines, to lower the oxygen tension in spleen and bone marrow,[37] but their mechanism of action *in vivo* is still uncertain.[38] The degree of protection they afford is limited. Thus, the effect of

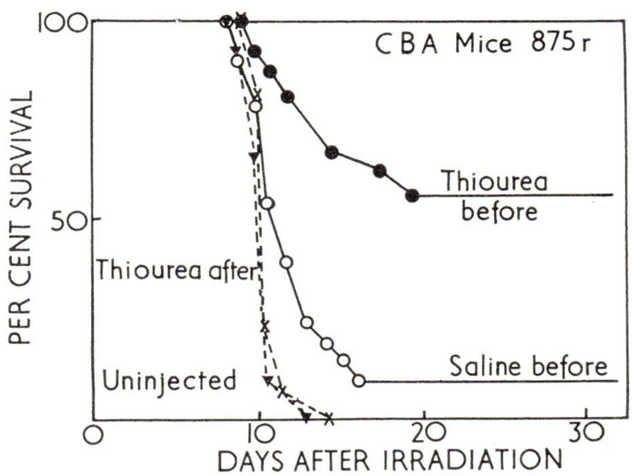

26/FIG. 9.—Survival of CBA mice after whole-body irradiation with 875 rads.

●——● 2 ml. of 0·28 M thiourea intraperitoneally a few minutes before irradiation.
×- - - -× 2 ml. of 0·28 M thiourea intraperitoneally a few minutes after completion of irradiation.
○——○ 2 ml. of 0·15 M saline intraperitoneally a few minutes before irradiation.
◄——► Uninjected. (After Mole.[7])

thiourea that is shown in FIG. 9 is only equivalent to a reduction of about 15 per cent in the dose of radiation, because the dose-mortality curve is steep[7], and all the substances are ineffective if given a few minutes after irradiation has been carried out.

The effects of large doses of radiation on animals are often increased by infection and normally mitigated by repair. When Gram-negative bacteria in the intestinal tract of rats were suppressed by the non-absorbable antibiotics neomycin and polymyxin B the animals survived exposure to 550 rads (though not to 650 rads) of X-rays, whereas 550 rads was uniformly lethal to untreated animals.[39] The finding that good results were obtained by shielding the spleen from radiation was followed by the discovery that protection was given by injections of spleen and bone marrow after exposure, the depleted blood-forming tissues being colonised by cells derived from those which had been injected.[40] The repair of radiation damage by grafts of bone marrow cells is also considered in Chapter 41. It has been reported that combined treatment with AET before irradiation, bone marrow immediately after, and streptomycin for ten days to suppress infection can triple the LD_{50} for irradiated mice. Important though they are, the results of these experiments do not justify the hope that human populations can be adequately protected from the effects of massive total-body doses of ionizing radiation.

CONCLUSION

Although much remains to be learned about the complex changes that radiation can cause in the animal body, progress has clearly been made in tracing the origin of these changes to cells and intracellular structures. Some of the cellular changes, such as an inhibition of mitosis, are apparent almost immediately, while others may be hidden for many generations.

If the immediate damage to the cell has not been too severe, a partial or complete recovery may appear to occur. The regeneration of tissues that have been grossly injured is a striking feature of the histological changes observed in an animal after irradiation, and the fate of the animal, in the first few weeks, seems to depend on the amount of destruction and the rate of repair.

Unfortunately, the visible recovery of a damaged tissue carries no guarantee that all the cells are normal. The sterility produced by irradiation is sometimes only temporary, but when fertility returns there may be mutant genes in some of the germinal cells. The change which has made a cell the potential source of a malignant tumour may not be revealed for many years.

It seems likely that damage to chromosomes represents a part of the injury caused by radiation to somatic cells. However, it is by no means certain that direct chromosome breakage is a main cause of the acute effects of radiation on animals. Disorganisation of enzyme systems, rather than inactivation of individual enzymes, is perhaps responsible for these effects.

In the higher animals, as in *Drosophila* and much simpler organisms, some of the effects of radiation can conveniently be regarded as a consequence of one or several ionizations in a sensitive target. But effective ionizations do not appear to be limited to those which occur in organic structures themselves. The immediate aqueous environment of such structures, in which radiation produces oxidising free radicals, exerts an influence which cannot be neglected.

It is perhaps surprising that an agent which brings about the ionization of atoms in a non-specific manner should produce such well-defined biological effects. The fact that the higher animals are more sensitive to radiation than many viruses or unicellular forms of life is understandable, because the integrity of an animal tissue depends not only on the cellular units themselves, but on their organisation, and because the functioning of one tissue may be co-ordinated with that of another. But the reasons for the great differences in sensitivity between one cell and another are by no means fully understood.

Whatever the mechanisms by which radiation exerts its various biological effects, the effects themselves are not unique. Dividing bacteria are more sensitive than resting ones to a number of antibiotics and synthetic drugs. Many chemical substances are able, under certain conditions, to prevent cell division without preventing cell growth. Chemical substances, like radiation, can induce malignant tumours after a long latent period. The gene-mutations produced by radiations do not appear to differ qualitatively from those that occur spontaneously, or those that are produced by the mutagenic mustard gas and the nitrogen mustards. An understanding of the biological effects of radiation is clearly bound up with the solution of wider biological problems.

REFERENCES

1. LAWRENCE, J. H., and TENNANT, R. (1937). *J. exp. Med.*, **66,** 667.
2. CRONKITE, E. P., and BRECHER, G. (1952). *Ann. Rev. Med.*, **3,** 193.
3. OUGHTERSON, A. W., LEROY, G. V., LIEBOW, A. A., HAMMOND, E. C., BARNETT, H. L., ROSENBAUM, J. D., and SCHNEIDER, B. A. (1951). *Medical Effects of Atomic Bombs.* Oak Ridge, Tenn.: Office of Air Surgeon, N.P. 3037, U.S. Atomic Energy Commission Tech. Information Service.
4. WARREN, S. (1961). *The Pathology of Ionizing Radiation.* Springfield, Ill.: Charles C. Thomas.
5. LEROY, G. V. (1947). *J. Amer. med. Ass.*, **134,** 1143.
6. BLOOM, W., Ed. (1948). *Histopathology of Irradiation from External and Internal Sources.* (National Nuclear Energy Series.) New York: McGraw-Hill.
7. MOLE, R. H. (1951). *J. Chim. phys.*, **48,** 258.
8. BUCKTON, K. E., JACOBS, P. A., COURT-BROWN, W. M., and DOLL, R. (1962). *Lancet*, **2,** 676.
9. TROWELL, O. A. (1952). *J. Path.*, **64,** 687.
10. HOLMES, B. E. (1956). In *Ciba Foundation Symposium on Ionizing Radiations and Cell Metabolism.* Eds. WOLSTENHOLME, G. E. W., and O'CONNOR, C. M. London: J. & A. Churchill.
11. LATARJET, R. (1951). In *Symposium on Radibiology. The Basic Aspects of Radiation Effects on Living Systems.* Ed. NICKSON, J. J. New York: John Wiley & Sons.
12. DAVIES, D. R., and EVANS, H. J. (1965). In *Advances in Radiobiology*, Vol. II. Eds. AUGMENSTEIN, L. G., MASON, R., and ZELLE, M. New York: Academic Press.
13. BOND, V. P., FLIEDNER, T. M., and ARCHAMBEAU, J. O. (1965). *Mammalian Radiation Lethality. A Disturbance in Cellular Kinetics.* New York: Academic Press.
14. LINDOP, P. J., and ROTBLAT, J. (1961). *Proc. roy. Soc. B*, **154,** 332.
15. COURT-BROWN, W. M., and DOLL, R. (1957). *Leukæmia and Aplastic Anæmia in Patients Irradiated for Ankylosing Spondylitis.* Medical Research Council Report 295. London: H.M.S.O.
16. BOREK, C., and SACHS, L. (1966). *Nature* (*Lond.*), **210,** 276.
17. AUB, J. C., EVANS, R. D., HEMPELMANN, L. H., and MARTLAND, H. S. (1952). *Medicine* (*Baltimore*), **31,** 221.
18. SEARLE, A. G. (1967). Progress in Mammalian Radiation Genetics. In *Radiation Research* 1966. (Proc. Third Internat. Cong. of Radiation Research.) Amsterdam: North-Holland Pub. Co.
19. SNELL, G. D. (1933). *J. exp. Zool.*, **65,** 421.
20. KOLLER, P. C., and AUERBACH, C. A. (1941). *Nature* (*Lond.*), **148,** 501.
21. RUSSELL, W. L., RUSSELL, L. B., and KELLY, E. M. (1958). *Science*, **128,** 1546.
22. MULLER, H. J. (1955). *Science*, **121,** 837.
23. *Recommendations of the International Commission on Radiological Protection* (1965). Oxford: Pergamon Press.

24. Medical Research Council (1960). *The Hazards to Man of Nuclear and Allied Radiations.* (2nd Rep. Med. Research Counc.). London: H.M.S.O.
25. MULLER, H. J. (1950). *J. cell. comp. Physiol.*, **35**, Suppl. 1, 9.
26. MULLER, H. J. (1950). *Amer. Scientist*, **38**, 33.
27. Min. of Health (1960). *Radiological Hazards to Patients.* (2nd Rep. Adrian Comm.). London: H.M.S.O.
28. FOWLER, J. F., MORGAN, R. L., SILVESTER, J. A., BEWLEY, D. K., and TURNER, B. A. (1963). *Brit. J. Radiol.*, **36**, 188.
29. GRAY, L. H., CONGER, A. D., EBERT, M., HORNSEY, S., and SCOTT, O. C. A. (1953). *Brit. J. Radiol.*, **26**, 638.
30. THOMLINSON, R. H., and GRAY, L. H. (1955). *Brit. J. Cancer*, **9**, 539.
31. CHURCHILL-DAVIDSON, I., FOSTER, C. A., WIERNIK, G., COLLINS, C. D., PIZEY, N. C. D., SKEGGS, D. B. L., and PURSER, P. R. (1966). *Brit. J. Radiol.*, **39**, 321.
32. HEWITT, H. B. (1962). In *The Scientific Basis of Medicine Annual Reviews*, p. 305. London: The Athlone Press.
33. GRAY, L. H. (1957–58). *Lectures on the Scientific Basis of Medicine*, Vol. VII. London: The Athlone Press.
34. BACQ, Z. M. (1951). *Experientia (Basel)*, **7**, 11.
35. HOLLAENDER, A., and KIMBALL, R. F. (1956). *Nature (Lond.)*, **177**, 726.
36. ORD, M. G., and STOCKEN, L. A. (1959). *Ann. Rev. nuclear Sci.*, **9**, 523.
37. DiSTEFANO, V. (1964). *Ann. N.Y. Acad. Sci.*, **114**, 588.
38. SCOTT, O. C. A. (1963). *Ann. Rev. Med.*, **14**, 371.
39. ROSOFF, C. B. (1963). *J. exp. Med.*, **118**, 935.
40. FORD, C. E., HAMERTON, J. L., BARNES, D. W. H., and LOUTIT, J. F. (1956). *Nature (Lond.)*, **177**, 452.

Chapter 27

PATHOGENICITY AND VIRULENCE OF MICRO-ORGANISMS

BY G. P. GLADSTONE

I

THE GERM THEORY OF DISEASE AND THE RELATIONSHIP BETWEEN HOST AND PARASITE

FROM very early times it was realised by some peoples that diseases could be spread from person to person by direct contact and indirectly by contact with the clothing and dwellinghouse of a sick person. This was well recognised by the Jews, for in Leviticus precise instructions were given to the priest to isolate lepers, burn their clothing, scrape away the plaster from the walls and even demolish their houses. Mixed up with these laudable attempts at hygiene were many sacrificial rites and ceremonies to which equal weight was given. In the first chapter we saw that extraordinary ideas were held in ancient times concerning the causation of disease, and it is not surprising that not all ancient physicians acknowledged the idea of contagion. Epidemic disease, at first attributed to the wrath of supernatural powers, was later regarded by the physicians of ancient Greece as caused by climatic, cosmic and tellurian natural phenomena. Hippocrates, for instance, made no distinction between contagious and non-contagious disease. He was, indeed, said to have extinguished the plague of Athens by lighting fires as an atmospheric corrective. The weight of authority in the pronouncements of Hippocrates and Galen had an immense influence on subsequent thought and the idea of contagion practically disappeared during the Dark Ages. In the early Middle Ages great epidemics of disease swept through Europe, such as the Black Death in 1347–49. These could not fail to impress all alike with their mode of spread and there was a gradual return to the belief that a sick person could transfer his illness to others. Boccaccio in the introduction to the *Decameron* (1350), in which the actors were supposed to be people who had fled from Florence into the country at the time of the Black Death (1348), says:

> "Such . . . was the quality of the pestilential matter as to pass not only from man to man but . . . that anything belonging to the infected if touched by any other creature would certainly infect and kill that creature in a short space of time. . . . The rags of a poor man just dead, being thrown into the street and two hogs coming by at the same time and rooting amongst them, . . . in less than an hour turned round and died on the spot." *

Galenic-Hippocratic dogmatism, although still lingering on into the seventeenth century, in reality received a death blow in the year 1546. In that year Fracastoro (1483–1553) (FIG. 1) published his celebrated *De Contagione*. In this

* If this is a true account, *Past. pestis* must have changed its habits considerably since that time!

small volume of seventy-seven pages he made extremely accurate clinical observations of infectious diseases and their mode of spread, and may be said to have laid the foundation for the germ theory of disease, although it was more than one hundred and thirty years before bacteria were discovered.

According to Fracastoro, epidemic disease was spread by "seminaria" or seeds, either directly from person to person, or via objects which had been in contact with an infected person (fomites). Seminaria could be carried in the air and spread disease "at a distance". This effect he likened to the "halitus" of an

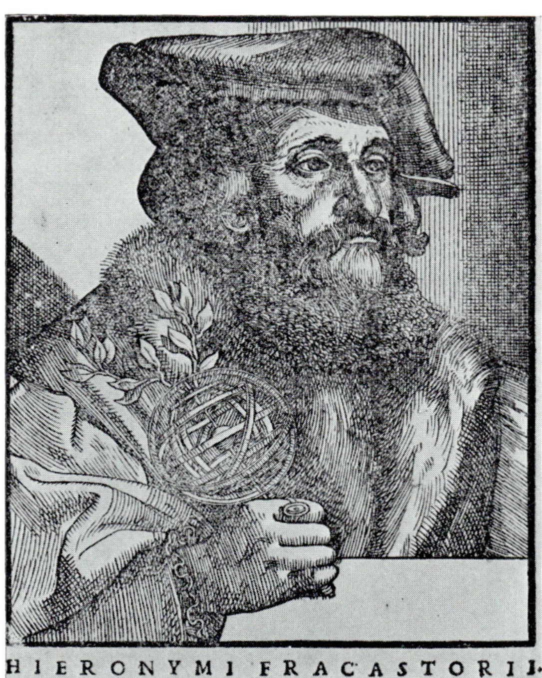

27/FIG. 1.—Girolamo Fracastoro (1483–1553)

"A number of prints, portraits and statues purporting to reproduce the features of Fracastoro have survived. They differ so greatly from each other that it is hard to believe they represent the same man." (Singer and Singer.[1]) This portrait is generally considered the most authentic. It appears as frontispiece to Fracastoro's astronomical work *Homocentrica* and was engraved when he was about 50 years old.

onion which produces "a watery discharge in the eye". It has been questioned whether he regarded these seminaria as living. There is no doubt that he believed them capable of "multiplying and propagating their like", but he regarded their origin as being sponaneous in the "humour" of the disease process.

The idea that living creatures were concerned in the causation of disease, which had been put forward at various times, received new life from the work of Fracastoro, and Kircher (1602–80) wrote a number of treatises on the subject purporting to show microscopic organisms in pathological effluvia under a magnifying-glass. Bulloch[2] has concluded, however, that his descriptions are too vague to be of any value.

Leeuwenhoek (1632–1723) in a letter to the Royal Society in 1683 gave the first undoubted description of bacteria, which he obtained from the scrapings of his teeth. However, nearly two hundred years elapsed before bacteria were proved to have anything to do with disease. Meanwhile, a paper appeared in London in 1720 by Benjamin Marten entitled *A New Theory of Consumptions* which, because of its almost uncanny anticipation of the germ theory of disease, deserves quoting. It not only revived the ideas of Fracastoro and related his seminaria to the living animalcules of Leeuwenhoek and possibly to others too small to be seen under the microscope, but for the first time suggested that infectious diseases might have specific causes. Marten wrote:

> "For how can we better account for the regular types [that] the Small pox, Malignant, and all other Continual and Intermitting Fevers as well as many other Distempers keep, and the peculiar attributes and crises, etc. they have, than by concluding they are severally caused by innumerable Animalculae, or exceeding minute animals that variously offend us according as their species are different and as their peculiar shape and parts are more or less injurious to our fluids and solids." (Singer.[3])

Although his theory was remarkably accurate, he had of course no evidence to support it.

Agostino Bassi (1773–1856) (FIG. 2), a lawyer with a keen interest in scientific pursuits, was the first person to demonstrate a micro-organism as the specific cause of an infectious disease. In 1835 he described a fungus as the cause of muscardine, a disease of silkworms. He showed that it was transmissible probably by "seeds" in food and by direct contact, although he was unable to grow it outside the body. This work was carried out under a great handicap as Bassi so injured his eyesight that he became half blind.

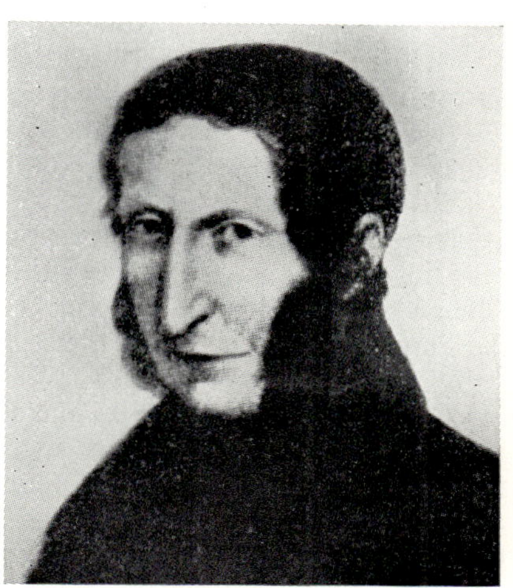

27/FIG. 2.—Agostino Bassi (1773–1856). (Frontispiece to *Opere di Agostino Bassi*. Pavia 1925.)

Although Pasteur's (1822–95) (36/FIG. 2) studies on fermentation and later on the silkworm disease *pébrine* led him to the view that specific germs were responsible for specific diseases, it is to Robert Koch (1843–1910) (42/FIG. 3) that we owe the complete establishment of the germ theory of disease. His work on anthrax in 1876 was in every way a masterpiece of planned experiment, careful technique and accurate observation. He infected mice with the blood of sheep dead of anthrax; carried the infection twenty times from mouse to mouse, showing in each case the presence of rod-shaped organisms in the blood; isolated the organism in pure culture in serum, and transmitted the disease by means of the pure culture. He showed that an allied organism from putrid blood, although resembling the anthrax bacillus closely, would not cause anthrax. In this work and the subsequent monograph on the *Ætiology of Traumatic Infective Diseases* (1878), Koch established the specific nature of bacterial disease.

Koch's Postulates: *The evidence required before a particular microbe can be regarded as the cause of a particular disease.*

Although the acceptable criteria for regarding a bacterium as the cause of a particular disease were deduced from purely theoretical considerations by Henle in 1840, they are rightly attributed to Koch, who produced the experimental basis for them.

(1) The first postulate demands the presence of the particular microbe in every case of the disease. In the words of Koch,[4] translated by Watson Cheyne, "A thoroughly satisfactory proof [of the parasitic nature of a disease] can only be [obtained] when we have succeeded in finding the parasitic micro-organisms in all cases of the disease in question, when we can further demonstrate their presence in such numbers and distribution that all the symptoms of the disease may thus find their explanation and finally when we have established the existence for every individual infective disease of a micro-organism with well-marked morphological characters".

In 1883 Koch described his method for obtaining pure cultures of bacteria by "plating out", a method which, apart from modifications made by Koch himself, has not been altered to the present day. He was then able to add two other criteria[5] (1884):

(2) That the organism must be capable of being grown outside the body in pure culture for a number of generations: "to determine whether formed elements . . . present in the lesion . . . show any sign of possessing independent life . . . it is necessary to isolate the parasites. . . ."

(3) " . . . then to produce the disease anew with all its characteristic features by introducing the parasite alone into a healthy organism." It may be added that the parasite should be capable of being isolated from animals affected by the experimental disease and should be shown to possess the same characters.

We know now that it is not possible to satisfy all these ideal conditions in every case in which a micro-organism is the cause of disease.* Our technique may not be adequate to observe or isolate the organism in every case, especially when it is present in small numbers or associated with other bacteria. Moreover the implied corollary that the organism should not be present in healthy individuals completely breaks down when the problem of the healthy carrier is considered (see below). Although most bacteria and many viruses have been isolated and cultivated, some, such as the leprosy bacillus and a number of viruses, have never been grown apart from the host, but there is no doubt of the ætiological role of these organisms. The leprosy bacillus is present in every case of the disease, usually in enormous numbers, and its distribution is in the lesions observed. No one doubts that it is the cause of leprosy, although it has never been grown in sustained culture and experimental disease has never been produced in animals in spite of claims to have obtained restricted growth in the tissues of mice.[7]

* For a general discussion on Koch's postulates see Fildes and McIntosh.[6]

The third postulate, the production of disease by the inoculation of an organism into healthy individuals, cannot always be satisfied owing to the lack of an experimental animal susceptible to infection. Strictly the postulate demands the production of the identical disease in the same species of animal from which the pure culture of the organism was in the first place derived. Clearly this would be a very sound proof of its causative role. As we are dealing largely with human infections, we have to rely on other species of animal for artificial induction of disease. These may be insusceptible, or may succumb to a disease quite unlike that occurring in man. However, if the experimental disease has characteristic and recognisable features, and if the organism obeys the first two postulates in the experimental animal, i.e. if it is present and distributed according to the observed lesions and can be isolated in pure culture, the third condition is adequately met. Again, "distribution according to the observed lesions" must not be applied too rigidly. There are organisms which produce disease by settling locally at some point in the body and manufacturing potent poisons which circulate to the rest of the tissues. Lesions in which no organism can be demonstrated will then be produced at a distance. Diphtheria is such a disease, and because of his inability to apply completely the postulates of his master, Loeffler[8] exercised great caution in putting forward the claim that he had isolated the causative bacillus.

We have now a useful addition to Koch's postulates which is discussed in Chapter 36: agglutination of a suspension of bacteria by the blood serum of an infected individual. Use was made of this phenomenon by Shiga,[9] who clearly identified the causative organism of dysentery which bears his name, from among a number of other morphologically identical bacteria in the fæces of a dysentery patient. It was the only organism that was clumped by the patient's serum. Such a test is not universally applicable, however. For some time a particular strain of *Proteus vulgaris* (X19) isolated from the urine of a patient with typhus fever[10] was regarded as the causative organism of typhus, because it was agglutinated not only by the blood serum of the patient from whom it was isolated, but by that of all cases of typhus tested, and not by normal serum. However, this organism obeyed none of Koch's postulates, being absent with few exceptions from these patients and never giving rise to disease in experimental animals. There are undoubtedly antigens common to this organism and *Rickettsia prowazeki*, the proved cause of typhus. Whether this circumstance is fortuitous or whether there is some close link between the two organisms is still a point of controversy.

Finally, there is one class of bacterial disease in which all Koch's postulates break down. It is toxic food poisoning due to *Cl. botulinum* or *Staph. aureus*. The organisms themselves need not be present in the body, for the disease is produced by the ingestion of toxins formed during the growth of these organisms in the food. The disease is thus not an infection by the organisms, which may in fact be dead, but a toxæmia due to the very potent poisons they have produced; it is to be classed in the same category as ergot poisoning.

Pathogenicity and Virulence

In the past, these two terms have been used somewhat loosely to denote the ability of a micro-organism to produce disease and are often regarded as synonymous. However, there is a distinct advantage in following the suggestion of Miles[11] who confines the term "pathogenicity" and "pathogenic" to denote a general ability of an organism to produce disease without specifying the conditions. On the other hand, he reserves the term "virulence" and "virulent" for the ability to produce disease under certain specified conditions. The conditions which may affect virulence are: the strain of micro-organism, the susceptibility of a particular host, the route of entry of the organism and certain other environmental factors such as temperature. Virulence, moreover, implies degree. For example, a strain of a bacterial species able to produce disease in a certain set of circumstances with a small number of organisms is said to be more virulent than another strain which requires a larger number of organisms. A third strain which fails to produce disease with a still larger number is called relatively avirulent under the conditions used. Yet all three strains are from a pathogenic species. Again, a pathogenic organism may be virulent for one host but avirulent for another, or it may be virulent by one route but not by another.

General Host-Parasite Relationship

Before considering the validity of the corollary implied in Koch's first postulate, that pathogenic germs should not be found in healthy tissues, it would be convenient to consider host-parasite relations in general. In the words of Theobald Smith, parasitism is "a compromise or truce between two living things accompanied by predatory processes whenever opportunity is offered by one or the other party".[12] It is not to the advantage of the parasite to destroy its host and there are in fact many examples of this harmonious relationship between two organisms. It is indeed possible that this close association is a very widespread phenomenon, but that it remains unrecognised except in those cases where the parasite is of a size and shape sufficiently distinct from the cells or subcellular elements of the host to make it clear that it is of exogenous origin. Sometimes it may be recognised by a disease which the parasite produces either in its own host when the harmonious balance is upset, or in hosts of other species when it is transferred to them.

An association between two living entities without apparent damage to either partner is a phenomenon found in all forms of life from the lowest to the highest evolutionary stage. It may range from the intimate contact represented by lysogeny in bacteria, in which the nucleic acid of the "parasitic" temperate phage is incorporated into the genome of the host cell, to the loose connection shown by surface colonisation of the skin and mucous membranes by bacteria and other ectoparasites.

The so-called "episomes" of bacteria represent a stage slightly less intimate than lysogeny. Episomes are intracellular agents defined by Jacob and Wollman[13] as genetic elements of exogenous origin which may be either integrated wilth the genome of the cell or free in the cytoplasm. Certain temperate phages, e.g. lambda of *E. coli*, the sex fertility factor F of "male" bacteria and the agents determining the formation of colicines are of this kind.*

The many non-injurious parasites infecting the protozoa are still less intimately connected with the host cell.[14] For instance, the chloroplasts present in

*It may be questioned whether episomes are strictly parasites. In the absence of a strict definition of 'parasite', there seems no valid reason to put them in a different category.

Paramœcium bursaria and certain other protozoa have been shown to be algæ. The parasites are recognised by their green colour and can be obtained in a free-living condition. There is no suggestion that they ever harm the cell but, on the contrary, by providing nutrients by photosynthesis, they are probably beneficial. Another type of parasite is found in the so-called "killer" strains of *Paramœcium aurelia*. This is a small rickettsia-like body, the "kappa" particle, which does not harm its host but which secretes a toxin, paramœcin, toxic to strains not possessing kappa (non-killer strains). Kappa protects its host from the effects of this toxin, for if kappa is removed from the cell, the latter becomes as sensitive as non-killer strains to the action of the toxin.[15, 16]

Inapparent parasitism is perhaps more frequently encountered in the insects and other arthropods than in any other group of animals. In these animals, organisms resembling bacteria or rickettsiæ not only live inside the cells of their hosts, but can be transmitted from parent to offspring in the germ cells. So close is the association between parasite and host, that some workers have doubted whether they are separate organisms. However, in some cases the parasite has been demonstrated, either by its ability to produce disease when transferred to other hosts, as for instance with certain of the rickettsiæ responsible for diseases of man, or by its cultivation apart from the host.

The vertebrates, including man, may also harbour micro-organisms as inapparent infections, which do no damage to the host (for refs see 18, 19). For instance, it has been clearly established over the last decade that a large number of viruses may inhabit the cells of the body without causing any ill effects. Many of these have never been shown to produce disease in the species of animal from which they were taken, and they would have been unrecognised were it not for the evidence of multiplication and cytopathic effects on cells in tissue culture. Some of these so-called "orphan viruses" (viruses in search of a disease) however, have not been shown to be associated with disease, e.g. diarrhœa, respiratory disease and meningitis.

Under the heading of inapparent intracellular parasitism, we may include an infection of mice which has unique features namely lymphocytic choriomeningitis (LCM). This infection will be considered in more detail in Chapter 40 in which its connection with autoimmunity is discussed. It may be stated here that the virus parasitises the cells of many organs of the mouse without having any direct ill effect on the cells. Mice infected from their mothers *in utero* harbour large amounts of virus throughout life without suffering any symptoms. They are immunologically tolerant to the virus, producing no antibodies or delayed hypersensitivity reactions to it. Infection *ab initio* in the adult mouse, however, is followed by the development of antibodies and the infiltration of organs by lymphocytes, with secondary cellular damage leading to death. There is strong evidence that this cytopathic action is the result of a delayed hypersensitive autoimmune reaction to the tissues brought about by the formation of new antigens in the cell following infection by the virus[20] and not to any cytopathic action of the virus itself.

The Healthy Carrier

This term is used for an individual (man or animal) who, while remaining healthy himself, harbours pathogenic organisms which are capable of being transferred to others and producing disease. The term might be extended to cover also the carriage of organisms potentially dangerous to the carrier himself (endogenous infection). We may classify the carrier state into:

(1) *Commensalism.*—Among the more or less permanent bacterial residents (commensals) of the body surfaces, there are a number of pathogenic organisms which are prevented from causing disease only by the integrity of the body integument and certain self-sterilising activities of the skin, mucous membranes and conjunctiva. Some of these potentially pathogenic organisms are found so invariably that they may be regarded as part of the resident flora. *Str. viridans*, *Actinomyces* sp., *H. influenzæ* and certain of the anærobic fusiform bacilli are nearly always present in the mouth and throat, and *Cl. tetani* and *Cl. welchii* are common inhabitants of the intestine. *E. coli*, universally present in the intestine, may at times invade the tissues and produce disease. *Staph. aureus* is found in the anterior nares of about 50 per cent of the population. The pneumococcus is also present in the nasopharynx of about 50 per cent of individuals, but, except during epidemics, the prevalent strains are usually those that do not give rise to epidemic disease and are probably of low virulence for man.

Some of these commensals may be potentially dangerous for the carrier himself. For instance, in subacute bacterial endocarditis due to *Strep. viridans* the organism enters the blood stream from the mouth following a tooth extraction. Normally this organism is rapidly removed and does no damage, but if there is a congenital abnormality of the heart valve or an old rheumatic lesion of the valve it may settle on the endothelium and produce septic vegetations and bacteriæmia. Actinomycosis is another example due to passage of *Actinomyces israeli* from the mouth into the tissues through a break in the integument.

(2) *Incubationary carriage.* This is a condition of unstable equilibrium in which the pathogenic organism has gained access to the tissues and has been recognised in the incubation period of the disease before it has grown sufficiently or produced sufficient damage to the body to make disease evident. For instance, in enteric fever, it is sometimes possible to find *Salm. typhi* in the blood, and even in the fæces, before the onset of the disease.

Under this heading we may also place the so-called *slow virus infections* of animals, infections in which the incubation period may extend over several months or years.[21] During this time in many of these diseases active multiplication of the virus is taking place in the body and, if the virus has access to the external environment, the animal must be regarded as a potential source of infection, e.g. in scrapie.[22, 23] Scrapie is a natural disease of sheep affecting the central nervous system particularly the cerebellum and hypothalamus. In recent years the disease has been successfully transmitted to mice.[24] The mice suffer from a disease very similar to the natural disease in sheep, so enabling some of the conditions determining infection to be investigated. The incubation period is several months during which the mouse appears healthy. However, there is a progressive multiplication of the infecting agent ("virus") throughout this time, first in the spleen and lymph nodes where it persists in large amounts and then in the thymus and salivary glands extending to the lungs and intestine and finally to the spinal cord. It gradually increases in amount in the CNS until symptoms appear in 5–6 months. During this time there seems to be no evidence of a defence response on the part of the host. It is possible that the formation of protective antibody is inhibited by the excessive production of "virus" in the lymphoid tissue (immunological paralysis, Chapter 41). Alternatively, the "virus" may not be antigenic, possibly owing to an absence of capsid protein. That it differs from the known viruses is shown by its unusual resistance to heat, formalin and proteolytic enzymes.

Visna virus infection is another disease of the central nervous system of sheep in which the incubation period may be as long as several years.[25] The virus multiplies slowly in the organs of the sheep throughout this period and appears in the spinal fluid, blood and saliva. However, unlike scrapie, the virus stimulates the production of high titres of neutralising antibody. It is not clear why the disease should progress to death in the presence of antibody.

Certain of the viruses causing tumours in animals may be included in the category of slow virus infections.[26] Their peculiar latency and pathogenicity are discussed in Chapter 24. Until more is known about the mode of transmission of these viruses and the factors determining the production of tumours, it is impossible to state whether carriers of latent virus are dangerous.

(3) *Convalescent carriage.*—This is a condition in which the organism persists in the tissues after the disease is at an end. The parasite is localised, and its noxious effects neutralised, but the body defences have failed to eliminate it completely. For example, following at attack of typhoid fever, the infection may persist in the gall bladder, a condition which is epidemiologically important because of the continued excretion of typhoid bacilli in the fæces.

We may include under "convalescent carriers" those individuals who have become infected, but whose infection has remained subclinical and unrecognised. Nevertheless they continue to harbour the pathogenic organism and disseminate it to others. In epidemics of many diseases such carriers are common and may outnumber the true clinical infections by as much as a hundred-fold, as is found, for instance, in epidemics of poliomyelitis. They are, therefore, of great importance epidemiologically as they are not readily recognised and isolated. Examples of diseases spread by such carriers are: meningococcal meningitis, streptococcal and staphylococcal respiratory infection and diphtheria, and a number of viral infections such as poliomyelitis, infectious hepatitis and homologous serum jaundice in man. In all these infections organisms are carried on sites from which they can be readily disseminated to other individuals.

In poliomyelitis, for example, individuals have been shown to harbour the virus in their intestines for weeks without any evidence of disease, and are undoubtedly a potential source of danger in the spread of infection.[27] Carriers are not confined to man. Rabies virus may persist in the vampire bat as an inapparent infection and infect man, and many arboviruses have their reservoir in birds from which the virus is transmitted by arthropod vectors to man. The demonstration that psittacosis virus may be carried in healthy birds as an inapparent infection has proved of great importance in the control of the disease in man. Infection in the bird occurs early in life, or even congenitally, and may persist for at least a year.[28] During this time the virus may be excreted from the nasal passage and from the cloaca in a fully virulent state, so that the bird is a highly dangerous carrier and may pass on infection to man or to other birds. The bird itself suffers no ill effects, but may succumb to the disease if kept under unhealthy conditions.

There are two well-recognised examples in which persistent convalescent carriage may lead to clinical disease in the carrier himself: herpes simplex virus infection and Brill's disease. Herpes virus infects young children giving rise to stomatitis. After the child's recovery the virus remains latent in the cells of the mucous membrane of the mouth and lips and persists into adult life, probably spreading from cell to cell as new cells are formed and old cells desquamated. Some external stimulus, e.g. the development of a cold or fever, appears to light up the infection and the carrier develops herpes labialis. Brill's disease, due to *Rickettsia prowazeki* is a mild form of endemic typhus occurring among immigrant Polish and Russian Jews in the North-Eastern coastal towns of the U.S.A. There is evidence that these individuals have had in the past a clinical or subclinical infection with the virus which has persisted in an inapparent state and, under appropriate conditions, lights up as a clinical disease.

The examples of inapparent infections in vertebrates quoted above make it clear that even pathogenic organisms may grow in the tissues without necessarily causing disease. There is a dynamic equilibrium between parasite and host. The factors upsetting the equilibrium may be environmental, by which the resistance of the host is lowered or the growth of the parasite is favoured, or intrinsic, for example the mutation of the parasite.

It may be possible to explain some of the puzzling features of the epidemiology of influenza in man in terms of the disturbance of an equilibrium between parasite and host by some environmental factor. In many cases epidemics start from a number of centres with little or no possibility of intercommunication; this was seen in the outbreak in Sardinia in 1949. It has been suggested that a latent infection with the virus is present in a number of individuals in these centres, and that some external factor, for example a climatic one, affects all of them simultaneously, starting an outbreak of the disease.

Increased activity of the parasite, or mutation to a more virulent form, may explain the upset in the equilibrium between parasite and host without the intervention of an external factor. Certain of the pneumonites viruses of mice may be present as a latent infection in the lungs without any apparent signs or symptoms. Serial intranasal inoculation of extract of lung has in time led to the development of typical disease. The serial passage has selected a more virulent parasite so that it eventually overcomes the host's efforts to keep it in check, and disease results.

Summary

The contagious nature of certain diseases was not recognised by all ancient peoples, and the first clear conception of it was that of Fracastoro in 1546.

Leeuwenhoek described bacteria in 1683, but it was not until the latter half of the nineteenth century that Pasteur and Koch related them to disease. Robert Koch (1876) fully established the germ theory of disease and laid down certain conditions to be satisfied before an organism can be regarded as the cause of a particular disease. These criteria, known as Koch's postulates, demand that the organism shall be found in all cases of the disease in question and its distribution be in accordance with the lesions observed; that the organism can be isolated from the lesions and grown in pure culture apart from the body; and that the pure culture can produce the identical disease in another animal. A further useful criterion is the demonstration of agglutination of the causative organism by the patient's serum.

Pathogenicity is distinct from virulence. Pathogenicity is the ability to produce disease without specifying the conditions. Virulence is the capacity to produce disease in a given set of circumstances. Various degrees of virulence may be found depending on conditions associated with both the host and the parasite, but the organisms are either pathogenic or not.

Living organisms at all stages of evolution may harbour parasitic exogenous genetic elements which may be intimately integrated with the genome of the cell as in "lysogeny" or may be detached as free living organisms as in "commensalism", the parasitisation of the surface of the skin and mucous membranes of vertebrates with bacteria. Between these extremes all degrees of association between parasite and host may be found without harmful effects to either.

The carrier state (inapparent infection) is the harbouring of a pathogenic micro-organism potentially capable of spreading to others and producing disease. The term may be extended to cover carriage of organisms potentially dangerous to the carrier himself. The carried organism may be a normal inhabitant of the body surfaces, or be present during the incubation period of a disease in the carrier or, more usually, following recovery from a clinical or subclinical attack of the disease in the carrier, with persistence of the organism at a site from which it can be disseminated to others (convalescent carrier). Recurrence of the disease may occur in the persistent carrier many years after infection.

REFERENCES

1. SINGER, C., and SINGER, D. (1917). *Ann. med. Hist.*, **1,** 1.
2. BULLOCH, W. (1938). *The History of Bacteriology*. London: Oxford Univ. Press.
3. SINGER, C. (1913). *The Development of the Doctrine of* Contagium vivum 1500–1750. London: Private print.
4. KOCH, R. (1878). *The Ætiology of Traumatic Infective Diseases*, translated by W. Watson Cheyne. New Sydenham Society, London 1880, p. 21.
5. KOCH, R. (1884). *The Ætiology of Tuberculosis*, translated by S. Boyd in *Microparasites in Disease*. Ed. WATSON CHEYNE, W., New Sydenham Society, 1886, p. 65.
6. FILDES, P., and MCINTOSH, J. (1920). *Brit. J. exp. Path.*, **1,** 119.
7. REES, R. J. W., WATERS, M. F. R., WEDDELL, A. G. M., and PALMER, E. (1967). *Nature (Lond.)*, **215,** 599.
8. LOEFFLER, F. (1884). *Mitt. k. GesundhAmte*, **2,** 421. (English abstract by T. W. Hime in *Microparasites in Disease*. Ed. W. WATSON CHEYNE, New Sydenham Society, 1886, p. 445).
9. SHIGA, K. (1898). *Zbl. Bakt.*, **23,** 599.
10. WEIL, E., and FELIX, A. (1916). *Wien. klin. Wschr.*, **29,** 33, 974.
11. MILES, A. A. (1955). *Symp. Soc. gen. Microbiol.*, **5,** 1.
12. SMITH, T. (1934). *Parasitism and Disease*. Princeton: Princeton Univ. Press.
13. JACOB, F., and WOLLMAN, E. L. (1958). *C.R. Acad. Sci. (Paris)*, **247,** 154.
14. DROOP, M. R. (1963). *Symp. Soc. gen. Microbiol.*, **13,** 171.
15. BEALE, G. H. (1954). *The Genetics of* Paramœcium aurelia. London: Cambridge Univ. Press.
16. SONNEBORN (1959). *Advanc. Virus Res.*, **6,** 229.
17. BROOKS, M. A. (1963). *Symp. Soc. gen. Microbiol.*, **13,** 200.
18. KOPROWSKI, H. (1952). *Ann. N.Y. Acad. Sci.*, **54,** 963.

19. Walker, D. L., Hansen, R. P., and Evans, A. S., Eds. (1958). *Symposium on Latency and Masking in Viral and Rickettsial Infections.* Minneapolis: Burgess Publishing Co.
20. Hotchin, J. (1962). *Cold Spr. Harb. Symp. quant. Biol.*, **27,** 479.
21. *Monograph of the National Institute of Neurological Dis. and Blindness* (1965). **2**. Washington D.C.: U.S. Govt. Printing Office.
22. Hourrigan, J. L. (1965). Ref. 21, p. 263.
23. Morris, J. A., Gajdusek, D. C., and Gibbs, C. J. (1965). Ref. 21, p. 273.
24. Chandler, R. L. (1961). *Lancet*, **1,** 1378.
25. Thormar, H. (1965). Ref. 21, p. 335.
26. Eddy, B. E. (1965). Ref. 21, p. 369.
27. Brown, G. C., Francis, T., and Ainslie, J. (1948). *J. exp. Med.*, **87,** 21.
28. Meyer, K. F. (1942). *Medicine* (*Baltimore*), **21,** 175.

Chapter 28

PATHOGENICITY AND VIRULENCE OF MICRO-ORGANISMS

BY G. P. GLADSTONE

II

COMMUNICABILITY

THERE are three conditions determining the production of disease by micro-organisms: (1) The organism must be capable of being transferred from a source of infection to the surface of a new host and, unless carried directly into the tissues through a break in the integument, must be able to survive on the surface for at least a short time. This condition may be called *Communicability.* (2) The organism must be able to pass through the integument, either through the intact tissue or through an accidental breach, and to find the right conditions for growth in the body tissues, and must also be resistant to those reactions of the host which might lead to its destruction. This condition, called *Invasiveness,* is discussed in Chapter 29. (3) *Pathogenic action.* The organism must be capable of damaging the tissues. We have seen in the last chapter that the mere presence of the microbe in the body tissue does no harm. Disease is the manifestation of some chemical activity of the microbe, whether directly by the production of toxins (Chapter 30), or more indirectly by bringing about conditions leading to self-intoxication by the tissues (Chapter 39), or possibly by competing for nutrients required by the host.

In this chapter we shall consider *Communicability.* Coburn[1] reserves this term for the transference of the organism from a source of infection to a new host and uses the term "infectivity" to denote the establishment of the organism on the body surface. Since these two factors are not readily distinguishable in most cases, both will be included here under the term "communicability".

A consideration of the factors determining the spread of pathogenic organisms from a source of infection to a new host belongs more to the realm of Epidemiology than that of Pathology. However, a knowledge of how bacteria are disseminated, how they reach and survive on the body surfaces, and by what route they get into the tissues is essential for the understanding of invasiveness. No apology will be made, therefore, for discussing the facts here.

INTRINSIC FACTORS IN COMMUNICABILITY

There has been much conflict of opinion as to whether some intrinsic property is possessed by certain strains of micro-organisms which determines their ability to spread from person to person; that is, whether there exist so-called "epidemic strains" differing from others in their greater ability to spread to new hosts.[2] Such intrinsic factors, if they exist, might be a capacity to withstand desiccation, to survive and grow in vectors, or to survive on the surface of the body. Perhaps the clearest evidence in favour of the existence of epidemic strains is that of Greenwood and Topley and their co-workers[3] in their studies on experimental epidemiology in mice. Some strains of both *Past. muriseptica* and *Salm. typhi murium*, which appeared to be identical in other characteristics, differed considerably in their ability to produce epidemics by natural spread from mouse to mouse. This difference in communicability was not related solely to difference in virulence, that is in ability to produce disease when introduced directly into the tissue, although clearly virulence must play a part since the criterion of spread was the production of disease. Similar observations have been described by Webster and Clow[4] in pneumococcal infection, and by Coburn, Evans, and Nathan[1] in streptococcal infection, in mice.

These observations may well apply to natural epidemics of human disease.[5] It is well known that in some epidemics the microbe spreads rapidly among the human population at risk, whereas in others, due to the same species of microbe, the spread is more limited. Such variation is found, for example, in the hospital epidemics of staphylococcal infections and presents one of the most important challenges to the epidemiologist. Even when the extrinsic factors prevalent in an epidemic, such as the increased numbers of organisms disseminated, the nature of the source of infection and the ease with which the organisms can spread from it are taken into account, there appears to be some intrinsic property of certain hospital strains of staphylococci which allows them to spread widely among the population at risk in contrast to others which remain more confined.

As the spread of infection is generally assessed by the ability to produce sepsis, one of these factors must be virulence. There is little doubt that organisms isolated from infected persons and carriers during an epidemic are more virulent than those isolated in inter-epidemic periods, and hence fewer organisms need be transferred to set up disease. In organisms such as hæmolytic streptococci and meningococci this is reflected in the presence of surface antigens lacking in those isolated in inter-epidemic periods. Certain hospital strains of staphylococcus, without apparent change in antigenic structure, are also more virulent than others. Babies colonised with these strains developed more than 20-fold more clinical infections than those colonised with other strains.[6]

Virulence, however, is not the only factor. If spread of infection is assessed, not by clinical disease, but by bacteriology, wide-spread infections of carriers with heavy contaminations of their environment may occur with strains which fail to produce a single clinical case of disease (for refs. see 7, p. 67). Even certain strains of the usually virulent phage type 80/81 may spread extensively from the nasal mucosa of one individual to that of another without causing sepsis. It would seem, therefore, that in staphylococcal epidemics in man as in the experimental infections of Greenwood and Topley, communicability or infectivity is an attribute distinct from virulence.

What are the characters likely to be associated with communicability? How do "hospital" epidemic strains of staphylococci, for example, differ from strains not epidemic and from those isolated in other environments? There is no doubt that a major difference between such strains is in antibiotic resistance. Most, although not all, hospital epidemics of staphylococcal sepsis are brought about by strains resistant to penicillin and often to other antibiotics as well. Although it is easy to understand how such strains could be selected in a patient treated with penicillin or other antibiotic, it is not clear at first sight how antibiotic resistance could play a part in the spread of infection to individuals who have never received the antibiotic. The explanation appears to lie in the observations of Gould[8] that extensive use of penicillin in a closed hospital environment causes a considerable contamination of the environment with the drug including areas of the body liable to be colonised with staphylococci. As we shall see when we consider colonisation of organisms on the body surfaces, the presence of antibiotics in such sites may result in suppression of the natural flora and allow resistant strains to gain a foothold. White[9] found that the penicillin resistant type 80/81 colonised the anterior nares in greater numbers and more persistently than sensitive strains, but whether this was related to its resistance to pencillin was not established.

The ability of the epidemic strain to survive outside the body in a dried state and preserve its infectivity and virulence is another factor determining communicability. Rountree (ref. 7, p. 67) noted that epidemic hospital strains of staphylococci dried on cotton or wool fabrics survive for considerably longer periods than other strains.

There are probably many other intrinsic factors determining communicability at present unknown.

Extrinsic Factors in Communicability

Let us consider some of the extrinsic factors determining the transference of micro-organisms to a new host. They may be summarised as follows:

A Reservoir of Infection

The reservoir of infection in human disease is usually either a patient suffering from the disease or a healthy human carrier, but many human diseases are carried by animals which may or may not show signs of disease themselves. Sometimes the patient is his own source of infection, the organism being present as a normal commensal somewhere on the body surface, and being transferred to another site by direct or indirect contact. For example, puerperal sepsis may be caused by a streptococcus from the throat of the patient herself. The commensal may also invade the tissues at the site which it has colonised, for example the invasion of the blood stream through a tooth socket by *Str. viridans*, a normal inhabitant of the mouth (Chapter 27).

The source of infection may be unconnected with a living host, for example soil contains *Pseudomonas pyocyanea* and many pathogenic species of the clostridia which may contaminate wounds.

The effectiveness of a reservoir is determined by the number of organisms it contains and their ability to leave the reservoir. Completely closed infections are clearly not communicable, whereas sites of infection which communicate with any of the passages open to the exterior, such as the respiratory and intestinal tracts, are potential sources from which disease may be communicated to others.

The Vehicle, or Mode of Transmission

The methods of transference from the source of infection to a new host are as follows:

(*a*) *Transmission by direct contact.*—The most important diseases clearly acquired by direct contact are the venereal diseases. Examples of infection transferred directly from animals are rabies from the bite of a rabid dog, rat-bite fever, and anthrax which is acquired by handling infected animals or their products. Examples from non-living sources are infection of wounds by soil carrying clostridia responsible for tetanus and gas gangrene, and the infection of burns by dust contaminated with *Pseudomonas pyocyanea.*

(*b*) *Congenital transmission.*—Infection may be transmitted to the progeny either at the ovum stage, when it may become infected from either parent, or from the mother later in fœtal life, when the organism either passes directly from the maternal to the fœtal blood, or forms a lesion in the placenta from which the fœtus is infected.

There does not appear to be any known example in human pathology of infection taking place directly through the germ cells, but in animals a number of examples are known. *Salm. pullorum*, the cause of bacillary white diarrhœa of chickens, can be transmitted through the egg which may be infected on its way down the oviduct or from the sperm of the cock. Examples of the transmission of parasites through the eggs of arthropods have been mentioned in Chapter 27, and are considered further in a later section.

The passage of infection from the blood of the mother to that of her young is by no means as common as might be supposed from the close association between the mother and her fœtus.The placenta appears to be a barrier even when the organisms are present in the mother's blood. However, the barrier is not always effective and there are many examples of the passage of organisms particularly viruses from the mother to her fœtus.[10] Perhaps the most documented is the passage of rubella virus during the first three months of pregnancy leading to abnormalities in the newborn, particularly congenital cataract, mute deafness and cardiac disease. Sometimes the fœtus is infected without the mother showing any signs of clinical disease. This occurs not only with rubella but with variola, varicella and serum hepatitis.[11] On the other hand the reverse may occur: a healthy child may be born by a mother suffering from smallpox.

Congenital syphilis is the classical example of a bacterial disease in man transmitted *in utero*. The treponemata may pass directly from the maternal circulation to that of the child, or a lesion in the placenta may occur from which large numbers of organisms may infect the fœtus.

Listeria monocytogenes is another bacterium which is transmitted *in utero* leading to *granulomatosis infantiseptica*, a disease which is invariably fatal. Very rarely tubercle bacilli may be transmitted, but only following the development of a tuberculous lesion in the placenta.

(*c*) *Transmission by objects which have been in contact with an infected person* (*fomites*).—This mode of transmission depends on the ability of the organism to survive outside the body, possibly in a desiccated state. Organisms such as *Treponema pallidum*, and *Br. tularensis*, which have little ability to survive are not likely to be transmitted by fomites. On the other hand, *B. anthracis*, *Myco. tuberculosis*, *Str. pyogenes*, the virus of foot and mouth disease and smallpox virus may be so transmitted. Downie[12] has shown that this last can survive in dried crusts for more than a year. A striking example of the spread of smallpox by fomites occurred in Brighton in 1950[13] when three laundry workers contracted the disease after sorting the dirty linen from an individual who was not at the time suspected of having the disease. Lavatory seats have been implicated in the transmission of infection usually on insufficient grounds. Hutchinson,[14] however, has shown that seats may become contaminated with Sonne dysentery bacilli from droplets from the pan formed at the time of flushing. The infection may then be transferred to the hands.

There is a great deal of evidence to suggest that the hands are an important link in the dissemination of bacteria from the respiratory tract, particularly from the nose and perhaps also from the perineum. Hamburger and Green[15] found that enormous numbers (in one case 21,000,000) of hæmolytic streptococci could be recovered from the hands of nasal carriers of these organisms and appreciable numbers from the hands of throat carriers. The hand contamination was shown to be from the handkerchief at the time of blowing the nose. Rubbo and Benjamin[16] also inculpated the hands as vehicles of transfer. They heavily contaminated the nasal fossæ of two subjects with *Serratia marcescens*. One subject was then allowed to go about his daily occupation but to avoid touching any part of his face during the experimental period (1 hour), whereas no restriction was placed on the other subject. Various sites of the body and clothing were then swabbed and cultured. In the subject whose activities were limited, only the skin immediately round the nose showed contamination, but in the other, the organism was found on every site sampled and was most numerous on the hands. When the mouth had been contaminated, dissemination was less, but the organism could still be recovered from the hands.

The contamination of the skin round the nose and the upper lip with nasal secretion must be of regular occurrence, and surveys of the habits of individuals show that there are numerous chances of contamination being transferred to the hands. Thus Hare and Thomas[17] found that nine students touched their mouth or nose a total of no fewer than 120 times in the course of a single hour's lecture, and a dye which fluoresced in ultraviolet light instilled into the nostrils was found on the fingers and on every object handled (see also Ref. 18).

(d) Transmission by food, water, and milk.—Food and milk frequently harbour pathogenic germs responsible both for intestinal diseases such as typhoid, paratyphoid, food poisoning, and dysentery and for general diseases such as tuberculosis, brucellosis, poliomyelitis, and scarlet fever. Food may become contaminated from the animal producing it; for example, ducks' eggs and the meat from pigs and cattle may harbour salmonellæ and cause food poisoning; cow's milk may harbour bovine tubercle bacilli or brucellæ. Food also may become contaminated from a human carrier who is excreting an intestinal pathogen in his fæces—usually salmonella or shigella—or in his nasal mucus—often a staphylococcus—and transferring the organism to foods from his hands which easily become contaminated from these sources. The means by which hands become contaminated with fæcal organisms was well demonstrated by Hutchinson.[14] In one outbreak of Sonne dysentery in nursery schools she was able to recover the causative organism from the hands of up to 50 per cent of the children. Although the hands might have picked up the organism from the lavatory seats, the most likely method of contamination was shown to be from the use of toilet paper. Double thicknesses of five different brands of toilet paper were wrapped over the fingers, which were then lightly pressed onto stools containing Sonne

dysentery bacilli. In all but one of fifteen tests, the organism could be cultured from the fingers.

Transmission by food and milk, of course, depends on the ability of the organism to survive in these media. Some organisms not only survive but grow readily in food and milk, and the prevalence of intestinal infection in tropical countries is probably associated with the rapid growth of intestinal pathogens in food brought about by the high temperatures. Even in temperate climates, however, the danger of bacterial growth in food is very real. In outbreaks of food poisoning due to the staphylococcus, salmonella or *Cl. welchii*, it is frequently found that the food has been allowed to stand for some time in a warm place before consumption. The number of pathogenic organisms originally present is often too small to cause disease, but the organisms may grow several-fold in a few hours. Many of the war-time consignments of spray-dried eggs from the U.S.A. were found to harbour salmonella organisms which were often resistant to light cooking.[19] The egg powder could generally be eaten with impunity if cooked immediately after it had been reconstituted with water, the number of organisms resisting cooking being too few to cause disease. If, however, the reconstituted egg was allowed to stand for some time before cooking and eating, infection often resulted.

Hæmolytic streptococci do not multiply to any extent in milk. The comparatively rare milk-borne epidemics of disease due to these organisms have not resulted from inoculation of the milk by droplets of saliva or mucus from a human case or carrier, which would be unlikely to infect the milk with sufficient numbers to produce disease. They have followed superficial infection of the udder of the cow. The usual form of mastitis in the cow is due to *Str. agalactiæ* which is innocuous to man, but sometimes the udder gets infected from the hands of a milker carrying *Str. pyogenes*. From such an infection large numbers of organisms may be passed into the milk.

Because of the inability of most organisms to survive for any length of time in water, particularly if clear and free from organic matter, water-borne disease is limited to that produced by organisms which can infect in comparatively small numbers, e.g. cholera and typhoid. Salmonellæ, other than *Salm. typhi*, seldom produce water-borne epidemics owing to the relatively large numbers required to infect. Since *Salm. typhi* does not usually survive for long in clear water, water-borne disease is usually the result of continual leakage of small numbers of organisms into the water supply, often from defective sewers. Infection may take place by drinking infected water, or it may be more indirect by the use of contaminated water for washing vegetables or utensils used for storing milk. Oysters from estuaries and water-cress from beds contaminated with sewage have resulted in several outbreaks of typhoid fever. Some infections are acquired by bathing; for instance, leptospirosis may result from bathing in water contaminated with rat urine containing *Leptospira icterohæmorrhagiæ*. The leptospira is thought to enter through the conjunctiva or possibly the respiratory mucous membrane. Poliomyelitis has also been transmitted by bathing, the source of the virus being a sewage outflow.

(*e*) *Arthropod vectors.*—The diseases most commonly transmitted by arthropod vectors are those due to viruses and rickettsiæ, but bacterial diseases, e.g. recurrent fever, bubonic plague and oroya fever are also spread in this way with multiplication of the bacterium in the tissues of the vector. Arthropods may also be responsible for the spread of typhoid, dysentery, cholera, tularæmia and anthrax by mechanical transmission of the bacterium on their body surfaces without multiplication.

Viruses and rickettsiæ invade the tissues of the vector and multiply in its cells and may persist throughout its life span. Sometimes, the parasite may pass through the germ cell and infect the larvæ, nymphs and adults of a new generation as occurs for instance with certain rickettsiæ in the tick and mite.

In recent years, more than 200 so-called arboviruses have been described. These are viruses producing a viræmia in one or more vertebrate species from which blood-sucking arthropods, usually culicine and anophiline mosquitoes, but also ticks and mites, become infected. The viruses multiply in the cells of the vector which can then transmit the infection by inoculation directly into the blood of a susceptible vertebrate at the next meal. Tick-borne arboviruses, such as those responsible for tick-borne encephalitis, have been shown to be present in the salivary glands of the tick in high concentration and are transmitted during the lengthy hours of sucking. This process may be so prolonged that a viræmia may develop and the tick become secondarily infected by the same blood meal.

The tissues of the tick seem to be admirably adapted for the growth of many different varieties of rickettsiæ. Some of these are normal harmless inhabitants of the tick. Others, such as *R. rickettsii* and *Coxiella burneti* are responsible for diseases in man. In the tissues of the tick these organisms grow profusely, reaching a titre which may be as much as 10^9 mouse LD_{50}. They are excreted in the coxal fluid and fæces of the tick, and infection in man may take place, not only from the bite, but also from scratching the infected fæces into the skin.

The successful transmission of infective disease to man by arthropods may involve a highly complex ecological association between micro-organism, vector or vectors, animal reservoir, favourable environmental conditions and susceptible human subject. This is particularly evident in the mosquito-borne virus diseases. Many of these viruses may be carried by more than one species of mosquito and produce inapparent viræmia in a variety of animal species. It is, therefore, often difficult to sort out the essential chain by which man eventually becomes infected. This is illustrated by carriage of St. Louis encephalitis virus by three species of Culex in the Western United States which feed on almost any vertebrate in their environment. Birds are known to develop a sufficiently high degree of viræmia for the further passage of the virus to man, but whether other vertebrates or other species of mosquito known to harbour the virus, can carry on the cycle is not known.[20] The cycle ends with man himself as the viræmia in man is insufficient to infect fresh vectors. Similar difficulties are encountered in the transmission of yellow fever. *Ædes ægypti* is known to transmit yellow fever virus from primate to man or from man to man, but the virus has been isolated from at least six other species of mosquito. The extent to which these species feed on other animals in the environment has received little attention.

Although the passage of *R. rickettsii* to a vertebrate host is dependent on the tick, *Coxiella burneti* is more usually transmitted in other ways, e.g. in dust and excrement of animals. The mite-borne rickettsiæ are usually transmitted by the bite of the mite larvæ which are infected either at the previous generation, the infection passing through the adult and egg, or at the larval stage. Neither viruses or rickettsiæ survive in the tissues of the mite for the same length of time as in the tick.

The viruses and rickettsiæ mentioned so far are harmless for their vectors in spite of the large numbers often found in their tissues. However, *R. prowazeki*, the cause of epidemic typhus, produces a fatal disease in the louse. It might be thought, therefore, that the louse was a dangerous carrier for only a short time. However, the rickettsiæ survive in the dead louse and in its fæces, infection from these contaminated sources by scratching being considered more likely than from the bite. Rarely *R. prowazeki* may infect ticks, producing a fatal disease in the vector similar to that in the louse.[21]

The carriage of *R. mooseri* in the rat flea is also short lived, but here it is the parasite that succumbs being only able to survive in the flea for a few hours.

(*f*) *Spread by air*.—From time immemorial epidemics have been attributed to pestilential air. "Noxious effluvia" exhaled by the sick and "miasmata" from putrefying marshes were regarded as important causes of disease, and the term malaria (bad air) is a vestige of the belief that the disease was transmitted in this way. We have seen that Fracastoro in his studies on contagion considered air an important vehicle of infection. Although he likened contagion spread by air to the "exhalation of an onion", it is not to be thought that he considered the disease-producing agent as volatile. He thought of his seminaria as particulate bodies.

Pasteur,[22] during his studies on spontaneous generation, clearly demonstrated that air contained microscopic germs which caused putrefaction and fermentation. Lister,[23] realising the possibility that germs of disease were spread in the same way, developed his famous technique of antiseptic surgery, attempting to kill airborne germs by spraying the air with carbolic acid. Tyndall[24] emphasised the importance of airborne dust in the carriage of germs. With the work of these pioneers before them, the early bacteriologists did not dispute the possibility of germs being carried by air. In fact it was regarded as axiomatic, the only controversy being whether droplets from the mouth or dust from dried secretions carried the germs. In the first two decades of this century, however, following failure to recover organisms from the nose and throat on culture plates exposed more than a few feet from a person who was coughing or sneezing, ideas underwent a change. Airborne infection came to be regarded as of minor importance, much greater weight being given to direct and indirect contact, although large droplets expelled from the mouth were regarded as possible factors, in, for instance, the spread of tuberculosis. Bacteria which remained suspended in the atmosphere were considered as too few to influence the spread of disease. In 1933 W. F. Wells[25] published an account of an effective apparatus for the bacteriological sampling of air. In this and his subsequent papers (summarised in Ref. 26), he clearly demonstrated that droplets expelled during coughing and sneezing would not necessarily fall to the ground; if small enough they would evaporate rapidly, leaving the solid material contained in them airborne for long periods. Bacteria in these droplets, therefore, would not be detected by agar plates exposed on the ground. This work stimulated intensive research into the part played by air in the spread of infection, research which shows no signs of abating as shown by the numerous reviews, monographs and symposia published in recent years (see, for instance, refs. 7, 27, 28, 29, 30).

There are many anomalous features of airborne infection that still await elucidation. The subject is of sufficient importance to merit consideration in some detail.

How do bacteria and viruses become airborne?

There are two ways: (*a*) by expulsion from the respiratory passages of a person harbouring the organism in the respiratory tract, and (*b*) on particles of dust thrown into the air from the ground, from solid objects and in detritus from the skin.

Bacteria from the respiratory tract can become directly airborne only in association with droplets of mucus or saliva from the nose or mouth. That the air expired in quiet respiration is usually sterile was first shown by Tyndall and has been confirmed many times. Duguid,[31] however, using a delicate technique noted that an average of about two bacteria-containing particles were expelled every five minutes from the nose in quiet nose breathing and pointed out that, although this appears to be few, it adds up in the course of a day to an appreciable number. On the other hand, there is general agreement that any form of nasopharyngeal activity expels enormous numbers of droplets into the air. Talking, particularly when enunciating those consonants in which lip movements and a more or less explosive emission of the breath are involved, for example, f, p, t, s, gives rise to airborne droplets ranging in numbers from a few dozen to a few hundred depending on the emphasis given to the sound. It is, however,

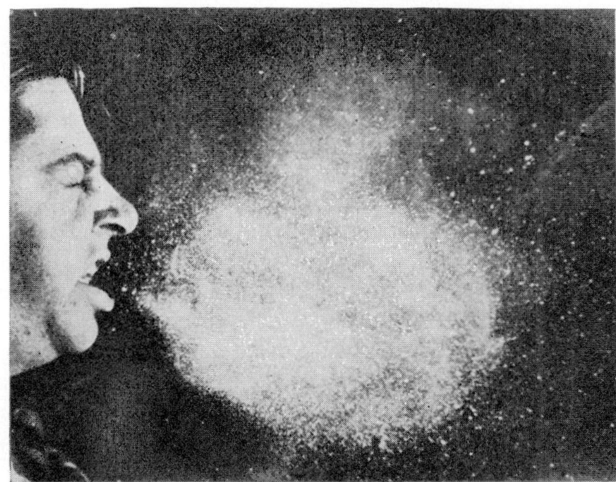

28/FIG. 1.—Droplets expelled during a sneeze. (From Jennison.[32])

coughing and particularly sneezing which are mainly responsible for the expulsion of airborne droplets. In the latter they are produced mainly from the saliva in the front of the mouth, but also from the nose. In FIG. 1 40,000 particles have been voided, but as many as 10^6 droplets have been noted.[31] If the sneezer has a head cold the droplets may be accompanied by long strings of mucus as in FIG. 2.

What is the fate of the expelled droplet?

This depends on its size. The droplet is formed by the atomisation of secretion in the air stream. Its size will therefore be governed by the velocity of

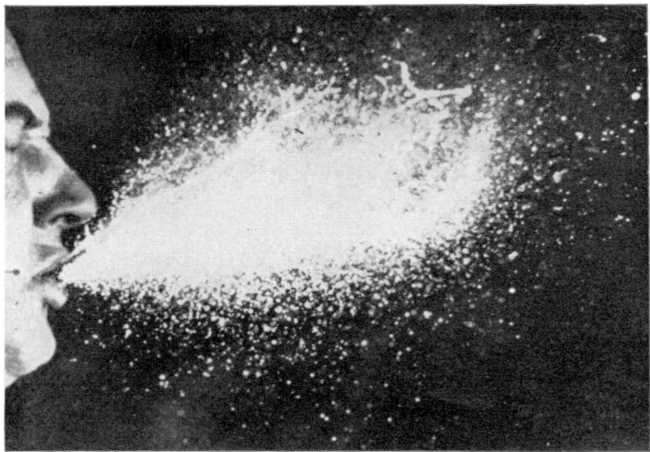

28/FIG. 2.—Droplets and strings of mucus expelled during a sneeze by an individual suffering from a head cold. (From Jennison.[32])

the air stream, and the viscosity, chemical composition and particulate inclusions of the secretion. It has been estimated that a diameter of 10μ is the minimum droplet size producible from water atomised in a high-speed air stream of 100 metres/second or greater. It is possible that in coughing and violent sneezing velocities at the glottis may reach this figure. As the viscosity of mucus and saliva is higher than that of water it is improbable that particles as small as 10μ in diameter are formed initially. Attempts have been made to measure the size of particles as expelled from the mouth, by allowing them to impinge on glass plates. Even if there is rapid evaporation a mark is left on the plate which gives some idea of the size of the droplet. In coughing and talking various investigators have found droplets ranging from 10 to 1,000μ, the commonest size being about 50 to 200μ.[26, 32, 33] If smaller particles than these are formed they are lost by evaporation before they reach the plate. Direct measurement of particles emitted from a sneeze has been made from photographs, as in FIG. 1. These give figures of the same order of magnitude, but again many of the smaller particles may have disappeared by evaporation before the photograph could be taken. Indeed, it has been shown by cinematograph studies that all droplets produced from a sneeze have disappeared in 0·26 sec., before they have travelled a distance of two feet.[32] In this time, the smaller particles of 50μ or less have evaporated and the larger particles have fallen to the ground.

The relation between the rate of evaporation and particle size below 100μ is shown in Table I. Although these results refer to water, comparable results would be obtained with saliva or mucus. With these small particles the rate of evaporation is not materially affected by temperature or humidity. As shown in the Table, even at 75 per cent humidity very rapid drying of the particles occurs. With particles above 100μ diameter, Wells[35] has shown that in still air at 22° C. particles of diameter 200μ dry in 5·2 seconds, 500μ in 32 seconds, 1,000μ in 129 seconds and 2,000μ in 515 seconds. The fate of a droplet, therefore, is determined

28/TABLE I

TIME TAKEN FOR EVAPORATION OF WATER DROPLETS SHOWN IN RELATION TO SIZE AT 15° C.

Droplet Diameter μ	*Per cent Relative Humidity* 0	25	50	75
	secs.	*secs.*	*secs.*	*secs.*
1	$0{\cdot}29 \times 10^{-4}$	$0{\cdot}39 \times 10^{-4}$	$0{\cdot}58 \times 10^{-4}$	$1{\cdot}18 \times 10^{-4}$
2	$1{\cdot}16 \times 10^{-4}$	$1{\cdot}55 \times 10^{-4}$	$2{\cdot}3 \times 10^{-4}$	$4{\cdot}7 \times 10^{-4}$
5	$7{\cdot}3 \times 10^{-4}$	$9{\cdot}7 \times 10^{-4}$	$1{\cdot}5 \times 10^{-3}$	$2{\cdot}9 \times 10^{-3}$
10	$2{\cdot}9 \times 10^{-3}$	$3{\cdot}9 \times 10^{-3}$	$5{\cdot}8 \times 10^{-3}$	$1{\cdot}2 \times 10^{-2}$
20	$1{\cdot}16 \times 10^{-2}$	$1{\cdot}6 \times 10^{-2}$	$2{\cdot}4 \times 10^{-2}$	$4{\cdot}7 \times 10^{-2}$
90	0·25	0·3	0·5	1·0

(After Henderson.)

by whether its diameter is more or less than a threshold value of about 100μ. Droplets of this size or smaller do not have time to reach the ground but evaporate almost instantaneously, leaving behind a dried particle which may be as little as 1μ or less in diameter. Such a dry, shrunken particle, which Wells has called a "droplet nucleus", tends to remain airborne, being held up by currents of air. Droplet nuclei not less than the size of a bacterium (about 1μ) may contain bacteria which, if they are able to survive in the desiccated state, often remain alive in the air for a long time. Droplets greater than 100μ are likely to fall to the ground before much evaporation has taken place, being too heavy to remain airborne. In photographs of sneezes it is often possible to note a downward trajectory of the larger particles, though they are expelled further than the smaller ones. They dry on reaching the ground, and any particulate organisms they contain, as well as salts and other matter in solution, lie as dust.

Dust containing bacteria of animal origin may also be formed from dandruff, hair, skin squames, dried sputum, and so on. Dust particles may become airborne and join the droplet nuclei suspended in the atmosphere (known as indirect airborne carriage). They are coarser than the droplet nuclei and do not remain suspended for so long, but long enough to be important potential vehicles of the more hardy pathogenic bacteria. For instance, dust from skin squames may have a diameter of 8–16μ and settle at the rate of only 1–2 feet per minute in still air.[27] In turbulent air they might remain airborne for long periods of time. Their importance in the dissemination of staphylococci is discussed in a later section.

Are bacteria from the nose and mouth in fact found suspended in the atmosphere?

Various methods have been devised for the bacteriological sampling of air. These range from procedures giving qualitative data, such as the exposure of nutrient agar plates which collect infected particles large enough to settle by gravity, to apparatus designed for quantitative estimations of organisms more or less permanently airborne.

The early device for quantitative sampling of airborne bacteria designed by Wells has been largely replaced by the "slit-sampler" of Bourdillon, Lidwell and Thomas[36] which, in this country, has become the apparatus of choice. A known volume of air is drawn through a slit so arranged that it lies along the radius of an agar plate at a fixed distance from the surface of the agar. A band of air of the dimensions of the slit impinges radially on the surface of the plate. The plate can be made to rotate on its axis at a known speed which can be varied. Particles in the air carrying bacteria stick to the surface of the agar and after suitable incubation can be counted as colonies. However, colony counts do not give a true estimate of the number of bacteria in the air, as each particle giving rise to a colony may contain more than one bacterium. In order to estimate the size of particles and the mean number of bacteria they contain, Andersen[37] devised an apparatus which allows a differential impingement of particles on a series of culture plates according to the size of particle. The air is allowed to pass at a constant rate sequentially through a series of perforated plates of diminishing pore size, each immediately suspended over a culture plate. The jet velocity of the air increases as the pore size diminishes which will have the effect of depositing the particles in order of size as their inertia overcomes their aerodynamic drag. Particle size and distribution at each level was determined by measuring microscopically impinged particles of Carnauba wax from an aerosol.

Such methods have shown that many normal inhabitants of the mouth may be found in true airborne particles, in airborne dust and in large droplets precipitated immediately after coughing, talking and sneezing. For instance, Williams and his colleagues,[38] in their surveys of aerial contamination in primary schools in Southall, showed that certain types of non-pathogenic streptococci which could only have come from the mouth were present in appreciable numbers in droplets or droplet nuclei small enough to be sterilised by U.V. radiation. These salivary streptococci appear to have the same importance in assessing aerial contamination from the respiratory passages as *E. coli* has in assessing fæcal contamination of water supplies.[39] If they are present, then there is a potential danger that pathogenic organisms from the respiratory tract may also be present, even if they are not readily detected.

In order to determine whether organisms from the throat and nose as well as from the mouth are disseminated, Duguid[31] contaminated various sites of the respiratory tract with *Serratia marcescens*—an organism easily recognised by the blood red colonies that it produces. He found that relatively few droplets expelled during coughing originated from the nose and throat, most coming from the front of the mouth. Not all agree with this observation.[40] Rubbo and Benjamin,[16] however, have confirmed the importance of the saliva as a source of droplets, and noted that individuals who secrete a large amount of saliva disseminate organisms more effectively than individuals who secrete less. The administration of atropine, which inhibited salivation, considerably lessened the number of organisms issuing from the mouth.

Are pathogenic organisms found in air?

In spite of widespread contamination of air in public places frequented by healthy people, pathogenic bacteria can rarely be isolated from it. It was generally expected that the overcrowded, poorly ventilated air-raid shelters, in which people regularly slept during certain periods of the last war, would provide ideal conditions for the spread of epidemic respiratory disease. However, not only was there no epidemic disease, but Pulvertaft[41] failed to find pathogenic bacteria, such as hæmolytic streptococci and pneumococci, in the air in tests carried out over nearly a year. Even in barracks, where every soldier carried meningococcus in his nasopharynx, he failed to find the organism in the air. A similar observation was made by Rubbo and Benjamin[16] using subjects who were known to be throat carriers of hæmolytic streptococci. The carriers were asked to sing and cough in a closed room while the air was sampled bacteriologically, but, although numerous mouth organisms were collected, a hæmolytic streptococcus was hardly ever found. The results were similar with nasal carriers. Hare and Thomas[17] found that five nasal carriers of *Staphylococcus aureus* failed to contaminate the air of a cubicle by sneezing, coughing and talking and only did so by "snorting", a form of activity not usually indulged in by civilised people. Even in hospitals and sanatoria, in which the air might be expected to house pathogenic bacteria, remarkably few have been isolated from the air provided care has been taken not to stir up dust. Where plates and slides were placed directly in front of the mouth of carriers of hæmolytic streptococci,[15] and of patients with scarlet fever, faucial diphtheria or open tuberculosis,[42] comparatively few pathogenic organisms were collected. However, surveys of the still air of primary schools[38] and hospital wards[43, 44] have clearly shown a small but persistent airborne contamination with hæmolytic streptococci and staphylococci in particles small enough to be sterilised by U.V.L. It would be unwise therefore to dismiss entirely the importance of carriage of these organisms in droplet nuclei in the spread of infection, since the small numbers present might be more than compensated by their persistence. Moreover, concomitant viral respiratory infection may greatly increase the number of droplet nuclei containing nasal staphylococci. Eichenwald and his colleagues[45] noted that a small minority of newborn babies who carry staphylococci in their noses caused explosive outbreaks of staphylococcal infection in the nursery, and, after discharge, in the family unit. These "cloud" babies, so called from the extensive aerial contaminations observed in their environment, showed no overt signs of staphylococcal disease, but suffered from viral respiratory infections common in hospitalized newborn infants. That the source of infection was directly from the respiratory tract was suggested by the small size of the particles (about 5μ), and the failure to prevent dispersal by enclosing the infant's body in a plastic bag, a procedure which is successful in limiting the spread of infection from infants suffering from impetigo. However, it is still not certain that the infective particles were true droplet nuclei, since desquamation of mucosal epithelial cells is common in viral respiratory infections, and it is possible that staphylococci become associated with such cells and become dispersed in the same way as on dried skin scales, the smaller size of the particles than those of skin squames being explained by the lack of keratinisation of the mucosal cells.

The tubercle bacillus from individuals with open pulmonary tuberculosis is probably dispersed in the air in fine droplets which remain airborne as droplet nuclei. It is possible that the failure to recover tubercle bacilli from the air of hospitals and sanatoria, noted above, may be due to technical difficulties of culture, for, if cultural methods are replaced by exposure of guinea-pigs, evidence of aerial contamination from patients with open tuberculosis can be obtained. Riley and his colleagues[46] noted that when air from single bedrooms housing such patients was drawn through a chamber containing a number of guinea-pigs, 15 per cent of the patients were shown to have dispersed their tubercle bacilli in sufficient numbers and on sufficiently small particles to set up tuberculous foci deep in the lungs of the guinea-pigs. It was estimated that one particularly infective patient dispersed some 60 infective particles per hour. As these particles had to traverse considerable distances from the patient to the guinea-pig, it is likely that they were in the form of permanently airborne droplet nuclei. This is supported by epidemiological evidence as discussed in a later section.

Because of the difficulty of demonstrating airborne viruses, there is no direct evidence of the presence of viruses in droplets or droplet nuclei. However, there is indirect evidence which is discussed later.

Let us now consider the contamination of air by bacteria in *dust*. It has repeatedly been shown that dust harbours pathogenic germs. Hæmolytic streptococci can be isolated from the dust of wards in which patients with scarlet fever are being nursed, and in outbreaks of puerperal fever the particular type of streptococcus responsible has often been found in the dust of the lying-in-ward. In the same way tubercle bacilli can be found in the dust in wards of sanatoria.[35]

It has been frequently noted that respiratory carriers of a pathogenic organism may contaminate their bedding, clothing and skin with the organism, which may subsequently become airborne in dust from these sources, following the slightest activity on the part of the carrier.[17, 47] From the observations of Hare[48] that organisms expelled from the respiratory tract are mostly contained in large droplets which fall rapidly, a possible source of contamination of dust is the precipitation and drying of these droplets. However, some observations of Duguid and Wallace[47] on the aerial contamination of the environment by two nasal carriers, suggest that this is not the main source of contamination. Carrier 1 was made to undertake physical activity wearing ordinary clothes, with a mask over mouth and nose; and Carrier 2 was made to sneeze violently wearing dust free sterile clothing and no mask. Under the first set of conditions contamination by *Staph. aureus* was found in every one of 15 experiments. Under the second, no staphylococcus was found in 12 out of 15 tests, and in the remaining three the numbers were negligible. It would seem, therefore, that contamination of the air is not directly from droplets moist or dry. The recent observations of Lidwell, Williams and their colleagues (see ref. 29, p. 116, 268) have shown that aerial contamination with staphylococci is from skin squames. Davies and Noble[49] for instance, noted a close correlation between the number of staphylococci dispersed into the air in a hospital ward and the number of skin squames collected from the air. When particles from the air were allowed to impinge on nutrient agar and observed microscopically, the micro colonies of staphylococci that grew out were, with a single exception, associated with skin scales. Staphylococci probably do not grow on the skin, except in moist areas such as the perineum. Other areas of skin become contaminated from areas where the organism can grow, of which the anterior nares and the perineum are the most important. Hare and Ridley[50] found that perineal carriers were particularly effective dispersers. The infection is carried to the skin from these sites, probably on hands and perhaps on clothing, and the contaminated skin squames are dispersed into the air from friction, in dust from clothing and even in droplets of water in the act of washing[17] and taking a shower[27].

We have already seen that the size of these particles is of the order of about 8–16μ in diamater, too large to penetrate deep into the air passages, but of a size readily filtered off in the nasal fossæ. They might well be responsible, therefore, for the spread of the carrier state by colonisation of the anterior nares. This is particularly likely in newborn infants who become colonised with staphylococci within a few weeks of birth. Although no doubt some of those developing the carrier state are infected from the hands of carriers, a proportion become infected under conditions which preclude direct contact.

Infected skin squames may also be responsible for contamination of bedding. Since 1940, when van der Ende and his colleagues[51] first demonstrated with the slit sampler the dispersal of pathogenic streptococci during operations of bed making, great prominence has been given to dust from bedding as the source of aerial contamination in hospital wards. On the basis of these results they recommended the impregnation of blankets with oil, a procedure which considerably reduced the number of streptococci in the air.[52] However, these procedures, although preventing aerial dissemination, add to the danger of carriage by contact. Rubbo and his colleagues (ref. 7, p. 231) noted a much higher count of staphylococci on contact plates from the surface of oiled than from that of unoiled blankets, and drew attention to the greater danger of contamination and spread on the hands, particularly if they are moist. They point out, that in any case, blankets are unlikely to play the major role in aerial contamination by dust, because ward dust consists mainly of cellulose fibres, wool dust being too gross in size and weight to remain airborne for long. Cotton fibres on the other hand fragment to a mean diameter of 18μ and, although settling in still air at a rate of 1–2 feet per minute, were light enough to be kept airborne by convection currents. By sampling air at different heights in a room, using the Andersen sampler, they showed that staphylococci could be recovered at all levels, and were associated with particles 10–20μ in size containing no wool. These particles, which they call "fibre" nuclei, arise from cotton fabrics such as cotton blankets, sheets and pillow slips, but also from the surface of wool blankets when covered by a clean counterpane, dispersion being brought about by friction between the surfaces of the two textiles. Friction between the bed clothes and gauze dressings may also play a part in disseminating bacteria. Rountree and her colleagues[53] showed a dramatic fall in staphylococcal cross infection in a surgical ward when gauze dressings were replaced by plastic seal dressings. Friction may also explain the dissemination in dust from the clothes of nasal carriers of staphylococci even when a sterile gown is worn.[17]

What evidence is there that airborne bacteria and viruses produce disease?

This can be considered under two headings: (1) experimental in animals; (2) epidemiological.

(1) *Evidence from animal experiments.*—Various forms of apparatus have been devised for exposing animals to airborne clouds of bacteria and viruses.[54] These have ranged from the artificial "sneezer" producing particles of all sizes to various forms of apparatus like that of Henderson,[34] which produce ærosols of particles only a few microns in diameter which dry almost instantaneously to

form droplet nuclei. In most of these methods the animal is so placed that only the nose and mouth are exposed to the cloud.

There is no doubt that animals can readily be infected with a host of different agents of disease by such artificial clouds. Tubercle bacilli, pneumococci, streptococci, brucellæ, anthrax bacilli and pasteurellæ have all been used with success, as well as such viruses as those of influenza and mouse pneumonites. The effective dose, as calculated by the number of organisms in the ærosol and the volume of air inspired in a given time, is often quite small. An important factor is the size of the particle. This not only determines the site in the respiratory tract at which the particles are arrested, but also the number retained. Numerous investigations have been made on the filtering efficiency of the nasal passages. For particles greater than 5μ the nose is a highly efficient filter, largely because the high velocity of the air, and the centrifugal force due to the sudden change in direction of the air-stream as it passes through the tortuous nasal passages, cause the particles to impinge on the moist adhesive surface of the mucous membrane. As the air passes down the respiratory tract, its velocity gets less and impingement of contained particles progressively diminishes. In the lung alveoli, where the velocity is zero, particles no longer impinge but may settle. It is mainly the finer particles of about 1μ in size that reach the lung, but many of these are expelled in the expired air. That some particles, often less than 1μ in diameter, are retained in the lung is evident from the colour and mineral content of the lungs after many years of life.

As the larger particles are filtered off early in their passage down the respiratory tract any that contain pathogenic bacteria should tend to produce upper respiratory disease, such as tonsillitis, middle ear disease and sinusitis, whereas true lung infections should be caused by small particles. This is fully borne out by animal experiment.

Infection can be transmitted from man to animal, animal to animal, and animal to man by coughing or sneezing directly into the respiratory pathway. Bourdillon and Glover[55] used a ferret infected with influenza (donor) to infect other ferrets (recipient), a spray being produced by the sneezing of the donor which contained particles of about 17μ by the time it reached the recipient, the larger particles having sedimented during passage through the air between the animals.

That animals can be infected from airborne contaminated dust was shown a long time ago by Chaussé.[56] Guinea-pigs exposed to dust brushed from the clothing, bedding or handkerchiefs of tuberculous patients readily succumbed to disease.

(2) *Epidemiological evidence.*—Evidence as to the means of transmission in air has been collected indirectly, mainly by introducing procedures which will limit one or other form of airborne infection—droplet, droplet nucleus or airborne dust—and noting the effect on the incidence of cross infection.

The chance of moist droplets passing directly from one person to another depends on the nearness of the two individuals. By increasing the distance between individuals in a population at risk, and noting the effect on cross infection, it should be possible to assess the importance of this mode of transmission. Glover[57] noted that men sleeping in barracks in adjacent beds tended to carry the same type of meningococcus in the nasopharynx. When beds were separated by more than three feet the carrier rate fell. He considered that the spread was due to unconscious coughing during sleep, aided by the common habit of sleeping with the mouth open, producing direct droplet spray infection. Following the introduction of Glover's method of spacing out beds, no case of cerebrospinal meningitis was reported in the Caterham barracks in 1917, where heavy epidemics had previously taken place. Wannamaker[58] reported a similar find with carriers of hæmolytic streptococci. Occupants of adjacent beds carried the same type of hæmolytic streptococcus. The carrier rates fell rapidly as the distance between the beds was increased. Since spacing of beds would have no effect on contamination by droplet nuclei or dust, which would be evenly dispersed, it must be concluded that in these cases direct droplet spray was responsible for the transfer of infection. Others, however, have not been so successful in relating carrier rates to the spacing of beds.[59] Certainly the distance between beds appeared to play no part in the spread of staphylococcal infection in a surgical ward (ref. 29, p. 268).

There is little doubt that many virus diseases such as influenza, the common cold and infections due to adenoviruses and respiratory syncytial virus, as well as the specific exanthemata, measles, mumps, chicken-pox and smallpox are spread by airborne carriage, but we are still ignorant of the means by which this is brought about. Certainly in most of these diseases the virus is present in the pharyngeal washings at the most infectious stages and, therefore, likely to be spread by droplets. However, except in smallpox, the virus does not appear to persist in the environment, no further cases developing once the patient has been isolated. Persistent droplet nuclei and dust are therefore unlikely vehicles of transfer, infection probably taking place by direct droplet spray from person to person. However, Wells and his colleagues[60] claim to have reduced cross infection in classrooms and children's hospitals by irradiating the upper air, a procedure which might be expected to kill bacteria and viruses airborne in droplet nuclei but is less likely to affect organisms in droplets and dust. This has not been the general experience, however, in spite of the fact that irradiation considerably reduces the number of normal mouth organisms in the air.[61]

It is difficult to escape the conclusion that in pulmonary tuberculosis, where the primary lesion is in the lung alveoli, infection must be brought about by the inhalation of tubercle bacilli on minute particles such as droplet nuclei. We have already seen that guinea-pigs can be infected from air containing such particles dispersed by patients with open pulmonary tuberculosis. Experimentally, animals may be infected with three to five "bacillary units" which penetrate deep into the lung, but less readily with larger numbers on coarser particles (Chapter 42). In man, pulmonary tuberculosis is relatively uncommon, so it is difficult to assess the effect of ultraviolet irradiation of the air on the spread of infection. Lurie[62] has, however, succeeded in reducing natural spread in rabbits by irradiating the air between adjacent cages.

The role of airborne dust in the spread of respiratory infection has been assessed by observing the effect of the dust-laying techniques described above on the incidence of respiratory disease in closed communities such as army barracks, and on cross infection in hospital wards. In spite of some favourable reports,[63] most authorities agree that these techniques have not in general lessened the incidence of the common respiratory diseases. Loosli and his colleagues,[64] for instance, found no difference in the incidence of streptococcal nasopharyngitis among recruits housed in "oiled" and "unoiled" barracks. Further, Lemon and his colleagues[65] described an outbreak of streptococcal infection due to a dangerous carrier who succeeded in heavily contaminating barracks, the organism being recovered from 84 per cent of beds. Removal of the carrier immediately ended the epidemic, in spite of the fact that the environment remained heavily loaded with the organism for some time.

Wannamaker[58] attempted to assess the importance of dust on the carrier rate of hæmolytic streptococci in the respiratory tract by issuing blankets heavily contaminated with streptococci to one group of men and sterile blankets to another group. No significant difference in the subsequent carrier rate was noted. Rammelkamp, Wannamaker and their colleagues[66] (see also ref. 30, chapter 2) found subsequently that even the insufflation or planting on the pharyngeal mucous membrane of dried secretion from individuals suffering from streptococcal sore throat failed to produce infection, and they concluded that the organisms, although remaining viable, had lost their infectivity by drying, being probably destroyed by phagocytes before they could start to grow.

It is conceivable that viruses such as those of variola, and obligate parasites such as psittacosis which remain infective in the dried state, may be spread by airborne dust. In the Brighton epidemic of smallpox mentioned earlier, inhalations of dried exudate might have been responsible for infection of laundry workers. Dried excreta from birds with psittacosis may be responsible for the spread of infection to man.

If there is doubt about the importance of airborne dust in the spread of respiratory disease, there is little doubt about its importance in the spread of surgical sepsis, particularly in burns, in which large areas are exposed to infection, and in operation wounds. Colebrook and his colleagues (for ref. see 30, chapter 2) in their pioneer work on the aseptic dressing of burns, noted that bacteria pass readily through gauze dressings covering, for example, an infected burn, and become airborne in dust. By the introduction of forced ventilations with filtered air to give 20 changes of air per hour, not only was there a reduction in the bacterial count in the air but also a significant reduction in cross infection with streptococci, staphylococci and *Ps. pyocyanea.* Similar observations were made in operating theatres in which as many as 40–50 bacteria per cu. ft. of air is not unusual. Airborne dust was responsible for most of this contamination as shown by the high sedimentation rate in exposed plates. It was estimated that about 300 contaminated particles an hour, many of which contained staphylococci, were falling on sterile tables and equipment (for ref. see 30, Chapter 5). The introduction of a ventilation system such as that used in the burn clinics, brought about a 10-fold reduction in aerial contamination accompanied by a similar reduction in sepsis.

In Summary.—Bacteria from the respiratory passages may become airborne in the act of talking, coughing and sneezing, on droplets of saliva and mucus. Rapid drying of the smallest particles leads to carriage of bacteria on dried particles called droplet nuclei which remain more or less permanently airborne. It is difficult to find pathogenic bacteria associated with droplet nuclei, but there is strong evidence that they may play a part in dissemination of pulmonary tuberculosis. Large droplets fall to the ground and dry. Dust from these, from dried sputum, and, in the case of staphylococci, particularly from skin squames may become secondarily airborne. Pathogenic bacteria in a hospital environment are regularly found in airborne dust. Dust laying techniques have not modified bacterial respiratory infection, but the continual elimination by forced ventilation with clean air has contributed to the fall in the incidence of sepsis in operating theatres and burn clinics. There are still many factors in the carriage of bacteria by air not yet understood.

Factors determining the Establishment of the Organism on the Body Surface

We have already seen (Chapter 27) that the body surfaces, skin and mucous membranes of the upper respiratory tract and alimentary canal of man and animals are colonised by resident bacterial flora. These become established soon after birth, are characteristic of different regions of the body and are very difficult to remove or change. The establishment of other organisms in these sites which, if they are pathogenic, is often a prerequisite to invasion, is met with considerable resistance not only from certain self-sterilising factors produced by the host, but even more from the presence of these resident flora. We may summarize briefly the factors resisting colonisation of a foreign intruder as follows:

Host Factors

Skin.—The keratinised intact skin is not a likely site for bacterial growth. However moist areas of skin and the crypts of the sweat and sebaceous glands are more suitable and indeed are colonised by bacteria such as diphtheroids and *Staphylococcus albus.* The skin in such areas has a self-sterilising action for many other bacteria including pathogenic organisms such as *Streptococcus pyogenes* and *C. diphtheriæ.* One of the factors involved in this action is undoubtedly the long chain unsaturated fatty acids which Burtenshaw[67] showed to be present in alcohol and ether extracts of skin and which he found lethal to *Strep. pyogenes. Staph. aureus* was resistant, which may explain the persistence of this organism on the skin of carriers (for further discussion on the defence mechanisms of the skin see ref. 68)

Mucous membranes and conjunctiva.—The continual mechanical flushing with secretion is probably one of the most important mechanisms for removing foreign invaders. The conjunctiva, mouth, nasal mucosa and upper respiratory tract are continually washed with tears, saliva or mucus which converges at the glottis and passes to the stomach. Any diminution of secretion or interference with its flushing action assists bacterial colonisation, e.g. the development of ascending parotitis along Stensen's duct in water deprivation, or the predisposition to chronic bronchitis due to metaplasia of the ciliated epithelium of the bronchi, the cilia having an important function in assisting the flow of mucus up the bronchi and trachea.

Low pH.—It has long been recognised that the acidity of the stomach is an important bactericidal mechanism. However, the fact that intestinal pathogens such as *Salm. typhi* and *V. choleræ* can infect after passing through the stomach shows that the so-called "gastric germicidal barrier" is not completely effective. Considerable variation in the acidity of the gastric juice is found not only between different individuals but at different times in the same individual. Moreover, if the pathogenic organisms are contained in large boluses of food or are imbibed with large amounts of water, they fail to reach the low pH required for killing.

Lysozyme.—Fleming's lysozyme, a protein of low molecular weight, is found in tears, nasal secretion, saliva and extracts of various organs. It breaks down certain polysaccharides in the cell wall of some bacteria, and thus brings about their lysis. It is selective in its action and probably helps to determine the character of the flora in the conjunctival sac, where it is present in particularly high concentration. Although present in extracts of skin, it probably plays no part in determining the skin flora, since it is inactivated by small amounts of acid. Colebrook[69] showed that *M. lysodeikticus*, an organism highly susceptible to lysozyme, persists on the skin for longer periods than the less susceptible *Str. pyogenes*. Goldsworthy and Florey[70] showed that lysozyme is present in the mucus of the intestine of some species of animals, but absent from that of others. Whether it has any effect in determining the intestinal flora is not known. In general, pathogenic bacteria are less susceptible to lysozyme than non-pathogens and it is doubtful whether it plays much part in preventing colonisation by pathogenic organisms.

Mucin.—Mucus from the respiratory mucous membrane contains a mucopolysaccharide to which influenza virus can become adsorbed[71] and thereby the virus is prevented from attaching itself to the mucopolysaccharide receptors of the respiratory epithelial cells. What importance, if any, the mechanism may have in protection against infection of the respiratory mucosa is not known.

Antibodies.—Both antibacterial and antiviral antibodies may be present in mucus, though at a considerably lower titre than in the blood. Francis[72] has shown that neutralising antibodies against influenza virus A may be present in the nasal secretions of normal individuals, but again we are uncertain about their protective role. The presence of antipneumococcal antibodies in the blood does appear to limit the carriage of pneumococci on the mucous membrane.

It has recently been shown that antibody globulin similar in type to IgA of the blood and specific for certain bacteria, red blood cells and viruses may be present in appreciable amounts in saliva, intestinal and nasal mucus and even tears (see ref. 73). These antibody globulins have the characters of the IgA of the blood except that they differ in molecular size and antigenic structure and are probably produced locally. Local synthesis in the parotid gland has in fact been demonstrated using fluorescent antibody. They may contribute to the bactericidal action of saliva and mucus on Gram-negative organisms, but this is rendered less likely from the fact that they apparently fail to fix complement.

Other factors.—Other bactericidal factors have been described in saliva and mucus of the respiratory and alimentary tract, but their nature has not yet been elucidated.

Bacterial.—Inhibition of the growth of foreign invaders by resident bacteria may take different forms. In some cases metabolic products of the resident organisms are inhibitory to the growth of the invader. For instance, the low pH of the vaginal mucus (pH 4·0–4·4) is due to the fermentation of glycogen by the resident *L. acidophilus* which suppresses the growth of other organisms. Similarly, the intestinal contents of the breast-fed infant are acid as the result of fermentation of the lactose of human milk by *Lactobacillus bifidus*, and this probably helps to protect the infant against the organisms responsible for infantile diarrhœa.

Antibiotics and other inhibitory substances may be formed by resident flora active against the invader, but apart from the possibility of the production of H_2O_2 by salivary streptococci active against diphtheria bacilli, none has been clearly defined. In other cases well-adapted species may simply "crowd out" others less able to grow in a particular site. As Wilson and Miles[74] have said, the efforts of a new species of bacterium to establish itself might be likened to an attempt to grow a new plant by scattering a few seeds in a field already occupied by other plant associations.

That such suppression of the growth of one species by another is possible may be demonstrated by applying locally an antibiotic which is active against some but not all of the resident species. For instance, the application of penicillin or aureomycin to the throat suppresses many of the local organisms, particularly Gram-positive cocci such as *Str. viridans*, and sometimes is followed by the development of Gram-negative bacilli and fungi which are not normally found there in any quantity. In fact continued application has sometimes led to severe fungal infections of the throat, which usually clear up as soon as the natural flora is allowed to develop again. In a similar way the systemic administration of antibiotics may encourage resistant organisms to flourish. A number of cases of acute staphylococcal enterocolitis have been reported following the systemic use of some of the broad-spectrum antibiotics such as aureomycin. Some patients have died, and antibiotic-resistant staphylococci often in pure culture, have been isolated from the intestinal tract—frequently along its whole length—and sometimes from the respiratory tract as well. Such cases of "staphylococcal cholera", almost unknown before the introduction of antibiotics, can only be due to suppression of the intestinal flora which apparently normally prevent undue growth of staphylococci.

The reverse procedure—the deliberate seeding of staphylococci of low virulence on the mucous membranes of newborn babies to prevent the natural colonisation of virulent hospital strains—is now being practised with some success. Eichenwald and his colleagues[75] inoculated the nasal mucosa and umbilical stump of newborn infants with a coagulase positive staphylococcus (502-A) of low virulence before these sites had a chance to become colonised with other strains, and assessed the subsequent colonisation with phage type 80/81 and other hospital staphylococci in these and in an equal number of controls. Of 108 infants successfully colonised with 502-A only 4·6 per cent became colonised with hospital staphylococci, whereas of 143 controls 39 per cent became colonised. Later, he extended the procedure to adults in an attempt to replace dangerous strains resident in carriers with the harmless strain. Although 502-A failed to obtain a foothold or replace the resident strain when implanted on the nasal mucosa, it did so after the resident strain had been suppressed with oxacillin. Once established, it generally persisted for several weeks with complete suppression of the original strain. Such examples of "bacterial interference" open up new approaches to the treatment of the chronic carrier state.

Microbes do not always compete with each other for establishment on the body surface. Sometimes they act synergistically. It is now known that certain strains of hæmolytic streptococci are unable to establish themselves in the respiratory tract of animals unless the mucous membrane is previously infected with influenza virus.[1, 76]

Summary

Three conditions are necessary for an organism to produce disease: (1) It must be *communicable*, i.e. capable of transfer from a patient or carrier to a new host. (2) It must be *invasive*, i.e. able to penetrate the body integument, either through the tissue or a breach in it, find the right conditions for growth, and protect itself from the defensive mechanisms of the host. (3) It must be *pathogenic*, i.e. able to damage the body tissues by the production of toxin or other means. The present chapter is concerned with communicability.

The conditions determining communicability are (i) those connected with the biological properties of the organism (intrinsic), and (ii) those connected with the environment (extrinsic).

The intrinsic biological property of an organism which determines its communicability may be distinct from virulence, that is its ability to produce disease when in the body tissues. Some strains of a particular organism disseminate rapidly among the population at risk but are no more virulent than other strains which remain more localised. Probably many factors are involved. There is suggestive evidence that antibiotic resistance is important in a hospital environment in which widespread contamination of the environment by the antibiotic has the effect of suppressing the natural flora of the body surfaces and selecting antibiotic resistant strains. Resistance to desiccation may be another factor.

The extrinsic factors are (1) the nature of the reservoir of infection, the number of organisms present and the possibility of their becoming disseminated from it; (2) the means of transfer by which germs are carried to a host; and (3) the suitability of the body surfaces for colonisation. The reservoir of infection may be a patient or animal suffering from the disease, a human or animal carrier, or a non-living source. The means of transfer may be by direct or indirect contact. Direct contact may be from the outside environment or by congenital transmission through the ovum or via the placenta, either directly from maternal to fœtal blood or via a placental lesion. Indirect contact may be by infected objects (fomites), water, food, milk, arthropods, or air. Transfer by indirect contact depends on the ability of the organism to survive and perhaps grow outside the body. There is strong evidence that the hands are important in the carriage of pathogenic organisms from nasal secretion and fæces.

The ability of food and milk to act as culture media for pathogenic bacteria is often the factor determining intestinal infection, particularly food poisoning. Pathogenic germs may be carried by arthropods, mechanically on the feet or in the intestines, or the germs may invade and grow in the tissues of the arthropod. Infection is transferred by bites, or by the host's scratching the infected fæces of the arthropod into the skin.

There is no direct, but much indirect, evidence that air plays an important role in the transfer of pathogenic germs in natural infections in man and animals. The means by which organisms are carried in the air, however, are in dispute. Bacteria may be carried in the air in droplets of saliva or mucus from the mouth or nose. Infection may be transferred (1) directly in such droplets from the respiratory tract of one person to that of another, or (2) the droplet may dry, and remain suspended in the atmosphere for long periods of time and infect persons at a considerable distance from its original source, or (3) the droplet may fall to the ground, dry, and become secondarily airborne as dust. Dust may become infected from skin scales also, e.g. by staphylococci. Attempts to assess the importance of each of these means of transfer have been made by epidemiological investigations, bacteriological sampling of air and dust, animal experiments, and the use of methods of eliminating one or other of these means to transfer, e.g. by ventilation, irradiation, or by dust-laying techniques. No general conclusion is possible, but it is likely that the importance of each means of transfer depends on the nature of the infection. For example, pulmonary tuberculosis is likely to be spread by droplet nuclei, staphylococcal infection by skin squames in dust and meningococcal meningitis and certain viral respiratory diseases by droplets. Dust and/or droplet nuclei also plays a part in the dissemination of staphylococci and *Ps. pyocyanea* in surgical sepsis of burns and operation wounds as shown by the successful results of forced ventilation.

Colonisation on the body surfaces is in many cases a prerequisite to infection. This depends on local conditions. There are "self-sterilising" machanisms of the integument which prevent colonisation. These are (1) *mechanical:* the washing away of the bacteria by secretions, and their removal by coughing, deglutition, peristalsis, and desquamation of surface epithelium; (2) *chemical:* the destruction of the organisms by acid and more specifically by unsaturated fatty acids; (3) *biological:* the destruction by lysozyme and possibly other bactericidal substances in secretions; (4) the antibiotic and "crowding out" action of certain resident bacteria.

REFERENCES

1. Coburn, A. F., Evans, J., and Nathan, J. (1954). *Brit. J. exp. Path.*, **35**, 270.
2. Coburn, A. F., and Pauli, R. H. (1941). *J. exp. Med.*, **73**, 551.
3. Greenwood, M., Hill, A. B., Topley, W. W. C., and Wilson, J. (1936). *Spec. Rep. Ser. med. Res. Coun. (Lond.)*, No. 209, p. 144. H.M.S.O.
4. Webster, L. T., and Clow, A. D. (1933). *J. exp. Med.*, **58**, 465.
5. Coburn, A. F., and Young, D. C. (1949). *The Epidemiology of Hæmolytic Streptococcus.* Baltimore: Williams and Wilkins Co.
6. Fekelty, F. R., Buchbender, L., Shaffer, E. L., Goldberg, S., Price, H. P., and Pyle, L. P. (1958). *Amer. J. pub. Hlth.*, **48**, 298.
7. Williams, R. E. O., and Shooter, R. A., Eds. (1963). *Infections in Hospitals.* Oxford: Blackwell Scientific Publications.
8. Gould, J. C. (1958). *Lancet*, **1**, 489.
9. White, A. (1961). *J. clin. Invest.*, **40**, 23.
10. Sever, J., and White, L. R. (1968). *Ann. Rev. Med.*, **19**, 471.
11. Stokes, J., Berk, J. E., Malamut, L. L., Drake, M. E., Barondess, J. A., Baske, W. J., Wolman, I. J., Farquhar, J. D., Bevan, B., Drummond, R. J., Maycock, W. d'A., Capps, R. B., and Bennett, A. M. (1954). *J. Amer. med. Ass.*, **154**, 1059.
12. Downie, A. W., and Dumbell, K. R. (1947). *Lancet*, **1**, 550.
13. *Lancet* (1951). **1**, 169.
14. Hutchinson, R. I. (1956). *Mth. Bull. Minist. Hlth. Lab. Serv.*, **15**, 110.
15. Hamburger, M., and Green, M. J. (1946). *J. infec. Dis.*, **79**, 33.

16. Rubbo, S. D., and Benjamin, M. (1953). *J. Hyg.* (*Lond.*), **51,** 278.
17. Hare, R., and Thomas, C. G. A. (1956). *Brit. med. J.*, **2,** 840.
18. Andrewes, C. H. (1950). *New Engl. J. Med.*, **242,** 235.
19. Report (1947). *Spec. Rep. Ser. med. Res. Coun.* (*Lond.*), No. **260**, H.M.S.O.
20. Reeves, W. C. (1965). *Ann. Rev. Entomol.*, **10,** 25.
21. Řeháček, J. (1965). *Ann. Rev. Entomol.*, **10,** 1.
22. Pasteur, L. (1922). *Œuvres de Pasteur*, **2,** 210. Paris: Masson et Cie.
23. Lister, J. (1868). *Brit. med. J.*, **2,** 53, 101, 461, 515; (1869). *ibid.*, **1,** 301.
24. Tyndall, J. (1883). *Essays on the Floating-matter of the Air in Relation to Putrefaction and Infection.* London: Longmans, Green & Co.
25. Wells, W. F. (1933). *Amer. J. publ. Hlth.* **23,** 58.
26. Wells, W. F. (1955). *Airborne Contagion and Air Hygiene.* Cambridge, Mass.: Harvard Univ. Press.
27. Williams, R. E. O. (1960). *Bact. Rev.*, **30,** 660.
28. Riley, R. L., and O'Grady, F. (1961). *Airborne Infection.* New York: Macmillan.
29. Gregory, P. H., and Monteith, J. L. Eds. (1967). *Symp. Soc. gen. Microbiol.*, **17,** London: Cambridge Univ. Press.
30. Williams, R. E. O., Blowers, R., Garrod, L. P., and Shooter, R. A. (1966). *Hospital Infection*, 2nd edit. London: Lloyd-Luke.
31. Duguid, J. P. (1945). *Edinb. med. J.*, **52,** 385.
32. Jennison, M. W. (1942). *Ærobiology*, p. 108. Washington, D.C.: Amer. Ass. Advanc. Sci.
33. Duguid, J. P. (1945). *J. Hyg.* (*Lond.*), **34** 471.
34. Henderson, D. W. (1952). *J. Hyg.* (*Lond.*), **50,** 53.
35. Wells, W. F. (1934). *Amer. J. Hyg.*, **20,** 611.
36. Bourdillon, R. B., Lidwell, O. M., and Thomas, J. C. (1941). *J. Hyg.* (*Lond.*), **41,** 197.
37. Andersen, A. A. (1958). *J. Bact.*, **76,** 471.
38. Williams, R. E. O., Lidwell, O. M., and Hirch, A. (1956). *J. Hyg.* (*Lond.*), **54,** 512, 524.
39. Williams, R. E. O., and Hirch, A. (1949). *J. Path. Bact.*, **61,** 138; (1950). *Lancet*, **1,** 128.
40. Hamburger, M., and Robertson, O. H. (1948). *Amer. J. Med.*, **4,** 690.
41. Pulvertaft, R. J. V. (1947). *Brit. med. J.*, **2,** 517.
42. Duguid, J. P. (1946). *Brit. med. J.*, **1,** 864.
43. Lidwell, O. M., Noble, W. C., and Dolphin, G. W. (1959). *J. Hyg.*, (*Lond.*), **57,** 299.
44. Shooter, R. A., Smith, M. A., Griffiths, J. D., Brown, M. E. A., Williams, R. E. O., Rippon, J. E., and Jevons, M. P. (1958). *Brit. med. J.*, **1,** 607.
45. Eichenwald, H. F., Katsevalor, O., and Fosso, L. A. (1959). *Amer. J. Dis. Child.*, **98,** 432; (1960) **100,** 161.
46. Riley, R. L., Mills, C. C., O'Grady, F., Sultan, L. U., Wittstadt, F., and Shivpuri, D. N. (1962). *Amer. Rev. resp. Dis.*, **85,** 511.
47. Duguid, J. P., and Wallace, A. T. (1948). *Lancet*, **2,** 845.
48. Hare, R. (1946). *Brit. med. J.*, **1,** 868.
49. Davies, R. R., and Noble, W. C. (1962). *Lancet*, **2,** 1295.
50. Hare, R., and Ridley, M. (1958). *Brit. med. J.*, **1,** 69.
51. van den Ende, M., Lush, D., and Edward, D. G. ff. (1940). *Lancet*, **2,** 133.
52. van den Ende, M., and Spooner, E. T. C. (1941). *Lancet*, **1,** 751.
53. Rountree, P. M., Harrington, M., Loewenthal, J., and Gye, R. (1960). *Lancet*, **2,** 1.
54. Rosebury, T. (1947). *Experimental Airborne Infections.* Baltimore: Williams & Wilkins.

55. Bourdillon, R. B., and Glover, R. E. (1948). *Spec. Rep. Ser. med. Res. Coun. (Lond.)*, No. **262,** p. 297. H.M.S.O.
56. Chaussé, P. (1914). *Ann. Inst. Pasteur*, **28,** 771.
57. Glover, J. A. (1920). *Spec. Rep. Ser. med. Res. Coun. (Lond.)*, No. **50,** p. 133. H.M.S.O.
58. Wannamaker, L. W. (1954). In *Streptococcal Infections.* Ed. McCarty, M., Symp. N.Y. Acad. Med., No. **7,** Chapter 12. New York: Columbia Univ. Press.
59. Armstrong, C., Fotheringham, J. C., Little, C.J.H., and Thompson, T. O. (1931). *J. roy. Army. med. Cps.*, **57,** 321.
60. Wells, W. F., Wells, M. W., and Wilder, T. S. (1942). *Amer. J. Hyg.*, **35,** 97.
61. Medical Research Council (1954). *Spec. Rep. Ser. med. Res. Coun. (Lond.)*, No. **283,** H.M.S.O.
62. Lurie, M. B. (1944). *J. exp. Med.*, **79,** 559.
63. Wright, J., Cruickshank, R., and Gunn, W. (1944). *Brit. med. J.*, **1,** 611.
64. Loosli, C. G., Lemon, H. M., Robertson, O. H., and Hamburger, M. (1952). *J. infect. Dis.*, **90,** 153.
65. Lemon, H. M., Loosli, C. G., and Hamburger, M. (1948). *J. infect. Dis.*, **82,** 72.
66. Rammelkamp, C. H., Morris, A. J., Catanzaro, F. J., Wannamaker, L. W., Chamovitz, R., and Marple, E. C. (1958). *J. Hyg. (Lond.)*, **56,** 280.
67. Burtenshaw, J. M. L. (1942). *J. Hyg. (Lond.)*, **42,** 184.
68. Rothman, S., and Lonencz, A. L. (1963). *Ann. Rev. Med.*, **14,** 215.
69. Colebrook, L. (1930). *Min. Hlth. Interim. Rep. Dep. Comm.* "Maternal Mortality and Morbidity" Appendix D.
70. Goldsworthy, N. E., and Florey, H. W. (1930). *Brit. J. exp. Path.*, **11,** 192.
71. Florey, H. W. (1954). *Proc. roy. Soc. B*, **143,** 147.
72. Francis, T., Jr. (1940). *Science*, **91,** 198.
73. Tomasi, T. B., Tam, E. M., Solomon, A., and Brendergast, R. M. (1965). *J. exp. Med.*, **121,** 101.
Tomasi, T. B., and Bienenstock, J. (1968). *Advanc. Immunol.*, **9,** 1.
74. Wilson, G. S., and Miles, A. A. (1964). *Topley and Wilson's Principles of Bacteriology and Immunity*, 5th edit. p. 2462. London: Edward Arnold.
75. Eichenwald, H. F., Shinefield, H. R., Borsi, M., and Ribble, J. C. (1965). *Ann. N.Y. Acad. Sci.*, **128,** 365.
76. Glover, R. E. (1941). *Brit. J. exp. Path.*, **22,** 98.

Chapter 29

PATHOGENICITY AND VIRULENCE OF MICRO-ORGANISMS

By G. P. Gladstone

III

INVASIVENESS

In the last chapter we considered how bacteria and viruses are communicated from a source of infection to a new host and some of the factors affecting their colonisation of the body surface. We have now to discuss certain factors determining their invasion and growth in the body tissues.

Penetration of the Skin and Mucous Membranes

Micro-organisms may cause disease by growing on the surface of the body and producing toxic substances which are absorbed into the body. This is found for instance in cholera, where the vibrio grows in the lumen of the intestine producing potent toxins, but the organism does not penetrate beyond the basement membrane. More usually, however, penetration of the integument, with or without local injury, is a prerequisite for the production of disease.

It is generally agreed that bacteria and probably viruses will not pass through a perfectly intact skin and that some measure of trauma is necessary even if it damages only the most superficial layers of the epidermis. For instance, certain dermotropic viruses such as vaccinia virus will not parasitise the skin unless the cornified epithelium has been damaged, but only very slight pressure is needed to produce the necessary trauma. Mucous membranes, on the other hand, do not present such an impermeable barrier, although considerable differences are found between different species of bacteria and viruses in their ability to invade and in the extent of their penetration. Influenza virus, for instance, parasitises the cells of the respiratory mucous membrane. It does not penetrate further, but desquamation and rupture of these cells liberates virus into the lumen and it is then able to infect other cells, so bringing about lateral extension rather than deep penetration.

The penetration of vaccinia virus through the olfactory mucous membrane has been studied by Yoffey and Sullivan[1] in the cat, monkey and rabbit. They cannulated the cervical lymphatic duct and examined the issuing lymph after virus particles had been instilled into the nose. The virus was recovered, but only after 12 or more hours' delay. This finding, together with evidence of an inflammatory reaction in the nasal mucosa, suggested that parasitisation of the cells of the mucous membrane was a preparatory step but that, unlike the influenza virus, the vaccinia virus then penetrated farther and reached the lymphatics. Poliomyelitis, on the other hand, although a much smaller virus, could not be recovered from the lymph, and apparently could not parasitise the epithelial cells. Nevertheless the central nervous system of monkeys can be regularly infected with this virus by instillation into the nose. It would appear that the virus passes from the nasal mucosa to the brain along the olfactory nerves. No virus could be recovered from the blood, and section of the olfactory tracts prevented infection.* F. K. Sanders,[2] working with viruses allied to poliomyelitis, demonstrated the passage of virus along nerve axons. He pointed out that this is not really an anomaly, for the axon is merely a prolongation of the nerve cell which may be up to a metre in length. The virus may thus invade the cell at this distance from the site of multiplication. In experimental infections, poliomyelitis virus invades the olfactory hairs, which are exposed on the surface of the olfactory mucous membrane. Schulz, Warren, and Drinker[3] showed that virulent pneumococci also passed through the nasopharyngeal mucous membrane of the rabbit, from which they apparently entered the lymphatics, since they could be isolated from the cervical lymph before they reached the blood stream.

The classical observations of Ørskov and his colleagues[4, 5] in tracing bacteria in the tissues following ingestion leave no room for doubt that many pathogenic bacteria pass through the intact intestinal mucosa. After mice had been fed with broth cultures of *Salm. typhi murium* and *Salm. enteritidis*, both natural pathogens for the mouse, the organisms appeared in the mesenteric glands in 22–30 hours. With such feeding experiments it is unusual to find evidence of a local lesion suggesting the point of entry. Even an organism like *B. anthracis*, which produces a well-marked local lesion when it enters through an abrasion in the skin, fails to show any evidence of infection in the intestinal mucosa when the disease is acquired by ingestion, as for example in cattle.

Attempts were made by Florey[6] to obtain histological evidence of penetration of bacteria through the intestinal mucosa. He first used certain non-pathogenic bacteria isolated from the air and made direct observations of their fate when placed on the surface of the mucous membrane of loops of ileum of cats and rabbits. He observed that they were rapidly removed from the surface of the villi by the efficient clearing mechanism previously described (Chapter 28). There was no evidence that any organisms passed through the cells but some were observed for a time in the striated borders, until washed out by mucus secreted by the cells (6/PLATE F). In the colon, however, where there are no villi, the mechanism was less efficient and coliform bacteria could be observed in the mucus at the bases of the crypts. With the pathogenic organism *B. ætrycke* (*Salm. typhi murium*), Florey obtained a very different picture. There was considerable desquamation of epithelial cells and an exudation into the lumen of phagocytic cells which rapidly engulfed the organisms. Bacteria were found inside apparently normal epithelial cells and seemed to pass from these into the stroma. Phagocytes in the stroma also contained bacteria, but whether they had engulfed organisms in the lumen and returned with their load of bacteria, or whether they had taken up free bacteria in the stroma, could not be determined. It was suggested that passage was both through the cells (though how the organisms penetrated the cell was unknown) and between the cells, and possibly also by carriage in returning phagocytes.

* Although experimental infection can be produced through the nasopharynx, the evidence is against this route in natural infection in man, since the olfactory bulbs of fatal cases usually neither show lesions nor contain virus.

These results are in contrast to the general experience mentioned above that no local lesion associated with penetration is obtained. Florey's conditions, however, were very different from those of feeding experiments. He used relatively large numbers of *Salm. typhi murium* (a "milky suspension") containing the toxic O antigen (Chapter 30) and applied them to a limited area of mucous membrane. The local concentrations of toxin therefore would be very high and might well account for the inflammatory reactions. These would not be so evident in feeding experiments where the organisms would not only be diluted with the bowel contents, but would be dispersed over a much wider area.

How far an inflammatory reaction assists penetration is uncertain, for with two other pathogenic organisms, *Erysipelothrix monocytogenes* (*Listeria monocytogenes*) and *Myco. tuberculosis bovis*, Florey found no histological evidence of penetration, even after the epithelial cells had been artifically damaged, although it is well established that tubercle bacilli do pass through the intestinal wall within a short time after infection. Ørskov and Jensen for instance, isolated tubercle bacilli from the cervical and mesenteric glands of guinea-pigs 2–8 days after the organisms had been given by mouth. There has been a general failure to obtain any indication as to the point of entry, even with large infecting doses, the ulceration of the intestine commonly observed in animals infected by feeding being a late phenomenon and secondary to the establishment of the organism in the tissues.

It would appear from Florey's observations that non-pathogenic organisms are incapable of passing through the wall of the ileum, although it is possible that they may do so through that of the large intestine. That this does not apply to avirulent strains of normally pathogenic species, however, has been shown by Maaløe,[7] who found that penetration of the wall of the small intestine occurred equally well with two strains of *Salm. typhi murium*, of which only one was subsequently able to survive and grow in the body tissues and produce disease. Nevertheless, both organisms contained the O antigen and were therefore equally toxic and this might have been the factor determining penetration.

The spirochætes, *Treponema pallidum* amd *Leptospira icterohæmorrhagiæ* readily pass into the tissues without forming any immediate lesions at the point of entry. Probably the latter organism passes through the conjunctiva, as guinea-pigs can be infected by instillation into the conjunctival sac. However, passage through the nasal or respiratory mucous membrane may also be possible, the organism being carried down the lacrimal duct in the tears.

To Summarise: There is abundant evidence that bacteria and viruses can pass through intact uncornified epithelium, but the mechanism by which they get through is very little understood. In the case of viruses, preliminary parasitisation of the cells of the integument seems to be necessary. Probably this is not true of bacteria, though we know very little about their means of penetration and how far it is related to their virulence or toxicity.

Spread in the Body

The subsequent spread of the organisms in the tissues depends not only on factors connected with the host, such as the anatomy of the portal of entry, its lymphatic drainage and vascular supply, but also on factors connected with the organism. Bacteria and viruses vary very much in the extent to which they spread in the body quite apart from anatomical considerations. Reference has already been made to those viruses which remain confined to the cells of the integument and to *V. choleræ* which never penetrates beyond the basement membrane of the intestinal epithelium.

Cl. tetani shows no ability to spread, being confined to the point at which it has been deposited by a penetrating foreign body.

C. diphtheriæ is a slightly more invasive organism producing local tissue damage and is found in the submucous tissue of the tonsil and upper respiratory tract but very rarely extends beyond the local lesion. *Staph. aureus*, which often enters the body through a break in the epithelium at the base of a hair follicle, usually remains localised as in a boil, but may spread in the tissues invading the lymphatics or the blood stream. *Str. pyogenes* has a greater tendency to spread in the tissues both by contiguity, producing such spreading infections as erysipelas or cellulitis, or along lymphatic channels. A still more invasive organism is *B. anthracis* which may spread by contiguity, but in highly susceptible animals invariably invades the blood stream. In an animal dead of anthrax it is common to find the capillaries throughout the body containing large numbers of bacilli. *Treponema pallidum* is one of the most invasive organisms known; five minutes after application to the scarified skin of the scrotum of guinea-pigs it is found in the local inguinal glands,[8] and from there spreads throughout the body.

There are many gaps in our knowledge concerning the factors that determine whether an organism spreads in the tissues. In the sections following, some of these factors will be discussed.

Factors influencing the Ability to grow in the Host's Tissues

Obviously an essential factor in the establishment of the parasite is that it should find in the host's tissues the right conditions for growth, quite apart from its need to survive in face of the defensive resistance of the tissues of the host.

Over the past 30 years, great advances have been made in our understanding of the nutritional requirements and metabolic pathways of bacteria, including many of those pathogenic to man and animals. However, attempts to relate the growth requirements of pathogenic bacteria *in vitro* to their growth and production of disease *in vivo* have met with only partial success (for reviews see ref. 9). Pathogenic organisms require very much the same factors for growth as the animal body. Many of them have remarkable powers of adapting themselves to their environment. They are likely to find all their basic requirements in the tissues; indeed extracts of animal organs are the chief ingredients of standard media used for growing pathogenic bacteria. Non-pathogenic bacteria are, in general, even less exacting in their growth requirements, so that the problem, considered on the grounds of nutrition, is not why do pathogenic germs grow, but rather why do not non-pathogenic germs grow as well, or at all, in the body.[10] Lewis[11] suggests that the limiting factor determining growth may not be the supply of nutrients but the necessity to have them in a balanced proportion, and that what is a balanced proportion for one organism may not be so for another. Numerous examples may be quoted of media unable to support the growth of a micro-organism, not because they lack essential growth factors but because they contain chemically similar nutrients in unbalanced proportions, excess of some competitively inhibiting the utilisation of others. The balance may be restored, either by reducing the concentration of the former or by increasing the concentration of the latter. Thus *B. anthracis* growing in a chemically defined medium is inhibited if large amounts of serine or leucine are present; growth may be restored by decreasing the concentration of these amino acids or by adding more of threonine or valine respectively, which reverse the inhibition.[12] Braun has obtained some evidence that factors of this kind may operate *in vivo*.[13] He noted that the growth of a strain of *Salm. typhi murium* of low virulence was suppressed if large amounts of threonine were present, whereas the growth of a strain of high virulence was unaffected. By infecting guinea-pigs with mixtures containing a few virulent and many less virulent organisms, and at the same time injecting threonine, the virulent organisms were rapidly selected and the animals died more rapidly than controls without threonine.

Artificially produced auxotrophic mutants of a pathogenic organism, that is mutants requiring to be given preformed a growth factor readily synthesised by the parent (prototrophic) strain, have been shown to have lost the virulence of the prototroph if the growth factor is one not readily supplied by the host. Virulence, however, can be restored by supplying the missing factor. This phenomenon was first recorded by Bacon and his colleagues[14] using the experimental infection of mice with mutants of *Salm. typhi* requiring *p*-amino benzoic acid (PABA). PABA is not found free in mouse tissues but is present as part of the molecule of folic acid. Folic acid as it exists in the tissues will not support the growth of "PABA-less" mutants and hence such mutants fail to grow in the tissues.[15] Virulence could be restored, however, by adding PABA. Similar observations have been made by Furness and Rowley[16] with "purine-less" mutants of *Salm. typhi murium* and by Garber and his colleagues with "purine-less" mutants of *Klebsiella pneumoniæ* (for ref. see 17). The former authors were able to restore the ability to synthesise purines and at the same time virulence by phage transduction, that is by lysogenisation with phage from a prototrophic strain which, in the process of transference of phage transferred also the missing gene for purine synthesis. Garber noted that "purine-less" mutants of *K. pneumoniæ*, but not mutants possessing other nutritional deficiencies, lacked virulence for mice infected by the intraperitoneal route. It was found that peritoneal fluid was deficient in purines in a form assimilable by the organism, whereas it contained all the nutritional requirements for the other mutants.

It might be argued that these examples are artificial laboratory curiosities which have no place in nature. However, a natural purine dependent, mouse avirulent strain of *Salm. typhi* has been isolated from a human carrier.[18]

A direct relation between infection and the presence of an essential growth factor was observed by Keppie, Smith and their colleagues (see ref. 19) in their studies on brucellosis. They noted that the placentæ of animals susceptible to infection (e.g. cattle, sheep, goats and pigs) contained erythritol, an important growth factor for brucellæ, whereas those of species resistant to infection were devoid of this substance.

In considering the relation between growth *in vivo* and the nutritional requirements of bacteria, Dubos[10] has pointed out that the changed conditions of the tissues as the result of inflammation must be taken into account. The increased glycolytic activity of inflammatory cells produces an area in which the lactic acid and CO_2 concentrations may be high with a corresponding fall in oxygen tensions. It is possible that strains of bacteria having identical growth requirements when tested under optimal conditions *in vitro* may show gross differences in an inflammatory focus *in vivo*. Moreover, the host environment must not only be adequate for growth but must be adequate for the synthesis of those factors, considered later in this chapter and in Chapter 30, which enable the organism to survive in the face of the defensive factors of the host and to damage the tissues (e.g. surface antigens, capsules and toxins). Inflammation may provide such conditions. For instance, the high concentrations of HCO_3^- in an inflammatory focus may be responsible for the production of capsules by *B. anthracis in vivo* as has been found *in vitro*.

There is another approach to the problem of the relationship between the growth of the organism *in vitro* and its ability to grow in the tissues: the effect on infection of altering the composition of the diet of the host. Since, however, many of the factors essential to the bacterial cell are also essential to the host, the complexities inherent in such an approach may be readily appreciated.[20]

Sometimes a factor in the diet may enhance virulence. Many years ago, Hitchings and Falco[21] noticed that mice fed a certain natural diet were 100,000 fold more susceptible to experimental Type I pneumococcal infection than others fed a defined diet. The factor determining this difference was found to be Mn^{++}. Further investigations by Fischein and Braun (see ref. 22) showed that Mn^{++} in the presence of certain breakdown products of DNA had the effect of selectively stimulating the growth of virulent (smooth) pneumococci of Types I and II at the expense of their avirulent (rough) mutants. The mechanism involved in this selection, however, is obscure.

Temperature is one of the most important factors influencing growth in the tissues (for review see Ref. 23).

Pasteur was the first to suggest that the optimal temperature for growth of the parasite must have some relation to the temperature of the host. In his classical experiments he showed that anthrax developed in the usually resistant fowl if the bird was immersed in cold water. Following this work, many attempts have been made to influence infection by artificial alterations in the body temperature, by either chilling or warming. Frogs and lizards, by warming, have been infected with anthrax and plague respectively, and the artificial fever required to cure syphilis in the rabbit has been related to the thermal death point of *Treponema pallidum*. This may have some bearing on the fact that the condition of patients with certain forms of neuro-syphilis, particularly dementia paralytica, can often be greatly improved by fever induced artificially. The physiological effects on the body defence mechanism of such gross alterations in body temperature must, however, be taken into account, and in many cases it is difficult to assess whether the effect is on the organism or on the body.

Temperature relationships may play a part in infection by *Myco. ulcerans*. This organism is responsible for the production of localised ulcers in the exposed skin of the limbs of man, and always remains in these superficial lesions. Its optimum temperature was found to be 33° C., little or no growth taking place at 25° C. or 37° C.[24] It is likely that its growth on a superficial surface exposed to the air, and its failure to invade the deeper structures, are related to its requirement for a relatively cool temperature for growth. Another organism of like nature, *Myco. balnei*, also produces skin ulcers but these are less severe than those produced by *Myco. ulcerans*. When injected intraperitoneally in various animals it seems to confirm the importance of temperature in determining the extent of the resultant disease. In cold-blooded animals, it produces a generalised fatal infection; in mice and hamsters, the infection is localised to the exposed parts such as the scrotum, tail, nose and foot pads; and the more hyperthermic chicken is unaffected.[25]

Another example of a relation between temperature and the ability of the parasite to grow in the tissues is shown in infection in rabbits by Type III pneumococcus. Rich and McKee[26] and Enders and Shaffer[27] showed independently that only certain strains of this organism would produce a fatal infection in rabbits and that these were the strains able to grow at 41° C., a temperature attained by the rabbit in fever. Strains unable to grow at this temperature produced a local infection, but rapidly died out as the body temperature rose above a critical level. This work was extended by Muschenheim and his colleagues,[28] who showed that the temperature sensitive strains which failed to kill rabbits under normal conditions did so when the temperature of the rabbit was artificially reduced.

Lwoff[22] has called attention to the importance of temperature in the growth and survival of viruses in tissue culture. He noted that the yield of poliovirus growing in human KB cells at 40° C. was 250 times less than at 37° C. The difference was not due to an effect on the host cells. He applied this observation to the experimental infection of mice with poliovirus. A high proportion of mice kept at 36° C., which raised their body temperature by about 2° C., survived a dose of virus which killed all of a control group kept at 20° C. Further work showed that there was a correlation between the virulence of strains of poliovirus and their ability to grow at fever temperatures. Using the Sabin attenuated vaccine strain in tissue culture, the yield at 40° C. was less than 1/1000 of that at 37° C.; with a strain of low virulence (K.P.) the fall was about a hundredfold, and the yield of the highly virulent Mahoney strain was only reduced by a factor of 10. In further work (see ref. 30) Lwoff showed that the thermosensitive factor appeared to be at that stage in the development of the virus associated with the formation of polymerase, necessary for the replication of viral RNA.

In contrast to poliovirus, some virus infections are promoted by a raised temperature. The virus of herpes simplex grows in monolayer culture at 31° C. producing plaques which are limited in size. At 37° C., however, the plaques increase greatly in size and contain giant cells. It has been suggested that the raised temperature of the skin in fever may activate the virus dormant in the cells to produce giant cells which enable the virus to spread from cell to cell without coming into contact with antibody present in the blood. An attack of herpes labialis is the result.[31]

H ion concentration.—Although the pH of the normal tissues is that found optimal for most pathogenic organisms, in an inflammatory area acid resulting from glycolysis may lower the pH to 6·5. Dubos has shown that, although this pH is not low enough to kill or prevent the growth of many organisms, the lactic acid produced may be bactericidal on its own account, particularly under the conditions of lowered O_2 tension found in inflamed tissues.[10] He noted that the BCG attenuated strain of tubercle bacillus was more susceptible than the virulent strain to lactic acid. As both strains are taken up by monocytes when they enter the tissues, attempts to explain their difference in virulence on the basis of their difference in susceptibility to lactic acid must take into account the intracellular environment.

Both strains grow initially inside the monocyte without let or hindrance, perhaps due to the lack of an inflammatory reaction in the early stages of infection. With the development of inflammation and an increased metabolic and glycolytic activity of the monocyte, the growth of the BCG strain is inhibited but not that of the virulent strain. It is possible that this may be due to a differential susceptibility of the two strains to a raised intracellular concentration of lactic acid. However, although there is no doubt that resistance to tuberculosis increases with the increased metabolic activity of the monocyte (Chapter 37), its association with glycolysis and intracellular lactic acid is still highly speculative Some indirect evidence that extracellular lactic acid may be protective is given by the well known fact that, when glycolysis is deranged, as in diabetes, and keto-acids largely replace lactic acid, staphylococcal and tuberculous infections are more prevalent and more extensive. Dubos and Weiss have found that keto-acids are not only less toxic to tubercle bacilli and staphylococci than lactic acid, but will reverse the toxicity of lactic acid.[10]

Virus growth is also affected by H ion concentrations. Lwoff[29] showed that there was a critical value of about pH 6·9 below which the yield of poliovirus in tissue culture was greatly reduced. Highly virulent strains appeared to be less affected by pH than those that were less virulent. He believes that the ability of strains to grow in the presence of the low H ion concentration of an inflammatory exudate may be an important factor in virulence.

Oxidation-reduction potential.—Perhaps the clearest relationship between certain requirements of organisms and their ability to grow in the body was shown by Fildes[32] in his classical work on the pathogenesis of tetanus. It had long been known that washed spores of *Cl. tetani* would not germinate in the tissues of the guinea-pig and produce disease, although this animal is highly susceptible to tetanus. If the spores were injected together with soil or with certain ionisable calcium salts, germination occurred and tetanus developed. Fildes found that the same thing would occur if the spores were injected into areas of necrotic tissue or into a testicle whose blood supply was cut off by ligation, and showed that calcium produced such areas of necrosis. He found that no germination of spores occurred *in vitro* unless the Eh of the medium was lowered to + 0·01v., a point at which methylene blue is in the reduced condition. The Eh of the normal tissues of the guinea-pig was estimated at about + 0·12v., but in necrotic areas, or in the tissues of guinea-pigs maintained at lowered oxygen pressures, the Eh dropped to a level at which germination could occur, and tetanus developed. Other anærobes also have similar requirements. Those forming toxins that cause necrosis of tissue, such as *Cl. welchii*, can establish suitable conditions for their own growth once a small nidus of necrosis has allowed germination to start. Diffusion of tissue-destroying enzymes, such as lecithinase and collagenase, produced by the organism, perhaps assisted by solution of the hyaluronic acid cementing substance of the connective tissue by hyaluronidase, allows the organism to multiply on an ever advancing front. The typical spreading lesion of gas gangrene is the result.

With the strict ærobes such as the tubercle bacilli, a lowered oxidation reduction potential has the reverse effect, inhibiting rather than increasing infection. The centre of a caseous area which is practically anærobic is largely devoid of tubercle bacilli, but in the wall of a tuberculous cavity in the lung which is exposed to the air, enormous numbers of tubercle bacilli may be present.

Species, organ, and cell specificity.—One of the most puzzling features about bacterial and viral infection is the host specificity which is often found, and for which no reason has been discovered. For instance, the leprosy bacillus will grow only in human tissues apart from some restricted growth in mice under highly artificial conditions (Chapter 27). As no one has ever been successful in growing this organism adequately *in vitro* we know nothing of its growth requirements. However, we cannot say the same about the gonococcus whose only host is man. We know its growth requirements and they are relatively simple.

Not only do organisms have a selective affinity for the tissues of particular animals, but they may also have an affinity for particular tissues, and even for particular cells, of the same animal. This is only partly determined by anatomical relationships. The meningococcus and pneumococcus colonise the same area of mucous membrane in the nasopharynx, but the pneumococcus and not the meningococcus can then pass further down the respiratory tract to produce pneumonia. The factors determining the essential difference in the mode of spread of these organisms are not understood.

Dubos has thrown some light on the difference in selective localisation of tubercle bacilli in the organs of the rabbit and guinea-pig.[10] If virulent bovine tubercle bacilli are injected intravenously into guinea-pigs, or even directly into renal tissue, the kidneys remain free from infection. In contrast, the kidneys of the rabbit are extremely susceptible. Dubos showed that spermine oxidase was present in guinea-pig but not in rabbit kidney, and that the oxidative deamination of the polyamines spermine and spermidine of normal tissue by this enzyme resulted in the production of a substance having marked tuberculocidal properties in high dilution. This substance has since been identified as a dialdehyde. It apparently acts by inhibiting protein synthesis.[33]

Sometimes organ localisation is associated with a factor which acts by stimulating the growth of the pathogen rather than by depressing the bactericidal action of the tissues. Selective localisation in the tubules and pelvis of the kidneys of *Corynebacterium renale* in cattle and *Proteus mirabilis* in man may be related to the stimulating effect of urea on the growth of these organisms. Their toxic effect on the kidney is probably due to ammonia formed by the action of urease on urea (see ref. 19).

Animal viruses vary widely in host specificity. Some, like poliovirus, are restricted to certain cells of man and higher primates. Others, like the arboviruses, parasitise a large range of host cells. Some viruses, e.g. rabies, are restricted to a particular type of cell, but the cell can be that of almost any mammal. There is no doubt that the possession of a particular type of receptor to which the virus can become attached is an important factor in viral tropism. This was first shown with influenza virus which adsorbs to the surface of cells of the respiratory mucous membrane at receptor sites containing N-acetylneuraminic acid. Destruction of these sites with neuraminidase from *V. choleræ* prevents adsorption of virus (see ref. 34).

Holland and his colleagues[35] investigated the adsorption of poliovirus to susceptible cells *in vitro*. They noted that cells grown in tissue culture from animals susceptible to the virus adsorbed virus which then underwent multiplication producing cytopathic lesions in the culture, whereas cells in tissue culture from animals not susceptible failed to adsorb virus, to produce detectable amounts of virus progeny, or to show cytopathic changes. The cell receptors appeared to be protein associated with lipoprotein of the cell membrane. That the difference between susceptible and resistant cells depended on the possession of a specific receptor to which the viral protein coat becomes attached was shown when viral nucleic acid devoid of the capsid protein was used as the infective agent. The cellular and host tropism almost completely disappeared, cells, organs or whole tissues of almost any mammal being readily infected. It would seem, therefore, that many different cells have the capacity to support the growth of poliovirus once it can enter the cell, but lack the type of receptor on the cell surface which allows the necessary preliminary attachment of the intact virus. Because virus receptors are formed on cells in tissue culture, it does not necessarily mean that these receptors are present in the cell *in vivo*. This was shown by Holland[35] who noted that the failure of monkey kidney cells, which support the growth of poliovirus in monolayer cell culture, to become infected *in vivo* or in organ culture was due to the lack of virus binding material in homogenates of whole organs. It is suggested that loss of the normal contact relationships between cells, as is found in monolayer cultures, "de-differentiates" the cell, produces receptors and enables the cell to become susceptible to the virus. It would seem that loss of cellular differentiation is an important factor in determining the ability of a virus to infect cells. Poliovirus or adenovirus quickly destroyed undifferentiated human or monkey kidney cells but had no effect, for instance, on explant cultures of the differentiated ciliated respiratory epithelium.

In contrast, the possession of receptors for a particular virus does not necessarily mean that the cell is capable of supporting the growth of that virus. The red blood cell of certain species of animals have receptors for the influenza and other myxoviruses to which the viruses readily become attached and bring about the phenomenon of hæmagglutination.[34] However, the red cell is unable to support the growth of these viruses and no penetration of virus and replication of viral nucleic acid takes place.

Resistance to the Defence Mechanisms of the Host

There are two ways by which micro-organisms can be killed in the body of the host: (1) destruction inside phagocytes following phagocytosis, and (2) destruction by antibacterial substances in the body fluids including antibodies and complement. Contributing to these effects, without themselves killing the organisms, are the various other functions of antibody: localisation by agglutination, assistance of phagocytosis by opsonisation and prevention of adsorption of viruses to susceptible cells (see Chapter 37). Micro-organisms can overcome these mechanisms by producing substances that will (*a*) hinder phagocytosis, (*b*) resist intracellular destruction, (*c*) neutralise the antibacterial substances in the body fluids and (*d*) facilitate spread through the tissues or counter attempts at localisation. However, it is a mistake to regard factors produced by the microbe in the body as necessarily assisting the microbe, or factors produced by the host as necessarily assisting the host. As we shall see, the organism may produce enzymes which destroy its own antigens which protect it against the body defences[36]; on the other hand, the phagocyte may not destroy the organism, but may help it to spread, and protect it from the antibacterial action of the body fluids.

Bacterial antigens and haptens.—The production on the bacterial surface of antigens and haptens is one of the most important factors acting in all the ways indicated above. The antigens may be present in the form of a loose gel round the bacterial surface, that is as a capsule; or they may be more intimately bound to the cell structure, like the surface somatic antigens in the cell wall of Gram-negative bacteria.

The presence of these substances on the surface of the cell makes it difficult for the phagocyte to ingest the bacterium. The virulence of the pneumococcus, for instance, is almost entirely dependent on the ability of its polysaccharide capsule to hinder and, in certain circumstances, to prevent phagocytosis. Rough mutants which have lost the ability to form a capsule are rapidly engulfed and killed by phagocytes, but if the phagocytes of the body are destroyed the rough organism has all the potential virulence of the smooth organism. Rich and McKee[37] showed that, if a rabbit was largely deprived of its leucocytes by injections of benzene, rough pneumococci would produce a fatal infection. Where the surface antigen or hapten is readily liberated from the organism into the body tissues, it may help the organism to survive by uniting with antibody in the tissue fluids. In fatal cases of pneumococcal pneumonia in man large amounts of capsular polysaccharide have been isolated from the lungs. The union of this material with antibody will prevent agglutination and hinder opsonisation of the organism. The ability of this hapten to protect capsulated pneumococci against phagocytosis in antibody-leucocyte mixtures and to enhance their virulence in experimental infections has been repeatedly demonstrated. Free capsular polysaccharide may inhibit phagocytosis even under conditions in which the capsule on the organism is relatively ineffective. Wood and his colleagues[38] have shown that, on a fibrinous surface, capsulated organisms may be taken up by phagocytes without opsonisation ("surface phagocytosis", see Chapter 4). However, with certain strains of Type III pneumococcus, which produce large amounts of free polysaccharide capsular material, the leucocytes are caught in the slime and are not able to take up the organisms.

In contrast to the capsules of capsulated organisms, the somatic surface antigens and haptens of non-capsulated Gram-negative bacteria, for example the salmonellæ, are firmly bound to the cell. However, there is evidence that even here these substances may be liberated into the environment, where they not only inhibit the opsonic action of antibody, but also its ability to sensitise the organism to the bactericidal action of complement.

With *Streptococcus pyogenes* the antigen which is most closely associated with virulence is a protein (M protein), which is present on the surface of the organism and acts like the capsule of the pneumococcus in hindering phagocytosis. From some strains of streptococci the M protein is readily liberated into the culture medium, and if the same thing occurs in the animal body, it might be thought, on the analogy of the liberation of polysaccharide from the capsule of the pneumococcus, that these strains would be highly virulent. The reverse, however, appears to be the case. Olarte[39] found that those strains that retained the M protein were more virulent for mice than those strains from which it was easily removed. It is possible that the liberation of M protein was not due (as in the case of the Type III pneumococcus mentioned above) to an excessive production of the antigen, but to the removal of a limited amount already formed, leaving the coccus in a naked condition vulnerable to the defences of the host. The factor determining the liberation of M protein from these strains has not been identified, although the work of Elliott[40] strongly suggests that a proteolytic enzyme produced by the streptococci themselves is responsible. From many strains of *Str. pyogenes* he isolated a proteinase in a crystalline form and showed that it was formed autocatalytically from an inactive precursor. This enzyme attacked the M protein on the streptococcal cell, first liberating it into the medium and subsequently destroying it. The production of M protein and proteinase by these strains appeared to be mutually exclusive, for when the conditions were optimal for the production of proteinase, little or no M protein was found in the cell. Strains which produced proteinase had very low virulence for the mouse, but the interesting observation was made that when they were passed twenty times serially through the mouse their virulence was increased about ten million times and coincident with this increase in virulence was the complete suppression of the production of proteinase and the appearance of M protein in the organism.

Hyaluronic acid is another substance produced by some strains of *Str. pyogenes* and Group C hæmolytic streptococci which is present in the form of a capsule, but unlike the M protein is not antigenic. Although undoubtedly of importance in connection with the virulence of Group C streptococci, some controversy has arisen with regard to its importance for that of *Str. pyogenes*. The work of Rothbard,[41] however, has shown that it has a definite, although small, effect in increasing the resistance of these organisms to phagocytosis and enhancing their virulence, and this has been confirmed by Wood.[42] As with the proteinase and M protein, the production of hyaluronidase by some strains precludes their production of hyaluronic acid (see below); with other strains, a capsule is produced early in growth, but is subsequently destroyed by the enzyme produced later.[43]

It is a common finding that the serial passage of pathogenic bacteria through susceptible animals enhances their virulence. This is generally attributed to the selection of variants able to survive and grow more rapidly in the body tissues, and these are usually strains which, as in the case of the *Str. pyogenes* quoted above, contain a full complement of the surface somatic antigens associated with virulence. Braun[13] studied the conditions for the selection of smooth variants from mixed smooth and rough populations of *Brucella suis*. He showed that a thermostable breakdown product of the action of DNase of smooth strains on DNA, and probably identical with 6-furfurylaminopurine, kills rough but not smooth strains. We have already noted a similar phenomenon with the pneumococcus. Breakdown products of DNA acting in the presence of Mn^{++} selected smooth (capsulated) strains of pneumococci from mixtures with rough strains, but here the selection was the result of stimulation of the growth of the smooth strain rather than inhibition of the rough strain. How far the selection of smooth strains of *Brucella* and pneumococcus operates *in vivo* is not known, but the effect of feeding diets containing Mn^{++} in enhancing the virulence of pneumococci in mice in experimental infection, noted above, suggests that it may play a part.

Staphylocoagulase and clumping factor.—The production of coagulase is generally considered to be a characteristic attribute of pathogenic staphylococci distinguishing them from the non-pathogenic strains. This substance acting in the presence of a thermolabile factor in human or rabbit plasma converts fibrinogen to fibrin. Highly purified prothrombin can take the place of this factor, and it is generally thought that the clotting of fibrinogen in the presence of coagulase is brought about by thrombin activated by coagulase. Unlike the conversion of prothrombin to thrombin in the natural clotting of blood, however, plasma factors V and VII and Ca^{++} are not required.

A bound form of coagulase, the so-called *clumping factor,* is present on the surface of most coagulase-positive staphylococci. This is antigenically quite distinct from coagulase, but acts like it in converting fibrinogen to fibrin which deposits on the surface of the organisms and causes them to adhere in a network of fibrin.

There has been much discussion on the possible mechanism whereby these agents could contribute to virulence (see ref. 44). The early observations of Wilson Smith and his colleagues[45] suggested that fibrin in the vicinity of the organisms prevented phagocytosis. However, coagulase-negative organisms artificially held in a mass of fibrin are readily ingested by polymorphs which pass into the fibrin network. Indeed, the observation of Wood on "surface phagocytosis"[38] (see Chapter 4) make it clear that fibrin, far from interfering with phagocytosis, actually enhances it, enabling leucocytes to engulf organisms which without it are not taken up. It is more likely that clumping factor plays a secondary role in increasing the effectiveness of some of the extracellular toxins produced by staphylococci. Pathogenic staphylococci differ from non-pathogenic, not only in producing coagulase and clumping factor, but also in producing a host of extracellular enzymes and toxins some of which are lethal for leucocytes (see below). It would seem that clumping of staphylococci producing these toxins might have the effect of increasing the local concentration of toxins and destroying leucocytes migrating into the clumped mass of cocci. Some evidence for this hypothesis was obtained by Kapral[46, 47] who noted that staphylococci (strain 18Z) possessing clumping factor injected intraperitoneally into mice were immediately clumped due to the formation of surface fibrin from fibrinogen in the peritoneal fluid. Over the next 3 hours, the clumped cocci became surrounded by polymorphs which, however, were unable to penetrate the mass of organisms presumably due to their destruction by leucocidal toxins. If the same number of organisms were injected in a large volume of fluid, clumping did not occur and the mouse survived. A mutant of this strain lacking coagulase and clumping factor, but producing as much toxin as the parent strain, was not clumped but was rapidly engulfed by polymorphs, the concentration of leucocidal toxin in the vicinity of single cocci probably being insufficient to kill the leucocyte.[47] However, Kapral and his colleagues[48] found that when inoculated intravenously into mice and rabbits, this mutant was just as virulent as the parent strain. It seems, therefore, that these factors are not essential for virulence, a conclusion supported by the discovery of another mutant of 18Z which produced both factors but was avirulent for rabbits.[48]

A small minority of staphylococci produce a capsule and are highly virulent for mice (see ref. 49). These capsulated staphylococci grow diffusely in plasma soft agar and apparently lack clumping factor,[50] but still produce soluble coagulase. It is possible that the capsule obscures the former, since a mutant lacking the capsule is clumped by plasma. We have here, therefore, naturally occurring highly virulent strains where virulence is not dependent on a functional clumping factor. As with other capsulated organisms, these strains owe their virulence primarily to the resistance to phagocytosis offered by the capsule.

It has been claimed that soluble coagulase inhibits the bactericidal action of serum for staphylococci (for refs. see 51). However, the evidence is not convincing.[52]

Leucocidins.—Soluble toxins that destroy leucocytes are found particularly in staphylococci and streptococci. Pathogenic staphylococci produce at least three leucocodins, two of which are identical with α and δ hæmolysins (see Chapter 30). The third is a non-hæmolytic toxin discovered by Panton and Valentine in 1932 which acts specifically on polymorphs and monocytes of man and rabbits and has no action on the white cells of other species or any other cell.[53] It has been purified and shown to consist of two synergistic thermolabile proteins, antigenically distinct and inactive singly.[54]

Two of the streptococcal leucocidins are probably identical with the O and S hæmolysins. A third, identified as DPNase and produced only by Group A, C and G β-hæmolytic streptococci appears to act on the phagocyte only after the organism has been engulfed.[55]

How far leucocidins are responsible for the virulence of staphylococci and streptococci is still not determined. However, since the leucocyte represents the main if not the only mechanism that the animal body possesses for removing these organisms, it is likely that they may be important.

Ability to withstand destruction inside Leucocytes

Some pathogenic organisms (e.g. the pneumococcus) once they have been taken up by phagocytes are rapidly destroyed and digested in the phagocytic vacuole by lysozomal enzymes (see Chapter 4). Their virulence depends on resistence to phagocytosis. On the other hand the so-called facultative intracellular parasites, e.g. *Myco. tuberculosis*, *Brucella* and *Listeria*, are readily taken up by macrophages irrespective of their virulence. It is their subsequent fate inside the macrophage that determines virulence. For instance, as we have seen, virulent tubercle bacilli are engulfed as readily as the BCG strain, but survive and grow inside the macrophage, whereas BCG organisms after a period of survival and growth are destroyed. We have already considered the possible role of lactic acid in this differential susceptibility. The subject is considered further in Chapter 37. Intermediate between these extremes are organisms like *Staphylococcus aureus*.

There has been some controversy whether the virulence of staphylococci resides in their resistance to phagocytosis or in their resistance to intracellular destruction after engulfment.[56, 57] It would appear that both are important. The ability of the organism to produce lethal toxins for the phagocyte within and without the cell might be a common factor. However, other factors play a part. The surface antigens, particularly the capsule of capsulated strains but also cell wall antigens (e.g. teichoic acid) are certainly of importance in preventing phagocytosis.[56] Once the organism is engulfed, it may continued to survive for some hours. It is doubtful, however, whether staphylococci resemble the facultative intracellular parasites and grow inside macrophages.[57] Where growth has been observed (for refs. see 58) the cell is probably already dead, presumably killed by toxins produced intracellularly. Intracellular survival, however, is not necessarily contingent on destruction of the phagocyte. There is some evidence that teichoic acid in the wall of the engulfed staphylococci may be a factor in preventing intracellular destruction[49, 59] (Chapter 37). Host factors also play a part. Macrophages from individual rabbits vary considerably in their ability to destroy intracellular staphylococci, those from newborn rabbits being particularly refractory.[57] These differences were not dependent on antibodies or other humoral factors. However, as discussed in Chapter 37, there is some evidence that the macrophage itself may be stimulated to increased metabolic activity by certain organisms leading to their intracellular destruction (cellular immunity).

Bacterial Factors opposing Localisation

Hyaluronidase. Many Gram-positive bacteria (e.g. streptococci, staphylococci, pneumococci, *Cl. welchii, Cl. septicum*) possess an enzyme, hyaluronidase, that promotes diffusion in tissues by breaking down the hyaluronic acid polysaccharide that constitutes the tissue-cementing substance.[60] The action of this enzyme is most striking—McClean has compared the different rates of diffusion of intradermally injected saline and hyaluronidase with the "different behaviour of a drop of water when placed upon glazed and upon blotting paper".[61]

It might be expected that hyaluronidase would aid infection by promoting the spread of the organism and of any toxins or enzymes produced by it, but so many factors are concerned that it is difficult to assess the role of the enzyme in natural infection. It is true that injection of hyaluronidase may assist the spread of an experimental staphylococcal infection, but this may or may not bear any relation to the amount of hyaluronidase actually produced by the organism.[61] In experimental *Cl. welchii* infections the enzyme would seem to play little part, as Evans has shown that antihyaluronidase has no protective effect.[62] When hyaluronidase is injected experimentally its effect on invasiveness depends on the virulence of the organism and the size of the infecting dose. When the infecting dose is small and the organism relatively avirulent the enzyme may disperse the organisms, so that they come into more intimate contact with the phagocytes and antibacterial substances of the body fluids, and become so dispersed that their toxic products cannot reach a concentration high enough to cause tissue damage. Under these conditions hyaluronidase can prevent an infection becoming established and the body actually benefits from the lack of localisation of the organism. On the other hand, when the dose of invading organisms is large or their virulence high, hyaluronidase helps in invasion.

Hyaluronidase may affect the invasiveness of an organism in another way. We have seen that the possession of the enzyme by *Str. pyogenes* precludes the possession of the hyaluronic acid capsule, one of the factors associated with virulence, and that in fact it has been possible to protect mice against streptococcal infection by the injection of hyaluronidase.

Streptokinase.—Streptococci and staphylococci produce fibrinolytic substances known as streptokinase and staphylokinase respectively, streptokinase being the better known. These kinases act by converting an inactive constituent of normal plasma, plasminogen, into an active proteolytic enzyme, plasmin, which digests fibrin clots or attacks fibrinogen and renders it non-coagulable. Plasma also contains a plasmin inhibitor which is sufficient to combine with the small amount of free plasmin that is normally present, but not with the additional amount of plasmin released by the bacterial kinases. To what extent in the course of natural disease the kinases effectively promote the digestion of the fibrin barrier that forms around a focus of inflammation is not known, but it has been suggested that streptokinase is an important factor in the tendency of streptococcal inflammation to spread.

Streptokinase and streptodornase (the streptococcal desoxyribonuclease) have come into clinical use as aids in the removal, or "enzymatic debridement", of clotted exudates, for example in the pleural cavity.

Proteolytic enzymes.—Many pathogenic as well as non-pathogenic bacteria produce proteolytic enzymes but how far these are concerned in their virulence is not known. *Cl. welchii* and *Cl. histolyticum* produce collagenases which break down the collagen framework of muscle, leaving the muscle fibres intact.[64, 65] Anticollagenase, however, plays no part in the protection of animals against experimentally induced gas gangrene.[66] Nevertheless, it has frequently been observed that cases of gas gangrene are particularly severe when *Cl. histolyticum* is among the infecting organisms. In such cases the muscle may be digested down to the bone and it is not clear whether the severity of the disease is due directly to the toxicity of the *Cl. histolyticum* protease, or to its action in promoting the spread of the other infecting organisms, or to its supplying nutrients to these organisms by digesting the flesh of the patient.

Practically all the pathogenic clostridia produce proteolytic enzymes and these can be differentiated according to whether or not they are inhibited by normal serum. It may be significant that the proteases of the non-invasive clostridia (e.g. *Cl. botulinum, Cl. tetani*) are inhibited by normal serum whereas those of the invasive organisms (e.g. *Cl. welchii, Cl. septicum*) are not.[67]

Some strains of streptococci produce an inactive precursor, or zymogen, of a proteolytic enzyme which is autocatalytically converted to the active enzyme by a trace of active enzyme in a manner similar to the trypsinogen-trypsin conversion.[50] Its ability to destroy the M protein of the organism and its relation with virulence have already been considered.

The absence of local toxicity to the host's cells.—We have already considered how a local inflammatory area may provide conditions unfavourable for the growth of micro-organisms. In addition, the inflammatory reaction helps in the localisation and destruction of bacteria (Chapter 4) by bringing phagocytes and plasma to their vicinity, and this may explain why some of the organisms that produce little or no local damage at the time of entry, and consequently no inflammatory reaction, are not localised but rapidly invade the whole body; for example *Treponema pallidum* can be found in many tissues of the body a few hours after infection, whereas the local chancre does not appear for about four weeks. On the other hand organisms forming a powerful necrotoxin, such as staphylococci, produce a marked local inflammatory reaction and are localised after infection. Obviously lack of toxicity to host cells is of limited importance and cannot explain invasiveness in every case. Strains of organisms of equal toxicity may possess very different powers of spreading in the tissues (*cf.* Maaløe[7]) and organisms with little toxicity may not spread.

Summary

Factors determining the production of disease by micro-organisms are (1) their ability to colonise on the surface of the body (considered in Chapter 28); (2) their ability to pass through the integument; (3) their ability to find the right condition for growth in the tissues and (4) their ability to counter the defence mechanism of the host.

A few organisms such as *V. choleræ* produce disease without the necessity to penetrate the integument. Other organisms must pass into the tissues. The undamaged skin is probably resistant to penetration. Bacteria and viruses pass through the mucous membrane, but the latter only if they are able to parasitise the cells of the integument first. It is not known how they pass through. Considerable variation is found between micro-organisms in the extent of their spread in the body tissues. This may be along preformed channels or may be by contiguity. Survival in the body depends on the ability of the body tissues to provide an environment suitable for the growth of the organism. In this connection such conditions as temperature, pH, oxidation-reduction potential and presence of growth factors are discussed, but very often the differential susceptibility of different animals to the invasion of micro-organisms cannot be related to any known growth conditions. With viruses the presence of receptors on the surface of susceptible cells is an essential condition for their parasitisation. In addition to their finding the right environment for growth, organisms must be able to counter the defence mechanisms of the body. The presence of surface somatic antigens and haptens on the bacterial cell inhibits phagocytosis, intracellular destruction and the bactericidal action of antibody-complement mixtures. The production of leucocidins which destroy leucocytes, and the secretion of various enzymes acting on substrates in the body prevent localisation and assist the spread of organisms through the tissues.

REFERENCES

1. Yoffey, J. M., and Sullivan, E. R. (1939). *J. exp. Med.*, **69,** 133.
2. Sanders, F. K. (1953). *Symp. Soc. gen. Microbiol.*, **2,** 297. London: Cambridge Univ. Press.
3. Schulz, R. Z., Warren, M. F., and Drinker, C. K. (1938). *J. exp. Med.*, **68,** 251.
4. Ørskov, J., and Moltke, O. (1928). *Z. ImmunForsch.*, **59,** 357.
5. Ørskov, J., and Jensen, K. A. (1931). *Z. ImmunForsch.*, **70,** 146.
6. Florey, H. W. (1933). *J. Path. Bact.*, **37,** 283.
7. Maaløe, O. (1948). *Acta Path. microbiol. scand.*, **25,** 414, 755.
8. Kolle, W., and Evers, E. (1926). *Dtsch. med. Wschr.*, **52,** 1075.
9. Symposium of the Society of General Microbiology (1964). **14**. London: Cambridge Univ. Press.

10. DUBOS, R. J. (1954). *Biochemical Determinants of Microbial Diseases.* Harvard Univ. Monogr. Med. Pbl. Hlth., **13,** Chap. 2. Cambridge, Mass: Harvard Univ. Press.
11. LEWIS, R. W. (1953). *Amer. Naturalist,* **87,** 273.
12. GLADSTONE, G. P. (1939). *Brit. J. exp. Path.,* **20,** 189.
13. BRAUN, W. (1956). *Ann. N.Y. Acad. Sci.,* **66,** 348.
14. BACON, G. A., BURROWS, T. W., and YATES, M. (1951). *Brit. J. exp. Path.,* **32,** 85.
15. WOODS, D. D., and FOSTER, M. A. (1964). Ref. 9, p. 30.
16. FURNESS, G., and ROWLEY, D. (1956). *J. gen. Microbiol.,* **15,** 140.
17. GARBER, E. D. (1960). *Ann. N.Y. Acad. Sci.,* **88,** 1187.
18. FORMAL, S. B., BARON, L. S., and SPILMAN, W. (1954). *J. Bact.,* **68,** 117.
19. KEPPIE, J. (1964). Ref. 9, p. 44.
20. CLARK, P. F., MCCLUNG, L. S., PINKERTON, H., PRICE, W. H., SCHNEIDER, N. A., and TRAGER, W. (1949). *Bact. Rev.,* **13,** 99.
21. HITCHINGS, G. H., and FALCO, E. A. (1946). *Proc. Soc. exp. Biol.* (*N.Y.*), **61,** 54.
22. FISCHEIN, W. (1960). Ref. 17, p. 1054.
23. BENNETT, I. C. (1960). *Bact. Rev.,* **24,** 16.
24. MACCALLUM, P., TOLHURST, J. C., BUCKLE, G., SISSONS, H. A. (1948). *J. Path. Bact.,* **60,** 93.
25. LINELL, F., and NORDEN, A. (1954). *Acta tuberc. scand.,* Suppl. 33.
26. RICH, A. R., and MCKEE, C. M. (1936). *Bull. Johns Hopk. Hosp.,* **59,** 171.
27. ENDERS, J. F., and SHAFFER, M. F. (1936). *J. exp. Med.,* **64,** 7.
28. MUSCHENHEIM, C. (1943). *J. infect. Dis.,* **72,** 187.
29. LWOFF, A. (1959). *Bact. Rev.,* **23,** 109.
30. LWOFF, A. (1962). *Symp. Quant. Biol.,* **27,** 159.
31. HOJZAN, M. D., ROIZMAN, B., and TURNER, T. R. (1960). *J. Immunol.,* **84,** 152.
32. FILDES, P. (1929). *A System of Bacteriology,* **3,** 298. Medical Research Counc. London: H.M.S.O.
33. BACHRACH, U., and PERSKY, S. (1964). *J. gen. Microbiol.,* **37,** 195.
34. BURNET, F. M. (1951). *Physiol. Rev.,* **31,** 131; (1952). *Ann. Rev. Microbiol.,* **6,** 229. GOTTSCHALK, A. (1957). *Physiol. Rev.,* **37,** 66; (1959). *The Viruses,* Vol. 3, Chap. 4. Eds. BURNET, F. M., and STANLEY, W. M. New York: Academic Press.
35. HOLLAND, J. J. (1964). Ref. 9, p. 257.
36. STAMP, LORD (1955). *Lectures on the Scientific Basis of Medicine* 1953–54, **3,** 279. London: Univ. Lond. The Athlone Press.
37. RICH, A. R., and MCKEE, C. M. (1934). *Bull. Johns Hopk. Hosp.,* **54,** 277.
38. WOOD, W. B., Jr., SMITH, M. R., and WATSON, B. (1946). *J. exp. Med.,* **84,** 387.
WOOD, W. B., Jr., and SMITH, M. R. (1949). *J. exp. Med.,* **90,** 85.
WOOD, W. B., Jr. (1953). *The Harvey Lectures* 1951–52. Ser. **47,** p. 72. New York: Academic Press.
39. OLARTE, J. (1948). *J. Immunol.,* **58,** 15.
40. ELLIOTT, S. D. (1945). *J. exp. Med.,* **81,** 573.
ELLIOTT, S. D., and DOLE, V. P. (1947). *J. exp. Med.,* **85,** 305.
ELLIOTT, S. D. (1950). *J. exp. Med.,* **92,** 201.
41. ROTHBARD, S. (1948). *J. exp. Med.,* **88,** 325.
42. WOOD, W. B., Jr. (1960). *Bact. Rev.,* **24,** 41.
43. MACLENNAN, A. P. (1956). *J. gen. Microbiol.,* **15,** 485.
44. TAGER, M., and DRUMMOND, M. C. (1965). *Ann. N.Y. Acad. Sci.,* **128,** 92.
45. SMITH, W., HALE, J. H., and SMITH, M. M. (1947). *Brit. J. exp. Path.,* **28,** 57.
HALE, J. H., and SMITH, W. (1945). *Brit. J. exp. Path.,* **26,** 209.
46. KAPRAL, F. A. (1965). Ref. 44, p. 259.
47. KAPRAL, F. A. (1966). *Postepy Mikrobiol,* **5,** 297.

48. Li, I. W., and Kapral, F. A. (1962). *J. infect. Dis.*, **111,** 204.
Karas, E. M., and Kapral, F. A. (1962). *J. infect. Dis.*, **111,** 209.
49. Mudd, S. (1965). Ref. 44, p. 45.
50. Kœnig, M. G., and Melly, M. A. (1965). Ref. 44, p. 231.
51. Ekstedt, R. D. (1965). Ref. 44, p. 301.
52. Cybulska, J., and Jeljaszewicz, J. (1966). Ref. 47, p. 261.
53. Gladstone, G. P., and van Heyningen, W. E. (1957). *Brit. J. exp. Path.*, **38,** 123.
54. Woodin, A. M. (1960). *Biochem. J.*, **75,** 158.
55. Bernheimer, A. W., Lazarides, P. D., and Wilson, A. T. (1957). *J. exp. Med.*, **106,** 27.
56. Mudd, S., Yoshida, A., Li, I. W., and Lenhart, N. A. (1963). *Nature* (*Lond.*), **199,** 1200.
57. Kapral, F. A. (1965). Ref. 44, p. 285.
58. Rogers, D. E. (1966). Ref. 47, p. 279.
59. Li, I. W., and Mudd, S. (1965). *J. Immunol.*, **94,** 852.
Mudd, S. (1968). *Topics in Medicinal Chemistry*, **2,** 247. Eds. Rabinowitz, J. L., and Myerson, R. M. New York: John Wiley & Sons.
60. Chain, E., and Duthie, E. S. (1940). *Brit. J. exp. Path.*, **21,** 324.
61. McClean, D. (1930). *J. Path. Bact.*, **33,** 1045.
62. Evans, D. G. (1943). *J. Path. Bact.*, **55,** 427.
63. Miller, J. M., White, B. H., and Long, P. H. (1953). *Lancet*, **1,** 220.
64. MacFarlane, R.G., and MacLennan, J. D. (1945). *Lancet*, **2,** 328.
65. Bidwell, E., and van Heyningen, W. E. (1948). *Biochem. J.*, **42,** 140.
66. Evans, D. G. (1947). *Brit. J. exp. Path.*, **28,** 24.
67. Smith, L. De S., and Lindsley, C. H. (1939). *J. Bact.*, **38,** 221.

Chapter 30

PATHOGENICITY AND VIRULENCE OF MICRO-ORGANISMS

BY W. E. VAN HEYNINGEN

IV

BACTERIAL TOXINS

IT must be pointed out once again that the ability of an organism to grow in the body is not the same thing as the ability to produce disease. We are in fact exceedingly ignorant of this latter subject. There are, however, some harmful effects of infection that can be traced with varying degrees of precision. In the course of their invasion of the host many pathogenic bacteria produce an array of substances that are toxic to the host or assist in the invasion, or combine both functions. These are the *bacterial toxins*, among which are the most formidable poisons known. Their production by the organism is independent of the host and may take place in cultures growing *in vitro*. It is often assumed that such toxins account for the harmful effects of most, if not all, infectious diseases, but in fact the harmful effects of only three diseases, namely diphtheria, tetanus and botulism, can be ascribed with certainty to bacterial toxins. (The red rash of scarlet fever is directly due to the scarlet fever toxin of the hæmolytic streptococcus, but this is hardly a harmful condition.) In most cases it is difficult to define with any certainty the part that a bacterial toxin may play in an infectious disease; on the other hand, there are hardly any other established explanations for the harmful effects of infectious diseases. We will discuss the criteria for judging the pathogenic role of toxins at the end of this chapter.

The first known bacterial toxin was diphtheria toxin. Its presence in culture filtrates of the diphtheria bacillus was suggested in 1887 by Loeffler and its existence established in 1888 by Roux and Yersin. In 1890 tetanus toxin was discovered by von Behring and Kitasato and by Knud Faber, and in the same year von Behring and Kitasato showed that the serum of animals injected with sublethal doses of diphtheria and tetanus toxins contained specific antitoxins that neutralised the toxins and protected animals against them. In 1869 von Ermengen discovered botulinus toxin. These are some of the more important discoveries in the history of bacteriology and immunology. In the years that immediately followed, medical research was dominated by the idea that toxins were responsible for the harmful effects of all infectious diseases and that the answer to them lay in antitoxic immunity. Although these hopes were not realised the discoveries that were incidental to the research led to a considerable expansion in the knowledge of immunology.

Exotoxins and Endotoxins

The bacterial toxins as far as we know, are either simple proteins or polymolecular complexes of phospholipid, polysaccharide and protein. There are several differences between these two types of toxin, which are usually known (for convenience) as exotoxins and endotoxins respectively: (1) The exotoxins are almost all derived from Gram-positive organisms, although a few are produced by Gram-negative organisms; the endotoxins are all derived from Gram-negative organisms. In general, the exotoxins are in fact extracellular and the endotoxins intracellular, but this is not a hard- and fast-rule; sometimes Gram-positive organisms produce toxins both extra- and intracellularly, and sometimes the toxins of Gram-negative organisms can be recovered from filtrates of autolysed cultures. The endotoxins constitute part of the cell wall of Gram-negative organisms. In smooth variants they are identical with the somatic O antigens on the surface, but they also exist in rough variants, possibly in less accessible situations. (2) The exotoxins are much more toxic than the endotoxins. (3) The exotoxins have specific pharmacological actions, whereas the effects produced by the endotoxins are all the same irrespective of the organisms from which they are derived. (4) The exotoxins are more heat-labile than the endotoxins. (5) The exotoxins are completely neutralised by their homologous antitoxins in stoicheiometric proportions, whereas the endotoxins are only partially neutralised (if at all) even in the presence of excess antibody. (6) The exotoxins can be toxoided, that is, made non-toxic but still capable of stimulating the production of antibodies that combine with toxin and toxoid and neutralise toxin. The endotoxins cannot be toxoided.

We will see later in this chapter that the toxic component of all endotoxins is a small-molecular lipid, which for present purposes we may regard as a "passenger" within the larger complex. In essence, therefore, some of the differences between the endotoxins and exotoxins are those that we may expect between small-molecular substances and proteins.

EXOTOXINS

Toxicity of Exotoxins

Table I lists exotoxins produced by the principal toxinogenic pathogenic Gram-positive bacteria; Table II lists some properties of the bacterial toxins that have been purified. The protein megacin from *Bacillus megatherium* has been included because it is toxic to at least one form of life, namely certain other bacteria, although it is apparently not toxic to animals.

Comparative Toxicity

It is not really possible to make meaningful comparisons of the toxicities of various poisons when different breeds of animals of different species, sexes, ages, weights and susceptibilities are treated by different routes by different workers at different times in different laboratories in different countries with poisons having different actions on different tissues. In Table II an attempt is made to arrive at a very rough comparison of the toxicities of some bacterial toxins with some other poisons. It will be seen that some of the bacterial exotoxins differ in toxicity by orders of magnitude from the non-protein poisons and the endotoxins. As a purely theoretical and largely meaningless exercise it may be calculated that the lethal dose of the bacterial neurotoxins (tetanus, botulinum,

30/Table I

Exotoxins Produced by the Principal Toxinogenic Pathogenic Gram-positive Bacteria

Corynebacterium diphtheriæ [Diphtheria in man.]: Shick toxin, lethal, dermonecrotizing.

Staphylococcus aureus (*Micrococcus pyogenes var. aureus*) [Pyogenic infections in man and animals.]: (1) Alpha-toxin, lethal, dermonecrotizing, hæmolytic; (2) Beta-toxin (phospholipase C), lethal, hæmolytic; (3) Gamma-toxin, lethal, hæmolytic; (4) Epsilon-toxin, hæmolytic; (5) Hyaluronidase, spreading factor; (6) Staphylocoagulase, coagulates plasma; (7) Staphylokinase, fibrinolytic; (8) Enterotoxin, emetic; (9) Leucocidin, kills leucocytes.

Streptococcus pyogenes [Scarlet fever, tonsillitis, pyogenic infections, etc. in man.]: (1) Dick toxin, non-lethal, erythrogenic; (2) Streptolysin-O, lethal, cardiotoxic, hæmolytic; (3) Streptolysin-S, lethal, hæmolytic; (4) Hyaluronidase, spreading factor; (5) Streptokinase, fibrinolytic; (6) Streptodornase, desoxyribonuclease.

Bacillus anthracis [Anthrax in man and animals.]: A complex œdema-producing toxin.

Clostridium botulinum [Botulism in man and animals.]: (1–6) Six type-specific neurotoxins; (7) Hæmagglutinin.

Clostridium œdematiens [Gas gangrene in man; black disease and bradsot in sheep; bacillary osteomyelitis in buffaloes.]: (1) Alpha-toxin, lethal, dermonecrotizing; (2) Beta-toxin (phospholipase C), lethal, hæmolytic, dermonecrotizing; (3) Gamma-toxin (phospholipase C), lethal, hæmolytic, dermonecrotizing; (4) Delta-toxin, hæmolytic; (5) Epsilon-toxin (lipase), lethal, hæmolytic; (6) Zeta-toxin, hæmolytic.

Clostridium septicum [Gas gangrene in man; blackleg and braxy in sheep.]: (1) Alpha-toxin, lethal, hæmolytic; (2) Beta-toxin, desoxyribonuclease.

Clostridium sordellii [Gas gangrene in man.]: (1) An œdema-producing toxin; (2) A hæmorrhagic toxin.

Clostridium tetani [Tetanus in man and animals.]: (1) Tetanospasmin, neurotoxic; (2) A non-spasmogenic neurotoxin; (3) Tetanolysin, lethal, hæmolytic, cardiotoxic.

Clostridium welchii [Gas gangrene and enteritis necroticans in man; lamb dysentery, struck and infectious enterotoxæmia in sheep.]: (1) Alpha-toxin (phospholipase C), lethal, hæmolytic, dermonecrotizing; (2) Beta-toxin, lethal; (3) Gamma-toxin, lethal; (4) Delta-toxin, lethal; (5) Epsilon-toxin, lethal, dermonecrotizing; (6) Eta-toxin, lethal (?); (7) Iota-toxin, lethal, dermonecrotizing; (8) Theta-toxin, lethal, hæmolytic, cardiotoxic; (9) Kappa-toxin (collagenase), lethal, proteolytic; (10) Lamda-toxin, proteolytic; (11) Mu-toxin, (hyaluronidase), spreading factor; (12) Desoxyribonuclease.

dysentery) is 1 mg. for 1 million Kg. of living matter, or 4 oz. for the entire human population of the world.

Species susceptibility.—There may be great variations in the susceptibility of various species of animals to a given bacterial toxin. Thus the guinea-pig is 100 times more susceptible to diphtheria toxin than the mouse; the rabbit 1000 times more susceptible to dysentery toxin than the mouse. Moreover, different samples of the same toxin may vary in their relative toxicity to different species. Thus some samples of type B botulinus toxin are 6000 times more toxic to guinea-pigs than mice, whereas other samples show only a 3-fold difference; some samples of tetanus toxin are 350 times more toxic to guinea-pigs than mice, others only

30/TABLE II

TOXICITY OF BACTERIAL ENDO- AND EXOTOXINS COMPARED WITH SOME OTHER POISONS (THE REPORTED VALUES OF TOXIC DOSES HAVE BEEN ROUNDED OFF).

Poison	*Chemical nature*	*Molecular weight*	*Toxic dose* (μg)	*Toxicity (per unit weight test animal) compared with strychnine*
Strychnine	$C_{21}H_{22}O_2N_2$	334	10 (lethal, mouse)	1
Tetrodotoxin (fish poison)	$C_{11}H_{17}O_8N_3$	319	0·2 (lethal, mouse)	50
Crotactin (snake poison)	protein	?	1 (lethal, mouse)	10
Ricin (plant poison)	protein	36,000	0·1 (lethal, mouse)	100
Bacterial endotoxins	protein-poly-saccharide-lipid	+1,000,000	100 (lethal, mouse)	0·1
			200 (lethal, sensitive strain rabbit).	5
Botulinum A toxin (crystalline)	protein	1,130,000	0·000,02 (lethal, mouse)	500,000
Botulinum B toxin	protein	1,000,000?	0·000,02 (lethal, mouse)	500,000
Botulinum D toxin	protein	1,000,000?	0·000,01 (lethal, mouse)	1,000,000
Tetanus toxin (crystalline)	protein	67,000	0·000,02 (lethal, mouse)	500,000
Cl. welchii Epsilon toxin	protein	40,500	0·1 (lethal, mouse)	100
Diphtheria toxin (crystalline)	protein	72,000	0·05 (lethal, guinea pig)	5,000
Dysentery neurotoxin	protein	82,000	0·002 (lethal, rabbit)	500,000
Staphylococcal leucocidin:				
F Component (crystalline)	protein	32,000	0·004 } /ml	
S Component (crystalline)	protein	38,000	0·004 } /ml (lethal, macrophages)	
Staphylococcal enterotoxin	protein	24,000	2 (emesis, monkey)	
Staphylococcal Alpha toxin	protein	44,000	1 (lethal, mouse)	10
Staphylococcal Delta toxin	protein	68,000	2/ml (50% hæmolysis of 1% red cells)	
Streptococcal erythrogenic toxin	protein	27,000	0·000,000,5 (skin reaction, man)	
Bacillus megatherium megacin	protein	51,000	0·01/ml (inhibits bacterial growth)	

3 times. Such differences can also be seen at the cellular level; the *Cl. welchii* Alpha and *Cl. œdematiens* Gamma toxins both are phospholipases C; the Alpha toxin lyses sheep red blood cells rapidly and horse red cells slowly; the Gamma toxin *vice-versa*, but both toxins hydrolyse the phospholipids extracted from sheep and horse red cells at the same rate. Similar phospholipase toxins from three strains of *Cl. bifermentans* are per unit of *in vitro* enzymic activity 9, 60 and 70 times less toxic and less hæmolytic than the *Cl. welchii* phospholipase.

Oral Toxicity

The lethal doses for animals that have been discussed so far refer to doses administered parenterally. It is often assumed that the bacterial exotoxins,with the exceptions of botulinus toxin and staphylococcus enterotoxin, are not toxic by mouth. It has been supposed that the toxins are destroyed in the gut by the digestive enzymes or under the conditions of pH. However, it has been shown that such toxins as diphtheria toxin and tetanus toxin are in fact toxic by mouth provided a big enough dose is given. The lethal dose by mouth is many thousand times that of the parenteral dose, with the result that it becomes difficult in practice to introduce such a large dose into experimental animals by the oral route. The ratio of the oral and parenteral lethal doses of botulinus toxin is smaller than that of tetanus toxin. There is some evidence that botulinus toxin passes through the wall of the gut, either unchanged or in the form of toxic fragments (see below).

The Assay of Exotoxins

Exotoxins may be assayed by measuring their biological potency or their antibody-combining power. Leaving aside measurements of enzymic activity in the few special cases of toxins that are known to be enzymes (e.g. phospholipases, see below), the measurement of biological potency generally consists in determining the least dose that will produce a certain effect within a certain time, such as killing a certain proportion of experimental animals, hæmolysing a certain proportion of red cells, producing a certain-sized area of necrosis in the skin, etc. These assays have the advantage that they measure the biological acitivity of the toxins, and the disadvantage of the inaccuracy that is inherent in measurements involving a group of animals, red cells, etc. which vary in individual susceptibility. In assays of antibody-combing power the toxin is titrated against antitoxin and the biological effect is used qualitatively rather than quantitatively as an indicator of toxin excess. But such an indicator may not be necessary; many toxin-antitoxin complexes flocculate when toxin and antitoxin are mixed in certain proportions, and it so happens that in most cases neutral or near-neutral mixtures flocculate faster than more toxic or more antitoxic mixtures. Flocculating toxins can be assayed without external indicator by determining that amount of toxin that flocculates first with a given amount of antitoxin. Assays of antitoxin combining power have the advantage of greater accuracy, but the disadvantage that they measure the total antigenic potency of the toxin preparation which is likely to include toxoid (inactivated toxin that is still antigenic, see below).

The Nature of Exotoxins

The exotoxins all appear to be proteins. None of the purified exotoxins so far examined has been reported to be a protein conjugated with a prosthetic group, but the discussion below will show that in some other respects the exotoxins are complex:

Protoxins

Several exotoxins are secreted into the culture media as inactive protoxins. These include *Cl. botulinum* types A, B and E toxins and *Cl. welchii* Epsilon and Iota toxins. The inactive protoxins are converted into active toxins by proteolytic enzymes which may be present in the culture fluids, or in the gut of animals ingesting the toxins. Under the conditions of culture these protoxins may not be fully activated, possibly owing to a deficiency of proteolytic enzymes in the culture fluids, or to the presence of inhibitors of proteolytic enzymes. The protoxins resemble the zymogens trypsinogen and pepsinogen which are converted to active enzymes by proteolytic enzymes which split off small fragments of the inert precursors.

Dissociation and Aggregation

The molecular weight of botulinus toxin seems to vary from about 70,000 to about 1,000,000. It has been shown that the type A molecule, with a molecular weight of about 1,000,000 will dissociate under certain conditions of pH and ionic strength into particles with a molecular weight of about 70,000, some of which are atoxic and some more toxic than the original preparation (with no gain in total toxicity.) It was also shown that when botulinus type A toxin with a sedimentation coefficient of 17·9 was ingested by rats, particles with a sedimentation coefficient of 7 appeared in the lymph. There are suggestions of even smaller fragments of botulinus toxin. When the purified type E toxin was partially digested with trypsin some of the toxicity of the preparation would diffuse through dialysing membranes.

Tetanus toxin molecules, on the other hand, appear to aggregate readily when the toxin is in a purified state. It may form inactive and active dimers.

Complexity

Some bacterial toxins appear to be complexes of two or more separate proteins.

Staphylococcal leucocidin.—The most striking example is the staphylococcal leucocidin which kills rabbit and human leucocytes with characteristic changes in morphology. This toxin has been shown to consist of two proteins, the F and S components, both of which have been crystallized (see Table II). These components are inactive singly, but together they act synergistically.

Staphylococcal Alpha toxin.—The hæmolytic staphylococcal Alpha toxin may be a complex of antigenically and biologically indistinguishable proteins. An apparently homogeneous preparation of the complex could be resolved by electrophoresis in a density gradient into four components that did not differ strikingly in biological properties.

Anthrax toxin.—Anthrax toxin appears to consist of three distinct synergistically active protein components. Factor I is not toxic when injected alone but together with factor II it evokes œdema in the skin of the rabbit and kills mice. The mixture of factors I and II is less lethal per unit of œdema-producing activity than the crude toxin, and this led to the demonstration of a third factor. Factor III differs serologically from factors I and II, is nonlethal by itself or when mixed with factor I, but is lethal when mixed with factor II, and increases the lethality of mixtures of factors I and II per unit of œdema-producing activity.

Plague toxin.—The toxicity of the plague bacillus appears to be due to a mixture of two components which are unequally divided between the material extractable from the cell and the cell wall material.

Diphtheria toxin.—There is evidence that diphtheria toxin may not be a single protein. Crystalline toxin preparations showed only one line on immuno-diffusion against antisera from horses hyperimmunized against crude toxin,and antisera from horses immunized against the crystalline toxin gave only one line against crude toxin. But if the crystalline toxin was partially denatured by heating or by treatment with alkali, the single diffusion line would separate into four lines; if the crystalline toxin was partially digested with pepsin or trypsin, three lines were obtained. The new separated lines all showed reactions of identity with the original single line.

It is possible that crystalline diphtheria toxin, although immunologically and kinetically homogenous, is not chemically homogenous. It may be a mixture or complex of several molecular species rather than a single molecular species. The preparations of crystalline toxin that have been isolated in many laboratories all over the world are consistently similar, and even if these preparations are mixtures of molecular species they have a constancy which must be significant in the physiology of the diphtheria bacillus. The whole complex is diphtheria toxin.

The Antigenicity of Exotoxins

The exotoxins are antigenic (i.e. they stimulate the production of antibodies when introduced into suitable animals in a suitable way) and they are neutralized by the antitoxins thus formed.

Neutralization by Antitoxin

It does not always follow that a biologically active protein antigen should be neutralized by its homologous antibody. Thus the antisera to many enzymes do not neutralize, or only partly neutralize, their enzymic activity; for example, urease-antiurease floccules may retain 80 per cent of the enzymic activity. Other enzymes, e.g. the bacterial lecithinases, are completely inhibited *in vitro* by their homologous antibodies. Whether or not an antibody neutralizes an enzyme's activity appears to be fortuitous. The antibody-combining site and the "active centre" of an enzyme are not the same, and they may or may not be close together; if they are close, neutralization of the enzyme's activity may be due to mechanical obstruction of the active centre by the antibody.

It is a matter of fact that the actions of all the known bacterial exotoxins are inhibited by their homologous antitoxins, and this, together with the observation that many enzymes are not inhibited by their antibodies, led some workers to believe that there was a fundamental immunological difference between toxins and enzymes. However, the action of antitoxins on toxins is generally observed *in vivo* and in these circumstances other factors besides toxin, substrate and antitoxin come into play. The toxic enzyme urease is an interesting case in point. Antiurease inhibits urease only 20 per cent *in vitro* but nevertheless it completely protects rabbits against the lethal effects of the enzyme. It is known that the presence of circulating antibody promotes the rapid elimination of an antigen. Phagocytosis of a toxin-antitoxin complex, even when it is not in the form of a visible precipitate, may be important, but it cannot be the only factor because antitoxin may neutralize toxin in situations when there are no phagocytes. Thus it may inhibit the action of hæmolytic toxins on washed red blood cells. In these cases it is possible that the toxin-antitoxin complex may not be able to penetrate barriers that are open to the unimpeded toxin. In this connexion it is interesting that diphtheria toxin inhibits protein synthesis by HeLa cells and by extracts from these cells (see below), and that diphtheria toxin-antitoxin floccules retain a significant toxicity against cell-free extracts although the action of the toxin against intact HeLa cells (and of course the whole animal) is neutralized by antitoxin.

Toxoids

Toxins may spontaneously lose their toxicity without losing their antigenicity, i.e. they may still stimulate the production of antibodies which combine with both the toxic and atoxic proteins and neutralise the toxin. This was first noticed by Ehrlich who gave the name of "toxoid" to the detoxified antigen. Toxoiding is not confined to toxins—it may also take place with enzymes, and presumably the structural changes which take place during toxoiding also take place in proteins which are not known to have toxic or enzymic properties.

Toxin can be toxoided by treatment with formaldehyde, and by numerous other agents, including hexamethylene-tetramine, ketone, nitrous acid, iodine, ascorbic acid, carbon disulphide and pepsin. In general toxoiding is carried out by incubating the toxin solution with 0·1–0·2 per cent formaldehyde at pH 6 to 9 at 37° C. for several weeks. The process of toxoiding is nearly complete within a few days but prolonged treatment is necessary to ensure the complete detoxification demanded for antigens destined for human use. Prolonged toxoiding tends to reduce first the power to stimulate the production of antibodies and then the power to combine with antibodies.

Passive and Active Immunization

Animals may be protected against the effects of bacterial toxins by passive or active immunization. This subject is dealt with fully in Chapter 37.

Humans who have survived an attack of diphtheria are generally immune to the disease for life, but not so the survivors of tetanus. The reason for this is that the amount of tetanus toxin that will kill is far less than the amount that is necessary to produce active immunity.

Factors Affecting Toxinogeny

Culture Media

Culture media that promote good growth of a particular toxin-producing bacterium are not necessarily toxinogenic. Generally a number of factors have to be carefully controlled, such as the pH, the organic and inorganic constituents and (sometimes) the gas phase. Toxinogenic factors of culture media are rarely identified, probably because the work that is entailed is not only difficult but extremely tedious.

In the case of anthrax it is not possible to demonstrate production of all the components of the complex toxin in a laboratory culture medium; one of the non-toxic components is readily produced *in vitro* but the complete toxin is only found in the body fluids of heavily infected experimental animals.

Effect of iron.—The production of at least five bacterial toxins (scarlet fever, tetanus, *Cl. welchii* Alpha, diphtheria and dysentery) is inhibited when there is more than a low level of iron (0·1–1·0 mg. Fe/1.) in the culture medium. With some strains of *Cl. tetani* toxin production is greatest at very low concentration of iron, but with others iron has no inhibitory effect and indeed is added to promote bacterial growth. The iron content of the culture medium affects both the metabolism and Alpha toxin production of *Cl. welchii*, but these two effects do not appear to be connected. Toxin production by *Corynebacterium diphtheriæ* is inhibited at concentrations of iron above 0·1 mg. Fe/1. In cultures at this level of iron, toxin production does not take place until the end of the logarithmic growth phase, when the exogenous supply of iron has presumably been exhausted. The difference in virulence between the *gravis* and *mitis* strains of the diphtheria bacillus is probably connected with the effect of iron on toxin production. The high iron content of the body tissues is unfavourable for toxin production, but less so for *gravis* strains than for *mitis*; on the other hand, *mitis* strains produce more toxin than *gravis* strains in media containing a critically low concentration of iron. *Gravis* strains grow more rapidly than the *mitis* strains in media containing much iron, and so produce a thick pellicle in still cultures, or a thick diphtheritic membrane in the throat. The outermost layer of growing organisms in these membranes will produce toxin since they are deprived of iron because it will have been removed by the layer of organisms nearer to the source of nutrients. Although *mitis* strains produce less toxin in natural infections they can produce more toxin in properly controlled laboratory cultures. This is because they are capable of more abundant growth than *gravis* at the low concentrations of iron that favour toxin production. In fact the PW8 strain that is used throughout the world for toxin production is a *mitis* strain.

Diphtheria cultures secreting toxin into the medium also secrete porphyrin. Under appropriate circumstances it can be shown that above the critical level of 0·1 mg. Fe/1., for every 4 atoms of iron added to the culture medium 4 less molecules of porphyrin and 1 less molecule of toxin are produced. These proportions of iron, porphyrin and protein are the same as those in cytochromes and it has been suggested that in the absence of iron the diphtheria bacillus is incapable of synthesizing cytochrome *b*, but still synthesizes the porphyrin and protein moieties, which are secreted. The protein moiety may be related to the toxin. We will return to this subject in the section on lysogeny and toxinogeny.

The production of the highly lethal so-called neurotoxin of *Shigella dysenteriæ* is also inhibited by iron, at concentrations above 1 mg. Fe/1. In this case, however, toxin production does not take place at the expense of cytochrome production; on the contrary, toxin production and cytochrome synthesis increase with iron concentration up to 1 mg. Fe/1., and below this level all the iron in the medium is incorporated into bacterial cytochrome. It is only when the iron is in excess of that required for cytochrome synthesis that toxin production is inhibited.

Animal Passage

On repeated sub-culture most toxinogenic organisms lose their capacity to produce toxin and therefore it is generally necessary to refer to a freeze dried specimen of a culture that is known to produce toxin. Some workers favour infecting animals and re-isolating the organisms, but this passage of the organisms through animals does not seem to be in vogue today.

Lysogeny and Toxinogeny

Lysogeny and toxinogeny appear to be related in a number of cases, viz., staphylococcus toxin, Streptococcus toxin, *Bacillus cereus* toxin, and, particularly, diphtheria toxin.

There are toxinogenic and non-toxinogenic strains of *Corynebacterium diphtheriæ*. A non-toxinogenic strain of the diphtheria bacillus when infected with a temperate phage is converted to a stable state of lysogeny and toxinogeny. All toxinogenic strains of the bacillus are lysogenic, i.e., they carry a prophage, but not all lysogenic strains are toxinogenic, because not all corynebacterial phages are toxinogenic, and moreover some bacilli which become lysogenized by a toxinogenic phage do not become toxinogenic. Reversion to non-lysogeny always means reversion to non-toxinogeny.

Interesting studies have been made of the protein produced by non-toxinogenic strains of the diphtheria bacillus under conditions in which toxinogenic strains produce toxin. When cultures of non-lysogenic and lysogenic strains were transferred to an iron-free medium they entered into the declining phase of growth and measureable amounts of porphyrin and protein were secreted within 1 to 2 hours. Both strains produced the same amount of porphyrin and protein. In the case of the lysogenic strain, this protein was toxic, antigenic and largely monodisperse; in the case of the non-lysogenic strain it was non-toxic, non-antigenic, and polydisperse. Possibly the non-lysogenic strain contains a factor, perhaps a protease, that breaks down the monodisperse toxin into a polydisperse mixture of non-toxic, non-antigenic fragments.

The theory about the relationship between toxin and cytochrome protein (see above) has not yet been proved, but nothing that is known about the relationship of phage to toxin is inconsistent with it. Some of the polydisperse protein material produced by non-lysogenic strains of the diphtheria bacillus in the absence of iron may be derived from the protein moiety of cytochrome-*b*.

Biological Actions of Exotoxins

Toxins with Dermonecrotizing Activity

Some exotoxins produce an area of necrosis when injected into the skin and this has been taken to mean that these toxins are generally cytotoxic. Other toxins act on specific tissues, organs or cells, and yet others act on non-cellular material such as collagen fibres and the soluble components of plasma.

Oxygen-labile action on red blood cells.—Most of the dermonecrotizing toxins of the anærobic clostridia, and of the staphylococci, are hæmolytic (and lethal). There are oxygen-stable and oxygen-labile hæmolysins. The oxygen-labile hæmolysins include the Theta toxin of *Cl. welchii*, the tetanolysin of *Cl. tetani*, the pneumolysin of the pneumococcus and streptolysin-O of the hæmolytic streptococcus. They have several properties in common in spite of their diverse sources. They are reversibly activated by reducing agents, irreversibly inactivated by cholesterol, and serologically related, i.e. any one of them is neutralised by the antitoxin to any of the others. These hæmolysins are interesting not only because of their common immunological properties but also because their biological activity resembles that of the saponins: (1) Both types of substance are lethal, hæmolytic and cardiotoxic. (2) The hæmolytic activity of both types is inhibited by cholesterol. (3) A single dose of streptolysin-O has no effect on the frog's heart, except that it releases an inhibitory substance which is heat-stable, non-dialysable and chloroform-soluble. If the inhibitory substance is washed away the heart is sent into systolic contracture by a second dose of streptolysin-O. Pneumolysin and tetanolysin have the same effect. (4) Mice injected with the O-labile hæmolysins, or with saponin, rapidly develop a temporary resistance specifically to lethal doses of both types of substances. (5) Mice can be protected against streptolysin-O by previous injection of cholesterol. These observations suggest that possibly the oxygen-labile hæmolysins may have a common hæmolytically active prosthetic group that acts as a hapten.

Oxygen-stable action on red blood cells.—Hæmolysis by several of the oxygen-stable hæmolysins, viz. staphylococcal Alpha and Beta toxins, *Cl. welchii* Alpha toxin, *Cl. septicum* Alpha toxin, streptococcal streptolysin-S, is preceded by an induction or "silent" period during which the hæmolysin acts upon the cells but no hæmolysis takes place. The hæmolysis that follows the induction period cannot be stopped by antitoxin—it is spontaneous and independent of the hæmolysin. The spontaneous lysis of toxin-treated cells can be prevented by agents which protect the cells from osmotic shock, such as sucrose and polyethylene glycol.

Staphylococcal Beta toxin and *Cl. welchii* Alpha toxin are "hot-cold" hæmolysins. Red cells incubated at 37° C. with low concentrations of these toxins do not hæmolyse if kept at 37° C. but hæmolyse as soon as they are cooled. Cells treated with staphylococcal Beta toxin are also lysable at 37° C. by a number of substances including, apparently, glycerol, broth constituents, lipases and proteases, but they are no longer susceptible to lysis by the Alpha toxin.

Action on other cells.—*Staphylococcal toxins.* Staphylococcal Alpha toxin is toxic to rabbit polymorphs and human blood monocytes, but not to human polymorphs. It attacks rabbit platelets, liberating protein and other substances. It produces cytopathic changes in cultures of various mammalian cells. It lyses *B. megatherium*, *S. lutea* and *Strep. viridans* and spheroplasts of *E. coli*. It breaks down isolated lysosomes, liberating degradative enzymes. The Alpha toxin also acts on smooth muscle, producing a contraction. Staphylococcal Beta hæmolysin attacks platelets as well as red cells; the Delta hæmolysin produces cytopathic changes in a number of cell lines of human and animal origin.

Diphtheria toxin.—Diphtheria toxin also produces cytopathic changes in various cell lines of human and animal origin and it can be calculated that 200 to 400 molecules of toxin will kill one cell. The cytopathic effects of diphtheria toxin on tissue cultures follow some time after profound chemical changes have taken place. Protein synthesis is completely inhibited within about 90 min. of the addition of toxin to a culture of HeLa cells, whereas cytopathic effects first became visible in a few cells after 4 hours. The action of the toxin is probably not on the cell membrane as the uptake of radioactive potassium by monkey kidney cells is normal for several hours in the presence of a saturating dose of toxin, and there is no leakage of radioactive phosphorus from intoxicated cells.

The effect of diphtheria toxin on the synthesis of protein by a cell-free system extracted from HeLa cells has been studied. Such extracts readily synthesise protein under appropriate conditions and this protein synthesis is rapidly inhibited in the presence of a low concentration of diphtheria toxin.

Toxins with Specific Actions

Neurotoxins.—Tetanus and botulinum toxins produce marked and characteristic neurological symptoms and they appear to act exclusively on nervous tissue. On autopsy of animals dying of tetanus and botulism, even after massive doses of toxin, there are no gross or microscopical (or even electron-microscopical) signs of lesions in any tissues or cells.

Botulism.—Botulinum toxin causes a flaccid paralysis. It acts on the peripheral nervous system by suppressing the output of acetylcholine at cholinergic synapses. At the skeletal neuromuscular junction the toxin causes a reduction of the frequency of miniature end-plate potentials without changing their mean amplitude, thus having a presynaptic action. During botulinum intoxication the entire muscle membrane becomes susceptible to applied acetylcholine in the same way as a chronically denervated muscle.

Tetanus.—Tetanus toxin causes a spastic paralysis. It acts mainly on the central nervous system and it is now reasonably clear, after a debate of many years, that it reaches the anterior horn cells of the spinal cord by travelling up the regional motor nerve trunks. Like strychnine, it acts by suppressing synaptic inhibition. It is not known whether it affects the as yet unidentified inhibitory transmitter. Although the main action of the toxin is central there is evidence that it may have a peripheral influence as well. Such peripheral action would generally be masked by the central effects. Thus both botulinum and tetanus toxins paralyse the cholinergic nerve of the *spincter pupillæ* of the eye.

Dysentery toxin.—The so-called neurotoxin of *Shigella dysenteriæ* is as potent as tetanus and botulinum neurotoxins and produces symptoms of flaccid paralysis similar to those of botulinum toxin. But it produces such symptoms only in the rabbit, which is the most susceptible species. In other species (e.g. rats, hamsters) it does not produce neurological symptoms, but it affects the blood vessels of various organs. In the rabbit the affected blood vessels appear to be confined to the central nervous system, particularly the cervical enlargement of the spinal cord. As a result of this vascular damage there is a secondary destruction of motor nerve cells, but the neurological symptoms are probably due to pressure resulting from œdema in the spinal cord. The toxin therefore should be considered as a hæmorrhagic toxin whose action is confined to blood vessels, since it is not generally cytotoxic as judged by the skin test.

Dick toxin.—The streptococcal erythrogenic toxin (Dick toxin) is another hæmorrhagic toxin with a highly specialized site of action. As little as 0·000,000,5

μg. of this toxin will produce an erythematous flush when injected into the skin of a sensitive human subject, and yet the toxin appears to be without lethal action in experimental animals.

Staphylococcal enterotoxin.—The staphylococcal enterotoxin causes emesis when introduced into the gut of humans and rhesus monkeys, and both species rapidly acquire a resistance to the toxin. The mode of action of the toxin is entirely unknown, but it is not generally cytotoxic.

Staphylococcal leucocidin.—The action of the staphylococcal leucocidin (the Panton-Valentine leucocidin) appears to be limited to macrophages and polymorphonuclear leucocytes of certain species. In leucocidin-treated leucocytes there is first a loss of cell motility, then a withdrawal of pseudopodia. The cytoplasmic granules lose their orderly streaming and are subject to Brownian movement. After a few minutes the cells become spherical but not greatly swollen, and most of the granules disappear. The remaining granules then become closely applied to the cell wall. There is no disruption of the cell. Protein is released and this protein is not derived from the soluble protein of the cell, but from the granules. This release of granule protein is probably the result of depolarization of the leucocyte cell membrane.

The Action of Exotoxins at the Molecular Level

In only a few cases is there an understanding of the mode of action of bacterial exotoxins at the molecular level, that is, where it is known what the chemical nature is of the substances they act upon, and what change they bring about in those substances. In these few cases it has been shown, not surprisingly, that the toxins are enzymes.

Phospholipases.—It is now evident that a number of the so called classical bacterial exotoxins are phospholipases—enzymes that break down the phospholipids in one way or another. The phospholipids comprise sphingomyelin and derivatives of phosphatidic acid:

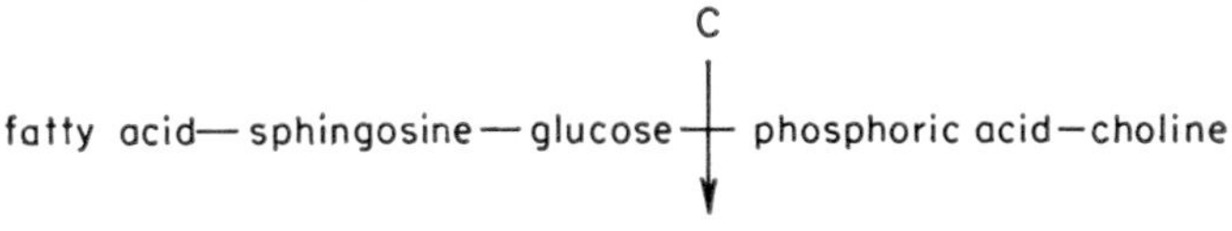

C

fatty acid— sphingosine — glucose ↓ phosphoric acid — choline

sphingomyelin

and

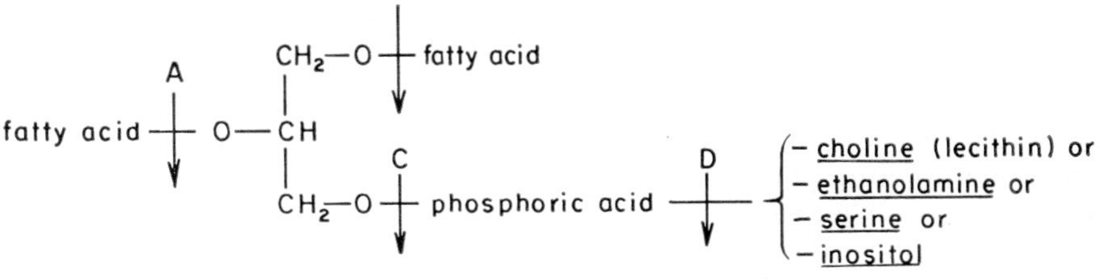

B

A CH$_2$—O ↓ fatty acid

fatty acid ↓ O—CH

C D

CH$_2$—O ↓ phosphoric acid ↓ { – choline (lecithin) or – ethanolamine or – serine or – inositol }

phosphatidyl –

Phospholipases occur in animal and plant tissues as well as bacteria. They have been classified according to the phospholipid bonds they attack. Phospholipase A splits off a fatty acid residue from the 2-carbon atom of the glycerol residue of phosphatidyl choline (lecithin)/ethanolamine/serine/inositol, leaving the surface-active lysophosphatides. The fatty acid on 1-carbon atom of phosphatides and lysophosphatides is split off by a phospholipase B, or lysophospholipase. Phospholipases C split off the phosphoryl choline/ethanolamine/serine/inositol residues from phosphatides, leaving a diglyceride; they may also split off the phosphorylcholine residue from sphingomyelin, leaving cerebroside. The only known phospholipase D (from certain green plants) splits off the basic residue of phosphatides.

Phospholipase C, Clostridial.—The *Cl. welchii* Alpha toxin has been shown to be a phospholipase C. At first it was thought to attack only phosphatidyl choline, and not phosphatidyl ethanolamine, phosphatidyl serine or sphingomylein. However it has since been shown that when the *Cl. welchii* Alpha toxin is allowed to act upon mixtures of phospholipids it will hydrolyse these other phospholipids as well.

Phospholipases C are also produced by a number of other clostridia, viz. *Cl. œdematiens* (Beta and Gamma toxins), *Cl. hæmolyticum* (Mu toxin) *Cl. bifermentans*, and probably *Cl. sordellii*, *Cl. chauvœi*, *Cl. sporogenes*, *Cl. centrosporogenes* and *Cl. tertium*. The phospholipases of *Cl. welchii* and *Cl. œdematiens* are antigneically distinct, but there are antigenic relationships between the phospholipases of *Cl. œdematiens* Beta toxin and *Cl. hæmolyticum* Mu toxin, and between the *Cl. welchii* and *Cl. bifermentans* enzymes.

Phospholipase C, ærobic sporing bacilli.—Bacillus anthracis, *B. mycoides* and particularly *B. cereus* also produce phospholipases C that attack all the phospholipids in the pure state. The action of these enzymes on free phosphatides (but not on phosphatides in the form of lipoprotein) is inhibited by normal serum.

Phospholipase C, Staphylococcal.—Recently the presence of two phospholipases C in staphylococcal filtrates has been demonstrated: (*a*) an enzyme attacking phosphatidyl inositol and lysophosphatidyl inositol, and (*b*) an enzyme attacking sphingomyelin and lysophosphatidyl choline. The sphingomyelinase appears to be identical with the Beta toxin and it is suggested that the particular sensitivity of the sheep red cell to this toxin is due to its comparatively high content of sphingomeylin. The enzyme attacking the inositol phosphatides is always present in cultures producing the Alpha toxin but apparently is not identical with this toxin. In addition, a phospholipase A is found in filtrates of $\alpha\beta$ strains of the staphylococcus when the Beta hæmolysin (sphingomyelinase, lysophospholipase) activity is high. Since the product of phospholipase A is lysophosphatide, the continuous destruction of this product might favour the production of phospholipase A. The action of phospholipases from various sources (viz. *Cl. welchii*, *B. cereus*, staphylococci and snake venom) is greater on native than on pure phospholipids and it may therefore be that the activity of these enzymes *in vitro* bears little relation to their action under native conditions.

Other enzymic actions.—Some bacterial products attack the soluble constituents of body fluids, the interstitial material of cells and the reticular scaffolding of muscle. These include the proteolytic enzymes streptokinase and staphylokinase which convert the inactive pro-enzyme plasminogen into the active enzyme plasmin that digests fibrin and prevents the clotting of blood; staphylocoagulase that causes the clotting of blood; the enzyme hyaluronidase, or spreading factor, that depolymerises hyaluronic acid, the cementing substance of cells; and the enzyme collagenase (e.g. the Kappa toxin of *Cl. welchii*) that breaks down the scaffolding of muscle without attacking the fibres themselves.

It is likely that these enzymes assist the organisms in their invasion of the host, but it is difficult to decide whether they should be considered as toxins in the classical sense. They probably would not have been so considered by the early discoverers of bacterial toxins because their contribution to the toxicity of bacterial filtrates is small in comparison with the other toxins in such filtrates.

The fixation of tetanus toxin by nervous tissue.—Despite the extreme potency of botulinum and tetanus toxins, their easily recognizable symptomatology, and the restricted sites of their action, we know little or nothing about the chemistry of their actions. In the case of tetanus toxin it is possible that its fixation by nervous tissue (the Wasserman-Takaki phenomenon of 1898) might provide an avenue of approach towards the chemical investigation of its action: Of the number of toxins, enzymes and other proteins tested, only tetanus toxin appears to be fixed. Determination of the toxin-fixing capacity of subcellular fractions of brain has shown that the capacity of nerve-ending particles (synaptosomes) to fix toxin is high while that of mitochondria and microsomes is low. When the synaptosomes were disrupted by osmotic shock and then refractionated, their toxin-fixing capacity was found to be due to synaptic membranes, the synaptic vesicles having an exceptionally low toxin-fixing capacity.

On chemical fractionation of nervous tissue it was found that ganglioside fixed the toxin. Gangliosides are water-soluble lipids apparently complexed in nervous tissue (perhaps as mixed micelles) with water-insoluble substances such as cerebrosides and the toxin-fixing capacity of ganglioside is greatly enhanced when it is complexed with a certain proportion of cerebroside, which is itself incapable of fixing toxin.

It is not yet known what the significance of the fixation of tetanus toxin by nervous tissue or ganglioside may be, or whether this fixation is, or is not, essential for the lethal action of the toxin. It is clear, however, that the fixation itself is not the lethal event. Fixation of toxin by nervous tissue, or by ganglioside/cerebroside is independent of temperature, but the lethal action of the toxin seems to be dependent on the temperature, as experiments with frogs maintained at different temperatures have shown. This would appear to rule out the suggestion that the toxin, in fixing to a ganglioside/cerebroside patch in a susceptible site acts merely by blocking the action of a substance such as a synaptic transmitter. The toxin must bring about some chemical change, and the potency of the toxin suggests an enzymic action, or an effect on an enzymic action, but so far it has not been possible to demonstrate any enzymic action of tetanus toxin on ganglioside, whether in simple solution of ganglioside in buffer, or in brain homogenates or slices.

ENDOTOXINS

The endotoxins are toxic components of the cell wall of many pathogenic and non-pathogenic (smooth and rough) strains of the enteric group of bacteria (e.g. typhoid, dysentery, coli bacteria). Many of the non-pathogenic species are normal inhibitants of the gut. Under the conditions of infection these toxic substances are set free and may produce various toxic manifestations: fever, leucocytosis, stimulation of various hormone and enzyme systems, especially proteolysis (fibrinolysis), and activation of the reticulo-endothelial system. Higher doses of toxin caused a marked leucopenia, breakdown of defence mechanisms, severe cellular injury of the lungs, kidneys, digestive tract, etc. and hæmorrhagic reaction. These reactions of endotoxins are non-specific, that, is, the endotoxins all cause the same reactions irrespective of their parent organisms.

The endotoxins are powerful antigens, stimulating the production of antibodies that are specific for the surface antigens of the bacterial species from which the endotoxins are derived. These antibodies do not neutralise the endotoxins.

The endotoxins have a complex composition. Boivin originally showed that the toxicity of smooth strains of the enteric group of Gram-negative organisms was due to a complex containing phospholipid and polysaccharide which he was able to extract with trichloracetic acid. The complex, which had a lethal dose of about 0·1 mg. for the mouse, could be extracted only from smooth variants, not from rough, and strains that were devoid of the complex were thought not to be toxic. (In fact, however, many rough strains of Gram-negative enteric bacteria are as toxic as smooth strains and produce the same toxic effects.) Besides accounting for all the toxicity of the organisms the complexes also proved to be identical with the dominant O somatic antigens. They were precipitated by antibacterial sera and on injection into rabbits readily stimulated the production of antibodies that precipitated the toxins and agglutinated the organisms, thus showing that the toxic antigens are situated on the surface of the cells. In recent years toxic substances, similar in constitution to the O antigens, but differing immunologically, have been extracted from rough strains.

Boivin believed that the toxic O antigen was a complex of phospholipid and polysaccharide, but Morgan, who extracted *Salm. typhi* and *Sh. shigæ* with diethylene glycol, showed that it contained protein as well. His complex accounted for from 5 to 7 per cent of the total dry weight of smooth variants and contained from 5 to 12 per cent phospholipid, from 50 to 55 per cent polysaccharide and from 17 to 25 per cent protein. When rough variants were treated in the same way only 0·2 per cent of the dry weight was extracted.

For present purposes we need not concern ourselves further with the phospholipid component ("lipid B"), as it can be removed with formamide without affecting the antigenicity or toxicity of the remaining polysaccharide-protein complex. When this residue is hydrolysed with weak acid, it yields an acidic conjugated protein and a degraded, non-viscous polysaccharide; on alkaline hydrolysis it yields an amphoteric unconjugated protein and a viscous undegraded polysaccharide. The undegraded polysaccharide is a hapten controlling the immunological specificity of the O antigen. The polysaccharide from any organism and the conjugated protein of any other organism can be recombined to yield the O antigen, the specificity being determined by the polysaccharide, e.g. *Salm. typhi* conjugated protein combined with *Sh. shigæ* undegraded polysaccharide yields *Sh. shigæ* O antigen.

We now know something about the toxic component of the endotoxins. According to the method of hydrolysis the toxicity may reside either with the undegraded polysaccharide or the conjugated protein; the undegraded polysaccharide is a lipopolysaccharide, and the conjugated protein a lipoprotein. A lipid residue ("lipid A"), with which the toxicity appears to be associated is shared by the polysaccharide and the protein, and remains attached to the former on alkaline hydrolysis and the latter on acid hydrolysis:

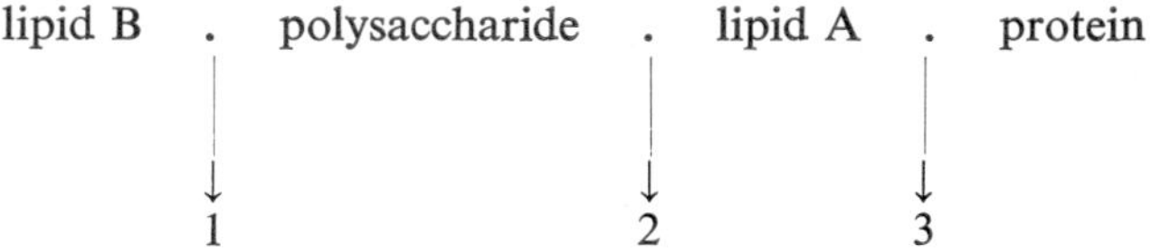

Bond 1 cleaved by formamide; bond 2 by acid; bond 3 by alkali.

The endotoxin complexes are probably even more complex: gentle extraction of *Brucella melitensis* with dilute pyridine yields a particle with very high molecular weight containing additional loosely bound lipid and phospholipid resides:

[lipid . phospholipid. (lipid B . polysaccharide . lipid A. protein)]n

The toxic lipid A appears to be a polyglucosamine phosphate to which long chain fatty acids are bound by ester and amide linkages.

The endotoxins exist as cell wall components of both rough and smooth strains of enteric organisms. The polysaccharide component consists of several different kinds of monosaccharide units, and in smooth strains it contains additional 3, 6-dideoxyhexose units (e.g. colitose, abequose, paratose, tyvelose) not present in rough strains. These additional hexose units account for the O-antigenic specificity of the smooth strains, and, possibly, for the greater ease with which endotoxins are extracted from smooth strains.

THE ROLE OF TOXINS IN DISEASE

What are the criteria for judging that a toxin is responsible for the harmful effects of an infectious disease? Ideally they are fulfilled when: (*a*) the organism is known to produce a toxin; (*b*) virulent variants produce the toxin and avirulent do not; (*c*) injection of the toxin separately from the germs produces symptoms that mimic the disease; (*d*) the infecting organism produces the disease without multiplying profusely or spreading extensively, the blood is sterile, and organs at a distance from the seat of infection are affected; (*e*) the disease can be prevented by immunization against the toxin.

It is clear that a toxin may play a pathogenic role without fulfilling all these criteria. We shall now examine them in more detail.

(*a*) *Toxin production.*—A failure to demonstrate toxin production *in vitro* does not necessarily mean that the organism is incapable of producing a toxin. It is seldom easy to find the correct conditions for the production of a particular toxin, and these are not necessarily the same as the conditions for luxuriant growth of the organism. The wrong strain of organism may be employed, or the wrong culture medium, or the wrong test animal, and it may be extremely difficult to hit upon the right combination. For example, if a non-lysogenic rather than a lysogenic strain of the diphtheria bacillus were used, or if a lysogenic strain were grown in a medium containing a concentration of iron normally encountered in culture media, or if the filtrate of a lysogenic culture in iron-free medium were injected into mice rather than guinea-pigs, it would not seem that there was such a thing as diphtheria toxin. Even after exhaustive attempts to demonstrate toxin production *in vitro* have failed it may still be unwise to assume that a toxin may not be produced under the natural conditions of infection. The case of anthrax illustrates this point. For many years investigators attempted to demonstrate toxin production in order to account for the pathogenesis of this disease, but always without success. Nevertheless it has been shown that in infected guinea-pigs the organism does indeed produce a toxin, but this can only be found *in vivo* in the plasma of animals in which the number of organisms in the blood has reached at least three million chains per ml.

(*b*) *Virulent variants.*—Absence of correlation between virulence and toxin production does not necessarily mean that the toxin does not produce harmful effects. This is largely because other, comparatively non-toxic, factors can determine virulence, as the following examples show. Rough strains of *Sh. shigæ* produce an extremely potent neurotoxin but are avirulent because they lack the O antigen. In *Cl. welchii* virulence is generally correlated with Alpha-toxin production, but some feeble toxin producers are virulent and some active toxin producers are avirulent. In the staphylococci virulence is associated as much with the non-toxic coagulase as with the toxic Alpha hæmolysin.

(*c*) *Mimicry of the natural disease.*—This criterion is relevant only when the toxin is practically the sole pathogenic agent of the disease, and therefore fits only botulism, tetanus, diphtheria and the rash of scarlet fever. In other cases the harmful effect produced by more than one toxin acting together, and by the other pathogenic agencies, will confuse the issue; and this will be further complicated by the peculiar features which result from the variation in the organs particularly attacked by different bacteria.

(*d*) *Restricted growth.*—Ideally the organism that produces harmful effects by means of a toxin remains localized at its portal of entry into the body and there manufactures its poison which is transmitted to distant organs and tissues. On the other hand, it cannot be assumed that the organism that spread extensively in the body, and even produces septicæmia, does not produce toxins.

(*e*) *Protection by immunization.*—The diseases whose pathogenicity is entirely due to toxins (e.g. diphtheria, tetanus) are preventable by active immunization and prophylactic passive immunization against the toxin. But protection against a disease by immunization against a toxin cannot be taken as proof that the toxin is responsible for the pathogenic effects of the disease. The role of the toxin may be purely aggressive, and the action of the antitoxin concerned with preventing the organism from establishing and extending a foothold, rather than with neutralizing a toxic factor.

It is instructive to consider the case of gas gangrene, where *Cl. welchii*, and other clostridia grow and produce toxins in the tissues of the host and the host is in a state of shock. A similar state can be induced in experimental animals by injecting cell-free filtrates of cultures of the toxinogenic organisms. But in clinical gas gangrene no toxin is detectable systemically and systemic antitoxin is ineffective. Yet amputation of the affected limb brings immediate relief and apparently removes a source of shock-producing substances. It is conceivable that these shock-producing substances may be degradative enzymes (or may arise from the action of such enzymes) from the lysosomes in the tissue of the host. It has in fact been found that some bacterial toxins release degradative enzymes from lysosomes, and this may have wider consequences and may be important in understanding the immediate consequences of the fundamental action of some toxins, if not the fundamental action itself.

REFERENCES

For a recent review on endotoxins see *Bacterial Endotoxins* (1964). Ed. Landy and Braun, New Brunswick, The Institute of Microbiology, Rutgers, The State University for exotoxins see VAN HEYNINGEN, W. E., and ARSECULERATNE, S. N. (1964). *Ann. Rev. Microbiol.*, **18,** 196; for histotoxic clostridia see MACLENNAN, J. D. (1962). *Bact. Rev.*, **26,** 177; for toxins in bacterial classification see OAKLEY, C. L. (1954). *Ann. Rev. Microbiol*, **8,** 411; for assay of toxins see VAN HEYNINGEN, W. E. (1960). Hoppe-Seyler/Thierfelder *Handbuch der physiologisch- und pathologisch-chemischen Analyse*, Heidelberg, Springer-Verlag, 10 Aufl. **10,** 785; for tetanus and botulinum toxins see WRIGHT, G. P. (1955). *Pharmacol. Rev.*, **7,** 413; for the prevention and treatment of tetanus see ECKMANN, L., Ed. (1967). *Principles on Tetanus.* Bern: Hans Huber.

Chapter 31

VIRUSES AND VIRAL INFECTION

1. THE NATURE OF VIRUSES AND THEIR GROWTH

BY M. L. FENWICK

Definition of a Virus

A virus is the ultimate form of intracellular parasite, stripped to the barest essentials required for its own propagation. It has no metabolic or respiratory systems of its own and depends for its reduplication upon the enzymes and metabolic machinery that it finds inside its host cell. The virus behaves in some respects as a micro-organism which requires a very rich and complex medium—the interior of a living cell—before it can thrive and multiply. On the other hand it resembles in some ways a giant molecule and, like many proteins, can be purified to crystalline form.

1. It is very small, between 20 and 200 mμ across as compared to about 1 μ (1,000 mμ or 10^{-6} metres) for a bacterium and about 10 μ for an animal cell. Consequently viruses pass through filters that retain bacteria.

2. It need contain only one sort of nucleic acid, either deoxyribonucleic acid (DNA) or ribonucleic acid (RNA), whereas all living cells contain both. At the same time although no virus has yet been shown to possess both DNA and RNA, there is no logical reason to exclude such a possibility.

3. As mentioned above, it has no metabolic system and depends upon its host cell for the energy and ingredients needed in the synthesis of new virus particles. It contributes, in the form of a code contained in its nucleic acid, only the essential information to determine the design of these particles.

4. A virus particle does not grow in size or divide by binary fission like a bacterium. Instead it first disintegrates, releasing its nucleic acid, and this process is followed by the synthesis within the host cell of the viral components which are finally assembled to form new virus.

There are a number of small infectious agents which, like viruses, are obligate intracellular parasites, but unlike them possess both DNA and RNA and multiply by binary fission. These include the rickettsiæ, which cause Rocky Mountain spotted fever and typhus fever, and the agents of psittacosis, of lymphogranuloma venereum and of trachoma.

31/FIG. 1 (*see opposite*).—Electron micrographs and models of virus particles.
(A) Herpes virus particle without its outer envelope. (From Wildy *et al.*[6])
(B) Model of herpes virus showing the icosahedral arrangement of 12 pentagonal and 150 hexagonal morphological units or capsomers. (From Wildy *et al.*[6])
(C) Vaccinia virus. (From Nagington & Horne.[7])
(D) Bacteriophage T2. The outer sheath of the tail has contracted revealing the inner tube. Tail fibres can be seen. (From Brenner *et al.*[8])
(E) Adenovirus type 5 showing the tailed capsomers at the corners of the icosahedron. (From Valentine & Pereira.[9])
(F) Model of adenovirus constructed from 252 spheres, 12 of which represent the tailed pentagonal capsomers. (From Dr. R. C. Valentine.)

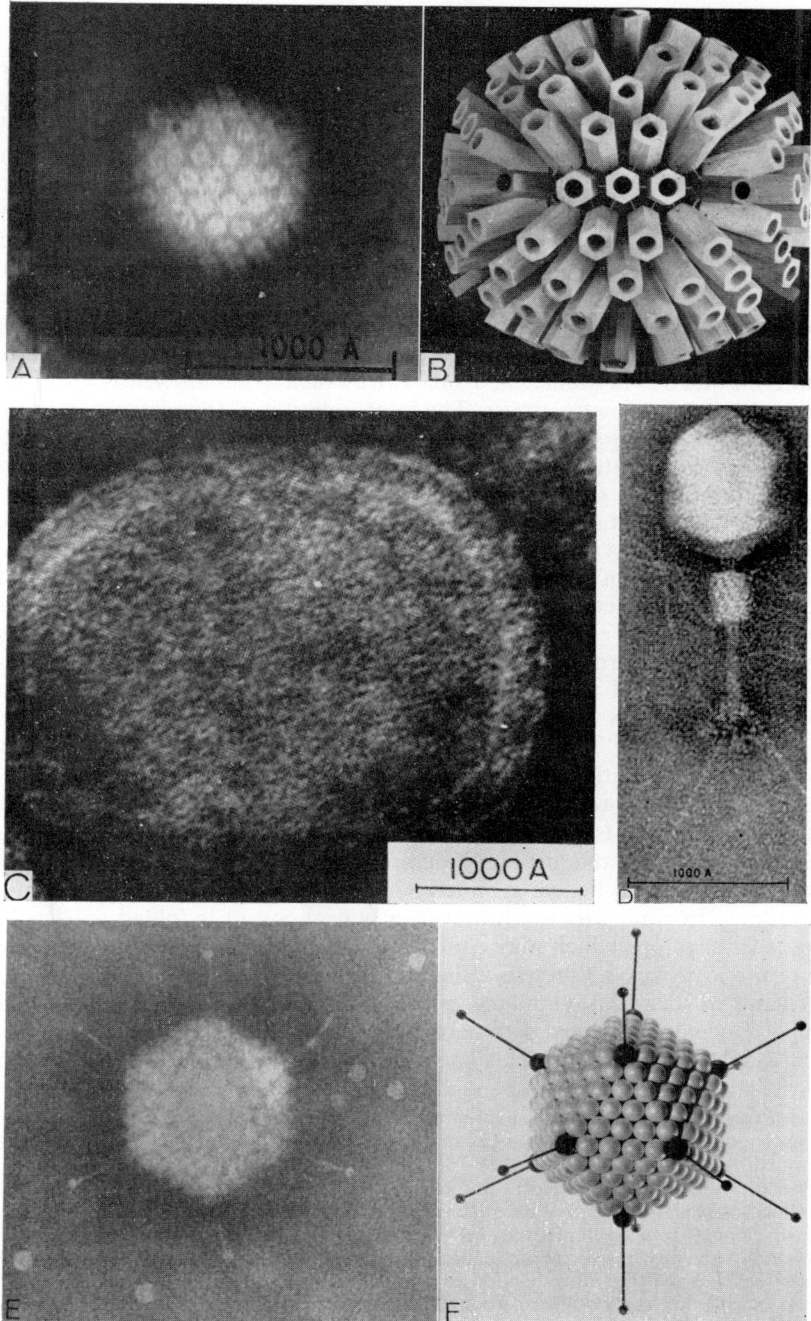

31/Fig. 1.

Structure

The techniques of X-ray diffraction and electron microscopy (in particular the use of "negative staining") have yielded, within the past decade, much information about the structure of virus particles. Negative staining involves treating the virus with heavy ions, frequently phosphotungstate, which penetrate the crevices on the surface and are opaque to the electron beam. The viral protein and nucleic acid on the other hand are relatively transparent, so that under the high magnification of the electron microscope the particle stands out in light tones against a dark background, with "shadows" of phosphotungstate emphasizing its surface structure. Magnifications of up to 500,000 times can be achieved with some electron microscopes. At this magnification a spherical protein molecule of molecular weight 36,000 appears on the microscope screen as a disc about 2 millimetres in diameter; a small virus such as poliomyelitis virus would appear about 1 centimetre across. The interpretation of the pictures in terms of detailed structure is sometimes complicated by the fact that since the electron microscope concentrates on a plane of focus which is much thicker than a virus particle, it therefore shows simultaneously both "front" and "back" of the particles if both are stained with phosphotungstate. Some electron micrographs of negatively-stained viruses are shown in FIGS. 1 and 2.

The nucleic acid of a virus is always surrounded and protected by a protein coat known as the "capsid". In some cases this central complex is itself surrounded by an outer envelope. The capsid is made of a single type, or a small number of types, of protein molecule packed in a regular array which determines the size and shape of the virus particle. There are two distinct ways in which the protein molecules can be packed, creating structures with either "helical" symmetry or "cubical" symmetry. In the former case the molecules are arranged side by side in a continuous tightly-packed spiral chain forming a cylindrical tube such as that of tobacco mosaic virus (FIG. 2 E, F). The nucleic acid of tobacco mosaic virus is a single chain which fits into a groove between the turns of the protein helix and probably determines the overall length of the virus particle. Viruses with helical symmetry in their capsids are thus rod-shaped or filamentous. In some viruses, however, a helical capsid is folded and enclosed in an outer envelope which may confer a more spherical overall shape, as in the case of the myxoviruses such as influenza virus (FIGS. 2C, 2D).

Viruses with cubical symmetry, on the other hand, are shaped like spheres or regular polyhedra. Cubical symmetry is defined by the existence of mutually perpendicular axes about which a body may be rotated so as to present a number

31/FIG. 2 (*see opposite*).—Electron micrographs and models of virus particles.

(A) Bacteriophage øX 174, with only 12 capsomers in its capsid. Two empty capsids have been penetrated by the negative stain. (From Tromans, W. J. and Horne, R. W.[37])

(B) Poliomyelitis virus. (From Horne and Nagington.[10])

(C) Influenza virus showing irregular shape and size of particles and spikes projecting from the outer envelope. (From Hoyle, Horne and Waterson.[11])

(D) Model of a myxovirus such as influenza or mumps, showing the helical capsid enclosed in its outer envelope. (From Horne and Wildy.[1])

(E) Sections of tobacco mosaic virus rods (full length 300 mμ). (From Horne and Nagington.[10])

(F) Model of tobacco mosaic virus showing the RNA lying in a groove between the helically arranged capsomers, which in this case are single protein molecules. (From Klug and Caspar.[12])

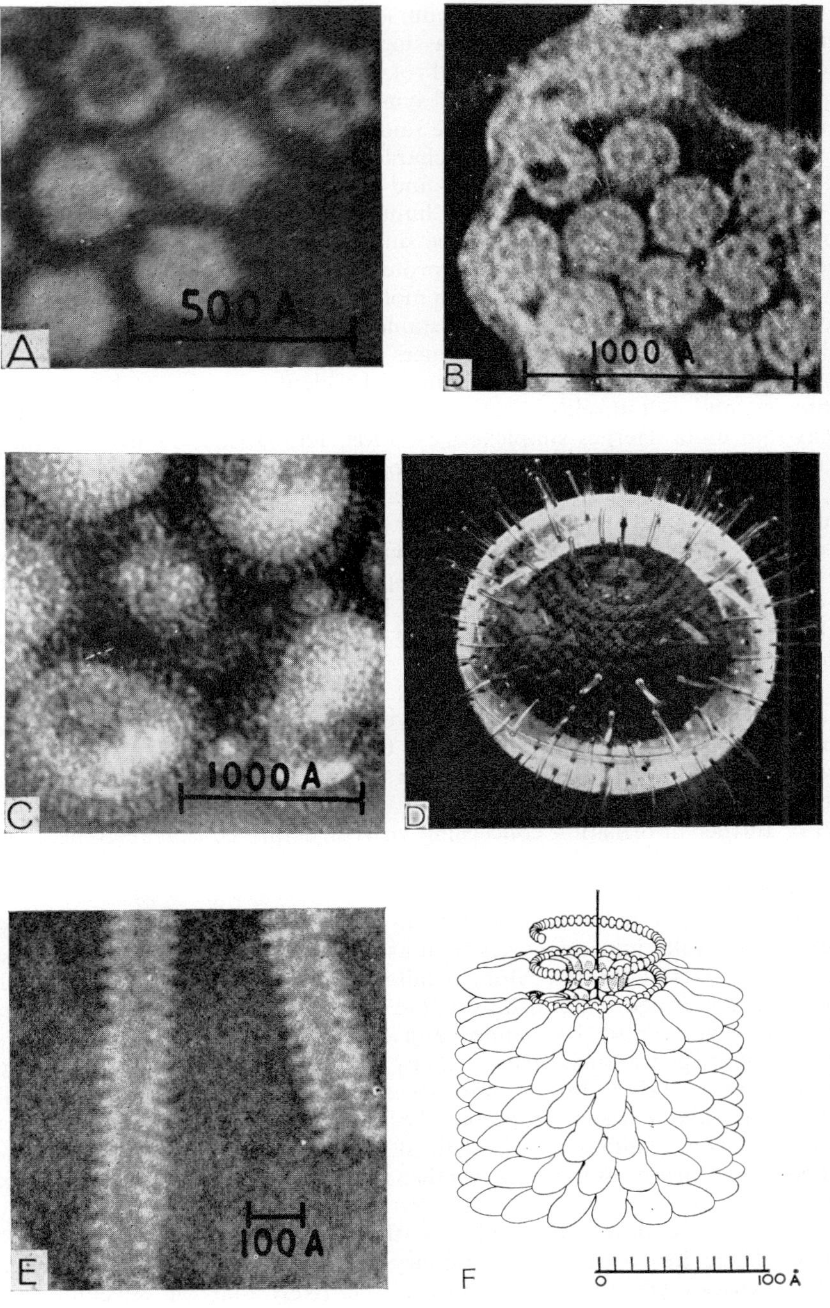

31/Fig. 2.

of identical appearances during the course of one revolution. Thus a cube has four-fold symmetry about an axis passing through the mid-points of opposite sides; there are also axes of three-fold rotational symmetry passing through two opposite corners, and axes of two-fold symmetry passing through the mid-points of opposite edges. A cube is therefore said to have 4:3:2 symmetry. A number of viruses have the 5:3:2 symmetry characteristic of the regular dodecahredon (12 pentagonal faces and 20 corners) and icosahedron (20 triangular faces and 12 corners) and such capsids can be built from multiples of 60 identical non-symmetrical subunits (which might be single protein molecules) or from intermediate numbers of units (groups of protein molecules) with various degrees of symmetry. It is these groups of protein molecules which are often distinguishable in electron micrographs of negatively-stained virus particles. They are sometimes called morphological units or "capsomers". For example the tiny bacteriophage øX 174 (FIG. 2A) appears to be built of 12 identical units each with 5-fold symmetry, and poliomyelitis virus (FIG. 2B) is thought to have 12 five-fold and 20 six-fold units. Herpes simplex virus (FIGS. 1A, 1B) has 12 five-fold (at the corners of the icosahedron) and 150 six-fold units, and adenovirus type 5 (FIGS. 1E, 1F) has 12 five-fold units with tails and 240 six-fold units. The capsids of viruses with cubical symmetry are often stable in the absence of their central core of nucleic acid. Empty shells of many viruses have been observed with their nucleic acid cores replaced by phosphotungstic acid in negatively-stained preparations (e.g. FIG. 2A) but it is not known whether they can be built up without nucleic acid or whether they are degradation products of mature particles.

Finally there are viruses, so far only observed among the bacteriophages, whose capsids display both types of symmetry—cubical in the head, which contains the nucleic acid, and helical in the tail, by means of which the virus attaches itself to its host cell and through which the nucleic acid passes into the cell (FIG. 1D).

For further information concerning virus structure consult references 1–3.

Classification

Early attempts at the classification of viruses were based on type of host. They fell naturally into categories such as animal (usually mammalian), insect, plant and bacterial viruses. More detailed knowledge of their structures has sometimes confirmed relationships within these groupings, for instance a great many plant viruses are rod-shaped and contain RNA, whereas there are no known rod-shaped animal viruses; many bacterial viruses have a head and a tail and contain DNA. But as more viruses are discovered and more detailed information about their properties becomes available, similarities emerge between viruses in different host-defined categories and it is now generally accepted that viruses are viruses whether they prefer to grow in beasts or bacteria.

Virus classification is desirable but the ideal system is still a matter for debate.[4] There are no known evolutionary relationships between viruses, or even between viruses and (other) organisms. It is likely that the development of cellular organisms preceded the appearance of the viruses that parasitise them and the viruses may perhaps have been derived originally from normal cellular constituents modified to give them their infectious qualities. One approach to the problem of classification is to assign an order of importance to certain selected viral properties and subdivide the viruses progressively according to each selected property in turn. Such systems have the practical advantage that they are easily comprehended and are relatively easy to memorise. They are open to the criticism that they are too rigid, and based upon a hierarchy of properties which may conceivably be upset by new knowledge, necessitating a complete or partial reorganisation of the system. It has been questioned, for instance, whether the type of nucleic acid (DNA or RNA) is of primary importance in classifying a virus: some other property, such as molecular weight of the nucleic acid, might be more fundamental. These doubts have led to the proposal that a classification based on a large number of properties with no hierarchy, each being given the same emphasis, should be allowed to evolve gradually as information accumulates. Nevertheless a hierarchical system will have mnemonic value as well as displaying many of the relationships between viruses. The following properties have been suggested as the basis of such a classification:

1. Type of nucleic acid (DNA or RNA).
2. Presence or absence of an outer envelope surrounding the capsid.
3. Symmetry of the capsid (helical, cubical or complex).

Table I shows the categories into which some well-known viruses fall when arranged according to these properties. Choice of a different hierarchical order of the same properties would not, of course, affect the compositions of the final groups but would change their relative positions in the table. Some of the groups so obtained had already been given names on grounds of morphological or host-range similarities—herpes and pox viruses, myxoviruses, arboviruses, picorna viruses. The myxoviruses have irregular shapes. They have been divided into two subgroups according to the diameter of the nucleoprotein helix within the envelope (9 mμ in subgroup 1 and 18 mμ in subgroup 2) and the intracellular site of multiplication (nucleus in 1; cytoplasm in 2). The arboviruses are so named because they are borne or transmitted by arthropods, such as insects. They are otherwise a rather heterogeneous and poorly characterised group. Vesicular stomatitis and rabies viruses have a characteristic bullet-like shape with one flat and one rounded end. The picorna viruses are the small (pico) RNA viruses. Reovirus, with its relatively large double-stranded RNA, does not fit very comfortably into this group. Adeno (certain types), polyoma and Rous sarcoma are oncogenic, i.e. cancer-producing, viruses.

Mechanisms of Virus Growth

The essential characteristic of a virus is that it carries the information needed to direct the manufacture of identical copies of itself. This information is in the form of a chemical code contained in the structure of the nucleic acid of the virus. It concerns the synthesis not only of identical molecules of nucleic acid, but also of proteins (and perhaps other components as well) from which new virus particles can be assembled.

What the virus lacks is the machinery for translating the code it carries into the form of new molecules, and this machinery it finds in good working order in the living cell that it infects. It is therefore not surprising that the mechanisms

31/Table I

Classification of Virus

			Group Name		*Dimensions* mμ	*Approx. mol. wt. of nucleic acid* × 10^6	*Host*
DNA	Env	Com	Pox	Vaccinia (cowpox)	250	160 (D)	Cow
DNA	Env	Com	Pox	Variola (smallpox)	250		Man
DNA	Env	Cub	Herpes	Herpes simplex	180	50 (D)	Man
DNA	Env	Cub	Herpes	Varicella (herpes zoster, chickenpox)	180		Man
DNA	Nak	Com		Phage T2	Head 100 × 80 Tail 110 × 20	130 (D)	*E. coli.*
DNA	Nak	Com		Phage λ	Head 54 Tail 140 × 12	30 (D)	*E. coli.*
DNA	Nak	Cub		Tipula	120	150 (D)	Insect
DNA	Nak	Cub		Adeno	70	23 (D)	Man
DNA	Nak	Cub		Warts	55		Man
DNA	Nak	Cub		Polyoma	45	3·4 (D)	Mouse
DNA	Nak	Cub		Phage øX 174	30	1·7 (S)	*E. coli.*
DNA	Nak	Hel		Phage fd	800 × 5	1·5 (S)	*E. coli.*
RNA	Env	Com		Rous sarcoma	75	10 (S)	Hen
RNA	Env	Com		Rabies	180 × 75		Dog
RNA	Env	Com		Vesicular stomatitis	180 × 65	3–4 (S)	Cattle
RNA	Env	Cub	Arbo	Western equine encephalitis	53		Man, bird *via* mosquito
RNA	Env	Cub	Arbo	Yellow fever	38		Man, *via* mosquito
RNA	Env	Hel	Myxo 2	Mumps	150–500		Man
RNA	Env	Hel	Myxo 2	Measles	120–250		Man
RNA	Env	Hel	Myxo 2	Rubella	100–300		Man
RNA	Env	Hel	Myxo 2	Newcastle disease	120–180	7 (S)	Hen
RNA	Env	Hel	Myxo 2	Distemper	115–160		Dog
RNA	Env	Hel	Myxo 1	Influenza	80–120	2 (S)	Man
RNA	Nak	Cub	Picorna	Reo	60	10 (D)	Mouse, etc.
RNA	Nak	Cub	Picorna	Polio	27	2 (S)	Man
RNA	Nak	Cub	Picorna	Colds	27		Man
RNA	Nak	Cub	Picorna	Foot and Mouth	24	2 (S)	Cattle
RNA	Nak	Cub	Picorna	Turnip yellow mosaic	25	2 (S)	Turnip
RNA	Nak	Cub	Picorna	Phage f2	24	1 (S)	*E. coli.*
RNA	Nak	Hel		Beet yellow	1,250 × 10		Beet
RNA	Nak	Hel		Tobacco mosaic	300 × 17	2 (S)	Tobacco

Abbreviations: Env = enveloped; Nak = naked; Cub = cubical; Hel = helical; Com = complex; S = single strand; D = double strand.

by which virus-specific materials are produced in the infected cell are closely similar to those operating in an uninfected cell in the course of its normal growth and metabolism: in general the differences between cellular and viral biochemical pathways lie in details rather than in fundamental principles.

However, there are a few instances of viral components for which there is no known counterpart in the normal cell. In these cases an abnormal biochemical mechanism must be introduced and the virus achieves this by carrying in its nucleic acid the information necessary to determine the synthesis of a new enzyme which in turn catalyses the abnormal reaction. Detailed reviews of the biochemistry of virus growth may be found in references 2, 3, 5.

As we have seen, the major, and sometimes the only, constituents of viruses are nucleic acid (DNA or RNA) and protein, and it may be profitable at this stage to recall some of the principles involved in the biosynthesis of these materials in normal cells.

Normal Cells

DNA occurs in normal cells in double-stranded form, the two strands being cross-linked by many relatively weak hydrogen bonds between specific pairs of bases—adenine pairs with thymine and guanine with cytosine. The two strands are thus complementary in their base sequences, and the sequence of either define the sequence of the other (see FIG. 3). The synthesis of new DNA requires a

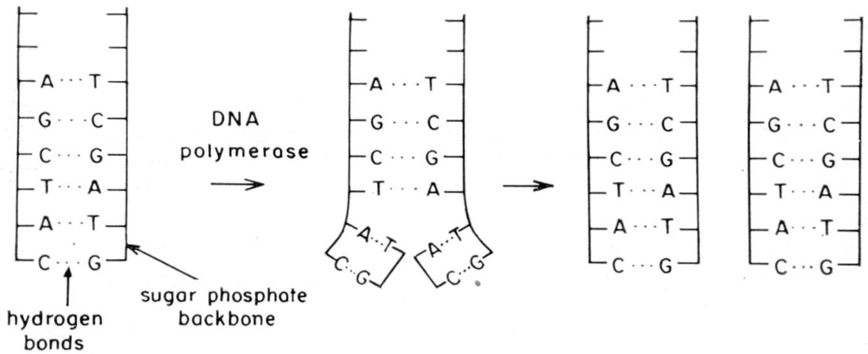

31/FIG. 3.—Mechanism of replication of DNA. The complementary strands of the template are separated, one being found in each of the daughter duplexes.

DNA template and an enzyme, DNA polymerase. The template is copied by the progressive separation of its two strands and the formation of a complementary strand parallel to each by the stepwise addition of the appropriate deoxyribonucleotides. The final result is that the two strands of the original template remain intact but they are separated, one being found in each daughter molecule as illustrated in FIG. 3. Nearly all of the DNA of animal cells is found in the chromosomes in the nucleus; a small quantity, of uncertain function, is in the mitochondria of the cytoplasm.

RNA has only been found in single-stranded form in normal cells although folding of the chains permits base pairing between complementary regions of a chain. Cellular RNA is synthesised with the help of the enzyme RNA polymerase which, like DNA polymerase, requires double-stranded DNA as a template. In this case only one strand of the DNA is transcribed by base-pairing into RNA and uracil replaces thymine in the new RNA strand, pairing with

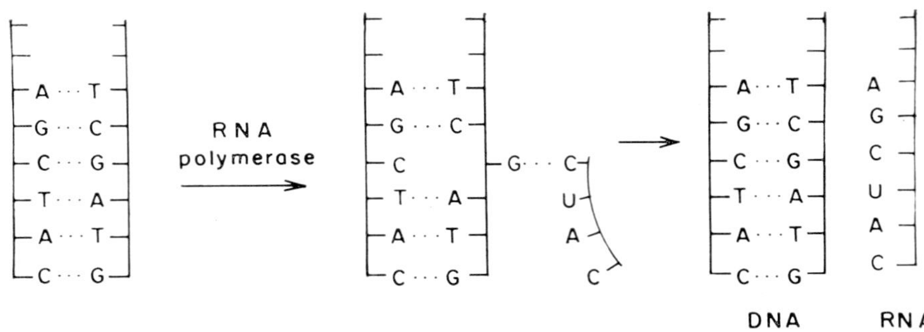

31/Fig. 4.—Mechanism of synthesis (transcription) of RNA from a DNA template. The number and exact nature of the links between the growing RNA strand and the DNA strands is not certain, but the DNA duplex finally remains intact and only one of its strands is transcribed.

adenines in the template strand of the DNA. The new RNA strand is finally released, leaving the DNA template intact as shown in Fig. 4. Most, if not all, RNA synthesis occurs on DNA templates in the nucleus of animal cells, although the bulk of the total RNA is found in the ribosomes of the cytoplasm.

The synthesis of protein, i.e. the formation of long chains of covalently linked amino-acids, requires the direction of an RNA template or message (which in turn has been transcribed from a DNA template using RNA polymerase). Before being incorporated into protein, free amino-acids are attached to RNA molecules—"transfer RNA"—and a slightly different molecule is required for each species of amino-acid. The transfer RNA acts as an adaptor or translator of the message contained in the RNA template. It probably possesses a special triplet of bases at a critical point in its structure which recognises by

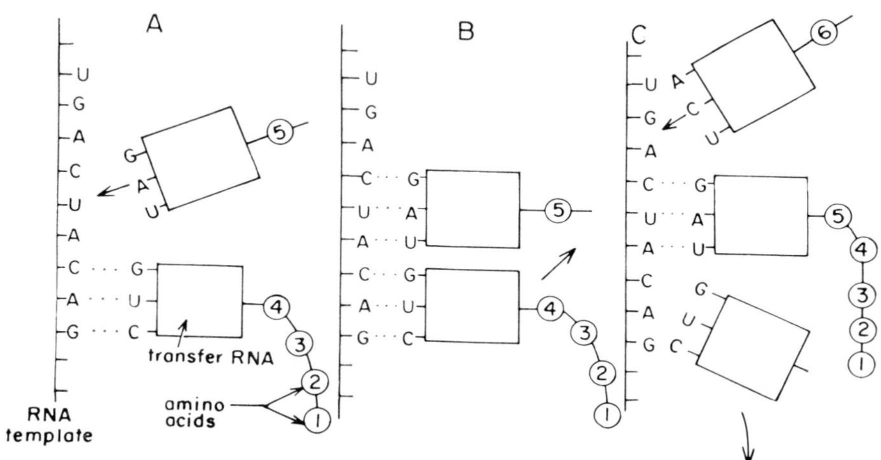

31/Fig. 5.—Mechanism of protein synthesis using an RNA template. Triplets of nucleotide bases are recognised by transfer RNA which positions the next amino-acid (A, B) in order that the growing protein chain may be linked to it (C).

base-pairing a complementary triplet in the template RNA (FIG. 5). In this way the message is read progressively from one end, probably as a series of three-letter (nucleotide) words, each being translated into a one-letter (amino-acid) word. Each amino-acid in turn appears to be linked to the growing chain as it is freed from its transfer RNA, and then the next triplet is read. The ribosomes, small particles with a complicated structure of RNA and protein, play an essential part in protein synthesis, but their exact function and relationship to the RNA message is not yet clear.

Virus Growth Cycles

We now turn to the consideration of cells infected with viruses. One principle that is probably common to all viruses is that the nucleic acid alone, if introduced intact into the host cell, can initiate infection leading to the formation of complete virus particles. All other components of the mature virus particle are concerned only with protecting the nucleic acid or assisting its penetration into the host. Thus all virus growth cycles resulting in the formation of infective progeny can be broadly divided into the following six phases:

1. *Adsorption.*—The virus must have some affinity for the host cell. Usually there are specific sites at the surface of the cell to which the virus adheres and if these are masked or changed no infection can occur. The presence or absence of specific viral receptors probably accounts for much of the host cell specificity of viruses. For example it has been shown that the host specificity of poliovirus can be altered by changing its protein coat. This was accomplished by infecting tissue culture cells "A" with poliomyelitis and Coxsackie viruses simultaneously. Coxsackie is structurally very like poliovirus, but unlike polio, is able to infect a second type of cell "B". Under the appropriate experimental conditions the doubly infected "A" cells were found to contain new virus particles composed of poliovirus RNA coated with Coxsackie virus protein. These hybrid particles, like Coxackie virus, could infect cells "B" although the progeny of such an infection were normal poliovirus particles. Thus this type of experiment (as well as earlier ones with mixed particles of tobacco mosaic virus) also demonstrates that while the protein coat controls adsorption it is the nucleic acid of the infecting virus that determines the composition of both nucleic acid and protein of the progeny. In fact it may be that any viral nucleic acid, if it could be introduced into the cell by artificial means, would direct the formation of mature progeny virus in any living cell. Of course this could only happen if the code relating nucleotide triplets to specific amino-acids is the same in all cells. There have indeed been reports of the successful infection of bacteria with the nucleic acids of animal viruses but the evidence for such phenomena cannot yet be regarded as conclusive.

2. *Penetration.*—The adsorbed virus, or at least its nucleic acid, must be able to penetrate the cell wall.

3. *Stripping.*—The outer coat or coats of the virus must be removed in order to expose the nucleic acid in a form in which it can transmit its information. This may occur simultaneously with penetration or later, inside the cell.

4. *Synthesis.*—The components needed for the construction of new virus

particles, often several hundred per infected cell, are synthesised using small precursor molecules obtained from the medium in which the cells are grown, or in some cases by the breakdown of host macromolecules.

5. *Maturation.*—The newly synthesised viral components are assembled into virus particles.

6. *Release.*—The progeny virus leaves the cell in search of another host. In some cases release rapidly follows maturation, the new virus particles leaking steadily out as they are completed. In other cases the progeny particles accumulate inside the cell until they are released in a burst at the end of the cycle as the cell disintegrates.

Two other terms are commonly used in describing the growth cycles of viruses. The early substantial loss of infectivity following adsorption, probably corresponding to stripping, is known as "eclipse". The time elapsing between eclipse and the beginning of maturation (i.e. the first appearance of new intracellular virus) is usually called the "latent period".

Particular Viruses

We will now analyse in a little more detail the growth cycles of two DNA and two RNA viruses, taking as examples a bacterial and an animal virus of each type in order to show the basic similarities between apparently quite different systems. Much information has been obtained by the study of viruses (bacteriophages or simply "phages") that attack bacteria. The advantages are that the bacterial hosts grow very quickly in suspension in liquid media, they are easily infected and rapidly produce a high yield of progeny virus which is stable and can be purified. Infectious virus particles are detected by their cell-killing ability. A mixture of bacteria and phage, appropriately diluted, is spread evenly on the surface of nutrient agar jelly. Each phage particle infects a bacterial cell and soon kills it, liberating several hundred progeny particles which diffuse to the surrounding cells and infect and kill them. The killed cells disintegrate and are no longer able to scatter light, so that after several cycles of infection, taking perhaps 8 hours, clear circular patches a millimetre or more in diameter appear in the milky white layer of bacteria. Each patch or "plaque" has been initiated by a single phage particle, and by counting the plaques the concentration of virus in the original sample can be determined and expressed as a number of plaque-forming units per millilitre. Similar techniques have more recently been developed for the study of animal virus systems. Susceptible mammalian cells are grown in tissue culture in liquid media (Fig. 6), with a generation time of about 24 hours as compared to about 1 hour for bacteria, and plaque-forming units can be detected (Fig. 7) although the plaques in this case may take several days to develop. The differences between bacterial and animal virus systems are mostly related to the host cells. The bacterial host for example has a tougher cell wall, lacks a well-defined nuclear membrane and has a higher rate of metabolism.

DNA bacteriophage.—T2 is one of a much-studied group of seven "T" (originally standing for type) phages of the colon bacillus *Escherichia coli.* They possess a distinct head and tail, both made of protein, and a single enormous molecule of double-stranded DNA is enclosed in the head. The host bacteria have a rigid cell wall surrounded by a thin lipoprotein membrane in which are found specific receptors for the adsorption of T2 (other phages adsorb at different sites and do not compete with T2). The tail of the phage consists of a central tube surrounded by a sheath with six fibres attached at its distal end (FIG. 1D). When phage particles are added to a suspension of bacteria at neutral pH and in the right salt concentration they diffuse in all directions until collision with a bacterium results in adsorption of the phage tail fibres to the host cell receptors. In general, the rate of adsorption of virus by cells is directly proportional to the concentration of cells and follows first order reaction kinetics if the number of available adsorption sites is much greater than the number of virus particles. The tail of the phage carries an enzyme, lysozyme, which attacks and weakens the rigid cell wall at the point of adsorption. Then an unknown stimulus triggers the sudden contraction of the outer sheath of the phage tail, thrusting the tip of the inner tube through the weakened wall of the bacterium. The phage DNA—tightly packed within the head—now unwinds and is threaded intact through the narrow central channel in the tail core into the host cell.

Within a few minutes of the penetration of the phage DNA the synthesis of bacterial RNA and protein stops and the DNA of the bacterium begins to disintegrate. After 6 minutes' incubation at 37° C. the first new phage DNA can be detected, conveniently distinguishable from cellular DNA by its possession of the unusual base hydroxymethyl cytosine. At 10 minutes new viral antigen (protein) can be detected by precipitation with specific anti-viral antiserum and the first mature plaque-forming units appear, terminating the latent period, at about 15 minutes after infection. During the early part of the latent period a small quantity of a new type of RNA is produced and a number of new enzymes concerned with nucleic acid metabolism are made. The probable sequence of events is that the infecting phage DNA acts as a template for the transcription of virus-specific RNA molecules using the pre-existing RNA polymerase enzyme of the host, as illustrated in FIG. 4. These RNA molecules carry the messages which in turn direct the synthesis (see FIG. 5) of various enzymes required for the production of new phage DNA and its precursors, and possibly also for a protein that destroys the host DNA. The infecting DNA is then copied by the mechanism previously described for cellular DNA (FIG. 3). Some of the daughter molecules are used for the transcription of further RNA templates which carry the codes for the various structural proteins of the phage. Eventually a pool of 20–30 of the giant DNA molecules accumulates and they begin to fold up into a very compact form aided by protein binders. The packing problem is considerable since a molecule 0·06 mm. (i.e. 60,000 mμ) long and 2 mμ wide has to be confined within a phage head of about 80 mμ internal diameter. Finally maturation starts as head protein molecules are assembled in regular array around the condensed DNA molecules and tail structures are built and attached.

DNA animal virus.—Vaccinia virus (as well as infecting cows, amongst other animals, and giving them cow-pox) will multiply in cultured human cells known as HeLa, a much more convenient system for the study of growth mechanisms. The nucleic acid of vaccinia is similar to that of T2, a double-stranded DNA molecule of molecular weight about $1{\cdot}6 \times 10^8$ daltons (T2 DNA is about $1{\cdot}3 \times 10^8$), and so we may expect a basic similarity in the growth mechanisms of the two viruses although they differ greatly in structure (FIGS. 1C, 1D). The DNA of vaccinia comprises only about 6 per cent of its weight, the rest being made up of lipid materials (6 per cent) and protein (88 per cent) whereas T2 is composed of approximately 50 per cent DNA and 50 per cent protein.

The first obvious difference between the growth cycles of the two viruses is in the mechanisms of adsorption and penetration. Vaccinia has no tail for adsorption nor apparatus for injection of its DNA. Such complicated machinery is unnecessary because of the ability of animal cells to engulf and absorb particulate matter from the surrounding medium. The virus adsorbs to the cell surface, probably attached by magnesium ion bridges, and is taken intact into the cell by an invagination of the cell wall. Stripping of the DNA occurs in two stages. The first stage appears to be mediated by a cellular enzyme, present at the time of infection, which breaks down the outer coat of lipid and protein. The second stage, however, is prevented if an inhibitor of protein synthesis is added at the time of infection—it presumably depends upon the formation of a new protein. It has been suggested that a component of the virus liberated during the first stage of stripping induces the production of a cellular enzyme which catalyses the second stage. Such a mechanism would explain the observation that although virus particles that have been heated before infection do not undergo the second stage of uncoating, if a normal particle of a related but distinguishable strain of virus is present in the same cell both normal and heated viruses proceed to multiply. The heated virus yields an inactive inducing component but if a normal particle is present the enzyme which it induces acts on the partly stripped heated virus also and both grow.

The whole of the growth cycle is far slower than in the case of bacteriophage. Penetration and uncoating occupy the first hour at 37° C. during which time the rate of cellular DNA synthesis in the nucleus falls markedly, possibly also in response to the early liberation of viral protein. The first new viral DNA is detected in the cytoplasm at about 2 hours but new infective particles do not appear until 7 hours after the initiation of infection and increase to a maximum at about 20 hours.

A new type of RNA is made in the cytoplasm of the cell from $1\frac{1}{2}$ hours after infection. This synthesis is distinct from the essentially nuclear RNA synthesis occurring within the normal cell and probably represents transcription of viral messenger RNA from the infecting DNA. It is presumably catalysed, as in the case of phage T2, by a pre-existing cellular RNA polymerase or else by an enzyme carried into the cell by the virus itself. The resulting RNA templates direct the synthesis of new enzymes, including a new DNA polymerase, enabling replication of the viral DNA to start in the cytoplasm. The initiation of DNA synthesis is in turn the signal for the cessation of early enzyme synthesis—if DNA synthesis is inhibited, enzyme formation continues uninterrupted. Presumably other RNA templates, including those transcribed from progeny DNA molecules, direct the production of structural components. Virus particles are assembled and finally released when the cell disintegrates as a result of the drastic interference with its own metabolism.

RNA bacteriophage.—All the RNA-containing phages of *E. coli* so far isolated (such as phages f2, MS2, R17) are small and spherical in shape, about 24 mμ in diameter, tailless and contain a single strand of RNA of molecular weight about 1×10^6. They will infect only male bacteria because they can adsorb only to a special type of fibre found exclusively on male cells. This is probably the same fibre by which the male forms a link with a female cell and along which the male chromosome passes into the female during mating. The adsorbed virus is thought to release its RNA into the central channel of the fibre whence it passes into the male bacterium. For a brief period as it passes from its protective coat to the safe interior of the host cell the viral RNA is susceptible to attack by added (i.e. extracellular) ribonuclease, an enzyme which catalyses the breakdown of naked RNA. The cell now contains a foreign RNA template which insinuates itself into the bacterial protein-making apparatus and codes the synthesis of virus-specific proteins. The only one that has so far been identified apart from virus coat protein is a new RNA polymerase, which helps catalyse the replication of the viral RNA by a process which seems to be unlike any occurring in the normal cell as it involves the copying of an RNA template (the viral RNA) without the participation of DNA. It is known that a double-stranded form of RNA with complementary base pairing can be extracted from infected cells. The new polymerase first makes a (minus) strand complementary to the infecting viral (plus) strand and then new plus strands are built on this double-stranded template, each newly synthesised plus strand displacing its predecessor into free single-stranded form. The viral RNA is made up of some 3,000 nucleotides which, if it is all used as template for protein synthesis at a ratio of 3 nucleotides per amino-acid, would be enough to define protein molecules with a combined molecular weight of about 120,000. The main coat protein (molecular weight 14,000), a stabilising structural protein (about 35,000) and the viral RNA polymerase, of uncertain size, probably represent the total information carried by this relatively small RNA molecule.

Coat protein begins to accumulate soon after the start of RNA replication, at about 15 minutes, and the first mature plaque-forming units appear at about 25 minutes, reaching a maximum of up to 1,000 particles per cell by 60 minutes.

RNA animal virus.—The small spherical RNA-containing animal viruses are very slightly bigger than the RNA phages, 27 mμ in diameter, and contain about twice as much RNA in a single strand of molecular weight 2×10^6. Poliomyelitis virus is one of this class and like vaccinia it grows well in HeLa cells, the first progeny maturing at about 3 hours after infection, rising to several hundred plaque-forming units per cell at 6 hours.

An initial weak electrostatic attachment to the cell surface is followed by a stronger binding, reversible only at low pH, and then the virus particle is probably ingested like vaccinia before being stripped of its protein coat. Consequently, in contrast to the case of the RNA phage (above), the RNA of poliovirus is at no stage exposed to attack by extracellular ribonuclease enzyme. The earliest observed effect of infection is a fall in the rate of cellular RNA synthesis shortly followed, within the first hour, by a similar fall in protein synthesis. It has been reported that both of these effects are caused by proteins coded by the viral RNA. Soon a new RNA polymerase enzyme is produced and replication of viral RNA begins (also probably within the first hour) by the same mechanism, involving double strand formation, as in the RNA phage system. Some of the progeny RNA molecules may also express their messages, stepping up the production of viral coat protein, and finally virus particles are built up, withdrawing protein from the pool to coat the RNA molecules. This process of maturation permits "phenotypic mixing", a common phenomenon among viruses. If a cell is infected with two types of poliovirus at once (or polio and Coxsackie as mentioned above under "Adsorption") both contribute coat protein molecules to the pool and the progeny RNA molecules become coated with a mixture of both types of protein (which can be detected by their reaction with type-specific antisera).

It will be particularly interesting to know how the amounts of various viral proteins synthesised are controlled. For instance, much more coat protein seems to be made than RNA polymerase. A possible explanation is that the coat message is situated at the beginning of the viral RNA molecule and the polymerase message at the end, and that there is always a chance that some accident will prevent the reading of the entire chain from beginning to end. Or it may be that coat protein specifically suppresses the production of other viral proteins.

Clearly there are as many different growth cycles as there are viruses and susceptible cells. There are large and complicated RNA viruses, and no doubt small and relatively simple DNA viruses; there are viruses with single-stranded DNA and others with double-stranded RNA. However, the above examples illustrate many of the general principles involved and the sort of variations that may be expected.

Non-lytic Infection

The growth cycles described in the previous paragraphs are *lytic*, i.e. they result in the lysis or dissolution of the host cell. Finally we will consider briefly some cell-virus interactions which do not cause the death of the cell; instead the virus comes to terms with the cell and confers on it certain new hereditary properties. Such a situation arises when bacteria are "lysogenised" or when animal cells are "transformed" by viruses.

Lysogeny.—When a bacterial culture is infected by a "temperate" phage (such as λ), as distinct from a "virulent" phage (such as T2), a small proportion of the bacteria are not killed and in the surviving cells the DNA of the phage is inserted into the DNA of the bacterial chromosome, which is broken to accommodate it. The phage in this state is known as the *prophage*—it has no detectable infectivity and is automatically replicated every time the bacterial chromosome divides, so that the daughter cells also contain the prophage. Such cells are *lysogenic* and may be detected by virtue of the facts that (i) they appear to make a repressor substance which makes them immune to lytic infection by another phage particle of the same type as the first, and (ii) they may be *induced* by various shock treatments which probably serve to reduce the level of the repressor. The result of induction is the initiation of a lytic cycle of infection, leading to the death of the cell and the release of much progeny phage.

Sometimes the induced prophage carries with it a neighbouring section of the host's DNA, which is then built into a mature phage particle. When this particle infects and lysogenises another bacterium it brings with it, or *transduces*, the bacterial genes it has acquired, thus promoting a non-sexual type of genetic exchange.

In some cases a temperate phage confers on its host a new character which is not obviously transduced from a previous host. The process is then called simply "lysogenic conversion". A rare example of a practical use to man of a bacteriophage is the conversion of a non-toxinogenic strain of *Corynebacterium diph-*

theriæ to potentially toxin-producing forms by infection with a temperate phage. This is useful in the production of toxoid for immunisation.

Transformation.—A phenomenon that is possibly related to lysogenisation occurs when certain cultured animal cells are infected with polyoma virus, a virus which causes tumour growth in mice. A small proportion of the animal cells survive the infection but they are altered in appearance and have lost the regular growth pattern that is characteristic of normal cultured cells. Instead they grow randomly, forming piles of cells, and these *transformed* cells will initiate tumours if inoculated into animals. These phenomena are considered in more detail in a later section.

Tumours in hens and cell transformation *in vitro* are also caused by Rous sarcoma virus. This is more difficult to visualise since the virus contains RNA and not DNA—i.e. a message for protein synthesis rather than a piece of chromosome-like material. Presumably some mechanism other than direct incorporation of the viral nucleic acid into a host chromosome must operate in perpetuating the virus's influence. It has been suggested that a new virus-specific DNA is made in the infected cell and that this is then integrated, although this would involve the hitherto unknown process of RNA-directed DNA synthesis.

Having discussed the growth of viruses within individual cells we now turn to a consideration of the wider effects of infection when the host cells form part of an animal.

2. FUNDAMENTAL MECHANISMS IN VIRUS DISEASE

BY J. F. WATKINS

The pathological effects of bacterial infection arise mainly from the effects of bacterial toxins upon a variety of cells of the host. The pathological results of viral infection, on the other hand, arise partly from the effects of virus particles upon the cells they have invaded, and partly from reactions of the host. The kind of disease a particular virus infection produces in the host depends on three groups of factors:

A. The nature of viral damage in host cells.
B. The nature of virus invasion of the body.
C. The nature of the host reaction.

THE NATURE OF VIRAL DAMAGE IN HOST CELLS

This is most easily understood by considering the changes viruses produce in cells in culture. The techniques of cell culture are summarised in FIG. 6, from which it will be seen that the end-result of most techniques is the production of a monolayer of cells on a glass surface, which may be the side of a bottle or tube, or a glass coverslip. When a cell in such a monolayer is infected with a virus, one of four possible results will ensue, depending on the properties of both the virus and the cell. These results can be described by the terms degeneration, fusion, transformation, and abortive infection. The first two constitute the "cytopathogenic effect" of the virus, usually abbreviated to "CPE".

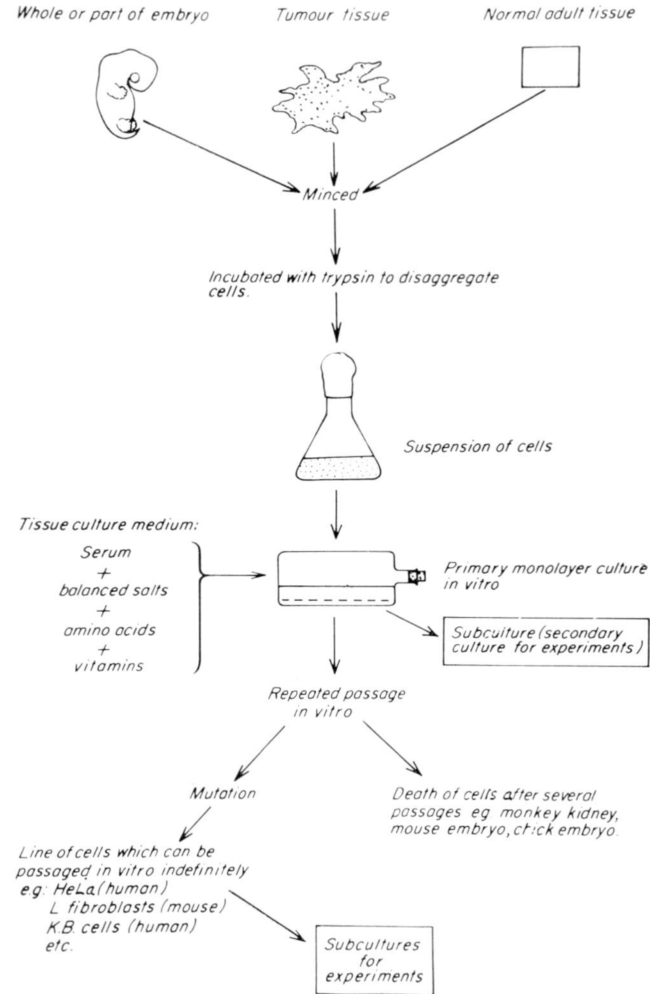

31/FIG. 6.—The basic steps involved in cell culture.

Degeneration

This is the dissolution of a cell as the result of virus development within its nucleus or cytoplasm. Important examples of rapid degeneration (often called "lysis") are given by poliomyelitis virus infection of monkey kidney cells, Coxsackie virus infection of HeLa cells, and certain arbovirus infections of chick embryo fibroblasts. Slower destruction occurs in cells infected, for example, with myxoviruses, poxviruses and adenoviruses. To the naked eye, this type of CPE appears as the removal of cells from the glass surface into the medium. An elegant demonstration of the effect of a single virus particle and its progeny upon a monolayer culture can be given by using the technique of plaque formation.[13] A cell culture growing as a monolayer in a Petri dish is infected with a highly diluted suspension of a suitable virus, which is allowed one hour to adsorb to the cells; the fluid medium is then replaced by medium mixed with agar, which sets, and the culture is incubated at 37° C for two to seven days, depending on the virus-cell system in use. A layer of agar containing neutral red, a vital dye, is then poured over the culture. The neutral red penetrates the first agar layer, and is taken up by living cells only. Circular plaques of unstained cells are seen (FIG. 7), each representing the development of a single virus particle, and invasion of the surrounding cells by its progeny, an invasion limited to contiguous cells by the agar overlay. This technique provides a highly accurate method of assaying the infectivity of a suitable virus suspension. Just as in an infected cell culture, where progeny virus can pass through the medium to infect surrounding cells, so, in virus infection of tissues, spread to neighbouring cells will occur.

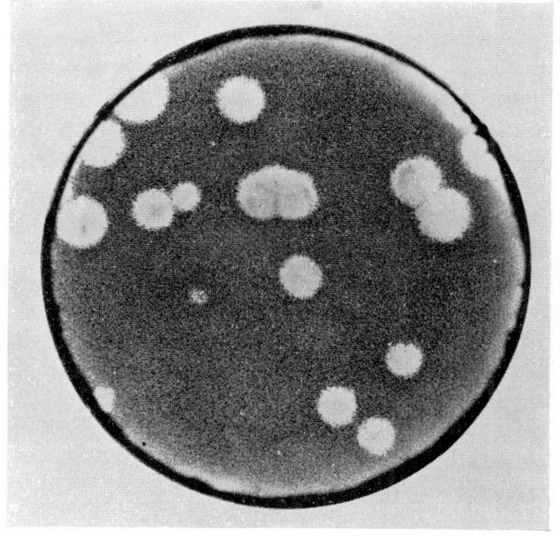

31/FIG. 7.—Plaques formed by foot-and-mouth disease virus on a monolayer of pig kidney cells. The surviving cells have taken up stain, enhancing the contrast. (By courtesy of Mr. R. Burrows, Animal Virus Research Institute, Pirbright.)

Microscopically, those infected cells which remain attached to the glass show various alterations, depending on the severity of the destructive process, and the stage of virus development which has been reached. At the end of the process the cells are degenerate, and rounded, with pyknotic nuclei, but at earlier stages of virus development the nucleus or cytoplasm may show characteristic changes. One of these changes is due to the development of "inclusion bodies", which are areas of cytoplasm or nucleus with abnormal staining properties. Examples of animal viruses which form inclusion bodies are, among RNA viruses, polimyelitis virus and yellow fever virus, which form intracytoplasmic inclusions, and, among DNA viruses, the poxviruses, which form intracytoplasmic inclusions, and adenoviruses and herpes simplex virus, which form intranuclear inclusions (FIG. 8). For many years there was discussion about what inclusion bodies represented. As a result of the application of more powerful techniques, such as electron microscopy and the use of radio-active isotopes, it has come to be recognised that in most cases inclusion bodies are the site of virus synthesis. Thus, Horne and Nagington[10], using negative staining, with phosphotungstate,

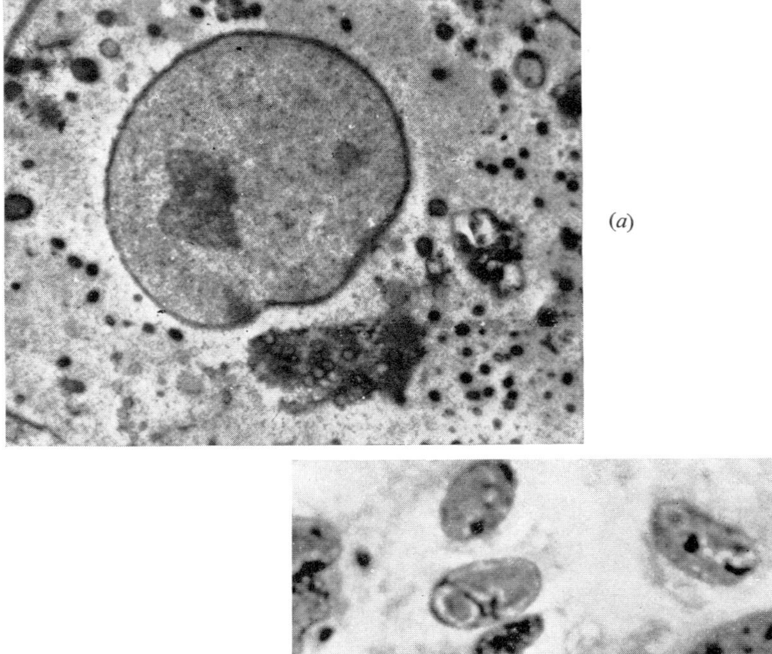

(*a*)

(*b*)

31/Fig. 8.—Inclusion Bodies in Infected Cells.

(*a*) Cell of the chick chorioallantoic membrane infected with vaccinia, showing the nucleus and a cytoplasmic site of virus production.

(*b*) Nuclear inclusion bodies in HeLa cells infected with herpes simplex virus.

of HeLa cells infected with poliomyelitis virus, were able to show the presence of virus particles in intracytoplasmic inclusions about 1 μ in diameter (Fig. 2B). Cairns[14] studied the development of vaccinia virus in KB cells, using thymidine labelled with tritium to show DNA synthesis, and fluorescent antibody to show the synthesis of virus proteins. His findings indicated that each infecting virus particle in the cytoplasm of a cell infected with several particles starts a separate centre of synthesis of DNA and protein. By about nine hours after infection the centres begin to run together. Because the vaccinia inclusions visible with the light microscope in stained cells, the so-called "Guarnieri bodies" (FIG. 8), have been shown by many workers to be Feulgen positive, and later, to contain elementary bodies, there is no reason to doubt that they represent the actual sites of virus synthesis. Similar considerations apply to the intranuclear inclusions of herpes simplex virus, which can be demonstrated by suitable fixation and staining, and of adenoviruses.

Why should a cell die as a result of virus infection? It is possible to conceive of a cell remaining alive, and growing, with a virus multiplying in its cytoplasm or nucleus, and examples of this kind of coexistence can be found. Several biochemical consequences of viral infection are known which show at least what sort of disturbance could kill the cell. For example, Baltimore and Franklin[15] have shown that mengovirus shuts off RNA synthesis in L cells within minutes of infection, probably by coding for a non-structural virus protein that inhibits DNA-dependent RNA polymerase. Poliomyelitis virus has been shown to produce a similar effect. Other experiments suggest that the cytopathic effect of poliomyelitis virus depends on the synthesis of viral capsid proteins, and that the effect of these proteins on the cell is manifest an appreciable time before the inhibition of RNA synthesis alone could cause death. There is evidence-that structural components of mature poliomyelitis virus may inhibit cellular RNA and protein synthesis when cells are infected with very large amounts of virus, and viral RNA synthesis is prevented by guanidine, an inhibitor of poliomyelitis virus growth[16]. Adenoviruses have a toxic effect on HeLa cells which appears long before the virus has completed its growth cycle[17]; this effect appears to be due to a cytotoxic protein which inhibits the synthesis of macromolecules by the cell. The effects of infection of rabbit kidney cells with pseudorabies virus, a member of the herpes group, have been studied by Kaplan and co-workers.[18] They found that infection was followed by a progressive decrease in cellular DNA synthesis, accompanied by a progressive increase in viral DNA synthesis; there was also evidence that specific proteins, synthesised between 4 and 7 hours after infection, caused a leakage of protein from the cell. The killing of a cell by a virus may therefore be a complex process, involving interference with several cellular mechanisms.

Fusion

Many viruses display a cytopathogenic effect which enables them to infect a neighbouring cell without passing to the exterior. A cell infected in culture with such a virus develops, during the latent period, the ability to fuse with its uninfected neighbour, so that progeny virus can pass directly into fresh cytoplasm. This process may continue in the cell culture until a syncytium is formed, which may have hundreds of nuclei. Eventually the multinucleate cell will degenerate and come off the glass. Herpes simplex, measles, varicella and parainfluenza 1 are some of the viruses which show this phenomenon in culture. An illustration of a syncytium formed by herpes simplex virus in HeLa cells is given in FIG. 9. The process of infection in the recruited cells is the same as in the primarily infected cell, with intranuclear inclusion formation in the case of herpes simplex virus. The property of forming multinucleate cells may not be present in all strains of a particular virus, and variants which have lost the ability to cause fusion can often be isolated from giant-cell forming strains.

The mechanism of virus-induced fusion is unknown. Fusion may at times occur between uninfected cells. For example, the Langhans giant cells seen in tuberculous lesions are formed by fusion of macrophages; binucleated cells, probably formed by fusion, are seen in regenerating rat liver after damage with carbon tetrachloride. Phagocytosis, or pinocytosis, involves a local fusion of two arms of cytoplasm to form a vesicle. The effect of infection with certain

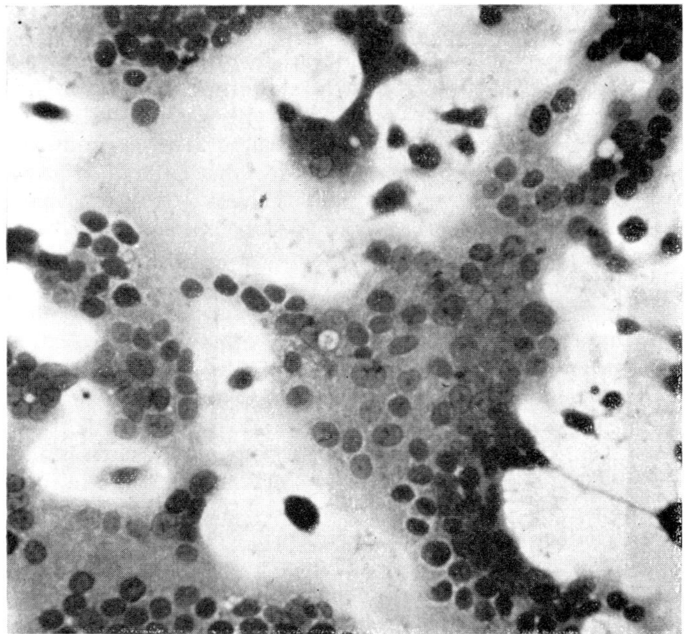

31/FIG. 9.—Syncytium formed by fusion of HeLa cells infected with herpes simplex virus.

viruses may therefore be to accentuate, or unmask, a normal property of the plasma membrane; or the virus may bring about fusion by some mechanism quite different from that in normal cells. Fusion of cells after infection with herpes simplex virus occurs about four hours before new virus can be detected, so that the phenomenon is not due to the direct action of virus particles on the cell surfaces involved. If viral DNA synthesis is inhibited by 5-iodo-2-deoxyuridine, an analogue of thymidine, no fusion occurs, although virus capsids are formed. This suggests that progeny DNA is important in fusion, possibly by coding for late proteins which affect the cell surface. Evidence from several sources suggests that the breakdown of lysosomes, with release of enzymes such as phosphatases, may be involved in fusion.

Multinucleate cells are not confined to cell cultures. They can also be found, for example, in the vesicles of herpes simplex infection. Their possible significance in the pathology of virus disease is discussed below.

Transformation

The discovery that cells in culture could develop new properties as a result of infection with certain viruses arose from the study of virus-induced tumours in animals. Since such tumours are discussed elsewhere, this account of transformation will ignore the historical sequence of events, and deal with transformation as simply another form of *in vitro* cell-virus interaction. In cell cultures transformation is detected by a change in the morphology and growth characteristics of cells, and in the whole animal by the production of tumours, from which *in vitro* cultures can be derived. As a rule, no infectious virus can be detected in transformed cells. Transformed cell lines have been produced by polyoma virus, certain adenoviruses, and a virus isolated from primary cultures of monkey kidney, in which it produced vacuolisation of cells, which led to its being called "Simian vacuolating agent". As it was the fortieth of many vacuolating agents it is now called by the abbreviation, "SV40" (see ref. 19 for a review). Certain RNA tumour viruses, such as Rous sarcoma virus, can also produce transformation in cell cultures.

All the important facts about transformation can be illustrated by a summary of the results obtained with polyoma virus. This virus was isolated by Gross in 1953 (see ref. 20), from inbred mice which had a high incidence of leukæmia. The virus was not responsible for the leukæmia, but its injection into suckling mice led to the development of a variety of tumours. Other workers found that the virus would grow in mouse embryo cells in culture, producing degenerative changes. Stewart and Eddy christened the virus "polyoma". Transformation of cells in culture by the virus was first described by Vogt and Dulbecco,[21] who infected secondary hamster embryo cells with large amounts of virus. The cells were not destroyed by the virus, which did not multiply, and heavy whorls of cells, made up of many layers, developed within a few weeks of infection. With passage, these cells gradually replaced the original cells. The transformed cells were more elongated than normal, grew in a random, criss-cross pattern, unlike normal cells, which were aligned in parallel bundles, and gave rise to tumours when injected into isogenic hamsters. No infectious virus could be found in the cells or the culture medium, and no infectious DNA could be isolated from the cells. Treatment of the cells by methods known to cause reactivation of lysogenic bacteriophage (see *Lysogeny*, above) failed to induce the production of infectious virus, and no virus capsid protein could be detected by fluorescent antibody. Recently, however, the presence of complete viral DNA in cells transformed by polyoma or SV40 virus has been demonstrated by biochemical methods.[35] Infectious SV40 virus has been recovered from several transformed lines by cell hybridisation.[36]

Many workers have shown that some at least of the properties of transformed cells are produced by information present in the viral genome. Adult hamsters show no ill effects after inoculation with infectious polyoma virus, but develop antibodies to the virus. These immunised animals do not develop tumours after injection of suitable numbers of isogenic transformed cells, indicating that the transformed cells are rejected because they have a "transplantation" antigen. Sera from tumour-bearing hamsters can detect a nuclear antigen in transformed mouse embryo cells when employed in fluorescent antibody or complement-fixation techniques. This nuclear antigen has been called the "T" antigen. The simplest explanation for these findings is that at least some of the virus genome is present in the transformed cells, where it controls the synthesis of at least two new proteins. The relationship between these proteins and transformation is still an open question.

Abortive Infection

This result of some virus-cell associations is included in order to emphasise the fact that all cells do not support growth of all viruses. Failure of a virus to produce any infectious progeny in cells may arise from a failure to penetrate, as with poliomyelitis virus and L strain mouse fibroblasts, or from failure of complete virus to develop once its nucleic acid has entered the cell. The ability, or inability, or a virus to develop in lines of cells defines the "host range" of the virus. Some virus components may be synthesised during abortive infection, and cells may show signs of damage. For example, Aurelian and Roizman[22] described the results of infection of dog kidney cells in culture with large inocula of herpes simplex virus. The cells produced viral antigen, interferon, and small amounts of DNA characteristic of herpes DNA, but no particles with the physical characteristics of herpes simplex virus. The cells showed some signs of infection, such as rounding and cell fusion, and there was a reduction in the numbers of cells able to multiply. Influenza virus in HeLa cells is another example of abortive infection. After large inocula cell damage is produced, and viral antigens can be detected.[23]

The pathological significance of abortive infection is that cells which cannot support virus growth may nevertheless be damaged or destroyed by infectious virus which has been produced by susceptible cells elsewhere in the body.

The Nature of Virus Invasion

The surface of the body, for the purposes of discussing infection, can be considered as composed of those cells which are accessible to direct attack from the environment. Not only the skin, but also the entire linings of the alimentary tract, the respiratory system, and the urogenital system are, in this sense, parts of the body surface. The cross-section of an idealised animal body shown in Fig. 10 makes this clear. Within the body the cardiovascular and lymphatic systems can be considered as two interconnected cavities; the cerebrospinal fluid is contained in a cavity separate from these. The rest of the body is composed of the cells which make up the various organs and tissues. In order to infect the body a virus particle must begin by infecting surface cells, or by being injected through the body surface by, for example, a mosquito bite. The infection may be limited to the surface, or the virus may pass, *via* the lymphatic system and the blood, to the cells of the various organs. The latter course of events may be termed "sequential infection", since a sequence of viral growth cycles is required before the characteristic pathology of the disease develops. A classification of viruses of man, according to whether they usually set up a surface or sequential infection, is given in Table II. It should be added that in theory, and occasionally in fact, a virus which usually sets up a surface infection may go on to set up a

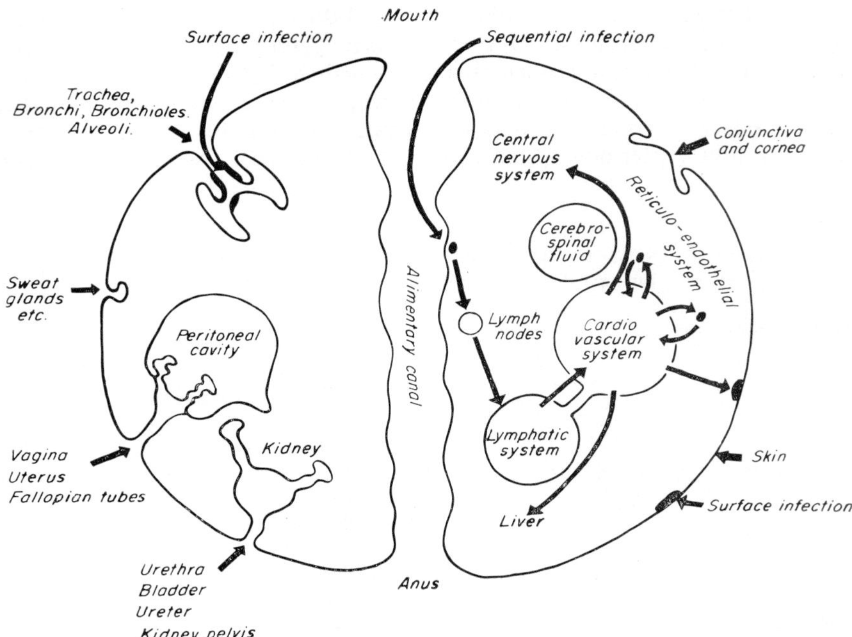

31/FIG. 10.—Cross-section of an idealised animal body, to illustrate the notion of "surface" and "sequential" infection.

sequential infection, and a virus which requires sequential infection to produce its characteristic disease may fail, for several reasons, to penetrate beyond the surface. Thus, from the time of the initial invasion to the time when there is sufficient destruction of target cells to produce the symptoms of a particular disease, there will be a period of time varying from a few days, in surface infections, to many days, even weeks or months, in sequential infections. This period is called the "incubation period" of the disease.

These generalisations may now be illustrated by some specific examples.

Influenza

This disease is caused by influenza virus of man, a member of the Myxovirus group. The envelope of influenza virus consists of lipoprotein, some at least of which is probably of host cell origin, together with an enzyme, neuraminidase, whose substrate is neuraminic acid, a component of the sialic acids which form the prosthetic group of many mucoproteins of the cell surface. Because of its ability to agglutinate erythrocytes of chickens and some other species, by adsorbing to the neuraminic acid on their surfaces, with consequent linking together of individual erythrocytes to form clumps, this component of the virus envelope is called "hæmagglutinin". When the virus has been inhaled it adsorbs to the sialic acid receptors on the surfaces of cells lining the upper respiratory tract, the trachea, and the larger bronchi. The RNA-protein helix then enters the cytoplasm, possibly by phagocytosis, possibly by fusion of the viral envelope with the cell membrane. There follows a period during which the viral RNA is replicated in the cell nucleus, and the viral hæmagglutinin is made in the cytoplasm. The components are assembled at the cell surface, which, at the end of the latent period, contains the hæmagglutinin, and complete virus is released from the cell by a process of budding. The result is death of the cell about twenty-four hours after adsorption of virus to its surface. The progeny virus is

31/TABLE II

SOME VIRUSES INFECTING MAN, ARRANGED ACCORDING TO WHETHER THE "TYPICAL" DISEASE INVOLVES SURFACE OR SEQUENTIAL INFECTION

1. **Surface infections**

Target cells	*Virus*
Skin	Molluscum contagiosum
	Wart
	Herpes simplex
Oropharynx and nasopharynx	Some Coxsackie A types
	Common cold viruses
	Influenza
	Adenovirus
Respiratory epithelium	Influenza
	(Psittacosis and related "viruses")
Alimentary epithelium	Echovirus
	Reovirus
Conjunctiva and cornea	Adenovirus
	Herpes simplex
	(Trachoma)
Urogenital tract	None known

2. **Sequential infections**

Target organ	*Route of entry*	*Virus*
C.N.S.	Alimentary epithelium	Poliomyelitis
		Coxsackie virus
	Skin (monkey bite)	Herpes B.
	Skin (animal bite)	Rabies
	Skin (arthropod bite)	Arbovirus types
	Unknown	Herpes zoster (varicella)
Liver	Alimentary epithelium	Infectious hepatitis
	Skin (mosquito bite)	Yellow fever
Myocardium	Alimentary epithelium	Coxsackie B types
Skin	Oropharynx	Smallpox
		Measles
		Rubella (German measles)
Lymphoid-macrophage system	Unknown	Glandular fever

then carried through the mucus lining the respiratory tract, a process probably facilitated by its neuraminidase, until it can enter another healthy cell. In this way many respiratory epithelial cells are killed. Death of cells triggers the development of acute inflammation in the lining of the respiratory tract, and provides an area in which secondary infection with such bacteria as *Staphylococcus aureus* can occur. The process is brought to an end by processes which are discussed in a later section. There is no evidence of productive infection of cells outside the respiratory epithelium during an attack of influenza. The generalized, toxic symptoms which occur during the disease have been attributed to abortive infection of cells elsewhere in the body by virus which has entered the blood stream. Influenza thus displays the characteristics of an almost pure surface infection, with a short incubation period of one or two days.

Poliomyelitis

The pathogenesis of this disease has largely been determined by studies in chimpanzees by Sabin and Bodian, and their co-workers. The subject has been reviewed by Westwood.[24] As the disease in chimpanzees is similar to that in man, the probable sequence of events in the latter species can be described with confidence. After the virus has been ingested it adsorbs to cells lining the ileum and possibly also the oropharynx, and enters the cells, probably by phagocytosis. Multiplication in these cells is followed by spread to neighbouring epithelial cells, and possibly lymphoid cells in the Peyer's patches, so that a surface infection is set up. At this stage virus can pass into the environment by excretion in the fæces. Pharyngitis and slight pyrexia may also occur. Virus then passes to the regional lymph nodes, where another cycle of infection occurs, and then to the blood, to produce viræmia. By spreading in the blood stream virus reaches systemic lymph nodes and the brown fat depots, and undergoes more cycles of replication. The infection frequently goes no further, but occasionally virus passes, *via* the blood stream or along nerves, to the anterior horn cells of the spinal cord. Virus replication in the motor neurones leads to a series of cytological changes including chromatolysis, or dissolution of the Nissl granules, pyknosis of nuclei, and sometimes development of inclusion bodies, ending with death of the cell and loss of function. There is evidence that the process may not go to completion in all affected motor neurones, in which case the cell may recover normal function. For the development of paralytic poliomyelitis, therefore, a sequence of developmental cycles is required. This explains the long incubation period of the disease, which ranges from 7 to 20 days, with a median value of 12 days.

Smallpox

The understanding of this disease has been increased by the studies of Fenner[25] on an analogous disease of mice, called ectromelia. He injected ectromelia virus into the foot-pads of mice, and followed its appearance in various organs. His findings are summarised in FIG. 11. In smallpox the initial invasion probably occurs in the nasopharynx, where multiplication of virus must be minimal, because no symptoms are produced. Virus then passes to the regional lymph nodes, where multiplication occurs, then to the reticulo-endothelial system *via* the blood (primary viræmia). After another cycle of multiplication in cells of the reticulo-endothelial system virus enters the blood stream again (secondary viræmia), and is carried to the skin, mucous membranes and other organs. When the virus reaches the skin, about twelve days after the initial infection, multiplication in epithelial cells produces foci of necrotic cells and vesicle formation.

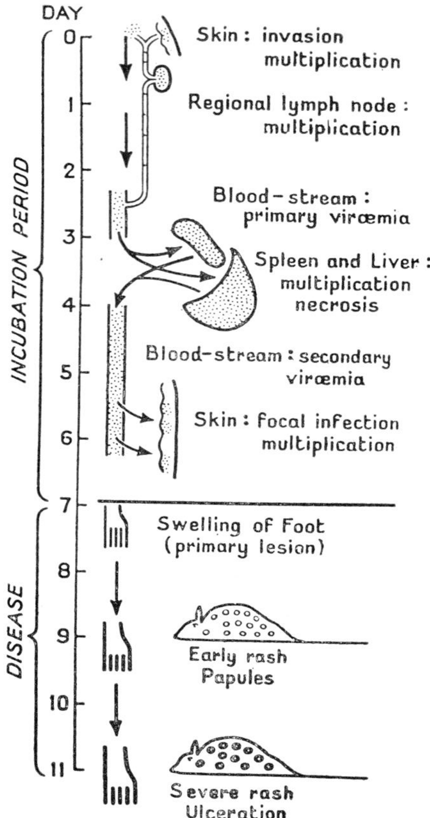

31/FIG. 11.—The spread of ectromelia in the mouse. (From Fenner.[25])

These foci constitute the rash of smallpox, and are also the means of release of virus into the environment.

Rabies

This disease illustrates another kind of sequential infection. The virus is introduced into the body by the bite of a rabid animal, which secretes virus in its saliva. It probably multiplies locally, and then travels along the nerves to the central nervous system, where invasion of cells leads to an encephalitis and the appearance of the characteristic symptoms. There is some evidence that the virus can spread from the brain by the peripheral nerves, to set up focal infections in muscles and salivary glands. The incubation period is usually about 8 weeks, but may be as long as a year, and is probably determined by the distance between the entry wound and the central nervous system.

Yellow Fever

Virus is introduced into the body by the bite of an infected mosquito. There may be some multiplication at the site of infection, followed by spread to lymph nodes and the blood stream. The target organ is the liver, in which the virus produces foci of mid-zonal necrosis of parenchymal cells, often with characteristic inclusions.

The Nature of the Host Reaction

The pathology of a virus disease depends, as we have seen, on the type of damage the virus produces in host cells, and on whether invasion is limited to surface cells, or a sequential infection develops. The extent of the damage caused by the first factor, and the ability of a virus to spread beyond the body surface will obviously depend, not only upon its own properties, but also upon the reactions which infection triggers in the host. These reactions, and the way in which they influence viral infection, will now be discussed.

Antibody Formation

Neutralising antibody.—The proteins which form the virus capsid and envelope are treated like any other proteins by the immunological mechanisms of the body; that is, they are antigens, and provoke the formation of antibodies. The sources of the viral antigen may be virus particles which have been phagocytosed by insusceptible phagocytes, virus particles which have lost their infectivity before they can enter susceptible cells, or non-infectious virus material which is produced by infected cells, by errors of translation or assembly, at the same time as they produce infectious virus. Thus, if serum is taken from a convalescent patient, and mixed with a suspension of the virus which caused the disease, the treated virus is unable to infect experimental systems, such as cell cultures, fertile hens' eggs, or animals, in which the untreated virus can produce characteristic changes, or death. Such a serum is said to contain "Neutralising Antibody". The most important single fact for understanding the role of neutralising antibody in disease is that if virus is added to susceptible cells before the addition of antibody, the cells will be infected, but if antiserum is added before virus, infection will not occur. In other words antibody cannot neutralise virus once the latter has entered the cell. FIGURE 12 shows a HeLa cell culture

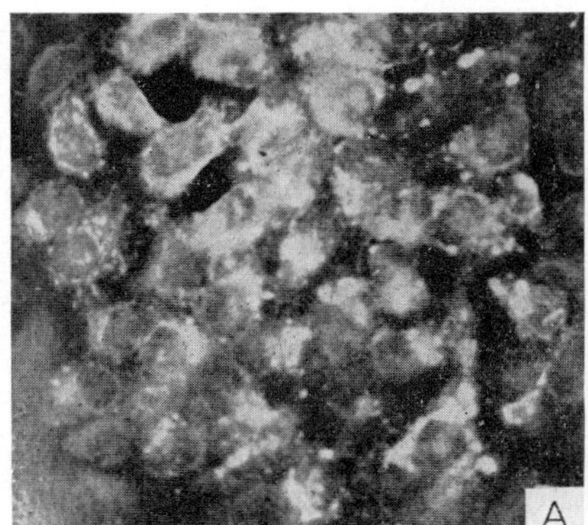

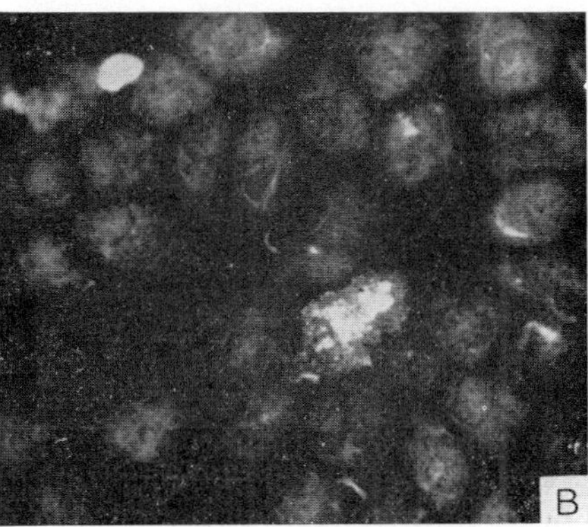

31/FIG. 12.—Inhibition of the spread of Newcastle disease virus in the presence of neutralising antibody 24 hours after infection of a monolayer of HeLa cells. (*A*) Cluster of infected cells to which virus has spread from a single central infected cell. Viral antigen is detected by its attachment of fluorescent antibody. (*b*) Similar culture infected and then incubated in the presence of anti-viral serum. The virus has remained localised in the isolated cell originally infected. (From Wheelock and Tamm.[26])

infected with Newcastle Disease virus of fowls, and subsequently incubated in the presence or absence of neutralizing antibody.[26] Infected cells were detected by fluorescent anti-viral antibody. In the presence of antibody cell-to-cell spread did not occur, since progeny virus was immediately neutralised, and the only cell showing evidence of virus growth was the one infected before the addition of antiserum. Prevention of virus spread in this way can obviously contribute to recovery from virus disease, but, as we shall see later, recovery is not a simple process completely explicable by the action of antibody. In addition, it should be borne in mind that many cells will be irreversibly damaged before blood levels of antibody are high enough to prevent cell-to-cell spread. By the time clinical symptoms appear, such as paralysis in poliomyelitis, or a rash in the viral exanthemata, or jaundice in yellow fever, most of the cells liable to infection have been infected. The appearance of neutralising antibody in the blood, as a result of its formation, or passive introduction as pooled gamma-globulin, or convalescent serum, will not be of much help to the patient. On the other hand, if large amounts of neutralising antibody are given early in the incubation period, before virus has reached the target organ, the progress of the disease may be interrupted.

Since antibodies cannot reach infected surface cells until some degree of increased capillary permeability has been produced by an inflammatory reaction, one might predict that prophylactic active immunisation against such diseases will not be completely effective, and would be more likely to produce an attenuated form of the disease than to prevent it altogether. This is indeed the case. On the other hand, since sequential infections require a viræmic phase for development of the disease, in which virus will come into immediate contact with antibodies, one might predict that active immunisation against such diseases will be highly effective, and this prediction is also correct.

Some viruses can cause persistent infection in the presence of large amounts of circulating antibody. These viruses have the property of causing the cell which they infect initially to fuse with its neighbours, so that progeny virus can pass directly into fresh cytoplasm. One such virus is herpes simplex, whose persistence is shown by the recurrence of vesicles ("cold sores"), usually at mucocutaneous junctions, such as the lips, in individuals with neutralising antibody in their blood. Limited spread by giant-cell formation may explain this "latent infection". Measles, mumps and varicella (chickenpox) viruses can also provoke giant-cell formation, and it is possible that a continued latent infection of the kind described may be responsible for the lifelong immunity observed after infection by these viruses. It has been conjectured that varicella virus may persist in dorsal root ganglia, since herpes zoster ("shingles"), which is caused by varicella virus, can occur, possibly as a recrudescence of a latent infection, many years after an attack of chickenpox.

In addition to their formation in virus disease, neutralising antibodies can be produced by active immunisation with inactivated, or live attenuated virus. The commonest inactivating agent is formalin, which destroys the ability of viruses to multiply, without affecting the antigenicity of the proteins involved in neutralization. Attenuated viruses are obtained from virulent strains by selection of mutant strains which have lost the invasive powers of the wild-type, while retaining its antigenicity. The use of attenuated strains has the advantage that the immunising dose is greatly increased by the limited multiplication of the virus. Inactivated viruses used for immunisation include poliomyelitis, influenza and rabies viruses. Live attenuated viruses include poliomyelitis, vaccinia, yellow fever and measles. For reasons given above, active immunisation is useless once infection has started, except in rabies. Because the incubation period of this disease is so long, active immunisation with killed virus may produce sufficient antibody before the virus reaches the central nervous system to prevent the spread of virus once it has reached the target cells.

Neutralising antibody is like any other antibody, in that neutralising activity is found in the gamma-globulin fraction of the serum proteins. If the serum is further fractionated by ultra-centrifugation, neutralising antibody can be found in the 19S macroglobulin (IgM), the 7S globulin (IgG), and in a heterogeneous group of molecules in the 7S to 15S fractions. The latter group has been designated as IgA antibody. Neutralising activity may not appear in all fractions simultaneously. For example, 19S neutralising antibody to poliomyelitis virus appeared in rabbits within about 8 to 12 hours after inoculation.[27] In studies on human volunteers experimentally infected with adenoviruses, IgM, IgG, and IgA neutralising antibodies appeared at about the same time, one to three weeks after infection.[28] IgG and IgA antibody persisted for at least fifty weeks in one of the volunteers. IgM antibody persisted for 14 weeks in volunteers inoculated with live virus, but only 4 weeks after inoculation with viral protein alone. Tokumaru[29] found that the initial response to herpes simplex infection was characterised by an early increase in IgM antibody, followed in about 3 weeks by a predominance of IgG and IgA. IgA antibody has biological properties differing from those of IgM and IgG antibodies, in that it appears in higher concentrations in nasal and parotid secretions, and colostrum. Skin sensitising antibodies (reagins) are found exclusively in the IgA fraction. The general picture that emerges from these and similar studies may be expressed, for didactic purposes, as follows: IgM neutralising antibody appears before, or simultaneously with, IgG and IgA antibodies, depending upon the species studied. It persists only as long as viral antigen is present in the animal, so that inactivated virus only elicits temporary synthesis, while live virus leads to prolonged formation. IgG and IgA neutralising antibodies may persist for at least a year, even when immunisation is carried out with inactivated virus. IgA antibody is more variable in its appearance than IgG, and may only be produced in low titres, or not at all, in some individuals. It may play an important role in protecting mucous membranes from infection.

The precise mechanism by which neutralising antibody prevents infection is not known. It does not simply prevent adsorption of virus to the cell surface, by coating binding sites in the viral capsid or envelope, because virus which has adsorbed to cells may still be neutralised by the addition of antiserum. Insusceptibility of adsorbed virus to neutralisation is taken to indicate that virus has penetrated the cell. Thus, the antibody attached to a virus particle may prevent penetration by inhibiting phagocytosis or, if the virus-antibody complex can enter the cell, antibody may somehow inhibit the breakdown of the viral capsid, and so prevent release of nucleic acid into the cytoplasm.

Serological typing of viruses can be carried out with neutralising antibody. For example, adenoviruses have a common antigen which can be detected by complement-fixation tests, but antibody to one strain of adenovirus may not neutralise another strain. By performing cross-neutralisation tests adenoviruses can be subdivided into several antigenic types whose biological properties may also differ. Poliomyelitis virus can be divided into three types, so that antibody against one type will not neutralise the other two. For this reason poliomyelitis vaccines must contain all three types. Influenza viruses of man can be subdivided by complement-fixation tests into three groups, A, B and C. Viruses in Group A can be subdivided into three types, A, A1 and A2, by using the fact that neutralising antibody against one type will inhibit agglutination of fowl erythrocytes by that type (hæmagglutination-inhibition), but not by the other two types.

Complement-fixing antibody.—If a suspension of virus particles is used as the antigen, neutralising antibody will, of course, show complement-fixation in a complement-fixation test. But viruses may contain several different proteins, all of which will elicit antibodies. Many of these antibodies are not capable of neutralising, since they are not specific for the proteins in the virus coat which are involved in the neutralisation reaction. Such antibodies can be detected by complement-fixation with fractions of virus ("soluble antigens") as antigens, and they may be important in the serological typing of viruses. As there is no evidence that such antibodies are important in understanding the pathology of virus disease, they will not be discussed further.

Interferon

In 1957, Isaacs and Lindenmann[30] reported a curious observation they had made while studying viral interference, which is the inhibition of multiplication of a virus by previous or simultaneous treatment with certain other viruses, which may be infective or inactivated. They added heat-inactivated Influenza A virus to pieces of chorio-allantoic membrane in a culture medium, and incubated the mixture overnight. Next day the medium from the treated chorio-allantoic membranes was removed and added to fresh chorio-allantoic membrane, together with infective influenza virus. When the second mixture was incubated it was found that no multiplication of virus occurred, although the virus multiplied in chorio-allantoic membranes in normal culture medium. That is to say, the medium in which the chorio-allantoic membrane and heated virus had been incubated contained a substance, or substances, which could prevent the development of influenza virus in susceptible cells. Isaacs and Lindenmann named this material "Interferon".

Subsequent studies by many workers have shown that interferon is a low molecular-weight protein which is produced by cells in response to a large number of substances, including RNA and DNA viruses, bacterial cells and endotoxins, rickettsiæ, nucleic acids, and a polyanionic polysaccharide called "statolon". Interferon is produced not only by cells treated with virus inactivated by ultraviolet light, heat, or formalin, but also by cells infected with viruses. Interferon produced by one type of virus will inhibit replication of a number of unrelated viruses. That is, it is not virus-specific. On the other hand, while interferon made in the cells of one species will inhibit viral multiplication in other cells from the same species, it will not, in general, inhibit multiplication in the cells of other species. That is, it is host-specific. Interferon does not affect extracellular virus, virus adsorption, intracellular release of viral nucleic acid from its protein coat, or virus release. Studies with inhibitors of DNA, RNA and protein synthesis have shown that cellular DNA-directed RNA synthesis is required for interferon formation, and indicate that interferon, in turn, induces the synthesis of a second protein, which is ultimately responsible for the inhibition of viral growth in cells treated with interferon. The subject has been reviewed by Wagner.[31]

A hypothesis to explain the action of interferon has been put forward recently by Marcus and Salb.[32] These workers isolated ribosomes from normal chick embryo cells and from chick embryo cells which had been treated with interferon. They then studied the complexes (polysomes) formed between these ribosomes and RNA from Sindbis virus or normal cell "messenger" RNA. The evidence suggested that viral RNA could be translated in polysomes formed with ribosomes from normal cells, but not in polysomes formed with ribosomes from interferon-treated cells. Normal chick messenger RNA, on the other hand, could be translated in polysomes formed with ribosomes from both sources. They suggest that the second protein induced by interferon is a "translation inhibitory protein", which functions by binding to ribosomes and inhibiting translation of viral RNA, while permitting translation of cell messenger RNA. While this hypothesis may some day have to be changed, it has the merit of being the only one in existence which relates the action of interferon to current ideas about cellular control mechanisms. It leaves unanswered the questions of how viruses induce the formation of interferon, and how interferon induces the synthesis of the translation inhibitory protein.

Studies on whole animals, usually mice, indicate that circulating interferon appears in the serum after intravenous or intrapulmonary injection of large doses of certain viruses. Passively injected, or actively induced, interferon has been found to protect mice against challenge with certain arboviruses and vaccinia virus. Interferon has been found in the serum of humans after viral infection or immunisation with live virus vaccines. Human and animal leucocytes have been found to release interferon after viral infection. Observations of this kind have led to the suggestion that circulating interferon may play a role in terminating viral infections, and to the hope, so far unrealised, that it may be used as a chemotherapeutic agent in the treatment of virus diseases.

Other Host Reactions

While there is strong evidence that the presence of neutralising antibody can prevent, or weaken, the establishment of viral infection, there is doubt whether the appearance of circulating neutralising antibody plays an important part in recovery from a primary virus infection. Onset of recovery from virus infection before neutralising antibody has risen to levels capable of protection has been observed, for example, in infection with vaccinia, influenza and poliomyelitis viruses. In addition, not only are there theoretical reasons, outlined above, for supposing that administration of large amounts of antibody would be of little or no use in fully developed virus diseases, but failure of such administration to alter the course of the disease has frequently been observed, for example, in progressive vaccinial infection of man, measles, poliomyelitis and rabies. Furthermore, individuals suffering from agammaglobulinæmia and hypogammaglobulinæmia, in whom production of antibodies is greatly diminished, or totally absent, have been observed to recover normally from infection with vaccinia and measles viruses. Other factors must therefore be involved in recovery from viral diseases. These factors have been reviewed by Baron[33], and include interferon production (already dealt with), delayed hypersensitivity, pyrexia, the development of local acidity at the site of infection, and local decrease in oxygen tension.

The possibility of a contribution by delayed hypersensitivity, which implies a cell-mediated mechanism, to recovery, is largely theoretical. Such experimental evidence as exists does not, on the whole, support the idea. For example, guinea-pigs whose ability to form antibody, as well as to develop delayed hypersensitivity to vaccinia virus, was abolished by X-irradiation and methotrexate, recovered as rapidly as control animals from skin infection with vaccinia virus.[34] Hypersensitivity of the immediate type, that is, an allergic reaction to viral proteins,

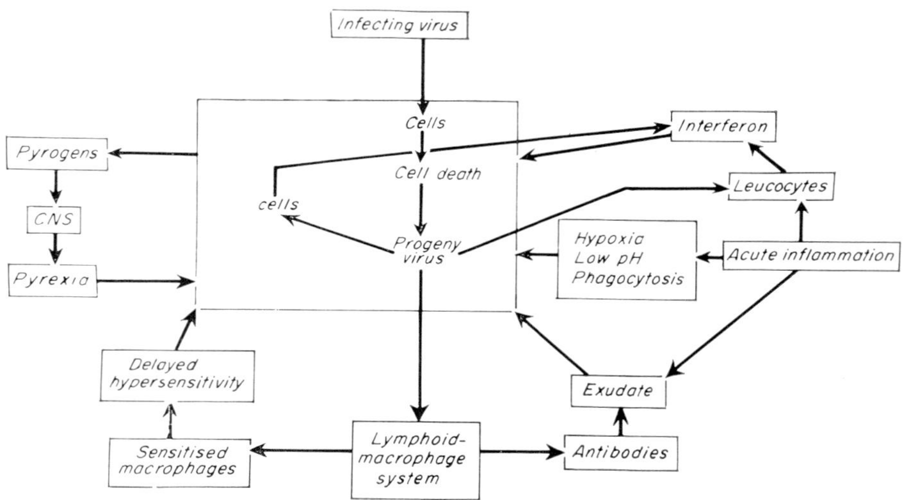

31/FIG. 13.—Host reactions to a focus of virus infection.

may be partly responsible for the acute inflammation which arises at the site of viral infection. Such a reaction, while contributing to the pathological picture of the disease, could also have the effect of accelerating the access of neutralizing antibodies to the site of infection. Skin rashes in viral exanthemata, such as smallpox and measles, are considered by some to arise partly as a result of an allergic reaction to foci of virus multiplication in the skin.

An influence of body temperature on recovery has more experimental evidence to support it. Correlations have been found, for example, between the optimal temperature for development of poliomyelitis strains in culture, and their virulence for monkeys; the strains with lower optimal temperatures were less virulent. Artificial induction of high temperatures has been found to hasten recovery of mice from infection with encephalomyocarditis virus. The pyrexia which develops during virus disease may well play a part in terminating the infection. The suggestion that local acidity aids recovery comes from observations on the lowering of the pH at the site of acute inflammation, and on the known inhibitory effects of lowering the pH on the growth of certain viruses in cell culture. Similar kinds of observation lie behind the idea that local hypoxia is involved in recovery from infection.

The most sensible picture to carry in your mind is one in which all these mechanisms, antibody formation, hypersensitivity reactions, pyrexia, interferon, and local acidity and hypoxia may be involved in recovery from infection. The relative contribution of each mechanism will depend on such factors as the characteristics of the individual host animal, the size of the infecting dose of virus, and the characteristics of the strain of virus producing the infection. The complexity of the reactions involved is illustrated in FIG. 13, which sets out the theoretical host reactions to a focus of virus infection, and their possible interreactions. It will be seen that the reactions are negative feedback loops affecting the focus. Increase in cell destruction and in progeny virus increases the strength of the efferent arms; this results in an increase in the strength of the afferent arms, all of which tend to decrease the amount of virus present in the focus. The end result is a damping process ending, if successful, in a return to normal conditions.

REFERENCES

1. HORNE, R. W., and WILDY, P. (1961). *Virology*, **15**, 348.
2. Cold Spring Harbor Symposia on Quantitative Biology (1962). Vol. 27. Basic mechanisms in animal virus biology.
3. HORSFALL, F. L., and TAMM, I., Eds. (1965). *Viral and Rickettsial Infections of Man*, 4th edit. Philadelphia: J. B. Lippincott. [An excellent series of articles on a wide range of virological subjects.]
4. Proceedings of the 9th International Congress of Microbiology, Moscow (1966). Symposium E.1. Classification of viruses.
5. LEVINTOW, L. (1965). *Ann. Rev. Biochem.*, **34**, 487; WITTMANN, H. G., and SCHOLTISSEK, C. (1966). *Ann. Rev. Biochem.*, **35**, 299.
6. WILDY, P., RUSSELL, W. C., and HORNE, R. W. (1960). *Virology*, **12**, 204.
7. NAGINGTON, J., and HORNE, R. W. (1962). *Virology*, **16**, 248.
8. BRENNER, S., STREISINGER, G., HORNE, R. W., CHAMPE, S. P., BARNETT, L., BENZER, S., and REES, M. W. (1959). *J. molec. Biol.*, **1**, 281.
9. VALENTINE, R. C., and PEREIRA, H. G. (1965). *J. molec. Biol.*, **13**, 13.
10. HORNE, R. W., and NAGINGTON, J. (1959). *J. molec. Biol.*, **1**, 333.
11. HOYLE, L., HORNE, R. W., and WATERSON, A. P. (1961). *Virology*, **13**, 448.
12. KLUG, A., and CASPAR, D. L. D. (1960). *Advanc. Virus Res.*, **7**, 225.
13. DULBECCO, R. (1955). *Physiol. Rev.*, **35**, 301.
14. CAIRNS, J. (1960). *Virology*, **11**, 603.
15. BALTIMORE, D., and FRANKLIN, R. M. (1962). *Proc. nat. Acad. Sci. (Wash.)*, **48**, 1383.
16. HOLLAND, J. J. (1964). *J. molec. Biol.*, **8**, 574.
17. PEREIRA, H. G. (1958). *Virology*, **6**, 601.
18. KAMIYA, T., BEN-PORAT, T., and KAPLAN, A. S. (1965). *Virology*, **26**, 577.
19. DEFENDI, V. (1966). *Progr. exp. Tumor Res. (Basel)*, **8**, 125.
20. GROSS, L. (1961). *Oncogenic Viruses*. Oxford: Pergamon Press.
21. VOGT, M., and DULBECCO, R. (1960). *Proc. nat. Acad. Sci. (Wash.)*, **46**, 365.
22. AURELIAN, L., and ROIZMAN, B. (1964). *Virology*, **22**, 452.
23. HENLE, G., GIRARDI, A., and HENLE, W. (1955). *J. exp. Med.*, **101**, 25.
24. WESTWOOD, J. C. N. (1963). *Virus Pathogenicity*, Chapter 7. In *Mechanisms of Virus Infection*. Ed. WILSON SMITH. New York: Academic Press.
25. FENNER, F. (1948). *Lancet*, **2**, 915.
26. WHEELOCK, E. F., and TAMM, I. (1961). *J. exp. Med.*, **113**, 301.
27. SVEHAG, S.-E., and MANDEL, B. (1964). *J. exp. Med.*, **119**, 1.
28. LEHRICH, J. R., KASEL, J. A., and ROSSEN, R. D. (1966). *J. Immunol.*, **97**, 654.
29. TOKUMARU, T. (1966). *J. Immunol.*, **97**, 248.
30. ISAACS, A., and LINDENMANN, J. (1957). *Proc. roy. Soc. B*, **147**, 258.
31. WAGNER, R. R. (1965). *Amer. J. Med.*, **38**, 726.
32. MARCUS, P. I., and SALB, J. M. (1966). *Virology*, **30**, 502.
33. BARON, S. (1963). *Advanc. Virus Res.*, **10**, 39.
34. FRIEDMANN, R. M., BARON, S., BUCKLER, C. E., and STEINMULLER, R. I. (1962). *J. exp. Med.*, **116**, 347.
35. WESTPHAL, H., and DULBECCO, R. (1968). *Proc. nat. Acad. Sci. (Wash.)*, **59**, 1158.
36. WATKINS, J. F., and DULBECCO, R. (1967), *Proc. nat. Acad. Sci. (Wash.)*, **58**, 1396.
37. TROMANS, W. J., and HORNE, R. W. (1961). *Virology*, **15**, 1.

Chapter 32

THE NATURE OF ANTIGENS AND ANTIBODIES

By E. P. Abraham

INTRODUCTION

When the body recovers from certain infectious diseases it becomes more resistant to the organism that infected it. This increased resistance is known as acquired immunity. Depending on the nature and severity of the infection, it may be weak and transient, or substantial and lifelong.

The immunity acquired in this way is often associated with the appearance in the blood stream of substances called antibodies, which combine specifically with the infecting organism or with a toxin that it produces. Immunity to some diseases had been produced artificially, by inoculation with harmless forms of pathogenic organisms, before the characteristic properties of antisera were known. The first clear evidence of the formation of antibodies appears to have been provided in 1890 by von Behring and Kitasato, who showed that the sera of animals which had received repeated injections of small amounts of tetanus toxin or diphtheria toxin had acquired the property of specifically neutralising these toxins. Five years later Bordet described the agglutination of bacteria by the sera of animals into which the bacteria had been injected; and in 1897 Kraus observed that the serum of an animal which had acquired immunity to the plague bacillus, or the cholera vibrio, formed a precipitate when mixed with the filtrate of a culture of the organism concerned.

The immunological reactions that were discovered at the end of the nineteenth century were subsequently shown to be examples of a more general phenomenon. A large variety of foreign cells and simpler entities, such as protein molecules, having no connection with infectious disease, were found to stimulate the formation of specific antibodies when introduced parenterally into the body. Antibodies are not restricted to the serum but may be found in other body fluids and tissues, and immunology now includes the study of allergies and of tissue transplantation. Substances that stimulate the formation of antibodies, and react with them specifically, are called *antigens*. Conversely, a substance that appears in the body in consequence of the parenteral administration of an antigen, and that reacts specifically with that antigen, is called an *antibody*.

Antigens and antibodies are sometimes named in a manner descriptive of the reaction between them. When the antigen is a soluble substance, such as a protein foreign to the body, it may combine with the corresponding antibodies in the antiserum to form a precipitate. The antibodies may then be called precipitins. When the antigen is a constituent of foreign cells, such as bacteria, or erythrocytes from another species of animal, the combination of antigen and antibody causes the cells to agglutinate. The antibody may then be called an agglutinin and the antigen an agglutinogen. These terms were introduced when the nature of antibodies was obscure. It is now clear that a single antibody can be involved in either the formation of a precipitate or the agglutination of cells, according to the situation of the specific antigen with which it reacts. Moreover, many incomplete antibodies are known to exist, which combine with antigen but do not form precipitates.

It was only after the value of immunology to medicine was already well established that progress began to be made in understanding the nature of the phenomena involved. Many of the fundamental problems are chemical ones. The nature of antigens and antibodies, and of the forces that govern the specific reaction between them, are clearly questions that must be answered in molecular terms. Progress in this direction has been greatly facilitated by the fact that the problems may be studied *in vitro* and by general advances in the chemistry of complex molecules. But a knowledge of the structure of antibodies is also required for an understanding of the mechanism by which a specific antibody is synthesised in the body. This important biological question has facets which bring it into the province of molecular biology and of genetics.

THE NATURE AND SPECIFICITY OF ANTIGENS

Although it is not possible to define precisely the chemical properties that are necessary for a molecule to be antigenic, two general points appear to be established. Firstly, size is important. Antigens are large molecules, having a molecular weight in most cases of more than 10,000, and adsorption of a substance on particles of collodion, charcoal or kaolin sometimes increases its antigenicity (Chapter 34). The antigenicity of proteins seems to increase with increasing molecular weight. Among a series of dextrans, which consist of glucose residues joined mainly by 1:6 linkages, antigenicity was only detected in compounds with a molecular weight of 35,000 or more.[1] Secondly, an antigen is a substance which is foreign to an individual in which it can stimulate the production of antibody.

These statements require some qualification. Synthetic amino-acid copolymers with molecular weights of about 4,000 can act as antigens.[2] The smallest molecule so far reported to be antigenic (in guinea-pigs) is the trinitrophenyl derivative of the antibacterial polypeptide bacitracin, with a molecular weight of 1928,[3] although the question arises whether this reactive peptide forms an antigen by combination with body protein. Although the protein in an animal's own circulation is not antigenic for that animal this does not apply to all body proteins and so-called autoantibodies have been obtained to protein of the lens of the eye, the thyroid gland, and milk (see Chapter 40).

The molecules of many antigens consist partly or entirely of protein, but a peptide structure is not essential for antigenicity, at least in some species. Certain carbohydrates of high molecular weight, such as the dextrans produced by micro-organisms, the capsular polysaccharides of virulent pneumococci, and the blood group substances A and B are antigenic in man, though apparently not in the rabbit.[4, 5]

DETERMINANTS OF SPECIFICITY

Protein antigens.—Proteins vary in their antigenic power. Ovalbumin is a good antigen and hæmoglobin is a poor one. Gelatin is non-antigenic in rabbits.

Extensive investigations have been made of the specificity of native protein antigens and of the way in which this specificity is altered by chemical changes in the molecule.

The antibodies formed against protein antigens have a high degree of specificity. Thus, if antisera are prepared in rabbits against one of the blood proteins, such as the serum albumin, of a number of other animal species, each antiserum will react more strongly with the particular protein used in its preparation than with any other. A given antiserum will also react with the serum albumin of related animals, but the intensity of the reaction will decrease as the zoological relationship becomes more distant. This behaviour reflects an increasing chemical difference in proteins of the same type from animals of decreasing similarity. When different types of protein are compared, such as the chemically distinct serum albumin and serum globulin, they show no serological relationship even if they are taken from the same animal.

If a minor chemical change in a protein is sufficient to influence its antigenic specificity, the existence of an enormous number of distinct protein antigens becomes readily understandable. Proteins contain amino-acid residues joined by amide linkages into a polypeptide chain, which in its fully extended form has the structure:

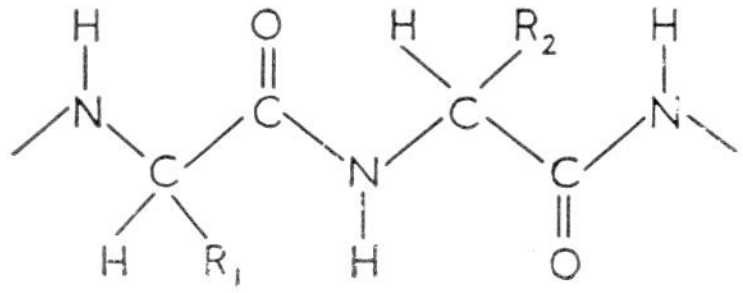

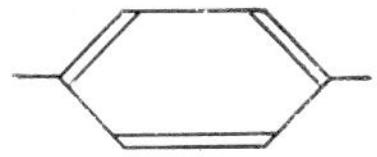

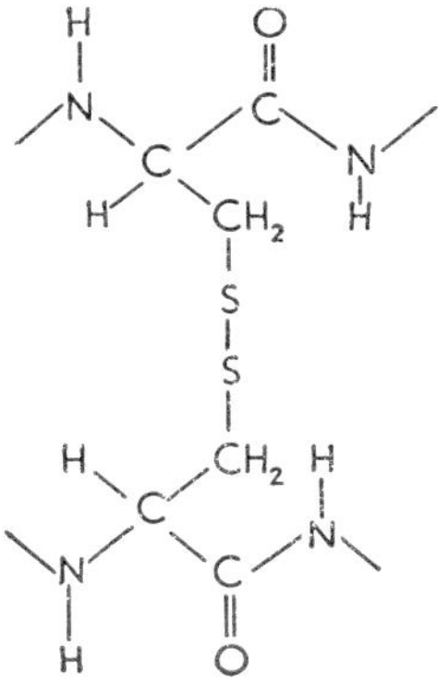

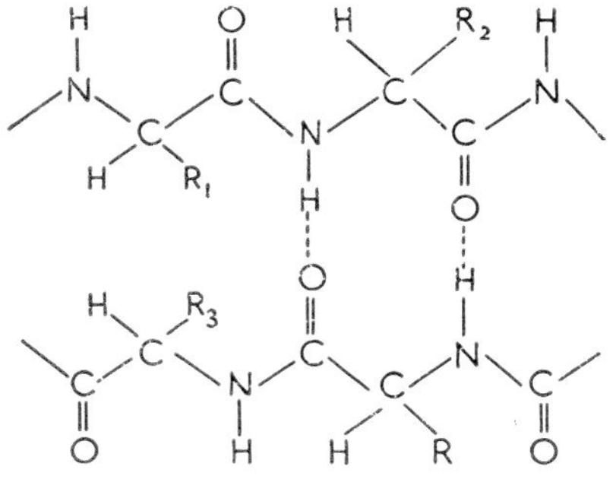

The side groups R_1, R_2, . . . , attached to the backbone of the peptide, depend on the amino-acids present, and may include acidic, basic and neutral radicals. For example, with glutamic acid $R = CH_2CH_2COO^-$, with lysine $R = CH_2CH_2CH_2CH_2NH_3^+$, with leucine $R = CH_2CH(CH_3)_2$, and with tyrosine $R = CH_2$—⟨benzene ring⟩—OH. Since there are more than twenty naturally occurring amino-acids the number of arrangements that are formally possible in a long chain is very large indeed. Moreover, a protein molecule does not consist merely of a long polypeptide chain. Parts of a chain may be joined, or one chain may be linked to another, through the sulphur atoms of cystine residues, or through hydrogen bonds between $>C{=}O$ and $>NH$ groups, as shown in the structures on page 934. Thus, superimposed on the primary structure determined by the sequence of amino-acid residues in the peptide chain there may be a secondary structure, due to a coiling or folding of the chains into specific configurations held together by hydrogen bonds, and a tertiary structure due to the way in which the folded chains are cross-linked by disulphide bonds and packed into a protein molecule. When proteins are denatured hydrogen bonds are broken and their polypeptide chains are partly uncoiled.

Information has been obtained from studies with both native and chemically modified proteins about the factors on which antigenic specificity depends.

The role played by aromatic amino-acid residues in influencing antigenicity received attention at an early stage. Gelatin, which contains no tyrosine or tryptophan and very little phenylalanine, is non-antigenic in some species. When a sufficient number of the tyrosine residues in a molecule of an antigenic protein are changed, by reaction, for example, with iodine, the immunological properties of the protein are markedly altered.

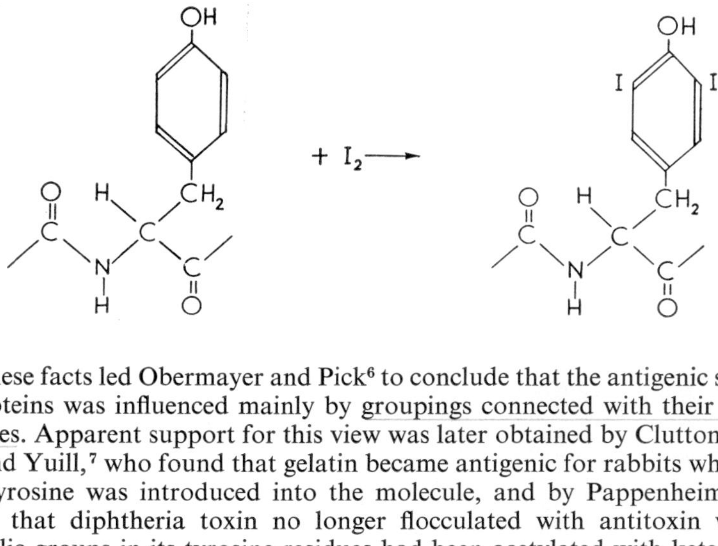

$+ I_2 \longrightarrow$

These facts led Obermayer and Pick[6] to conclude that the antigenic specificity of proteins was influenced mainly by groupings connected with their aromatic residues. Apparent support for this view was later obtained by Clutton, Harington and Yuill,[7] who found that gelatin became antigenic for rabbits when glucosido-tyrosine was introduced into the molecule, and by Pappenheimer,[8] who found that diphtheria toxin no longer flocculated with antitoxin when the phenolic groups in its tyrosine residues had been acetylated with ketene. However, a different explanation of the failure of gelatin to act as an antigen was suggested by Haurowitz.[9] He postulated that an antigen molecule must have rigidity, and that in gelatin, with its abnormally high content of glycine residues which are devoid of projecting side chains, rotation is possible around the longitudinal axis of the peptide. This view has been supported by Sela and Arnon,[10] who found that the introduction of a number of L-cyclohexylalanyl residues into gelatin yielded products which were relatively strong antigens.

While aromatic residues may make a significant contribution to the antigenic behaviour of some proteins, they are certainly not the only factor of importance, for chemical changes that do not affect aromatic rings can greatly alter serological properties. For example, Landsteiner (FIG. 1) found that when the acid groups were esterified with methyl alcohol the resulting protein derivatives had lost their capacity to react with antisera for the unchanged proteins.

$$-\mathrm{CO{-}NH{-}CH(CH_2CH_2COOH){-}CO}- \longrightarrow -\mathrm{CO{-}NH{-}CH(CH_2CH_2COOCH_3){-}CO}-$$

Hence, these groups appeared to play at least as important a part as tyrosine residues in governing antigenic behaviour. On the other hand, reaction of some of the amino groups of a protein with formaldehyde may cause only a relatively small change in serological properties, even though other biological properties are greatly affected.

Although no single amino-acid residue is alone responsible for antigenic properties, the latter are governed by a smaller unit than the whole protein molecule. A molecule of protein antigen is able to combine with more than one molecule of antibody, the number increasing with the molecular weight of the antigen (Chapter 33). Ovalbumin, with a molecular weight of 40,000, can combine with five molecules of its specific antibody. Consequently, there are at least five "active patches" or "determinants" in the molecule. An interesting attack on the problem of the nature of protein determinants was begun by Landsteiner.[11] He obtained peptides from silk, by partial hydrolysis with hydrochloric acid, which combined with antibody. These peptides appeared to have molecular weights between 600 and 1,000 and to consist of not more than 12 amino-acids. More recently it has been found that a fragment of bovine serum albumin, which is formed when the protein is digested with chymotrypsin and which has a molecular weight of about 12,000 is able to combine with rabbit anti-bovine-serum albumin.

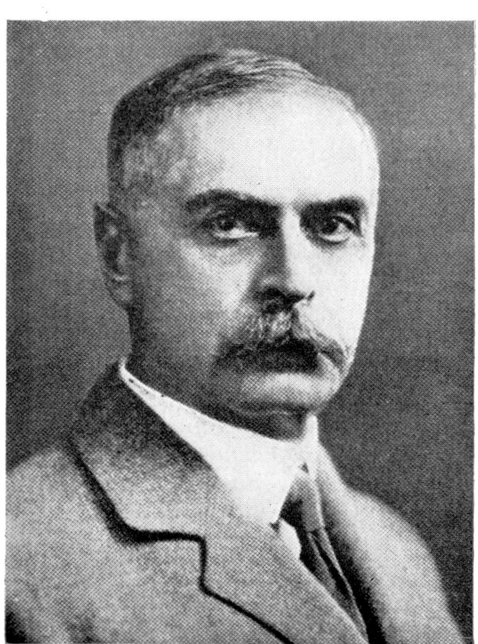

32/FIG. 1.—Karl Landsteiner (1868–1943).

The secondary and tertiary organisation of the proteins, which involves folding and packing of the polypeptide chains, appears to play a part in determining antigenic specificity. Thus, proteins may show a considerable change in serological properties on denaturation; antisera to native proteins generally react much less strongly with the same proteins denatured by heat, and in some cases antibodies have been obtained by injecting a denatured serum protein from one animal into another animal of the same species.

These findings indicated that many factors, including size and shape and the chemical nature of side chains in amino-acid residues, could affect the antigenic behaviour of a given protein. But the complexity of protein molecules, and the difficulty and labour involved in the determination of a complete protein structure hindered the acquisition of more precise information by studies of the native proteins themselves. Well-defined progress has been made, however, by somewhat different approaches which have depended on the changes that occur in the serological properties of proteins when they are combined with simpler substances of known constitution and on the fact that synthetic polypeptides may be antigenic.

Synthetic conjugated protein antigens.—Obermayer and Pick had found in 1906 that when proteins were treated with iodine their original antigenic specificity was partly or completely lost, but that they gained a new specificity which was shared by other proteins treated in the same way. Antibodies formed by immunising an animal with one iodinated protein would react with a whole series of other iodinated proteins. It appeared that iodotyrosine residues in a protein could dominate its antigenic behaviour if they were present in sufficient number. This work indicated that it would be possible to introduce into proteins new chemical structures which would determine their antigenic properties, but the modifications that could be brought about by procedures such as iodination were restricted in scope, and little further advance was made on these lines for a number of years.

In 1917, however, Landsteiner[11] began an important series of investigations into the properties of antigens that had been made by coupling diazonium compounds with proteins. By this reaction it was possible to synthesise conjugated antigens whose specificity was largely determined by simple chemical groups of known structure. Groups which govern the specificity of an antigen are now known as determinant groups.

When diazonium salts are mixed with proteins in aqueous solution they react mainly with the tyrosine and histidine residues, forming coloured azo compounds which contain the same kind of linkage as that present in the simple azo dyes. For example, each tyrosine residue couples with two molecules of benzene diazonium chloride in the positions *ortho* to the phenolic hydroxyl group:

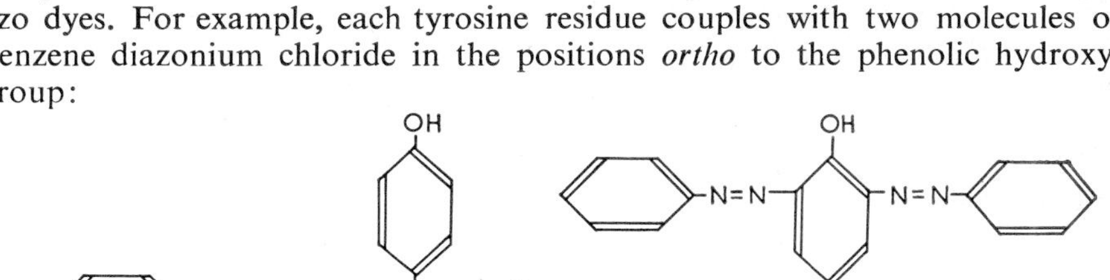

OH
2 N≡NCl + CH$_2$ → N=N N=N
CH$_2$
CH
NH CO

Diazonium compounds can be easily prepared by treating the hydrochlorides of aromatic amines with nitrous acid, the reaction occurring in the following way:

$$R{-}NH_3^+Cl + HONO \longrightarrow R{-}N{\equiv}NCl + 2H_2O$$

where R is an aromatic grouping.

By this technique, therefore, many different aromatic compounds could be coupled to proteins without much difficulty, and their effect on antigenic properties could then be determined.

Other methods of making conjugated proteins were subsequently used. For example, Pillemer, Ecker and Martiensen[12] coupled halogen derivatives, such as iodoacetic acid, α-bromopropionic acid and benzyl chloride, with free SH groups formed from cystine residues in keratin proteins on reduction with sodium thioglycolate.

$$\text{Protein}{-}\text{SH} + \text{R-X} \longrightarrow \text{Protein}{-}\text{S-R} + \text{HX}$$

Clutton, Harington and Mead[13] made use of the reaction of acid azides with α-amino groups to couple O-β-glucosidyl tyrosine with protein through a peptide bond:

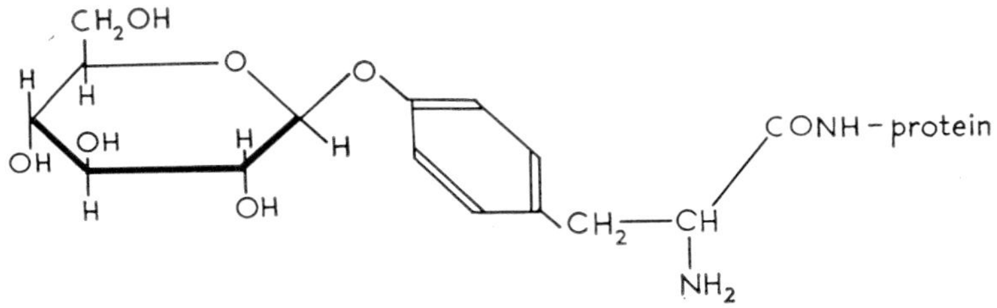

Coupling with diazo compounds, however, has been most commonly used, because it enables a large variety of conjugated antigens to be easily prepared, and there is no evidence that the method of coupling alters the essential nature of the results obtained.

Although a conjugated azo-protein has antigenic properties which are quite different from those of the protein used in its preparation, the protein specificity is retained to some extent, and it seems that both the azo groups and adjacent portions of the protein molecules form a part of the determinant structure. Overlapping reactions caused by the protein part of the antigen, however, can be excluded if the azo-antigens that are used for immunisation and for tests with the resulting antibodies are prepared from different proteins. Thus, horse serum azo-proteins can be used for immunisation and chick serum azoproteins for reactions with the resulting immune serum. In this way the reaction is made independent of the nature of the protein portion of the antigen, and it is possible to test the specificity of the azo component.

By coupling a variety of substituted aromatic amines to horse serum, and using the products to immunise rabbits, Landsteiner and his colleagues obtained precise information about the effect of a number of different chemical groups on antigenic specificity. Some groups conferred a new specificity on the antigen which seemed to be complete, but many others showed cross-reactions of varying intensity with groups of related chemical structure. It soon became clear that the chemical nature, shape, and size of the azo compound contributed to its influence on serological properties.

Polar groups which carry an electrostatic charge are strongly determinant. When coupling was carried out with aromatic amines containing free acid groups in the benzene ring, both the nature of the acid group and its position in the ring had a decisive influence on antigenic specificity. This is illustrated by Table I. Antisera formed against proteins coupled with *p*-aminobenzene sulphonic acid, for example, did not react with carboxylic acid antigens or even with an *o*-aminobenzene sulphonic acid antigen. The determining effect of arsonic acid radicals was exceptionally strong, since arsanilic acid serum reacted with a number of related substances containing the group AsO_3H_2 but with no other compounds. This has been attributed to the high electrostatic force exerted by the two negative changes of the arsonic acid group ($AsO_3^{=}$) in comparison with that exerted by the single charge of COO^- and SO_3^-. Later work by Haurowitz,[14] in which diazotised *m*-aminophenyl-trimethyl ammonium chloride $\left[=N-C_6H_4-N(CH_3)_3^+ Cl^- \right]$ was used for coupling, indicated that a positively charged quaternary ammonium ion, as well as a negatively charged acid group, is effective in determining specificity.

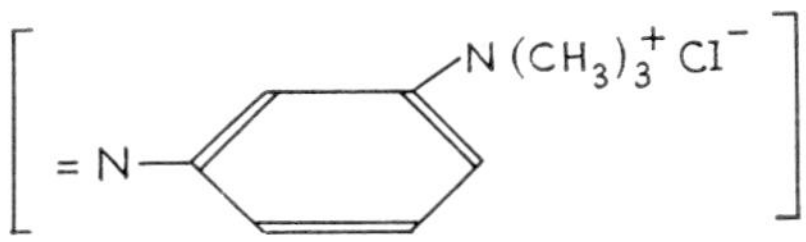

Substitution of the aromatic nucleus with relatively non-polar groups such as methyl, halogen and nitro, which do not carry a strong electrostatic charge, had a much smaller effect on specificity. An antiserum prepared against a compound containing non-polar groups generally showed cross reactions of varying intensity with most other compounds of the same type. The nitro group, however, which is more polar than halogen or methyl, seemed to have a somewhat stronger determining action than the latter.

The clear-cut change in specificity which occurred when an acid group was moved from one position to another in a benzene ring showed that antigenic properties depended not only on the kind of groups introduced into a protein but also on their arrangement in space. The importance of this arrangement was emphasised by the finding that optical isomers were serologically distinguishable. *Dextro*, *lævo* and *meso* tartaric acid were coupled to protein, in the form of their anilides, through an azo linkage:

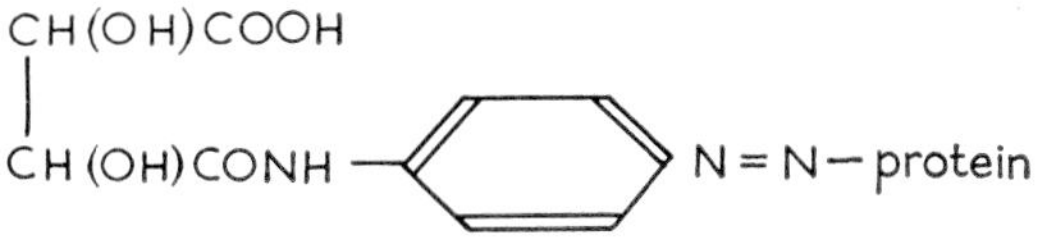

$$\begin{array}{l} CH(OH)COOH \\ | \\ CH(OH)CONH-C_6H_4-N=N-\text{protein} \end{array}$$

These isomeric acids differ from each other in the manner illustrated below, the heavily printed bonds being in front of the plane of the paper and the dotted ones behind.

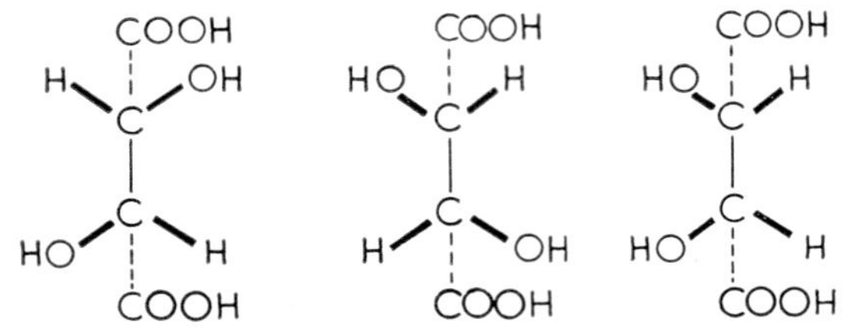

D-	L-	Meso
COOH H–C–OH HO–C–H COOH	COOH HO–C–H H–C–OH COOH	COOH HO–C–H HO–C–H COOH

The isomers could be distinguished by serological reactions. The *meso* antigen, which differed from both the D- and L-antigens in the configuration about only one asymmetric carbon atom, showed stronger cross reactions than the latter.

Various peptides were conjugated with proteins through their azobenzoyl derivatives, whose structure is illustrated by that given below for the derivative of glyclylycine.

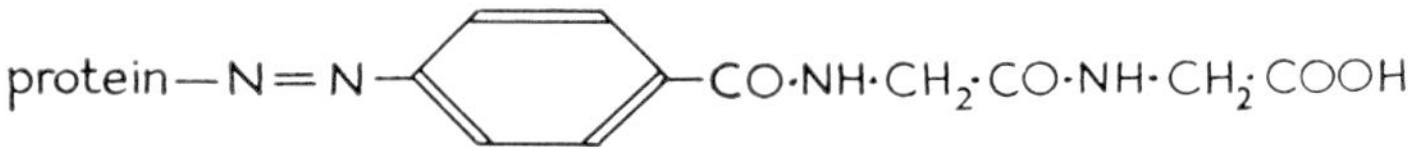

$$\text{protein—N=N—}C_6H_4\text{—CO·NH·}CH_2\text{·CO·NH·}CH_2\text{·COOH}$$

The specificity of four optically inactive dipeptides is shown in Table II. It is evidence that all four compounds reacted most strongly with the homologous antigens, but that each compound tended to show overlapping reactions with others in which the terminal amino-acid was the same. In other words, the

32/Table I

Effect of Polar Groups on Antigenic Specificity

(Data from Landsteiner.[11])

Antisera formed against	Tested against antigens made with: NH_2	NH_2, COOH (ortho)	NH_2, COOH (para)	NH_2, SO_3H (para)	NH_2, AsO_3H_2 (para)	NH_2, AsO_3H_2 (ortho)
NH_2	+ + +	O	O	O	O	O
NH_2, COOH (ortho)	O	+ + +	O	O	O	O
NH_2, COOH (para)	O	O	+ + +	O	O	O
NH_2, SO_3H (para)	O	O	O	+ + +	O	O
NH_2, AsO_3H_2 (para)	O	O	O	O	+ + + +	+

+ represents semiquantitatively the amount of precipitate formed.

32/TABLE II

EFFECT OF DIPEPTIDES ON ANTIGENIC SPECIFICITY

(Data from Landsteiner.[11])

ANTISERA FORMED AGAINST	TESTED AGAINST ANTIGENS MADE WITH			
	Glycyl-glycine	Glycyl-leucine	Leucyl-glycine	Leucyl-leucine
Glycylglycine	++±	O	O	O
Glycylleucine	O	++±	O	±
Leucylglycine	+	O	+++	O
Leucylleucine	O	+	O	++

32/TABLE III

EFFECT OF SIMPLE SUGARS ON ANTIGENIC SPECIFICITY

(Data from Avery, Goebel and Babers,[43] and Goebel.[44])

ANTISERA FORMED AGAINST	TESTED AGAINST ANTIGENS MADE WITH			
	α-glucoside	β-glucoside	β-galactoside	β-glucuronide
α-glucoside	++±	+	O	O
β-glucoside	+	+++	O	O
β-galactoside	O	O	++±	O
β-glucuronide	O	O	O	+++

specificity was largely determined by the amino-acid containing the free carboxyl group, so that with peptides, as with simple aromatic derivatives, negatively charged acid groups may have a predominant influence.

When tri- and pentapeptides of glycine and leucine were used, cross reactions frequently occurred between compounds having the same amino-acid at the free end of the chain, but other parts of the molecule were also important and the intensity of the cross reactions varied with the general similarity in structure. For example, the precipitates produced by a G_4L serum increased in the series L, GL, G_2L, G_3L, G_4L, where G = glycine, L = leucine.

The way in which carbohydrates affected antigenic properties, when they were coupled to proteins, became of particular interest when it was found that carbohydrates played an essential part in the structure of antigens present in pneumococci and a number of other cells.[4] In 1929 Avery and Goebel began a study of artificial compounds of this kind,[15] the sugar molecules being linked to protein through the benzene azo group. For example, sugars such as glucose and galactose were converted into *p*-amino-phenol-glycosides and the latter were diazotised and coupled with protein. The way in which glucose could be linked to protein is thus shown by (1) and (2).

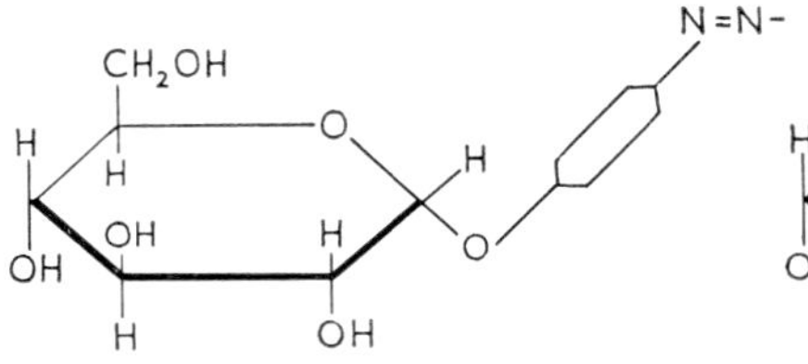

(1). α-glucoside 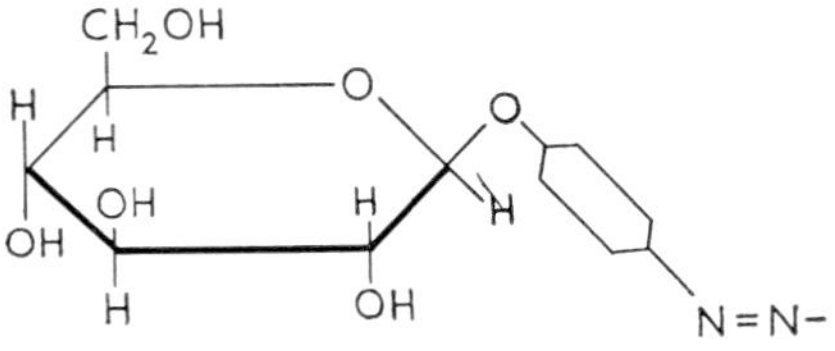 *(2). β-glucoside*

depending on whether there is an α- or β-glycosidic linkage between the sugar and the benzene azo group.

Among the carbohydrates tested in this way were the following:

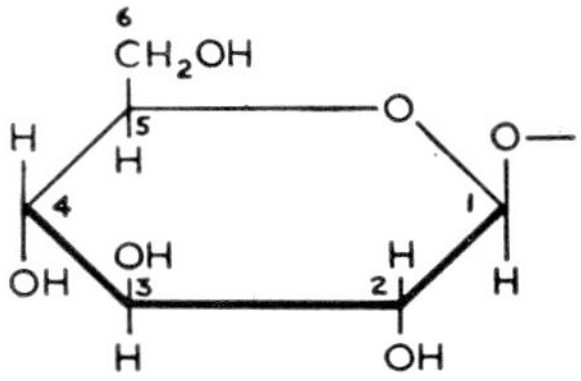

Glucose Residue 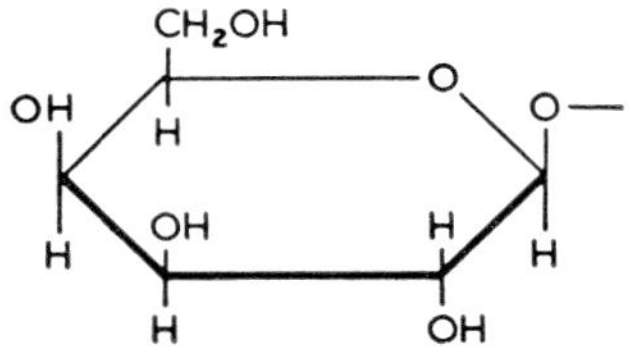 *Galactose Residue*

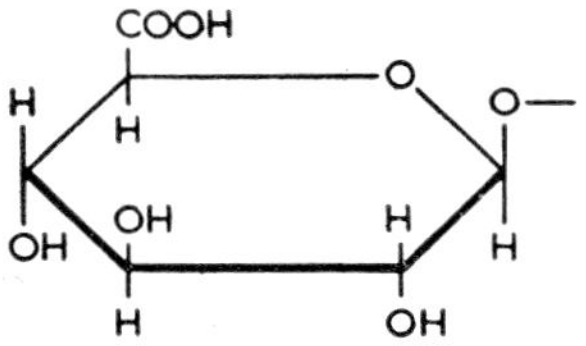

Glucuronic acid residue

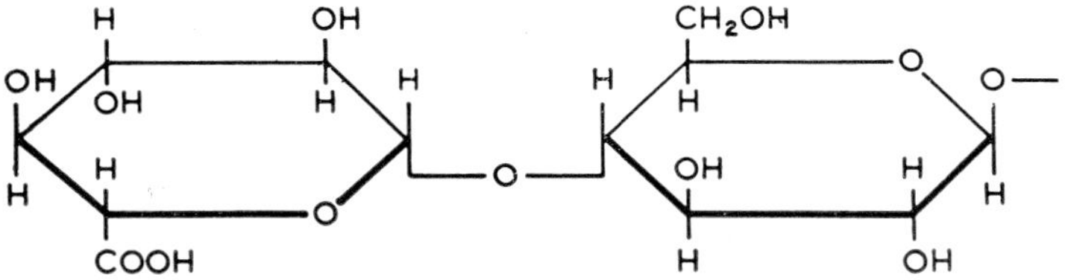

β-cellobiuronic acid residue

Some of the results obtained with the simple sugars are presented in Table III. The importance of stereo-isomerism is at once apparent, for glucose and galactose, which differ only in the configuration of the hydrogen and hydroxyl group round the fourth carbon atom, were clearly distinguished serologically. Moreover, the α- and β- forms of glucose could be differentiated, although in this case there was some cross-reaction. A further illustration of the strong influence of acid groups is provided by the fact that antisera to glucuronic acid were quite different from antisera to glucose.

With the disaccharides the relationships were rather more complicated, the intensity of cross reactions depending on similarity in molecular pattern as a whole, on the linkage of the two sugars, and particularly on the configuration of the terminal hexose. Antisera to cellobiuronic acid showed cross reactions with both glucose and glucuronic acid antigens; they also reacted with antigens made with gentiobiuronic acid, a disaccharide which contains glucose and glucuronic acid but differs from cellobiuronic acid in the position of the linkage between them.

Synthetic polypeptides.—Polymerisation of the N-carboxyanhydrides of one or several α-amino-acids, according to the scheme shown below, yields peptides composed of identical amino-acid residues, or random copoylmers, with molecular weights ranging from 1,000 to 10^6.

$$n\,\mathrm{HN{-}\overset{R}{\overset{|}{C}}H{-}CO}\ (\mathrm{OC{-}O}\ \text{ring}) \longrightarrow (-\mathrm{HN}-\overset{R}{\overset{|}{\mathrm{C}}}\mathrm{H}-\mathrm{CO}-)_n + \mathrm{CO_2}$$

Copolymers of certain amino-acids, such as L-glutamic acid, L-lysine, L-tyrosine and DL-alanine, or L-glutamic acid and L-lysine alone, are antigenic. It is believed that the antigenic sites are short L-amino-acid sequences in disordered, non-helical, regions of the polypeptide chains. A copolymer of D-glutamic acid and D-lysine did not elicit antibodies and did not react with antisera to the corresponding L-peptide.[16]

Inhibition Reactions. Haptens

Whether an antiserum reacts specifically with a given conjugated azoprotein can be determined by observing whether a precipitate forms when the two substances are brought together under appropriate conditions. An antiserum to an azoprotein commonly forms no precipitate when mixed with the protein-free azo component alone. Nevertheless, combination between the free azo component and the antibody can be shown to occur. The protein part of a conjugated antigen is necessary for the *production* of antibodies, possibly to hold a determinant group at a site involved in antibody formation, but it is not needed for a specific reaction with antibodies to occur. With the discovery of this fact it was established beyond doubt that antibodies could be directed towards relatively simple synthetic compounds of known constitution. Boyd[17] stated that from the point of view of the chemist this was probably the greatest single step forward ever taken in the study of immunology.

Substances which do not themselves stimulate the production of antibodies, but nevertheless react specifically with antibodies that can be formed against them when they are conjugated with a protein, have been called by Landsteiner *haptens*. Such substances probably determine the specificity of a number of antigens of medical importance.

Although precipitation is generally not observed, the combination of a free hapten and its corresponding antibody can easily be demonstrated, for when a hapten has combined with an antibody the latter no longer forms a precipitate on addition of homologous hapten-protein antigen. In other words there is a *specific inhibition of precipitation.*

Hapten-protein + antibody ——→ Hapten-protein-antibody precipitate.

Hapten + antibody ——→ Hapten-antibody complex.

Hapten-protein + Hapten-antibody complex ——→ no precipitate.

By the use of this reaction, a large number of simple synthetic compounds can be tested serologically without coupling them to proteins. The results obtained are in general agreement with those provided by precipitation reactions. They show quite clearly, however, that the area of the determinant structure that combines with antibody is not limited to a single group, even when the latter is an acid and exerts an exceptionally strong effect. For example, tyrosine azobenzene sulphonic acid inhibits more strongly than benzene sulphonic acid alone. Similarly, simple sugars are not inhibiting, while glucosides are, and the nitrobenzoyl derivatives of peptides inhibit more strongly than the peptides themselves. It appears that if two determinant groups, A and B, are close together in the antigen molecule they will stimulate the formation of anti-AB antibodies, but that if they are far apart they will act independently and give rise to two distinct kinds of antibody, anti-A and anti-B.[9]

CONCLUSION

It is clear that large molecules which are either peptide or polysaccharide in nature can be antigenic provided that certain structural requirements are met and among the latter may be some degree of rigidity. The reason for the apparent inability of copolymers of D-amino-acids to act as antigens is uncertain, though one possibility is that they fail to be transported to the site of antibody formation. Antibodies were formed preferentially to D-amino-acid residues in an antigen obtained by coupling poly DL-alanine to protein.

The specificity of an antigen is determined by the precise arrangements of certain groups in space, particularly those in exposed positions at the ends of peptide or polysaccharide chains. When such groups carry a positive or negative charge they exert a powerful determinant effect, but they may also consist of uncharged structures such as the side chain of a tyrosine residue or a simple sugar.

Because of the complexity of their structures the proteins supply a very large number of antigens with different determinant groupings. But a considerable variety of specific antigens is also found among naturally occurring polysaccharides. Thus, the capsular polysaccharides of pneumococci and the O-polysaccharides of salmonellæ are substances in which residues of D-glucose, D-galactose and L-rhamnose frequently occur. By changes in the linkages of these sugars and the substitution of one or another of them for an amino sugar, a sugar acid, a deoxy sugar, a polyol, or phosphoric acid, polysaccharides are obtained with more than one hundred different immunological specificities.[4] Human blood group substances obtained from normal secretions, such as saliva, gastric juice and ovarian cyst fluid, are glycoproteins, whereas those obtained recently from red cells themselves are glycolipids in which carbohydrate is linked through sphingosine to a fatty acid.[18] It is likely that in each case N-acetyl D-galactosamine and D-galactose respectively are important parts of the determinant group of substances A and B.

The ability of simple chemical substances to combine with proteins and act as haptens is responsible, in many cases, for drug allergies (see Chapter 40). For example, a small proportion of individuals are hypersensitive to penicillin. One of the antigens involved in this phenomenon is formed by reaction of penicillin, or a transformation product of penicillin, with amino groups of tissue protein to yield a penicilloyl derivative as shown below.[19]

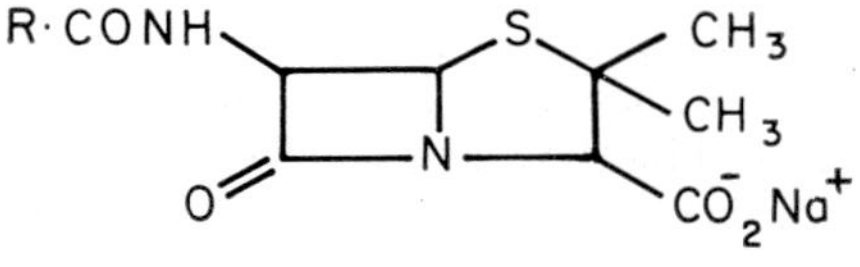

Penicillin

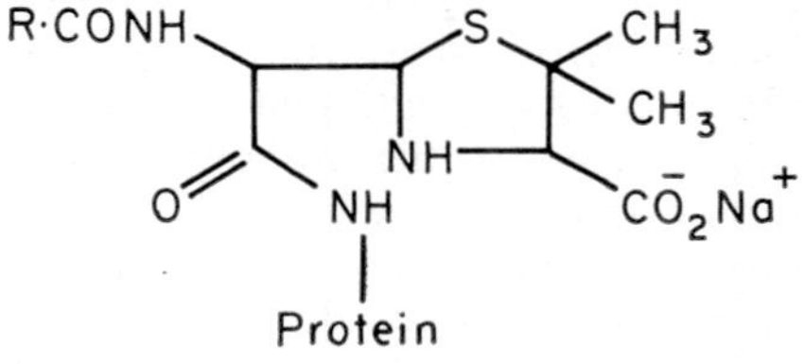

Antigen

THE NATURE OF ANTIBODIES

By 1910 antibodies were known to be associated with the serum globulin, for they had been found in the globulin fraction of immune sera precipitated by salts or alcohol. The nature of the antibodies themselves, however, was uncertain, and even in 1938 Marrack[20] wrote in a Report to the Medical Research Council that "controversy concerning the nature of antibodies centres round the question whether they are proteins or not". Nevertheless, Marrack was able to bring together much evidence that antibodies were in fact modified serum globulins and since 1938 it has become clear that this is so.

The difficulty of establishing the true nature of antibodies has been due in no small measure to the difficulty of purifying and characterising proteins, and to the complexity of the mixture of proteins in animal sera. The great advances that have been made during the last twenty years in the methods of studying macromolecules have made it possible to construct a much clearer picture than was formerly possible of the active constituents of immune sera.

Purification of Antibodies

The preparation of antibodies in a purified form is of clinical as well as theoretical importance, and has been the subject of extensive investigation. Two kinds of procedure have been used for purification. In the first the antibody fraction is concentrated by methods similar to those which have proved useful in purifying other proteins. In the second, the antibody is liberated from the specific precipitate that it forms with an antigen or hapten.

(1) As antibodies are concentrated in the globulin fraction of serum, the precipitation of the globulin proteins, with ammonium or sodium sulphate, is one preliminary step in their purification. Equally simple, though more specific, procedures can be used in a few cases to separate the antibody protein from a large proportion of the inert protein. For example, Northrop and Goebel[21] found that a preparation of Type I pneumococcus antibody which was completely precipitable by Type I polysaccharide could be obtained from immune

horse serum globulin by precipitation with 0·2 M acid potassium phthalate at pH 6. This preparation was fractionated by ammonium sulphate into three main parts and one of the fractions was obtained in a crystalline form. None of these fractions, however, was homogeneous and although they were all precipitated by the specific polysaccharide their protective value in animals was different.

Some antibodies, and particularly diphtheria antitoxin have been prepared in a highly active form on a large scale from antisera that have been partly digested by proteolytic enzymes. In 1939 Pope discovered that treatment of a solution of crude antitoxin for a short time with pepsin converted much of the inert protein into a form that was easily denatured by heat. The latter could be precipitated by heating at 59° C. and at pH 4·2 in the presence of ammonium sulphate, leaving the antibody in solution.[22] By this procedure, antibody preparations appear to have been obtained which contain less than 50 per cent of inert protein. Although the antibody is not inactivated by the digestion, however, it is undoubtedly broken down to a smaller molecule, and some change occurs in its biological as well as its physical properties.

Procedures for the purification of the human plasma proteins which depend on fractional precipitation with alcohol at low temperature and at a carefully controlled pH and concentration of salt were developed by Cohn and his colleagues at Harvard during the war of 1939–45. One of the results of this work was the production from pooled plasma of considerable quantities of γ-globulin fractions containing a number of antibodies to agents responsible for diseases common in man. These fractions contained twenty-five times as high a concentration of antibody as normal plasma, and in some cases showed titres comparable to those of the corresponding convalescent sera.

More recently wide use has been made of procedures developed by Sober and Peterson for the chromatographic separation of serum proteins. These depend on the elution of proteins from columns of diethylaminoethyl cellulose with solutions of gradually decreasing pH and increasing salt concentration. They enable globulin fractions to be obtained which contain all the antibody under study.[23]

(2) The purest preparations of antibodies have generally been obtained by decomposing the antigen-antibody precipitate. This has sometimes been done by dilute acid or alkali, sometimes by treatment with salt solutions, and sometimes by digesting the antigen in the precipitate by a protoelytic enzyme.

Antipneumococcus antibody has been liberated in several ways from the precipitate of antibody and specific polysaccharides. Felton[24] made use of the fact that the polysaccharides of Type I and Type II pneumococci formed insoluble calcium or strontium salts. Heidelberger and Kendall[25] found that a given amount of specific polysaccharide combined with less antibody in the presence of a high concentration of salt than under ordinary conditions. On treating the specific precipitate with 15 per cent sodium chloride, part of the antibody was dissociated and passed into solution. Up to 93 per cent of the protein in such solutions was precipitated by the specific polysaccharide, and it was thought to be nearly pure antibody.

Northrop[26] obtained a purified preparation of diphtheria antitoxin by treating the antigen-antibody precipitate with trypsin at pH 3·5. The antigen was digested, but a considerable proportion of the antibody, though modified, retained its acitivity. Various fractions were then obtained by precipitations with ammonium sulphate. In these fractions 90 per cent or more of the protein was precipitated by diphtheria toxin, but nevertheless they were not homogeneous and it appeared that at least two proteins were present that reacted with the toxin. One fraction was finally prepared which crystallised in thin plates but it had a lower molecular weight than the antitoxin prepared without enzymatic treatment. The antibody had therefore been changed by the trypsin in the course of its purification.

Singer, Fothergill and Shainoff introduced thiol groups into a protein antigen by allowing it to react with N-acetylhomocysteine thiolacetone. The specific precipitate of this antigen with antibody was dissociated by solution in water at pH 2·4 and the antigen precipitated by the addition of an organic mercurial which reacted with the thiol groups.[27]

Koshland, Englberger and Shapanka added a solution of the specific precipitate of antibody with an acidic antigen to a column of diethylaminoethyl cellulose, when the antigen was retained on the basic cellulose.[28] In other methods which have been developed for antibody purification a solution of the antibody is passed through a resin column to which the antigen or an appropriate hapten has been firmly bound by an amido or azo linkage.[29, 30] The antibody is adsorbed specifically and subsequently eluted by a solution of lower pH or a solution of the free hapten.

Heterogeneity of Antibodies

The work of Northrop and Goebel showed that antibodies formed against a single antigen in a single animal are not necessarily homogeneous. It is not surprising that a single antigen should stimulate the formation of several different antibodies, because antigen molecules may contain several different determinant groups. However, evidence was obtained that the immune serum to a given antigen may contain not merely two or three, but a considerable number of different antibodies. In some cases analysis by a physico-chemical method, such as partition chromatography, indicated the presence of a variety of antibody molecules.[31] In others, the evidence was serological. An immune serum to hen ovalbumin will react with goose ovalbumin, but when this reaction is finished it will still react with duck, guinea-hen, turkey or hen albumin. On the other hand, if it is allowed to react first with turkey ovalbumin it will subsequently react with hen ovalbumin but not with the ovalbumins of the remaining birds. By continuing the procedure it has been shown that hen antiovalbumin must contain at least five different antibodies. Similarly, equilibrium dialysis (see p. 952) revealed that the ability of a given hapten to displace a hapten of related structure from an antibody molecule declines as the degree of displacement increases. This indicated that the antibody combining sites are heterogeneous. The fact that differences in chromatographic behaviour did not appear to be correlated with differences in serological properties added to the complexity of this situation. It was suggested that the antibody globulin synthesised by different cells is not identical, and also that antibodies formed against a single determinant group may vary in the extent to which they are adapted to react with that group.

A great deal of progress has recently been made in this field by the application of powerful physico-chemical and immunological methods for the resolution and analysis of the serum proteins, by the discovery of reactions by which antibody molecules can be split into well-defined fragments and by the study of myeloma and Bence Jones proteins which appear in the serum and urine respectively of patients with myelomatosis.

Relation of Antibodies to Normal Serum Proteins

The Immunoglobulins

The Serum Proteins

The development of the ultracentrifuge by Svedberg and a moving boundary analytical electrophoresis apparatus by Tiselius enabled new information to be obtained about the nature of the serum proteins. In the ultracentrifuge a protein can be characterised by its sedimentation constant, which is the rate of sedimentation in a field of unit acceleration, and which depends on the size and shape of the molecule. If the sedimentation constant and diffusion constant are known, the molecular weight can be calculated. In the electrophoresis apparatus a protein can be characterised by its mobility in an electric field. Its mobility depends partly on its net electric charge, which is determined by the difference between the number of negatively charged acid groups and positively charged basic groups in the molecule.

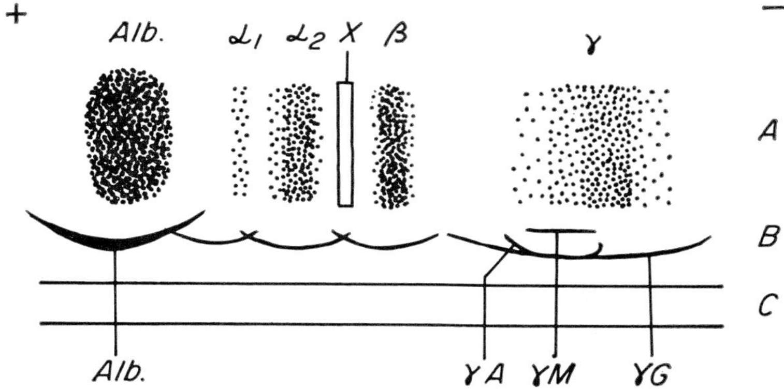

32/Fig. 2.—Illustration of results of electrophoresis of human serum in agar gel at pH 8·2. *A*: Stained protein after electrophoresis of serum introduced at X; *B: Some* of the arcs of precipitation after electrophoresis from an immune serum introduced into trough *C*. β and γ globulins have been carried towards the cathode, despite their negative charge, by endosmosis.

In the ultracentrifuge normal mammalian sera show two main components, corresponding to "albumin" and "globulin", with sedimentation constants (S_{20}) of about 4·5 and 7 respectively, and with molecular weights of about 69,000 and 160,000. In some sera, at least, there is also a small amount of a much larger globulin with an S_{20} of about 19 and a molecular weight of about 1,000,000.

A greater number of serum proteins can be recognised by electrophoretic analysis in solution by the moving boundary method. At a physiological pH where the proteins are negatively charged, the albumin migrates most quickly and is followed by three main globulin fractions which are known as α- β- and γ-globulin respectively. Electrophoresis on paper, in agar gel, or in starch gel has indicated that each of these globulin fractions is heterogeneous, and both electrophoresis and chromatography have indicated that the γ-globulin consists of a large family of structurally related proteins.

Further information about the variety of proteins present has been obtained by immunoelectrophoresis in which an immune serum to the serum subjected to electrophoresis in agar gel is placed in a trough cut parallel to the axis of migration. The immune serum and the proteins separated by electrophoresis diffuse towards each other and give rise to a series of arcs of precipitation when they meet.[32, 33] The types of protein revealed by electrophoresis in agar gel and a few of the large variety of proteins revealed by immunoelectrophoresis are shown in FIG. 2.

Immunoglobulins.—Early studies with immune sera in the boundary electrophoresis apparatus and the ultracentrifuge indicated that in man and the rabbit, at least, most antibodies were γ-globulins with an S_{20} of about 7 and a molecular weight of about 160,000. On immunisation, the amount of γ-globulin in the electrophoretic pattern was much increased (FIG. 3), and the close

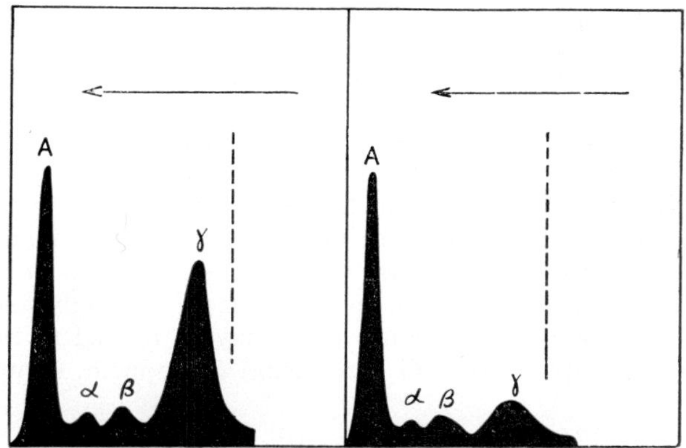

32/FIG. 3.—Electrophoretic pattern of an immune rabbit serum before (*left*) and after (*right*) removal of antibody. Dotted lines show initial position of boundaries; arrows direction of migration. "A" signifies albumin; α, β and γ designate α, β and γ globulins, respectively. Areas under the various peaks may be taken as proportional to the amounts of these components present. (After Boyd.[17])

association of this additional protein with the formation of antibody was shown by its diminution when the antibody is removed by precipitation with the corresponding antigen. However, when the horse was immunised against pneumococci, much of the antibody was often associated with a γ-globulin of higher molecular weight than the main γ-globulins, and a sedimentation constant of about 19. When the horse was immunised against diphtheria toxin, tetanus toxin, and other protein antigens, electrophoresis revealed that a new component had appeared which was not detected in the normal serum. This substance was called the T or β- component and migrated between the main β- and γ-globulins (FIG. 4).

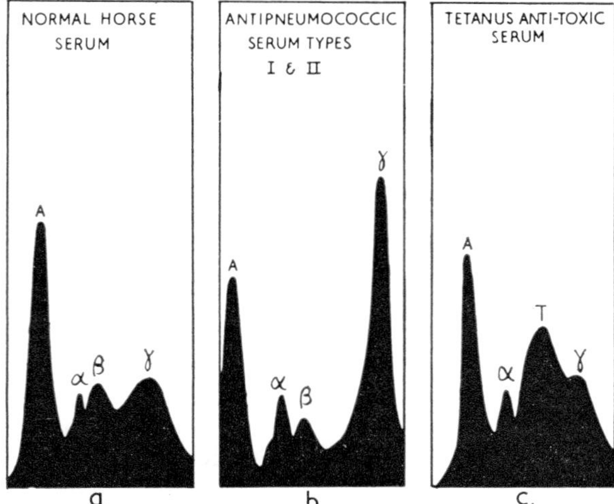

32/Fig. 4.—Electrophoretic Patterns of Normal and Immune Horse Sera

(*a*) Normal serum.
(*b*) Antipneumococcic serum, Types I and II.
(*c*) Tetanus antitoxic serum. (After Van der Scheer, Wyckoff and Clarke.[43])

It is now clear that antibody activity is present in three main classes of serum proteins which are known as immunoglobulins. The symbols recently proposed for the immunoglobulins of human serum, together with those used previously, are shown in Table IV.[34] Their sedimentation constants and behaviour on electrophoresis at pH 8·6 are shown in Fig. 5.[35] IgA, which was first detected by immunoelectrophoresis in human sera and was once thought to contain globulin with skin-sensitising antibody activity,[36] may be related to the T-globulin of horse sera (see Chapter 39). IgG is the main component, comprising 85–90 per cent of the total.

32/Table IV

Old and New Notation for Immunoglobulins

Old Symbols	*New Symbol*
γ, 7Sγ, or γ_2	IgG or γG
β_2A or γ_1A	IgA or γA
γ_1M, 19Sγ or γ-macroglobulin	IgM or γM

Structure of the Immunoglobulins

The immunoglobulins have a relatively high proportion of hydroxy and dicarboxylic amino-acid residues and also of proline residues. IgM contains about five times as much carbohydrate as IgG.

Substantial advances in our knowledge of the structure of the immunoglobulins have come from the finding that they can be split by papain and by reduction of disulphide bonds into well-defined fragments. When IgG is treated

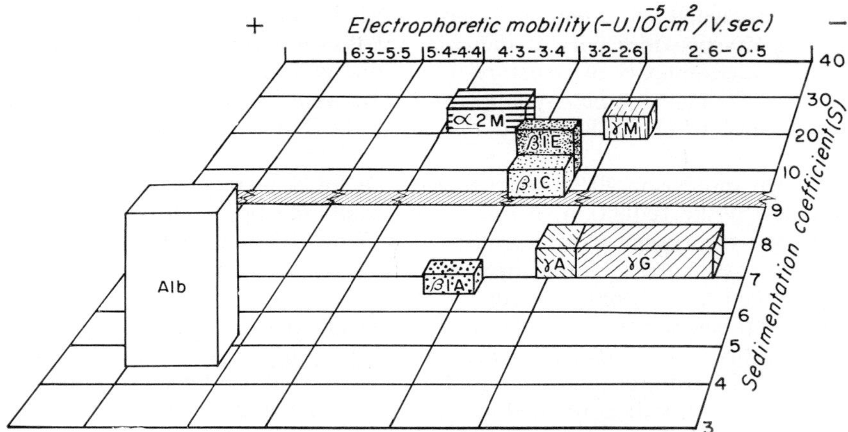

32/FIG. 5.—Pictorial description of the albumin and main immunoglobulins in human serum as revealed by sedimentation in the ultracentrifuge and moving boundary electrophoresis at pH 8·6. The many other serum proteins are not shown (data from reference 35).

with papain activated with cysteine it breaks into three pieces of approximately equal size. Two of these pieces (Fab-fragment) are very similar and contain an antibody site; the third, which can be obtained crystalline (Fc-fragment), contains no antibody site and is also quite different in other properties.[36] Reduction of IgG with mercaptoethanol in neutral solution splits a maximum of five disulphide bonds without any apparent change in molecular weight. But if the reduced product is dialysed against dilute acetic or propionic acid after its thiol groups have been protected by reaction with iodoacetamide it dissociates into two components which can be separated by chromatography on Sephadex.[36] These two components, with molecular weights of about 20,000 and 50,000 respectively are the peptide chains of IgG and are known as the light (L or B) chain and the heavy (H or A) chain. Two chains of each kind are present in the IgG molecule. Light chains, of which there are two antigenic types (K or I and L or II), are common to the three major classes of immunoglobulins, while the heavy chains determine the distinctive properties of each class. A proposed nomenclature for the different chains is shown in Table V.

32/TABLE V

NOTATION FOR THE LIGHT (L) AND HEAVY (H) CHAINS OF IMMUNOGLOBULINS

Immunoglobulin	*Light chain* *Type K*	*Light chain* *Type L*	*Heavy chain*
IgG	κ	λ	γ
IgA	κ	λ	α
IgM	κ	λ	μ

Although the different classes of immunoglobulins are not distinguished by their light chains, the latter are heterogeneous, showing about ten different components when subjected to electrophoresis in starch gel at pH 7 to 8. This heterogeneity provides part of the evidence that among the immunoglobulins "There is a complexity of structure in any one type which is unique in protein chemistry".[36] The complexity appears to be associated with an amino-acid heterogeneity which is largely confined to the N-terminal part of the light chains.[37]

Palmer and Nisonoff[38] have reported that IgG can be dissociated into half molecules by the reduction of one labile disulphide bond with mercaptoethylamine and subsequent treatment with acid. Thus the molecule appears to consist of two symmetrical fragments, each composed of two light and two heavy chains linked by disulphide bonds.

The number of sites on an antibody molecule at which combination occurs with an antigen or hapten is known as the valency of the antibody. This can be determined by equilibrium dialysis, in which a hapten is allowed to diffuse into a solution of antibody contained in a semipermeable bag. If a suitable hapten is used, such as p-iodo-benzoate labelled with radioactive iodine, the concentrations of hapten outside and inside the bag can readily be determined and thus the number of molecules of hapten which combine with one molecule of antibody. By this and other methods it has been concluded that the valency of a number of antibodies is two, a conclusion which is consistent with the finding that treatment of IgG with papain yields two fragments with a combining site.

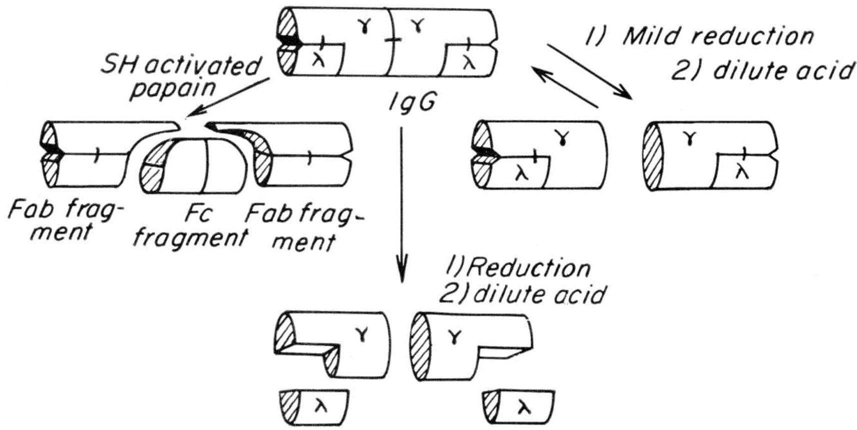

32/Fig. 6.—Types of models proposed by Edelman and Gally[39] for immunoglobulin IgG and subunits and fragments obtained from it. Vertical lines joining heavy chains (γ) to each other and to light chains (λ) represent disulphide bonds.

These and other data obtained from studies of IgG have led to the proposal of a topographic model for the antibody molecule of a type shown in Fig. 6[39]. In this model it is assumed that there is a combining site at each end of the molecule which involves both the γ and λ chains, although in other models the site has been associated only with the γ chain.

The light and heavy chains of IgG are held together by weak noncovalent interactions, as well as by disulphide bonds because these chains are only obtained in the free state when the molecule is treated with acid or other reagents, after reduction and because they can reassociate to form 7S molecules even when disulphide bonds are not reformed. And, since even γ and λ chains from different species can reassociate, the regions between the chains may have similar arrangements in all IgG globulins. Half molecules from IgG of two different species can reassociate to form hybrid molecules with one combining site for each of two different antigens.

Myeloma and Bence-Jones proteins

Multiple myeloma is commonly associated with a hyperglobulinemia and sometimes with the appearance of two types of Bence-Jones protein which can be distinguished antigenically. The myeloma proteins in the serum are related antigenically to the normal immunoglobulins, but they behave as though they are much more homogeneous than the latter and a much smaller degree of heterogeneity is shown by the light chains obtained from them. It is believed that this homogeneity arises from the fact that they are synthesised from a relatively homogeneous group of cells (see Chapter 35).

The Bence-Jones protein usually has a molecular weight of about 40,000 and yields material on reduction and alkylation which behaves like the light chains of serum immunoglobulins on electrophoresis. The light chain of an IgG myeloma protein is very similar to, and perhaps identical with, the chain from Bence-Jones protein of the same individual. Hence, it appears that Bence-Jones proteins consist of light chains devoid of heavy chains and that in their usual form they are light chain dimers.

In type K Bence-Jones protein leucine can substitute for valine at a single point in the carboxyl half of the peptide chain. This change is strongly correlated with certain antigenic differences which are sometimes found between the immunoglobulins of one individual and another (allotypes) and which are ascribed to a genetic factor known as Inv.[37] Inv activity is common to all classes of immunoglobulins and is associated with chains which are antigenically equivalent to type K Bence-Jones protein.

The antigen-combining site of antibody.—Although an immunoglobulin with specific antibody activity may resemble very closely one of the immunoglobulins without such activity it is clear that the antibody must have some peculiarity, in conformation or amino-acid sequence or both, at its active sites. The heavy chains of an antibody have been reported to inhibit specifically the reaction of the antibody with its antigen and they are almost certainly involved in the active site but other experiments have suggested that the light chains may also contribute.

A study of the ability of simple carbohydrate molecules of increasing size to inhibit the reaction of dextran with human antidextran antibody indicated that a hexaose represented the largest molecule to which the antibody-combining site could be complementary.[33] It has been estimated that an antibody may use between ten and twenty amino-acid residues for the definition of one combining site.

Recent experiments have tended to support the view, though they have not finally established it, that the specific nature of the combining site is associated with a specific sequence of amino-acids in this region of the molecule. A papain fragment of rabbit anti-bovine-serum albumin completely unfolded and lost its specific affinity for the antigen on standing in 7·5 M guanidine, but regained its affinity when dialysed in the absence of antigen. Thus its affinity appeared to be determined by the covalent structure of the molecule.[40] Rabbit antibodies to an acidic hapten (p-azobenzene arsonic acid) contained slightly more arginine and slightly less aspartic acid than corresponding antibodies to a basic hapten (p-azophenyltrimethylammonium). An antibody to a p-azo-β-phenyl-lactoside hapten contained slightly more aspartic acid and slightly less tyrosine than one to p-azobenzene arsonic acid.[28] An attempt was made to obtain information about the distribution of negatively charged groups on the active sites of antibodies to amino-acid copolymers containing positively charged lysine residues from studies of the ability of a series of methylene diamines to inhibit the antigen-antibody reaction. These studies indicated that negatively charged groups on the antibody site were 7–9Å apart, corresponding to adjacent side chains on the same side of an extended peptide chain, and that the essential differences in antibodies to different amino-acid copolymers lay in the primary structure.[42]

The three main classes of immunoglobulin which can have antibody activity, IgG, IgA and IgM, evidently have structural features in common. They are composed of two types of subunit, light and heavy peptide chains, held together by disulphide and non-covalent bonds and the heavy chains of one class of immunoglobulin differ from those of another. Within each class, however, there is a high degree of heterogeneity which has become increasingly apparent as new and sensitive procedures have been used to reveal it and this heterogeneity is associated, at least in part, with variations in the amino-acid sequence of the N-terminal portion of the light chains. An IgG immunoglobulin with antibody activity has two antigen-combining sites, probably placed symmetrically at two ends of the molecule. Detailed structures of such sites have not yet been elucidated but it seems that their specificity may be dependent on differences in primary protein structure. Whether or not this is so is important in relation to theories of antibody formation.

REFERENCES

1. Kabat, E. A., and Bezer, A. E. (1958). *Arch. Biochem.*, **78,** 306.
2. Sela, M., Fuchs, S., and Arnon, R. (1962). *Biochem. J.*, **85,** 223.
3. Nisonoff, A., and Thorbécke, G. J. (1964). *Ann. Rev. Biochem.*, **33,** 355.
4. Heidelberger, M. (1960). *Progr. Chem. Org. Nat. Products*, **18,** 503.

4(*a*). Westphal, O. (1960). *Ann. Inst. Pasteur*, **98,** 789.

5. Boyd, W. C. (1962). *Introduction to Immunochemical Specificity*, p. 36. New York: Interscience Publishers.
6. Obermayer, F., and Pick, E. P. (1906). *Wien. klin. Wschr.*, **19,** 23.
7. Clutton, R. F., Harington, C. R., and Yuill, M. E. (1938). *Biochem. J.*, **32,** 1111.
8. Pappenheimer, A. M. (1938). *J. biol. Chem.*, **125,** 201.
9. Haurowitz, F. (1949). 1st Int. Congr. Biochem. Cambridge. Abstracts of Communications, p. 459.
10. Sela, M., and Arnon, R. (1960). *Biochem J.*, **77,** 394.
11. Landsteiner, K. (1945). *The Specificity of Serological Reactions*, Rev. edit. Cambridge, Mass.: Harvard Univ. Press.
12. Pillemer, L., Ecker, E. E., and Martiensen, E. W. (1939). *J. exp. Med.*, **70,** 387.

13. Clutton, R. F., Harington, C. R., and Mead, T. H. (1937). *Biochem. J.*, **31,** 764.
14. Haurowitz, F. (1942). *J. Immunol.*, **43,** 331.
15. Avery, O. T., and Goebel, W. F. (1929). *J. exp. Med.*, **50,** 533.
16. Gill, T. J., Gould, H. J., and Doty, P. (1963). *Nature* (*Lond.*), **197,** 746.
17. Boyd, W. C. (1956). *Fundamentals of Immunology*, 3rd edit. New York: Interscience Publishers.
18. Watkins, W. M. (1966). *Science*, **152,** 172.
19. Levine, B. B. (1965). *Fed. Proc.*, **24,** 45.
20. Marrack, J. R. (1938). The Chemistry of Antigens and Antibodies. *Spec. Rep. Ser. med. Res. Coun.* (*Lond.*), No. 230. H.M.S.O.
21. Northrop, J. H., and Goebel, W. F. (1949). *J. gen. Physiol.*, **32,** 705.
22. Pope, C. G. (1939). *Brit. J. exp. Path.*, **20,** 201.
23. Sober, H. A., and Peterson, H. A. (1958). *Fed. Proc.*, **17,** 1116.
23(*a*). Levy, H., and Sober, H. A. (1960). *Proc. Soc. exp. Biol.*(*N.Y.*), **103,** 205.
24. Felton, L. D. (1932). *J. Immunol.*, **22,** 453.
25. Heidelberger, M., and Kendall, F. E. (1936). *J. exp. Med.*, **64,** 161.
26. Northrop, J. H. (1941). *J. gen. Physiol.*, **25,** 465.
27. Singer, S. J., Fothergill, J. E., and Shainoff, J. R. (1960). *J. Amer. chem. Soc.*, **82,** 565.
28. Koshland, M. E., Englberger, R. M., and Shapanka, R. (1964). *Science*, **143,** 1330.
29. Isliker, H. C. (1953). *Ann. N.Y. Acad. Sci.*, **57,** 225.
30. Karush, F., and Marks, R. (1957). *J. Immunol.*, **78,** 296.
31. Askonas, B. A., Humphrey, J. H., and Porter, R. R. (1956). *Biochem. J.*, **63,** 412.
32. Grabar, P., and Burtin, B. (1964). *Immuno-Electrophoretic Analysis*. London: Elsevier Publishing Co.
33. Kabat, E. A., and Mayer, M. M. (1961). *Experimental Immunochemistry,* 2nd edit. Springfield, Ill.: Charles C. Thomas.
34. *Bulletin of the World Health Organization* (1964). **30,** 447.
35. *Molecular Biology of Human Proteins* (1966). Vol. I. Schultze and Heremans, London: Elsevier Publishing Co.
36. Cohen, S., and Porter, R. R. (1964). *Advanc. Immunol.,* **8,** 287.
37. Milstein, C. (1966). *Nature* (*Lond.*), **209,** 370.
37(*a*). Putnam, F. W., Titani, K., and Whitley, E., Jr., (1966). *Proc. roy. Soc. B.*, **166,** 124.
38. Palmer, J. L., and Nisonoff, A. (1964). *Biochemistry*, **3,** 863.
39. Edelman, G. M., and Gally, J. A. (1964). *Proc. nat. Acad. Sci.* (*Wash.*), **51,** 846.
40. Buckley, C. E., Whitney, P. L., and Tanford, C. (1963). *Proc. nat. Acad. Sci.* (*Wash.*), **50,** 827.
41. Gill, T. J., King, H. W., Friedman, E., and Doty, P. (1963). *J. biol. Chem.*, **238,** 108.
42. Van Der Scheer, J., Wyckoff, R. W. G., and Clarke, F. H. (1940). *J. Immunol.*, **39,** 65.
43. Avery, O. T., Goebel, W. F., and Babers, F. (1932). *J. exp. Med.*, **55,** 769.
44. Goebel, W. F. (1936). *J. exp. Med.*, **64,** 29.

Chapter 33

THE ANTIGEN-ANTIBODY REACTION

BY E. P. ABRAHAM

ENOUGH has now been said about the properties of antigens and antibodies to provide a basis from which we can consider the nature of the reactions between them. To understand the reactions we must know not only what kinds of forces bind the antigen and antibody together, but also why these forces show such an extraordinary specificity.

HISTORICAL

The first theory about the formation and reactions of antibodies which deserves serious consideration was developed by Ehrlich, who suggested that antibodies were specific chemical groups, or side-chains, attached to cells, through which the latter absorbed their nutriment. He thought that the side-chains were blocked by combination with antigen, that the cell then responded by synthesising them in increased numbers, and that those in excess of cellular requirements were liberated as antibodies into the circulation. The theory had the merit of emphasising the chemical nature of the antigen-antibody reaction, but it pictured the reaction in too simple a form. Ehrlich believed that antigen and antibody combined irreversibly in a fixed proportion. It was soon found, however, that when equal amounts of an antitoxin were added successively to a given amount of toxin they neutralised a smaller proportion of toxin at each addition. Ehrlich was therefore forced to assume that toxins contained a variety of components which differed in their affinity for the antitoxins. an assumption which was not upheld by later work.

A different theory was introduced in 1903 by Bordet.[1] He recognised that an antibody could combine with an antigen in varying proportions, and that the amount of combination could be described by the same kind of equations as those which applied to adsorption. In consequence, he considered that serological reactions should be placed with adsorptive phenomena in a class apart from ordinary chemical reactions. Bordet's insistence on the fact that antigens and antibodies combine in multiple proportions was an important step forward, but too little was then known about the nature of intermolecular forces for precise ideas about the nature of the combination to be formulated.

In their original form these theories are now only of historical interest. But, before discussing more recent views of the nature of serological reactions, it is necessary to give an account of some of the fundamental facts that have been established about the reactions themselves, and to say something about the kind of forces that are now thought to be responsible for attracting one protein molecule to another.

THE COMBINATION OF ANTIGENS AND ANTIBODIES

PRECIPITATION AND AGGLUTINATION

The combination of an antigen and antibody is followed, under the right conditions, by some visible change such as precipitation or agglutination.

Precipitation occurs when the antigen is soluble, and agglutination when it is attached to the surface of a cell. The opinion has been held that precipitation and agglutination are secondary changes, and that they differ from the initial reaction in being non-specific in character. Whatever the nature of the visible changes, however, a great deal of information has been obtained about the specific antigen-antibody reaction by studying them in a quantitative manner. These quantitative studies were initiated largely by Heidelberger and Kendall.[2]

Precipitation

It is now firmly established that both the antigen and the antibody enter into the precipitate, and that they do so without any profound chemical alteration in their properties. Precipitation occurs rapidly under optimal conditions and may even be complete within a few seconds. Since it has sometimes been possible to dissociate antibody from the precipitate by the addition of salt solutions, it must be concluded that the reaction is reversible. The same conclusion can be drawn from the phenomena that are observed when antigen and antibody are mixed in different proportions.

When increasing amounts of antigen are added to a fixed amount of antibody the quantity of precipitate rises to a maximum and then falls, often eventually to zero. The composition of the precipitates formed under different conditions can be determined. If the amount of antigen in the precipitate is known, the amount of antibody can be estimated by analysing the precipitate for total nitrogen by a micro-Kjeldahl method. The total nitrogen minus the antigen nitrogen gives the antibody nitrogen. In the region where all the antigen is precipitated the amount of antigen in the precipitate is obviously equal to the amount that has been added. If all the antigen is not precipitated a special method must be found for determining it. This can easily be done when it contains some characteristic group, such as an azo-dye, a polysaccharide, an iodo-tyrosine residue, or a radioactive atom, which is not present in the antibody globulin. When the antigen is a simple protein, however, the amount that is not precipitated must be estimated by precipitin tests with a serum of known strength.

FIGURE 1 shows a typical curve giving the amounts of antibody precipitated from a rabbit antiserum by increasing amounts of the homologous antigen. In the zone OA, where antibody is in excess, antibody can be detected in the supernatant solution after the precipitate has been separated. To the right of B where antigen is in excess, the supernatant can be shown to contain antigen. In the region from A to B, which is called the equivalence zone, neither antigen nor antibody can be detected in the supernatant fluid.

It will be seen that the composition of the precipitate is not constant, but that the ratio of antibody to antigen decreases steadily from the zone of antibody excess to the zone of antigen excess. Consequently the antigen combines with antibody in multiple proportions. The compounds formed when there are equivalent amounts of antigen and antibody, or when antibody is in excess, give rise to precipitates, but the compounds formed in the presence of a large excess of antigen remain in solution. This behaviour is typical of the reactions between many antigens and antibodies; but it is not universal, for with horse antisera and simple protein antigens soluble compounds are formed when antibody, as well as antigen, is in excess. The reason for these differences in the solubility of compounds containing an excess of antibody is not yet clearly understood.

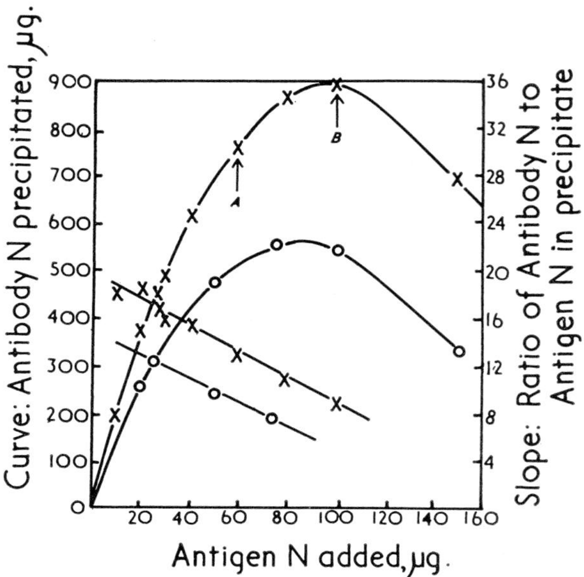

33/FIG. 1.—Amount of antibody N precipitated from a constant amount of anti-hen egg albumin serum by hen egg albumin and duck egg albumin and ratio of antibody to antigen in the precipitates. —x—x—x— Hen egg albumin; —o—o—o— duck egg albumin. (After Marrack.[24])

The precipitate formed when an antigen and antibody are mixed in equivalent proportions will redissolve on the addition of an excess of antigen. This behaviour can be readily explained if it is assumed that the reactions concerned are reversible. In some cases, however, it appears that a new equilibrium is reached only slowly on changing the concentrations of the reagents. Danysz observed in 1902 that if an equivalent amount of toxin is added to antitoxin in one step the mixture is non-toxic, but that if it is added slowly at intervals the mixture is generally toxic.[3] This "Danysz phenomenon" could hardly occur if the compounds formed with an excess of antibody rapidly came to equilibrium with further amounts of antigen.

When the molecular weights of antigens and antibodies could be determined, it became possible to estimate the molecular composition of specific precipitates. The interesting point has emerged that the higher the molecular weight of the antigen the larger is the number of antibody molecules with which it can combine. This is illustrated in the following table, in which R is the molecular ratio $\frac{\text{Antibody}}{\text{Antigen}}$.

33/TABLE I

VALUES OF ANTIBODY-ANTIGEN MOLECULAR RATIOS FOR PRECIPITATES FROM RABBIT ANTISERA*

Antigen	*Mol. wt.*	*R* *Equivalence zone*	*R* *Extreme antibody excess*	*R* *Antigen excess*	*R* *Soluble compound*
Egg albumin . .	42,000	2·5–3	5	2	1
Dye egg albumin† .	46,000	2·5–3	5	$\frac{3}{4}$	$\frac{1}{2}$
Serum albumin .	67,000	3–4	6	2	1
Thyroglobulin .	700,000	10–14	40	2	1

* This table is taken from Pauling.[25] † *R*-salt-azobiphenylazo egg albumin.

It appears from these results that the antigens are multivalent and that the number of combining sites which they have for antibody increases with their size.

Antigen-antibody reactions are usually studied at neutrality and in the presence of a physiological concentration of salt. As might be expected, any considerable deviation from these conditions is liable to affect the formation of the specific precipitate. For example, diphtheria toxin and antitoxin do not precipitate in the absence of salt, although they do combine, and precipitates have been found to dissolve when the pH is brought below 4·5 or above 9·5. These effects are undoubtedly caused by the changes brought about by inorganic ions in the electric charges of the protein molecules, and will be mentioned again in discussing the theories of serological reactions.

Precipitation in gels.—A good deal of attention has been given to the formation and analysis of antigen-antibody precipitates in gels. Oudin[4] showed that an antigen diffusing into agar containing the corresponding antibody produces a zone of precipitation which has a sharp advancing edge but a more diffuse tail due to the solubility of the precipitate in excess of antigen. Oakley and Fulthorpe[5] found that when a mixture of antigens is allowed to diffuse into a column of agar from one end and a mixture of the corresponding antibodies from the other, different lines of precipitation are produced where the different antigens and their antibodies meet. Under these conditions the position of a given line of precipitation depends partly on the concentrations of the reacting components and the procedure may thus be used for assessing antigen concentrations.

In general it appears that a specific precipitate in an agar gel does not constitute a barrier to the diffusion of antigens and antibodies that are serologically unrelated to the components of the precipitate. Ouchterlony[6] has developed a procedure in which antigens are placed in two different basins cut in an agar plate and allowed to diffuse towards antibody which is itself diffusing from a third basin (FIG. 2). If two different antigens are used (A_1 and A_2) precipitation occurs in two separate arcs (I) and this is known as a reaction of non-identity.

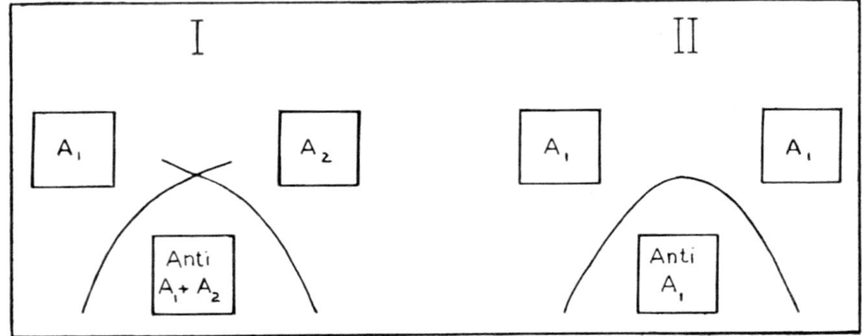

33/FIG. 2.—Illustration of lines of antigen-antibody precipitation obtained in agar gel by Ouchterlony's method. Antigen is designated by A and antibody by anti-A.

If two serologically identical antigens are compared the two arc-shaped lines of precipitation are confluent (reaction of identity, II).

A combination of electrophoresis and antigen-antibody reactions in agar gel, known as immuno-electrophoresis, has been considered in the preceding chapter.

Precipitation with Haptens

For the most part antibodies to conjugated azoproteins have been found to give no precipitate when mixed with the free hapten. In some cases, however, precipitates are formed. For example, Landsteiner found that antibodies formed against a protein coupled with suberanilic acid precipitated with the azo dye resorcinoldiazo-p-suberanilic acid $[(OH)_2C_6H_2(N{=}N{-}C_6H_4NHCO(CH_2)_6COOH)_2]$. Pauling and his colleagues found that simple compounds containing two or more arsonic acid groups formed precipitates with antibodies to conjugated antigens containing the phenylarsonic acid group.[7] It seems probable that the presence of at least two combining groups in a simple hapten is essential for precipitation to occur, since precipitates have never been observed when only one combining group is present. The presence of two such groups, however, may not be all that is required, for Hooker and Boyd[8] obtained no precipitates with a number of haptens containing two carboxyl groups. It has been suggested that the haptens which precipitate with antibodies in the free state are really aggregated in solution.

Agglutination

The reactions in which cells, such as red blood corpuscles or bacteria, are agglutinated by the appropriate antisera show a number of similarities to those in which soluble antigens give rise to a precipitate.

When increasing amounts of an antibody are added to a cell suspension the latter shows characteristic changes in behaviour. With the smallest quantities of antibody no agglutination occurs. As more antibody is added, a range of concentrations is reached over which the cells clump together. Finally, when an excess of antibody is present, in some cases agglutination again fails to occur.

Agglutination, like the precipitin reaction, is influenced by the pH and salt concentration of the solution. In the absence of salt it may not occur at all, and in the presence of a large amount of salt it is diminished. With high antibody concentrations agglutination takes place over a wide range of pH around neutrality. But as the antibody concentration is lowered the zone of agglutination becomes narrower and tends to shift towards the acid side of the neutral point. Under these conditions the reaction appears to merge into a non-specific agglutination caused by bringing the cells to their isoelectric point. At this point, which lies on the acid side of neutrality, the cells no longer have the normal charge which tends to keep them apart, and the forces between the cells themselves are greater than those between the cells and the water molecules with which they are surrounded.

The Combining Forces between Antigens and Antibodies

The way in which known chemical groupings have been found to influence antigenic specificity makes it clear that the forces involved in the combination of antigens and antibodies are chemical ones. Nevertheless, the combination cannot be due to the formation of new covalent bonds involving primary valencies. If this were so it would not be expected that the reactions would be so rapid, or that they would be reversible, and it would be inconceivable that so many different types of hapten, differing radically in their chemical properties, would play a part in the same general phenomenon.

It is therefore necessary to consider what other types of bond can be involved in the combination of different protein molecules, and what part they are likely to play in the antigen-antibody reaction. Among the factors which appear to be important are hydrophobic bonds, dispersion forces, hydrogen bonds and the Coulomb forces of electrostatic attraction between oppositely charged groups.[9, 10] Considered individually, all these forces are weak in comparison with those involved in covalent bonds, but if two large molecules were attracted by weak forces at many different points the linkage between them might be a relatively strong one.[11]

Hydrophobic bonds result from the fact that proteins contain non-polar side chains, such as those in residues of valine, leucine, isoleucine, alanine and phenylalanine. In an aqueous environment there is a tendency for such groups to adhere together, a gain in entropy resulting from their withdrawal from the aqueous phase. For a hydrophobic bond to be established, however, the non-polar groups concerned must be able to approach very closely to each other.

Dispersion forces, which are sometimes called van der Waals' forces, are general forces of intermolecular attraction and operate between molecules which have atoms in close contact. The nature of these forces was first recognised in 1930 by London. They are due to the fact that a molecule has an instantaneous dipole moment as the centre of negative charge of the rapidly moving electrons swings to one side or another of the centre of positive charge of the nuclei. This instantaneous dipole moment produces an instantaneous field which causes the electrons of any other molecule in the neighbourhood to move in such a way that there is a force of attraction between the second molecule and the first. The dispersion force between two interacting groups depends on the product of their electronic polarizabilities and for this reason will be greater, for example, for an iodine atom than a methyl group. It decreases very rapidly as atoms are separated and, consequently, when two molecules are in contact it is only those pairs of atoms which are themselves in contact which make a significant contribution to this type of attraction. In other words, the more closely the surfaces of two molecules can fit together the stronger will be the dispersion force between them.

The hydrogen bond, whose occurrence was first pointed out by Latimer and Rodebush in 1920, depends on the attraction of hydrogen attached to one electro-negative atom for an unshared pair of electrons of another electro-negative atom. In naturally occurring organic compounds the atoms bonded by hydrogen in this way are generally oxygen and nitrogen. For example, a C=O group will form a hydrogen bond with an –O–H or an N–H group in its vicinity in the following manner:

$$>C=O\ .\ .\ .\ H\text{–}O\text{–}$$
$$>C=O\ .\ .\ .\ H\text{–}N<$$

These bonds are somewhat more specific than dispersion forces because they are only formed between certain types of atoms and then only when one of the atoms can come into the appropriate position in space in relation to the other.

The Coulomb force between oppositely charged groups, such as the carboxyl ion ($RCOO^-$) and the ammonium ion (RNH_3^+) which are found in protein side chains, is given by the product of the two charges divided by the square of the distance between them and by the dielectric constant of the medium. In an aqueous medium, this force is greatly reduced by the high dielectric constant of water and, by itself, would be responsible for only a very weak attraction. However, when an ammonium ion and a carboxyl ion come close together, hydrogen bonds are formed between the hydrogen atoms of the former and the oxygen atoms of the latter, and these bonds in addition to the Coulomb attraction may produce a relatively stable complex.

The Nature of Antigen-Antibody Reactions

The Idea of Complementariness

Our knowledge of the way in which simple haptens determine antigenic specificity is compatible with the view that hydrophobic bonds, Coulomb forces, dispersion forces and hydrogen bonds all play a part in the combination of antigen and antibody.

The strong influence of charged polar groups in haptens indicates that Coulomb forces are sometimes important. Nevertheless, the combination of antigen and antibody cannot be considered in these cases to be merely a neutralisation of oppositely charged colloids, for at a physiological pH antibodies and most antigens are on the alkaline side of their isoelectric points and have a net negative charge. Moreover, the position of charged groups in haptens has been shown to be as important as their nature. It must therefore be concluded that groups such as carboxyl ions exert a powerful effect on antigenic properties because certain groups of opposite charge are so placed on the antibody molecule that there will be specific points of interaction when the antigen and antibody come close together. Grossberg and Pressman[12] obtained evidence that a negatively charged carboxyl group forms part of an antibody to the positively charged phenyltrimethylammonium ion. The combining site was destroyed when the carboxyl groups of the free antibody were esterified by reaction with diazoacetamide, but was damaged to a lesser extent when diazoacetamide was allowed to react with the antibody-hapten complex. In contrast, esterification of an antibody to a negatively charged hapten did not affect its combining power.

Coulomb attraction is not essential for antigen-antibody combination, because substances such as simple sugars, which contain no electric charges, have been found to act as determinant groups when conjugated with proteins. In such cases hydrophobic bonds, dispersion forces and sometimes hydrogen bonding must be presumed to play an important part. The influence that the spatial arrangement of these molecules has been found to have on antigenic specificity can be easily understood, because the forces involved are effective only between pairs of atoms so situated that they can be brought very close to one another.

The recognition of the importance of spatial arrangement in antigen and antibody molecules leads to an idea that was first put forward in a general form by Breinl and Haurowitz in 1930[13] and that was soon afterwards suggested independently by Alexander and by Stuart Mudd. This was the idea of complementariness in structure of antibodies and their homologous antigens. The combining sites of antigens and antibodies were assumed to have configurations complementary to each other. At these sites the atoms on the surface of the two molecules could fit very closely together, just as certain atoms in a substrate are thought to fit closely to specific atoms in the corresponding enzyme.

Simple illustrations of how this idea could account for antigenic specificity were given by Marrack. Thus, α-glucoside and β-glucoside haptens are serologically distinct. It will be seen that the binding face of an α-glucoside will be prevented, for steric reasons, from fitting closely to the binding face of an antibody complementary to the β-glucoside.

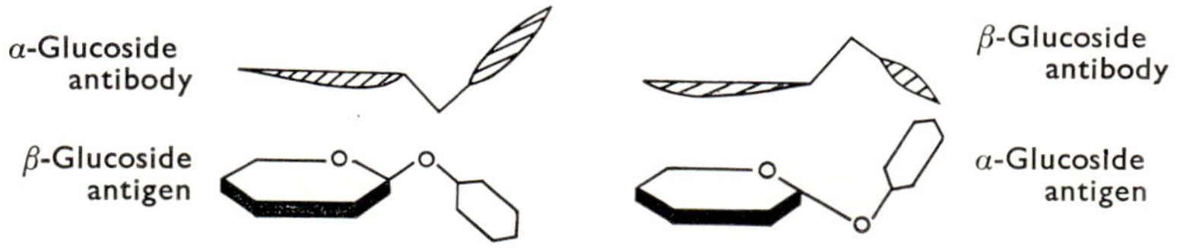

α-Glucoside antibody | β-Glucoside antibody

β-Glucoside antigen | α-Glucoside antigen

Similarly, the binding face on an antibody designed to fit oxanilic acid [—NH—CO—COO⁻] would not fit succinanilic acid [NH—CO—CH$_2$—CH$_2$—COO⁻]

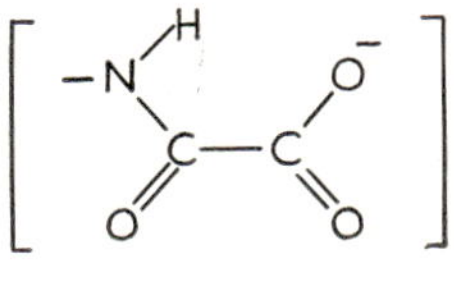

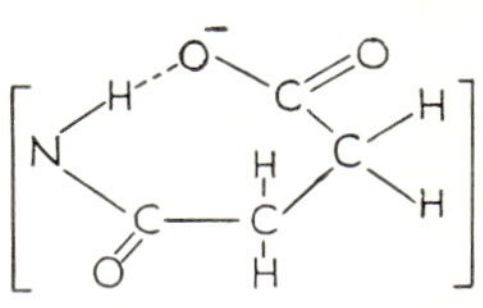

On the other hand, the cross reactions that occur between similar long chain anilic acids, such as adipanilic and suberanilic could be due to the flexibility of the chains, which would allow the carbonyl group and carboxyl ion of different compounds to be brought into similar positions in space.

Subsequently the concept of complementariness was adopted by Pauling, who imagined antigens and antibodies to fit together in the manner shown in FIG. 3, so that a firm combination results from the combined action of many weak short-range interactions. Pauling used the concept to explain a number of the facts that have been discovered about the specificity of haptens. Two examples will be given.

Landsteiner found that antibodies to the succinanilate ion ($C_6H_5NHCOCH_2CH_2COO^-$) reacted strongly with the *cis* maleanilate ion (I) but not with the *trans* fumaranilate ion (II).

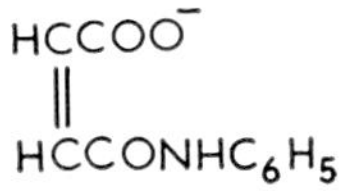

$$\begin{array}{c} HCCOO^- \\ \| \\ HCCONHC_6H_5 \\ \text{I} \end{array} \qquad\qquad \begin{array}{c} ^-OOCCH \\ \| \\ HCCONHC_6H_5 \\ \text{II} \end{array}$$

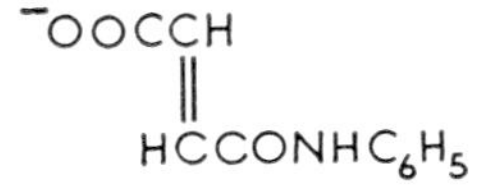

This was accounted for in the manner illustrated in FIGS. 4, 5 and 6. In FIG. 4 the succinanilate ion, in a configuration stabilized by a hydrogen bond between the imino group and an oxygen of the carboxyl group, is shown fitting into the combining regions of the homologous antibody. The antibody is assumed to have a positively charged ammonium ion in such a position that it approaches as closely as possible to the negatively charged carboxyl ion of the hapten, and also an > NH group capable of forming a hydrogen bond with the carbonyl group of the hapten. The maleanilate ion, shown in FIG. 5, is so similar to the succinanilate ion in shape that its carboxyl ion and carbonyl group can fit closely into the same combining regions of the antibody. With the extended fumaranilate ion, however, (FIG. 6) this is no longer possible.

Landsteiner also found that antibodies formed against a protein coupled with 4-chloro-3-aminobenzoic acid (III) reacted with 3-aminobenzoic acid (IV)

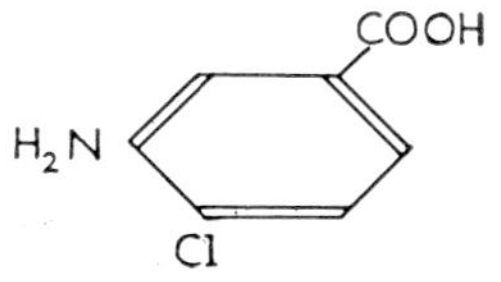

COOH
H_2N
Cl
III

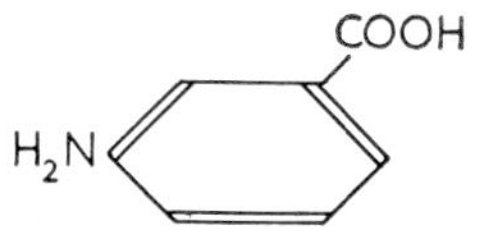

COOH
H_2N
IV

coupled to a different protein, but that antibodies formed against 3-aminobenzoic acid did not react with 4-chloro-3-aminobenzoic acid. A plausible explanation is that the 3-azobenzoic acid group can fit into an antibody cavity complementary to the larger 3-azo-4-chlorobenzoic acid group, but that the chlorine atom of the latter makes it too large to fit into a cavity designed for the 3-azobenzoic acid group.

In general a non-homologous hapten may be unable to show maximum affinity for an antibody because forces of steric repulsion, which arise from interpenetration of the electron clouds of different atoms, begin to operate on some part of it. Thus the remainder of the hapten may be prevented from

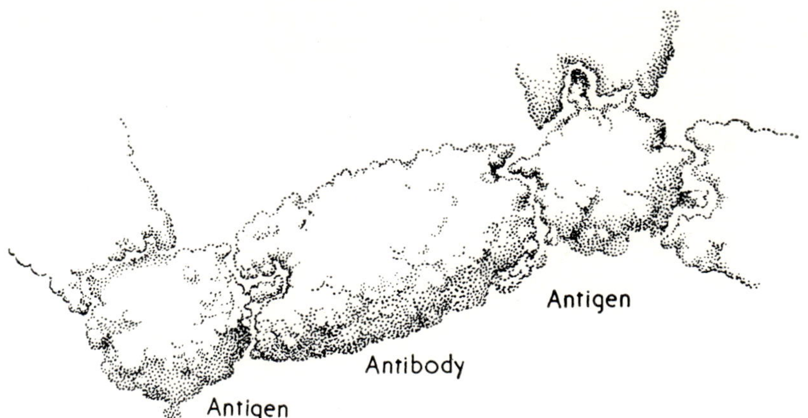

33/FIG. 3.—The postulated structure of a small portion of an antibody-antigen precipitate. (After Pauling.[26])

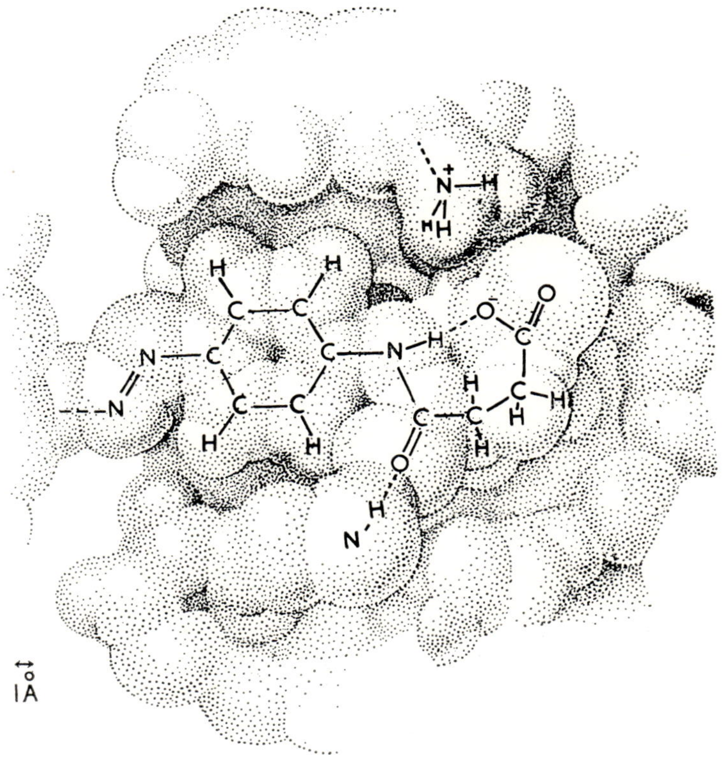

33/FIG. 4.—Hypothetical combining region of an anti-*p*-azosuccinanilate antibody. (After Pauling.[26])

making intermolecular contact unless there is a distortion of the antibody site. There appears to be a correlation between the degree of dilatation required to accommodate a given substituent in a hapten and the extent to which this substituent decreases binding affinity.[14]

It will be evident that the idea of complementariness allows a great variability in the force that binds different antigens and antibodies together, because

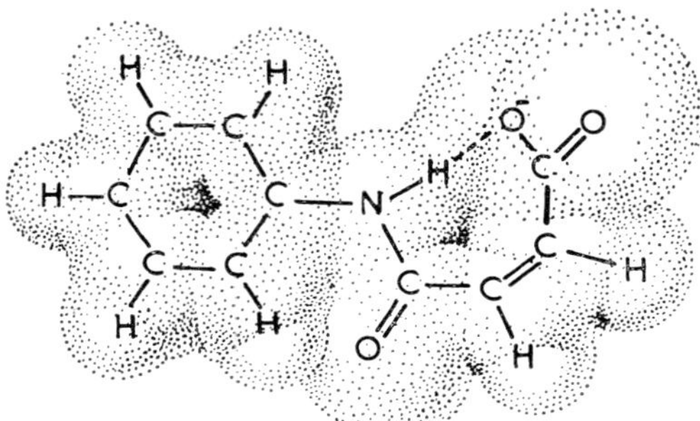

33/FIG. 5—The maleanilate ion, which combines strongly with the antibody shown in FIG. 4. (After Pauling.[26])

the force will depend on the area of the molecules that can be brought into contact, the exactness with which these areas can be fitted together, and the atomic groupings that they contain. It is thus possible to understand how antibodies can combine strongly with an homologous antigen and also show reactions of graded intensity with a series of compounds of related structure. No alternative idea has been suggested which will account for these phenomena of serological specificity in a satisfactory manner.

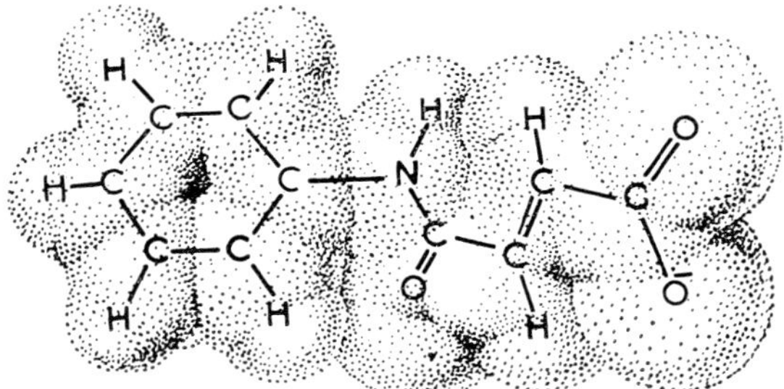

33/FIG. 6.—The fumaranilate ion, which has very small combining power with the antibody shown in FIG. 4. (After Pauling.[26])

The Initial Reaction

Extremely high rate-constants have been obtained for the combination of antibody with several homologous haptens. Since conformational changes would be expected to be relatively slow this suggests that little change in conformation occurred during binding.[15] However, the rate-constants obtained for the dissociation of the haptens are several orders of magnitude higher than those for the protein antigens, bovine serum albumin and insulin. It therefore appears that the latter are in a much less dynamic state of equilibrium with the antibody.

The association constants for haptens and antibodies vary over several orders of magnitude. A study of the association constants for the binding of purified antibody, homologous to the D-phenyl (*p*-azobenzoylamino) acetate group, to haptens of related structure indicated that a hydrophobic bond involving the phenyl group played an important role in the combination.[16] Similarly, a determination of the binding constants of 2:4-dinitrophenylacetate and 2:4-dinitrophenolate to purified antibody homologous to the ε-N-2:4-dinitrophenyllysyl group indicated that the $(CH_2)_4$ portion of the lysine residue in the latter made a significant contribution to the free energy of complex formation.

THE STRUCTURE OF ANTIGEN-ANTIBODY PRECIPITATES

The question now arises as to how the combination of antigen and antibody results in the formation of a precipitate or the agglutination of cells. Two rather different answers have been given to this question. In one, the phenomenon is considered as a non-specific aggregation of antigen-antibody complexes, comparable to the precipitation of normal cells or protein molecules which can be brought about by changes in pH or salt concentration. In the other, it is considered as a reaction depending on the same specific forces as those responsible for the initial antigen-antibody combination.

Bordet believed that antibody formed a layer on the surface of the antigen and so changed its properties that it flocculated in the presence of salts. He pointed out that the properties of the complex would vary with the amount of antibody it contained, and that it was thus possible to account for the absence of precipitation in the region of antigen excess. This theory was later elaborated in several ways. For example, Marrack suggested that precipitation might occur because hydrophilic polar groups of the antibody were turned towards polar groups of the antigen, and were thus no longer able to interact with the surrounding molecules of water. Boyd[17] suggested an "occlusion theory" in which the molecules of antibody were packed so tightly together on combination with the antigen that water molecules were no longer able to reach their polar groups.

In 1934 Marrack pointed out that if antibodies contained more than one combining site it would be possible for them to react with antigen molecules to form a framework, and that the latter could grow in size until macroscopic aggregates were precipitated. The formation of a precipitate would thus be due to the same forces as those involved in the specific combination of antigen and antibody. This theory was developed by Heidelberger[18] and later by Pauling.[19]

Pauling rightly assumed that antibodies are bivalent and antigens multivalent. This being so the first stage of the agglutination of cells can be illustrated by Fig. 7, and the framework of a specific precipitate can be imagined to have the kind of structure shown in Fig. 8. When combination occurs in optimum proportions the molecular ratio of antibody to antigen in the precipitate will be N/2, where N is the valency of the antigen. The larger the antigen molecule the greater will be the number of antibody molecules that can be packed around it, and thus the greater will be the maximum possible value of N. When the proportion of antigen is greater or less than the optimum the framework will be less compact, as shown in Figs. 9 and 10. In the presence of a large amount of antigen only small complexes will be formed, of the type shown in Fig. 11, and this provides a simple explanation of the absence of a precipitate in the zone of antigen excess. In the presence of a sufficient amount of antibody it would be expected that small soluble complexes would also be formed, and that they would finally be of the type shown in Fig. 12. In practice, however, it is only in

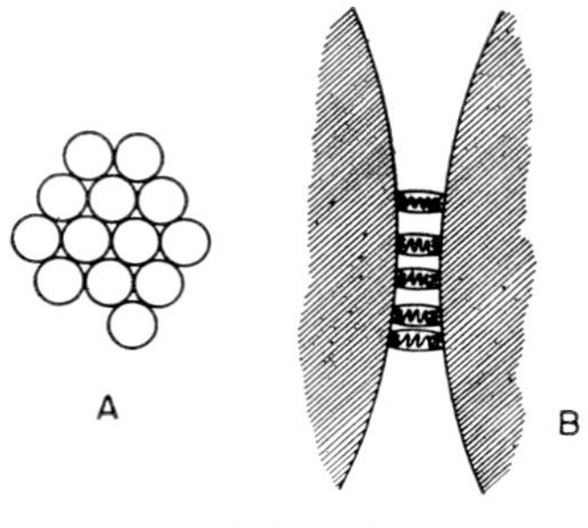

33/FIG. 7.

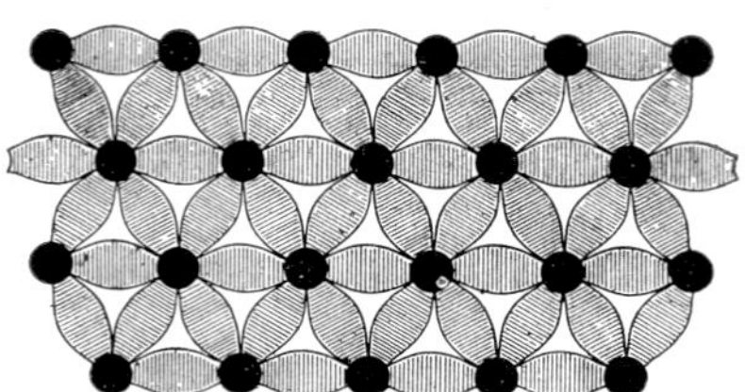

Portion of Antigen-Antibody Precipitate with all active regions saturated

Molecular Ratio $\frac{\text{Antibody}}{\text{Antigen}} = \frac{N}{2}$

N = Co-ordination Number of Antigen

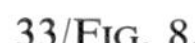

33/FIG. 8.

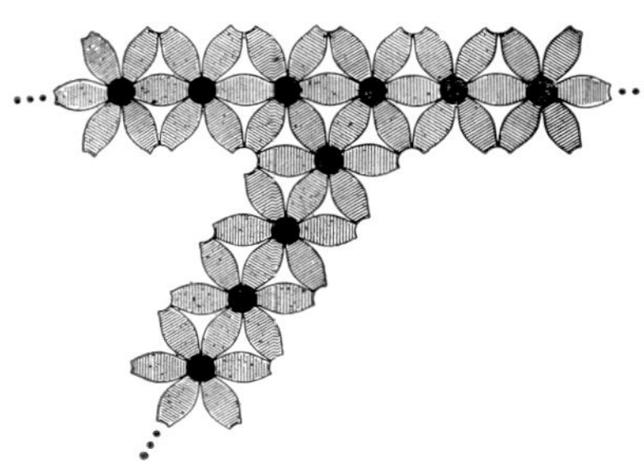

Portion of Precipitate with Excess Antibody
Molecular Ratio N-1

33/FIG. 9.

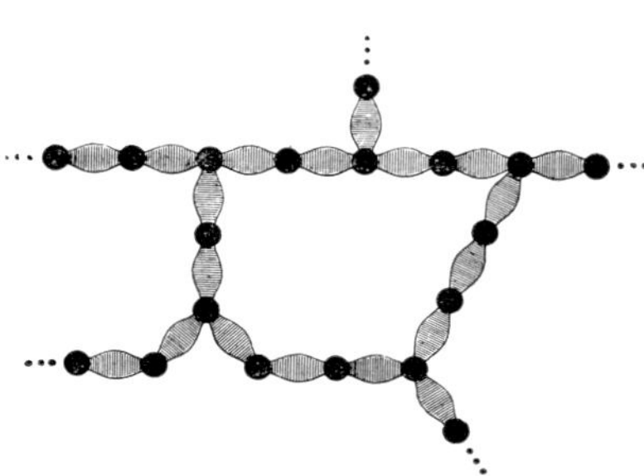

Portion of Precipitate with Excess Antigen
Molecular Ratio slightly greater than 1

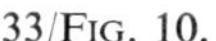

33/FIG. 10.

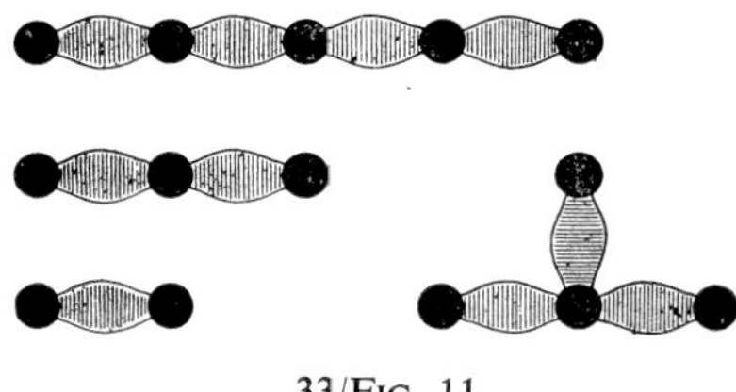

33/FIG. 11.

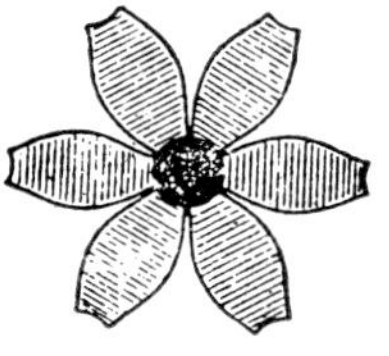

33/FIG. 12.

33/FIG. 7.—(*A*) Diagram representing agglutinated cells. (*B*) Diagram of the region of contact of two cells, showing the postulated structure and mode of action of agglutinin molecules.

33/FIG. 8.—A portion of an ideal antibody-antigen framework. One plane of the structure corresponding to the value twelve for the valence of the antigen molecules is shown.

33/FIG. 9.—A portion of an antibody-antigen network formed in the region of antibody excess.

33/FIG. 10.—A portion of the network formed in the region of antigen excess.

33/FIG. 11.—Representative soluble complexes formed with excess antigen.

33/FIG. 12.—A soluble complex formed with excess antibody.

(From Pauling.[25])

certain cases that no precipitate forms in the zone of antibody excess. The normal failure to obtain soluble complexes in this zone is not yet well understood: it may be due to the difficulty of saturating the multivalent antigens, or to the operation of factors such as those envisaged in the occlusion theory of Boyd.

A good deal of evidence has been obtained in support of the framework theory. In some cases separate clumps were formed when two morphologically distinguishable bacteria were mixed with their corresponding antibodies in the same solution and this could scarcely have resulted from a non-specific aggregation.[20] Clumps of pneumococci which had been agglutinated by an excess of antibody combined, on resuspension, with freshly added antibody and agglutinated once more to form larger aggregates. Hybrid antibodies, containing combining sites with different specificities, were obtained by reoxidation of a mixture of the fragments produced from purified antichick albumin and anti-bovine Ig on treatment with pepsin and reduction. These hybrids yielded mixed agglutinates of chicken and human erythrocytes when each type of cell was coated with one of the two homologous antigens. In contrast an artificial mixture of bivalent antibodies produced separate clumps.[21] Other experiments indicated that half molecules from rabbit anti-ovalbumin would recombine to give a precipitable antibody whereas hybrids with normal γ-globulin yielded products which were only able to block the reaction of anti-ovalbumin with antigen.[22]

To form a framework from an antibody and a hapten it is evident that the latter, as well as the former, must contain at least two combining groups. The fact that antisera to the *p*-azobenzene arsonate group only gave precipitates with substances containing two or more such groups was therefore consistent with the framework theory. Pauling and his colleagues[23] carried out an interesting experiment with a hapten containing two-different determinant groups, which showed clearly that both groups were involved in combination with antibody. The groups will be referred to as R and X. R was the p-azobenzene arsonate ion ($-N{=}NC_6H_4AsO_3^{=}$), and X the *p*-azobenzoate ion ($-N{=}NC_6H_4COO^-$). An antiserum against the R group was obtained by injecting a rabbit with an azo-protein containing R groups, and an antiserum against the X group was obtained from another rabbit in a similar manner. Two haptens were then synthesised which contained both R and X groups. The RX substances formed no precipitate with either anti-R serum or anti-X serum alone, but a large precipitate with a mixture of both antisera. The explanation is illustrated by the following reactions, in which r–r represents the binding groups of the anti-R serum and x–x the binding groups of the anti-X serum.

$$\text{r–r} + 2\text{RX} \longrightarrow \text{XR} \ldots \text{r–r} \ldots \text{RX} \quad (1)$$

$$\text{x–x} + 2\text{RX} \longrightarrow \text{RX} \ldots \text{x–x} \ldots \text{XR} \quad (2)$$

$$2(\text{x–x}) + \text{XR} \ldots \text{r–r} \ldots \text{RX} \longrightarrow \ldots \text{x–x} \ldots \text{XR} \ldots \text{r–r} \ldots \text{RX} \ldots \text{x–x} \quad (3)$$

The small soluble complexes formed in reactions (1) and (2) from single antisera contain no remaining valencies which enable them to grow larger. But in the presence of both antisera either of these complexes can grow indefinitely in the manner shown in (3) and finally form a precipitate.

It thus seems clear that a framework of antigen and antibody molecules is commonly present in an antigen-antibody precipitate. Nevertheless, the presence of non-specific substances, such as sodium chloride, may be necessary before it will occur. This may be connected with the fact that the small framework complexes formed in the early stages of the reaction would be negatively charged and the resulting force of electrostatic repulsion might prevent them from coming close enough to each other for larger aggregates to be formed. The cations of a salt would neutralise the negative charges of the complexes and thus lower the forces of repulsion. On this view non-specific forces would only play a secondary role in the formation of the framework itself.

REFERENCES

1. Bordet, J. (1903). *Ann. Inst. Pasteur*, **17,** 161.
2. Heidelberger, M., and Kendall, F. E. (1929), *J. exp. Med.*, **50,** 809.
3. Danysz, J. (1902). *Ann. Inst. Pasteur*, **16,** 331.
4. Oudin, J. (1949). *C. R. Acad. Sci. (Paris)*, **ccxxviii,** 1890.
5. Oakley, C. L., and Fulthorpe, A. J. (1953). *J. Path. Bact.*, **65,** 49.
6. Ouchterlony, Ö. (1953). *Acta path. microbiol. scand.*, **32,** 231; (1958). *Progr. Allergy*, **5,** 1.
7. Pauling, L., Campbell, D. H., and Pressman, D. (1941). *Proc. nat. Acad. Sci. (Wash.)*, **27,** 125.
8. Hooker, S. B., and Boyd, W. C. (1941). *J. Immunol.*, **42,** 419.
9. Kauzmann, W. (1959). *Advanc. Protein Chem.*, **14,** 1.
10. Karush, F. (1962). *Advanc. Immunol.*, **2,** 1.
11. Pauling, L. (1945). "Molecular Structure and Intermolecular Forces." In Landsteiner's *The Specificity of Serological Reactions.* Cambridge, Mass.: Harvard Univ. Press.
12. Grossberg, A. L., and Pressman, D. (1960). *J. Amer. chem. Soc.*, **82,** 5478.
13. Breinl, F., and Haurowitz, F. (1930). *Z. physiol. Chem.*, **192,** 45.
14. Pauling, L., and Pressman, D. (1945). *J. Amer. chem. Soc.*, **67,** 1003.
15. Day, L. A., Sturtevant, J. M., and Singer, S. J. (1963). *Ann. N.Y. Acad. Sci.*, **103,** 611.
16. Velick, S. F., Parker, C. W., and Eisen, H. N. (1960). *Proc. nat. Acad. Sci. (Wash.)*, **46,** 1470.
17. Boyd, W. C. (1942). *J. exp. Med.*, **75,** 407.
18. Heidelberger, M. (1939). *Bact. Rev.*, **3,** 49.
19. Pauling, L., Campbell, D. H., and Pressman, D. (1943). *Physiol. Rev.*, **23,** 203.
20. Topley, W. W., Wilson, J., and Duncan, J. T. (1935). *Brit. J. exp. Path.*, **16,** 116.
21. Fudenberg, H. H., Drews, G., and Nisonoff, A. (1964). *J. exp. Med.*, **119,** 151.
22. Nisonoff, A., and Palmer, J. L. (1964). *Science*, **43,** 376.
23. Pauling, L., Pressman, D., and Campbell, D. H. (1944). *J. Amer. chem. Soc.*, **66,** 330.
24. Marrack, J. R. (1950). In *The Enzymes*, Vol. 1, Pt. 1, Chap. 8. New York: Academic Press.
25. Pauling, L. (1940). *J. Amer. chem. Soc.*, **62,** 2643.
26. Pauling, L. (1948). *Endeavour*, **7,** 43.

Chapter 34

BIOLOGICAL FACTORS IN THE PRODUCTION OF ANTIBODIES

By G. P. Gladstone and E. P. Abraham

In the preceding chapters we have seen that antibodies are specialised serum globulins which are produced in response to the injection of certain macromolecules, usually proteins, known as antigens. Animals containing circulating antibodies, as the result of the injection of an antigen, are said to be *actively immunised.* Active immunisation can also result from accidental contact of antigens with the body tissues. This most commonly occurs following infection with micro-organisms.

On the other hand, animals may have circulating antibody as the result of an injection of serum from an actively immunised animal of the same or another species. They are then said to be *passively immunised* with homologous or heterologous antibody respectively. Passive immunisation can also be acquired naturally by the passage of antibodies through the placenta from the mother to the fœtus or through the colostrum to the newborn animal (Chapter 37). Although, as we shall see (Chapter 36), antibodies against certain bacterial and viral antigens, including toxins, are important agents in the defence of the body against infection, the term "immunised" need have no connection with protection against disease. It may, for instance, be used in connection with the production of antibodies against inert antigens such as egg albumin or serum globulin. A number of factors govern the production of antibodies during active immunisation. Some of the more important are now to be considered.

Time Relations of the Antibody Response After Single and Multiple Antigenic Stimuli

More than 50 years ago von Dungern[1] showed that the antibody response of an animal receiving an antigenic stimulus for the first time differed considerably from that of an animal which had previously encountered the antigen. Glenny and Südmersen[2] investigated this phenomenon further. They showed that when antigen (diphtheria toxoid) was injected for the first time there was a *latent* period before any antibody (antitoxin) appeared in the circulation, then a gradual increase of antibody to a low titre and then a slow fall though some antibody might remain for more than a year. This reaction to a single injection of antigen they called a *primary response.* A very different picture was obtained after a second injection. The immediate effect was a fall in circulating antibody because the antigen injected neutralised antibody already in the circulation. The fall was particularly marked if the injection was made directly into the blood stream. After the initial fall the titre rose rapidly to a maximum, 10–100 times the previous level. This was called the *secondary response.*

The secondary response was followed by a *phase of decline*, in which the curve representing the antibody titre fell steeply at first and then gradually flattened out to a level somewhat above that of the primary response. The secondary type of response could be produced a number of times in succession with a smaller rise each time until finally no increase occurred. In certain cases continued injections of antigen could even lead to a depression of the antibody response. A series of steps was thus produced, made up of an initial fall in antibody titre, a rise of diminishing extent at each injection and a decline, rapid with the earlier injections, but becoming less and less marked. The final level of antibody varied with the number of successive responses that had been produced.

Before considering the various phases in the immune response described by Glenny and Südmersen, it is necessary to note certain facts about the synthesis and heterogeneity of antibody globulin.

Synthesis of Antibody Gamma Globulin

Antibodies are newly formed gamma globulin molecules synthesised from the free amino-acid pool (for refs. see 3). They are not formed from more complex substances such as polypeptides. This is shown by experiments with isotopically labelled amino-acids, the labelled amino-acid being found in antibody actively acquired, irrespective of whether it is formed in the course of either a primary or secondary response, but not in antibody passively acquired. Such experiments have shown that the production of large amounts of antibody in the secondary response is not due to a release of preformed antibody from some cellular depot as was at one time believed. Synthesis continues throughout, even during the phase of decline, since the label continues to be incorporated into the globulin molecule for some time after the fall following the secondary response.[4]

Qualitative Differences in Antibody Globulin

In Chapter 32 the chemical and physical nature of the antibody globulin molecules was discussed. It was shown that antibodies may differ not only in the combining sites specifically orientated to the antigen, but also in certain physical properties. Three groups of antibody gamma globulin molecules were described: IgG with a sedimentation constant 7S, IgA with a constant 7–13S, and IgM with a constant of 19S. IgA differs from IgG and IgM in electrophoretic mobility, and IgA and IgM contain a higher proportion of carbohydrate than IgG. Within these groups further differences may be found. In fact the response to any one antigen may be the formation of a whole family of gamma globulin molecules with an overall orientation to the antigen but having differences in physiocochemical properties, affinity for antigen, specificity, ability to fix complement, to neutralise the biological activity of the antigen and to pass the placental barrier. The factors determining these differences are not fully known, but one factor would appear to be the time of formation of the antibody, whether it is formed as the result of a first contact with antigen (primary response) or after a second or subsequent contact (secondary response). In a consideration, therefore, of the kinetics of antibody formation we must consider also the quality of antibody formed.

The Kinetics of the Immune Response

Latent Period

This is the period which elapses between first contact with the antigen and the first indication of an immune response. Considerable variation has been described in its duration. A latent period of 4–6 weeks was found by Glenny following injection of diphtheria toxoid into a horse. Recent observations with particularly effective antigens, as for instance certain strains of phage (øX)[5] or certain animal viruses (poliovirus)[6], using sensitive methods for detecting antibody have shown that in certain circumstances the duration of the latent period can be reduced to a few hours. The possibility has even been raised that it might not exist at all,[6a] being an artifact determined by the failure to detect trace amounts of antibody at the beginning of the response. From observations made at the cellular level, it would appear that there is a true latent period and that it is probably determined by the time required for differentiation and mobilisation of antibody producing cells and perhaps also for the capture and "processing" of antigen in phagocytic cells (see Chapter 35).

The discrepancies observed in the duration of the latent period may be largely explained by the system used and the sensitivity of the test to detect an immune response. Some of the factors determining its duration are: (1) the nature of the antigen, particularly its physical state, whether it is part of a particulate body or is soluble; (2) its dose and (3) the route by which it is given.

Soluble antigens in general require a longer latent period to initiate an immune response than particulate antigens, particularly if they are injected into the blood stream. However, the very prolonged latent period obtained by Glenny with diphtheria toxoid is unusual and may be related to the rather insensitive methods he used for the measurement of antibody (by neutralisation of toxin as tested in the whole guinea-pig). Weigle[7], using soluble heterologous serum proteins labelled with I^{131} as antigen and a much more sensitive method of detecting the beginning of an immune response ("immune elimination" discussed in a later section), obtained a latent period of 6–13 days. This was in marked contrast with the latent period of 21–24 hours or even shorter obtained with phage øX and poliovirus mentioned above.

The dose of antigen is important. Large doses mask an early immune response as noted by Uhr and Finkelstein with øX phage (for refs. see 5.). On the other hand the dose can be too small. Taliaferro[8], using sheep red cells in rabbits, noted a progressively shorter latent period as the dose of antigen was increased.

The Rise of Antibody in the Primary and Secondary Responses

The early observations with soluble antigens obtained before the heterogeneity of antibody gamma globulin was realised showed a clear distinction between the exponential rise of antibody in the secondary response and the slow apparently non-exponential rise of the primary response (see ref. 9), as, for instance, in the observations of Glenny already noted.[2] On the other hand, there was general agreement that the rise of antibody using particulate antigens did not differ markedly in the two responses and that in each the rise was exponential.

Recent work (reviewed in ref. 5) has shown that when the rate of formation of each molecular species of gamma globulin is followed separately, little difference can be found between the two responses to both particulate and soluble antigens, the rate being in both cases exponential. The peak titre of antibody formed, however, may show gross differences. The failure to recognise the exponential rise in a primary response is probably due to differences in the time of appearance of the different immunoglobulins.

Primary response.—In most systems studied, the first antibody to be formed is a macroglobulin (19S type) whose rate of formation rises exponentially but tends to fall rapidly. Provided the dose is adequate, this is followed and overlapped by an exponential and more sustained rise in 7S antibody (FIG. 1) (Ref. 10). The picture may be still further confused by the appearance of other 19S

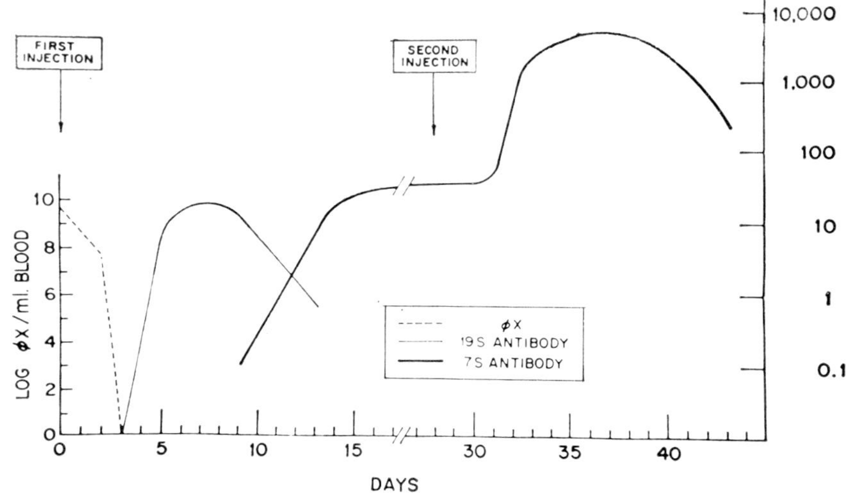

34/FIG. 1.—Antibody response to øX in the guinea-pig after two intravenous injections of 10^{11} øX phage particles administered 1 month apart. (After Uhr.[10])

or 7S exponential phases of serum antibody increase and if such differences are not recognised, as may happen, for instance, if the method of assay detects one class of antibody in preference to the other, the exponential nature of the primary response may be missed. This is more likely to occur with soluble antigens in which the magnitude of the 19S response is often small. Sometimes it is so small that it is difficult to detect. This may explain the failure of Nossal and his colleagues[11] to detect a 19S response with soluble "flagellin" (a protein from the flagella of a Salmonella species), whereas they obtained a good 19S response with whole flagella. On the other hand, small amounts of antigen may stimulate the production of 19S only. Uhr and Finkelstein[5] noted that a proportion of guinea-pigs injected with small doses of øX phage intraperitoneally produced a primary response of 19S antibody without detectable 7S type.

The exponential rise of a **secondary response** is much less difficult to interpret as it often consists mainly of a rise in 7S antibody, with only a small increase in 19S, to a peak titre some 10-fold or more higher than that of a primary response. There is usually a much shorter latent period, but the presence of residual antibody from the primary response makes it difficult to assess its duration and pre-existing antibody may also delay the antigenic stimulus (see later section). The secondary response is much less dependent on the nature of the antigen and its dose.

The antibody produced in a secondary response is not invariably of the 7S type. Nossal and his colleagues[11] noted that rats immunised with flagellin, which as we have seen failed to produce detectable 19S antibodies in a primary response, produced good titres of 19S antibodies as a secondary response. It would seem that a secondary response of 19S type depends on the absence of circulating antibody, particularly of the 7S type[12], at the time of injection of the second antigenic stimulus. Porter[13] obtained a good 19S secondary response to bovine and human serum albumin in rabbits 6 months after the primary injection, provided no residual circulating antibody was present. This inhibiting effect of antibody on the immune response is considered in a subsequent section.

Apart from a difference in physical characters, antibody formed in the two responses may differ qualitatively in other ways. There is a general tendency for antibody whether 19S (IgM) or 7S (IgG) to become more avid with the passage of time (i.e. to combine more firmly with antigen). This is even more marked with antibody formed in the secondary response, which as noted above, is usually 7S (IgG). With multiple injections of antigen, molecules of IgG are formed which have a still higher affinity and combining power for antigen—sometimes as much as 10,000 times greater than those formed initially.[14]

Plateau and Phase of Decline

The 19S antibody of a primary response, although the first to appear, is usually relatively short lived, and in a number of systems synthesis stops after a variable period of about 10 days to some weeks. The cause of cessation may be related to the elimination of antigen.[5, 6] Persistence of 19S antibody formation, however, has been described in some systems. For instance, antibody to O antigens of *Salmonella enteritidis* which is predominantly 19S in type, after an initial fall, may persist for at least 1 year.[15] It is more usual, however, to find that the antibody persisting in the circulation is 7S IgG in type. After an initial rise to a peak and fall, IgG usually persists for several months depending on the nature and initial dose of the antigen and the number of injections. Horses hyperimmunised with diphtheria toxoid have been known to contain antitoxin in their serum for 3–4 years.[16] It would appear that little or no administered antigen is necessary for continued synthesis of IgG but whether its persistence depends on residual antigen still present in the tissues is undecided.

The Establishment of Potential Immunity or Immunological Memory

The term "potential immunity" was first used by Glenny to denote the priming effect on the antibody forming mechanism brought about by a first contact with antigen which stimulates it to produce a much greater response to a second and subsequent contact. It has been largely superseded by the term "immunological memory".

Immunological memory without detectable antibody may be produced with very small doses of antigen. For instance, Nossal and his colleagues[11] using a highly sensitive test to detect antibody, noted that as little as 10^{-9} g. of flagella isolated from a salmonella species produced no detectable antibody, yet had "primed" the immune mechanism sufficiently to produce low but appreciable titres of antibody when the same amount was injected 6 weeks later. However, in common with others[17], they found that the immunological memory produced by such small doses was of poor quality, the titre of the secondary response being only 1/500 of that when the primary dose was increased to 10^{-5} g. of flagella.

A detailed analysis of the time of development of immunological memory has been carried out in rabbits and in mice by Coons and his colleagues.[18] They found that in mice the amount of antibody produced in a secondary response increased as the interval between injections of antigen was increased from 10 to 20 days and then tended to level off so that when the interval was 40 days or longer (up to 6 months) the secondary response stayed relatively constant. If a second dose of antigen is injected before the development of immunological memory, it may not only fail to produce a booster rise in antibody titre, but may actually produce a lower titre than if a single injection had been used.[19]

7S and 19S immunological memory.—In many systems, for example immunisation of guinea-pigs with øX phage antigen, persistent immunological memory seems to be confined to the 7S antibody response. Uhr and Finkelstein[5] using a very small dose of øX phage which only stimulates a 19S response, noted that a subsequent injection 1 month later gave a 19S response identical in magnitude and kind with the first response i.e. a typical primary response. Similar results were obtained with poliovirus by Svehag and Mandel.[6] These workers noted that if the dose of antigen were increased to give a 7S as well as a 19S primary response, a subsequent injection some weeks later produced a typical secondary response only of the 7S type, together with a primary response of the 19S type as if the animal had had no previous contact with the antigen. It is possible that the failure to obtain long lived immunological memory to Salmonella O antigen may be related to the sole production of 19S antibody in this system.[5]

However, it must not be supposed that long lived memory of the 19S type cannot be produced. We have already seen that a secondary response of the 19S type can be shown in certain systems particularly when 19S is the main if not the sole antibody response. Long lasting immunological memory of 19S type, although less often encountered, certainly exists.

Other Factors Influencing the Quantity and Quality of Antibody Gamma Globulins

We have already considered the influence of the stage in the immune response in determining the amount and quality of the antibody gamma globulin produced. Without analysing the stages of the immune response further, we may consider some of the other factors determining the overall production of immunoglobulin and their influence on its quality.

Nature of the Antigen

In Chapter 32 the factors determining antigenicity were discussed and it was shown that, in general, good antigens were large molecules likely to be retained in the body for long periods of time in the vicinity of antibody forming cells. Apart from molecular size, proteins vary in antigenicity for reasons unknown.

Thus ovalbumin with a molecular weight of 45,000 is an excellent antigen, whereas serum albumin with a molecular weight 69,000 is a poor antigen.

That retention of antigen is an important factor in stimulating and maintaining an immune response is shown by the response to pneumococcal polysaccharide. This substance is a highly effective antigen in man and in the mouse, a single injection of as little as 50 μg producing in man high titres of antibody within 2 weeks of injection which persist at a maximum value for 5–8 months and then only decline slowly. Heidelberger[20] noted that 20–50 per cent of the maximum titre was still present after 6 years. A booster dose given 2 years after injection failed to produce a secondary response, possibly because the antibody forming cells were still working at their full capacity. Associated with this unusual immune response is a peculiarly persistent retention of the antigen in the tissues. Coons[21] has shown by fluorescent antibody techniques that pneumococcal polysaccharide may be retained within the reticulo-endothelial and other cells of the mouse throughout its life span, probably due to the lack of any enzyme so far discovered in the mammalian body capable of breaking it down. The material appears to be nontoxic and quite bland, no inflammatory reaction being produced at the site of injection or in the regional lymph nodes.

The nature of the antigen may also determine the quality of antibody globulin. For example, pneumococcal polysaccharide in the horse produces mainly antibody globulin of the 19S type (IgM) whereas diphtheria and tetanus toxoid produce antitoxin of both IgG and IgA types. In the rabbit, as we have seen, the polysaccharide-lipoid-protein O antigen complexes of Gram-negative bacteria induce the formation of IgM antibodies, whereas flagellar antigens after an initial production of IgM type stimulate the production of IgG antibodies.

The physical nature of the antigen is also of importance. We have seen that the first antibody response to a primary injection of antigens on particulate cells such as those of bacteria, red cells and viruses is of 19S (IgM) variety, which appears early and rises to a high titre. On the other hand the response to a primary injection of a soluble antigen, also of the 19S type, is delayed and of low titre. The incremental increase in both cases, however, is exponential and of the same order. In order to relate the difference to the physical nature of the antigen, it is desirable that both the soluble and particulate antigens should be chemically identical. Nossal and his colleagues[11] achieved this by using flagellar antigen from a salmonella species existing in two physical states; (1) as native flagella (2) as soluble protein (flagellin). Both forms produced a good antibody response of identical immunological specificity, but whereas the response to a single injection of the particulate antigen (flagella) in rats was early, and high in titre, the response to soluble flagellin was delayed, and of a much lower titre. In this case the quality of the antibody was also different. The particulate antigen caused early IgM antibody followed later by antibody of the 7S type, whereas the soluble flagellin produced only the latter.

Adjuvants

Because of the more rapid and effective antibody response to particulate antigens, attempts have been made to increase the effectiveness of soluble antigens by adsorption onto particulate matter. In 1926, Glenny introduced alumina to increase the antigenicity of diphtheria and tetanus toxoid and his alum precipitated toxoid (APT) is the standard prophylactic used in this country for the immunisation of children. Glenny[22] showed that the rate of elimination of toxoid in the urine was slower with APT than with soluble toxoid.

Many other agents have since been used to enhance the antigenicity of a variety of substances and these so-called *adjuvants* have even been found to confer antigencity on non-antigenic substances such as penicillin (for review see ref. 23). Freund in 1937 introduced an adjuvant which has been used extensively in experimental immunisation in animals, but which is unsuitable for use in man, consisting of a suspension of dead tubercle bacilli or other acid fast bacilli in an oil-in-water emulsion, the antigen in the aqueous phase being emulsified in the mixture. This highly effective adjuvant acts not only by retaining antigen but also by producing granulomata rich in immunologically competent cells at the site of injection, and elsewhere in the body. Recently, White[24] has shown that the adjuvant effect depends on a peptide glycolipid in the acid-fast cell of unique composition known as Wax D. This consists of a monomolecular lipid layer containing equal amounts of mycolic acid (the substance determining "acid fastness") and polysaccharide with an attached peptide composed of diaminopimelic acid, D-glutamic acid and D and L alanine, the latter complex being similar in chemical composition to the mucopeptide of the cell walls of Gram-positive bacteria. Activity seemed to depend on the presence of this peptide since glycolipids lacking it were inactive.

Dose of Antigen

There have been numerous attempts to relate the amount of antibody produced to the amount of antigen injected. It has been estimated that at the time of maximum antibody formation about $2{\cdot}5 \times 10^7$ antibody molecules are formed by a single molecule of antigen.[25] The smallest dose of antigen giving an immune response depends on its nature, the route by which it is given, the species of animal used, whether it is given as a primary or subsequent injection and the sensitivity of the test used for detecting antibody. Some data of Nossal and his colleagues are of interest.[11] Using a highly sensitive bacterial immobilisation test for assay of antibody, they found as little as 10^{-8} g. of flagella injected into the foot pad of a rat produced appreciable amounts of antibody as a primary response. A dose as low as 10^{-9} g. was sufficient to produce a secondary response. The antibody resulting from these small doses whether produced by a first or second contact was all of the 19S (IgM) type.

Excessive doses of antigen depress antibody production and may bring on the condition of immunological paralysis discussed in Chapter 41.

The Route of Injection of the Antigen

The route by which the antigen is given will determine the particular lymphoid tissue first (or perhaps solely) stimulated. If introduced intravenously, the spleen is the organ mainly affected, whereas with subcutaneous injection it is the local lymph nodes. A comparison of the two routes, using diphtheria toxoid both in soluble form and adsorbed onto alumina (APT), showed a more effective immune response to soluble toxoid injected subcutaneously, but a better response to APT when given intravenously.[26] The quality of antibody may also differ according to the route by which the antigen is injected.

The Species of Animal. Phylogenetic Development of Immunogenesis

The most primitive animal capable of an immune response appears to be the lamprey[27], one of the higher cyclostome fish. It only reacts to a limited number of antigens, produces a single band of gamma globulin as demonstrated by immuno-electrophoresis and has only a primitive form of lymphoid tissue and no plasma cells. A stage lower in evolution, the hagfish, one of the lower cyclostomes, is quite incapable of producing an immune response and lacks lymphoid tissue, plasma cells and any form of gamma globulin. There appears to be a continuous spectrum of increasing complexity in immunogenesis from the lamprey, through the horned shark, which reacts to a wider range of antigens and has well developed lymphoid tissue but no plasma cells[28] and the chondreostean fish which possess plasma cells and have a much more sensitive immunological mechanism and a more lasting immunological memory. The next higher evolutionary stage is shown in the higher teleostean fish and amphibia and finally mammals and birds. Antibody globulin of the cold blooded animals seems to be mainly confined to a type of macroglobulin (IgM) whose specificity is much broader than that of the warm blooded animals. Sirotinin[29] for instance, found that goldfish, frogs and lizards failed to discriminate immunologically between horse serum and rabbit serum. That cold blooded animals are not devoid of ability to produce 7S antibody was shown by Uhr and his colleagues[30] using øX phage antigen incorporated into Freund's adjuvant.

The immune response in cold blooded animals is affected by temperature, little or no antibody being formed at low temperatures. Bisset[31] for instance, found no antibody response in frogs kept at 8° C. but antibody rapidly appeared when they were warmed to 30° C. and similar results were found by Uhr and his colleagues.[30] Sirotinin noted that frogs and reptiles produced antibody at summer temperatures but failed to do so in winter.

Although all species of mammals and birds make antibody globulin, both of the IgG and IgM types (and possibly of the IgA type although this antibody globulin has only been adequately studied in man), quantitative and qualitative differences are found in different species. We have already noted that anti-pneumococcal antibodies in the horse are of the 19S, IgM type. In the rabbit and in man they are mostly IgG in type. Chicken antibodies, which have a high proportion of IgM type have the peculiarity of only precipitating with antigen at high salt concentrations.[32]

The species used for immunisation may also affect the kinetics of the immune response particularly of the 7S antibody type. Uhr and his colleagues[5] using the same preparation of phage øX in rabbits and in man, noted that whereas in the rabbit 7S antibody was detected in 4 days with a rapid exponential increase, in man no 7S antibody appeared for approximately 2 weeks.

Age. Ontogenetic Development of Immunogenesis

In contrast to other serum proteins it is usually stated that gamma globulin is not formed in embryonic life. Animals such as man that receive maternal gamma globulin *in utero* are born with a concentration of gamma globulin equal to that in the maternal circulation. Almost immediately after birth this concentration falls reaching a low level in 3–10 weeks. With the development of the child's ability to synthesise its own gamma globulin, the concentration rises reaching adult levels of 600–1500 mg./100 ml. in 1–4 years.[27]

Is this apparent failure of the fœtus and newborn animal to produce appreciable amounts of gamma globulin due to an inherent inability to make antibodies or merely due to the segregation from antigenic stimuli in the security of the uterine environment?

Over the past years many attempts have been made to resolve this question by exposing the fœtus and newborn animal of many different species to a variety of antigenic stimuli. There is little doubt that the newborn animal and even the fœtus do possess the capacity to form antibody, although this capacity is poorly developed as compared with the adult and varies with the nature of the antigen and the species of animal.

Silverstein and his colleagues[33] have examined the ability of the fœtal lamb to make antibody to a variety of antigens injected *in utero* with and without Freund's adjuvant from 35 days gestation to normal term (150 days). These animals receive no gamma globulin from their mothers *in utero*, so that antibodies found in their serum are all self produced. The youngest animals immunised produced anti-phage antibodies within 6 days, even before functional lymph nodes and spleen were present, but after the first appearance of thymocytes in the primitive thymus. However, there was considerable variation in the time of response to different antigens, antibodies to ferritin and ovalbumin not being detected until after 65 and 25 days respectively and antibodies to diphtheria toxoid, *Salm. typhi* or B.C.G. not until several weeks after birth. Similar results were obtained in the rhesus monkey. The nature of the gamma globulin antibody produced in the fœtus was almost all of the IgM (19S) type. However, when Freund's adjuvant was used, gamma globulin of the 7S type was found in surprisingly large amounts, but only a small proportion of this was specific for the injected antigen. The nature of the residuum was undetermined.

Associated with this fœtal immune response were the changes in the lymph nodes and development of pyrinophilic cells as found in the adult (Chapter 35).

Similar results were obtained by Šterzl and his colleagues[34] in newborn germ-free piglets deprived of antibody from their mothers by withholding colostrum and immunised with a variety of particulate antigens. The antibody was solely of the 19S type, but when immunised *in utero*, a secondary response could be obtained soon after birth which was of the 7S type showing that immunological memory could be established *in utero*. Both the 19S and the 7S antibody, however, were of low combining capacity compared with those in the adult.

In man, the evidence that an immune response may occur *in utero* is more circumstantial. Infection *in utero* with *Treponema pallidium* or toxoplasma in the 5th or 6th months leads to the premature development in the fœtus of typical plasma cells.[33] In the cord blood of infants with congenital toxoplasmosis specific antibodies of the IgM type are found[35] which could only be of fœtal origin as this type of antibody fails to pass the placental barrier. Even in the normal child sensitive immunochemical techniques have shown the presence of small amounts of IgM in the cord blood and sera of infants within the first week of life.[36]

Many attempts have been made to immunise full term and premature infants at birth with variable results determined largely by the nature of the antigen. Whereas it is generally found that newborn infants fail to produce antitoxin to diphtheria toxoid even when allowance is made for the inhibitory effect of maternal antibody (see later section), both premature and full term infants produce antibody to virus antigens. Uhr and his colleagues[37] using øX phage as antigen noted that the antibody response in 11 premature infants was as good as that of 6 children 2–10 years of age. With a single dose of øX, 19S antibody appeared in the first week and increased to a maximum in 2–3 weeks with the appearance of 7S antibody. An efficient secondary response was obtained at 6 weeks. It is clear therefore, that, as in animals, the nature of the antigen plays an important part in determining the immune response in infants.

From the results of immunising fœtal and newborn animals recorded above, it is clear that the animal does not pass through a refractory stage as was believed at one time. However, the immune response in general is less efficient than in the adult in respect of quality and quantity of antibody formed and in its selectivity for only certain antigens. This is illustrated by the comparative ease with which a refractory state (immune tolerance, Chapter 41) can be produced by relatively small doses of antigen injected into the fœtus or, in some species, into the newborn animal. Such animals fail to develop sufficient antibody to eliminate the excess antigen which brings about the refractory state.

The time at which full maturation of the antibody forming system takes place varies in different species and with different antigens. Wolfe and his co-workers (for ref. see 27) noted that the immunological capacity in chickens was poorly developed at 4 weeks of age but increased rapidly in the next 2 weeks and in a year reached a level 4-fold higher than the level at 6 weeks.

The rate of development of immunogenesis in man has considerable importance in deciding when immunisation may be started effectively in children. Quite apart from the inhibitory effect of passively transferred maternal antibody considered in a later section, the administration of certain antigens before maturation of the antibody forming mechanism has fully developed may not only lead to no response, but there is at least a theoretical possibility that it may produce tolerance (Chapter 41). However, in no case so far recorded, apart from children suffering from hypogammaglobulinæmia (see later), has failure to respond at birth persisted into adult life.[38] Because of the poor response of infants to diphtheria prophylaxis in the first few weeks of life (for refs. see 27, 38) there has been a tendency to postpone immunisation in general until after the child is at least 3 months old. However, as we have seen, procedures that may be justified in diphtheria prophylaxis do not necessarily apply to other antigens. There is a practical need, for instance, to immunise infants as early as possible against whooping cough which is a particularly dangerous disease in the first few months of life. The evidence suggests that immunisation with pertussis vaccine is effective if started at 1 month but falls short of the response to immunisation at 3 months of age.[39] Other antigens which appear to be effective in early life are live (but not inactivated) poliovirus vaccine and, surprisingly in view of the poor response to diphtheria toxoid, alum precipitated tetanus toxoid. Osborn and his colleagues[40] noted that the levels of tetanus antitoxin in infants under 2 weeks of age given a single injection were not significantly lower than those produced by older infants. For the most part these early antibodies are of the IgM type. It is only later that they are replaced or accompanied by IgG.

Nutritional Factors

It has been found that the concentration of serum gamma globulin is maintained even in severe nitrogen starvation in which the serum albumin may be considerably depleted. This is illustrated in the disease known as *kwashiorkor* which is due to a dietary deficiency in protein, particularly in the essential amino-acid methionine. The disease occurs in young children and is characterised by a hypoalbuminæmia resulting in œdema and failure to grow. The production of gamma globulin is not decreased. On the contrary, in children suffering from infection, particularly common in this disease, the gamma globulin content of the serum may be increased three-to four-fold. We have, therefore, the anomalous condition of a serum albumin concentration reduced to a third and a gamma globulin concentration increased three-fold.[41] It would seem, therefore, that the gamma globulin is synthesised from the amino-acid pool at the expense of serum albumin and perhaps of other body proteins also.

A number of observations have been made on the effect of vitamin and other dietary deficiencies on the immune response, but with the exception of a diminished response where a deficiency of pyridoxine was correlated with a reduction of gamma globulin, the results have not been constant or well defined.

The Influence of Preformed Antibody on the Immune Response—Inhibitory Action

As long ago as 1909, Theobald Smith noted that an active immunity could be produced in guinea-pigs by the injection of diphtheria toxin neutralised with antitoxin, the efficacy of the mixture being related to the ratio of toxin to antitoxin that it contained. Under-neutralised mixtures, i.e. those giving some local reactions, were much more efficacious than neutral mixtures, and mixtures containing an excess of antitoxin "reduce the possibility of producing an active immunity and may extinguish it altogether" (Theobald Smith). This is the basis for the use of slightly under-neutralised toxoid-antitoxin floccules (TAF) in the active immunisation against diphtheria. Later, Glenny and Sudmersen[2] noted that antibody produced actively or injected passively depresses and may completely inhibit the immune response particularly when the antigen is injected directly into the circulation. This observation has been confirmed on many occasions since.

The mechanism of inhibition.—There is little doubt that, by uniting with the antigen, antibody blocks its capacity to stimulate the immune response. This is seen particularly when antigen in a soluble state is injected directly into the circulation. In addition to this "blanketing" action, antibody hastens the elimination of antigen from the body, and thus shortens the period during which antigen can stimulate the immune reaction. This effect has been studied on a number of occasions with labelled antigens, particularly by Dixon and his colleagues.[42] Using bovine gamma globulin labelled with I^{131} as antigen, they compared its rate of removal from the blood stream in normal, immunised, and irradiated rabbits with that of the animal's own gamma globulin similarly labelled and re-injected. In the normal rabbits, once equilibrium between the vascular and extravascular labelled proteins was established, the rate of metabolism as shown by the appearance of protein breakdown products containing I^{131} in the urine was of the same order for both proteins, but only over a period of 4 days after injection. Thereafter the antigenic bovine gamma globulin was eliminated at a greatly increased rate, none being detected after the seventh day (FIG. 2, curve C), whereas much of the animal's own labelled globulin, which did not act as an antigen, was still present after 11 days. Antibody was detected in the blood on the seventh day.

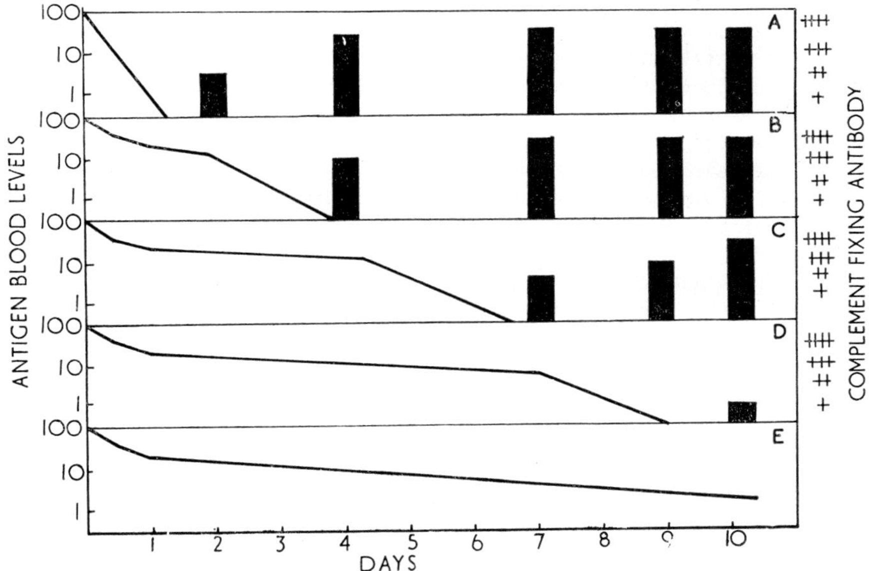

34/FIG. 2.—Showing the rate of elimination of antigen in relation to the antibody response in rabbits. Antigen: bovine γ-globulin marked with I^{131}. A = potentially immune animals with circulating antibody at the time of injection; B = potentially immune animals with no circulating antibody; C = normal animals not previously immunised; D = normal animals irradiated with 200r X-rays; E = normal animals irradiated with 500r X-rays. (From Dixon *et al.*[42])

In the immune rabbits, the rate of elimination and metabolism of the antigen was greatly increased, immediately when injected into animals having circulating antibody (FIG. 2, curve A), and in 2 days in animals immunised some weeks earlier, who were potentially immune, but whose circulating antibody had fallen to a level too low to be measured (Curve B). In both, a secondary immune response was observed.

In animals irradiated with 200 rads X-rays, the increased rate of metabolism of the antigen compared with that of the animals' own globulin was not established until 7 days (Curve D), and with animals irradiated with 500 rads, no increase in rate was observed (Curve E), In the former, but not in the latter, there was a small immune response in 10 days.

These results show clearly that the rate of elimination of antigen depends on the immune response to it. In animals already immune the rate of removal and metabolism of antigen is greatly accelerated; in normal animals the rate is slow to start with but becomes rapid as soon as the immune response is established; and in animals in which the immune response has been inhibited by X-irradiation the antigen is metabolised throughout at a rate no faster than that of the animals' own serum globulin. The increased rate of elimination of labelled antigen is a very sensitive test for an immune response as it can be observed even before circulating antibody can be detected ("immune elimination").

The next question is whether the rate of antigen elimination is directly dependent on the antibody titre. A clear relationship between antibody titre and antigen-elimination was established by the use of preformed antibody injected intravenously into normal rabbits who had been given a prior injection of antigen 2 and 3 days before. It was too early to expect an active immune response to the antigen, so that any change in the rate of elimination could be attributed to the antibody passively acquired. A sudden fall in circulating antigen followed each injection of antibody. This was probably due in the first place to a union of antibody with antigen and the removal of the complexes by the reticulo-endothelial system. Garvey and Campbell[43] showed that such complexes are filtered off in the sinusoids of the liver, probably by the Kupffer cells. However, estimations of small molecular products of protein breakdown marked with I^{131} in the blood, urine, and tissues showed that the elimination was also associated with a greatly increased rate of antigen catabolism. The rate of destruction appears, therefore, to depend solely on the antibody concentration at the time and not on any adaptation of the cells to catabolise the antigen more rapidly, for even if such adaptation had occurred in actively immunised animals it would have been lacking from those passively immunised.

When antigen unites with antibody *in vivo*, antibody as well as antigen is eliminated and destroyed. This is shown by experiments in which labelled rabbit antibody has been injected into rabbits followed by homologous antigen. This resulted in rapid elimination of the labelled antibody and the appearance of labelled breakdown products in the urine.[44]

The effect of 19S and 7S antibody on the immune response.—Investigations by Uhr and his colleagues[12] on the effect of passively administered antibody of each of these molecular species on the 19S and 7S primary responses to phage øX showed that 7S was much more effective in inhibiting both 19S and 7S primary responses in guinea-pigs. Passively administered 19S antibody depressed the subsequent 19S immune response but had no action on the 7S response. If 7S antibody were given 3 days after the injection of antigen during the exponential rise of 19S in a primary response, the further development of a 19S response was not only inhibited but was not followed by the usual 7S rise, and the development of 7S immunological memory did not take place. From the experiments of Dixon, the inhibitory effect was probably due to a premature elimination of antigen. This would result in cutting short a 19S response which, as we have seen, is dependent in this system on the continued presence of antigen. It would seem also that the loss of antigen had also affected the preliminary events leading up to the 7S primary response and the development of 7S immunological memory which apparently require an interval of time greater than 3 days for the antibody forming cells to be in contact with antigen. FIGURE 3 illustrates the effect of 19S and 7S antibody on the production of these antibodies.

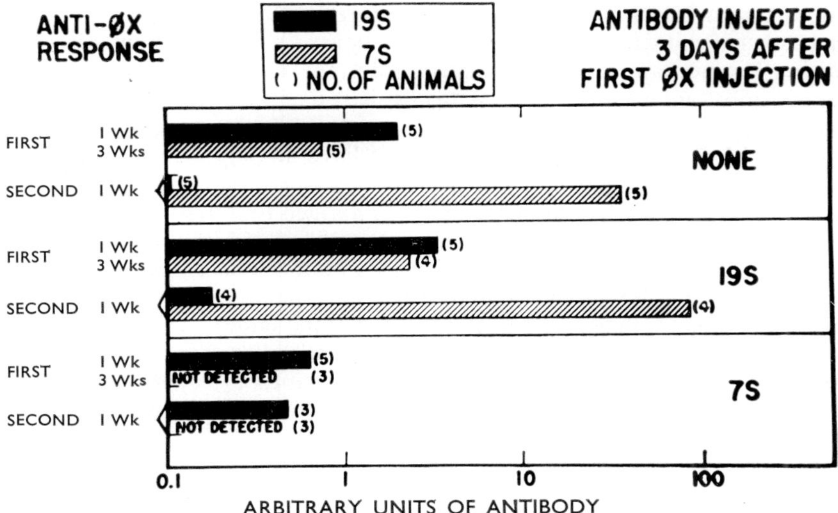

34/Fig. 3.—Inhibition of formation of antibody to øX by passively administered 19S and 7S antibody to øX. (After Finkelstein and Uhr.[12])

The progressively more avid 7S antibody produced after repeated injections of antigen is more effective in its inhibitory action than the less avid 7S of a primary response, presumably because it unites more firmly with antigen and thereby increases the rate of antigen metabolism and elimination. Uhr and Finkelstein[5] regard this inhibitory effect of 7S antibody as a "feedback" mechanism producing an equilibrium at a certain stage of immunisation and preventing over production of antibody.

The Influence of small Amounts of Antibody on the Immune Response—Stimulating Action

In spite of the general finding that circulating antibody depresses the immune response and leads to more rapid metabolism and elimination of antigen, the possibility that very small amounts of antibody may have the reverse effect has been raised as the result of comparing the immune responses of young piglets when fed, and when deprived of, colostrum, the only source of maternal antibody. With particulate antigens, little or no difference was observed[34, 45], but with soluble antigens (diphtheria and tetanus toxoids) the difference was marked, little or no antibody being produced if the pigs were deprived of colostrum, whereas high titres were found in pigs fed with it.[46] That specific antibody in the colostrum was responsible for the enhanced immune response was shown by feeding dilute antitoxic serum in place of colostrum. If the specific antitoxin was removed from the serum, the effect was abolished.

The factor determining whether antibody depresses or enhances the immune response probably depends on the concentration of antibody relative to the dose of antigen. This is supported by the observation of Terres and Wolins[47] who obtained an accelerated immune response to bovine serum albumin in mice if injected previously with rabbit antibody to bovine serum albumin, provided a concentration below the immunological equivalent of the dose of antigen was used, otherwise it depressed the immune response by immune elimination of the antigen. The mechanism of this enhancement is not fully understood. As enhancement is only found with soluble antigens, it is likely that union with antibody converts the antigen into one more nearly resembling a particulate antigen and assists in its retention in the body; but we have already seen that union with antibody is the very means by which antigen is removed and destroyed.The paradox is resolved when the proportion of antigen to antibody in the complex is taken into consideration. We have already noted that toxoid-antitoxin floccules (TAF) are a more effective antigen than toxoid alone, but only if the toxoid in the complex is "underneutralised" i.e. contains a proportion of toxoid to antitoxin greater than optimal. It is likely that the same consideration operates when small amounts of antibody unite with antigen *in vivo*. The retention of "underneutralised" in contrast to the rapid elimination of "neutralised" antigen-antibody complexes is discussed in Chapter 39 in connection with the mechanism of serum sickness.

Abnormalities in the Immune Response

So far we have considered the immune response of a normal immunologically competent animal to an antigenic stimulus. Like any other system of the body, however, the immune mechanism may go wrong. An abnormal response may take the form of a deficiency in the formation of gamma globulin: *hypogammaglobulinæmia*; the formation of abnormal types of gamma globulin: *dysgammaglobulinæmia*, or the mounting of an immune response to the antigens of the body itself: *autoimmunity* (discussed in Chapter 40).

Hypogammaglobulinæmia

This term is used to describe a number of pathological conditions in which there is a permanent deficiency in the concentration of gamma globulin in the serum accompanied by a tendency to develop infective disease of more or less severity. Since the discovery of this syndrome by Bruton[48] in 1952 in a boy who had an almost complete absence of gamma globulin in his serum and who suffered from 18 miscellaneous and severe infections within the first 4 years of life, numerous other instances have been described.

There appear to be at least 4 varieties of the disease which are summarised in Table I according to the data of Good and his colleagues.[49]

The most severe form is the *congenital sex-linked recessive* type of which Bruton's case is an example. The disease is confined to boys and consists of a failure to form antibodies, even under condition of intense antigenic stimulation, and an unusual susceptibility to most bacterial infections, but not to infections by facultative intracellular parasites (Chapter 37) or viruses. Such individuals have IgG globulin levels usually below 20 mg./100 ml. and IgA and IgM are absent. They entirely lack plasma cells and their lymphoid tissue is poorly developed. The thymus, however, appears normal, the number of circulating lymphocytes is normal and delayed type hypersensitivity reactions (Chapter 39) can be elicited as in normal persons.

The so-called *Swiss type* is another congenital form of the disease but involves both sexes.[50] In contrast to the sex-linked recessive type, this type involves the

34/TABLE I

TYPES OF HYPOGAMMAGLOBULINÆMIA

Type	*Sex*	*Type of Globulin Deficiency*	*Type of Infection Found*	*Lymphoid Tissue*	*Thymus*	*Plasma Cells*	*Ability to Show Delayed Hypersensitivity*
Congenital sex-linked	M	IgA and IgM absent IgG deficient	Bacterial	Poorly developed	Normal	Absent	Normal
Congenital Swiss type	M or F	—	Bacterial, fungal or viral	Deficient	Rarely neoplastic	Absent	Deficient
Ataxia telangiectasia	M or F	IgA mainly but also IgG	—	—	Deficient	—	—
Primary acquired	M or F	IgA, IgM and IgG	—	Deficient	Thymoma	Deficient	—

whole of the lymphoid tissue including the thymus which is greatly reduced in size and contains virtually no lymphocytes or Hassall's corpuscles. There is a profound lymphopenia. These patients usually die before 18 months of age with intercurrent infection not only bacterial but viral as well.

A type of immunological deficiency involving mainly a deficiency in IgA and to a lesser extent IgG is associated with cerebellar ataxia and oculocutaneous telangiectasis with unusual susceptibility to respiratory infection. This syndrome, named *ataxia telangiectasia*, is often associated with lymphocyte or reticular tumours. The thymus usually shows gross abnormality and the central lymphoid tissue is deficient. It has been suggested that the apparently unconnected manifestations of the syndrome are related through some deficiency in the development of mesenchymal tissue.[28]

Finally, *primary acquired hypogammaglobulinæmia* is a type of immunological deficiency occuring at any time of life from causes unknown.[51] It is often associated with benign thymoma which, it has been suggested,[28] is due to a secondary compensatory hyperplasia. *Secondary acquired hypogammaglobulinæmia* may result from granulomatous or neoplastic disease of the lymphoid tissue, e.g. Hodgkin's disease and chronic lymphatic leukæmia.

Gitlin and his colleagues[52] have drawn attention to a *transient type of hypogammaglobulinæmia* due to a prolongation of the normal inadequacy of gamma globulin synthesis in the first few weeks after birth. It is therefore restricted to early infancy. Two cases quoted by Gitlin failed to make gamma globulin 3–5 months after birth, and suffered from severe infections. After 5 months, however, the content of gamma globulin in the serum slowly rose to normal levels.

Dysgammaglobulinæmia

Under this heading are included a number of conditions in which one or more types of serum gamma globulin are increased in amounts and are abnormal in kind. These gamma globulins were thought to differ from the normal types of immunoglobulins in not appearing to possess antibody function. However, recently an abnormal gamma globulin from a patient with multiple myeloma has been shown to react specifically with a synthetic hapten, ε-dinitro-phenyl-L-lysine.[52a] Moreover, the fact that certain antigenic groups in these gamma globulins are identical with those in their counterpart types of normal immunoglobulin, indicates that dysgammaglobulinæmia is essentially a dysfunction in the formation of normal immunoglobulins.

There are two main types of the disease: (*a*) A type usually associated with *multiple myeloma*, (*b*) *Waldenström's macroglobulinæmia.*

Multiple myeloma is characterised by malignant plasma cell tumours in the bone marrow eroding and replacing the bone accompanied by an increase in the 7S gamma globulin either of the IgG or IgA types. In addition the urine may contain the so-called Bence Jones proteins. These proteins have a molecular weight of 20,000 (or more usually 40,000 as they tend to form dimers) and possess the property of precipitating on heating and redissolving on boiling, a property shared by the isolated L chains of 7S immunoglobulin. It was at one time thought that Bence Jones protein was an abnormal product but it is now known that small amounts are present in normal human plasma[53] and have been designated gamma L.

We have already seen (Chapter 32) that the normal 7S immunoglobulins of one individual are a heterogeneous collection of molecules divided primarily according to their antigens on the Fc fragment of the heavy chain (IgG and IgA); secondarily, according to the sequence of amino-acids in the C-terminal portion of the light chain (kappa and lambda); thirdly, according to allotypic markers (Gm I, II, III etc.); and finally into an unknown number of subtypes—according to the sequence of amino-acids on the N-terminal portion of the light chain—so large that no two molecules taken at random are identical. In contrast, the immunoglobulins from a patient with multiple myeloma are entirely homogeneous. We have, therefore, patients with either IgG or IgA immunoglobulins, but not both, each of which may be either kappa or lambda, but not both. Within these groups there are as many individual types as there are multiple myeloma patients, but no patient has more than one type.

It would appear that the disease is primarily a neoplasm of plasma cells, the secondary manifestations being the formation of a single type of 7S immunoglobulin often with excess production of the L chains of the same type which are excreted in the urine in the form of Bence Jones proteins.

Macroglobulinæmia.—This disease, first described by Waldenström[54] more than 25 years ago, is a condition in which the serum content of macroglobulin 19S is markedly increased. Like multiple myeloma, it is often associated with cytological proliferation in the bone marrow, but the predominant cell type is not the plasma cell but a lymphocytoid reticulum cell. Although the disease may progress and the patient die from cachexia and anæmia, the proliferating cells do not invade the bone and there is no bone pain. Sometimes the disease follows a benign course, the only signs being an increase in 19S macroglobulin, increased sedimentation rate and anæmia. A peculiar form of hæmorrhagic diathesis is often associated with the disease particularly bleeding from the mucous membrane of the nose, mouth and gums and also into the retina. The cause of the hæmorrhages is unknown but it has been suggested that the highly sticky macroglobulin covers the surface of the platelets and abolishes their normal functions.[55]

The macroglobulin has all the characters of the normal IgM except that it has not been shown as yet to have antibody function. Also, unlike normal IgM type macroglobulin, which consists of a heterogenous family of macroglobulins, the macroglobulin of this disease tends to be electrophoretically homogeneous and gives a narrow band on immunoelectrophoresis. As with IgG, IgA and Bence Jones proteins of multiple myeloma, the antigens on the L chains are either kappa or lambda but not both. Waldenström[56] interprets this homogeneity in pathological macroglobulin as being due to a pathological proliferation (neoplastic) of a single clone of cells, whereas the heterogeneity of IgM found in normal or immune sera is likely to be due to a physiological multiplication of many cell clones. A similar interpretation may apply to the findings of multiple myeloma.

H chain disease.—In multiple myeloma we saw that isolated L chains may be found in the serum and urine in the form of Bence Jones protein. A counterpart to this disease has been described in five patients in which a large quantity of an abnormal protein was present in the serum and urine with a sedimentation coefficient of 3·5S and was antigenically related to the H chains of IgG (for refs. see

57). This protein was first thought to be isolated H chains, but further analysis, using highly polar glycine solution to prevent aggregation, suggested that it was the Fc fragment of the H chain. In all five patients, the abnormal protein was antigenically homogeneous, none being found which cross reacted with IgA or IgM. Like the Bence Jones protein in multiple myeloma, the Fc fragment of IgG is apparently present in normal serum in a low concentration. Evidence obtained by feeding I^{131} to one of these patients showed that the disease was due to an over production of this fragment and not an increased degradation of normal IgG. Clinically the disease resembles multiple myeloma.

THEORIES OF ANTIBODY FORMATION

In the theory originally proposed by Ehrlich antibodies were regarded as normal cellular products that were formed in the absence of antigens but were produced in greatly increased amounts when antigens were present. The cell was supposed to react to the neutralisation of the preformed antibody with antigen by the production of antibody in excess (see Chapter 33). This theory lost favour for a time with the realisation that the number of different antibodies to be accounted for was extremely large. According to a theory elaborated later by Pauling[58] antibodies have the amino-acid sequences of normal globulins, but differ from the latter in that the specific conformation of their combining sites have been formed in the presence of an antigen, whose determinant groups have guided the folding of parts of the peptide chain into complementary configurations. Pauling's theory accounted for the heterogeneity of antibodies, but it threw little light on other immunological phenomena, such as immune tolerance and the striking difference between the primary and secondary response. Theories which assign to the antigen a less direct role in the formation of antibody thus began to be developed, some of which were closer in principle to the theory of Ehrlich than to that of Pauling.

Burnet and Fenner[9] proposed that the antigen does not modify the globulin molecules themselves but a self-duplicating unit in the cell from which these molecules are formed. In contrast, Burnet[59] later suggested that antibodies are formed by a population of cells in which new clones are constantly arising from somatic mutations. Enough clones were supposed to be produced to provide sites, in the cell population, that could react with every possible antigen. Reaction of an antigen with its complementary site in a cell at a stage of embryonic life was assumed to lead to cell death and immune tolerance. At a later stage of life the reaction was supposed to stimulate cell proliferation, so that a clone of cells which were all able to synthesise a specific antibody finally emerged.

A question of major importance in relation to the clonal selection theory is whether a single cell can produce more than one antibody. This question has not yet been decided. Nossal,[60] who prepared single cell suspensions from the popliteal lymph nodes of rats immunised with two or three different flagella antigens from strains of Salmonella, concluded that each antibody-producing cell can form only one antibody at a time. On the other hand, Attardi, Cohn, Horibata and Lennox,[61] who isolated single cells from the popliteal lymph nodes of rabbits immunised with two different strains of bacteriophage, reported that of 95 cells that were antibody-producers, 21 formed antibody against both antigens.

Theories which assume that the antigen in some way directs the formation of the antibody have been called by Lederberg[62] instructive theories and theories which assume the pre-existence of all possible antibodies have been called elective theories. The remarkable heterogeneity of the peptide chains of the immunoglobulins, about which we have learned a great deal in the last few years (see Chapter 32) has focused attention on two basic questions in this field: by what mechanism do the multiple differences in the amino sequences of this family of proteins arise; and are differences in amino-acid sequence responsible for the specific reactions of antibodies with their corresponding antigens? For the second question to be answered in the affirmative, the number of different amino-acid sequences must be sufficiently large to account for the enormous variety of antibody-combining sites.

The ability of certain strains of guinea-pig to make antibodies to hapten-polylysine conjugates, which is not shared by other guinea-pigs, or by pigs, mice, rats and rabbits, has been shown to be controlled by a dominant gene.[63] However, the level at which this control is exercised is uncertain.

A number of suggestions have been made to account for the variability of the light chains of the immunoglobulins. These include the accumulation of point mutations, hypermutability of a single gene, chromosomal rearrangements, and intrachromatid inversions of genetic material.[64] The problem is complicated by the need to explain how variations arise in the N-terminal portion of the light chains without comparable changes in their C-terminal portion (Chapter 32). This difference would be understandable if the two halves of the chain were synthesised separately on different templates and then linked together, but no evidence for such a process has been obtained.[65] However, Putnam, Titani and Whitley[66] have concluded that the variations in the amino-acid sequences of light chains are consistent with the presence of many genes for these chains, each of which could have arisen throughout evolution by duplication and independent mutation. The existence of repeated genes would presumably increase the chance that mutation would be non-lethal. Milstein[67] has considered the possibility that an enzyme may act as a mutagenic agent by producing cuts in specific stretches of DNA, resulting in a repeated process of damage and repair.

A vital question in relation to the problem of antibody synthesis is whether all the information required for the production of the specific conformations of biologically active proteins resides in the sequence of amino-acids in their polypeptide chains. Evidence in support of this view, based on the ability of an active conformation to reform rapidly after treatments which produce changes in tertiary structure, was obtained with a number of relatively small proteins containing single polypeptide chains.[68] In several cases similar evidence has been obtained with antibodies. Thus, Haber[69] found that an antibody fragment lost its capacity to combine specifically with antigen when its disulphide bonds were broken by reduction and non-covalent bonds were broken by the denaturing agent guanidinium chloride. But when the denaturing and reducing agents were removed by dialysis up to 27 per cent. of the original capacity to combine with antigen was restored. A similar result was obtained by Freedman and Sela[70] who found that DL-alanyl peptides could be attached to IgG without radically changing its antibody properties and that the resulting molecule, unlike the parent antibody, could be reduced in the presence of denaturing agents such as urea to give water-soluble products. Reoxidation of this material led to the restoration of about 25 per cent of the original antigen-binding capacity.

On the assumption that complete unfolding had, indeed, occurred in these experiments, the latter provide persuasive evidence for the hypothesis that the specific conformations of the combining sites of the antibodies concerned represent a pattern of folding which is determined only by the sequences of amino-acids in their peptide chains. If this hypothesis were accepted in a generalised form it would be difficult to imagine how the formation of antibody-combining sites could be dependent on the intervention of the antigen at the stage of protein synthesis, as they would be according to "instructive" hypotheses of the type proposed by Pauling, unless the antigen affected the translation of an RNA template. However, this objection to an "instructive" hypothesis would lose its force if the specific conformations of the antibodies used had been partly retained during the process of reduction and denaturation.

Two other questions are clearly of the first importance for a decision between an instructive and an elective theory. Is antibody formed only when antigen is present in antibody-forming tissue and is the antigen present in the antibody-producing cell or plasma cell, itself? The answers to these questions are still uncertain. In one study with large doses of an antigen labelled by a tritiated hapten the latter was detected in plasma cells by radioautography.[71] But a later investigation, in which a synthetic polypeptide trace-labelled with I^{125} was used in amounts no greater than that required to produce a response, did not confirm this result.[72] The antigen was injected in Freund's adjuvant into the hind foot pads of mice. Its localisation was studied by radioautography during intervals from 12 hours to 21 days in draining popliteal and flank lymph nodes and antibody-containing cells were detected by immunofluorescent staining. The radioautographs showed an intense deposition of antigen in the germinal centres of the lymph nodes, but grain counts which did not differ significantly from background in the antibody-containing cells. Provided that degradation with loss of the radioactive tracer had not occurred in the lymph nodes this result indicated that less than 15 molecules of antigen were present in each antibody-containing cell. Thus, these observations indicate that the amount of antigen taken up by antibody-producing cells may at least be very small; but they do not prove that no antigen is taken up by these cells at any stage.

Burnet and Fenner drew attention to analogies between antibody-formation and other cases in which the pattern of proteins synthesised by a cell may change, such as in cell differentiation, the synthesis of inducible enzymes, and drug resistance in micro-organisms. The acquisition of drug resistance is often associated with a change in the DNA of the cell, involving either a mutation in a chromosomal gene or the transfer of genetic material from a resistant cell to a sensitive one by a resistance transfer factor or a phage. Enzyme induction and cellular differentiation, however, can apparently occur without any change in chromosomal genes. As pointed out by Monod,[73] in both enzyme induction and antibody synthesis a protein is formed in greatly increased amount which is able to combine reversibly and in a stereospecific fashion with a small molecule, the latter being the substrate or inducer in one case and the hapten in the other. Cohn and Torriani[74] reported that the β-galactosidase induced in *E. coli* by certain β-galactosides is closely related to one of the normal proteins of the organism. The synthesis of this enzyme, like that of an antibody globulin, may therefore represent a variation on a pre-existing structural pattern. The induction of β-galactosidase by low concentrations of thiomethyl-β-D-galactoside shows a period of acceleration which is associated with the induction of a "permease" responsible for the transfer of galactosides into the cells.[75] The synthesis of the permease renders the cells "hypersensitive" to the inducer. Moreover, such cells may remain hypersensitive for a significant period when grown in the absence of the inducer, for the permease can be produced in considerable excess and be detected even when diluted among cells of the fourth generation. The cells are thus endowed with a "memory" of their early contact with the inducer which may be likened to the immunological memory that is manifested in the secondary response. Novick and Weiner[76] showed that at certain low inducer concentrations some cells in a population of *E. coli* become fully sensitive and others remain non-sensitive. This may be explained by the assumption that the chance contact of an appropriate portion of the cell with one, or only a few, molecules of inducer is sufficient to initiate the synthesis of permease. In these cells and their daughter cells inducer will be concentrated and more permease synthesised. Consequently sensitive and induced cells will come to be distributed in clones (all the cells in a clone stemming from the same original parent), as they would be if the properties concerned had arisen from mutations in the original population.

The discovery of the great variety of pre-existing gamma globulins has added emphasis to elective theories of antibody formation in recent years. Whether the heterogeneity of the immunoglobulins is sufficient to account for the number of different antibodies obtainable remains uncertain. But it provides, at least, a basis for great flexibility in tertiary structure. The possibility must be considered that an instructive mechanism, perhaps operating at the cytoplasmic level, is superimposed, in each case, on a protein whose appropriate amino-acid sequence is genetically controlled.

In summary, it is not yet possible to decide with certainty between elective and instructive theories. Elective theories are compatible with views which are commonly held about the mechanisms of protein synthesis, including the formation of inducible enzymes, and they have been elaborated to account for immunological memory. But some of these views have not been finally established, and whether a sufficient number of genes is available to account for all possible antibodies remains uncertain. An instructive theory can readily account for an almost inexhaustible number of different antibodies. But convincing evidence that antibody formation occurs only in the presence of antigen is lacking and the view that the tertiary structure of a protein is determined during its synthesis by reaction with a small molecule, such as a hapten, has not been generally accepted. A more precise understanding of the mechanism of antibody formation is likely to be associated with more detailed knowledge of the way in which the synthesis of cell protein in general is controlled.

Summary

The kinetics of the immune response depend on whether the tissues are exposed to antigen for the first time (primary response) or whether they have been exposed to antigen on previous occasions (secondary response). Each response consists of a latent period, rise of antibody to a peak or plateau and subsequent decline. The latent period of the *primary response* may vary from a few hours to several days, depending on the nature, dose and route of the antigen. The rise usually but not invariably involves two qualitatively different groups of antibody. A rise in macro immunoglobulin (19S) starts early, rises to a peak and falls with the elimination of antigen. This is overlapped and followed by a rise in 7S usually more sustained and not dependent on the continued presence of appreciable amounts, at least, of antigen. The rise in both cases is exponential, but the amount of antibody formed is small. A second dose of antigen produces a rise of antibody (*secondary response*) more rapid in onset which may reach a maximum value 10–100 times that of the primary response. The exponential rise of antibody in both responses, however, has the same slope. The secondary response may involve both molecular species of antibody if given before the decline of the 19S primary response, and before antigen of the first stimulus has been eliminated. Otherwise it is confined to the 7S response. Long lasting *immunological memory* (potential immunity), the capacity to give a secondary response to contact with antigen, is thus a property of the 7S antibody forming mechanism. However, exceptions are found in which only 19S response and 19S immunological memory occurs. Immunological 7S memory may be produced with small amounts of antigen giving apparently only a primary 19S response. With some antigens it takes time (30 or more days) to develop to a maximum. Antibody produced as a secondary and subsequent response is usually more avid than antibody produced earlier. Factors influencing the quantity and quality of antibody produced are the nature of the antigen particularly whether soluble or particulate, the dose, and the route of injection. In the evolutionary scale, the first animal to produce an immune response is the lamprey. Antibody produced by the cold blooded animals is of the 19S variety. In the individual animal, the age of development of an immune response depends on the species. Early antibody formation confined to 19S type may be produced in some animals such as the lamb *in utero*. Others do not develop an adequate mechanism until some weeks after birth. Full maturation of the antibody forming mechanism may take some weeks to develop. Nitrogen starvation (kwashiorkor) has little influence on the production of antibody. Preformed antibody causes an inhibition in immune response due to combination with antigen and increased metabolism and elimination of antigen. The increased rate of catabolism and elimination of labelled antigen is a sensitive indication of the development of an immune response ("immune elimination"). Animals with well established immunological memory may react to non-specific stimuli by an increased production of specific antibody ("anamnestic reaction").

Abnormalities in immunoglobulin formation occur naturally in man, and take the form of (1) deficiency in production involving all 3 types: IgM, IgA, IgG. (2) Formation of abnormal forms: (*a*) plasma cell tumour (myeloma, with increase in IgG or IgA with overproduction of free L chains (Bence Jones protein)), (*b*) macroglobulinæmia with overproduction of IgM of an abnormal form (*c*) "H chain disease", a rare disease in which the Fc fragment of the H chain is increased in amount.

The theories on the production of antibody may be divided into "instructive" in which the antigen directly influences the formation of the globulin molecule or its precursor and "elective" in which the antigen has a stimulating action on cells or subcellular entities forming a gamma globulin already orientated to the structure of the antigen. The theories are discussed in relation to our current knowledge of protein synthesis and it is concluded that it is not possible at the present time to decide with certainty between them.

REFERENCES

1. von Dungern, E. (1903). *Die Antikorper*, Jena.
2. Glenny, A. T., and Südmersen, H. J. (1921). *J. Hyg. (Lond.)*, **20,** 176.
3. Stavitsky, A. B. (1962). *Mechanisms of Antibody Formation*, p. 225. Eds. Holub, M., and Jarošková, L. Prague: Czech. Acad. Sci.
4. Schoenheimer, R., Ratner, S., Rittenberg, D., and Heildelberger, M. (1942). *J. biol. Chem.*, **144,** 541.
5. Uhr, J. W., and Finkelstein, M. S. (1967). *Progr. Allergy*, **10,** 37.
6. Svehag, S. E., and Mandel, B. (1964). *J. exp. Med.*, **119,** 1, 21.

6a. Litt, M. (1967). *Cold Spr. Harb. Symp. quant. Biol.*, **32,** 477.

7. Weigle, W. O. (1957). *Proc. Soc. exp. Biol. (N.Y.)*, **94,** 306.
8. Taliaferro, W. H., and Taliaferro, L. G. (1963). *J. infect. Dis.*, **113,** 155.
9. Burnet, F. M., and Fenner, F. (1949). *The Production of Antibodies*, 2nd edit. London: Macmillan & Co.
10. Uhr, J. W. (1964). *Science*, **145,** 457.
11. Ada, G. L., Nossal, G. J. V., and Austin, C. M. (1965). *Molecular and Cellular Basis of Antibody Formation*, p. 31. Ed. Šterzl, J. Prague: Czech. Acad. Sci.
12. Finkelstein, M. S., and Uhr, J. W. (1964). *Science*, **146,** 67.
13. Porter, R. J. (1966). *Proc. Soc. exp. Biol. (N.T.)*, **121,** 107.
14. Eisen, H. M. (1964–65). *Harvey Lect.*, **60,** 1.
15. Jackson, A. L., Koczot, F. J., and Landy, M. (1965). *Fed. Proc.*, **24,** 252.
16. Glenny, A. T. (1931). *System of Bacteriology*, **6,** 106. Medical Research Council. London: H.M.S.O.
17. Barr, M., and Glenny, A. T. (1946). *J. Hyg. (Lond.)*, **44,** 135.
18. Coons, A. H. (1965). Ref. 11, p. 559.
19. Good, R. A. (1965). Ref. 11, Discussion p. 615.
20. Heidelberger, M. (1953). *The Nature and Significance of the Antibody Response.* Ed. Pappenheimer, A. M., Jr. N.Y. Acad. Med. Symposium No. 5, p. 90. New York: Columbia Univ. Press.
21. Coons, A. H. (1953). Ref. 20, p. 200.
22. Glenny, A. T., Buttle, G. A. H., and Stevens, M. F. (1931). *J. Path. Bact.*, **34,** 267.
23. Munz, J. (1964). *Advanc. Immunol.*, **4,** 397.
24. White, R. G. (1965). Ref. 11, p. 71.
25. Hooker, S. B., and Boyd, W. C. (1931). *J. Immunol.*, **21,** 113.
26. Freund, J., and Bonanto, M. V. (1941). *J. Immunol.*, **40,** 437.
27. Good, R. A., and Papermaster, B. W. (1964). *Advanc. Immunol.*, **4,** 1.
28. Good, R. A., Finstad, J., Peterson, R. D. A., Kellum, M., and Sutherland, D. E. R. (1965). Ref. 11, p. 289.
29. Sirotinin, N. N. (1962). Ref. 3, p. 113.
30. Uhr, J. W., Finkelstein, M. S., and Franklin, E. C. (1962). *Proc. Soc. exp. Biol. (N.Y.)*, **111,** 13.
31. Bisset, K. A. (1948). *J. Path. Bact.*, **60,** 87.
32. Benedict, A. A., Brown, R. J., and Hersh, R. T. (1963). *J. Immunol.*, **90,** 399.
33. Silverstein, A. M., and Kraner, K. L. (1965). Ref. 11, p. 341.

34. ŠTERZL, J., MANDEL, L., MILER, I., and ŘÍHA, I. (1965). Ref. 11, p. 351.
35. EICHENWALD, H. F., and SHINEFIELD, H. R. (1963). *J. Pediat.*, **63,** 870.
36. WEST, C. D., HONG, R., and HOLLAND, N. H. (1962). *J. clin. Invest.*, **41,** 2054.
37. UHR, J. W., DANCIS, J., FRANKLIN, E. C., FINKELSTEIN, M. S., and LEWIS, E. W. (1962). *J. clin. Invest.*, **41,** 1509.
38. EVANS, D. G., and SMITH, J. W. E. (1963). *Brit. med. Bull.*, **19,** 225.
39. BARRETT, C. D., MCLEAN, I. W., MOLNER, J. G., TIMM, E. A., and WEISS, C. F. (1962). *Pediatrics*, **30,** 720.
40. OSBORN, J. J., DANCIS, J., and JULIA, J. F. (1952). *Pediatrics*, **9,** 736.
41. COHEN, S. (1963). *Brit. med. Bull.*, **19,** 202.
42. DIXON, F. J., TALMAGE, D. W., and MAURER, P. H. (1952). *J. Immunol.*, **68,** 693.
43. GARVEY, J. S., and CAMPBELL, D. H. (1954). *J. Immunol.*, **72,** 131.
44. MASOUREDIS, S. P., MELCHER, L. R., and SHIMKIN, M. B. (1953). *J. Immunol.*, **71,** 268.
45. ŠTERZL, J., VESELY, J., JILEK, M., and MANDEL, L. (1965). Ref. 11, p. 463.
46. SEGRE, D., and KAEBRELE, M. L. (1962). *J. Immunol.*, **89,** 782, 790.
47. TERRES, G., and WOLINS, W. (1961). *J. Immunol.*, **86,** 361.
48. BRUTON, O. C. (1952). *Pediatrics*, **9,** 722.
49. GOOD, R. A., MARTINEZ, C., DELMASSO, A. P., PAPERMASTER, B. W., and GABRIELSEN, A. E. (1963). *Immunopathology*, **3,** 177. Eds. GRABAR, P., and MIESCHER, P. A. Basle: Schwabe & Co.
50. WALDENSTRÖM, K. (1962). *Progr. Allergy*, **6,** 320.
51. WOLF, J. K. (1962). *New Engl. J. Med.*, **266,** 473.
52. GITLIN, D., JANEWAY, C. A., APT, L., and CRAIG, J. M. (1959). In *Cellular and Humoral Aspects of Hypersensitive States*, Chap. 10. Ed. LAWRENCE, H. S. New York: Hoeber-Harper.
52a. EISEN, H. N., LITTLE, J. R., OSTERLAND, C. K., and SIMMS, E. S. (1967). *Cold Spr. Harb. Symp. quant. Biol.*, **32,** 75.
53. BERGGARD, I. (1961). *Clin. chim. Acta.*, **6,** 545.
54. WALDENSTRÖM, J. (1944). *Acta med. scand.*, **117,** 216.
55. WALDENSTRÖM, J. (1965). *Advanc. metabol. Disorders*, **2,** 115.
56. WALDENSTRÖM, J. (1965). *Immunological Diseases*, Chap. 25. Ed. SAMTER, M. London: J. & A. Churchill.
57. FUDENBERG, H. H. (1965). *Ann. Rev. Microbiol.*, **19,** 301.
58. PAULING, L. (1940). *J. Amer. chem. Soc.*, **62,** 2643.
59. BURNET, F. M. (1959). *The Clonal Selection Theory of Acquired Immunity*. (Monogr. Walter and Eliza Hall Inst., Melbourne). London: Cambridge Univ. Press.
60. NOSSAL, G. J. V. (1960). *Brit. J. exp. Path.*, **41,** 89.
61. ATTARDI, G., COHN, M., HORIBATA, K., and LENNOX, E. S. (1959). *Bact. Rev.*, **23,** 213.
62. LEDERBERG, J. (1959). *Science*, **129,** 1649.
63. GREEN, I., PAUL, W. E., and BENACERRAF, B. (1966). *J. exp. Med.*, **123,** 859.
64. SMITHIES, O. (1963). *Nature* (*Lond.*), **199,** 1231.
65. PUTNAM, F. W., and TITANI, K. (1965). *Science*, **150,** 1485.
66. PUTNAM, F. W., TITANI, K., and WHITLEY, E. (1966). *Proc. roy. Soc. B*, **166,** 124.
67. MILSTEIN, C. (1966). *Proc. roy. Soc. B*, **166,** 138.
68. ANFINSEN, C. B. (1964). In *New Perspectives in Biology*. Ed. SELA, M. London: Elsevier Publishing Co.
69. HABER, E. (1964). *Proc. nat. Acad. Sci.* (*Wash.*), **52,** 1099.
70. FREEDMAN, M., and SELA, M. (1966). *J. biol. Chem.*, **241,** 2383, 5225.
71. ROBERTS, A. M., and HAUROWITZ, F. (1962). *J. exp. Med.*, **116,** 407.
72. MCDEVITT, H. O., ASKONAS, B. A., HUMPHREY, J. H., SCHECKTER, I., and SELA, M. (1966). *Immunology*, **11,** 337.

73. MONOD, J. (1959). In *Cellular and Humoral Aspects of Hypersensitive States*, Chap. 18. Ed. LAWRENCE, H. S. New York: Hoeber-Harper.
74. COHN, M., and TORRIANI, A. M. (1953). *Biochim. biophys. Acta*, **10,** 280.
75. COHN, M. (1957). *Bact. Rev.*, **21,** 140.
76. NOVICK, A., and WEINER, M. (1957). *Proc. nat. Acad. Sci.* (*Wash.*), **43,** 553.

Chapter 35

THE LOCALIZATION OF ANTIGENS AND THE SITES OF ANTIBODY FORMATION

By K. B. Roberts and J. L. Gowans

This chapter is concerned with the organs, the tissues, and the cell types which are responsible for the formation of antibodies. Our aim is to identify on a cellular level the sites where antibodies are produced in the immune animal.

Earlier in this century it was widely believed that antibody is formed in the cells of the reticulo-endothelial (RE) system. This conclusion was based largely on the assumption that the cells which take up antigen must also produce antibody. We shall begin, therefore, by considering what evidence there is that antigens are in fact localized in the phagocytic cells of the RE system. In this connection it is important to establish where soluble as well as particulate antigens become localized, since the RE system is often defined in terms of its phagocytic activity towards particulate or colloidal material.

LOCALIZATION OF ANTIGENS IN THE TISSUES

Use of Coloured Antigens

Antigenic azoproteins have been made by coupling synthetic dyes with a variety of purified proteins. McMaster and Kruse[1, 2] used a blue azoprotein, prepared by coupling bovine γ-globulin with an extremely diffusible blue dye, to study the localisation of a soluble antigen in mice. They argued that any breakdown of the azoprotein would lead to a rapid elimination of the dye and the absence of any staining of the tissues. This was in fact the case; the dye injected by itself, or as a mixture with the protein, was rapidly eliminated in the bile and in the urine, so that three hours after intravenous injection into mice no blue material could be detected in the tissues or in the blood plasma. On the other hand, the coupled azoprotein was retained for many weeks and immunological testing of the tissues showed that the coloured material in the cells was still antigenic. After intravenous injection, the distribution of the azoprotein in the tissues was similar to that of large molecular dyes, fine particulate matter, and bacteria. The Kupffer cells in the liver and the cells lining the sinuses in lymph nodes, especially in the mesenteric node, were particularly active in removing the blue antigen from the blood. Following intradermal injection, the azoprotein appeared predominantly in the draining lymph nodes, but only

35/Fig. 1 (*opposite*).—(*a*) and (*b*) are unstained and stained sections of the mesenteric lymph node of a mouse killed 48 hours after an intravenous injection of blue azoprotein. (× 13·5.)

(*c*) is the round nodule at the top of (*a*) as it appears, at a higher magnification and unstained, in a different section. (× 90.)

The black regions in the unstained section represent the azoprotein. The lymph follicles and lymphocytes in the medullary portion of the tissue contained no colour, although they were intimately surrounded by cells containing the coloured antigen. (From Kruse and McMaster.[2])

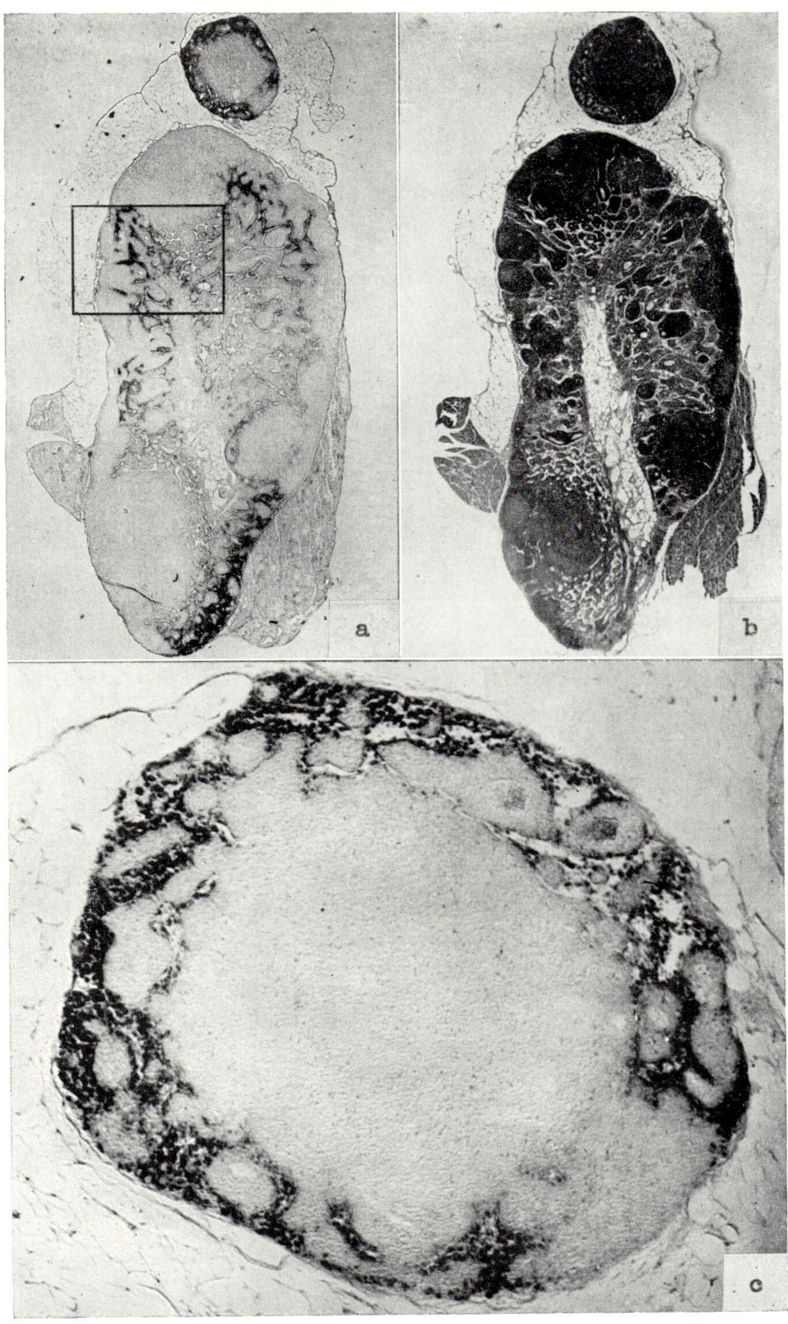

35/Fig. 1.

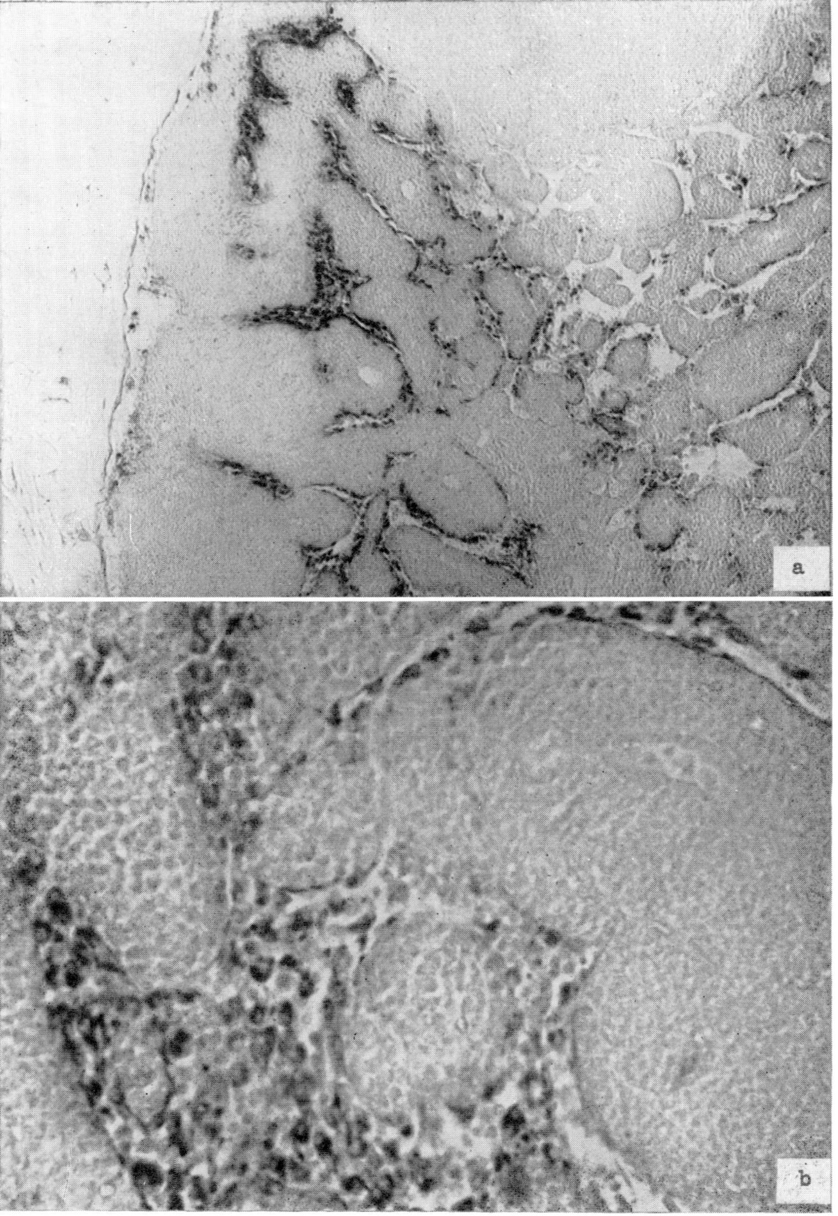

35/FIG. 2.—(*a*) The region included in the small rectangle drawn in Fig. 1(*a*). The blue antigen, black or dark grey in the photograph, stands out in the cells of the sinuses against the light grey of the lymphocytes. (×80.)

(*b*) A photograph of another unstained section of the same lymph node. (×350.) (From Kruse and McMaster.[2])

in the RE elements; it was not found in any of the lymphoid cells, even those next to macrophages containing blue protein (FIGS. 1 and 2). The dye was found in the cytoplasm, never in the nuclei. As an exception to its RE localisation, the protein was present in high concentration in the kidney tubular cells.

Use of Fluorescent Antibodies

An objection to the use of dye-coupled proteins in studies on antigen localization is that the coupling may affect the amount of protein taken up by the tissues and the time it persists in them. In a series of papers from Harvard, Coons and his associates have described the use of a method for locating antigen which avoids this complication.[3] They injected unaltered antigens of various kinds into animals and later prepared frozen sections of their tissues. On to these sections they poured the appropriate antibody which had been conjugated with a fluorescent dye. The antibody combined with the specific antigen and the precise location of the complex in the tissues was identified microscopically by its fluorescence in ultraviolet light. The slide could later be stained in the usual way for histological examination. They used soluble and particulate antigens and confirmed that the only cell type which invariably fixes antigen and in which antigen persists for any length of time is the RE phagocyte. For short periods after the injection of high doses of certain soluble antigens fluorescence was also detected in the lymphocytes of the spleen and lymph nodes; in addition, antigen actually penetrated into the nuclei of RE phagocytes and lymphocytes.[4, 5] These results with high doses of antigen differ in detail from those obtained with the dye-coupled proteins, but the significance of the differences is uncertain. The technique of locating and identifying antigens by means of fluorescent-labelled antibodies has wide applications in immunology.

Use of Radioactive Labels

Radioactive isotopes have been used in a number of studies to identify the sites of uptake of antigen. The most precise work has involved the injection of ^{125}I-labelled materials and their subsequent detection in the tissues by the technique of autoradiography. Humphrey and his colleagues used a synthetic polypeptide antigen which was labelled firmly with ^{125}I in its main antigenic determinants, so that it could be assumed with some confidence that the detection of radioactivity in autoradiographs implied the presence of antigen or its determinants in cells.[6] The technique is extremely sensitive and allows the detection of about 15 molecules of antigen in one cell. When the ^{125}I-labelled polypeptide was injected into the footpads of mice it became localized in the draining lymph nodes, in phagocytes lining the cortical and medullary lymph sinuses, in a manner identical to that revealed by the other studies we have considered. However, when the polypeptide was injected into mice in which circulating antibody had already been induced, an additional phenomenon was observed: antigen accumulated in striking amounts in some of the germinal centres of the nodes (FIG. 3).[6, 7] This follicular localisation has also been observed with other antigens, notably in studies with ^{125}I-labelled flagellin from *Salmonella adelaide*,[8] and it is thought that trapping takes place on or in a system of dendritic macrophages which make up a meshwork in the germinal centres. It apparently occurs only when specific antibody is already present in the animal; for example, it is not

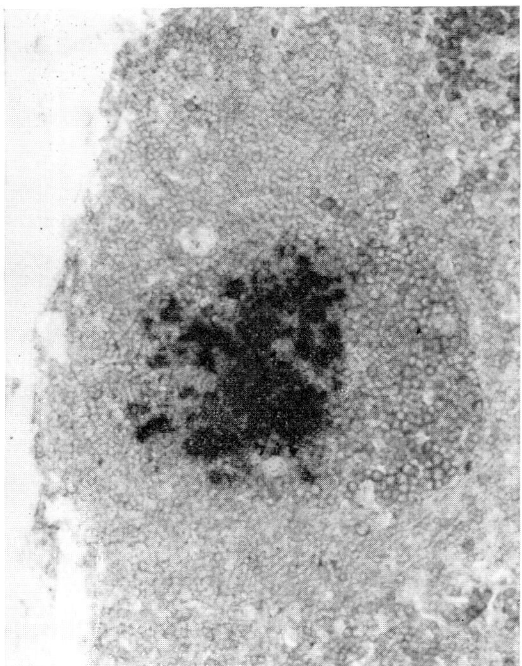

35/FIG. 3.—Germinal centre from the draining (popliteal) lymph node of an immunized mouse given a challenging injection of ^{125}I-labelled synthetic polypeptide antigen into the footpad. The autoradiograph shows the localization of the antigen (confluent, black autoradiographic grains) within a germinal centre. (From Humphrey *et al.*[7]).

seen following the injection of antigens into immunologically tolerant animals. When localization is observed in germinal centres after a first injection of antigen, as was the case in the studies on flagellin, it can be inferred that specific antibody was already present in the blood of the animal. Such "natural" antibody is almost certainly the result of previous contact with the antigen itself or one which cross reacts with it. Thus, follicular localization seems to be the consequence of immunization, not its initial cause. Antigen can persist for a considerable time in the follicles, and it has been suggested that it may serve to maintain the immune response. However, at present the significance of this interesting phenomenon is by no means clear.

Using radioactive labelling, it has been shown that a soluble protein injected intravenously into an animal having no corresponding antibody in the blood will at first disperse in the plasma; it then more slowly equilibrates with the whole of the extracellular fluids. The antigen is rapidly eliminated from the blood only when circulating antibody begins to be formed.[9] The rate of elimination of a radioactively-labelled antigen from the blood can be used as a measure of the immune response.

The whole problem of the retention of antigen in lymphoid tissue is of considerable theoretical importance for if antigens or their determinant groups do not persist for a long time, at least in small amounts, then direct template theories of antibody formation cannot be correct (see Chapter 34). Studies with ^{125}I-labelled antigens have shown that the cells which retain antigen in a lymph node are located some distance away from those which synthesize antibody.[6] The technique is sensitive enough to conclude that the number of antigenic determinant groups present in an antibody-forming cell must certainly be considerably less than the number of polyribosomes it contains. This makes it very improbable that antigen acts as a template upon which antibody molecules are synthesized.

Although a great deal is now known about the cellular localisation of injected antigens, there is no convincing evidence from studies either *in vivo* or *in vitro* that the R.E. phagocytes which take up antigen are the cells which go on to make antibody. The possible role of macrophages in the induction of antibody formation will be considered later.

Regional Location of Antigens

It may be appropriate here to summarize the regional location of antigen after various routes of injection, since this in turn will determine the main sites at which antibody is synthesized.

Intravenous.—After injection into the blood stream, antigens, particulate matter and certain colloidal dyes are located principally in the liver, the spleen and the bone marrow. These substances are also found to a lesser extent in the lungs, the adrenal and, with large doses, in some of the lymph nodes. The largest mass of R.E. cells in contact with the blood lies in the liver, so it contributes more than other tissues to the removal of foreign material from the blood stream. However, the liver only becomes involved in antibody formation when it is infiltrated by cells from elsewhere; most of the antibody formed after the intravenous injection of antigen, as we shall see, is synthesized in the spleen and bone marrow.

Intradermal injections are essentially injections into the lymphatics of the area. Following entry into the lymphatics, the antigen passes to the draining lymph nodes and is largely arrested there by the phagocytic cells lining the sinuses. It is possible, in some circumstances, for the antigen to pass beyond the draining nodes to those more centrally placed and even by way of the main lymph ducts into the blood stream to be distributed as described above. After subcutaneous injection, an antigen may, in part, be fixed locally while the rest finds its way either into the draining lymph nodes or into the circulation directly.

Into the peritoneal cavity.—Antigen injected intraperitoneally is probably absorbed mainly by the diaphragmatic lymphatics. French, Florey and Morris[10] have described, and illustrated in detail, the absorption of particles from the peritoneal cavity by the terminal lymphatics of the diaphragm. Apparently the mesothelial cells overlying these lymphatics separate to allow the passage of quite large particles. These then travel between or through the lymphatic capillary endothelial cells into the lymph vessels. The drainage of these lymphatics is into the lymph nodes of the chest. Material not fixed by these nodes will then pass into the blood via the large lymph vessels. Not all the antigen travels through the diaphragm; some is taken up by the macrophages of the omentum.

The Origin of Normal γ-Globulin

So far we have discussed the fate of injected antigen. We must now consider the experiments which attempt to locate the site of antibody formation by the demonstration of antibody in various organs, tissues, and cells.

Since circulating antibodies are contained almost exclusively in the γ-

globulin fraction of the blood plasma it is reasonable to start by enquiring where the normal globulin of the blood is synthesised. We must remember that the "normal" γ-globulin in the plasma almost certainly represents antibodies to the innumerable antigens encountered during life.

Miller and others[11] have shown by careful perfusion techniques that the liver of the rat is able to synthesize albumin, fibrinogen, and α- and β-globulins; no γ-globulin synthesis by the liver could be detected. The formation of γ-globulin was detected in the perfused rat carcase from which the liver was excluded, but the tissues involved could not be identified with certainty.

Ortega and Mellors[12] have adapted the fluorescent antibody technique to the study of the cellular origin of normal γ-globulin. They made an antibody to human γ-globulin in rabbits and coupled it with a fluorescent dye. This material was poured over frozen sections of human lymphoid tissue removed at operation. When examined under the microscope those cells which contained γ-globulin and consequently had taken up the specific antibody fluoresced in the UV light. γ-Globulin was found in mature and immature plasma cells including those containing Russell bodies. It was also found in certain cells of the germinal centres of lymphoid follicles. It was not found in primitive reticular cells or in small lymphocytes. It is relevant here to recall the absence of plasma cells and the poor development of germinal centres in the lymphoid tissues of patients with congenitally low levels of γ-globulin in their plasma.

"Normal" γ-globulin, then, unlike most other plasma proteins, is not made in the liver; it is formed in lymphoid tissue.

The Spleen and Lymph Nodes as Antibody Producers

Lymph nodes and spleen can produce antibodies. At least three different types of experiment lead to this conclusion. Firstly, large amounts of antibody can be extracted from these tissues. Secondly, these tissues, taken from immunized animals, can form antibody in tissue culture. Thirdly, cells from lymph nodes and spleen can continue to produce antibody when transplanted into suitable recipient animals.

Tissue levels of antibodies.—The first direct evidence for lymph nodes as antibody producers was provided by McMaster and Hudack.[13] They showed that the lymph nodes draining an ear injected with antigen have a higher antibody content than those of the control ear. This is not entirely convincing, for these draining lymph nodes are inflamed, and antibodies may accumulate in an inflamed area. McMaster and Hudack overcame this difficulty by injecting different antigens, bacterial vaccines obtained from closely related Salmonella organisms, into the two ears; at the height of agglutinin formation, they assayed antibody in the lymph nodes draining the two areas. "The concentration of each of the agglutinins was greatest in the lymph nodes on the side injected with the corresponding antigen and least in the lymph nodes of the opposite side. The concentration in the serum stood midway between the two. Had agglutinins been formed elsewhere than in the nodes, this distribution could not have occurred." This experiment has been repeated using, as antigens, alum-precipitated toxoids, viruses, bacteriophage particles, other bacteria and red blood cells. It has been shown in the mouse and the rabbit, and in various lymph nodes. Burnet and Lush,[14] for instance, inoculated rabbits and mice with bacteria, phage and viral antigens intranasally, into the foot-pad and into the cornea. In each case antibodies developed earlier and to a higher titre in the draining nodes than in the serum or other tissues.

Production of antibodies *in vitro*.—It has been known since the 1930s that splenic tissue taken from animals injected previously with antigen could release antibody *in vitro*. Many experiments have now shown that when cells from the spleen or lymph nodes of immunized animals are cultivated *in vitro* the antibody which can be detected in the medium is newly synthesized and is not simply released from a preformed pool. This conclusion is based on measuring the incorporation of radioactively labelled amino-acids into specific antibody during its formation *in vitro*.[15] The labelled antibody is recovered from the medium either by precipitation with specific antigen or by an anti γ-globulin serum.[16] It has also been detected by preparing autoradiographs after immuno-electrophoresis of the culture fluids.[17] Experiments on the synthetic capacity of lymphoid tissue *in vitro* have yielded other information. Thus, it has been shown that the bone marrow, in addition to the lymph nodes and spleen, synthesizes a considerable amount of antibody in immunized animals.[18] In another study sensitive methods were used to measure the affinity of antibodies synthesized by suspensions of lymphoid cells *in vitro* after primary or secondary injections of antigen had been given to the cell donors.[19] Following the injection of antigen into the rear footpad of rabbits, antibody of low affinity was made by cells from the draining lymph node, but none was made by the regional nodes draining the front legs. However, when such animals were challenged with a second dose of antigen in one of the front feet antibody of high affinity, typical of a secondary response, was rapidly formed by cells from the regional node. Primary immunization had apparently prepared the more distant nodes to respond to antigen in a secondary manner. The mechanism of this effect has not yet been worked out, but it is very likely due to the colonization of distant nodes by cells released from the primarily stimulated area, a point which we will discuss later.

In all these experiments the animals were injected with antigen before the lymphoid tissue was explanted into tissue culture. It is also possible to observe secondary responses *in vitro* by adding antigen to cultures of cells taken from primarily stimulated donors.[20] It is much more difficult to induce primary antibody formation *in vitro*, but, as we shall see later, some important successes have recently been reported.

Adoptive Antibody Formation

When suspensions of cells obtained from either the spleen or the lymph nodes of an actively immunized animal are injected into a suitable recipient animal antibody appears in its serum.[21] T. N. and S. Harris[22] have carried out experiments of this kind using cells from popliteal lymph nodes of rabbits. In one group of experiments a *Shigella* antigen was injected into the foot pad and cells from the draining lymph node were later transferred to rabbits that had received a sub-lethal dose of X-rays. When living cells were transferred anti-*Shigella* antibody appeared in the serum of the recipients, but when the cells were killed before transfer no antibody or insignificant amounts appeared. This was so even when the cells were killed by UV light or by mild heating, procedures that destroyed neither antigen nor antibody. The recipient could not respond to any transferred antigen because its antibody-forming powers had been depressed by X-irradiation. The obvious conclusion is that the transferred lymph node cells continued to synthesize antibody in the new host. This was shown unequivocally to be the case by employing donors and recipients which produced different, genetically determined γ-globulins, or "allotypes" (see Chapter 32). The anti-*Shigella* antibody in the blood of the recipient rabbits was identified as "donor" in origin by its reaction with an antiserum directed against the allotypic specificities of the donor's γ-globulins.[23] Immunity conferred by the activity of living, transplanted lymphoid cells is termed "adoptive" immunity. It is to be distinguished from "active" immunity in which the animal's own cells synthesize the antibody, and from "passive" immunity which is conferred by injecting preformed antibody.

Cells transferred from one animal to another of the same species usually have a limited expectation of life, for they will be destroyed after some days by the homograft reaction (Chapter 41). Therefore in many experiments on adoptive immunity, cells producing antibody are transferred to recipients which cannot mount a homograft reaction against them, for example X-irradiated animals or animals of the same highly inbred strain.

Mitchison,[24] for example, has demonstrated that spleen cells taken from actively immunized mice will continue to form antibody when transplanted into other mice. If the recipient animals are of the same inbred strain, then antibody continues to be formed for at least 4 months; the transplanted cells were still living and still producing antibody in the genetically identical tissues of the host. When the experiment was repeated using, as hosts, mice of a different strain, then antibody formation appeared to have stopped by the 5th day. The transferred cells in this case had been killed by a homograft reaction. If, in this second experiment, the hosts were previously immunized against cells of the donor, the homograft reaction was more rapid and antibody titres fell from the first day onwards.

Local Production of Antibody

Antibody is not formed exclusively in the spleen, lymph nodes and bone marrow. Some may be formed locally, at the site of injection of antigen, particularly if the antigen is injected in Freund's adjuvant or in an alum-precipitated form. These materials excite the formation of local granulomata: cells migrate from the blood into the injection site so that a small mass resembling a lymph node may form in the subcutaneous tissue or muscle. A large traffic of lymphocytes has been shown to pass from blood to lymph through a subcutaneous depot of Freund's adjuvant, emphasizing the resemblance to a lymph node.[25] In addition, the cells which synthesize antibody in the local granuloma are the same as those which do so in organized lymphoid tissue, namely plasma cells.[26] The way in which Freund's adjuvant enhances the production of antibody in animals is complex and is not related solely to local granuloma formation.

The submucosa of the small intestine of healthy animals is infiltrated with variable numbers of plasma cells and is a situation where local antibody formation occurs normally. Four classes of immunoglobulin have been detected in the plasma cells in the human gut, IgA, IgG, IgM and IgD, with the IgA-containing cells predominating.[27] The nature and location of the antigens which evoke these cells are not known. The antigens, possibly of bacterial origin, may stimulate the formation of plasma cells in the gut wall; or antigens may induce the formation of plasma cell precursors in the regional (mesenteric) nodes, from which they pass by way of the blood into the wall of the intestine.

The Cell Types involved in Antibody Formation

The spleen, lymph nodes and bone marrow, within which antibodies are synthesized, contain a complex mixture of cell types, We must now consider in detail which cells, among this mixture of types, are responsible for antibody formation. It might be expected that a study of the microscopic changes that occur in these organs after antigenic stimulation would identify the cells which take part in the formation of antibodies. However, these changes, as the following account illustrates, are very complex and involve several types of cell.

Ward, Johnson and Abell[28] showed that a single intravenous injection of a purified protein antigen into rabbits produced morphological changes in the spleen which were limited to the lymphoid follicles. The multiplication of "modified reticular cells" in the follicles coincided with the appearance of antibody in the blood. On the other hand, an examination of the rat spleen after a single intravenous injection of a particulate antigen showed a proliferation and differentiation of cells in the red pulp.[29] The principal cell involved in this change possessed a prominent nucleolus and abundant, basophilic cytoplasm. Ringertz and Adamson[30] have described the response of the regional lymph nodes of guinea-pigs to the repeated subcutaneous injection of a variety of antigens. During the first few days they noted a transient granulocyte response, a diffuse hyperplasia of the cortical lymphoid tissue, multiplication of reticulum cells and the formation of plasma cells in the medullary cords. The lymphoid hyperplasia was gradually replaced by an extensive formation of plasma cells extending into the cortex of the node. Large nodular centres appeared on the 10th day and eventually the major part of the node consisted of these nodular centres interspersed with a tissue rich in plasma cells.

These examples show that the histological changes in lymphoid tissue depend on whether single or multiple injections of antigen are administered, and possibly on the nature of the antigen and the species of animal used. It is clear that histological studies alone cannot unravel the precise cellular events which are essential for antibody production; it appears that lymphocytes, plasma cells and a range of more primitive cell types can all be involved to a varying degree.

Antibody Formation by Plasma Cells

The mature plasma cell has been described as "a round or, more commonly, oval cell with a strongly basophilic cytoplasm, often containing a juxta-nuclear light zone, and possessing an eccentrically situated nucleus with chromatin, somewhat clotted together and occasionally moulded into the shape of a cartwheel" (Fagraeus[31]). Such cells may occasionally be found in normal rabbits in the spleen, bone marrow, and kidney, but only in lymph nodes are any numbers seen in healthy animals. They are particularly associated, in pathological material, with chronic inflammation and with the special case of multiple myeloma. The latter is a condition in which multiple tumours composed of plasma cells occur in the bones and it is associated with hyperglobulinæmia. An unusual protein, "Bence-Jones" protein, is excreted in the urine in many cases of the disease. This protein is now known to comprise the immunoglobulin light chains which are produced in excess by the myeloma cells (see Chapter 32). One of the first suggestions that plasma cells synthesize antibodies came from this clinical association of myeloma with an increase in those plasma globulins among which antibodies are found. Later Bjørneboe, Gormsen and Lundquist[32] demonstrated an association between the high serum globulin during hyper-immunization of animals and the formation of plasma cells. In these experiments, mixtures of various pneumococcal antigens were given to produce very high levels of serum antibody globulin; plasma cells developed in the spleen, lymph nodes, liver and other organs and, surprisingly, in large numbers in the fat of the renal pelvis. This latter tissue, which resembled a plasma cell tumour in these animals, gave higher levels of tissue antibody than any other organ.

Fagraeus[31] developed these experiments. She first showed that a high level of globulin produced by passively immunizing rabbits did not of itself lead to plasma cell development; moreover large non-antigenic molecules, such as gelatin, did not influence the number of plasma cells to be found in various organs. Rabbits were then immunized intravenously with a variety of antigens and the histological appearances of the spleen correlated with the rise in titre during a secondary response. Side by side with the first appearance of antibody, in 2 or 3 days, there was a development in the spleen of what Fagraeus called "transitional cells". These cells possessed large, round nuclei containing several nucleoli and their cytoplasm was faintly basophilic. Later these cells diminished in size, the nucleus growing smaller, and the basophilia of the cytoplasm becoming more intense. The cytoplasm of this cell is thought to have high ribonucleic acid content, for it stains strongly with pyronine. The basophilic cell was called an immature plasma cell and its appearance coincided with the peak of the new formation of antibody. According to Fagraeus most of the immature plasma cells developed further into typical plasma cells. The transitional and the immature plasma cells described here tally in many respects with the cell previously called an acute splenic tumour cell, and described as forming in the red pulp of the spleen after an injection of an antigen or during the course of an infection. These were large mononuclear cells with a clear basophilic cytoplasm. Discussing its origin, Rich[33] says that motion-picture studies show that the type of locomotion is like a lymphoblast and not like that of monocytic cells. But Fagraeus has, on histological grounds, made out a case for the development of this cell from the RE system.

Fagraeus continued her experiments by studying the tissue titres of the spleen and the capacity of splenic fragments to produce antibodies *in vitro*. FIGURE 4 summarizes these results. It will be seen that, at a time when large numbers of immature plasma cells were found in the spleen, splenic fragments had a considerable capacity to form antibody in tissue culture. At this time the titre of antibody in the serum was rising at its fastest rate. Moreover the red pulp of the spleen, which contained the developing plasma cells was shown after careful dissection to produce antibody *in vitro*. The Malpighian corpuscles, consisting mainly of lymphocytes of various sizes, were unable to

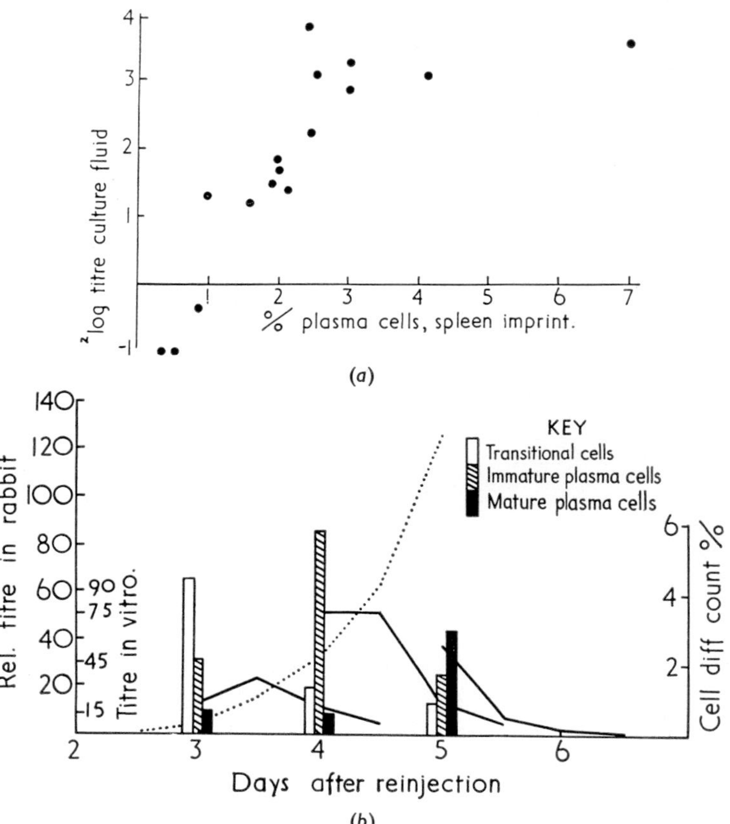

35/FIG.4.—(*a*) The relation between the numbers of plasma cells in the spleen and the antibody-forming capacity of splenic tissue pieces. Each dot denotes the arithmetic mean of 10–20 estimations from an equal number of cultures. About 0·2 mg. tissue was cultured in each tube for 24 hours.

(*b*) Antibody production *in vitro* in splenic tissue pieces in relation to the cytological picture in the spleen and to the serum titre of the rabbit.

.... relative increase in serum titre; ———— rate of antibody production *in vitro* in 12-hour intervals; cultures initiated on 3rd, 4th and 5th day respectively. (From Fagraeus.[31])

produce antibody in tissue culture. The evidence that Fagraeus presents suggests that antibodies are formed during the development of a plasma cell.

The appearance of plasma cells under the electron microscope shows that they possess an ultrastructure which fits them admirably for the role of antibody-forming cells. FIGURE 5 illustrates a plasma cell with its well developed endoplasmic reticulum and Golgi apparatus, structures known to be associated with rapid protein synthesis and secretion.

The most direct evidence for the production of antibody by plasma cells comes from the work of Coons and his associates.[34, 35] They devised a method for

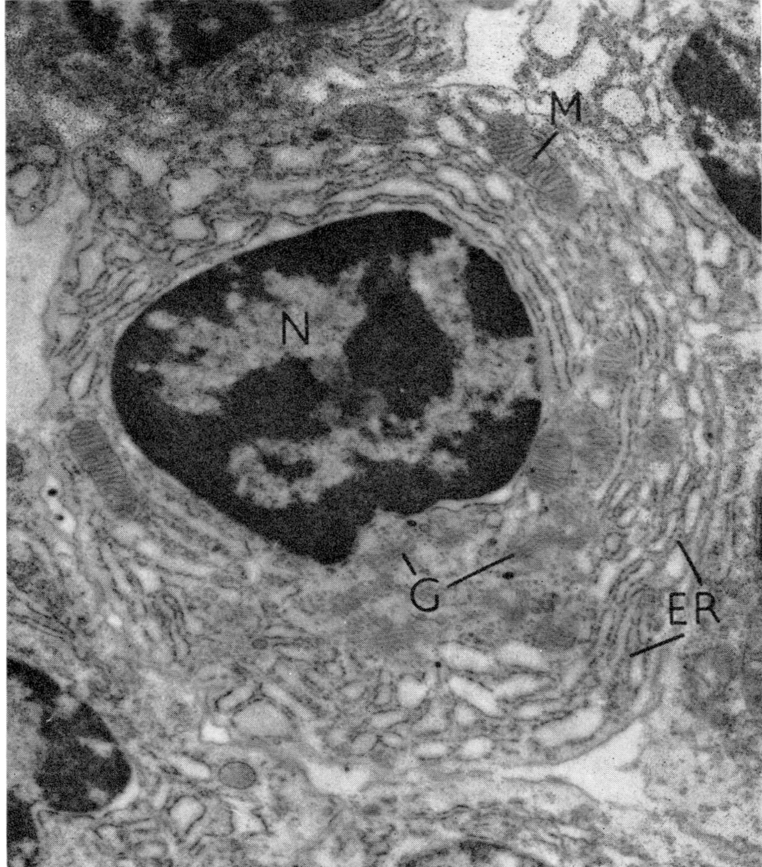

35/Fig. 5.—Electron micrograph of a plasma cell in a rat lymph node. The cytoplasm contains a Golgi apparatus (G) and a well-developed endoplasmic reticulum (ER) which are not seen in the small lymphocyte. The picture also shows a nucleus (N) and mitochondria (M). (×13,000)

the identification of cells containing antibody by elaborating their technique for the detection of antigen with fluorescent antibody. Frozen sections of tissue were flooded with a solution of antigen which was specific for the antibody to be detected. The antigen combined with the antibody wherever this was present in the tissue. The slide was then washed and treated with the specific fluorescent antibody which in turn combined with the added antigen. In this way three layers were built up: antibody in cells—antigen—fluorescent antibody. The cells containing antibody were finally detected by their fluorescence under the ultraviolet microscope (Fig. 6). Adjacent sections of the tissue were stained in the ordinary way for the histological identification of the fluorescent cells.

Coons[34] found that in rabbits, hyperimmunized with repeated injections of human γ-globulin or hen ovalbumin, the antibody was located in plasma cells

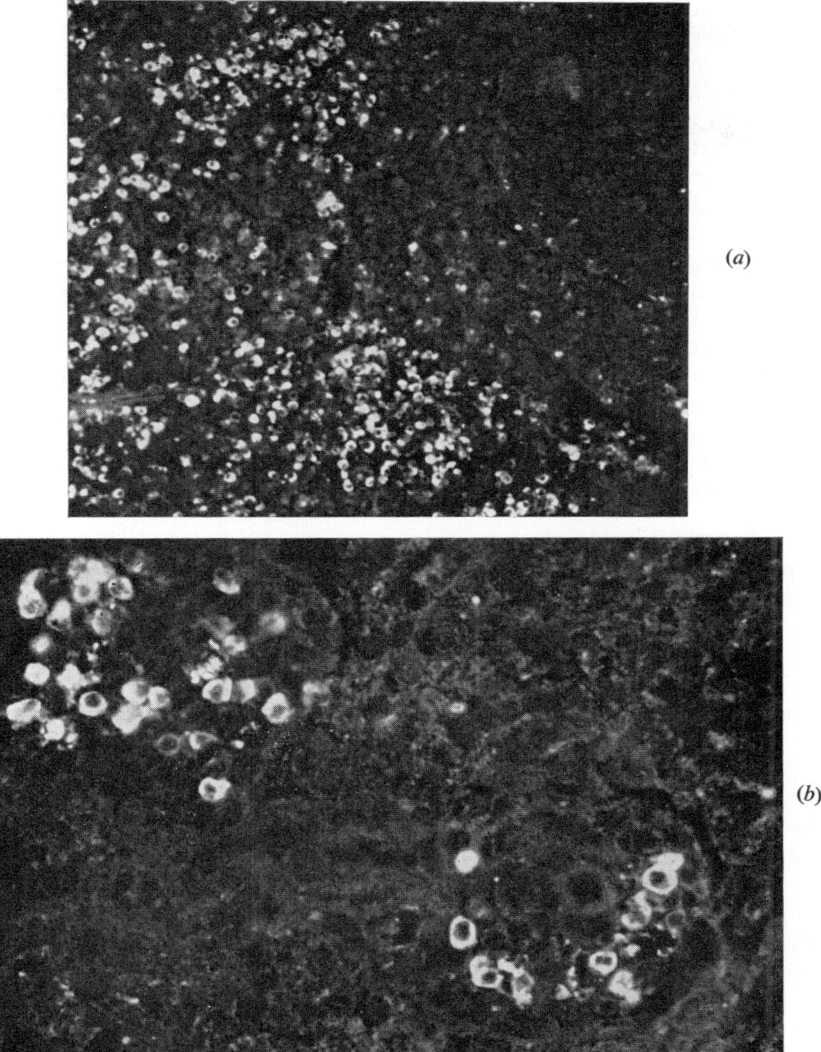

35/FIG. 6 (*a*) and (*b*) show the location of antibody-containing cells at the height of a secondary response to tetanus toxoid in the rat. The fluorescent areas identify the position of antibody in the cytoplasm of plasma cells. The method of immunofluorescence is described in the text. (*a*) Distribution of fluorescent cells in the red pulp of the spleen. The white pulp can be identified in the upper right-hand corner. (*b*) Fluorescent cells in the medullary cords of a lymph node. The cords, which run as finger-like projections into the medulla of the node, have been cut transversely in this section.

in the splenic red pulp, the medulla of lymph nodes, the submucosa of the ileum and the portal tracts of the liver. No antibody was detected in the Kupffer cells.

The application of this technique to the study of the primary and secondary response to diphtheria toxoid was particularly instructive.[35] The antigen was injected into the rabbit foot pad and the response in the draining popliteal lymph node was examined. After a single injection of antigen, antibody was first detected four days later in a very few cells, identified as immature plasma cells. The number of cells containing antibody had increased slightly by the seventh day but it remained at all times small. Coons drew attention to the disparity between the large number of cells taking up antigen after a single injection and the few cells that produced antibody. A second antigen injection, about five weeks after the first, gave a strikingly different result: four days later a profusion of antibody-containing cells was found in the medullary cords of the node and in areas adjacent to the follicles. The cells were again predominantly immature plasma cells many of which were in mitosis, together with some mature plasma cells. Coons concluded that the primary and secondary responses to antigen differ only in the number of cells producing antibody and not in their type.

Studies with Single Cells

Techniques have recently become available for identifying individual cells synthesizing antibody. In one of these, single cells have been isolated by micromanipulation from the regional lymph nodes of rats and incubated in minute drops of culture fluid.[36] The rats had been immunized with either bacteriophage or with a motile *Salmonella* organism. The release of antibody into the microdrops was determined either by the inactivation of phage particles introduced into the drop or by the immobilization of a few test bacteria which were introduced into the fluid after the presumptive release of antibody. These elegant experiments have shown that the great majority of cells forming antibody in both primary and secondary responses are plasma cells, although with the phage system a minority of the antibody-forming cells were identified by conventional microscopy as small lymphocytes. The main reason for undertaking these studies was to determine whether individual cells could synthesize two different antibodies when the animals from which they derived were immunized with two non-crossreacting antigens. The conclusion appears to be that individual cells will only make one antibody, and that technical difficulties make it uncertain that true "double producers" have ever been observed. It is important to realize that this experiment gives no information about the *potential* of individual cells to make more than one antibody; it simply shows that they will only synthesize one antibody at a time.

A simple method of identifying individual cells making antibody against sheep erythrocytes has been described by Jerne.[37] Spleen or lymph node cells from immunized animals are incorporated with sheep erythrocytes in a thin layer of agar in a petri dish and incubated for an hour or so at 37° C. During this time antibody is released from the cells and combines with the surrounding erythrocytes. Complement is then added and, after a further period of incubation, individual antibody-forming cells can be seen under the microscope lying in the centre of small clear areas formed as a consequence of red cell lysis. Again,

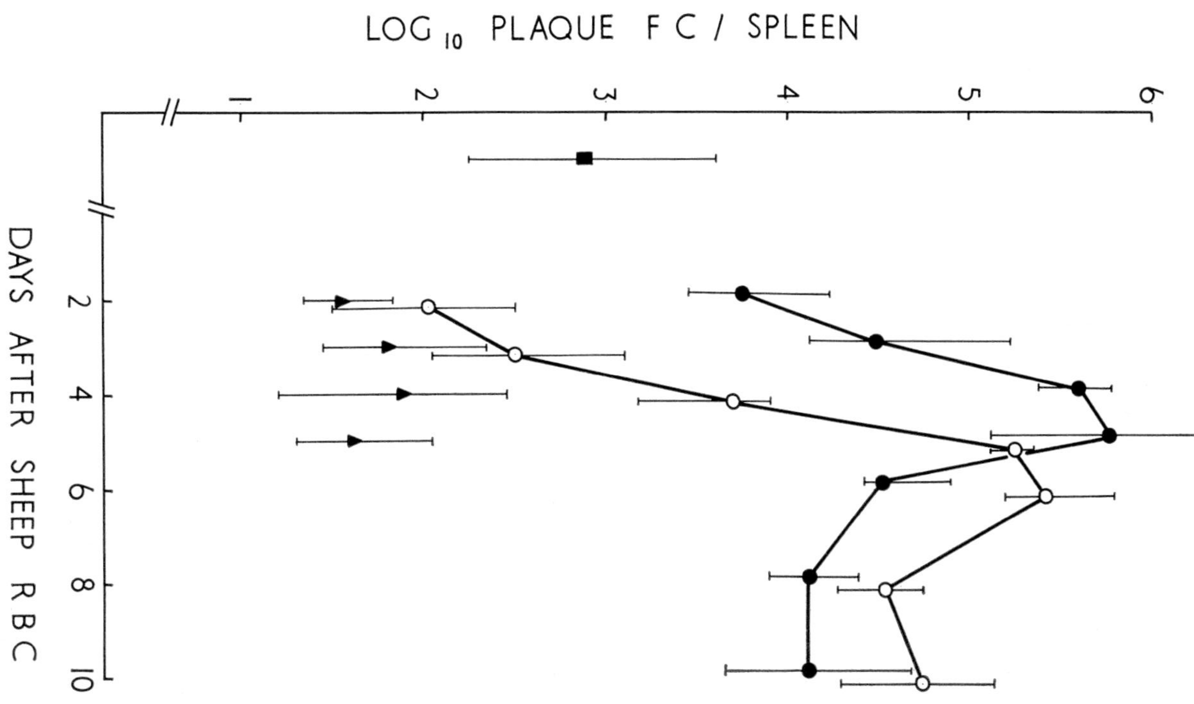

25/Fig. 7.—The primary immune response of rats to an intravenous injection of sheep erythrocytes, measured by counting the number of antibody-forming cells (plaque-forming cells) in the spleen.

●—● the response of normal rats. ○—○: the response of heavily irradiated rats given $2{\cdot}4 \times 10^8$ syngeneic small lymphocytes from normal rats at the same time as the antigen. The small lymphocytes restored the ability of the irradiated rats to respond to the antigen.

■: background level of PFC in normal, non-immunized rats.

▲: response of irradiated rats given antigen but no lymphocytes.

(From Ellis *et al.*, 1968.)

the majority of antibody-forming cells have been identified as plasma cells both under the conventional microscope and by electron microscopy.

The use of the Jerne plaque technique in following the antibody response to sheep erythrocytes (FIG. 7) has emphasized that the rise in the level of circulating antibody is associated with the rapid increase, by cell division, in the number of antibody-forming cells in lymphoid tissue. For about one day following the administration of antigen no DNA synthesis appears to occur in the precursors of the antibody-forming cells but, after this, the antibody response is grossly depressed if DNA synthesis is inhibited.[38]

We have already mentioned that when animals are immunized with more than one antigen, individual cells make antibody of only one specificity. It now appears that individual cells are further restricted to making only one molecular species of a particular antibody. Thus studies with fluorescent antibodies directed against the various immunoglobulin chains suggest that single cells make either κ or λ light chains and either α, γ or μ heavy chains.[39, 40] There is still doubt as to whether the same cell at different stages of its life history can make both 19S and 7S antibody, that is switch from μ to γ heavy chain synthesis.

Antibody Formation by Lymphocytes

The small lymphocyte is the predominant cell type in normal lymphoid tissue, and it is natural to suspect that it may be important in antibody formation. Harris and Ehrich[41] concluded that small lymphocytes synthesized antibodies from studies on the distribution of antibody in the efferent lymph draining the popliteal node of rabbits. After the injection of antigen into the foot pad they noted that there was first an impressive increase in the number of small lymphocytes in the popliteal node and that this was followed by an increase in the number of lymphocytes in the efferent lymph. The cells were found to contain more antibody than the lymph fluid in which they were suspended. It is now generally thought that the cells in lymph which were responsible for the formation of antibody in these experiments were not small lymphocytes but plasma cells and their precursors.[42] Experiments of a very similar kind have recently been carried out in sheep where, following the injection of small quantities of antigen into the lower part of the leg so that it was localized in the regional node, impressive numbers of large basophilic cells appear in the efferent lymph, and these were shown to be making antibody.[43] The cells which flow in the lymph from the regional node enter the blood and probably colonize lymph nodes elsewhere and are responsible for establishing a generalized immunity, because if a cannula is inserted into the efferent lymphatic and cells are drained away, no antibody appears in the blood. We have already mentioned how migrating cells may be responsible for preparing animals for secondary responses when antigen is localized to a single regional node. Of course, lymphoid tissue in many parts of an animal can also be made to engage in antibody formation if antigen is widely disseminated.

These experiments leave little doubt that many of the so-called large lymphocytes in the lymph and in blood are in fact antibody-producing cells or their precursors. In hyperimmune rabbits, suspensions of blood leucocytes, rich in large lymphocytes, have been shown to synthesize substantial amounts of antibody in culture.[45] Further, large lymphocytes, isolated from thoracic duct lymph and labelled *in vitro* with tritiated thymidine, have been identified in the tissues as typical plasma cells after transfusion into the blood.[46] On the other hand, it is now generally thought that small lymphocytes are not an important source of antibody; indeed their lack of the usual ultrastructural apparatus associated with protein synthesis and secretion does not make this conclusion surprising (FIG. 8). A few cells with the dimensions of small lymphocytes have been shown to release antibody in certain experiments, but the significance of these in immune responses is uncertain.

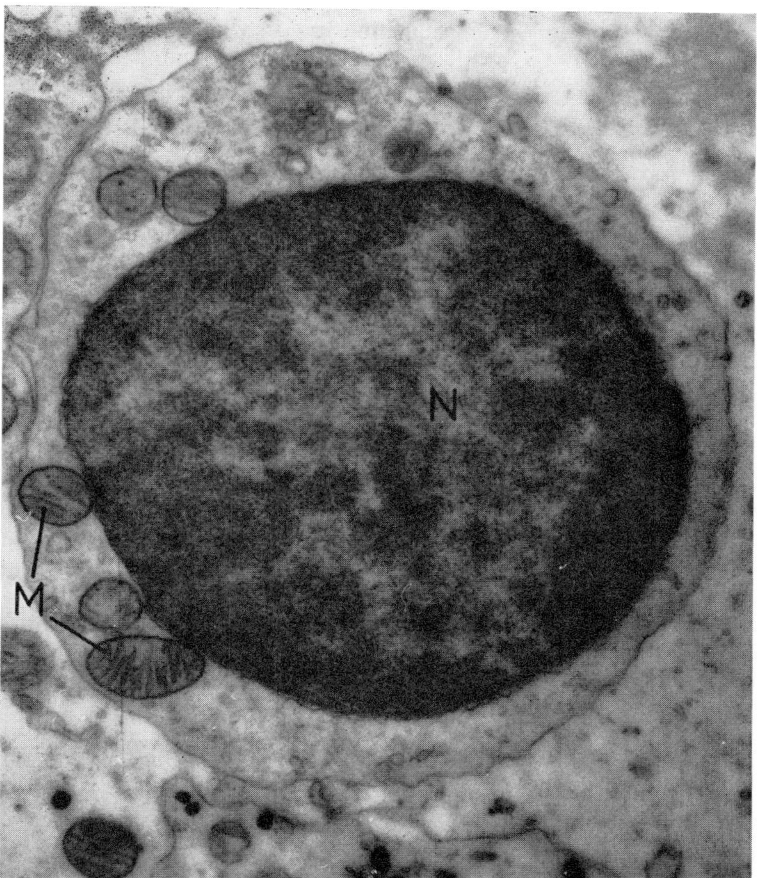

35/FIG. 8.—Electron micrograph of a small lymphocyte in a rat lymph node. The cell contains a nucleus (N), a few mitochondria (M), and some small vesicles. (×15,750)

Germinal Centres and Secondary Responses

The germinal centres of lymphoid follicles are composed of compact zones of large cells among which mitoses are frequently seen. It used to be thought that the products of these divisions were small lymphocytes but cell-labelling with tritiated thymidine has not yet confirmed this idea. Germinal centres are prominent in the lymphoid tissue of animals after immunization but are poorly developed or absent in hypogammaglobulinæmic patients and in germ-free animals. It is clear that germinal centres are involved in antibody responses but despite a great deal of study their precise role is not clear.[47]

Immunoglobulins and specific antibodies can sometimes be detected by immunofluorescence in germinal centres. The fluorescence usually occupies the whole centre and makes up a continuous, lacy framework in which the dark, non-fluorescing cell nuclei are embedded. The problem is to decide whether the antibody is synthesized locally in the centre, or made elsewhere and passively bound. The answer is not known, but the way in which passive immunization with antibody results in the localization of antigen in germinal centres (a phenomenon we have already discussed) suggests that passive binding may occur on at least some cells within the centres.

A popular view is that the dividing cells which compose germinal centres are formed as a consequence of primary immunization and that they "prepare" the animal in some way for the secondary response.[48] This hypothesis supposes that the cells are unable to synthesize antibody because the concentration of antigen has fallen to inadequate levels. However, they respond to a second injection of antigen by migrating from the centres and differentiating into plasma cells, which explains the final location of these in the red pulp of the spleen and the medullary cords of the lymph nodes. Unfortunately, there is, as yet, no direct evidence for this migratory process, although the association between the presence of germinal centres and the ability to mount secondary responses is well documented.

Immunized rats which are depleted of small lymphocytes by chronic drainage from a thoracic duct fistula still give normal secondary responses after challenge with antigen.[49] However, if the lymphocytes from the thoracic duct are injected into a heavily irradiated, non-immunized rat, it too will respond to antigenic challenge in a secondary manner.[50] This suggests that the faculty of immunological memory may be carried by two cellular mechanisms: dividing cells in germinal centres and circulating small lymphocytes. It is tempting to suggest that the dividing cells produce the small lymphocytes but, as mentioned above, there is no evidence for this view. The way in which small lymphocytes mediate secondary responses is discussed later.

Induction of Antibody Synthesis

The Role of Macrophages

We described in some detail the localization of antigens within the phagocytes of the RE system but left unanswered the question of whether the handling of antigen by phagocytes is an essential preliminary to the induction of antibody synthesis. Attempts have been made to answer this question by studying antibody formation *in vitro*.

Fishman and his colleagues persuaded macrophages in a rat peritoneal exudate to ingest bacteriophage particles. When ribonucleic acid (RNA) was extracted from the macrophages and incubated *in vitro* with fragments of lymph nodes (from non-immunized animals), small amounts of antiphage antibody appeared in the culture fluid; no antibody was formed when bacteriophage was added directly to the lymph node cultures.[51] It is still uncertain whether RNA from macrophages can instruct lymphoid cells to synthesize antibody in this system because the extracted "RNA" has been shown to be complexed with minute amounts of antigen or its determinants.[52] Certainly, such complexes of RNA and antigen are more immunogenic when injected into animals than the same quantity of native antigen alone,[52] but their relevance to the activities of living macrophages in the animal is quite unknown.

A primary response to sheep erythrocytes has been induced and carried to completion by incubating a suspension of spleen cells with the antigen *in vitro*; the cultures yielded substantial numbers of antibody-forming cells which were identified by the plaque assay.[38] There is some evidence that this response requires the activity of macrophages, since antibody formation to sheep erythroyctes can be induced *in vitro* with mixtures of macrophages and lymphocytes but not with lymphocytes alone.[53]

Secondary responses have been induced *in vitro* by incubating soluble antigens with cultures of lymphoid cells and the conditions for success appear to be much less demanding than for primary responses.[20] Whether this is related to the relative importance of macrophages in the two responses is not known.

The present evidence does not allow any generalisations about the necessity for macrophages during inductive events *in vivo*. However, it would be no surprise if particulate antigens, for example foreign erythrocytes or bacteria, had to be digested into a mixture of soluble antigenic components before they could stimulate lymphoid cells; nor if macrophages, by concentrating antigen on their surface, were particularly efficient at stimulating adjacent lymphoid cells. Histological observations provide some support for a collaboration between macrophages and lymphocytes: they are often seen in close contact in lymphoid tissue even, it has been alleged, to the point of establishing cytoplasmic bridges. Studies on antigen localization *in vivo* have not established that any particular class of macrophage or that macrophages in any particular location play a crucial role in antibody formation.

Antigen-sensitive Cells and Precursor Cells

An outstanding problem in cellular immunology is the identity of the ultimate precursors of plasma cells and their anatomical location at the moment of stimulation. It is generally agreed that plasma cells are derived from dividing precursors because they can be readily labelled with tritiated thymidine during the progress of an immune response *in vivo*.[54] It is also agreed that the earliest member of the plasma cell lineage in which antibody can be detected is a large, basophilic dividing cell called a "transitional cell' by Fragræus and a "plasmablast" by Coons. Cells at earlier stages than the plasmablast are difficult to identify because they do not contain antibody as a marker.

A number of cell types have been proposed as precursors of plasma cells. The older histological studies pointed to primitive reticulum cells in the splenic red pulp and in the lymph nodes. More recently there has been a debate as to whether the precursor is a dividing or a non-dividing cell at the time of stimulation; in more concrete terms, whether it is a large or a small lymphocyte.[55] The argument has been inconclusive but there is no fundamental reason why precursors should all be at identical stages of the cell cycle at the time of stimulation or, indeed, why there should be one lymphoid cell-type which is *the* plasma cell precursor. We have already suggested that in secondary responses plasma cells may come from the dividing cells in germinal centres and hinted that they may also come from small lymphocytes.

A further complication is the formal necessity to distinguish "antigen-sensitive" cells, which interact with antigen (or macrophage-processed antigen) to initiate the response, from the precursors which give rise ultimately to plasma cells. The simplest view would be that they are one and the same—that antigen-sensitive cells generate plasma cells—but this is not certain. The alternative is that they are distinct cell-lines which collaborate to put the response into effect. We must consider two sets of experiments.

The first concerns the role of small lymphocytes in the induction of antibody formation, a small lymphocyte in this context being defined as a cell in lymph with a diameter of less than 8μ and not synthesizing DNA when freshly isolated (see Chapter 5). There are two simple observations. (1) An injection of small lymphocytes from the thoracic duct of normal (non-immunized) rats will restore primary immune responsiveness to sheep erythrocytes in other rats whose immunological activity has been destroyed previously by a heavy dose of radiation; on the other hand, if the donor rat is made immunologically tolerant of sheep erythrocytes, then its lymphocytes possess no restorative capacity.[56, 57] (2) An injection of small lymphocytes from rats immunized some weeks previously with either tetanus toxoid[57] or a bacteriophage[50] will confer secondary immune responsiveness to the specific antigen on heavily irradiated rats; that is, the recipients respond in a secondary manner when challenged for the first time with antigen. In these experiments there is good evidence that the small lymphocytes which restore or transfer responsiveness are acting as antigen-sensitive cells. It has also been shown that in each response the antibody-forming cells which arise in the irradiated rat are the descendants of the injected small lymphocytes.[58] The obvious interpretation is that in both a primary and a secondary response in the rat, certain small lymphocytes can interact with antigen, start dividing and eventually produce the cells which synthesize antibody.

The second set of experiments also involved restoring immune responsiveness by injecting cells into unresponsive animals. Mitchell and Miller[59] thymetomized a group of adult mice, gave them a lethal dose of X-rays and then injected a suspension of bone marrow cells. The bone marrow cells protected against death from radiation, but in the absence of the thymus they did not restore the ability to make antibody. About two weeks later the mice were given an injection of lymphocytes together with an immunizing dose of sheep erythrocytes. The injection of lymphocytes restored the antibody response to normal but the antibody-forming cells were shown to be derived from the marrow and not from the lymphocytes. Mitchell and Miller concluded that the response of mice to sheep erythrocytes involves collaboration between two distinct cell lines: antigen-sensitive lymphocytes of thymus origin, and plasma cell precursors from the bone marrow.

One way of reconciling the two sets of experiments is to suppose that rat lymph contains two kinds of small lymphocytes, one coming originally from the thymus and the other from the bone marrow, and that they collaborate in lymphoid tissue during the induction of antibody-formation; but this is not the only possible explanation. Collaboration of this kind introduces an important new complexity into the subject but the notion is too recent to make further speculation profitable.

REFERENCES

1. McMaster, P. D., and Kruse, H. (1951). *J. exp. Med.*, **94,** 323.
2. Kruse, H., and McMaster, P. D. (1949). *J. exp. Med.*, **90,** 425.
3. Coons, A. H. (1952). *Symp. Soc. exp. Biol.*, **6,** 166.
4. Hill, A. G. S., Deane, H. W., and Coons, A. H. (1950). *J. exp. Med.*, **92,** 35.
5. Kaplan, M. H., Coons, A. H., and Deane, H. W. (1950). *J. exp. Med.*, **91,** 15.
6. McDevitt, H. O., Askonas, B. A., Humphrey, J. H., Schechter, I., and Sela, M. (1966). *Immunology*, **11,** 337.
7. Humphrey, J. H., Askonas, B. A., Auzins, I., Schechter, I., and Sela, M. (1967), *Immunology*, **13,** 71.
8. Nossal, G. J. V., Ada, G. L., Austin, C. M., and Pye, J. (1965). *Immunology*, **9,** 349.
9. Dixon, F. J. (1957). *J. cell. comp. Physiol.*, **50,** Suppl. **1,** 27.
10. French, J. E., Florey, H. W., and Morris, B. (1960). *Quart. J. exp. Physiol.*, **45,** 88.
11. Miller, L. L., and Bale, W. F. (1954). *J. exp. Med.*, **99,** 125.
    Miller, L. L., Bly, C. G., and Bale, W. F. (1954). *Ibid.*, 133.
12. Ortega, L. G., and Mellors, R. C. (1957). *J. exp. Med.*, **106,** 627.
13. McMaster, P. D., and Hudack, S. S. (1935). *J. exp. Med.*, **61,** 783.
14. *See* Burnet, F. M., and Fenner, F. (1949). *The Production of Antibodies.* 2nd edit., p. 54. Melbourne: Macmillan & Co.
15. Helmreich, E., Kern, M., and Eisen, H. N. (1961). *J. biol. Chem.*, **236,** 464.
16. Levine, H. I., Franklin, E. C., and Thorbecke, G. J. (1961). *J. Immunol.*, **86,** 440.
17. Hochwald, G. M., Thorbecke, G. J., and Asofsky, R. (1961). *J. exp. Med.*, **114,** 459.
18. Askonas, B. A., and Humphrey, J. H. (1958). *Biochem. J.*, **68,** 252.
19. Eisen, H. N. (1966). *Harvey Lect.*, **60,** 1.
20. Dutton, R. W. (1967). *Advanc. Immunol.*, **6,** 253.
21. Cochrane, C. G., and Dixon, F. J. (1962). *Advanc. Immunol.*, **2,** 205.
22. Harris, T. N., and Harris, S. (1960). In *Cellular Aspects of Immunity*, p. 172. Eds., G. E. W. Wolstenholme and M. O'Connor. London: J. & A. Churchill.
23. Harris, T. N., Dray, S., Ellsworth, B., and Harris, S. (1963). *Immunology*, **6,** 169.
24. Mitchison, N. A. (1957). *J. cell. comp. Physiol.*, **50,** Suppl.1, 247.
25. Morris, B. (1968). *Nouv. Rev. franc. Hémat.*, **8,** 525.
26. White, R. G., Coons, A. H., and Connolly, J. M. (1955). *J. exp. Med.*, **102,** 73.
27. Crabbé, P. A., and Heremans, J. F. (1966). *Gastroenterology*, **51,** 305.
28. Ward, P. A., Johnson, A. G., and Abell, M. R. (1959). *J. exp. Med.*, **109,** 463.
29. Wissler, R. W., Fitch, F. W., La Via, M. F., and Gunderson, C. H. (1957). *J. cell. comp. Physiol.*, **50,** Suppl. 1, 265.
30. Ringertz, N., and Adamson, C. A. (1950). *Acta path. microbiol. scand.*, Suppl. 86.
31. Fagraeus, A. (1948). *Acta med. scand. Suppl.* **204.**
32. Bjørneboe, M., Gormsen, H., and Lundquist, Fr. (1947). *J. Immunol.*, **55,** 121.
    Bjørneboe, M., Fischel, E. E., and Stoerk, H. C. (1951). *J. exp. Med.*, **93,** 37.
33. Rich, A. R., Lewis, M. R., and Wintrobe, M. M. (1939). *Bull. Johns Hopk. Hosp.*, **65,** 311.
34. Coons, A. H., Leduc, E. H., and Connolly, J. M. (1955). *J. exp. Med.*, **102,** 49.
35. Leduc, E. H., Coons, A. H., and Connolly, J. M. (1955). *J. exp. Med.*, **102,** 61.

36. Nossal, G. J. V. (1966). In *Methods in Cell Immunology*, Eds. Williams, C. A., and Chase, M. New York: Academic Press.
37. Jerne, N. K., Nordin, A. A., and Henry, C. (1963). In *Cell Bound Antibodies*, p. 109. Eds. Amos, B., and Koprowski, H. Philadelphia: Wistar Inst. Press.
38. Mischell, R. I., and Dutton, R. W. (1967). *J. exp. Med.*, **126,** 423.
Dutton, R. W., and Mishell, R. I. (1967). *J. exp. Med.*, **126,** 443.
39. Bernier, G. M., and Cebra, J. J. (1965). *J. Immunol.*, **95,** 246.
40. Cebra, J. J., Colberg, J. E., and Dray, S. (1966). *J. exp. Med.*, **123,** 547.
41. Harris, T. N., Grimm, E., Mertens, E., and Ehrich, W. E. (1945). *J. exp. Med.*, **81,** 73.
42. Ehrich, W. E., Drabkin, D. L., and Forman, C. (1949). *J. exp. Med.*, **90,** 157.
43. Hall, J. G., and Morris, B. (1963). *Quart. J. exp. Physiol.*, **48,** 235.
44. Hall, J. G., Morris, B., Moreno, G. D., and Bessis, M. C. (1967). *J. exp. Med.*, **125,** 91.
45. Hulliger, L., and Sorkin, E. (1963). *Nature* (*Lond.*), **198,** 299.
46. Gowans, J. L., and Knight, E. J. (1964). *Proc. roy. Soc. B.*, **159,** 257.
47. Cottier, H., Odartchenko, N., Schindler, R., and Congdon, C. C. (1967). *Germinal Centres in Immune Responses.* Berlin: Springer-Verlag.
48. Thorbecke, G. J., Asofsky, R. M., Hochwald, G. M., and Siskind, G. W. (1962). *J. exp. Med.*, **116,** 295.
49. McGregor, D. D., and Gowans, J. L. (1963). *J. exp. Med.*, **117,** 303.
50. Gowans, J. L., and Uhr, J. W. (1966). *J. exp. Med.*, **124,** 1017.
51. Fishman, M., and Adler, F. L. (1963). *J. exp. Med.*, **117,** 595.
52. Askonas, B. A., and Rhodes, J. M. (1965). *Nature* (*Lond.*), **205,** 470.
53. Ford, W. L., Gowans, J. L., and McCullagh, P. J. (1966). In *The Thymus: Experimental and Clinical Studies*, p. 58. Ciba Foundation Symp. London: J. & A. Churchill.
54. Schooley, J. C. (1961). *J. Immunol.*, **86,** 331.
55. Gowans, J. L., and McGregor, D. D. (1965). *Progr. Allergy*, **9,** 1.
56. McGregor, D. D., McCullagh, P. J., and Gowans, J. L. (1967). *Proc. roy. Soc. B*, **168,** 229.
57. Ellis, S. T., Gowans, J. L., and Howard, J. C. (1967). *Cold Spr. Harb. Symp. quant. Biol.*, **32,** 395.
58. Ellis, S. T., Gowans, J. L., and Howard, J. C. (1968). *Antibiot. et. Chemother.* (*Basel*), **15,** 40.
59. Mitchell, G. F., and Miller, J. F. A. P. (1968). *Proc. nat. Acad. Sci.* (*Wash.*), **59,** 296.

Chapter 36

ACQUIRED IMMUNITY: THE SEROLOGICAL REACTIONS OF BACTERIA

By G. P. Gladstone and E. P. Abraham

Introduction

It has been known from very early times that people who have suffered from certain infectious diseases are unlikely to contract the same diseases again. The infrequency of a second attack was noted particularly with smallpox, and nurses for patients with this disease were selected from those who had had it themselves. This observation led to the custom of infecting individuals artificially with smallpox, in the hope that it would produce a mild disease and protect against a severe natural attack. The practice of *variolation*, as it was called, is probably very old and no one knows its origin. It appears to have been carried out in China in the eleventh century, but it is doubtful whether it began there and, in view of the different methods used in different parts of Asia, Africa and the Balkans, it may have had more than one origin. The method employed in Greece in the eighteenth century was very similar to the method of vaccination used at the present time, and consisted in inoculating material from smallpox lesions through the skin by means of a needle scratch. In 1717, Lady Mary Wortley Montagu, the wife of the British ambassador in Turkey, introduced this method into Britain by having her two sons inoculated; the practice became fashionable and spread rapidly through Europe. However, variolation was dangerous, since, in place of the mild disease expected, a severe or even fatal attack of smallpox sometimes developed.

Edward Jenner (1749–1823) (Fig. 1) made his discovery of vaccination while practising variolation in his native village of Berkeley, in Gloucestershire. He was a pupil of John Hunter and learnt from him the value of accurate observations and planned experiment, and although he started his observations in 1775, it took him twenty years to convince himself of their accuracy. The account of his researches is best described in his own words[1]:

> " Among those whom in the country I was frequently called upon to inoculate, many resisted every effort to give them the smallpox. These patients I found had undergone a disease they called the Cow Pox contracted by milking cows affected by a peculiar eruption on their teats. On enquiry, it appeared that it had been known among the dairies [from] time immemorial and that vague opinion prevailed that it was a preventive of the smallpox. . . . I was struck with the idea that it might be practicable to propagate disease by inoculation, after the manner of the small-pox, first from the cow and finally from one human being to another. I anxiously waited some time for an opportunity of putting this theory to the test. At length the period arrived. The first experiment [May 14, 1796] was

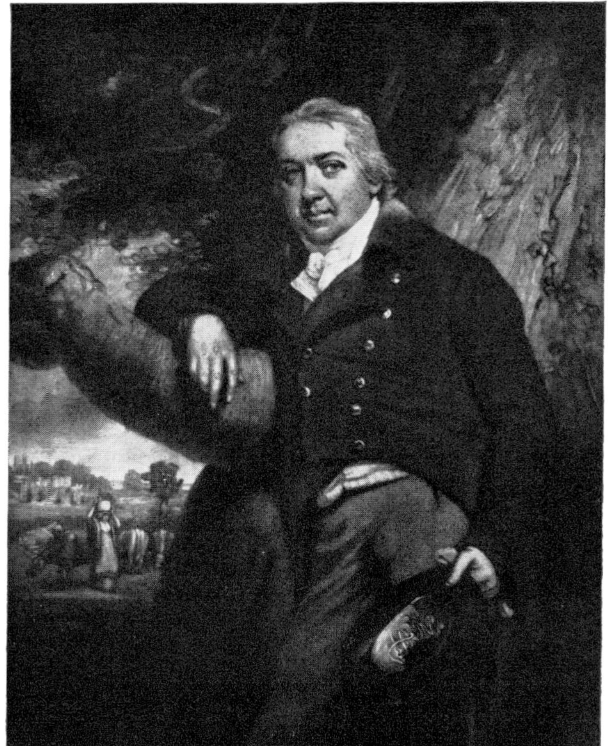

36/FIG. 1.—Edward Jenner (1749–1823). (From the mezzotint by Raphael Smith, R.A.)

made upon a lad of the name of Phipps in whose arm a little vaccine virus was inserted taken from the hand of a young woman who had been accidentally infected by a cow. Notwithstanding the resemblance which the pustule thus excited on the boy's arm bore to variolous infection, yet as the indisposition attending it was barely perceptible, I could scarce persuade myself the patient was secure from the smallpox. However, on being inoculated some months [July 1] afterwards, it proved that he was secure."

He obtained successful results in a number of other cases, and then sent a report to the Royal Society, "but the perusal of his cases and experiments produced no conviction whatever and he received a friendly admonition in reply that, as he had gained some reputation by his former papers [on the cuckoo] to the Royal Society, it was advisable not to present them one that would injure his established credit".[2] It is of interest to compare the attitude of the Royal Society to one of the greatest medical discoveries of all times, made by an established physician, with that afforded one hundred years earlier to Leeuwenhoek, the unknown linen draper of Delft, whose unconfirmed reports of microscopical observations were at once acclaimed and published by the Society as valuable contributions to knowledge. In spite of this and other rebuffs, Jenner continued to perform vaccination on a large scale and eventually succeeded in convincing the world that he had found a way of preventing one of its greatest scourges.

Jenner's discovery remained an isolated observation until eighty-four years later (1880), when Pasteur (1822–1895) (FIG. 2) accidentally discovered a prophylactic against chicken cholera. Cultures of the chicken cholera bacillus, which regularly infected chickens with a fatal disease, had been left in the laboratory over the summer vacation, and were then found to have lost much of their

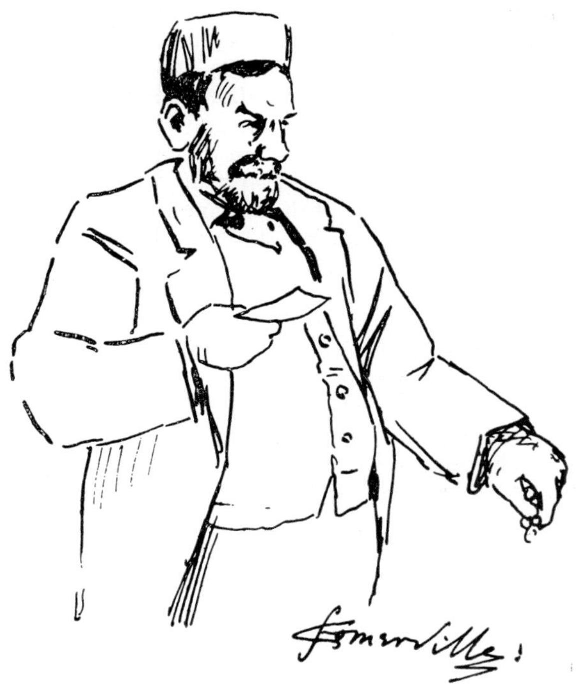

36/FIG. 2.—Louis Pasteur (1822–1895). Sketch drawn from life in his clinic at the rue d'Ulm, Paris, by Dr. Edith Œ. Somerville, D.Litt.

virulence. Fresh cultures were obtained, and although these regularly produced the disease in untreated chickens, they failed to infect chickens that had already been inoculated with the old cultures. Pasteur showed that the decrease in virulence was brought about by prolonged culture under aerobic conditions.[3] He at once saw the similarity between this observation and Jenner's discovery, and in honour of Jenner called his treatment "vaccination", a term which has been used ever since for the inoculation with bacteria, viruses, or their products, as a method of protection against infective disease. Six months later, he turned his attention to anthrax and noted the same phenomenon with this disease. His attenuated cultures were obtained by growing the anthrax bacillus in shallow layers at 42°–43° C. They then failed to infect cattle and sheep, but proved highly effective vaccines against the disease. Pasteur met the same scepticism as Jenner, but the famous experiment carried out at Pouilly-le-Fort in the presence of a large assembly of distinguished persons, when 25 sheep, 1 goat and 6 cattle were completely protected against a dose of virulent anthrax germs which killed all of a similar number of controls, fully established his claim. Swine erysipelas now engaged his attention. This time attenuation was effected by passing the organism serially through rabbits, when it lost its virulence for swine, but proved an effective vaccine.

Finally, Pasteur applied his principles of vaccination to rabies, but with the difference that vaccination was undertaken after infection had taken place from the rabid dog. The idea that vaccination could be undertaken during the incubation period after the virulent virus was already present in the body was against the medical opinion of the day, and, if Pasteur had not been successful, would hardly be accepted at the present day. The disease, however, has a long incubation period, usually greater than a month, and Pasteur believed it might be possible to bring about a refractory state, in the subjects bitten, by the use of vaccines before the infection became established.

The first step in the preparation of the vaccine was to shorten the incubation period, so that the virus would take a hold in the body as rapidly as possible. He achieved this by injecting serially into rabbits an emulsion of infected spinal cords from other rabbits, which reduced the incubation period to seven days, but at the same time increased the virulence of the virus. His next step was to attenuate this virulence, which he eventually did by drying infected spinal cords of rabbits in air, when the virus present in them became less and less able to infect as the time of drying was prolonged. He found that daily injections into dogs of emulsions of infected spinal cords of rabbits, dried for successively shorter periods of time, not only protected them from the virus contained in undried cords but also from disease acquired by rabid bites or from the injection of rabid saliva ("street virus"). What was even more important was the finding that vaccination started *after* the rabid bite completely protected the dog against the disease.

Pasteur's first human case was a nine-year-old boy, Joseph Meister, who had no less than fourteen bites on his hands, legs and thighs from a dog that was certainly rabid. On July 6, 1885, sixty hours after being bitten, this boy was inoculated over a period of ten days with thirteen injections of the emulsions of infected spinal cords dried for less and less time until finally a highly virulent virus was being given. The child suffered no ill effects and was therefore refractory, not only to infection from the original bites, but also to infection from virus of even greater virulence used for the later injections. Dubos[4] tells us the subsequent history of Joseph Meister. He became gate-keeper at the Pasteur Institute, and during the German occupation committed suicide rather than open to the German invaders the crypt where Pasteur is buried. The second case treated by Pasteur was that of the shepherd Jupille, who, seeing a dog about to attack some children, grappled with it, winding his whip about its muzzle and shattering its skull with his sabot. In the process he was severely bitter. The treatment was again successful, and Jupille's deed is commemorated in a bronze statue outside the Pasteur Institute.

The vaccines developed by Pasteur were all living though attenuated organisms, but it was soon found that in many cases dead vaccines could be used as well. The credit for this discovery is due to Theobald Smith

(1859–1934) who, together with Salmon (who gave his name to the *Salmonella*), showed that cultures of the bacillus of chicken cholera killed by heating at 58° C. for ten minutes protected pigeons against infection.[5]

These successes with both attenuated and dead organisms led to the widespread use of vaccines, under quite uncontrolled conditions, even in diseases which do not produce a lasting immunity against a second attack.

The next great advance was the discovery of antitoxins by von Behring[6] (1854–1917) (FIG. 3), made while he was endeavouring to obtain a killed vaccine against tetanus, the germ of which had been isolated by Kitasato the year before. Although Kitasato's name is associated with the discovery, the credit is apparently due entirely to von Behring. He used tetanus cultures detoxified with iodine trichloride. The serum of mice or rabbits which had received injections of these cultures possessed the remarkable property of making the toxin of the bacillus harmless. When this serum was injected into other mice they were protected against as much as 300 times the fatal dose of tetanus toxin. He called the substance in the serum which neutralised the toxin an antitoxin. A week later von Behring's second paper[7] appeared, in which he showed that the essential features of tetanus immunisation applied also to diphtheria. An important observation was that protection was specific, tetanus antitoxin affording no protection against diphtheria and *vice versa*.

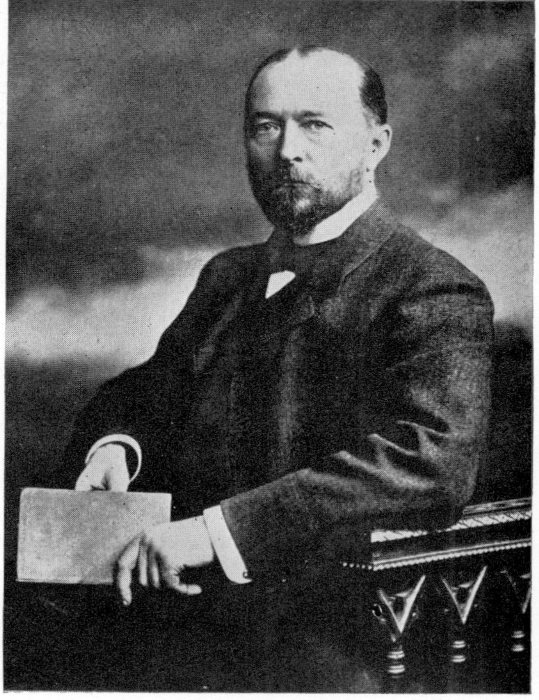

36/FIG. 3.—Emil A. von Behring (1854–1917). (From Mansch's *Medical World*.)

Paul Ehrlich[8] (1854–1915) (44/FIG. 4) now entered the field and demonstrated the formation of antitoxins against the non-bacterial toxins, abrin and ricin. Subsequently, during energetic researches carried out under very confined conditions, he investigated the reactions between toxins and antitoxins and laid down the principles and established the technique for their standardisation. The therapeutic value of antitoxin was soon recognised, and on Christmas night 1891 the first diphtheria patient was successfully treated.

The dramatic effect of antitoxin in the prophylaxis and treatment of diphtheria led to the hope that similar antitoxins might be prepared against the toxic effects of other organisms. Unfortunately, this was found to be so only in a limited number of infections. However, although antisera prepared by injecting bacterial cultures failed to neutralise the toxic properties of the cultures, they were soon found to have other properties which could be demonstrated *in vitro*. In 1893 Buchner[9] reported that fresh serum was able to kill certain bacteria but that it lost this property on heating at 55° C. He attributed the bactericidal action of serum to a heat-labile constituent which he called *alexine* (from αλεξειν = to ward off). A year later, Pfeiffer[10] described the dissolution of cholera vibrios by the fresh serum of guinea-pigs immunised with heated vaccines, and showed that the reaction was specific and could be correlated with protection against infection in both actively and passively immunised animals. In 1895, Bordet[11] showed that two factors were required for this reaction: one was a thermostable factor present in the antiserum, while the other, which appeared to be alexine, was inactivated by heating to 55° C. for half an hour and was present in normal serum. Alexine is now usually called *complement*, a term introduced by Ehrlich.

It was natural that such a direct lethal effect on the invading microbe should have strongly influenced ideas on the mechanism of immunity. Pfeiffer's observation gave strong support to the so-called "humoral" theory of immunity, which claimed that bactericidal substances present in the serum were responsible both for specific protection following immunisation and for the natural defence of the animal against infection. This theory was contrasted with the "cellular theory" of Metchnikoff,[12] who was equally convinced that phagocytosis by leucocytes was the important factor in protection and that any bactericidal substances present in the serum were derived from these cells. An enormous amount of work was expended by the proponents of the "humoral" and "cellular" schools in attempts to place the phenomena of immunity in one or other category. The controversy was eventually resolved by the work of Denys in Belgium and Almroth Wright in England, who demonstrated that humoral factors (opsonins) in the serum were necessary even in what appeared to be the purely cellular phenomenon of phagocytosis. Finally, Neufeld and Rimpau[13] showed that the amount of these humoral factors in the serum increased on immunisation, and that they failed to cause death of streptococci or pneumococci in the absence of leucocytes, but rapidly and specifically brought about phagocytosis when leucocytes were present.

The Nature of Immunity

In earlier chapters, the term "immune response" has been used to include any production of antibody to an antigen, which might or might not be associated with an infective agent. The term "immunity" is used here in a rather different sense, as the state of resistance to infective disease, irrespective of how this is brought about. *Innate immunity* denotes the resistance to infection found as an innate property of most animal species due to a number of causes apparently unconnected with the production of antibodies to the infecting microbe. It may be *relative* to the dose and virulence of the infecting organisms, e.g. the removal from the tissues of a few virulent or many avirulent organisms following their chance entry from the alimentary tract due to trauma. In some animal species it may be *absolute* due to many causes, some of which are discussed in Chapter 29, e.g. the inability of the animal's tissues to provide the right environment for the growth of the parasite and the insusceptibility of the tissues to the action of bacterial toxins. In contrast to innate immunity, *acquired immunity* is brought about actively by previous contact with the infecting microbe or its products, or *passively* by transfer of the serum (or sometimes cells) from an animal who has acquired active immunity.

We are concerned in this chapter with acquired immunity. Active immunity can be acquired naturally by an attack of the infective disease, or by an inapparent infection, or it may be acquired artificially by inoculation with vaccines. Passive immunity can be acquired congenitally, or by the injection of serum from actively immunised animals. It must be recognised that acquired immunity is a relative term. We have seen (Chapter 27) that the association of host and parasite is dynamic, and that an equilibrium may be established between them which may be upset in either direction, leading to disease on the one hand and destruction of the parasite on the other. Acquired immunity shifts the equilibrium between the host and parasite in favour of the former. Its effectiveness must be regarded as relative to the numbers and virulence of the invading microbes or the toxicity of their products.

Both in the normal and in the immune animal, bacteria are destroyed in the body by one or both of the mechanisms which were recognised by the early immunologists, namely extracellular destruction by antibacterial substances in serum and intracellular destruction in leucocytes after phagocytosis. In the immune animal, however, the mechanism by which this is brought about is not only greatly increased in effectiveness, but is specifically directed against a particular pathogenic microbe. In addition, a specific antitoxin may be present which neutralises the toxic properties of the microbe. This does not imply that there is no specific element in the normal body defences, but it is not so evident and non-specific factors are principally involved.

Serological Reactions of Bacteria

Before considering the specific factors involved in protection against bacterial infection, it is necessary to discuss effects on the bacterial cell following reactions between its antigens and their antibodies. Bacteria contain a large number of different antigens, but in the intact cell many of them are so situated that they do not form antibodies. It is the surface antigens which are most effective in stimulating the formation of antibodies. This is particularly evident where a very large surface of antigenic material is exposed, as in the flagella.

Immune Agglutination

Serum containing antibody against the surface antigens brings about clumping of the cells when mixed with a uniform suspension of bacteria in the presence of electrolytes. The clumping, known as immune agglutination, tends to be loose and flocculent when it involves the flagellar antigen, but to be relatively compact with surface somatic antigens. In some cases, as in O agglutination of *Salm. typhi*, the organisms in the clump appear to adhere at their poles, forming a reticulum (Fig. 4). The cause of agglutination is considered in Chapter 33.

Specific Capsular Reaction

The union of capsulated organisms with specific anticapsular antibody not only brings about agglutination, but also a change in the capsule which becomes

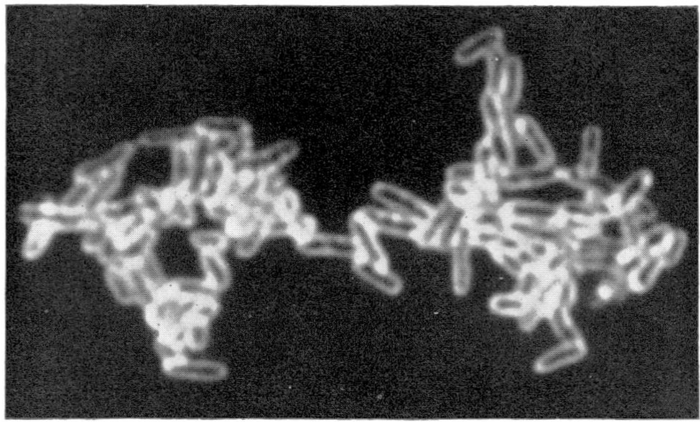

36/FIG. 4.—*Salm. typhi* O agglutination. Note end-to-end arrangement of bacilli. (Dark-ground illumination × 2600.)

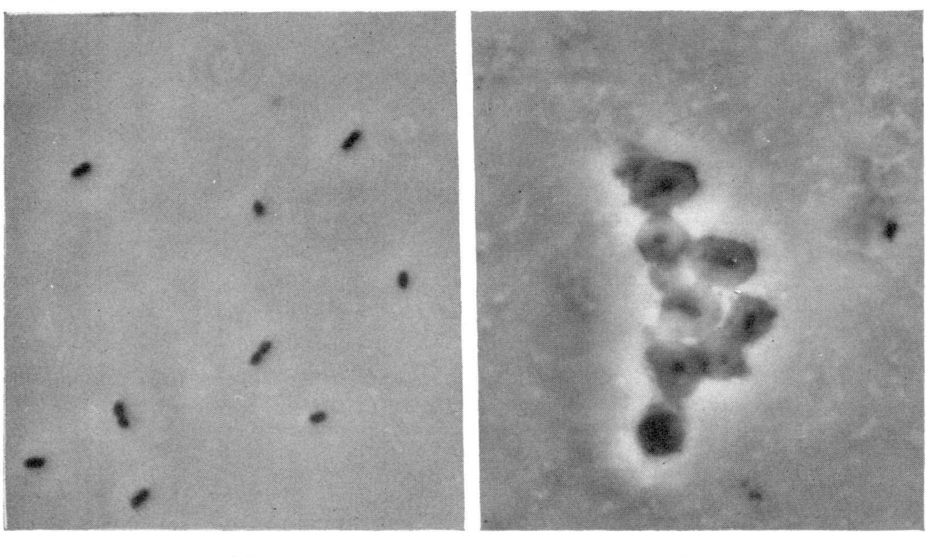

(*a*) (*b*)

36/FIG. 5.—THE SPECIFIC CAPSULAR REACTION WITH PNEUMOCOCCI TYPE III

(*a*) Before addition of antiserum.
(*b*) After addition of antiserum.
The capsule becomes readily visible and the cells are agglutinated. (Dark-phase contrast ×1100.)

opaque and readily visible in dark-phase contrast (FIG. 5). This reaction is generally called "The Neufeld Capsular swelling", or "Quellung" reaction. As Tomcsik[14] points out, these terms are misnomers since the reaction was first observed not by Neufeld, but by Roger, and swelling is not an essential feature; careful measurements in preparations in which the capsule can be demonstrated as nearly as possible in its native state have in most cases failed to show any increase in size. Where increase in size has been observed, it is a secondary phenomenon, that is probably the result of adsorption of complement[15] or of hydration.[16] The antigen-antibody reaction on which the phenomenon depends takes place within the capsule on the polysaccharide or polypeptide of which it is composed.

Bactericidal and Hæmolytic Action of Antibody and Complement

The lytic action of fresh guinea-pig antiserum on cholera vibrios (FIG. 6) described by Pfeiffer (see above) involves a primary union of antibody with one

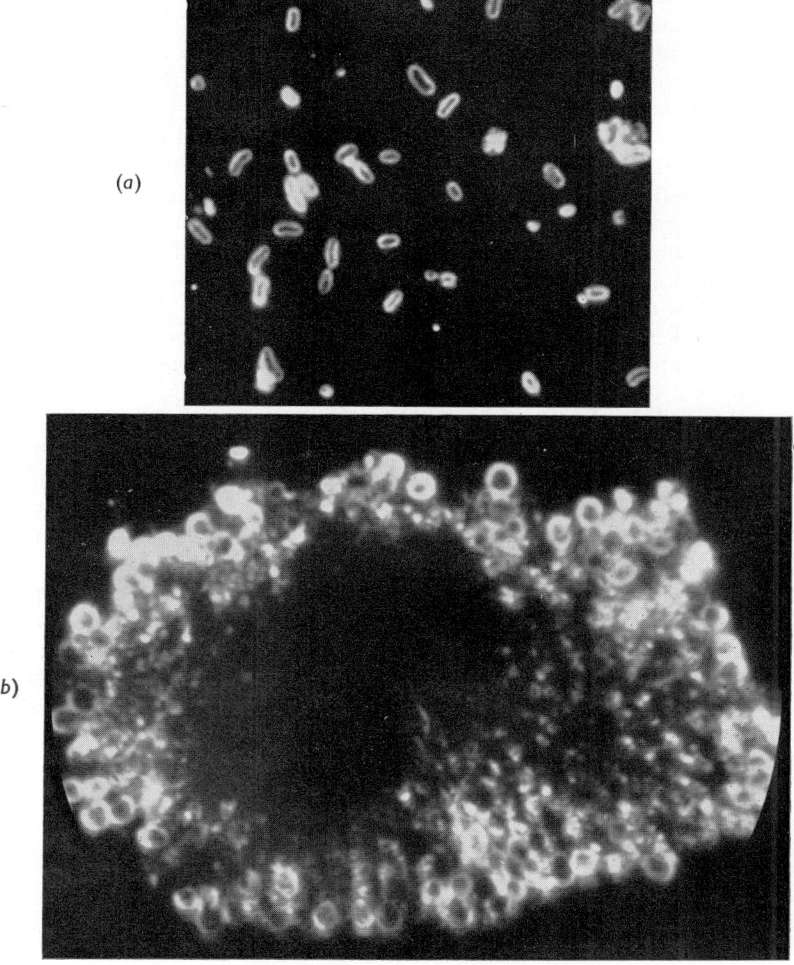

36/FIG. 6.—THE PFEIFFER PHENOMENON

(*a*) Normal *Vibrio choleræ*.

(*b*) *V. choleræ* after addition of fresh guinea-pig antiserum. Note agglutination, lysis of the organisms in the centre of the clump and swollen spherical organisms in the periphery. (Dark-ground illumination ×2100.)

of the surface antigens of the cell, followed by a secondary reaction with complement. Many other Gram-negative organisms and spirochætes may be killed in a similar way, with or without subsequent lysis, but Gram-positive organisms are resistant. Red blood corpuscles are also hæmolysed by antibodies to their surface antigens (so-called amboceptors), and complement, and since immune hæmolysis is easily measured it has been the subject of much investigation.

The nature of these reactions proved to be difficult to elucidate. Indeed, Heidelberger and Mayer[17] wrote in 1948: "It is happily a rare thing to find in scientific literature a vast body of writings so confusing and so mutually contradictory as those on the manifold activities of complement." The confusion was due in no small measure to the lability and complex nature of complement itself.

The components of complement.—Not long after its discovery, complement was shown to consist of at least two components. Ferrata found in 1907[18] that when guinea-pig serum was dialysed against distilled water a precipitate formed which could be separated from the solution and redissolved in saline. Neither the precipitate nor the remainder of the serum was active when added alone to a mixture of sheep red cells and their specific antibody, but the addition of both substances caused hæmolysis. The water-insoluble fraction, which had the properties of a euglobulin, became known as the midpiece of complement, and the soluble fraction as the endpiece. Both these components were inactivated by heating for a few minutes at 56° C.

Further work showed that two more components existed which were less labile to heat than midpiece and endpiece. In 1900 Von Dungern had reported that complement became inactive when treated with washed yeast cells, and in 1914 Coca[19] found that its activity could be restored, after this treatment, by the addition of serum in which both endpiece and midpiece had been destroyed by heating to 56° C. It followed that serum contained a third factor. Subsequently this factor was found to be largely precipitated with the midpiece on dialysis. A fourth component, which was inactivated by a short exposure to dilute ammonia, or hydrazine but not by yeast, was later shown to be present.[20]

Subsequently Pillemer[21] and his colleagues obtained more precise information about the nature of complement from the use of some of the modern techniques of protein chemistry. They suggested that midpiece, endpiece, third component and fourth component should be designated by the symbols C′1, C′2, C′3, and C′4 respectively. Some of the properties of these components are illustrated in the following scheme.

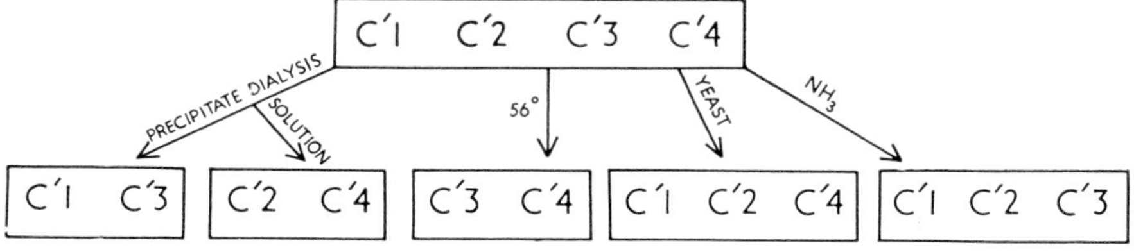

The relative amounts of the components are different in the sera of different species of animals. For example, the amount of C′3 is usually the factor which limits the activity of the guinea-pig complement, and the amount of C′2 that of human complement. Incomplete hæmolytic systems, each deficient in one of the four main components of complement have been widely used in qualitative studies. These systems are known as R reagents, R1, R2, R3 and R4 lacking C′1, C′2, C′3 and C′4 respectively.

After 1955 substantial advances were made in our knowledge of the chemical nature of the components of complement by the use of new methods for the separation and characterisation of proteins, including chromatography on ion-exchange cellulose and electrophoresis in gels.[22] This work has shown that components C′1, and C′3, at least, may themselves be complex. The four main components are considered here in the order in which they appear to react with sensitised red-cells.

C′1.—This component of guinea-pig and human complement is precipitated with the euglobulin fraction of the serum. Chromatography of an euglobulin of human serum on DEAE-cellulose, in a NaCl gradient in the presence of EDTA, yielded three fractions, named C′1q, C′1r and C′1s in order of their elution.[23] These fractions were inactive alone and were all required for the reconstitution of C′1 activity. The sedimentation rates of C′1q, C′1r and C′1s corresponded to 11S, 7S and 4S respectively, whereas the whole C′1 complex in normal serum showed a value of about 19S. It appears that C′1 dissociates into its subcomponents in the presence of EDTA and that these components can recombine to form a macromolecular complex.[24]

C′4.—A highly purified preparation of human C′4 was obtained from the pseudoglobulin fraction of serum by chromatography on triethylaminoethyl (TEAE) cellulose. From its behaviour on immuno-electrophoresis it was described as a β_{1E}-protein.

C′2.—Guinea-pig C′2 has been separated from the other components of guinea-pig complement by ion exchange chromatography on cellulose, but its degree of purity is uncertain.[23]

C′3.—Evidence has been obtained for the presence of five subcomponents in guinea-pig C′3. Chromatography of guinea-pig serum on DEAE cellulose yielded three protein fractions named C′3a, C′3b and C′3c respectively, which were all required for C′3 activity.[25] Independently, selective inactivation of C′3 indicated the presence of five factors, which migrated electrophoretically with the β-globulins.[23] Three of these factors, which behaved on Sephadex G-200 as 7S globulins, appeared to be identical with C′3a, C′3b and C′3c respectively.

Complement fixation and hæmolysis.—All four components of complement are required for the lysis of red cells, or bacteria, in the presence of their specific antibodies. Heidelberger and others showed that a variety of immune aggregates are able to adsorb protein nitrogen from sera containing complement. Subsequent experiments showed that the reaction of sensitised red cells with complement, or one of its components, which had been labelled with I^{131}, S^{35} or C^{14} resulted in the uptake of radioactive material. Antisera against one, or several, of the components of complement have been prepared and found to agglutinate sensitized cells. Hence it appears that the lytic action of complement depends on the fixation of a number, at least, of its components on the cell-antibody complex.

The fixation of complement during an antigen-antibody reaction is common, but not invariable and may vary with different types of antibody to the same antigen. The actual precipitation of an immune aggregate is not required for fixation; when pneumococcus Type II polysaccharide and rabbit antibody are mixed in dilutions so high that no visible precipitate is formed, the mixture will still fix complement. The presence of a specific antigen-antibody complex, however, does appear to be essential.

The lytic activity of complement is enhanced by small amounts of calcium and magnesium ions and is prevented if these ions are removed by chelation with EDTA. A variety of experiments have provided information about the order in which different components of complement react with the erythrocyte-antibody complex (EA) and the points in the sequence of reactions at which Ca^{++} and Mg^{++} are involved. The reaction of EA with C′1 leads to a complex designated EAC′1, which undergoes lysis in the presence of R1. The formation of EAC′1 appears to depend on the presence of Ca^{++}, but the way in which Ca^{++} exerts its effect remains to be determined. Reaction of EAC′1 with C′4 yields EAC′1,4 which is lysable by the R4 reagent. The formation of this complex occurs in the presence of EDTA and is thus independent of Ca^{++} or Mg^{++}. In contrast Mg^{++} is required for the conversion of EAC′1,4 to EAC′1,4,2. The latter undergoes lysis after reaction with C′3.

Further information about the sequence of events leading to immune hæmolysis has been obtained from kinetic studies by Mayer and others[26, 27] Under optimal conditions hæmolysis occurs after a short latent period, during which complement disappears from the extracellular fluid when present originally in a limited amount. Lysis is prevented if EDTA is added to the system at an early stage but not if the addition is made after about 5 minutes. Thus, two phases can be distinguished—a rapid early phase which is dependent on bivalent cations and a subsequent phase which is not. If the cells are washed at the end of the lag period they undergo lysis when suspended in saline without further addition of complement. This has led to the conclusion that the action of C′3 on EAC′1,4,2 is not contemporaneous with lysis but that it converts EAC′1, 4,2 cells into a new intermediate, designated E*, which spontaneously undergoes hæmolysis.

From the time of Ehrlich suggestions have been made that the lysis of sensitised cells in the presence of complement is caused by an enzyme. Although the nature of the final reaction which results in hæmolysis is still uncertain a number of observations have indicated that C′1 is the precursor of an esterase. Immune hæmolysis is inhibited by the esterase inhibitor diisopropylfluorophosphate (DFP). This can be attributed to the fact that DFP deprives EAC′1 cells of the ability to combine with C′4 and C′2. EAC′1,4,2 cells show esterolytic activity and, when treated with EDTA, material is released from them which can hydrolyse esters and also convert EA into EAC′1. It is thus possible that free C′1 is a proenzyme which is activated by fixation to antigen-antibody aggregates and that the resulting enzyme then acts on C′4 and C′2. These and other changes which may be involved in immune hæmolysis have been summarised in the following scheme:[24]

Intermediate complexes	*Biochemical event*
EA + C′1q + C′1r + C′1s $\xrightarrow{Ca^{++}}$ EAC′1	Generation of C′1 esterase
EAC′1 + C′4 $\longrightarrow$ EAC′1,4	Action of C′1 esterase on C′4
EAC′1,4 + C′2 $\xrightarrow{Mg^{++}}$ EAC′1,4,2	Action of C′1 esterase on C′2
EAC′1,4,2 + C′3a + C′3b + C′3c $\longrightarrow$ E*	
E* $\longrightarrow$ ghost + hæmoglobin	

It seems clear that immune hæmolysis is the final consequence of a series of reactions on the cell surface. The question arises whether lysis is due to the cumulative effect of damage at different loci and at different stages of the reaction sequence, or whether it can result from a transformation in a single area when the latter reacts with the last component of the C′3 system. The latter "one hit" or "non-cumulative" theory has received strong support from kinetic experiments by Mayer,[27] which indicate, for example, that the presence of a single EAC′1,4,2 site is sufficient to make a cell susceptible to lysis by C′3. Borsos, Dourmashkin and Humphrey have obtained direct support for the "one hit" theory.[28] Electron microscopy showed that the membranes of sheep erythrocytes lysed by rabbit antibody and guinea-pig complement contained pits or holes, 80–100Å in diameter, which were usually circular and were surrounded by a clear ring (FIG. 7). Sheep erythrocytes were prepared at the stage EAC′1,4,2 in which the number of active sites could be predicted from the theory of Mayer.[29] They were then treated with an excess of C′3 and the numbers of holes formed per unit area of membrane were counted. The numbers agreed closely with the predicted numbers of active sites.

By use of purified antibodies labelled with radioactive iodine it was estimated that the sheep red cell contained about 90,000 combining sites for 19S antibody and 600,000 for 7S antibody. Determinations of the amount of antibody required to cause 50 per cent lysis in the presence of excess of guinea-pig complement indicated that a single 19S antibody attached to a combining site may be sufficient to activate complement to produce a hole, but that two molecules of 7S antibody may be needed at neighbouring sites.[30] The formation of holes has been attributed to local damage to the lipid layer of the cell membrane, but the molecular basis of the change remains to be determined.

Bactericidal and bacteriolytic action.—Certain Gram-negative bacteria of the genera *Vibrio*, *Escherichia*, *Salmonella*, *Shigella*, *Hæmophilus* and *Brucella* are killed and, in some cases, lysed by complement following sensitisation with antibody to antigens of the cell surface. Gram-positive organisms and certain strains of *Salmonella* (*Salm. ballerup*, *Salm. typhi murium* and *Salm. paratyphi C*) are resistant. The earlier observations of Muschel[31] suggested that the difference in susceptibility between Gram-positive organisms and the susceptible Gram-negative organisms lay in the difference in structure of their cytoplasmic membranes. Recently, however, Muschel and his colleagues[32] showed that spheroplasts (that is cells in which the cell wall had largely been removed by lysozyme) of Gram-positive (*B. subtilis*) and of both resistant and susceptible Gram-negative organisms were equally susceptible to immune lysis. They conclude that it is not the nature of the cytoplasmic membrane but that of the cell wall which determines resistance. There is no doubt that among Gram-negative organisms the presence and nature of the surface antigens in the cell wall and slime layer are important. Organisms, whether of sensitive or resistant strains, that have lost their surface somatic antigens, the so-called rough variants (R), are particularly readily lysed by complement mediated by small amounts of anti-R antibody present in normal serum. The surface somatic O antigens (polysaccharide-lipoid-protein complexes) and particularly the "microcapsular" K antigens, e.g. Vi of *Salm. typhi* and *Salm. ballerup* (D-acetyl glucosaminuronic acid polymers), contribute to the resistance of strains con-

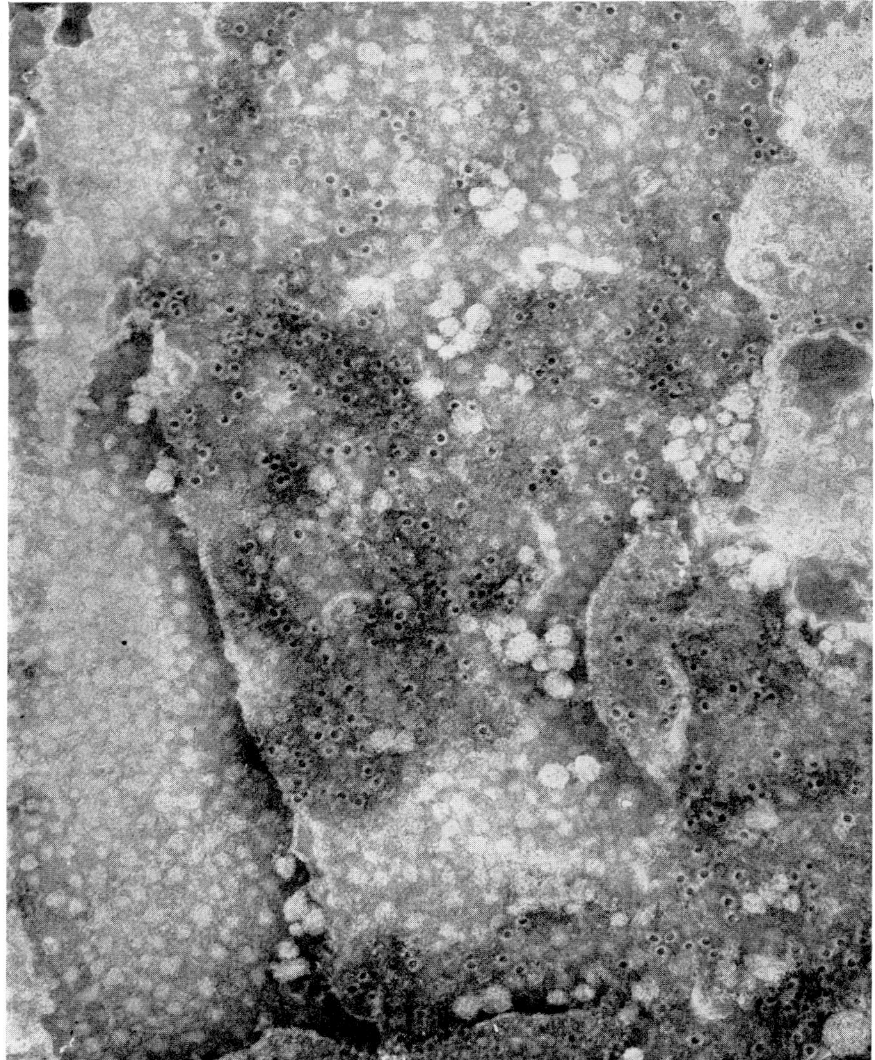

36/FIG. 7.—Electron micrograph showing a small area of an erythrocyte membrane fragment, after immune lysis with high concentrations of Forssman antibody and whole complement. Large numbers of "holes" in the surface of the membrane are illustrated. The "holes" appear black, being filled with phosphotungstate. Borsos *et al.*[28] (× 100,000.)

taining these antigens as shown by their greatly increased susceptibility when grown under conditions (e.g. at temperatures of 41° C.) in which these antigens are not formed.[33] Sometimes it is possible to overcome the resistance of certain of these strains by using a sufficient amount of antibody to their surface antigens. For instance, sensitisation of *Salm. typhi* may be effected by using relatively large amounts of antibody to both the "microcapsular" Vi and somatic O antigens.

Antibodies reacting with antigens foreign to the bacterial cell, but adsorbed on its surface, also sensitise the cell to the bactericidal action of complement.[34] However, anti-flagellar antibodies do not sensitise, possibly because the reaction with antigens of the flagella is too far removed from the cell soma.

Whether bacteriolysis or death of the organism without lysis takes place probably depends on the thickness and rigidity of the cell wall. Another factor would appear to be the presence of the enzyme lysozyme. We have already seen (Chapter 28) that this enzyme is present in mucus, and may play a part in preventing bacterial colonisation on the body surfaces. It is also present in many other body fluids and tissues but in concentrations unlikely to be bactericidal to pathogenic organisms. Amano and his colleagues (for refs. see 35), however, noted that concentrations of lysozyme as low as 5 μg/ml. had a synergistic action with antibody and complement, bringing about lysis under conditions in which in its absence only bactericidal action occurred. It would seem that the primary attack of complement on the cell after fixation to the cell wall following a surface antigen-antibody reaction is at the level of the cytoplasmic membrane.[36] The action of complement on the cell membrane may then cause death of the cell by leakage of essential metabolites from it, but the rigidity of the cell wall may preserve the structural integrity of the cell. The subsequent attack on the muco complex of the wall of the damaged cell by lysozyme may then be the factor determining lysis. Alternatively, lysozyme may act first, allowing complement to reach its essential substrate in the cytoplasmic membrane by removing much of the muco complex in the cell wall. Experimentally, it has not been possible to determine which of these ways is the more likely, because the synergistic action of lysozyme is shown both when it is added before antibody and complement and when it is added after.[31]

A special case of an absolute requirement for lysozyme in immune lysis has been described by Adinolfi and his colleagues.[37] Using IgA antibodies from human colostrum to certain strains of *E. coli*, they noted that both complement and lysozyme were required for lysis, whereas with antibodies from serum, which were IgM in type, complement alone was effective.

The sensitisation of bacterial cells to the bactericidal action of complement appears to depend on the amount of antigen present on the bacterial surface. Where this is very small, its union with antibody may not only fail to sensitise the cell but may interfere with sensitisation by another surface antigen-antibody reaction.[38] Where it is very large, sensitisation by antibody may also fail.[39] The nature of the antibody also appears to be important; chicken O antibody to *Salm. typhi*, although able to combine with O antigen, not only fails to sensitise the organism, but interferes with sensitisation by rabbit O antibody.[38]

These examples of interference may suggest a reason for an observation made many years ago by Neisser and Wechsberg.[40] Some antisera containing high titres of specific antibody failed to sensitise bacteria unless they were greatly diluted. It is possible that interfering antibodies are present in these sera and that sensitisation can be demonstrated only when their concentration is reduced by dilution, or that excessive amounts of antibody on the cell may interfere with either fixation of complement or its bactericidal activity. The latter suggestion is supported by the fact that the inhibitory zone (prozone) is narrowed by increasing the concentration of complement.[39]

Immune Opsonisation

The phenomenon of phagocytosis has been discussed in detail in Chapter 4, where it was noted that many organisms are not phagocytosed unless certain serum proteins are deposited on their surface, and that these opsonins, as they are called, are of more than one kind. There is no doubt that antibodies to the surface somatic and capsular antigens of many pathogenic organisms promote phagocytosis not only by blood leucocytes but by fixed phagocytic cells of the reticuloendothelial system. Very small amounts of antibody appear to be required for opsonisation by the latter cells *in vivo*. Benacerraf and his colleagues[41] found that as little as 0·01 μg of antibody nitrogen per 100 g. body weight was all that was required to opsonise 10^9 *E. coli* cells.

The role of complement in opsonisation has been extensively studied but is still controversial. The subject is well reviewed by Boyden and his colleagues.[42] It would appear that for adequate opsonisation by normal serum, the natural antibodies that it contains (see later section) are insufficient to opsonise bacteria alone. However, adequate opsonisation takes place if complement is present, the extra serum proteins of the complement being fixed to the surface of the sensitised cell as discussed in Chapter 4. Whether all or one or more components are required is still uncertain.

The claim that complement may opsonise without the need for antibody, made for instance by Šterzl and his colleagues[43] using serum from newborn germ-free piglets, cannot be substantiated, because the possible presence of natural antibody could not be excluded. On the other hand, there is no doubt that with an adequate concentration of antibody to the surface antigens of the bacterial cell, opsonisation may take place without added complement. Ward and Enders[44] for instance, noted that the same number of pneumococci were taken up by leucocytes in the presence of immune serum whether complement was present or not. With low levels of specific antibody complement may have a more important role. Biozzi and Stiffel[45] noted that removal of bacteria by the reticulo-endothelial system in the presence of immune serum was impaired in animals whose complement had been depleted, but could be restored by increasing the concentration of specific antibody.

Pondman and his colleagues[46, 47] have thrown some light on the role of complement in opsonisation by noting its dependence on the physical nature of the antibody globulin. Using a sheep red cell-anti-red cell system in rabbits, they noted that the specific antibody was present in both 7S (IgG) and 19S (IgM) types of immunoglobulin, and both types were effective in opsonisation. However, whereas 7S was effective without complement, 19S failed to opsonise unless complement was present. Since many of the so-called natural antibodies (see later section) are not only present in small amounts but are of the 19S type, Pondman's observation may be another reason why complement is required for opsonisation in normal serum.

Although complement was not required for the opsonisation of pneumococci by antibody, Ward and Enders[44] showed that it accelerated the reaction even when adequate antibody was present. Pondman also noted that it increased opsonisation of red cells by his 7S anti sheep red cell antibody. Moreover it determined the subsequent fate of the red cell in the leucocyte (see below).

Role of Antibody and Complement in Facilitating Intraphagocytic Destruction of Bacteria

In Chapter 4, the mechanism within the phagocyte leading to death of the ingested bacteria was discussed. We are concerned here with the possible function of antibody acting alone or with complement in accelerating or facilitating this process. One of the earliest observations implicating antibody in intracellular destruction of bacteria was made by Spink and Keefer[48] who noted that gonococci were taken up by leucocytes when suspended in saline but remained alive. In the presence of immune serum, however, they were rapidly killed. The result was somewhat invalidated by the fact that gonococci are susceptible to immune lysis by antibody and complement in the absence of cells, and under the conditions of the experiment, much extracellular lysis was in fact taking place. It is possible that destruction within the cell was merely a continuation of the process taking place outside.

Since many organisms are not phagocytosed in the absence of specific serum opsonins, it is not often possible to assess how far their subsequent intracellular destruction is dependent on their sensitisation by antibody or antibody plus complement. Jenkin[49] got over this difficulty by using a method of opsonisation not involving specific antibody. He noted that strains of *Salm. typhi murium* were readily taken up by mouse macrophages if treated with suspensions of phage to which they were resistant, but which were adsorbed to the bacterial surface. Serum was required in addition to phage, but not specific antibacterial antibodies, as all specific antibody could be removed from the serum by absorption without affecting phagocytosis. No destruction of the ingested organisms occurred. If, however, mouse serum not previously depleted of specific antibacterial antibody was used, rapid killing took place. Whether complement was involved was not determined. This recalls an early observation of Ward and Enders[44] who claimed that when pneumococci were opsonised with certain agents, but not with specific antibody, they resisted the usual rapid destruction inside polymorphs. Here, however, the opsonin was probably acting as a protective agent because pneumococci taken up by "surface phagocytosis" (see Chapter 4), that is under conditions in which no opsonin is required, are rapidly killed.[50]

In systems in which bacteria can be taken up by phagocytes without opsonisation, the effect of antibody or antibody plus complement on intracellular destruction can be studied without the complication due to its effect on phagocytosis. For instance Gelzer and Suter[51] used a strain of *Salm. typhi murium* which was phagocytosed by rabbit monocytes without the need for opsonins. In the absence of antiserum to the surface somatic antigens (anti-O), the ingested organisms not only survived but grew and ruptured the cell. When anti-O was present, but not anti-H (anti-flagellar antibody), little growth of the ingested organisms occurred and the monocyte was not damaged. The effect was obtained in the presence or absence of complement.

Mudd and his colleagues[52, 53] showed that fresh human serum not only increased phagocytosis of staphylococci by polymorphs, but also appeared to be necessary for intracellular destruction. They at first attributed this to antibody to a cell wall component (teichoic acid) acting in the presence of complement, since absorption of the serum with teichoic acid and inactivation of one or more components of complement both impaired phagocytosis and inhibited intracellular killing. However, in later work[53], absorption of antiteichoic acid serum from rabbits with teichoic acid in a quantity equivalent to the antibody titre failed to remove the activity. Moreover the activity of fresh human serum could also be removed by other cell wall components and even by *B. subtilis*. The active agent, therefore, would not appear to be specific.

It has been suggested that lysolecithin is formed intracellularly as the result of the interaction of complement with antigen-antibody complex, and that this would have the effect of releasing phagocytic lysozyme and other lethal factors into the phagocytic vacuole[54] from the lysozomes of the cell. Pondman[46] using his sheep red cell-rabbit macrophage system described above, noted that rapid lysis of sheep red cells took place in the macrophage if previously sensitised with 7S antibody in the presence of complement. No lysis took place if complement was absent. However, as extracellular hæmolysis was presumably occurring also, the work is open to the same criticism as that due to Spink and Keefer's observations on the gonococcus mentioned above, that intracellular hæmolysis was merely a continuation of extracellular lysis.

The intracellular death of some bacteria does not appear to be affected by immune serum. Certain of these, known as facultative intracellular parasites, are considered in Chapter 37. Others are not only phagocytosed in the absence of immune serum, but are rapidly killed as well. The K12 strain of *E. coli* is an example. Cohn[55] noted that rabbit polymorphs and macrophages engulfed and destroyed this organism with equal rapidity in the presence of either normal or immune serum, but the possibility that natural antibodies in normal serum were required was not excluded. He observed, however, that the subsequent degradation and digestion of the killed organisms which were labelled with P^{32} or C^{14}, depended on whether normal or immune serum had been present. Pretreatment with immune serum had the effect, not as might be expected of increasing the rate and extent of degradation, but of doing just the reverse, bringing about specific inhibition. It was suggested that this surprising result, so contrary to the usual enhancing effect of antibody on the catabolism of antigen *in vivo* (Chapter 34), was due to a possible protective effect of antibody globulin in preventing the lysozomal enzymes of the leucocyte from attacking bacterial substrates, a suggestion similar to that noted above to explain the observations of Ward and Enders on the protective effect of non-specific opsonins on intracellular destruction of pneumococci.

An acquired immune mechanism affecting the ability of macrophages to destroy intracellular bacteria, not involving antibody and complement, is considered in the section on Cellular Immunity in Chapter 37.

Neutralisation of Bacterial Toxins

Antitoxins to the so-called bacterial exotoxins have two attributes: they unite specifically with the toxin and they neutralise its toxic action in stoichiometric proportions. Anti-endotoxins, on the other hand, may unite specifically with the toxin, but fail to neutralise its toxic activity. The union of toxin and antitoxin has been considered in Chapter 37.

The mechanism by which antitoxins neutralise toxin is quite unknown. The toxic activity may be restored by dissociation of the toxin-antitoxin complex.

Serological Reaction of Viruses

Viruses may react immunologically like any other particulate body containing antigens, but, owing to their small size and intimate relation to the cells of their hosts, the reactions are technically much more difficult to demonstrate than those of bacteria. With relatively pure preparations of elementary bodies of a number of viruses, agglutination, opsonisation, complement fixation and precipitation of their soluble antigens have all been demonstrated. In addition, "neutralising" antibodies may unite with the virus particle and without killing it may prevent it from infecting new cells. This action is closely connected with the ability of antibodies to protect against virus infection, and is considered in Chapter 37.

Unity and Diversity of Antibodies determining Serological Reactions

The diversity of the secondary results following the union of antibody to the surface antigens of bacteria and other cells was at one time interpreted as necessarily due to the action of different antibodies and the terms precipitin, agglutinin, complement fixing antibody, bacteriolysin and opsonin were introduced to designate the antibody concerned. We now know that a single type of antibody globulin may be concerned in any or all of these reactions depending on the system used. These terms are therefore obsolete, but it is useful to retain them, not to designate the nature of the gamma globulin antibody, but to denote the particular type of reaction used to demonstrate it. On the other hand, previous chapters have made it clear that there may be a wide diversity of antibody globulin molecules differing in physicochemical structure, affinity with antigen, avidity (firmness of union with antigen) and specificity as the result of stimulation by a single pure antigen. We are beginning to sort out some of these antibodies, particularly those which differ in electrophoretic mobility, molecular weight and antigenicity (see Chapter 32). and to relate them to differences found in serological reactions. For instance, macromolecular antibodies IgM (19S) are less effective in fixing complement to red cell antigens than IgG (7S) but are much more effective in determining subsequent immune hæmolysis. Other examples are given in Chapters 38 and 39. Antibodies of the same immune patterns prepared in different animals may also differ in their serological reactions. An example was given above, where it was noted that antibody to *Salm. typhi* prepared in the rabbit was a bactericidin, whereas that prepared in the chicken was not.

Natural Antibodies and Non-specific Substances of like Nature present in Normal Serum

We have seen that the various serological reactions of bacteria which may be observed *in vitro* and the neutralisation of toxins and viruses are all conditioned by antibodies produced by immunisation. Before discussing the importance of these antibodies in the protection of immune animals (Chapter 37) against disease, let us consider certain substances which resemble antibodies in their action on bacteria, toxins, or viruses, but which are found in the sera of normal animals (including man) which have no history of being immunised, either artificially or by clinical infection, by homologous antigens.

Since 1893, when Buchner observed that the normal serum of the rat was lethal to certain bacteria, substances have been found in the sera of all vertebrates examined, and in many non-vertebrates, which have antibody-like activity demonstrable by one procedure or another against a vast array of antigens. The antigens include those of bacteria, viruses, fungi, metazoal parasites, red cells and even autologous cells not usually exposed in the circulation, as for instance spermatozoa. Many of these substances have the physicochemical characters of classical antibodies and give the same kind of reactions with antigens *in vitro*, but their origin and source are still uncertain. It is probable that they are heterogeneous in origin. Certainly there is strong circumstantial evidence that some arise by an unrecognised specific antigenic stimulus. For example, there is little doubt that the content of diphtheria antitoxin in the normal serum of man is the result of unrecognised contact with the diphtheria bacillus. The evidence for this has been ably assessed by Wilson and Miles.[56] Of particular interest is the possibility that the so-called non-toxigenic avirulent variants of *C. diphtheriæ* present in the throats of many normal individuals may produce minute amounts of toxin not demonstrable *in vitro* but sufficient to change a Schick-positive to a Schick-negative reactor.[57]

It is impossible, however, to relate the presence of all these so-called "natural antibodies" to specific antigenic stimuli, because individual sera may contain such a multiplicity of antibodies as to preclude the likelihood that they could have arisen by specific stimuli (for refs. see 58). Wilson and Miles[56] consider that they may be formed not by homologous but by heterologous stimuli. Common antigens are known to exist between commensal bacteria and pathogens, e.g. between coliform bacteria and Salmonellæ, and between enterococci and Shigellæ and the R antigen of rough coliform organisms may be common to the whole family of *Enterobacteriaceæ*. Also, animal tissues, red cells and bacteria may share antigens. Antibodies may thus be produced by one antigenic stimulus and be demonstrated by reactions with another cross reacting antigen. Even the isohæmagglutinins, that is the antibodies to A and B blood groups in man, which are thought by many to be genetically determined, may be the result of antigenic stimuli from blood group substances from the body fluids of other individuals.[59]

Evidence that the intestinal flora and other commensals influence the level and rate of synthesis of gamma globulin and, therefore, of natural antibodies, was obtained by Sell and Fahey[60] who noted that germ-free mice raised in a germ-free environment had a serum gamma globulin content of only 2 per cent of that of normal mice. Šterzl[43] attempted to deprive newborn piglets of all antigenic stimuli by using germ-free animals fed on a non-antigenic diet, reared under sterile conditions and deprived of colostrum, their only source of maternal antibody. In these circumstances, their gamma globulin level was extremely low, the small amount present being of low molecular size (2·7–5·1 S). He noted, however, that their serum was bactericidal in the presence of complement and opsonic for a number of Gram-negative bacteria, particularly rough strains. He claimed that these results were not the effect of antibody. However, as pointed out by Braun,[61] the amount of antibody which is required for sensitisation of rough organisms to the bactericidal action of complement is so small that it may not be detectable by other *in vitro* tests. Even under these rigid conditions, therefore, antibody production could not be excluded, and there is at least a possibility that it was formed without an antigenic stimulus. However, to establish a negative is difficult, and the alternative possibility that the piglets received antigenic stimuli in spite of the precautions used could not be altogether ruled out. The subject has great theoretical importance in deciding between an elective and instructive theory of antibody formation (Chapter 34). If it can be established that natural antibodies are products genetically derived without the requirement of an antigenic stimulus and accidentally orientated to a particular antigen, it would strongly support an elective theory. Unfortunately this is still far from possible.

Apart from the so-called natural antibodies considered in the last section, there are a number of agents in normal serum which kill, lyse and opsonise certain bacteria and neutralise certain viruses and which differ in several ways from antibodies. A large number of such agents have been described but only a few have been examined in any detail (for review see 35, 62).

One of the best characterised is **lysozyme**. We have already considered its presence in the granules of polymorphs (Chapter 4), and in the mucus and saliva (Chapter 28) of the body surfaces. We have also seen in this Chapter that its presence in serum may have a synergistic action on antibody-complement lysis of some Gram-negative bacteria. It is certainly a very potent enzyme in bringing about the destruction of cell walls of Gram-positive non-pathogenic organisms, but whether it is present in sufficient amounts in serum to have a direct effect on pathogenic organisms is doubtful, because most of these organisms are resistant to such concentrations. However, it may have more importance in the destruction of organisms within phagocytes.[63] Sensitivity may depend on cultural conditions, and the organism growing *in vivo* may be more susceptible than when grown *in vitro*. Certain strains of *B. anthracis*, for example, are completely resistant even to high concentrations of lysozyme, but become susceptible when grown in the presence of bicarbonate.[64]

Lysozyme is a strongly basic protein and will become adsorbed to the mucopolysaccharide and peptides of bacterial capsules. For instance, the glutamyl polypeptide capsule of *B. anthracis* binds lysozyme as shown by a pseudocapsular reaction visible with phase contrast. The capsulated bacillus which normally resists phagocytosis is now readily engulfed by polymorphs.[64] Lysozyme may therefore act as an opsonin. Whether it does so *in vivo*, however, is doubtful, as relatively large amounts are required.

Over the last 10 years prominence has been given to a substance found by Pillemer (for ref., see 65, 66) to be present in normal human serum and the sera of some animals and named **properdin** from *perdere* (to destroy). Pillemer discovered properdin while investigating the inactivation of C′3 component of complement by "zymosan", an insoluble carbohydrate fraction from yeast (see above). He showed that inactivation only took place above 20° C. and in the presence of magnesium ions. When zymosan was added to serum containing complement at 15° C. and then removed by centrifuging, no inactivation of C′3 occurred, but some change in the serum had taken place, since further addition of zymosan at 37° now failed to inactivate C′3. From the zymosan residue, protein was eluted, which constituted about 0·05 per cent of the proteins of the serum and which was at first thought to be a macroglobulin. On further purification, however, it proved to be a β globulin of molecular weight 230,000 with a sedimentation constant of 5·2 S[67]. A number of antibacterial and antiviral properties have been claimed for properdin acting in the presence of complement. Much of the work however, was carried out with partially purified properdin which was subsequently found to contain a 19S gamma globulin contaminant. It was found that many strains of seven species of Gram-negative bacilli and a strain of the non-pathogenic Gram-positive *B. subtilis* were killed (and some were lysed) when added to a mixture containing properdin, magnesium ions, and all four components of complement. This mixture—called the properdin system—also inactivated certain viruses. Properdin alone had no antibacterial or antiviral effect.

The resemblance between the action of the properdin system and that of the classical antibody-complement system in killing and lysing Gram-negative bacteria suggested that properdin might be a multispecific antibody (perhaps an aggregate of a number of homospecific antibodies) capable of reacting with a number of bacteria and sensitising them to the action of complement. It was suggested that it might be a natural antibody to zymosan, and its apparent non-specificity was explained as due to cross reactivity between zymosan and bacterial and viral antigens.[68] This idea was supported by the observation that adsorption of serum with large amounts of cell-wall stromata of sensitive bacteria at 0° C. selectively removed bactericidal activity against the homologous, but not the heterologous organisms.[69] The activity, however, could not be restored by the addition of purified properdin but was restored by a protein eluate, a 19S gamma globulin, from the cell stromata.[70] Moreover the recent purification of properdin and its characterisation as a β globulin with a sedimentation constant of 5·2 S, very different from that of immunoglobulins, and the further observation that it was antigenically distinct from IgG, IgA or IgM antibody globulin[70] argue against its being an antibody. This suggested that there were two systems in normal serum leading to bacteriolysis, a specific one involving normal antibody (19S IgM) and complement, and a non-specific one involving properdin and complement, but further studies have shown that both systems are inter-related. It would seem that for bactericidal or bacteriolytic action to take place in organisms sensitive to the properdin system, specific antibody, properdin and complement are all necessary. The earlier successful results with properdin and complement alone were probably due to unrecognised contamination with natural 19S gamma globulin antibody.

As antibody and complement are usually sufficient to kill or lyse bacteria without the necessity of added properdin, the role of properdin in the system described above is obscure. A possible explanation may be that the amount of specific normal antibody found in the serum for those organisms which require properdin, as well as antibody and complement, for lysis may be too small to sensitise the cell to the action of complement; the adsorption of properdin may then be necessary as an additional factor. As properdin is not fixed either to bacterial cells or to zymosan without prior adsorption of antibody, properdin could be likened to an extra component of complement. It is, however, quite distinct from the known components required, for instance for immune hæmolysis.[70]

The part played by properdin in the protection against natural infections in man and experimental infections in animals has been extensively studied but the results are conflicting.[71] The work for the most part has been carried out with crude eluates from zymosan, after treatment with serum, which contain in addition to properdin as we have seen, bacterial antibodies, and probably other antibacterial factors such as lysozyme. Before its role can be assessed, therefore, it will be necessary to repeat much of this work with the pure preparations of properdin which are now available.

Besides properdin and lysozyme, there are a number of other bactericidal substances in the blood and tissues which have received much less study. Some of these are non-specific, thermostable substances acting mainly on Gram-positive organisms, and do not require complement for their action. None of them has been obtained in a pure form, and we are uncertain of their mode of action. Many of them are strongly basic, and it has been suggested that they owe their bactericidal action to their ability to adsorb to acid substances on the bacterial cell. Two of these basic peptides with bactericidal properties have been obtained from animal tissues. One, having a high content of lysine, is bactericidal to *B. anthracis*, *Staph. aureus*, and hæmolytic streptococci; it also inactivates certain viruses.[72] The other, with a high content of arginine, is lethal to the tubercle bacillus.[73] These peptides are not normally found in serum, but Dubos suggests that they may be liberated from those tissues where the infectious agents are localised, as the result of tissue injury.[73]

It has long been known that the sera of the rat and rabbit contain bactericidal factors for *B. anthracis*, *B. subtilis*, and certain staphylococci. Myrvik[74] has shown that Ca ions are necessary for their action. They probably play little part in the protection of the animal against *B. anthracis* since, although the rat is relatively immune to infection, the rabbit (whose serum contains the factors in similar concentration) is relatively susceptible. Finally, bactericidal factors in human serum for coagulase-negative staphylococci have been described which also require Ca ions for their action and which appear to be different from any mentioned above. It has been claimed that they can be neutralised by a partially purified preparation of staphylococcal coagulase.[75]

Summary

The earliest record of immunisation against infections is "variolation", the deliberate infection of individuals with smallpox in the hope that a mild disease would be produced which would protect against a severe natural disease. Jenner in 1796 introduced "vaccination", the transmission of cowpox, which he found protected against smallpox. About a hundred years later, Pasteur developed living attenuated vaccines for chicken cholera, swine erysipelas, anthrax and rabies. Dead vaccines were found, by Theobald Smith and Salmon, to replace certain living vaccines. In 1890 von Behring discovered antitoxin.

The term "immunity", used in this chapter to mean resistance to infective disease, is determined by the nature, dose and virulence of the infecting organism as well as by the nature of the host and efficacy of the body defences. It may be an innate property of the host. Most animal species have an innate immunity to most pathogenic organisms relative to the properties of the invading organism; some have an absolute immunity due to various causes such as inability of their tissues to support the growth of the parasite or insusceptibility to the action of its toxins. Acquired immunity in contrast to innate immunity depends on the response to a previous contact with the infecting organism or its antigens (active immunity) or passage of certain antibodies (and sometimes cells) from an actively immune animal to another (passive immunity).

Antibodies reacting with antigens on the surface of bacterial cells may produce secondary reactions: agglutination in the presence of electrolytes, sensitisation to phagocytosis and to the lethal action of complement.

Complement is a complex entity consisting of at least four main components and at least two of these have been resolved into several subcomponents. The order in which the main components are fixed to a sensitised cell has been established, and lysis can apparently result from damage at a single locus. One component of complement is the precursor of an esterase and it is likely that the latter plays an enzymic role in the hæmolytic and bacteriolytic action of complement and antibody. However, the chemical nature of the reactions which occur is still unknown.

Bacteria are destroyed in the body either by the action of cell-free serum containing antibodies and complement in the case of certain Gram-negative bacteria, or ingestion and destruction by phagocytes in the case of Gram-negative and Gram-positive organisms. Lysozyme, an enzyme attacking mucopeptides of the cell wall, may have a synergistic action with complement in the destruction and lysis of susceptible Gram-negative bacteria sensitised with antibody to their surface antigens. Antibodies with or without complement may in certain cases assist the intracellular destruction of bacteria taken up by phagocytes. Neutralisation of bacterial toxins and prevention of viral attachment to susceptible cells are further properties of antibody that play a part in immunity.

Natural antibodies, that is antibodies present in the serum of normal individuals, may be the result of unrecognised specific stimuli or stimuli with antigens cross reacting with those used for their demonstration. Apart from antibodies, many less well defined factors have been described in serum and body tissues which have a lethal action on certain bacteria. Of these, properdin has been most studied. Properdin is a β globulin present in serum in a concentration of about 0·05 per cent of serum proteins with a sedimentation constant of 5·2 S. It is lethal to a number of antigenically unrelated Gram-negative bacteria and the Gram-positive *B. subtilis* in the presence of complement. There is evidence, however, that small amounts of specific natural antibody to the surface antigens of the susceptible bacteria are required. Properdin, therefore, may act like lysozyme in being synergistic in immune lysis involving specific antibody (19S) and complement. There is no evidence, however, that properdin is an extra factor of complement.

REFERENCES

1. Jenner, E. (1801). *The Origin of the Vaccine Inoculation.* London: Printed by D. N. Shury, Berwick Street, Soho.
2. Crookshank, E. M. (1889). *The History and Pathology of Vaccination*, Vol. **1**, p. 138. London: H. K. Lewis and Co.
3. Pasteur, L. (1933). *Œuvres de Pasteur*, Vol. **6**, p. 287. Paris: Masson et Cie.
4. Dubos, R. J. (1951). *Louis Pasteur*, p. 336. London: Victor Gollancz.
5. Salmon, D. E., and Smith, T. (1886). *Proc. biol. Soc.* (*Wash.*), **3,** 29.
6. von Behring, E., and Kitasato, S. (1890). *Dtsch. med. Wschr.*, **16,** 1113.
7. von Behring, E. (1890). *Dtsch. med. Wschr.*, **16,** 1145.
8. Ehrlich, P. (1891). *Dtsch. med. Wschr.*, **17,** 976, 1218.
9. Buchner, H. (1893). *Arch. Hyg.* (*Berl.*), **17,** 112.
10. Pfeiffer, R. (1894). *Z. Hyg. InfektKr.*, **17,** 345.
11. Bordet, J. (1895). *Ann. Inst. Pasteur*, **9,** 462.
12. Metchnikoff, E. (1905). *Immunity to Infectious Diseases,* translated by F. G. Binnie. London: Cambridge Univ. Press.
13. Neufeld, F., and Rimpau, R. (1904). *Dtsch. med. Wschr.*, **11,** 1458.
14. Tomcsik, J. (1956). *Bacterial Anatomy.* Symp. Soc. Gen. Microbiol., **6,** 41. Eds. Spooner, E. T. C. and Stocker, B. A. D. London: Cambridge Univ. Press.
15. Mudd, S., Heinmets, F., and Anderson, T. F. (1943). *J. exp. Med.*, **78,** 327.
16. Johnson, F. H., and Dennison, W. L. (1944). *J. Immunol.*, **48,** 317.
17. Heidelberger, M., and Mayer, M. M. (1948). *Advanc. Enzymol.*, **8,** 71.
18. Ferrata, A. (1907). *Berlin klin. Wschr.*, **44,** 366.
19. Coca, A. F. (1914). *Z. ImmunForsch.*, **21,** 604.
20. Gordon, J., Whitehead, H. R., and Wormall, A. (1926). *Biochem. J.*, **20,** 1028.
21. Pillemer, L. (1943). *Chem. Rev.*, **33,** 1.
22. Klein, P. C., and Wellensick, H. J. (1965). *Int. Rev. exp. Path.*, **4,** 245.
23. Lepow, I. H., Naff, G. B., Todd, E. W., Pensky, J., and Hinz, C. F. (1963). *J. exp. Med.*, **117,** 983.
24. Naff, G. B., Pensky, J., and Lepow, I. H. (1964). *J. exp. Med.*, **119,** 593.
25. Linscott, W. D., and Nishioka, K. (1963). *J. exp. Med.*, **118,** 795.
26. Mayer, M. M. (1961). In *Experimental Immunochemistry*, 2nd edit., p. 133 by Kabat, E. A., and Mayer, M. M. Springfield, Ill.: Charles C. Thomas.
27. Mayer, M. M. (1965). In *Complement*, p. 4. (Ciba Foundation Symp.) Eds. Wolstenholme, G. E. W., and Knight, J. London: J. & A. Churchill.
28. Borsos, T., Dourmashkin, R. R., and Humphrey, J. H., (1964). *Nature* (*Lond.*), **202,** 251.
29. Mayer, M. M. (1961). In *Immunochemical Approaches to Problems in Microbiology*, p. 268. Eds. Heidelberger, M., and Plescia, O. J. New Jersey: Rutgers Univ. Press.
30. Humphrey, J. H., and Dourmashkin, R. R. (1965). Ref. 27, p. 175.
31. Muschel, L. H. (1965). Ref. 27, p. 155.
32. Muschel, L. H., and Jackson, J. E. (1966). *J. Immunol.*, **97,** 46.
33. Nicolle, P., Inde, A., Diverneau, G. (1953). *Ann. Inst. Pasteur*, **84,** 27.
34. Adler, F. L. (1952). *Proc. Soc. exp. Biol.* (*N.Y.*), **79,** 590.
35. Skarnes, R. C., and Watson, D. W. (1957). *Bact. Rev.*, **21,** 273.
36. Bladen, H. A., Evans, R. T., and Mergenhagen, S. E. (1966). *J. Bact.*, **91,** 2377.
37. Adinolfi, M., Glynn, A. A., Lindsay, M., and Milne, C. M. (1966). *Immunology*, **10,** 517.
38. Adler, F. L. (1953). *J. Immunol.*, **70,** 69, 79.
39. Nagington, J. (1956). *Brit. J. exp. Path.*, **37,** 385, 397.
40. Neisser. M., and Wechsberg. F. (1901). *Münch. med. Wschr.,* **48.** 697.

41. BENACERRAF, B., SEBESTYEN, M. M., and SCHLOSSMAN, S. (1959). *J. exp. Med.*, **110**, 27.
42. BOYDEN, S. V., NORTH, R. J., and FAULKNER, . M. (1965). Ref. 27, p. 190.
43. ŠTERZL, J., MANDEL, L., MILER, I., and ŘÍHA, I. (1965). In *Molecular and Cellular Basis of Antibody Formation*, p. 351. Ed. ŠTERZL, J. Prague: Czech. Acad. Sci.
44. WARD, H. K., and ENDERS, J. F. (1933). *J. exp. Med.*, **57**, 527.
45. BIOZZI, G., and STIFFEL, C. (1962). In *Immunopathology*, **2**, 249. Internat. Symp. Basel: Schwabe and Co.
46. PONDMAN, K. W. (1965). Ref. 27, p. 216.
47. GERLINGS-PETERSEN, B. T., and PONDMAN, K. W. (1962). *Vox Sang.* (*Basel*), **7**, 655.
48. SPINK, W. W., and KEEFER, C. S. (1937). *J. clin. Invest.*, **16**, 169.
49. JENKIN, C. R. (1963). *Brit. J. exp. Path.*, **44**, 47.
50. WOOD, W. B. (1946). *J. exp. Med.*, **84**, 387.
51. GELZER, J., and SUTER, E. (1959). *J. exp. Med.*, **110**, 715.
52. MUDD, S., (1965). *Ann. N.Y. Acad. Sci.*, **128**, 45.
53. LI, I. W., and MUDD, S. (1965). *J. Immunol.*, **94**, 852.
53*a*. SHAYEGANI, M. G., and MUDD, S. (1969). *Bact. Proc.* In press.
MUDD, S. (1968). *Topics in Medicinal Chemistry*, **2**, 247. Eds. RABINOWITZ, J. L., and MYERSON, R. M. New York: John Wiley & Sons.
54. FISCHER, H. (1965). Quoted by Boyden *et al* in Ref. 42.
55. COHN, Z. A. (1963). *J. exp. Med.*, **117**, 27, 43.
56. WILSON, G. S., and MILES, A. (1964). *Topley and Wilson's Principles of Bacteriology and Immunity*, Chap. 48, 5th edit. London: Edward Arnold.
57. STEBBINS, E. L. (1940). *Amer. J. publ. Hlth.*, **30**, Suppl. 36.
58. BOYDEN, S. (1965). Ref. 43, p. 329.
59. WIENER, A. S. (1951). *J. Immunol.*, **66**, 287.
60. SELL, S. and FAHEY, J. L. (1964). *J. Immunol.*, **93**, 81.
61. BRAUN, W. (1965). Ref. 43, p. 369.
62. HIRSCH, J. G. (1960). *Bact. Rev.*, **24**, 133.
63. GLYNN, A. A., BRUMFITT, W., and SALTON, M. R. J. (1966). *Brit. J. exp. Path.*, **47**, 331.
64. GLADSTONE, G. P., and JOHNSTON, H. H. (1955). *Brit. J. exp. Path.*, **36**, 363.
65. PILLEMER, L. (1956). *Ann. N.Y. Acad. Sci.*, **66**, 233.
66. ISLIKER, H. (1958). In *Immunopathology*, Internat. Symp., **1**, p. 29. Eds. GRABAR, P., and MEISCHER, P. Basel: Schwabe & Co.
67. PENSKY, J., HINZ, C. F., TODD, E. W., WEDGWOOD, R. J., and LEPOW, I. H. (1964). *Fed. Proc.*, **23**, 505.
68. NELSON, R. A. (1958). *J. exp. Med.*, **108**, 515.
69. OSAWA, E., and MUSCHEL, L. H. (1960). *J. Immunol.*, **84**, 203.
70. WEDGWOOD, R. J. (1964). In *Immunological Methods*, p. 25. (Symp. Counc. Internat. Org. med. Sci.) Ed. ACKROYD, J. F. Oxford: Blackwell.
71. SHILO, M. (1959). *Ann. Rev. Microbiol.*, **13**, 255.
72. WATSON, D. W., and BLOOM, W. (1952). *Proc. Soc. exp. Biol.* (*N.Y.*), **81**, 29.
73. DUBOS, R. J. (1954). *Biochemical Determinants of Microbial Disease*, Chap. 2. Cambridge, Mass.: Harvard Univ. Press.
74. MYRVIK, Q. N. (1956). *Ann. N.Y. Acad. Sci.*, **66**, 391.
75. EKSTEDT, R. D. (1956). *J. Bact.*, **72**, 157.

Chapter 37

ACQUIRED IMMUNITY: HUMORAL AND CELLULAR FACTORS INVOLVED IN PROTECTION

By G. P. Gladstone

The ability of serum from actively immunised animals to confer on other animals specific protection against a number of infectious diseases shows clearly that antibodies play a part in acquired immunity. In the last chapter, we saw that the secondary results of the union of antibody with the antigens of micro-organisms led to opsonisation, bactericidal action mediated by complement, intracellular destruction, inactivation of viruses and neutralisation of toxins. It might be expected, therefore, that the protective action of immune serum is related to those antibodies which bring about these secondary reactions, and this has, in general, proved to be the case.

It is more doubtful whether immune agglutination contributes to protection. The mere clumping of bacterial cells together does not destroy them but may delay their spread through the tissues. Some evidence for this was obtained by Rich and McKee,[1] who showed that rabbits, actively or passively protected against pneumococcal infection and rendered leucopenic by injections of benzene, survived considerably longer than non-immune controls when challenged with a lethal dose of pneumococci, but eventually succumbed. At the challenge site the cocci were agglutinated, whereas in the controls they were dispersed. On the other hand, antibodies to the flagella of motile bacteria, which agglutinate the organism but have no other action, have no protective function, with the possible exception of antibodies to the flagella of *Cl. septicum*.[2]

Are antibodies the only factor involved in acquired antibacterial immunity? Can phagocytic cells become so altered by contact with the micro-organism or its antigens that they acquire an enhanced ability to dispose of the pathogen? With the resolution of the controversy between the cellular and humoral theories of specific protective immunity by the finding that committed antibody and uncommitted cell are both involved in the disposal of invading organisms by phagocytes, these questions might be considered to have been answered. Nevertheless, the possibility that, in the absence of antibody, cells might be specifically induced to destroy bacteria has been raised from time to time, but because of the difficulty of excluding the effect of antibody, it has received little attention. However, recent observations strongly suggest that phagocytes alone play an important part in immunity to certain infections involving the so-called facultative intracellular parasites mentioned in the last chapter. This subject of bacterial cellular immunity is considered in a later section of this chapter.

Antiviral immunity may also involve both humoral (antibody) and cellular mechanisms. Viruses are obligate intracellular parasites which invade many different kinds of parenchymal cells as well as the typically phagocytic cells of the blood and reticulo-endothelial system. Antibody can prevent entry of viruses, but once the virus is inside the cell any protective mechanism must be of cellular origin, since antibody cannot ordinarily penetrate into the cell.

We may classify acquired immunity as follows:

Antitoxic. Humoral: always involving antibodies (antitoxins).

Antibacterial (1) *Humoral*: involving antibodies. Uncommitted cells may also be required (phagocytosis).
(2) *Cellular*: not involving antibodies. Depending on committed phagocytic cells.

Antiviral (1) *Humoral*: involving antibodies acting on extracellular virus.
(2) *Cellular*: involving substances (interferons) produced within infected cells, and acting within the host cell producing it, and also in other cells.

In this chapter, some of the mechanisms involved in each type will be discussed and illustrated with examples, with the exception of antiviral immunity dependent on interferons which is considered in Chapter 31.

ANTITOXIC IMMUNITY

In diseases predominantly due to potent bacterial toxins, and in which the offending parasite does not invade the tissues to any extent, protection depends on the presence of antitoxin. In passively immunised animals, the titre of circulating antitoxin may be taken as a measure of their immunity. Actively immunised animals, however, have a potential capacity for rapidly forming more antitoxin in response to toxin ("immunological memory", see Chapter 34), so that in these animals immunity is greater than that indicated by their titre of circulating antitoxin.

Provided the rate at which toxin is produced is not too great, antitoxin is effective in preventing disease, even when injected after the organism has entered the tissues. The benefit of the prophylactic injection of tetanus antitoxin at the time of wounding was amply demonstrated in the First World War, and diphtheria antitoxin is also an effective prophylactic when given to persons who have been exposed to infection. Once sufficient toxin has been fixed to susceptible tissues to cause clinical symptoms, however, the amount of antitoxin that must be given is out of all proportion to the amount of toxin present because antitoxin fails partially or completely to neutralise fixed toxin (FIG. 1). In addition, Miles and Miles[4] have shown that toxins such as the α-toxin (lecithinase) of *Cl. welchii*, which increase the permeability of the blood capillaries, may, by causing a high pressure of intercellular exudate in the lesion, oppose the exudation of antitoxin-containing plasma, so that the antitoxin is prevented from reaching the site of infection. These factors, therefore, make it imperative to give antitoxin as early as possible in the course of the disease. Indeed, it might be argued that antitoxin, although used in therapy, acts in reality only as a prophylactic agent, since the benefit it confers is due almost entirely to the neutralisation of toxin in the free state while it is being produced by the invading organism.

The prophylactic used in the production of an active antitoxic immunity is a toxoid, which is often adsorbed on to an adjuvant (Chapter 34).

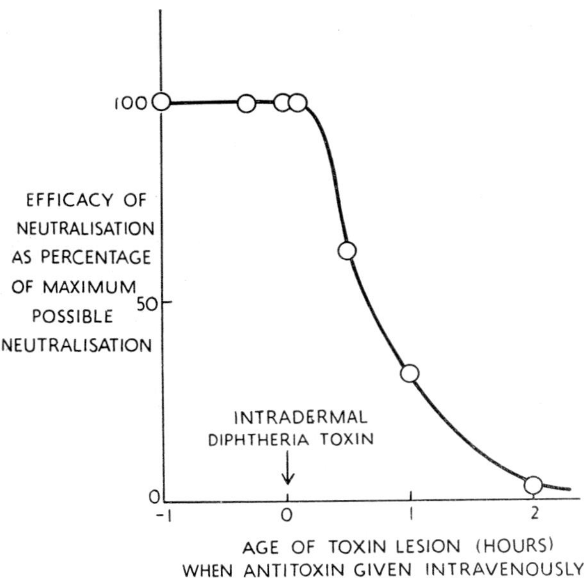

37/FIG. 1.—The decline in efficacy of intravenous diphtheria antitoxin administered at varying intervals after intradermal injection of diphtheria toxin in the guinea-pig. (From A. A. Miles.[3])

Has Antitoxic Immunity any Antibacterial Action?

It is possible that once the toxin produced by a bacterium has been neutralised, the normal basic immunity can deal with the parasite itself. Some toxins destroy leucocytes, and it is clear that the neutralisation of this leucocidal action may assist the body to overcome the invasion. The protective action of staphylococcal antitoxin has been ascribed to its antileucocidal action, but whether diphtheria antitoxin assists the elimination of diphtheria bacilli in the same way is doubtful. It has been claimed that diphtheria toxin has a lethal action on leucocytes, but this has not been substantiated by work in this department[5] in which human and guinea-pig leucocytes were subjected to as much as 100 Lf doses of pure crystalline toxin per ml. without being affected (see also ref. 6). However, Amies[7] suggests that toxin helps indirectly in the establishment of the bacilli in the tissues by an inhibitory effect on the inflammatory response. He showed that highly toxigenic diphtheria bacilli, when injected intracutaneously into guinea-pigs, at first proliferated locally without being taken up by leucocytes or producing an inflammatory reaction. It was only after the development of necrosis, brought about by the action of the toxin, that inflammation was observed. In contrast, when the same strain was injected into an animal protected with antitoxin, or when the organisms were washed free from toxin before injection or when a strain of less toxigenicity was used, an immediate inflammatory reaction took place and most of the bacteria were taken up by phagocytes and destroyed.

If toxin assists in the establishment of *C. diphtheriæ* in the tissues in the way

Amies suggests, it is possible to account for the more extensive bacterial invasion and infiltrating type of lesion found with *gravis* as compared with *mitis* strains solely on the basis of the known greater rate of toxin production by *gravis* strains under the conditions found in the animal tissues, without invoking other factors to explain the difference in virulence (for example, the possession by *gravis* strains of endotoxin, see ref. 8, or factors preventing their destruction by leucocytes[9]). Experimental evidence supporting this suggestion has been obtained by Scheibel[10] in guinea-pigs, using a technique for producing infection that simulated the natural disease in man. She found that toxoid gave a high degree of protection against infection with *gravis* strains and that the additional use of bacterial vaccines failed to improve the immunity.

A better-established example of antitoxic immunity directly preventing bacterial invasion is found in immunity to *Cl. welchii* and certain other anærobic bacteria which produce necrotising toxins. We have seen that, in *Cl. welchii* infections, the production of α-toxin is not only responsible for most of the pathological changes, but that it brings about the conditions that are necessary for the organism to grow in the tissues. We should expect to find, therefore, that antitoxin, by neutralising the α-toxin, would prevent *Cl. welchii* from becoming established in the tissues. Evans (for ref., see 11) has shown that this is in fact the case.

Immunity to anthrax is another example. Anthrax is a disease essentially invasive in character, the organisms spreading from the local lesion both by contiguity and, more usually, by the blood stream. It is common to find large numbers of bacteria in the blood in animals dying of the infection. At first sight, it might be thought that protection would depend on antibodies acting directly on the bacterial cell and determining phagocytosis, e.g. anticapsular antibodies. Although the capsule is undoubtedly a factor in the virulence of *B. anthracis*, antibody to the capsule has little protective action. Protection appears to depend on an antitoxin. Sixty years ago Bail noted that bacteria-free filtrates of œdematous lesions from animals dying of anthrax contained a thermolabile antigen which was highly effective in promoting protection against infection. This antigen is quite distinct from the capsule and it would appear that both are necessary for virulence. Non-capsulated variants may produce the antigen and such strains have proved effective as living vaccines. They are able to grow locally in the body tissues producing sufficient antigen to confer immunity, but being non-capsulated they are taken up by leucocytes and do not produce a generalised infection.

What is the nature of this antigen? As isolated from œdema fluid or produced in culture it has little toxicity. However, recent work by H. Smith[12] in this country, and Thorne[13] in America, has shown that œdema fluid and culture filtrates contain more than one extracellular antigen. They have isolated and purified, not only the "protective" antigen, but two other protein antigens which also appear to be non-toxic. However, the addition of one of these antigens to "protective" antigen results in a mixture which kills mice and produces an inflammatory reaction in the skin of guinea-pigs. It would seem that the anthrax bacillus produces two non-toxic components which become toxic when acting synergistically. One of these, however, is an effective antigen, producing antibody which not only protects against infection but neutralises the toxic action of the synergistic mixture. The link between the toxin and the invasiveness of the organism is still somewhat obscure, but there is suggestive evidence that the toxin acts particularly on the reticulo-endothelial cells and inhibits blood clearance.

Scarlet fever antitoxin is an example of an antitoxin which has no antibacterial action. It neutralises the erythrogenic toxin of *Str. pyogenes*, but has no effect on the invasiveness of the organism. Evidence for the neutralisation of toxin by antitoxin can be obtained *in vivo* by the intracutaneous injection of serum containing antitoxin in individuals with scarlet fever. Blanching of the rash occurs in the immediate neighbourhood of the injections (Schultz-Charlton reaction).

HUMORAL ANTIBACTERIAL IMMUNITY

This may be defined as acquired immunity to bacterial infection dependent on antibodies which act on structural surface antigens of the bacterial cell, with secondary effects leading to bacterial destruction. These secondary effects may be purely humoral, or may involve the cellular mechanism of phagocytosis and intracellular destruction.

Bacterial Capsules and Microcapsules

Where virulence is mainly related to a single structural antigen, as for instance the polysaccharide capsule of the pneumococcus (Chapter 29), it is usually possible to correlate protection with antibody to this antigen. Antibody to the type specific pneumococcal capsule will confer complete protection in mice against experimental infection with the same type of pneumococcus, but not against infection with other types, and there is a direct correlation between protection and the antibody titre of the serum. The protective effect of the serum is due to opsonisation and can be removed by precipitation with purified polysaccharide of the homologous type. Vaccines made from rough strains of pneumococci that have lost their capsular antigen will not confer protection.

With a few exceptions, the possession of a well-defined capsule in pathogenic bacteria is at least one factor determining virulence in that it enables the organism to resist phagocytosis. Antibody to the capsular antigen might therefore be expected to be important in protection. That this is not necessarily so has already been shown in immunity to anthrax. Another example is the failure of the capsular antigen of *Bordetella pertussis* to confer protection against whooping cough.[14] Sometimes it is possible to relate immunity to the so-called "microcapsular" antigens on the surface of the cell which are distinct from the cell wall but do not form a morphological capsule. The M protein of *Streptococcus pyogenes* is an example. Experimental acquired immunity in mice, and probably immunity in man, appears to depend on antibodies to the type specific M protein, which act like pneumococcal polysaccharide antibodies in opsonising the organism. Similarly, some degree of immunity to experimental *Salm. typhi* infection in mice may be conferred with antibody to the microcapsular Vi antigen which, as we have seen (Chapter 29), probably acts by sensitising the organism to the bactericidal action of complement as well as by opsonisation. A similar relationship has been found with antibodies to the somatic O antigen in the wall of the organism. However, prophylactic trials in man do not confirm the results of passive protection in mice, since significant but not spectacular immunity in man could be produced with vaccines which do not stimulate the production of Vi antibodies.[15] This discrepancy may be related to the difference in pathology between the experimental disease in mice and the natural disease in man, and suggests that a more realistic comparison should be made between immunity to typhoid in man (due to *Salm. typhi*) and immunity to natural typhoid in mice (due to *Salm. typhi murium*) which have a similar pathology. As cellular as well as humoral factors appear to operate in immunity to mouse typhoid, it is possible that such factors also operate in immunity to human typhoid (see below).

Immunity possibly dependent on many Antigens

Some bacteria possess such a vast array of antigens both structural and extracellular that it is often impossible to assign to a single antigen an essential role in immunity. For instance, immunity to staphylococcal infection, although certainly involving humoral antibodies as shown by the high susceptibility to infection of subjects with hypogammaglobulinæmia, is still obscure. In contradistinction to *Staphylococcus albus*, the coagulase-positive *Staphylococcus aureus* produces some 20 extracellular antigens, many of which have not been characterised, as well as complex structural antigens of the cell wall and surface. Because no single antigen has yet been found to produce effective immunity against infection, it is generally thought that staphylococcal immunity is multifactoral. Candidates for consideration are (1) the capsular antigen in those strains that produce capsules[16, 17]; (2) teichoic acid and other cell wall antigens[18]; (3) the surface protein antigen (Protein A) first described by Verwey[19, 20]; (4) coagulase[21]; (5) the Panton-Valentine leucocidin[22, 23]; and (6) α-toxin (for refs. see 24, 25). With the exception of the capsule which is effective against capsulated strains, none of these antigens is wholly protective alone. So far there is no data on the protective value of combinations of them.

Bordetella pertussis is another complex organism possessing 7 structural antigens having well-marked biological properties. However, probably only one of these is concerned in protection (for refs. see 26). Strains containing this antigen have been shown to be effective vaccines in prophylactic trials in man, but the antigen has still defied attempts at purification.

CELLULAR ANTIBACTERIAL IMMUNITY

We have already seen that certain bacteria known as the facultative intracellular parasites can be readily engulfed by phagocytic cells, usually without the need for opsonisation, and survive and even grow within the cell. Although both polymorphs and macrophages take up these bacteria, the phenomenon is most evident in the macrophage, since the polymorph is too short-lived for the fate of the intracellular organism to be observed for any length of time. The growth of the organism intracellularly may eventually lead to the death of the cell. Immunity to these infections can be acquired by previous infection, or by contact with bacteria or their products in the form of vaccines, but unlike the classical type of antibacterial immunity it cannot be related to the presence of antibodies, or, at any rate, antibodies existing in a free state. A classical example of the type of immunity in question is immunity to tuberculosis.

Immunity to Tuberculosis

Since the observations of Koch on the modified response of a tuberculous guinea-pig to reinfection (Koch phenomenon, see Chapter 39), extensive work has been carried out to determine whether a specific acquired immunity to tuberculosis does exist, and, if so, the mechanism on which it is based. No one doubts at the present time the existence of antituberculous immunity; the uncertainty lies in the mechanism. In spite of the fact that immunity to tuberculosis presents features that depart from the classical type of antibacterial immunity, there has been until recently a general disinclination to put it into a separate category (see, for example, ref. 27). Its study has been considerably complicated by the concomitant presence of delayed hypersensitivity (see Chapter 39), the chronic nature of the infection, the failure to relate protection to antibodies and the relatively low grade type of immunity produced. We may start with a brief description of the relevant facts.

In experimental superinfection in the guinea-pig, that is a second challenge with virulent tubercle bacilli in an animal already infected and suffering from a progressive disease, the bacilli at their route of entry tend to remain localised; their growth is inhibited and many are destroyed. In particular, they do not invade and produce lesions in the regional lymph nodes. This is in marked contrast to the fate of the organisms in the primary infection, which grow locally, invade and produce caseous lesions in the regional lymph glands, and from there spread to other organs resulting in a progressive disease from which the animal succumbs. We have here the anomalous situation of an animal who has acquired through a previous infection immunity to newly implanted organisms but not to those of the original infection. The explanation would appear to lie in the extreme susceptibility of the guinea-pig to the tubercle bacillus. Once the bacilli have become established in large numbers in the body in caseous lesions out of reach of the immune mechanism, they are unaffected. However, in more naturally resistant animals, as for example in man, provided the primary infection is not excessive, the development of immunity in the course of primary infection, e.g. in the lung, is shown, not only by the protection against the development of a secondary infection, but by the self-limitation of the primary lesion. It is the general experience that autopsies on subjects who have died from other causes often show a single encapsulated focus of infection (Ghon focus) which may have involved the peribronchial lymph glands but has not extended further. There are no other foci, even when the subject has been under special risk, for example a child in contact with a parent with open tuberculosis. As Rich[27] has pointed out, the lungs of such a child might be expected to contain multiple primary foci. It can only be concluded that the many tubercle bacilli, which must have been inspired subsequent to the development of the primary focus, have been destroyed. Even when immunity breaks down and progressive disease occurs, the nature of the disease is considerably modified compared with the rapid exudative disease of a non-immune subject.

Immunity to tuberculous infection in guinea-pigs and man may be produced by immunising with the attenuated strain of tubercle bacilli B.C.G. (Bacille-Calmette-Guérin), a bovine strain of fixed attenuated virulence. This strain multiplies *in vivo* but never leads to progressive disease. The use of this strain confers an immunity to superinfection comparable to that produced by infection with a virulent strain and allows experimental immunity to be studied without the guinea-pig succumbing to the primary infection. Dead organisms have also proved effective provided sufficient numbers are used.

Failure of antibodies to confer immunity.—There is no doubt that antibodies to the tubercle bacillus, demonstrable by agglutination, precipitation, hæmagglutination and complement fixation, are found in the serum in immunised animals. However, in no case has it been conclusively shown that protection can be conferred by passive transfer of serum, even when the antibody content of the blood of the recipient is maintained by repeated injection. Moreover, serum antibodies have not been shown to have any lethal or inhibitory action on the growth of tubercle bacilli in the presence of complement or phagocytic cells. Since tubercle bacilli are taken up by macrophages or polymorphs without opsonisation, antibodies are clearly not required for this purpose. The possibility that they may be required for subsequent intracellular destruction has been raised, but the evidence, to be discussed later, is against such action.

Although antibodies are not involved, there is a humoral factor present in inflammatory exudates of infected animals which appears to have a bacteriostatic action on the growth of tubercle bacilli both *in vivo* and *in vitro* and which is not found in normal animals. This was first demonstrated by Lurie[28], who placed inside the peritoneal cavity of normal and immune guinea-pigs and rabbits tubercle bacilli in silk bags impregnated with collodion, which were permeable to body fluids but not to cells. The bags were removed after 4–14 days for viable counts. In 9 experiments, he noted that the growth of the bacilli in the immunised animals was 4–190 times less than in the controls. The nature of the humoral factor is uncertain, but since the pH of the contents of the bag in the immunised animals was considerably lower than that in the controls, it has been suggested that inflammation brought about as the result of concomitant hypersensitivity was at least partly responsible for the difference.[29] Much of this low pH would be due to lactic acid produced by the inflammatory cells which has been shown to be tuberculostatic.[29]

Hypersensitivity and immunity in tuberculosis.—If humoral bacteriostasis mentioned above is the result of hypersensitivity, can immunity in general be merely a manifestation of hypersensitivity? The phenomenon of delayed hypersensitivity is discussed in detail in Chapter 39. Briefly, as it applies to tuberculosis, it is a specific increased reactivity of the tissues to the proteins of the bacillus brought about by infection, or by immunisation with attenuated living organisms, or by sufficient numbers of dead organisms, leading to a local inflammatory reaction at the site of contact of the tuberculoprotein, involving mononuclear cells. The question of its role in the pathology of tuberculosis is discussed in Chapter 42. Here we have to consider its possible role in immunity.

No factor in immunity to tuberculosis has received so much attention as the possible implication of hypersensitivity. The rapid localisation of the bacilli and failure to produce a tuberculous lesion on superinfection in the Koch phenomenon and its association with an inflammatory reaction at the site of the implanted bacilli, strongly suggested that the two were related and that the inflammatory reaction brought about by hypersensitivity to tuberculoprotein was the cause of the destruction of the bacilli. This view was widely held by the earlier workers and was developed, particularly in a series of papers by Krause (for refs. see 27). However, Rich in an able discussion of the problem occupying some 60 pages of his monograph[27] has produced cogent arguments for regarding the two as distinct. His conclusions are based on the observations briefly summarised below; but for a more detailed account his monograph should be consulted.

(1) There is no correlation between the degree of hypersensitivity and that of immunity.

It is possible to produce hypersensitivity in an animal in the absence of immunity. For instance, tuberculoprotein injected into a guinea-pig together with certain waxes from the bacillus sensitises the animal to tuberculoprotein but does not confer immunity.

(3) Hypersensitivity which develops concomitantly with immunity when guinea-pigs are immunised with B.C.G. is more short-lived and may be practically absent at a time when immunity is still apparent.

(4) Repeated intravenous injection of killed or attenuated tubercle bacilli is said to induce in guinea-pigs immunity without hypersensitivity.

(5) Acquired resistance both in man and in animals remains intact after sensitivity has been abolished by desensitisation with appropriate injections of tuberculin.

(6) Passive transfer of hypersenstivity can be achieved with buffy coat cells (probably lymphocytes) without transference of immunity (Chapter 39). The converse, namely the transference of immunity without hypersensitivity, however, has not been achieved.

(7) To the above we may add the claim of Weiss and Dubos[30] to have achieved immunity in guinea-pigs with methanol extracts of tubercle bacilli without producing hypersensitivity.

In spite of this clear distinction between immunity and hypersensitivity, it is difficult not to regard the acute inflammatory reaction of hypersensitivity as having at least some non-specific adjuvant effect on immunity, as for example in Lurie's experiment quoted above.

Moreover recent work of Mackaness and others (for refs. see 31) in connection with immunity to other forms of intracellular parasitism suggests that delayed hypersensitivity as a specific element in cellular immunity must not be dismissed too lightly. This work will be considered in connection with immunity to other facultative intracellular parasites in a later section (p. 1056).

So far no reference has been made to the difference in the fate of tubercle bacilli injected into normal and immune animals beyond the statement that, in immune animals, they tend to be localised, prevented from growing and eventually killed. In Chapter 42 in which the formation of the tubercle is described, it is stated that tubercle bacilli implanted into the tissues of normal animals are readily taken up by monocytes but are not necessarily destroyed in the cell. They often multiply intracellularly and kill the cell. The subsequent reaction to the small collection of tubercle bacilli forms the tubercle. In an animal with acquired immunity on the other hand, provided the numbers of bacilli implanted are not too great, the monocyte appears to have acquired the capacity, not only to inhibit the intracellular growth of the bacilli, but to destroy them. There is a general agreement that the basis for acquired immunity depends on the ability of the monocyte to destroy ingested tubercle bacilli, but there is still dispute about whether the cell itself is immune, whether humoral antibody promotes intracellular destruction or whether "cytophilic antibody" is concerned. This is a form of antibody firmly fixed to the cell, though presumably different from the specific factor, whatever its nature, that makes the cell hypersensitive.

Evidence for the importance of the immune monocyte or macrophage.—The first experimental evidence that cells themselves may become immune through contact with bacteria or their products without the participation of antibodies, was obtained by Lurie in his classical work on the survival and growth of tubercle bacilli in normal and immune monocytes in a situation out of reach of antibody.[32, 33] Macrophages from normal and immunised rabbits were infected *in vitro* with equal numbers of bovine tubercle bacilli and injected into the anterior chambers of the eye of albino rabbits, normal cells into one eye, immune cells into the other. In this situation they were out of reach of circulating antibody. After 10–20 days, viable counts were made on the bacilli from each eye. It was found that the number in the "immune" cells was 2–20 times smaller than in the normal cells.

Attempts were made to repeat the work in macrophages cultured *in vitro* where again the influence of immune serum could be excluded. Although Mackaness[34] could find no difference in numbers of bacilli growing in the two kinds of cells, this has not been the general experience (for refs. see 35). It would appear that, provided small numbers of organisms are used, there is a very significant reduction in the numbers of organisms in immune leucocytes compared with the numbers in normal cells in which the bacilli not only survive but multiply and destroy the cell.

What constitutes an immune monocyte? What mechanism has changed the normal cell into an immune cell?—These questions are still far from being answered. However, further investigations particularly by Mackaness (for refs. see 31, 36) have shown that the phenomenon is not confined to immunity to tuberculosis but appears to operate in other infections in which organisms are able to survive inside monocytes, that is in immunity to the facultative intracellular parasites. These include not only the *Mycobacteria*, but *Listeria*, *Brucella* and perhaps also *Salmonella*. Because these organisms grow more rapidly than tubercle bacilli they have been used in investigations on the conditions determining cellular immunity in preference to the tubercle bacillus.

Cellular Immunity in Infections due to Facultative Intracellular Parasites other than Tubercle Bacilli

As with immunity to tuberculosis, immunity to *Brucella* and *Listeria* infections depends essentially on the intracellular destruction of these organisms in phagocytes. Although brucellæ are subject to extracellular lysis with antibody and complement, antibody probably plays little part in protection, since immunity cannot be transferred passively with serum, and dead vaccines which produce high titres of antibody to the surface somatic antigens are ineffective. On the other hand, monocytes from guinea-pigs, rats and mice, immunised with living smooth strains of *Brucella abortus* or *melitensis*, greatly restrict the intracellular growth of these organisms *in vitro*, whereas normal monocytes have little effect and the organisms grow abundantly. The addition of antiserum to the medium in which either normal or immune cells were cultured had no effect.[37] Mackaness (for refs. see 31, 36) extended this work. He noted that mice immunised with an attenuated strain of *Br. abortus* (strain 19), not only produced peritoneal macrophages which inhibited and destroyed the organisms *in vitro*, but also rapidly eliminated the organisms from their tissues *in vivo* as shown by viable counts on liver and spleen. As brucellæ are taken up by the reticulo-endothelial cells of these organs, it would appear that the fixed phagocytic cells, as well as wandering macrophages, were also immune. Similar results were obtained with *L. monocytogenes* which produces a non-fatal disease in mice from which they recover. Monocytes from mice convalescent from infection kill *L. monocytogenes in vitro*, and the tissues eliminate the organisms of a new challenge infection rapidly, whereas early in the disease, before immunity has developed, the bacteria grow abundantly in both monocytes and tissues. The serum contains no humoral factor capable of protecting normal mice.

Is cellular immunity specific?—Mackaness noted that mice at certain stages of infection with *Br. abortus* not only elimated *Br. abortus* from their tissues, but also *L. monocytogenes* at an even greater rate than mice convalescing from infection with *L. monocytogenes* itself and *vice versa*. Further, mice immunised with the B.C.G. strain of tubercle bacilli were immune to infection with *L. monocytogenes*. *In vitro*, the peritoneal macrophages showed the same cross resistance. It would appear that this non-specific cross resistance between organisms having no antigenic relationship is a characteristic feature of acquired cellular immunity and is further evidence that it does not depend on specific antibody. However, a specific element can be demonstrated. Mackaness[36] noted that the peritoneal macrophages of mice 12 weeks after recovery from infection with *L. monocytogenes* lost much of their activity to destroy both *L. monocytogenes* and *Br. abortus*. If at this stage the mice were reinfected with *L. monocytogenes*, immunity was rapidly restored to its former level. The challenge inoculum grew briefly in liver and spleen and then died out and the peritoneal cells regained their activity against both *L. monocytogenes* and *Br. abortus*. This "recall", reminiscent of the secondary response in antibody formation, however, could not be achieved by reinfecting the mice convalescent from listerosis with *Br. abortus*, which grew in the tissues at the same rate and in the same numbers as in a normal mouse. Alternatively, the waning immunity of mice immunised with the living attenuated strain of *Br. abortus* could be recalled with *Br. abortus* but not with *L. monocytogenes*.

Cellular immunity dependent on continued antigenic stimulus.—In all these cellular immune reactions the amount and retention of bacterial antigen are important in determining the duration of immunity. With the exception of immunity to tuberculosis, dead vaccines are ineffective, probably because they are eliminated too rapidly. Living attenuated vaccine strains which are able to grow in the body, but which produce a self limiting inapparent infection, or small doses of virulent strains of organisms such as *L. monocytogenes* which multiply but do not produce a fatal infection, are required. Once the animal has eliminated the organisms from the tissues and the population of immune macrophages has been replaced with uncommitted cells, immunity wanes. Cellular immunity is, therefore, essentially an "infection immunity" lasting as long as the antigenic stimulus remains. The nature of this antigenic stimulus, however, is far from clear.

Cellular immunity in Salmonella infection.—Before considering the mechanism by which macrophages and reticulo-endothelial cells acquire immunity to the facultative intracellular parasites, we may study immunity to *Salmonella* infection as an example in which probably both humoral and cellular mechanisms operate. The term "humoral" here includes not only extracellular destruction mediated by complement, but opsonisation and intracellular destruction in so far as they are determined by antibody, whereas the term "cellular" is confined to an acquired ability of the macrophage to destroy the intracellular organism independently of antibody.

Immunity to *Salm. typhi murium* infection in mice has been extensively studied in recent years and, as it presents distinctive features which may throw light on cellular immunity in general, and immunity to typhoid in man in particular, we may consider it in some detail. *Salm. typhi murium* produces a natural disease in mice resembling typhoid fever in man. Strains of attenuated virulence exist which give rise to a symptomless infection in the liver and spleen. Phagocytosis by mouse macrophages usually requires opsonisation with antibody to a surface somatic antigen. Gelzer and Suter,[38] however, as already noted (Chapter 36) showed that with rabbit macrophages the main function of antibody was to assist intracellular destruction rather than opsonisation. Can a true cellular immunity exist in addition to or as a replacement for an immune mechanism based on antibody? This subject is still controversial. However, as with the earlier controversy between the proponents of "cellular" and "humoral" theories of immunity, a true solution may be found in a synthesis of the two views. Mouse typhoid like its human counterpart has characters very similar to other forms of infection by facultative intracellular parasites discussed earlier. The similarities may be summarised as follows:

(1) In spite of the apparent requirement for opsonisation by antibody *in vitro*, virulent organisms are taken up *in vivo* by the reticulo-endothelial cells of the liver and spleen although at a slower rate than when organisms pre-opsonised by antibody are injected[39] or when strains of low virulence are used. They grow in these cells and destroy them and may persist in these sites for weeks (chronic carrier state). They also survive and grow in peritoneal macrophages from normal mice. Mackaness[31] noted that 50 per cent of the infecting organisms taken up remained alive in these cells.

(2) Although dead vaccines produce high titres of antibody to the surface somatic O antigens, they give only a low grade immunity.[40] On the other hand living attenuated strains may protect against as much as 10,000 lethal doses of virulent organisms.[41] The vaccine strains grow in the R.E. cells and persist as an inapparent infection.

(3) Isolated peritoneal macrophages from immunised mice that have engulfed *Salm. typhi murium* dispose of these organisms with extreme rapidity. Mackaness[31] noted that all organisms engulfed were destroyed within 15 minutes.

This is in contrast to the 50 per cent survival in normal peritoneal macrophages mentioned above.

(4) Intracellular destruction is not specific. The cells from mice immunised with *Salm. typhi murium* will inactivate *L. monocytogenes* with equal rapidity and *vice versa.*

In spite of these similarities, there has been considerable reluctance to accept the view that immunity to experimental mouse typhoid is cell-determined, particularly by Rowley, Jenkin and their colleagues (for refs. see 42). These authors claim that the failure of heat-killed vaccines to protect, in spite of the development of O antibodies, is due to the destruction of a thermolabile protein antigen, shared with *Salm. paratyphi C, Salm. adelaide* and some other Gram-negative bacteria, and not to some property which the living organism confers on the macrophage.[42] This antigen appears to be different from the thermolabile factor 5 of the O antigen complex which is analogous to the thermolabile Vi antigen of *Salm. typhi.* Their main contention, however, against a pure cellular mechanism divorced from antibody, is the fact that protection can be conferred passively with serum, provided that a sufficient amount is used, and that it is from an animal actively immunised with living attenuated organisms or with vaccines in which the thermolabile protein antigen is not destroyed. Immunity, in fact, appeared to be directly related to the content of opsonins in the serum and persisted for 3 months after the vaccine strain could no longer be isolated from the liver and spleen. This is in contrast to immunity to other intracellular parasites, in which immunity wanes as soon as the organisms are eliminated. They explain the more rapid destruction in macrophages from the immune animal as due to a previous opsonisation of the organisms by antibody to the thermolabile antigen.

In spite of their emphasis on humoral-dependent immunity, however, they found that peritoneal macrophages from mice taken 14 days after immunisation with the living attenuated vaccine strain were superior in their bactericidal properties to macrophages from normal mice, a finding which directly supports a cellular theory. Moreover, these macrophages washed free from antibody, were as capable of transferring immunity to normal mice as was immune serum as shown by the rapid destruction of virulent organisms injected intraperitoneally into the recipient mice (FIG. 2). This immunity, however, is short-lived. Macrophages reaped some weeks later were no different from normal macrophages, although the mice were still immune.

Analysis showed that, as with the response to many other antigens (Chapter 34), the antibody response to immunisation with the living vaccine strain occurred in two phases. The first phase, which lasted over the period in which macrophages appeared to be immune, consisted of the formation of macroglobulin 19S antibody (IgM). This gave place to 7S globulin (IgG), and, at a time when the macrophages could no longer transfer immunity, the antibody in the serum was mainly 7S. Both 19S and 7S antibody were capable of passive transfer of immunity in serum. Further investigations showed that the ability of macrophages in the early stage of immunisation to transfer passive immunity was apparently related to the adsorption of 19S antibody on their surface. Urea eluates from "immune" cells were shown to contain a macroglobulin having the characteristics of 19S antibody and susceptible to mercaptoethanol

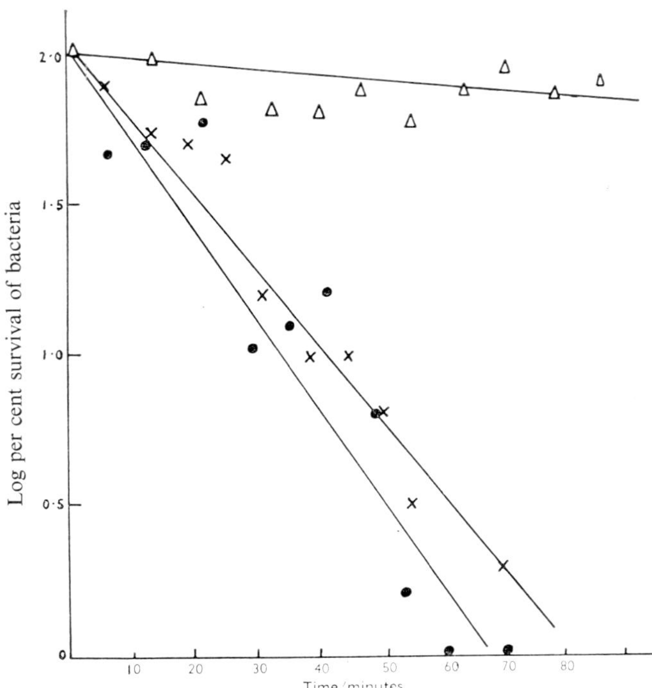

37/FIG. 2.—Passive transfer of intraperitoneal immunity to normal mice by either macrophages or serum obtained from mice previously immunised with a living attenuated strain of *S. typhi murium* M206. (From Rowley, Turner and Jenkin.[43])

△ - - △ Normal cells transferred.

x - - x Immune serum transferred.

● - - ● Macrophages from immune mice transferred.

These eluates appeared to be as capable as the cells themselves in transferring immunity to normal mice. In the later stages of immunisation, no 19S antibody could be eluted and the cells lost their immunity. 7S antibody, although present in the serum and capable of transferring passive immunity, did not apparently adsorb to macrophages. Jenkin and Rowley claim that the so-called cellular immunity in mouse typhoid is due to a cytophilic 19S macroglobulin antibody bound firmly to cells which acts, in common with free antibody, in opsonising the organism and, what is more important, in promoting intracellular killing. They see in this system a model for explaining cellular immunity in general as being due to bound antibody of the 19S type transferred with the macrophage and having such affinity with these cells that in many cases it cannot be found free in the serum, a suggestion reminiscent of that put forward to explain delayed type hypersensitivity (see Chapter 39). Similar views were expressed by Mackaness and Blanden in a recent review.[31] However, the lack of specificity of cellular immunity and the fact that persons suffering from hypogammaglobulinæmia who cannot form 19S antibodies "can develop the same degree of acquired immunity to tuberculosis and other intracellular infections as do normal individuals"[33] militates against this view.

Physiological Changes in the Immune Monocyte in Cellular Immunity

Whatever the mechanism involved, there is no doubt that a population of macrophages from the peritoneal cavity of animals with acquired cellular immunity against the diseases we have been considering differs from a population of normal cells not only in the increased ability to phagocytose and destroy ingested organisms but also in a greatly increased metabolic activity.[31, 33, 35] This is particularly noticeable in their enzymic content. Unlike the polymorph which, although it contains a large store of preformed enzymes in its granules, is unable to synthesise more once these have been liberated into phagocytic vacuoles, the macrophage has the capacity to synthesise enzymes continually. Macrophages from immune animals contain increased numbers of lysozomes and a greater content of lysozomal enzymes such as acid phosphatases. Moreover, they show a progressive increase in mitotic activity during the course of infection with living *L. monocytogenes* or the attenuated strain of *Br. abortus*[44] and are stimulated to a burst of mitotic activity by a second contact, e.g. following challenge with virulent organisms or even after contact with specific bacterial antigens. Normal mature macrophages seldom show mitoses and are not stimulated to divide by contact with bacteria.

This hyperactivity of peritoneal macrophages is not confined to infection with facultative intracellular parasites, but can be brought about by contact with a number of non-specific agents. Small amounts of "endotoxin", that is lipopolysaccharide from the walls of Gram-negative bacteria, are particularly effective. Moreover, the immune cell is stimulated to increased phagocytosis not only of specific bacteria but of non-specific non-living particles. This general hyperactivity may explain the non-specific factor in cellular immunity. However, there is, as we have seen in the "recall" of the immune state, a specific element as well and it is this that is still obscure.

Relation between Cellular Immunity and Delayed Hypersensitivity

In Chapter 39 the effect of specific antigen on cells, and in particular on macrophages sensitised to delayed hypersensitivity, is described. If the dose of antigen required to elicit the sensitive reaction is relatively large it has a destructive effect on the cell, inhibiting its migration and eventually killing it. If, however, the dose is small the reverse may occur, namely increase in cellular metabolic activity and stimulation to divide. For instance, macrophages from mice sensitised to bovine serum albumin by immunisation in Freund's complete adjuvant (Chapter 34), and subsequently challenged with the specific protein, incorporate tritiated thymidine into their DNA and undergo active mitosis.[45] Such an observation brings into focus once more the question whether delayed hypersensitivity might not be one of the factors concerned in the specific reaction of the immune monocyte to contact with the antigens of the infecting bacilli. Mackaness has pointed out that the conditions required to produce the cellular immune state are precisely those which lead to delayed type hypersensitivity, namely immunisation with living organisms. However, it cannot be the whole story. Although delayed hypersensitivity always developed during immunisation with *L. monocytogenes*, it did not run parallel with immunity. As already noted, immunity requires a sustained antigenic stimulus and wanes on elimination of the infecting organism. Hypersensitivity, on the other hand, may continue for many weeks (see ref. 31). As we have seen, Rich also found a lack of correlation between delayed hypersensitivity and immunity to tuberculosis, but he noticed that hypersensitivity could wane before immunity. Tubercle bacilli, however, are not eliminated as completely and effectively as *L. monocytogenes* or *Br. abortus* and it is possible that persistence in the tissues was sufficient to maintain immunity but not hypersensitivity. Unlike immunity to infection with the latter organism, which requires large numbers of bacteria to remain in the body, immunity to tuberculosis seems to be maintained by quite small numbers.

Summary of Cellular Antibacterial Immunity

Acquired immunity to facultative intracellular parasites, that is to organisms such as tubercle bacilli, *Br. abortus* and *L. monocytogenes*, which are taken up by macrophages and survive intracellularly, depends on a change in metabolic activity of the monocytes whereby they are mobilised more rapidly, undergo division, have a greater phagocytic activity and, particularly, inhibit the growth and bring about the death of engulfed bacteria. Free antibody apparently plays no part in this process. Apart from immunity to tuberculosis in which either living attentuated bacilli (B.C.G.) or dead organisms are effective, immunity is only brought about by living organisms which are taken up by the reticulo-endothelial cells of the tissues and only persists as long as the organisms remain in the body. Cellular immunity is non-specific, the "immune" monocyte not only destroying the specific organism but also antigenically unrelated bacteria. Waning immunity can be rapidly recalled by contact with the specific organisms used to produce it, but not by other facultative intracellular parasites, although, when immunity is once restored, these are as actively destroyed as the specific organism. Although delayed type hypersensitivity can exist in the absence of immunity, it is possible that it may play a part in the stimulation of the macrophage by a second contact with specific antigen.

Acquired immunity to mouse typhoid due to *Salm. typhi murium* can be transferred passively, not only by free antibody, but also by "immune" macrophages. The efficacy of the macrophage appears to depend on cellbound antibody of 19S type to a thermolabile antigen of the organism. This antibody can be eluted from the macrophage and probably acts not only by opsonisation but by sensitising the organism for intracellular destruction. There is as yet no evidence that other forms of cellular immunity can be related to the presence of cytophilic antibody on the macrophage.

IMMUNITY TO VIRUS DISEASES

There has been a tendency in the past to regard immunity to virus diseases as necessarily involving a different mechanism from that of immunity to bacterial diseases. This idea has been based largely on (1) the lack of correlation found in certain virus diseases between immunity and the production of antibody, (2) the early failure to produce immunity by the use of killed vaccines, and (3) the lifelong immunity which follows a single attack of certain virus diseases.

However, if due allowance is made for the peculiar nature of virus infections —the intracellular habitat of the parasite and its consequent protection from the defences of the host, and the tendency of many viruses to remain alive for long periods of time in the body cells and to spread from cell to cell without coming in contact with antibody in the serum—the differences between antiviral and antibacterial immunity are not as great as they appear at first sight. As with antibacterial immunity, immunity may be associated with antibody or may be due to a cellular mechanism analogous to the cellular immunity of facultative intracellular bacteria described in an earlier section of this chapter, but differing from it (*a*) in not depending on the macrophage although macrophages may be involved, and (*b*) in depending on the formation by the host cell of a special group of proteins known as "interferons".

Antiviral Immunity Dependent on Antibody

There is no doubt that antibody plays a large part in protection in many virus infections. This is shown by the correlation found between the content of antibody in the serum, the ability of the serum to confer passive protection on other animals and the removal of protection by absorption with virus. The efficacy of antibody can also be shown *in vitro*. Virus suspensions mixed with specific serum are unable to infect cells in tissue cultures, or on the chorio-allantoic membrane of the developing chick.

The Stage in Infection affected by Antibody and the Mechanism of Inhibition

In Chapter 31 the method by which animal virions enter cells and initiate infection was described in those virus infections in which it has been investigated. We may briefly summarise the salient facts. The virion, consisting of nucleic acid core and protein shell or capsid, adsorbs to the surface of a susceptible cell, probably by electrostatic attachment[46] to specific receptors. More efficient bonding then takes place. Transport into the cell by a mechanism known as "viropexis" then follows. This process consists of a flowing of the cell membrane over the adsorbed virus particle and fusion of the outer areas of the cell membrane so that the virion comes to be within a vesicle in the cytoplasm. The walls of the vesicle then disintegrate, accompanied or followed by disruption of the virions (with minor differences depending on the nature of the virus), and release of the viral core into the cytoplasm. The protein coat is degraded possibly by proteolytic enzymes, which in the case of vaccinia, seem to be induced in the cell by a protein of the virion itself.[47] The naked nucleic acid, which is the essential infecting unit of the virus, diverts the cell from the synthesis of its own cell substance towards synthesis of more viral nucleic acid and protein and new virus is formed and released. In some cases these sequential steps in the infection process may be by-passed. Naked viral nucleic acid of poliovirus, for instance, may be extracted by various methods[48] without destroying its infectivity. It is then able to pass into cells, not only those capable of being parasitised by the whole virion, but also into others normally resistant.

Antibody can only act by uniting with the complete virion, because the antigens of the virus are associated with its protein shell or capsid. It cannot therefore, inhibit infection by the naked viral nucleic acid[49] nor can it affect stages of infection subsequent to loss of the protein coat. Its possible actions would be to (1) prevent adsorption of virus to the surface of the cell, (2) neutralise virus after adsorption, and (3) inhibit engulfment.

A comprehensive discussion on the neutralisation of influenza virus is given by Fazekas de St. Groth.[50]

(1) *The effect of antibody on adsorption of the virus to receptors of the cell surface.*

The early work of Burnet and his colleagues on the neutralisation of viruses producing "pocks" on the chorioallantois of the developing chick, their later work on the inhibition of hæmagglutination by antibody to influenza virus, and the more recent work of Dulbecco and his colleagues[51] on the neutralisation of Western equine encephalomyelitis (WEE) and poliovirus, which produce "plaques" on monolayers of tissue culture cells, have established beyond question that antibody unites with free virus and prevents its union with host cells. However, there are certain features about the interaction of viruses and antibody which still require explanation. For instance, there is a conflict of opinion about whether the complex of antibody and virus is freely reversible. Burnet and Fazekas de St. Groth and their colleagues concluded from their observations on a number of viruses producing pocks on the chorioallantois, and others causing hæmagglutination, that, at any rate initially, the complex was freely reversible by such mild procedures as simple dilution, although a firmer union may follow later (for ref. see 50). On the other hand, Dulbecco and his colleagues,[51] using their plaque technique on mono layers of cells infected with WEE and poliovirus, were equally convinced that the union was sufficiently firm to be unaffected by dilution, and was only dissociated by the addition of a large excess of virus inactivated by ultraviolet light. Both groups of workers have found a certain residuum of virus that resists neutralisation even in the presence of excess antibody. Burnet[52] has pointed out that any system of viral antibody titration involves three intrinsically variable participants: antibody, virus particle and indicator host cells, and considerable variation may result in any neutralisation tests, not only with different systems, but also on different occasions within one system. Although antibody of both 19S and 7S types is capable of neutralising poliovirus[53] considerable heterogeneity in affinity and avidity exists in any population of antibody molecules. Virus particles and host cells are no less variable with respect to affinity of virus cell receptors for antibody and their number and sites on the cell.

The recent work of Lafferty[54, 55] on the reaction between influenza virus and its antibody titrated on tissue culture cells, not only illustrates this heterogeneity but also clarifies the issue concerning the reversibility of the virus-antibody complex. In common with earlier workers, (e.g. ref. 56) he noted that virus and antibody react in two stages: initial union freely dissociable by dilution, with complete restoration of infectivity, followed after a prolonged interval of time (150 minutes) by a much firmer union in which only 0·1 per cent of the virus particles were recoverable on dilution. The fall in infectivity could not be related to aggregation. The secondary stabilising reaction, however, was not irreversible, because treatment with ultrasonic vibration followed by dilution to prevent recombination brought about dissociation. Analysis of the kinetics of the stabilising reaction showed that it took place in three stages. An initial lag, which became more pronounced as the serum concentration was reduced, was followed by a rapid exponential inactivation at a rate proportional to the serum concentration. Finally, the neutralisation curve flattened out leaving a residual fraction of virus particles not inactivated as described by previous workers. As the residual noninactivated virus was present even when antibody was in great excess, it was concluded that a small proportion of virus particles united with antibody but failed to form a stable combination with it. Lafferty attributed this to a union with a non-avid type of antibody. That the size of the unneutralised residuum depended on the antibody and not on the virus, was shown by the extreme variability obtained when different antisera were used to neutralise the same virus suspension. Further investigation on the nature of the stabilising secondary reaction between virus and antibody showed that monovalent fragments of antibody globulin, fractions I and II (Fab), obtained by Porter's method of papain digestion (Chapter 32) united with virus as effectively as untreated divalent antibody, but the union was completely reversible on dilution and

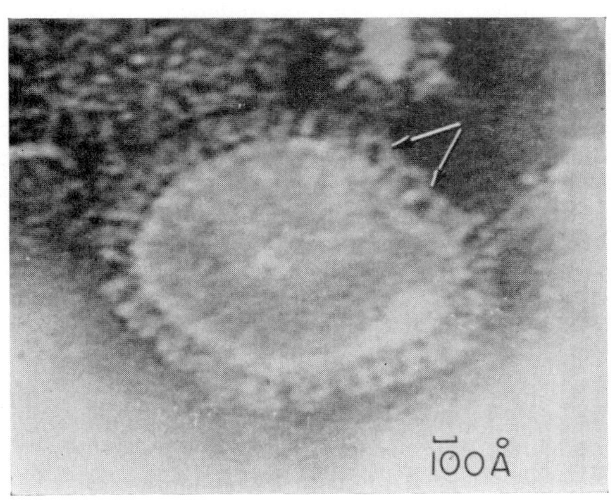

37/FIG. 3.—The two-site attachment of antibody by both valencies to influenza virus observed when the virus reacts with low concentrations of antibody. (From Lafferty and Oertelis.[55])

failed to stabilise with time. It would seem, therefore, that both valencies were required for stabilisation. Lafferty suggested that the two stages, initial easily reversible union and less easily reversible stabilisation, were determined according to whether one or both valencies of the antibody molecule united with the surface of a viral particle. The reversible combination was thought to be brought about by attachment of an antibody molecule by one of the two valencies; stabilisation by a further attachment of the other valency. This hypothesis was tested by direct observation in the electron microscope. In a stabilised mixture of viral particles and low concentrations of antibody, single molecules of antibody were shown as "loops" attached at both ends to the same virus particle (FIG. 3). With higher concentrations, bridges of antibody could be observed between adjacent viral particles. When the concentration of antibody was very high, the antibody molecules were so tightly packed on the surface of the virus that there was room for attachment by one valency only. It is suggested that this may account for an increase in the non-neutralised (dissociated) fraction observed when vaccinia virus reacts with very high concentrations of antibody. However, this was not observed by Dulbecco and his colleagues[51] with WEE and poliovirus, who noted that the proportion of WEE virus remaining unneutralised fell with increasing concentrations of antibody while that of poliovirus remained unchanged. It is possible that the less firm union at high concentration was offset by the increased neutralising ability of the high concentration.

According to Lafferty, the main factor determining the presence of an unneutralised fraction of virus was union with a non-neutralising (non-avid) type of antibody. Analysis showed that a higher proportion of unneutralised virus was present when an electrophoretically fast moving gamma globulin antibody fraction was used for neutralisation than when a slower moving fraction was used. The antibody fractions were not characterised further. There was no evidence that the fast moving fraction was univalent.

The amount of antibody globulin required to prevent adsorption of a single viral particle might be expected to depend on the size of the virus relative to the size of the antibody molecule assuming that the sites at which attachment takes place to the cell receptors are distributed over the surface of the virus. Fazekas de St. Groth[50] has pointed out that antibody attached to the virus probably acts by steric hindrance over a much wider area than the mere point of attachment of virus to the cell receptors. He has calculated that an antibody molecule would "shade" about 20 per cent of the surface of an influenza virus attached with the long axis radially. If both valencies are united with a single virus particle as Lafferty has described, a larger proportion of the surface of the virus might be expected to be "shaded".

(2) *The effect of antibody on virus after adsorption to the host cell.*

Although antibody will prevent virus from being adsorbed to a susceptible cell, a distinction must be made between its action in preventing adsorption and its action in preventing infection. The amount of antibody preventing infection, although related to that preventing adsorption, need not necessarily be identical with it. Rubin and Franklin[57] found that one antibody equivalent per viral particle (Newcastle disease virus, NDV) was all that was required to prevent infection of chick embryo cells, but several antibody equivalents were required to prevent adsorption. Similarly, Dulbecco and his colleagues found that WEE and poliovirus were neutralised by one antibody molecule per virus particle, whereas Mandel[58] found that an amount of antibody sufficient to neutralise poliovirus would not prevent its adsorption to HeLa cells provided sufficient time was allowed for adsorption to take place.

Once adsorption has taken place, virus is still capable of being neutralised by antibody provided it is added at an early stage or at a low temperature. This has been well established for influenza virus,[59] poliovirus[60, 61, 62], Newcastle disease virus (NDV)[63] and vaccinia.[64] If the temperature is raised, a much more stable union of virus with the cell membrane takes place. Poliovirus can then no longer be neutralised by antibody although some degree of neutralisation of influenza, NDV and vaccinia virus is still possible. The irreversible stage probably represents commencing penetration, but may take place with isolated membranes of susceptible cells in which no evidence of "penetration", i.e. degradation of capsid protein and release of RNA, is found.[62]

(3) *The effect of antibody after engulfment of virus by susceptible cells.*

There is no doubt that virus once it has been engulfed and is present in the cytoplasmic vesicle cannot be neutralised by antibody, although it still possesses its protein capsid. Even virus particles, which have already united with antibody and which, in spite of this, have become adsorbed to the cell, can be engulfed. Dales[65] using electron microscopy noted that some vaccinia virus particles after being exposed to antibody could be taken up by susceptible cells in a way similar to untreated virus. The virus particle was observed within the cytoplasmic vesicle surrounded by a fuzzy coating attributed to antibody. No further penetration and stages in viral development, however, occurred and all trace of virus had disappeared in 6–8 hours with concomitant degradation of viral DNA. Silverstein and Marcus[63] also noted that, although most NDV virus particles adsorbed to a susceptible cell were eluted when treated with antibody, a few that escaped elution were engulfed. These failed, however, to develop further and presented an abnormal appearance within the vesicle in the electron microscope. On the other hand, influenza virus coated with labelled antibody failed to become engulfed by susceptible cells.[66]

Viruses in Macrophages

Although most viruses when "neutralised" by antibody, either before or at the time of adsorption to susceptible cells, do not reach the stage of engulfment, examples were cited in the last section of viruses which, in spite of union with antibody, were engulfed. The "opsonised" virus then failed to develop further. This is analogous to the effect of opsonisation in bringing about destruction of some bacteria inside phagocytes (p. 1037). It is pertinent to enquire whether this rather exceptional effect of antibody in preventing viral development, which operates in susceptible cells not normally regarded as phagocytic, plays a more important role when the virus particle is taken up by phagocytic cells. There is no doubt that many viruses which cause infections in which viræmia is a prominent feature may be demonstrated in blood leucocytes by fluorescent antibody. Although polymorphs are known to engulf viruses in the blood (e.g. experimental ectromelia virus in mice), they appear to play little part in their destruction, the virus often being able to be recovered in a fully infective state. The polymorph may even protect viruses from the neutralising action of antibody.

The macrophage and particularly the fixed reticulo-endothelial cells of the liver and spleen, however, are in a different category. These cells may not only engulf viruses non-specifically as they do any other particulate foreign matter in the blood, but may also act as the specific host cell for virus infection. They may thus have a dual role, as a phagocyte and as a host cell.

There is no doubt about the first role, namely the ability to take up viruses and bring about their destruction. Mims[67] noted that the avirulent C.L. strain of vaccinia is readily taken up by the Küpffer cells in mouse liver a few minutes after intravenous injection. Within 1 hour, no antigen could be detected by fluorescent antibody and it failed to reappear. Similar results were obtained with subtoxic doses of influenza, myxoma, NDV and vesicular stomatitis viruses in the mouse and ectromelia in the rat, all of which are avirulent for the particular host when injected intravenously.

The second role, the reverse of the first, namely the ability of macrophages to act as host cells and contribute to the establishment of the virus in the body, has been studied mainly with pox viruses. Mims[67] noted that ectromelia virus was rapidly taken up by the Küpffer cells of mouse liver. Five minutes after intravenous injection 90 per cent of the virus was in the liver. Fluorescent antibody studies showed that after a fall in the amount of antigen in the cell attributed to "eclipse", virus reappeared in the Küpffer cells and also spread to the hepatic cells eventually leading to death. He claimed that infection of the hepatic cells was preceded by infection of the Küpffer cells. Some interesting observations were made when the same experiment was carried out in mice specifically immunised against ectromelia. Instead of the usual action of antibody in preventing adsorption of the virus, and consequently its uptake by the host cell observed in other cells, the Küpffer cells engulfed the virus as if no antibody were present. The eclipse phase followed as in cells from a non-immune animal. However, virus failed to reappear, there was no subsequent infection of hepatic cells, and the animals survived. That specific antibody was concerned in this change in the infection pattern was demonstrated when virus was mixed with immune rabbit serum and injected intravenously into normal mice. The antibody-virus complexes were taken up by the Küpffer cells as could be shown by fluorescent antibody to rabbit gamma globulin. The complexes then gradually disappeared until they were no longer observable by fluorescent antibody and virus failed to reappear. These results clearly show that even when the macrophage is a susceptible host cell for a specific virus, it can switch over to its more usual function of a phagocytic cell with intracellular destruction of the virus when the virus is opsonised by antibody.

It has been generally believed that phagocytosis "is of no real significance for the outcome of virus infections"[68] and may actually assist in spreading viruses particularly if they can multiply in the phagocyte. Although this may be true of many virus infections, the experiments of Mims quoted above suggest that this view has to be modified in selected cases. These experiments were carried out in the intact animal under conditions difficult to control. Clearly further work is required particularly with macrophage suspensions cultured *in vitro*.

Inaccessibility of Antibody as a Factor Modifying Acquired Immunity to Virus Infection

The correlation between acquired immunity to virus infection and the presence of circulating antibodies to the virus depends on the ready accessibility of virus to antibody before it becomes attached to its host cell. This is most evident when the virus is introduced directly into the blood stream, for instance by a blood-sucking arthropod. In other cases correlation may break down. There may be little immunity with a high serum content of neutralising antibody, or alternatively, immunity may be of a high order with little detectable antibody. Herpes simplex infection in man is the classic example of a persistent infection in which appreciable serum antibody titres are present. Most adults are infected with this virus, which, for the most part, remains latent in the cells of the mucous membrane of the lips. From time to time, however, overt infection takes place and the infected individual acquires an appreciable titre of herpes antibody. Yet this does not eliminate the virus or prevent further attacks. The most probable explanation is that infection is maintained by passage of virus from cell to cell, but with sufficient virus becoming extracellular to maintain the titre of antibody. Most of the virus, however, is out of reach of antibody. Influenza is another virus infection in which virus is, at any rate partially, out of reach of antibody. It has been found that ferrets, in spite of having high titres of antibody in their serum, may still be infected by the intranasal route. In this instance, the relative inaccessibility of the virus to antibody is not due to the continued cellular habitat of the virus, but to the fact that virus in the respiratory mucus is not exposed to antibody in the serum. When antibody is instilled intranasally it gives good protection against infection. Nevertheless the respiratory mucus contains 5–10 per cent of the titre of circulating antibody which may explain why systemic vaccines for influenza are efficacious. In viral infections in which local multiplication is followed by generalised viræmia and parasitisation of other cells, the development of humoral immunity may effectively prevent generalised spread without having any effect on the local infection. Infection of the cells of the alimentary tract with poliovirus is an example. Virus may continue to be excreted in the fæces for long periods of time in spite of a high content of circulating antibody, yet antibody in the blood effectively prevents it from extending to nerve cells.

The apparent converse, namely an effective immunity in the apparent absence of antibody is also found. This is probably a reflection of the relatively small amounts of antibody which are effective in preventing viral attachment to sensitive cells. In some viral diseases it is possible to transfer immunity passively with antiserum with a content of antibody below the level at which it can be detected *in vitro*. In other cases the tissues containing the susceptible cells may have an appreciable concentration of antibody without a detectable concentration in the blood.

CELLULAR IMMUNITY IN VIRUS INFECTIONS. THE PRODUCTION OF INTERFERONS

In many cases of so-called cellular immunity in virus diseases, antibody-dependent protective immunity has not been adequately excluded. However, evidence is accumulating that a true cellular immunity not involving antibody may play a part in acquired immunity to virus diseases. This immunity depends on the production by the susceptible cell of a class of substances called *interferons* quite distinct from antibody. The subject is discussed fully in Chapter 31 and will not be considered further here.

NATURALLY ACQUIRED PASSIVE IMMUNISATION: PASSAGE OF ANTIBODIES FROM MOTHER TO YOUNG

Antibodies may be transferred from the mother to the offspring in two ways: (1) *in utero*, (2) via the colostrum or the milk after birth. The route depends to a large extent on the nature of the animal (for refs., see 69 and 70). The transmission *in utero* was originally thought to be always via the placenta, since an inverse relationship was noted between the number of layers of tissue in the placenta separating the fœtal and maternal circulation in different animals and the passage of antibodies. Thus the ungulates, which have four or more layers, obtain no antibody *in utero*, whereas rabbits, apes, and man, which have but one, obtain most of their antibody in this situation. Largely through the work of Brambell and his colleagues, however, this relationship is now known to be invalid. In work extending over 20 years (summarised in ref. 71), they made a thorough investigation into the transmission of immunoglobulins in the rabbit, which receives all its antibody *in utero*, and showed that the passage of antibody to the fœtus occurs, not via the placenta, but via the uterine cavity, through the yolk sac and into the vitelline veins. They devised a technique for investigating the passage of different proteins by injecting them into the uterine lumen and noting their appearance and concentration in the fœtal blood. Gamma globulins from different species were differentiated, either by isotopic markers, or as antibodies of different specificity. They noted a highly selective transmission to the fœtus: homologous (maternal) gamma globulin passed readily, human, guinea-pig and dog less readily and, finally, horse and bovine gamma globulin only to a small extent. Only traces of other serum proteins were transmitted. Of the various molecular species of gamma globulin, IgG (7S) and IgM (19S) passed through equally readily, a somewhat surprising result in view of the retention of IgM by the human placenta and gut of the mouse and rat (see below). Hartley[72] also described a differential passage of antibody from different species in the guinea-pig, in which the mechanism of transfer is similar to that of the rabbit, horse diphtheria antitoxin being much less readily transmitted than antitoxin from the guinea-pig itself.

The different rates of transmission of gamma globulin from different species appear to depend on the nature of the Fc fragment of the molecule (see Chapter 32). Hartley[72] had previously shown that pepsin-refined horse or guinea-pig antitoxin, in which the Fc fragment is destroyed, failed to pass from the maternal to the fœtal circulation in man and the guinea-pig respectively. This was confirmed by Brambell with pepsin-refined rabbit antitoxin in rabbits, using his technique of intra-uterine injections. In support of this he found that the Fab fragments were also not transmitted. In contrast, the isolated Fc fragment of IgG obtained by Porter's method of papain digestion, when injected into the uterine lumen passed to the fœtus almost as readily as the whole IgG molecule.

Rats and mice receive some of their antibody *in utero* by the same route as in the rabbit and guinea-pig, namely from the uterine lumen into the yolk sac and vitelline veins, but towards the end of pregnancy, fœtal rats may also imbibe antibody globulin from the amniotic fluid.[73] However, the greater part of the antibody received from the mother is transmitted after birth via the milk. Maternal antibodies are secreted in the milk throughout lactation and the wall of the small intestine of mice and rats is permeable to antibody globulin up to 16–20 days of age. As in the ungulates (see below), it probably reaches the circulation via the lymphatics. A rather abrupt cessation of permeability takes place at about 20 days in the rat. Bangham and Terry[74] noted that 14-day-old rats fed gamma globulin labelled with I^{131} absorbed 90 per cent of the protein in 3 hours, whereas 21-day-old rats absorbed only 0·5 per cent. The change in permeability has also been demonstrated in a dramatic way by Bessis.[75] He fed to 20-day-old rats a drop of rabbit serum containing antibodies to rat red blood corpuscles. Death from acute hæmolytic anæmia occurred within 24 hours. Massive doses of the antibody administered to 25-day-old rats, however, had no effect.

The passage of serum proteins through the gut wall of the rat and mouse shows a selectivity similar to the passage of proteins through the yolk sac of rabbits and guinea-pigs. Macroglobulin 19S antibody, however, which is transmitted through the yolk sac of rabbits, is not transmitted through the gut wall of the rat. Heterologous gamma globulin is transmitted less readily than homologous globulin, and only small amounts of serum albumin[74] pass into the circulation. As with the yolk sac of the rabbit, the Fc, but not the Fab, fragments of gamma globulin are transmitted through the gut wall of the mouse and rat.

The mode of transmission has received considerable investigation. It would seem that both the yolk sac endoderm of the rabbit, and the intestinal tract endoderm of the rat, absorb very much more protein than eventually appears in the circulation of the offspring. In the rat, there seems to be a saturation point beyond which no increase in the amount fed has any effect on the amount appearing in the circulation. Moreover, although differences are found in the rate and amount of gamma globulin from different species appearing in the blood, this selectivity does not operate at the stage of absorption by the endoderm. Hemmings[76] noted that 83–93 per cent of gamma globulin, irrespective of its source whether from the rabbit or ox, was absorbed within 24 hours by the yolk sac endoderm of rabbits, but only 12 per cent of rabbit and 5 per cent of bovine gamma globulin eventually reached the circulation. The cells must, therefore, catabolise much of the protein they absorb. Evidence for such degradation was obtained by Bamford[77] using I^{131} labelled gamma globulin placed in isolated intestinal sacs *in vitro*. Free labelled iodide appeared in the mucosal fluid.

There is evidence that the gamma globulin that eventually finds its way into the circulation in young rodents has undergone changes during its passage through the cells. Morris[78] fed rabbit anti-brucella serum to young rats. This serum contained complete antibodies of both IgM and IgG types. IgM was not transmitted and the IgG had changed from a complete to an "incomplete" type, a non-agglutinating type only demonstrable by Coombs antiglobulin reaction, that is, by adding anti-rabbit globulin to brucellæ sensitised by the incomplete rabbit antibody. If we can argue from this system to transmission through the placenta of man, these results may have significance in explaining the selective transmission of incomplete Rh antibodies in hæmolytic disease of the newborn (Chapter 40).

Transmission of gamma globulin through the intestinal wall of rats and mice appears to be competitive. Morris (for ref. see 71) noted that in the mouse, transmission of gamma globulin from one species was inhibited by feeding with gamma globulin from another species, the amount required for inhibition being inversely proportional to the amount transmitted. He showed that the inhibitory effect was due to the Fc fragment.

Hartley[79] first drew attention to the similarity between the selective transmission of antibody, and its selective absorption to cells in passive anaphylaxis, which is discussed in Chapter 39, and suggested that both processes depended on attachment of the protein to specific receptors in or on the cell. The similarities have been summarised by Brambell[80]: both involve only gamma globulin molecules; both are selective; both depend on the Fc fragment of the antibody molecule and both can be reversed or inhibited by gamma globulins, or their Fc fragments, of other species, the same approximate quantitive relation being found in the amount required to inhibit and the amount required to sensitise or be transmitted. In one instance, however, the analogy apparently breaks down. Reagin antibodies on which anaphylactic sensitisation of man depends (Chapter 39) are not transmitted. However, the difference here might be in the high affinity of reagin antibodies for cells and for macroglobulins in the serum from which they are not easily released. Their retention would thus prevent transmission. Brambell has suggested that the mechanism of transmission depends initially on a non-selective pinocytosis of serum proteins which, in fact, can be demonstrated in the pinocytic vacuoles of rat endodermal cells. A great part of the protein is then digested by the enzymes of the lysozomes of the cell. He postulates that specific receptors adapted to the Fc part of the H chain of the homologous gamma globulin molecule and sited in the walls of the pinocytic vacuoles (and hence originally on the membrane of the microvilli) combine with homologous gamma globulin and so protect it from degradation (Fig. 4). Heterologous gamma globulins will unite with these receptors in so far as their Fc fragments resemble that of the homologous type. As the pinocytic vesicle

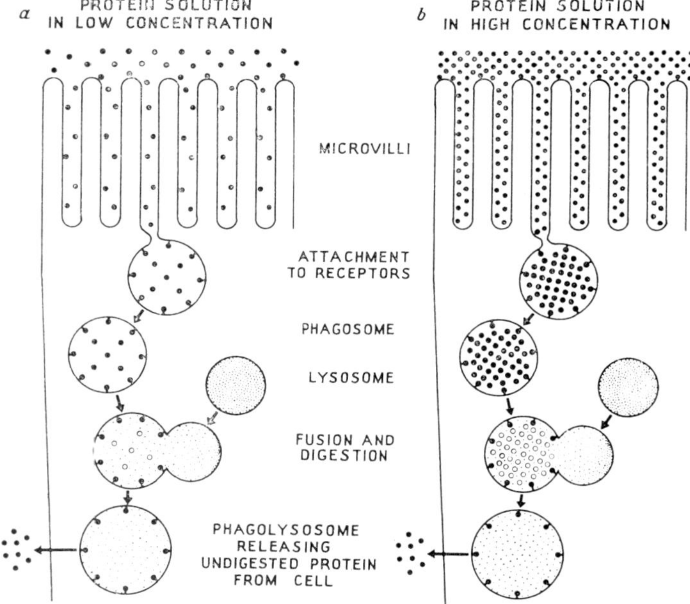

37/Figs. 4.—Possible mechanism by which gamma globulin is transmitted through the intestinal mucosa of the rat or mouse. A constant amount of gamma globulin molecules irrespective of the concentrations adsorb to receptors on the microvilli, and hence on the phagosomal surface, and are thereby protected from lysozomal enzymes. These are subsequently released into the circulation.

(*a*) Low concentrations; (*b*) high concentrations of gamma globulin. The amount released is constant provided the receptors are saturated. (From Brambell.[71])

reaches the deeper layers of the cell, the globulin is released into the intercellular fluid from which it reaches the blood stream via the lymphatics. Two factors would thus affect transmission: (1) the amount and rate of gamma globulin catabolised, dependent on its concentration and (2) the affinity of the gamma globulin for receptors on the endodermal cells, not dependent on concentration provided the receptors are saturated. With respect to the first, Brambell has shown that the half-lives of 7S IgG from different species were directly correlated with their ability to pass through the rabbit yolk sac endoderm.

A similar mechanism may operate in ungulates which receive all their antibody globulin after birth through the colostrum from which it passes through the endoderm of the small intestine into the lymphatics. Permeability of the intestinal endoderm, however, only persists for 36 hours, no more antibody being transmitted although the milk continues to contain it.

The cause of the sudden cessation in transmission at 16–20 days in the rat and mouse and at 36 hours in the ungulates is still not understood. However, in the mouse and rat, it appears to be related to a sudden rise in alkaline-phosphatase activity of the duodenal cells. Premature induction of this increase in phosphatase with corticosteroids led to a premature cessation in transmission (for ref. see 71).

In man it is generally assumed that transfer takes place via the placenta, and indeed Brambell himself points out that the method of transfer found in the rabbit is here precluded on morphological grounds. However, he is inclined to the view that transfer may not be through the placenta, but by a more roundabout route involving the amniotic fluid and fœtal gut.[81] Whatever the route, some selective mechanism operates, as in the rabbit, since some antibodies are transferred and others are retained.[79] Moreover, the cord blood of the fœtus often contains a higher titre of antibodies than the maternal blood, although both contain the same concentration of other plasma proteins.[82]

There is little doubt that the passage of antibody from the mother results in the immunity of the newborn animal to a number of diseases in the first few weeks of life. The importance of antibodies in the colostrum in protecting calves from colibacillosis has been emphasised by Ingram.[83] A method commonly used for the protection of lambs against lamb dysentery due to *Cl. welchii* type B is to immunise the sheep actively during pregnancy, so that antitoxins may be imbibed in the colostrum by the lamb. Passage through the placenta of diphtheria antitoxin protects the human infant in the first few weeks of life and renders it Schick negative. As with other forms of passive immunisation, the protection is only transient.

Summary

Acquired immunity may depend on antibodies or may be determined by cells (macrophages) in the absence of antibodies. *Antitoxic immunity* is solely determined by antitoxin in the serum which neutralises the toxin and prevents a damaging effect on cells. It may or may not also have an antibacterial action, i.e. preventing spread of the organism in the tissues (e.g. infection with *Cl. welchii* and *B. anthracis*). *Antibacterial immunity* may be (*a*) *humoral*, depending on antibodies to the surface antigens of the bacteria which sensitise them to the action of complement, or to phagocytosis and destruction within phagocytes.

The agglutinating reaction of serum antibodies may delay infection, but has no destructive actions on the bacteria; (*b*) *cellular*, depending on a change in the macrophage enabling it to destroy facultative intracellular parasitic bacteria such as *Myco. tuberculosis*, *Listeria*, *Brucella* and perhaps *Salmonella* more rapidly and completely. Cellular antibacterial immunity depends on an increased metabolic activity of the phagocyte and has not so far been related to cell-bound antibody except in immunity to *Salm. typhi murium* in mice which seems to depend on a cell-bound 19S antibody to a thermolabile antigen of the organism. Cellular immunity is not entirely specific, unrelated bacteria being as readily destroyed by the immune macrophage as the specific organism used for the production of immunity. However, the recall of immunity after waning is specific. With a few exceptions, notably immunity to tuberculosis, cellular immunity is an "infection immunity". That is it is produced by infection with living organisms, virulent or attenuated, and wanes on elimination of the organisms. It is still uncertain what mechanism is involved in cellular immunity, and whether it is related to delayed type hypersensitivity in which metabolic changes in the macrophage are also found.

Immunity to virus diseases may also involve humoral and cellular factors. *Antiviral antibody* unites with the virion and prevents its attachment to susceptible cells. It may also prevent its penetration after attachment. A residuum of virus not neutralised by excess antibody may be due to union with a non-avid type of antibody. Phagocytes probably play a secondary role in viral immunity. Phagocytosis may not destroy the virus and may even lead to its dissemination particularly if the phagocyte is a host cell for virus multiplication. However, in a few cases, notably pox virus infection in mice, coating of virions with antibody may bring about intracellular destruction in Küpffer cells. *Cellular immunity* in virus infections is mediated by substances produced by the infected cell known as "interferons". These are considered in Chapter 31.

Antibodies pass from mother to her young (1) *in utero*, either via the yolk sac and vitelline veins (rabbit, guinea-pig) or via the placenta (man) or (2) after birth in the colostrum (ungulates) or in the milk (rats, mice). The yolk sac endoderm of the rabbit and the endodermal cells of the intestine of ungulates and of young rats and mice show a differential permeability to gamma globulin from different sources and of different physical states. The differential permeability in the rat endodermal cells is probably due to union of the selected globulin, perhaps on a site on the Fc part of the molecule, to receptors in the pinocytic vacuoles of the cell which protect it from catabolism. Subsequently it is released unchanged, whereas the non-selected proteins are destroyed. Loss of permeability occurs in 16–20 days in the mouse and rat and in 36 hours in the ox.

REFERENCES

1. Rich, A. R., and McKee, C. M. (1934). *Bull. Johns Hopk. Hosp.*, **54,** 277.
2. Henderson, D. W. (1937). *Brit. J. exp. Path.*, **18,** 224.
3. Miles, A. A. (1951–52). In *Lectures on the Scientific Basis of Medicine*, Vol. **1**, Chap. 10. (British Postgraduate Medical Federation.) London: Univ. of London, The Athlone Press.
4. Miles, A. A., and Miles, E. M. (1943). *Brit. J. exp. Path.*, **24,** 95.
5. Glencross, E. J. G. (1956). Personal communication.

6. McLeod, J. A., and McLeod, J. W. (1961). *Brit. J. exp. Path.*, **42,** 179.
7. Amies, C. R. (1954). *J. Path. Bact.*, **67,** 25.
8. MacLennan, J. D. (1951). *Recent Advances in Bacteriology*, Chap. 13, 3rd edit. Ed. Dible, J. H. London: J. & A. Churchill.
9. Orr-Ewing, J. (1946). *J. Path. Bact.*, **58,** 167.
10. Scheibel, I. (1950). *Brit. J. exp. Path.*, **31,** 442.
11. van Heyningen, W. E. (1950). *Bacterial Toxins*, Chap. 2. Oxford: Blackwell Scientific Publications.
12. Smith, H. (1964). *Symp. Soc. gen. Microbiol.*, **14,** 1.
13. Thorne, C. B. (1960). *Ann. N.Y. Acad. Sci.*, **38,** 1024.
14. Evans, D. G., and Adams, M. O. (1952). *J. gen. Microbiol.*, **7,** 169.
15. *Bulletin of the World Health Organization* (1964). **30,** 447.
16. Fisher, S. (1960). *Aust. J. exp. Biol. med. Sci.*, **38,** 339.
17. Morse, S. I. (1962). *J. exp. Med.*, **115,** 295.
18. Li, I. W., and Mudd, S. (1965). *J. Immunol.*, **94,** 852.
19. Verwey, W. F. (1940). *J. exp. Med.*, **71,** 635.
20. Stamp, Lord, and Edwards, H. H. (1964). *Brit. J. exp. Path.*, **45,** 264.
21. Boake, W. C. (1956). *J. Immunol.*, **76,** 89.
22. Součková Štěpánová , J., Gladstone, G. P., and Vaněček, R. (1965). *Brit. J. exp. Path.*, **46,** 384.
23. Mudd, S., Gladstone, G. P., and Lenhart, N. A. (1965). *Brit. J. exp. Path.*, **46,** 455.
24. O'Antona, D. (1958). C. R. Quatrième Congrès internat. Stand. Biol. Brussels., p. 3.
25. Elek, S. D. (1959). *Staphylococcus Pyogenes*, Chap. 11, London: E. & S. Livingstone.
26. Munoz, J. J. (1963). *Bact. Rev.*, **27,** 375.
27. Rich, A. R. (1951). *Pathogenesis of Tuberculosis.* Oxford: Blackwell Scientific Publications.
28. Lurie, M. B. (1939). *J. exp. Med.*, **69,** 555.
29. Dubos, R. J. (1954). *Biochemical Determinants of Microbial Diseases.* Cambridge, Mass.: Harvard Univ. Press.
30. Weiss, D. W., and Dubos, R. J. (1956). *J. exp. Med.*, **103,** 73.
31. Mackaness, G. B., and Blanden, R. V. (1967). *Progr. Allergy*, **11,** 89.
32. Lurie, M. B. (1933). *J. exp. Med.*, **57,** 181.
33. Lurie, M. B. (1964). *Resistance to Tuberculosis.* Cambridge, Mass.: Harvard Univ. Press.
34. Mackaness, G. B. (1954). *Amer. Rev. Tuberc.*, **69,** 495.
35. Suter, E., and Ramseier, H. (1964). *Advanc. Immunol.*, **4,** 17.
36. Mackaness, G. B. (1964). *Symp. Soc. gen. Microbiol.*, **14,** 213.
37. Holland, J. J., and Pickett, M. J. (1958). *J. exp. Med.*, **108,** 343.
38. Gelzer, J., and Suter, E. (1959). *J. exp. Med.*, **110,** 715.
39. Jenkin, C. R., and Rowley, D. (1959). *Nature* (*Lond.*), **184,** 474.
40. Greenwood, M., Topley, W. W. C., and Wilson, J. (1931). *J. Hyg.* (*Lond.*), **31,** 257.
41. Jenkin, C. R., Rowley, D., and Auzins, I. (1964). *Aust. J. exp. Biol. med. Sci.*, **42,** 215.
42. Jenkin, C. R., and Rowley, D. (1965). *Aust. J. exp. Biol. med. Sci.*, **43,** 65.
43. Rowley, D., Turner, K. J., and Jenkin, C. R. (1964). *Aust. J. exp. Biol. med. Sci.*, **42,** 237.
44. Khoo, K. K., and Mackaness, G. B. (1964). *Aust. J. exp. Biol. med. Sci.*, **42,** 707.
45. Forbes, I. J., and Mackaness, G. B. (1963). *Lancet*, **2,** 1203.
46. Philipson, L. (1963). *Progr. med. Virol.*, **5,** 43.

47. Joklik, W. K. (1965). *Progr. med. Virol.*, **7,** 44.
48. Schaffer, F. L. (1962). *Cold Spr. Harb. Symp. quant. Biol.*, **27,** 89.
49. Alexander, N. E., Koch, G., Mountain, I. T. M., Sprunt, K., and van Damme, O. (1958). *Virology*, **5,** 172.
50. Fazekas de St. Groth, S., (1962). *Advanc. Virus Res.*, **9,** 1.
51. Dulbecco, R., Vogt, M., and Strickland, A. G. R. (1956). *Virology*, **2,** 162.
52. Burnet, F. M. (1960). *Principals of Animal Virology*, Chap. 11, 2nd edit. New York: Academic Press.
53. Svehag, S. E., and Mandel, B. (1964). *J. exp. Med.*, **119,** 1. 21.
54. Lafferty, K. J. (1963). *Virology*, **21,** 61, 76.
55. Lafferty, K. J., and Oertelis, S. (1963). *Virology*, **21,** 91.
56. Burnet, F. M. (1936). *Aust. J. exp. Biol. med. Sci.*, **14,** 247.
57. Rubin, H., and Franklin, R. M. (1957). *Virology*, **3,** 84.
58. Mandel, B. (1962). *Cold Spr. Harb. Symp. quant. Biol.*, **27,** 123.
59. Fazekas de St. Groth, S. (1948). *Nature* (*Lond.*), **162,** 294.
60. Mandel, B. (1961). *Virology*, **14,** 316.
61. Fenwick, M. L., and Cooper, P. D. (1962). *Virology*, **18,** 212.
62. Holland, J. J., and Hayer, B. H. (1962). *Cold Spr. Harb. Symp. quant. Biol.*, **27,** 101.
63. Silverstein, S. C., and Marcus, P. I. (1964). *Virology*, **23,** 370.
64. Joklik, W. K. (1964). *Virology*, **22,** 620.
65. Dales, S. (1965). *Progr. med. Virol.*, **7,** 1.
66. Mims, C. A. (1961). Aust. Soc. Microbiol. Meeting. Brisbane, p. **4** (quoted in Ref. 50).
67. Mims, C. A. (1964). *Bact. Rev.*, **28,** 30.
68. Burnet, F. M. (1960). *Principles of Animal Virology*, Chap. 10, 2nd edit. New York: Academic Press.
69. Brambell, F. W. R., Hemmings, W. A., and Henderson, M. (1951). *Antibodies and Embryos*. London: Univ. of London, The Athlone Press.
70. Evans, D. G., and Smith, J. W. G. (1963). *Brit. med. Bull.*, **19,** 225.
71. Brambell, F. W. R. (1966). *Lancet*, **2,** 1087.
72. Hartley, P. (1949). *Mth. Bull. Minist. Hlth. Lab. Serv.*, **7,** 45.
73. Anderson, J. W. (1959). *Amer. J. Anat.*, **104,** 403.
74. Bangham, D. R., and Terry, R. J. (1957). *Biochem. J.*, **66,** 579, 584.
75. Bessis, M. (1947). *Rev. Hémat.*, **2,** 114.
76. Hemmings, W. A. (1957). *Proc. roy. Soc. B*, **148,** 76.
77. Bamford, D. R. (1966). *Proc. roy. Soc. B*, **166,** 30.
78. Morris, I. G. (1965). *Proc. roy. Soc. B*, **163,** 402.
79. Hartley, P. (1951). *Proc. roy. Soc. B*, **138,** 499.
80. Brambell, F. W. R. (1963). *Nature* (*Lond.*), **199,** 1164.
81. Brambell, F. W. R., Brierley, J., Halliday, R., and Hemmings, W. A. (1954). *Lancet*, **1,** 964.
82. Barr, M., Glenny, A. T., and Randall, K. J. (1949). *Lancet*, **2,** 324.
83. Ingram, P. L. (1964). *Symp. Soc. gen. Microbiol.*, **14,** 122.

Chapter 38

REACTIONS TO EXOGENOUS ALLERGENS: ANAPHYLAXIS

BY G. P. GLADSTONE

IN the last two chapters we have been considering reactions of the body to the presence of foreign antigens which are essentially of benefit to it. We have seen that antibodies when produced in adequate quantity, can react with soluble antigens bringing about their rapid elimination; they can also neutralise toxins, clump, opsonise and bring about phagocytosis of foreign cells including bacteria and, in certain cases, cause death or lysis of cells, mediated by complement. Unfortunately, the production of antibodies does not invariably lead to these beneficial results. It may have the reverse effect when the body cells experience an antigen for the second time, resulting in severe symptoms and even death, although the antigen may have been quite innocuous on the first occasion. This phenomenon, whereby an *immunological* response is the cause of reactions damaging to the body cells, is called *hypersensitivitiy* or *allergy*.*

Hypersensitivity can occur in a large number of conditions, some produced artificially, others occurring naturally and a number associated with infective disease. The relationship between the hypersensitive state and the production of antibodies is, in certain cases, quite evident. In other cases antibodies have not so far been detected and the immunological basis for the conditions can only be inferred indirectly. It is possible that in all infective disease of long enough duration to allow an immunological response, symptoms due to hypersensitivity to bacterial or viral products are present, superimposed on those due to the direct toxic and other effects of the organisms themselves.

We will start by considering hypersensitivity produced artificially where its relationship to the production of antibodies can be clearly demonstrated, a condition known as *anaphylaxis*. The term is compounded from the Greek and implies that the guarding (φίλαξις) is reversed (ἀύα). It was first used by Richet[1] (FIG. 1) in 1902 for a phenomenon best described in a translation from his own words.

> " During a cruise on Prince Albert of Monaco's yacht, the Prince . . . suggested to P. Portier and myself a study of the toxin production of *Physalia* [the jelly-fish known as 'Portuguese Man-of-War'] found in the South Seas. On board the Prince's yacht, experiments were carried out proving that an aqueous glycerine extract of the filaments of *Physalia* is extremely toxic to ducks and rabbits. On returning to France, I could not obtain any *Physalia* and decided to study comparatively the tentacles of *Actinaria* [sea anemone]. . . . While endeavouring to determine the toxic

* The term "allergy" was introduced by von Pirquet to denote any altered capacity of the body to react to a foreign substance, and as such could include immune reactions. It is usually limited to hypersensitive reactions as defined above. Some, however, restrict its use to certain forms of hypersensitivity, particularly that associated with infective disease. It is probable that all forms of hypersensitivity have a common basis, so no distinction will be made between the two terms, and they will be used synonymously.

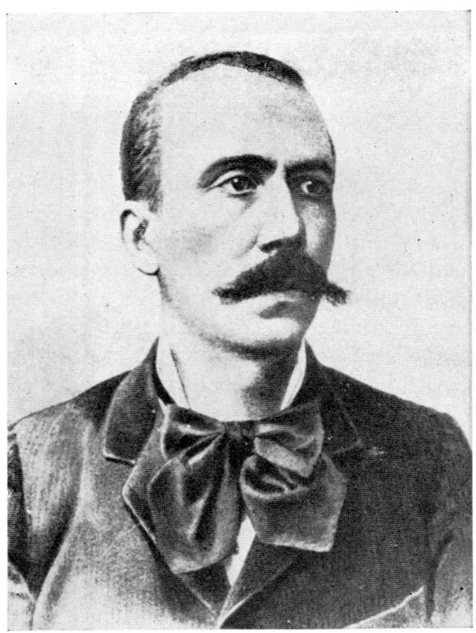

38/FIG. 1.—Charles Robert Richet (1850–1935).

dose [of extracts], we soon discovered that some days must elapse before fixing it; for several dogs did not die until the fourth or fifth day after administration or even later. We kept those that had been given insufficient to kill, in order to carry out a second investigation upon these when they had recovered. At this point an unforeseen event occurred. The dogs which had recovered were intensely sensitive and died a few minutes after the administration of small doses. The most typical experiment, that in which the result was indisputable, was carried out on a particularly healthy dog. It was given at first 0·1 ml. of the glycerin extract without becoming ill; twenty-two days later, as it was in perfect health, I gave a second injection of the same amount. In a few seconds it was extremely ill; breathing became distressful and panting; it could scarcely drag itself along, lay on its side, was seized with diarrhœa, vomited blood and died in twenty-five minutes."

Richet was using a toxic protein and the effect might well have appeared to be due to an increased sensitivity to the toxin. That this was not so was shown by Theobald Smith who, in the same year that Richet made his observations, discovered independently a similar phenomenon in guinea-pigs used for assaying diphtheria antitoxin. Animals injected with neutral mixtures of toxin and antitoxic serum, to which they were indifferent, became acutely ill and often died immediately after the same neutral mixture was injected some days later. He did not publish his results but communicated them verbally to Ehrlich two years later, and Otto[2] in Ehrlich's laboratory investigated what he named the "Theobald Smith phenomenon" further. He showed that it was independent of both toxin and antitoxin in the mixtures, the phenomenon being readily produced with normal horse serum.

Subsequent work has clearly defined the conditions that determine whether an animal will develop the state of anaphylaxis or, as it is sometimes called, anaphylactic shock.

Active Sensitisation

To bring about a state of anaphylaxis, the animal must have previously experienced the antigenic protein. After the first administration of the antigen, certain changes take place in the body which is then said to be sensitised to that particular antigen. It is essential for sensitisation that the antigen reach the body cells in an unaltered state, and sensitisation is most readily brought about, therefore, by parenteral injection, although inhalation and even ingestion may be effective. Much of the ingested protein may be destroyed in the alimentary canal, but the mucous membrane is apparently permeable to some extent to unchanged protein, and since incredibly small amounts of antigen will sensitise the guinea-pig (for example 1 μg. of egg albumin or 0·000001 ml. of horse serum), it is only necessary for small quantities such as these to escape digestion and pass through the mucous membrane of the alimentary tract.

The size of dose required for sensitisation depends on the species of animal. The very small doses mentioned above are effective in guinea-pigs, which are the most easily sensitised animals known, but are quite ineffective in rabbits and dogs. On the other hand, if the dose is too large, sensitisation may be greatly delayed or may not occur. In some animals, for instance the rabbit, two or more doses at frequent intervals may be necessary.

It is usually stated that a complete antigen must be used for sensitisation and that it must be foreign to the cells normally in contact with the blood stream. Gelatin, for example, which is not an antigen, will not sensitise, but when it is made antigenic by the introduction of aromatic diazonium groups or glucosides containing tyrosine, it is effective. Guinea-pigs can be sensitised with their own lens protein, since it does not normally come into contact with the blood stream. The statement that only complete antigens can sensitise requires modification, however, in the light of Landsteiner's work[3] on sensitisation by simple chemical compounds. This work is considered in Chapter 40. Briefly, he showed that many simple chemical compounds will sensitise guinea-pigs when injected intracutaneously or applied in some other way to the skin. There is evidence that this sensitisation is brought about because the chemicals become linked to proteins of the body forming complete antigens which depend for their specificity on the original chemical, and for their antigenicity on the body protein.

The Development of Anaphylactic Shock

Anaphylactic shock takes place when a second injection of the antigen is given after a certain period of time. This latent period varies with different species and with the degree of sensitisation. A period of at least 8–10 days is always required and with some species 3–4 weeks, but once this period has elapsed highly sensitised animals may remain capable of being shocked for an indefinite period. Shock is only produced if the antigen is given in a relatively high concentration. Doses larger than those needed for sensitisation must be given, and generally—in some species always—the requisite concentration can only be reached by giving the antigen directly into the circulation.

An important point about anaphylaxis is its *immunological specificity.* The material used to produce shock must be identical or have a close immunological relationship with that used for sensitising. Unlike the sensitising agent, however, it need not be a complete antigen or have any particular ability to form an antigen by conjugation with protein *in vivo.* Haptens that carry the groups determining the specificity of the sensitising antigen, and are of sufficient molecular size, will induce shock in animals sensitised with the complete antigen and may be as effective as the antigen itself. Parts of the hapten molecule containing the specific radicle, but too small to induce shock, may nevertheless specifically *inhibit induction of shock* by the whole antigen, just as they can inhibit the precipitation reaction. Tillett, Avery and Goebel[4] found that guinea-pigs sensitised to *p*-aminophenol glucosido- or galactosido-protein complexes were not shocked when the isolated sugar was injected, but that the sugar specifically inhibited shock to the whole antigen. The refractory state, however, did not last more than a few hours after injection of the sugar.

It might be expected that as simple chemicals can sensitise after uniting with proteins in the body they could produce shock in the same way; but this is apparently not the case, at any rate in experimental anaphylaxis in animals, although unconjugated drugs may induce shock in man (Chapter 40). Anaphylactic shock can be produced by the injection of protein conjugates of these substances, but even a highly reactive substance such as picryl chloride cannot produce shock in experimental animals when injected alone. Arsphenamine, which has been much used in the treatment of syphilis, is an exception. Both sensitisation and shock can be induced by this substance without any previous linkage to protein, in both cases presumably because it conjugates with body protein.

Shock in Different Species

We have seen that animal species differ in the ease with which they can be shocked and in the dose needed for sensitisation. They differ also in the symptoms, signs and pathological lesions of shock. Indeed one of the difficulties in obtaining a unified concept of anaphylaxis has been the protean character of shock as seen in different animal species. Whereas the blood pressure in the rabbit and guinea-pig rises, at any rate initially, in the dog it falls progressively. The guinea-pig dies from asphyxia with signs of acute respiratory distress, whereas the rabbit dies of acute right heart failure. The dog dies of circulatory failure following segregation of much of its blood in the liver, the systemic blood pressure sometimes falling to a few cm. of mercury.

We believe now that the main manifestations of anaphylactic shock can be accounted for by two tissue changes—contraction of smooth muscle and damage to capillary endothelium—and that the differences between species, wide though they appear to be, are due to relatively minor factors. These factors, and also some concomitants of shock that seem to need a different explanation, will be discussed after the pathological picture in different species has been described.

Guinea-pig

Here the main symptoms are attributable to contraction of bronchial muscle, which is particularly well developed in the guinea-pig throughout the lung. Within a few minutes of the intravenous injection of a shocking dose of antigen, the animal shows signs of severe respiratory distress. It is because of the ease with which they can be sensitised and their dramatic response when shocked that guinea-pigs have been used more than any other animal in the study of anaphylaxis.

When bronchial muscle contracts it is expiration that is particularly difficult; this is seen in asthma in human beings. A guinea-pig in anaphylactic shock has an acute attack of asthma with intensely laboured respiration. It becomes deeply cyanotic and usually dies in about ten minutes.

The picture seen post-mortem corresponds with the physiological effects (FIG. 2). The lungs are over-inflated and do not collapse when the thorax is opened or even when they are cut into pieces. Microscopically, the bronchioles

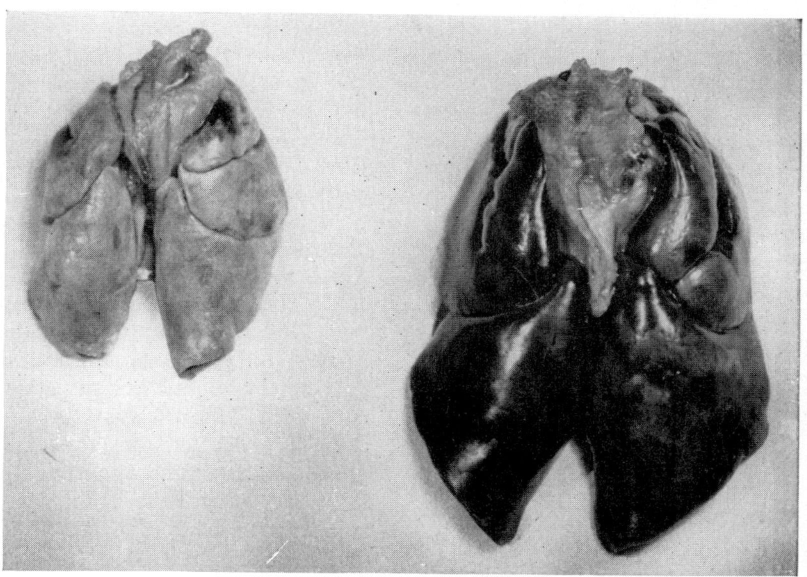

38/FIG. 2.—Lung of guinea-pig killed by anaphylactic shock (*right*) compared with lung of normal guinea-pig.

are almost closed by folds of mucosa thrown up by the muscle contraction (FIG. 3) and there is œdema of the interstitial tissue round the bronchial tree. In the body generally there is congestion of the mucous and serous membranes, sometimes with hæmorrhages. Miles (see ref. 5) has shown that there is also an increase in permeability of all the skin capillaries, and Burrage and his co-workers,[6] using a technique which enabled them to observe living tissue microscopically, noted changes also in the liver very similar to, but much less marked than, those in the dog described in the next section.

Dog

The predominant signs of shock in the dog are quite different. Death seldom takes place in less than 1–2 hours even in the most severe shock and quite often the animal recovers completely. The most prominent symptom is prostration and weakness, due to a profound fall in the systemic blood pressure, which may sink to 40 or 50 mm. mercury and

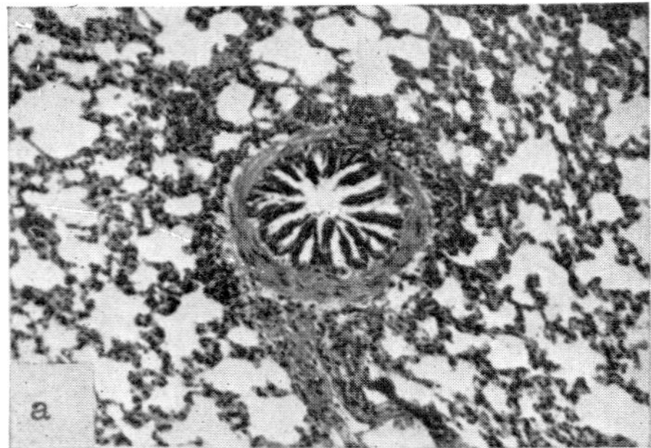

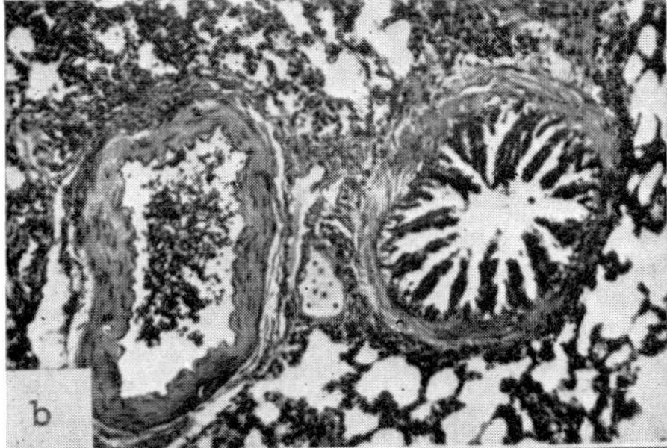

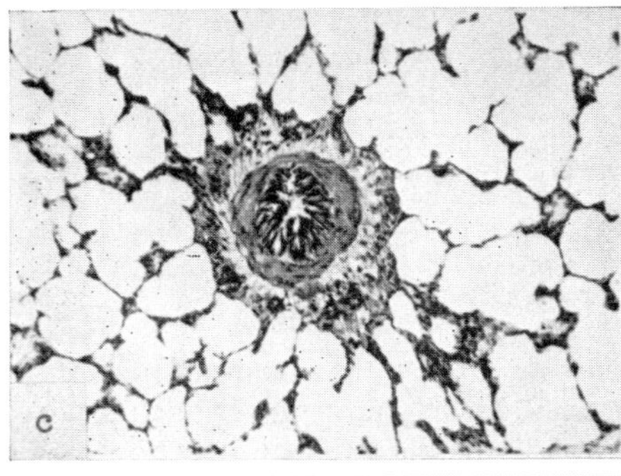

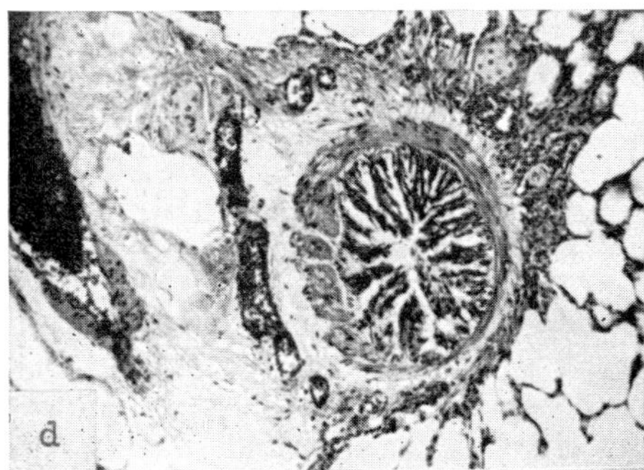

remain at that level till the animal dies or recovers (FIG. 4).

This startling fall in systemic blood pressure is due to segregation of a large part of the circulating blood in the liver. If the abdomen is opened during the period of prostration, the liver is seen to be very much swollen, deep purple and of woody hardness. Weil[7] calculated that about 60 per cent of the total blood volume could be accommodated in the liver, apart from that which accumulated in the congested intestines.

There has been a good deal of discussion about the exact means by which a large part of the blood that enters the portal system is prevented from leaving it in this condition. Most agree that contraction of some part of the hepatic venous system is concerned. Thus the symptoms in the dog, so different from those in the guinea-pig, are fundamentally due to the same cause, the contraction of smooth muscle.

Simonds[9] states that among 22 species of animals that he examined, the dog had the most highly developed musculature in the walls of the hepatic veins, but he gives no further details of this observation. Bauer and his co-workers[10] noted that the musculature of the hepatic veins at their exit into the inferior vena

38/FIG. 3.—CONSTRICTION OF BRONCHIOLES IN ANAPHYLACTIC SHOCK IN THE GUINEA-PIG

(*a*) and (*b*) sections of normal lung.

(*c*) and (*d*) sections of lung of shocked animals.

Note almost complete obliteration of lumina of bronchioles, and distension of the alveoli. (From Dixon and Warren.[8])

cava was so well developed in the dog that it formed sphincter-like structures, and they believed that closure of these accounted for the effects of shock. However, Simonds and Brandes[11] showed that mechanical obstruction at these sites did not lower the systemic blood pressure to the same extent as did anaphylaxis. It seems more likely, as the experiments of Maegraith and his colleagues[12] suggest, that there is spasmodic contraction of the muscle of the whole hepatic venous tree which can come on and pass off quite quickly. The rapidity

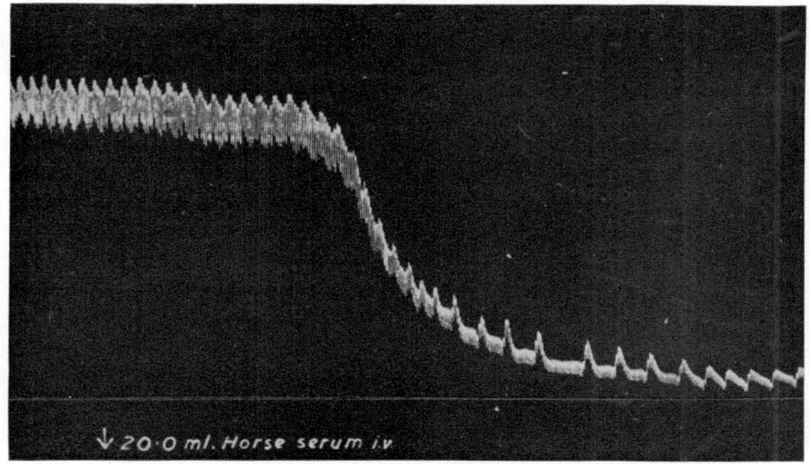

38/FIG. 4.—Blood pressure tracing of dog during anaphylactic shock.

with which changes in the liver occur in shock has been well demonstrated by the histological studies of Dean and Webb[13] who found that within 10–12 seconds of the start of anaphylactic shock the liver sinusoids were dilated and congested, and that in one minute there were already extensive hæmorrhages round the central veins of the lobules, with signs of damage to the neighbouring liver cells. Engorgement increased up to fifteen minutes and then began to subside. They failed, however, to find direct evidence for contraction of the hepatic veins and, in spite of the rapidity with which the lesions developed, favour an alternative view that congestion of the liver is due to direct damage to the walls of the sinusoids followed by hæmorrhage and pressure on the intra- and sublobular veins. Although this may be a contributory factor, the rapidity of local congestion and the subsequent restoration to normal suggests a spasmodic reaction as the more likely determining factor.

Not only is the liver the main organ to show changes in the shocked dog, but it is apparently responsible for most if not all of the pathology of shock. Manwaring[14] demonstrated that shock could be prevented if the liver was excluded by ligature. Moreover, if the liver from a sensitised dog was united with a normal dog by parabiosis, the latter underwent shock when injected with the appropriate antigen. Symptoms were also produced in a normal dog when blood taken from the liver immediately after shock was injected, but not when systemic blood was used. He concluded that the liver was not only the organ which suffered the most damage in shock, but it was also responsible for producing a toxic substance which caused the shocked condition. The importance of the liver in the causation of anaphylactic shock in the dog has been confirmed more than once. Waters and Markowitz,[15] however, claim to have produced shock in hepatectomised dogs, although less readily than in normal animals. Their dogs were very highly sensitised and it would appear that in such animals, as Manwaring himself showed, the liver is not absolutely indispensable.

The appearances of other organs are those which might be expected, congestion and hæmorrhages in the intestine being prominent. Manwaring, Beattie and McBride,[16] however, thought that there was more œdema and necrosis of the intestine than could be accounted for by portal obstruction, and suggested that spasm of the intestinal muscle occurred. In the lungs, polymorphonuclear leucocytes accumulate in the capillaries as they do in the guinea-pig.[17]

Rabbit

The rabbit also presents distinctive features. Usually more than one sensitising dose of antigen is required and even then sensitisation may fail. Grove[18] found about 25 per cent of rabbits resistant to sensitisation. Death is caused by acute right heart failure, the right heart being enormously dilated, and this is due to an intense contraction of the branches of the pulmonary artery. However, it is not only the pulmonary artery that contracts. Vallery-Radot[19] has shown by arterioradiograph a general arterial constriction throughout the body and a characteristic feature of anaphylaxis in the rabbit is the sudden blanching of the ears due to constriction of the peripheral arterioles. These vascular reactions have been observed directly by Abell and Schenck[20] using chambers in the rabbit's ear. Within two-and-a-half minutes after an intravenous injection of a shocking dose of horse serum all the arterioles had undergone intense contraction, obliterating their lumina. This lasted for about five minutes, after which there was a gradual return to normal.

Man

The production of anaphylactic shock in man is described in Chapter 39, where it is considered in relation to other forms of hypersensitivity.

Changes in the Blood in Anaphylaxis

In all animals the blood becomes less coagulable in anaphylactic shock, and may remain fluid *in vitro* for two or more days. Jaques and Waters[21] have demonstrated that in the dog this is the result of the liberation of heparin from the liver. In other species, heparin is apparently not released, although certain metachromatic material, probably a sulphated mucopolysaccharide with no action on clotting time, is found in the blood.[22]

Leucopenia in the peripheral blood is another constant feature and is due to the accumulation of leucocytes in the capillaries of the lungs.

A fall in the number of circulating platelets is also found, and this may contribute to the diminished coagulability of the blood. The platelets appear to be segregated with the leucocytes in the lungs. In the dog they are also found in the liver. As we shall see, in the rabbit they may play an important part in the causation of anaphylactic shock.

It has long been known that complement is removed or considerably depleted from the blood in anaphylactic shock. Evidence is accumulating that this may have significance in the causation of anaphylactic shock in some species (see p. 1100).

Passive Sensitisation

The antigenicity of the sensitising agent, the identity or immunologically specific relationship between this and the shocking agent and the time required for sensitisation all point to the involvement of antibody in the anaphylactic reaction. This is made quite conclusive by the finding that sensitisation can be transferred passively. Consideration of passive transfer will involve us in a consideration of the relationship between anaphylaxis and immunity.

The transference of sensitivity with the serum from one animal to another has been noted from the earliest days. Doerr and Russ[23] showed that the degree of sensitivity produced by the transferred serum was related to its content of antibody, as shown by precipitation reactions with the specific antigen. Serum from an animal that had been highly immunised with successive closely spaced doses of antigen, and shown to contain a high concentration of antibody, was more effective than serum from an animal that had received few injections of antigen and in which the antibody content was low.

Nature of Antibody Transferring Anaphylactic Sensitisation

Although most workers agree with Doerr and Russ in finding a close correlation between passive anaphylactic sensitisation and the content of precipitating antibody in the serum, anomalies have been found which can now be largely clarified in the light of recent work on the physico-chemical nature of gamma globulin. Before discussing this work, it will be convenient to consider a system which has been used extensively in the study of passive anaphylaxis and in which a close correlation between immune precipitation *in vitro* and passive anaphylactic sensitisation *in vivo* has been obtained, namely the passive transfer of rabbit antibody to guinea-pigs. There is little doubt that in this *heterologous* system, that is the transfer of serum from an animal of one species to that of another, antibody bringing about sensitisation is the same as that demonstrable by precipitation reactions with antigen. The relationship has been extensively studied by Kabat and his colleagues[24, 25, 26] They noted that although passive sensitisation was correlated with precipitation, the former was a much more sensitive test for antibody than the latter, the rabbit antiserum being capable of being diluted to a level below the limit of visible precipitation while still being able to sensitise. Further work showed that, in addition to antibody demonstrable by direct precipitation with antigen, the so-called "incomplete" rabbit antibody, that is antibody which fails to precipitate with antigen alone but co-precipitates with an antigen-antibody complex[27] is also capable of sensitising guinea-pigs.

In the heterologous system considered above, the antibody globulin involved whether "complete" or "incomplete" is the classical 7S type IgG.[28] The same type of antibody is probably concerned in the passive sensitisation of guinea-pigs by human antiserum. However, not all heterologous antisera will transfer sensitisation. Horse, sheep, pig, goat and chicken antiserum fail to sensitise[29] although, as we shall see, their gamma globulins are quite as readily fixed to guinea-pig tissues as are rabbit and human gamma globulins.

It is in the *homologous* system, that is sensitisation by antisera from an individual of the same species, that anomalies arise. It has been known for a very long time that human homologous sensitisation, whether actively acquired or passively transferred from one individual to another, depends on a special type of antibody globulin known as "reagin" (considered in detail in Chapter 39). Recent work has shown that analogous types of antibody exist in other animals e.g. the guinea-pig, rabbit, mouse, rat and dog and are responsible for homologous sensitisation in these species.[30] The subject is closely connected with the ability of antibody to become fixed to cells, and the mechanism of sensitisation as studied in isolated tissues will be considered further in a subsequent section (p. 1088).

Latent Period for Fixation of Antibody

Before shock can be induced in a passively sensitised animal, a latent period is necessary. Using the heterologous system described above, viz. passive sensitisation of guinea-pigs with rabbit antibody, Benacerraf and Kabat[31] have shown a quantitative relationship between the dose of antibody transferred and the duration of the latent period; with 2·0 mg. of antibody nitrogen, immediate shock could be obtained; with 1·02 mg. the latent period was 30 minutes; and with 0·24 and 0·12 mg. it was 1 and 2 hours respectively. The latent period required with the smaller doses is probably related to the time required for fixation of the antibody to the tissues. With the larger doses, in which no latent period was apparently required, a different mechanism may operate involving an antigen-antibody reaction in the circulation (see p. 1094).

The concentration of antibody in the circulation after passive transfer also determines the dose of antigen required to produce shock. Using rabbit antibody passively transferred to guinea-pigs, Kabat and Landow[25] showed that the amount of antigen required for the shocking dose was about fifty times that giving optimal precipitation with the amount of antibody in the blood stream. In other words, it is essential that an amount of antigen is present in the circulation at the time of shock many times over and above that which is "neutralised" by circulating antibody. (For a review of the quantitative relations of antigen and antibody in anaphylaxis, see ref. 24).

Site of Antigen-Antibody Reaction

We have seen that anaphylactic shock can be produced in two ways. Firstly, it will occur if antigen is injected and several days are allowed to elapse while antibodies are being formed, after which a shocking dose of antigen is given. Secondly, it will occur if ready-made antibody is injected (passive sensitisation) followed by antigen a few hours later. Thus, for the production of shock two components, antigen and antibody, must be present in the body, and it must be presumed to depend on some reaction that takes place between the two. Much controversy in the past has centred round the question whether the antigen-antibody reaction causing shock takes place in the circulation or on the cells. The "humoral" theory postulated that a toxic substance, "anaphylotoxin", was liberated into the circulation as the result of an antigen-antibody reaction taking place in the blood. This theory was largely based on the production of shock following the injection of antibody-antigen mixtures, or serum in which antigen-antibody reactions had been allowed to take place. It was found, however, that this was not a specific effect, for the injection of normal serum treated with certain agents, for instance barium sulphate, talc, inulin, kaolin, or agar, produced much the same symptoms. A number of other so-called "anaphylactoid" agents such as peptone can also produce very similar symptoms. There are certainly features shared by both anaphylactic and anaphylactoid shock and there is little doubt that common factors operate in both conditions, possibly by activating a serum protease producing vaso-active peptides (p. 1103).

The alternative ("cellular") theory is that shock is brought about by the union of antigen to antibody which is fixed to cells. Toxic substances are then released from the cells as the result of the reactions, and these are the immediate cause of the manifestation of shock. As we shall see, these two theories are not mutually exclusive, and modern ideas suggest the implication of both cellular and humoral factors in anaphylaxis, their relative importance being determined by the particular manifestation of the anaphylactic reaction and the nature of the animal concerned. We will consider first those cases where anaphylaxis is mainly due to a union of antigen with antibody fixed to tissues.

Reactions due to Union of Antigen with Antibody fixed to Tissue Cells

There is no doubt that antibody can become fixed to cells, and the union of antigen with this fixed antibody can bring about some of the reactions of anaphylaxis. Two reactions involving fixation of antibody to tissues have been used extensively for the study of the mechanism of anaphylaxis: (1) *passive cutaneous anaphylaxis*; (2) *Schultz-Dale* reaction.

Passive Cutaneous Anaphylaxis (PCA)

If a small amount of antigen is injected intracutaneously into a sensitised dog, rabbit, guinea-pig or rat, and at the same time a vital dye is injected intravenously, a local area of skin at the site of injection of the antigen rapidly becomes coloured due to an increase in capillary permeability brought about by a local anaphylactic reaction. By injecting a small amount of antibody intracutaneously into a normal animal, sensitisation can be confined to an area of skin. Sensitisation takes 2–6 hours to develop and can be demonstrated by injecting antigen into the same site and the vital dye intravenously, or the antigen can be injected intravenously with the dye. The reaction is very sensitive, 0·003 μg. of antibody being able to sensitise.[72] A similar reaction can be obtained in man (*cf.* Prausnitz-Küstner reaction, see Chapter 39), but here the increased capillary permeability is so marked that a weal appears, and there is no need to use a vital dye. Wealing is not found in guinea-pigs, rats or rabbits.

Schultz-Dale Reaction (S-D)

That manifestations of shock can be demonstrated in isolated tissues was clearly shown by the discovery of Schultz,[32] which was further developed by Dale,[33] that unstriped muscle taken from sensitised animals and washed free from circulating antibody would show contraction *in vitro* in the presence of antigen, just as smooth muscle does *in vivo* in general anaphylactic shock. The reaction has been shown, for instance, with small pieces of guinea-pig intestine (Schultz), guinea-pig uterus (Dale), and strips of bronchus and pulmonary artery from guinea-pigs and rabbits respectively (Grove[34]), but not apparently strips of bronchus from the rabbit.

The strip of smooth muscle, often guinea-pig uterus, attached to a kymograph lever and bathed in a fluid to which substances for test can be added has become a recognised tool for the immunologist. The trivial name for the apparatus is the "uterus bath" and the general phenomenon described above is known as the Schultz-Dale (S-D) reaction (FIG. 5). The S-D reaction can be obtained with the uterine horns not only of sensitised guinea-pigs, but also of highly immunised animals in which there is much circulating antibody. However, the tissue must be washed free from excess antibody, since the S-D reaction is inhibited by free antibody unless the amount of antigen added is greatly in excess of that required to neutralise it. This is in conformity with Kabat's observation that, at any rate in the guinea-pig, circulating antibody prevents general anaphylaxis unless an amount of antigen is used many times in excess of that of the circulating antibody.[25]

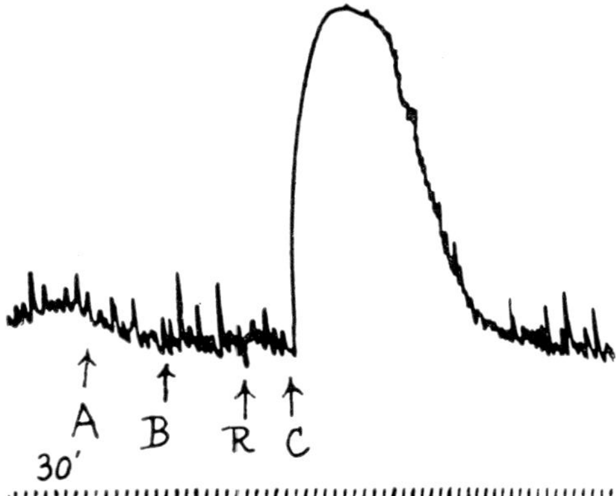

38/FIG. 5.—The Schultz-Dale reaction, with the uterus of a guinea-pig sensitised to horse serum. At A, 1/500 sheep serum added; at B, 1/500 cat serum; at R, the bath was washed out with Ringer's solution and at C, 1/2500 horse serum added. The uterus contracts only on the addition of the antigen to which it has been sensitised. (From Dale.[33])

The S-D reaction may also be carried out with the uterus from passively sensitised guinea-pigs. As in passive sensitisation in the living animal, a latent period must elapse between the time of the administration of the serum and the removal of the uterus, evidence that the latent period represents the time required for the fixation of antibody to the tissue cells.

Adsorption of Gamma Globulin to Cells. Its Relation to Sensitisation

An interesting development of the S-D reaction was the finding that the guinea-pig uterus from normal animals can be passively sensitised by perfusion with, or even simply by soaking in, Ringer's solution containing antibody[35]. As in general passive sensitisation a latent period of some hours was required, although apparently in certain circumstances this might be shortened to a few minutes.[35]

In recent years, the adsorption of antibody globulin to tissues and its relation to sensitisation has been extensively studied *in vitro* (for refs. see 36 and 37). Several workers have shown that rabbit gamma globulin labelled with I^{131}, whether antibody or normal gamma globulin, is readily adsorbed to strips of guinea-pig ileum, minced lung and mesentery. Once adsorbed the globulin cannot be removed by washing, but may be eluted by solutions of unlabelled gamma globulin but not by alpha, or beta globulins or serum albumin. The process of adsorption depends on time and concentration, and occurs at 0° C., suggesting that it is unlikely to be due to an active uptake by cells. There is a tendency for the union to become firmer with time, possibly due to a displacement of homologous gamma globulin already adsorbed before removal of the tissue from the body.[36]

The degree of sensitisation brought about by adsorption of antibody gamma globulin to guinea-pig tissues has been investigated by the S-D reaction (using a strip of ileum), and by passive cutaneous anaphylaxis (PCA) in the skin of the intact animal. Two other mechanisms, which will be considered later, have also been used: viz. liberation of histamine from chopped sensitised lung and degranulation of mast cells. Irrespective of the concentration of antibody used, maximum sensitisation occurred in lung tissue when less than 1 μg. antibody globulin/g. wet weight had been adsorbed[38], and in the ileum when 0·8 μg./g. wet weight was adsorbed.[39] Moreover, sensitisation, in contrast to adsorption, depended on the temperature at which adsorption had taken place and appeared to require considerable activation energy.[40]

A further distinction between adsorption and sensitisation is shown by the difference in sensitising capacity of antibodies from different species, all of which are adsorbed. Horse, rat and fowl antibodies are adsorbed to guinea-pig lung, but fail to sensitise, whereas those from man, rabbit, monkey, guinea-pig and dog are both adsorbed and do sensitise.[29] As we have seen, the same distinction is found in general passive anaphylaxis and also in PCA sensitisation. It is possible that different sites on the tissues are occupied by these two groups of gamma globulins. The difference is also reflected in their ability to inhibit or reverse sensitisation of guinea-pig tissues by antibody. Whereas 100, 500 and 5,000 times as much non-specific gamma globulin from guinea-pig, rabbit and man respectively were required to inhibit the PCA reaction in the guinea-pig using rabbit antibody, a concentration of 50,000 times as much horse gamma globulin failed to inhibit.[41] Similar results were found using reactions in isolated tissues.[36]

The high ratio between the amount of non-specific gamma globulin required to inhibit sensitisation and the amount of specific gamma globulin required to sensitise, even when these globulins are from the same animal, suggests that antibody gamma globulin has a much greater affinity for tissues than non-specific gamma globulin. Since much, if not all, gamma globulin probably consists of antibody molecules to several unrecognised antigens, it is improbable that the selectivity depends on the nature of the antibody (antigen-combining) groups on the molecule. Recent progress in the knowledge of the different types and physico-chemical structure of gamma globulin antibodies has confirmed this suggestion. Of the three fractions I, II, III obtained by Porter (see Chapter 32) on papain digestion of antibody gamma globulin, fractions I, II (Fab fragments) containing the antibody (antigen combining) groups are unable to sensitise guinea-pig skin to PCA[42] and other guinea-pig tissues.[29] Of the three groups of gamma globulin molecules differing in physico-chemical properties (Chapter 32), the heavy 19S (IgM) antibodies fail to sensitise possibly because their fraction III (Fc fragment) differs from that of the 7S antibodies that are able to sensitise. Recent investigations into the ability of the other two groups of gamma globulins, IgA and IgG (both 7S), to sensitise have revealed further heterogeneity in the gamma globulin molecules and a complex situation is found depending on the species of animal used and whether the antibody globulin is fixed to homologous or heterologous tissues (for refs. see 30, 43). In the guinea-pig we have already seen that general passive sensitisation by *heterologous* (rabbit) antibody is dependent on IgG. Similarly, sensitisation of isolated tissues by heterologous (rabbit) antibody is also dependent on IgG. However, *homologous* sensitisation of guinea-pig tissues by guinea-pig antibody is brought about, not by IgG, but by a form of antibody gamma globulin having more resemblance to IgA in electrophoretic mobility but differing from it in having a low carbohydrate content. Typical IgA has not so far been found in the guinea-pig and this atypical IgG antibody has been designated IgG_1, or "anaphylactic antibody".[30] It has been shown to be responsible, not only for general anaphylactic sensitisation, but also for PCA in guinea-pig skin[44] and sensitisation of guinea-pig lung as demonstrated by antigen-induced histamine release.[45] The slower migrating IgG (designated IgG_2), which contains the same specific antigen combining groups on its Fab fragments as those of IgG_1 but different Fc fragments, not only fails to sensitise, but will block sensitisation by IgG_1. Guinea-pig IgG_2 behaves like a classical antibody in fixing complement and sensitising antigen coated erythrocytes to lysis by complement whereas IgG_1 has neither of these properties. It would appear, therefore, that the earlier suggestion that sensitising antibodies are confined to those able to fix complement with antigen[46] is now no longer tenable.

The system in the mouse is very similar to that in the guinea-pig, but in the rat, dog and in man homologous sensitisation depends on types of gamma globulin having even greater differences from the classical IgG. The nature and properties of these sensitising antibodies in man (called reagins) are considered in Chapter 39.

Summarising.—There are at least two distinct groups of antibody gamma globulins concerned in passive sensitisation (to general anaphylaxis, PCA or of isolated tissues): (1) The classical IgG_2, demonstrable by complement fixation and precipitation, sensitises guinea-pig tissues when derived from certain heterologous species, e.g. the rabbit and man, but fails to sensitise when derived from the guinea-pig. On the contrary it may block sensitisation. (2) The second group represented by IgG_1 (guinea-pig and mouse) or special "reagin" like antibodies (rat, dog and man) has a faster electrophoretic mobility, does not fix complement and, in the case of man, shows other differences listed in Chapter 39. This gamma globulin is responsible for sensitisation of homologous tissues. Yet a third group from cow, horse, rat and chicken is adsorbed by guinea-pig tissues but fails to sensitise.

These anomalous results can be explained by the nature of the Fc fragment of the gamma globulin molecule. IgG_2 antibodies of those species that will sensitise guinea-pig tissue (rabbit, monkey, dog, man) have by chance the structure in their Fc fragment appropriate for sensitisation which, in the

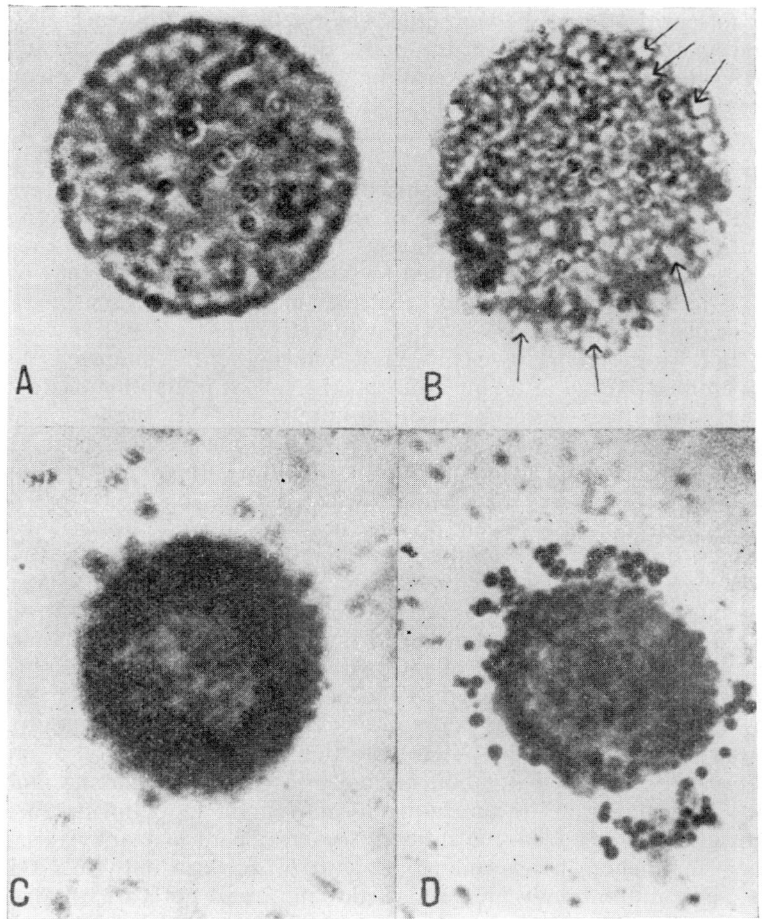

38/FIG. 6.—THE EFFECT OF ANAPHYLACTIC REACTION ON MAST CELLS

Sensitised mast cell from the peritoneal cavity of the rat.
A and C before contact with antigen;
B and D after contact with antigen.
Note vacuolation in C and granules outside the cell in D.
A and B phase contrast × 580;
C and D stained with toluidine blue × 460. (From Mota and Dias da Silva.[66])

guinea-pig itself, is normally the characteristic of IgG_1 antibodies. This structure is presumably lacking in the IgG antibodies of those species that fail to sensitise (horse, rat and fowl).

CELLULAR SITE OF ADSORPTION OF GAMMA GLOBULIN

The site at which antibody gamma globulin unites with and sensitises the tissues is not known. It appears to be on the cell surface rather than on structures within the cells.[46] Humphrey and Mota[29] suggest that the site of adsorption leading to sensitisation is the *mast* cells. These cells are found widely distributed in connective tissue throughout the body, being particularly numerous in the muscle layers of the guinea-pig uterus and ileum[46] and in the liver, pleura, lung and mesentery. Direct evidence that mouse mast cells adsorb heterologous globulin was obtained by White and his colleagues[47] using fluorescent antibody as a direct stain for globulin. They found that a fast moving guinea-pig globulin fraction (probably IgG_1 as it sensitised guinea-pig skin to a PCA reaction) specifically adsorbed to mast cells in frozen sections of mouse tongue, an observation suggesting that heterologous tissues may sometimes be sensitised by guinea-pig IgG_1, normally limited to sensitisation of homologous tissue.

It has been repeatedly demonstrated that mast cells from sensitised tissues lose most of their granules on contact with antigen *in vitro* and *in vivo* and no longer stain with toluidine blue (Fig. 6). It is likely that this damage is due to an antigen-antibody reaction taking place on the cell or in its immediate vicinity. However, an antigen-antibody reaction known to take place in and cause damage to vascular endothelium does not lead to mast cell damage although mast cells are found only a few microns distant from vascular endothelium. This was shown by Humphrey and Mota[29] who prepared antibody to Forssman antigen, a heterophilic antigen present in the vascular endothelial cells of guinea-pigs. Injection of this antibody into guinea-pigs caused extensive damage to vascular endothelium with gross œdema and rapid death but without signs of anaphylactic shock. When added to isolated tissues it failed to produce a positive S-D reaction, cause damage to mast cells or liberate histamine from guinea-pig lung (see ref. 29). It might be objected that failure to produce these reactions was due to the reversal of the normal procedure for demonstrating anaphylactic reactions, i.e. the addition of free antibody to fixed antigen. Humphrey and Mota, however, met these objections by showing that a positive S-D reaction can be obtained if rabbit antibody to guinea-pig gamma globulin is added to normal ileum. The guinea-pig normal gamma globulin adsorbed to the tissue reacts with the added free antibody (reversed passive anaphylaxis. Fig. 7).

The phenomenon of *reversed passive anaphylaxis* can only be produced if both antigen and antibody are gamma globulins, and both are obtained from species whose antibody globulin can sensitise. Thus reversed passive sensitisation to S-D reaction could not be obtained with horse gamma globulin followed by rabbit anti horse gamma globulin, although *direct* passive sensitisation (when

38/Fig. 7 (*see opposite*).—Diagram Showing the Effect of Different Antigen/Antibody Reactions on or Near the Mast Cell

(1) Direct anaphylactic reaction. Guinea-pig mast cell (MC) sensitised with homologous anaphylactic antibody (IgG_1) which is adsorbed by its Fc fragment to a specific site on the cell. The union of allergen (A) with the Fab parts of the adsorbed gamma globulin molecule brings about damage to the mast cell.

(2) The failure of IgG_2 to sensitise the mast cell probably because the site of adsorption is different from that of IgG_1.

(3) Forssman antibody (FA) unites with Forssman antigen (FG) on the vascular endothelial cell (EC) and complement (C). Although this causes disruption of endothelial cells by immune lysis, the mast cell in the immediate vicinity is unaffected.

(4) Reversed passive anaphylactic reaction. Anti-guinea-pig IgG_1 (Gab) unites with antigenic groups on the Fc part of IgG_1 adsorbed to the mast cell and complement, resulting in damage to mast cell.

MC
A
A
IgG1
1
MC
A
A
IgG2
No effect on mast cell
2
MC
EC
EC
FA
FG
FG
C
C
No effect on mast cell
3
IgG1
IgG1
C
Gab
MC
MC
C
4

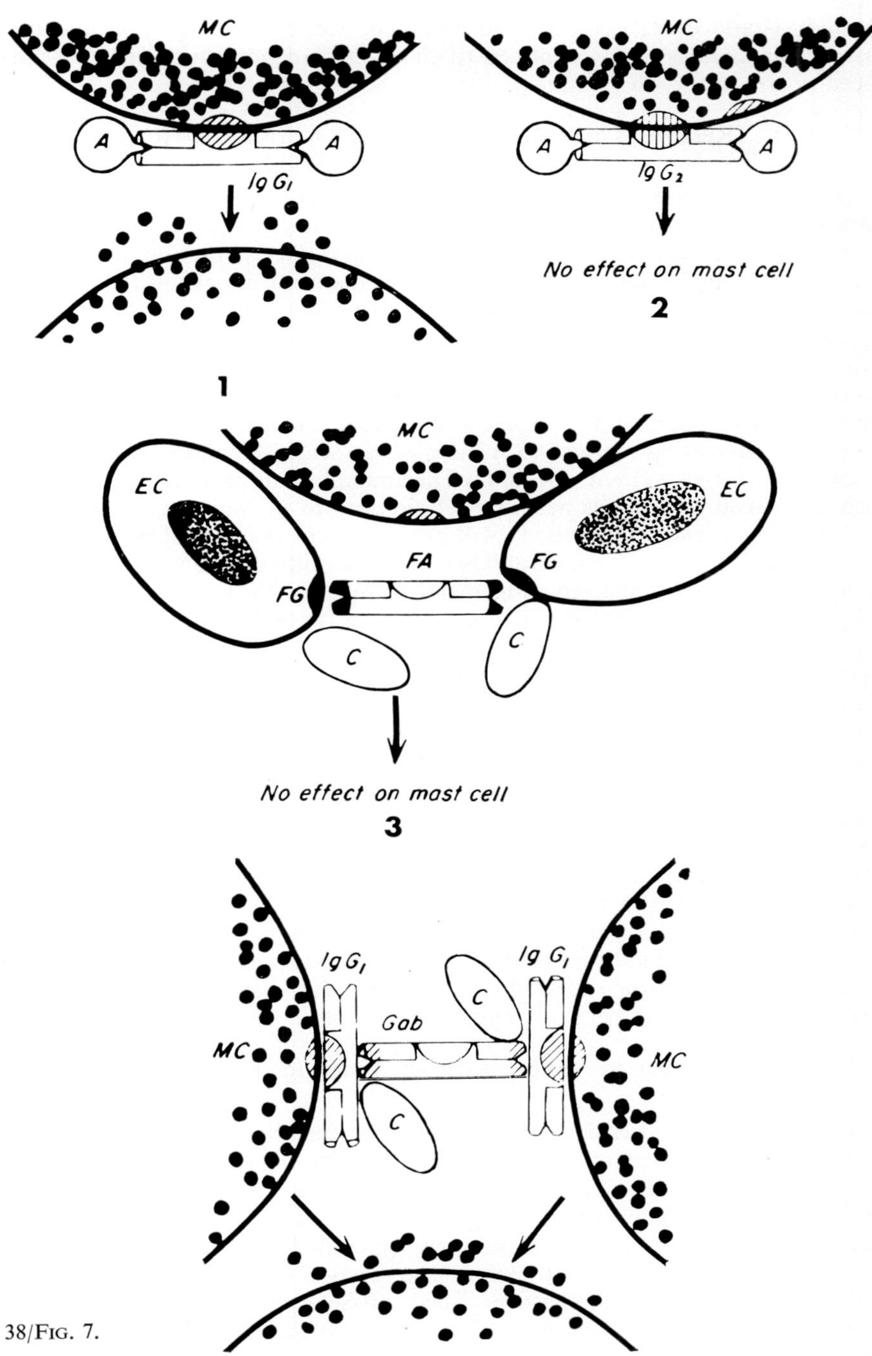

38/Fig. 7.

antibody is added first) could be so obtained. The demonstration of reversed passive anaphylaxis is not confined to the S-D reaction. Shock may be produced *in vivo* in the whole animal.

Reactions due to the Union of Antigen with Antibody in the Circulation

Although antibody may be fixed to certain tissues of the rabbit as it is in the guinea-pig, and a S-D reaction obtained with such tissues (e.g. sections of pulmonary artery), it would appear that an antigen-antibody reaction taking place in the blood rather than on any fixed tissue is the most important factor determining shock in the rabbit. The evidence for this may be summarised as follows: (1) the rabbit suffers from a general vasoconstriction of the systemic vessels rather than from a disturbance of any particular viscus, although the pulmonary arteries appear to be particularly affected. (2) Active sensitisation is only effective after several doses of antigen have been given, and there is an appreciable amount of circulating antibody. (3) In passively sensitised animals, shock may be induced without a latent period. (4) The amount of antigen inducing shock in passively sensitised animals bears no relationship to the amount of circulating antibody, i.e. circulating antibody will not "protect" the animal however little antigen is given. (5) In shocked rabbits with a high titre of antibody, as much as 90 per cent cent of the injected antigen may be found in the vessels of the lungs.[48] It has been suggested that this is present in the form of immune precipitates, which are formed in the circulation and are filtered off in the lung capillaries together with clumps of platelets and leucocytes.[49] These may act mechanically as emboli blocking the micro-circulation in the lungs and contributing to the obstruction to the pulmonary arterial system and congestion of the right heart.[50, 51] In addition, there is evidence, discussed later, that platelets play an important role in the causation of shock in the rabbit, and it is likely that the essential antigen-antibody reaction occurs in the vicinity of circulating platelets in contrast to that in the guinea-pig which involves the fixed mast cells. Even in this species, however, in certain circumstances union of antigen and antibody in the circulation may be a more important factor in the causation of shock than the more usual union of antigen with fixed tissue antibody. As noted above, if large amounts of antibody are used to sensitise guinea-pigs passively, shock may be produced by antigen injected immediately after the introduction of the antibody, i.e. no latent period is required for fixation of antibody.

Local Reaction due to Antigen-Antibody Union in the Circulation—Arthus Phenomenon

In 1903, a year after Richet had described anaphylactic shock, Arthus[52] observed a marked local inflammatory reaction following repeated subcutaneous injections of non-toxic antigen into rabbits at 6-day intervals. The first injection produced no effect; later injections induced erythema and œdema and still later injections areas of necrosis, which slowly separated and after several weeks were replaced by areas of cicatrisation. The reaction could be elicited even if a fresh site was used for each injection. Abell and Schenck[20] watched the vascular changes leading to this phenomenon in ear chambers, the antigen being introduced directly into the moat of the chamber. The first application produced the constriction of arterioles noted in general anaphylaxis. Subsequent applications gave rise to slowing of the blood stream in veins and capillaries with adherence of leucocytes to the walls of the vessel and to one another, followed by exudation of plasma, and blocking of many of the vessels by emboli of leucocytes. The condition gradually returned to normal. Further applications of antigen produced greater degrees of damage to capillary endothelium with extravasation of blood into the tissue spaces. Eventually there was destruction of the vessel walls followed by the compensatory formation of new vessels. Such changes in any tissue would lead eventually to the necrosis seen macroscopically in extreme cases of the Arthus phenomenon.

The Arthus phenomenon is not produced only in the skin. It can be elicited by local application of antigen to any tissue of a sensitised rabbit so far examined.[53] Thus local application of the antigen to the lungs by inhalation causes congestion, with the histological picture of pneumonia, and application to the brain may occasion neuro-muscular disturbances.

The Arthus phenomenon is most easily elicited in rabbits, but it can also be produced in other animals. It has been shown that this is correlated to some extent with the efficiency with which the animal produces precipitating antibody (for refs., see 54). It is not readily elicited in guinea-pigs which are poor producers of precipitating antibody, but it can be demonstrated in these animals following passive sensitisation with rabbit antibody. Kabat has shown that the conditions for the passive Arthus phenomenon differ in a number of ways from passive anaphylaxis: (1) sensitisation could only be transferred with precipitating antibody, "incomplete" non-precipitating antibody, which, as we saw, was effective in general anaphylaxis, was ineffective in Arthus sensitisation; (2) a latent period was not required; (3) horse antibody was as effective as rabbit in transferring Arthus sensitisation, although it failed to sensitise to general anaphylaxis or to P.C.A.; (4) the amount of antibody required for Arthus sensitisation was greatly in excess of that required for general anaphylactic sensitisation. Ovary and Bier[55] noted similar differences between local anaphylactic and Arthus sensitisation. They also showed that antihistamine drugs had no action on the Arthus phenomenon, suggesting that histamine plays no part. 5-HT is also not involved, since pre-treatment with reserpine which releases both histamine and 5-HT has no action on the Arthus phenomenon.[78]

The mechanism underlying the Arthus phenomenon is still obscure. It is certainly determined by an antigen-antibody reaction, but a reaction involving the precipitating type of antibody, which is free in the circulation and not fixed to tissue cells. It is improbable, however, that the phenomenon is due solely to the formation of an immune precipitate *in vivo*,[56] although this may be a contributing factor because there is evidence that an immune precipitate may be found in affected vessels.[49] There is little doubt that the blocking of blood vessels by leucocytic emboli is the main cause of the necrosis. Stetson[57] believes that the phenomenon in all its manifestations is due to the toxic action on vascular endothelium of the products of glycolysis of collections of leucocytes which collect in the peripheral vessels in the area of an Arthus reaction to such an extent as to lead to a leucopenia in the general circulation. He showed that the Arthus phenomenon could not be obtained in animals rendered leucopenic by the use of nitrogen mustard. The reason for the clumping of leucocytes and their collection in the area of an Arthus reaction is obscure, but it has been suggested that they are chemotactically attracted to components of complement fixed to the antigen-antibody precipitate. However, clumping of leucocytes is not confined to the Arthus phenomenon. We have already seen that clumping of platelets, and leucocytes with them, and their removal by the lung capillaries, occurs in general anaphylactic shock and it also occurs following the injection of anaphylactoid agents. It would seem that it is a factor common to a number of stress reactions, whether involving an immune complex or not.

Reactions brought about by Preformed Antigen-Antibody Complexes

We have already seen that the argument of the proponents of the humoral theory of anaphylaxis, that shock was produced by a reaction of antigen and antibody in the circulation, was supported by the observation that shock resembling anaphylaxis could be brought about by injecting into the circulation antigen-antibody precipitates, or serum treated with such precipitates. However, large doses were required, and further work suggests that the antigen-antibody complex was merely acting as a non-specific "anaphylactoid" agent. When *small* doses of soluble antigen-antibody complexes, formed in the region of antigen excess, were injected into mice[58] and guinea-pigs,[59] shock was induced after a latent period of 15 minutes.[60] Such complexes also produced a positive S-D reaction on the uterus of the unsensitised guinea-pig after a latent period of about one minute.[61] As the proportion of antibody to antigen was increased and the complex became insoluble, the effect fell off, until a *neutral* complex (i.e. having equivalent amounts of antigen and antibody) failed to produce a reaction. As with passive sensitisation, the nature of the antibody in the complex appears to be important, rabbit but not chicken antibody being effective.[62] This fact distinguishes anaphylaxis from another biological action of these complexes, namely the production of the lesions of experimental serum sickness in the walls of arteries discussed in Chapter 39 where the subject is considered in relation to serum sickness in man. In experimental serum sickness the source of antibody is not important.[62]

It is possible to look on anaphylaxis brought about by these complexes as a special case of passive anaphylaxis, the antibody gamma globulin of the complex becoming attached to tissues and carrying with it the antigen necessary for the induction of shock. If the complex is too large, as in immune precipitates, the antibody may be prevented from reaching its site of sensitisation.

The Role of Histamine in Anaphylaxis

It was early recognised that the signs and symptoms of anaphylactic shock bear a striking resemblance to histamine poisoning, and it has now been established with some certainty that the release of histamine from an inactive or inaccessible state is, at any rate, one of the factors involved in the manifestation of anaphylaxis. Reference has already been made to the release of histamine from sensitised guinea-pig lung by antigen *in vitro* as an indicator of anaphylaxis in isolated tissues. It remains to consider where histamine is made and stored and how it is released.

Presence of Histamine in Mammalian Tissues

It is now well established that histamine is present in mammalian tissues in a preformed state. The concentration varies in different organs and in different species. There appears to be some correlation between the histamine content of an organ and the number of mast cells it contains, much of the stored histamine in the body being in fact found in these cells. Mast cells contain an active histidine decarboxylase and there is strong evidence that the histamine contained in the cell is formed in the cell itself.[63] When C^{14} labelled histidine is incubated with a suspension of cells from rat peritoneal fluid containing mainly mast cells, C^{14} labelled histamine is formed and bound in these cells. There is no valid evidence that the cell stores histamine made elsewhere in the body, because the addition of large amounts of unlabelled histamine does not reduce the rate of formation and binding of labelled histamine which it would do if the cell stored exogenous histamine. Similar results were obtained *in vivo*. When C^{14} labelled histidine was injected into a dog with a mast cell tumour, Bloom and his colleagues[64] were able to isolate labelled histamine 24 hours later from the tumour. Histamine, however, is not confined to mast cells. In guinea-pig and human blood, it is mainly found in the basophils (which are allied to, but not identical with, mast cells) and, in rabbit blood, in the platelets. In certain tissues, such as the gastro-intestinal tract, histamine may be found in areas which are devoid of mast cells, e.g. the parietal cell region of the stomach and the deeper layers of the mucosa. There is some evidence that histamine is not stored in these localities, but is produced *de novo* at the time of application of a variety of stimuli including that leading to anaphylactic shock. Schayer[63] has described an inducible form of histidine decarboxylase which he believes to be present in vascular endothelium, and which is capable of being activated by an outside stimulus with extreme rapidity. He suggests that it may normally have a function as a regulator of the micro-circulation, but excessive stimuli may produce sufficient amounts of histamine to be demonstrated pharmacologically. He contrasts the *formation* of this "intrinsic" histamine with the *liberation* of "extrinsic" histamine from mast cells, terms first used by Dale in much the same connection.

The form in which histamine is held in the mast cell in an inactive state is still controversial. Its presence in the large metachromatic granules of the cell is now well established. The granules also contain heparin, and there is some evidence that histamine, a basic amine, exists in the granule in ionic combination with this acidic mucopolysaccharide (for refs. see 36). In view of the diverse substances and stimuli that liberate histamine from mast cell granules, however, e.g. the polyamine 48/80, trypsin, saponin, detergents, hypotonic saline, trauma and a variety of other stimuli, linkage with heparin cannot be the only factor. The granule is surrounded by a fine membrane 60Å thick visible in the electron microscope[65] and it is possible that the integrity of the membrane is another factor contributing to the retention of histamine.

Liberation of Histamine from Tissues in Anaphylaxis

That histamine is released into the blood and lymph in general anaphylactic shock in many animals, noted more than 30 years ago, is now fully established. Its liberation from isolated sensitised tissues, e.g. guinea-pig and human lung, dog's liver and rabbit and human blood cells (in which the platelets and basophils respectively probably represent the main source of stored histamine) can also be demonstrated when antigen is added to these tissues *in vitro*. As noted above, the liberation of histamine from chopped sensitised guinea-pig lung on the addition of antigen, and its detection by its ability to contract guinea-pig ileum, is a convenient system to investigate anaphylactic reactions *in vitro*. Using this system, Austen and Humphrey[37] have summarised the conditions for the liberation of histamine in anaphylaxis as follows: (*a*) the reaction requires Ca^{++} ions; (*b*) it is temperature-dependent; (*c*) it requires an unknown factor present in the tissues which is destroyed when heated at 45° for 25 minutes; (*d*) it requires SH groups; (*e*) it is highly sensitive to changes in the NaCl concentration, hypertonic saline decreasing and hypotonic saline increasing histamine release; (*f*) it needs a glycolytic mechanism as energy source, but is not dependent on cytochrome-mediated ærobic metabolism. Evidence is presented that the reaction depends on the activation of an esterase by the antigen-antibody reaction which can be inhibited by di-isopropyl fluorophosphate (DFP).

Degranulation of Mast Cells in Anaphylactic Reactions

The observations on the conditions for the release of histamine in anaphylaxis noted above can be directly correlated with the conditions determining the degranulation and disruption of sensitised mast cells by antigen. The phenomenon has been described morphologically by Mota and Dias da Silva.[66, 67] Using mast cells from the peritoneal cavity of actively sensitised rats, they noted that within a few seconds after the addition of antigen, the cell slightly increased in size and then suddenly became vacuolated with successions of vacuoles appearing and disappearing giving it a bubbling appearance (FIG. 6). On occasions, extrusion of granules was noted but without loss of continuity of the cell membrane. The final result was a loss of regular outline, large empty spaces being seen among the remaining granules.

Because of the ease with which suspensions of mast cells can be obtained from the rat in high concentration, they are admirably suited for the study of passive sensitisation and its relation to histamine release and mast cell damage by antigen. Unfortunately certain anomalies are found in the type of antibody able to sensitise rat tissues. As noted above, the rat resembles man in having a special reagin type of antibody determining homologous sensitisation, the so-called "mast cell lytic" antibody.[68] As in man, this is present in rats, actively sensitised under special conditions, in such small amounts that there is no possibility of correlating its content with mast cell sensitisation and antigen-induced histamine liberation. However, the presence of homologous gamma globulin on the rat mast cell can be detected indirectly by making use of reversed passive sensitisation, i.e. *antibody*-induced histamine release when rabbit antibody to rat gamma globulin is added to the rat mast cell. The mechanism by which histamine is released in this system, however, differs in certain ways from that involved in the antigen-induced classical type of anaphylactic reaction. The differences are discussed in the section "The role of complement" (p. 1100).

Enzyme Activation in Histamine Release from Mast Cells

From the early days of the discovery of histamine, the view that it was released in anaphylaxis by the activation of a proteolytic enzyme has been widely held. Before it was realised that histamine existed in the tissues in a free or loosely bound state, the only source of histamine envisaged was from protein. It was thought that histamine was formed from the decarboxylation of histidine after extensive proteolysis, either of the antigen, or of body proteins. Subsequently it was believed that histamine was bound to the cell by an amide link, and was released when the link was split by a peptidase. Crystalline trypsin certainly releases histamine from tissues or blood cells. However, as noted above, the agents that liberate histamine from tissues are so diverse that this observation loses much of its weight.

Many attempts have been made to relate the release of histamine in anaphylaxis to the activation of a serum or tissue protease, particularly the activation of serum plasminogen to plasmin. The evidence is conflicting and has been well reviewed by Austen and Humphrey.[37] They conclude that plasmin, or a tissue fibrinolytic enzyme, is either not activated, or, if activated, plays no part in the release of histamine in general anaphylaxis or in anaphylactic reactions in isolated tissues. However, this does not preclude the possibility that other types of serum and tissue enzymes are activated, and, in fact, Austen and Humphrey,[37] as noted earlier, have produced strong evidence for the activation of a chymotrypsin-like esterase in anaphylactic reactions involving chopped guinea-pig lung.

As mast cells, at least in the guinea-pig and rat, are probably both the site of the antigen-antibody reaction and also the source of histamine, they might be expected to contain an enzyme or enzymes responsible for the release of histamine. Mast cell enzymes have been studied in some detail particularly by Benditt and his colleagues[69], who found a chymotrypsin-like peptidase in the mast cells of rat, mouse, rabbit, dog and man. This enzyme splits the acetylated esters of tyrosine, tryptophan and phenylalanine but fails to split the synthetic arginine ester TAME (p-toluene-sulphonyl-l-arginine methyl ester) and is inhibited by DFP, so distinguishing it from a trypsin type of enzyme. Humphrey and his colleagues (for refs. see 37) suggested that this enzyme was activated in anaphylactic reactions involving the mast cell. They extended their observations on the activation of chymotrypsin in direct anaphylactic reactions in chopped guinea-pig lung, in which the system was too complex to determine the origin of the enzyme, to suspensions of isolated rat mast cells, making use of reversed passive sensitisation with rabbit anti-rat gamma globulin described above. However, as we shall see, this system is hardly comparable, since the mechanism of histamine release in *reversed* anaphylactic reactions, unlike that of *direct* anaphylactic reactions, appears to involve complement and probably the activation of C′1 proesterase (C′1p).

Other enzymes, such as diphosphopyridine nucleotidase (DPNase) and phospholipases A and C have been suggested as being concerned in histamine release but on insufficient grounds. There is no valid evidence that they play a part either in anaphylactic-induced histamine release or in mast cell disruption.

The release of histamine from sensitised rabbit *platelets* into the plasma, when antigen is added to whole blood or platelet suspensions in plasma, may also be enzyme dependent, but the evidence is not so strong as in the systems involving the mast cell.

The Role of Complement in Histamine Release

In direct anaphylactic reactions.—The greatly reduced titre of complement in the blood in systemic anaphylaxis, its fixation by antigen-antibody reactions and its known cytotoxic action naturally led to the view that complement might be concerned in cell damage, when adsorbed to an antigen-antibody complex, either in the circulation or on a cell surface.

In Chapter 36 evidence was presented showing that the initial step in the hæmolytic action of complement was the activation of the proesterase C′1p to the active esterase C′1a which sets in motion the complex steps involving the other components and leading to lysis. There is no doubt that some of the conditions determining the release of histamine by antigen from sensitised chopped lung of the guinea-pig appear to be those also concerned in the activation of C′1p, e.g. the requirement for Ca^{++}, inhibition by DFP and thermolability. However, recent evidence is strongly opposed to the participation of complement, at least in the direct (antigen-induced) anaphylactic reactions that have been studied in detail. The evidence, as it applies for instance to the liberation of histamine from chopped sensitised guinea-pig lung, may be summarised as follows:

(1) The isolated sensitised tissue may be washed free from serum complement without impairing its ability to release histamine on the addition of antigen. It might be argued that tissue bound complement was responsible. However, it has yet to be shown that complement can be bound to sensitised tissues in the absence of antigen.

(2) The anaphylactic release of histamine is prevented if the tissue is heated to 45° C. for 30 minutes, a temperature well below that required to inactivate complement.

(3) Although it was at one time thought that antibody capable of sensitising tissues was that involved in the fixation of complement[46] recent work, as noted in an earlier section, has made it clear that, at any rate in anaphylactic reactions in guinea-pig tissues, the type of homologous antibody (IgG_1) sensitising the tissue does not fix complement. The slower moving homologous gamma globulin (IgG_2) which does fix complement will not sensitise the tissues.

(4) Although immune hæmolysis mediated by complement and the release of histamine are both inhibited by DFP, differences are found when other inhibitory agents are used. SH inhibitors prevent histamine release but have no action on immune hæmolysis, and the pattern of inhibition by phosphonate esters is different in the two systems.[70] On the other hand, certain dibasic acids, e.g. succinate and maleate, enhance the release of histamine but not immune hæmolysis.

This evidence makes it clear that the activation of one or more components of complement is not responsible for the release of histamine in the direct anaphylactic sensitisation of guinea-pig tissues, that is where antibody (actively induced or passively administered) is fixed to the tissue and the reaction is induced by added antigen.

It is well known that, besides the red cell, complement will disrupt or lyse a variety of other cells when sensitised by antibody to antigens of their cell structure and there is reason to believe that the same system operates as in lysis of the red cell.[71] It is pertinent to enquire whether complement can release histamine in circumstances where it is known to produce cellular damage namely in immune lysis of histamine containing cells. So far no information is available whether mast cells can undergo immune lysis when sensitised by antibody to some structural antigen, and if they do, whether they release histamine (see 70). Gocke and Osler[72], however, obtained positive evidence with rabbit platelets which are rich in histamine. They noted that platelets sensitised by monkey anti-rabbit platelet serum, in the presence of fresh guinea-pig serum as the source of complement, were not only lysed, but released their histamine. Preheating the guinea-pig serum to 56° for 30 minutes, or the addition of the chelating agent EDTA which removed Ca^{++}, considerably depressed the amount released. It is legitimate to assume that the active agent was complement.

In reversed passive anaphylactic reactions.—In Chapter 36 we saw that immune hæmolysis could be brought about by complement when the red cell is sensitised by antibody not only to structural antigens of the cell surface, but also to extraneous antigens adsorbed to its surface. Similar results are found with platelets and nucleated cells. In reversed passive anaphylactic sensitisation, which, as we have seen, is an anaphylactic reaction induced when anti-gamma globulin is injected *in vivo*, or added to tissues to which gamma globulin is bound, the situation is closely parallel. If the mast cell, as seems likely, binds homologous, or less readily, heterologous, gamma globulin (acting as an extraneous antigen), antibody to such gamma globulin might be expected to sensitise the cell to the action of complement. This is in fact what is found. Austen, Humphrey and their colleagues (for refs. see 37) using suspensions of rat mast cells to which rabbit anti-rat gamma globulin and guinea-pig complement were added, noted that the cells underwent all the changes already noted as characteristic of direct anaphylactic reaction with degranulation and liberation of histamine. The guinea-pig complement, although not absolutely necessary, greatly enhanced the effect which was abolished by heating at 56° for 30 minutes. There is no reason to believe that the mechanism involved was different from the cytopathic action of complement following its fixation to an antigen (rat globulin)-antibody (rabbit anti-rat globulin) complex on the surface of the mast cell. The antibody concerned was the classical complement-fixing IgG_2 type of gamma globulin.

Summarising.—From these results it would appear that there are two similar but distinct immunological methods of releasing histamine from the same type of cell: (1) direct anaphylactic sensitisation with antibody, either as homologous IgG_1, or heterologous IgG_2, and addition of its matching antigen. This involves activation of an esterase probably from within the mast cell itself without the participation of complement; (2) reversed passive sensitisation brought about by preliminary adsorption of the animal's own anaphylactic type (IgG_1) immunoglobulin (or IgG_2 type from another animal) onto the tissues. These globulins then act as antigens and unite with a matching antibody to them, which is of the IgG_2 class and capable of fixing complement. One or more components of complement are fixed and activated. It would appear that when gamma globulin is acting as an antibody and is adsorbed to the mast cell surface, complement is not required for the release of histamine by antigen, even when that antibody is of the classical complement-fixing IgG_2 type (e.g. when heterologous rabbit antibody is used to sensitise guinea-pig tissues). On the other hand, when it is acting as an antigen (irrespective of whether it is "anaphylactic type" (homologous) or "classical type" (heterologous)), complement is involved in the release of histamine by anti-gamma globulin of the classical type. These observations are represented schematically in FIG. 7.

Inhibition of Anaphylactic Reactions with Histamine Antagonists

Numerous attempts have been made to protect animals against anaphylactic shock by the injection of synthetic drugs having a pharmacological action antagonistic to that of histamine (antihistamines). Large numbers of antihistamines are known, and evidence for histamine release has been sought by noting the effects of these drugs on the manifestations of anaphylaxis in guinea-pigs. Although complete suppression of shock was seldom obtained, there was a significant decrease in mortality and in the acute symptoms. The S-D reaction is also inhibited by these drugs. However, it has generally been found that the concentration of antihistamines necessary to inhibit the S-D reaction is far larger than that found necessary to abolish equivalent muscular contractions due to histamine. This has been explained in two ways: it has been pointed out that in the S-D reaction, the antihistamine to be effective must reach the site at which histamine is released in sufficient concentration to neutralise the liberated histamine. Histamine added from without, however, is not concentrated in the vicinity of sensitive cells and can therefore be more readily neutralised. Alternatively, or perhaps in addition, the muscular contractions in the S-D reaction may be due only partially to histamine, other substances responsible for muscle contraction being released at the same time. It is known that, whereas many antihistamine drugs at low concentrations are relatively specific in their antagonistic action on histamine, at higher concentrations they are much less specific. Thus, it is likely that at high concentrations antihistamines may inhibit muscular contractions due to substances other than histamine.

ROLE OF OTHER FACTORS

Although from the considerations in the last section it can be said with some certainty that histamine plays an important part in anaphylactic shock, there is little doubt that it is not the only factor involved. We have already seen that *heparin* is liberated from the liver of the shocked dog and this, together with the fall in platelet count, is responsible for the lack of coagulability of the blood. If, as seems likely, histamine and heparin are loosely combined in the mast cell, the liberation of one may be accompanied by the liberation of the other. However, this is not invariable, and it has been suggested that where they are not found free together, the heparin, a relatively large and poorly diffusible molecule, after release has become bound to the cement substance of connective tissue to which it is known to have an affinity. In the liver there is relatively little connective tissue, and heparin is released with histamine into the lymph of the thoracic duct.

Although the over-all picture of anaphylactic shock resembles that of histamine shock, there are a number of observations that cannot be readily fitted into it. For instance, it has been observed that the uterine muscle from a sensitised guinea-pig, when so poisoned with histamine that it no longer reacts to it, still contracts when antigen is added to the kymograph bath.[73] Another observation, which cannot be fitted into the histamine theory, is the difference between the effect of histamine and antigen on the uterus of the sensitised rat; whereas histamine causes relaxation, antigen causes contraction.[74] Thirdly, we have already noted that antihistamines fail to abolish entirely the manifestations of anaphylaxis, or do so only when doses are used which are no longer specifically inhibitory for histamine.

The first demonstration that a factor other than histamine may be involved in anaphylactic shock is that of Kellaway and Trethewie.[75] They showed that the perfusate from the lungs of guinea-pigs during anaphylactic shock contained in addition to histamine a "*slow-reacting substance*" (SRS-A) which, as its name suggests, produced a slower and more prolonged contraction of muscle than histamine. It also causes contraction of the rat uterus which is relaxed by histamine. This factor has been further studied by Brocklehurst and his colleagues[76], who perfused the isolated lungs of sensitised guinea-pigs through the pulmonary arterial tree with Tyrode solution containing the antigen and collected the perfusate in fractions. The first fractions contained histamine which gave the typical rapid contraction of the guinea-pig ileum that was reversed by mepyramine. Later fractions contained increasing amounts of SRS-A, which gave a slow type of muscular contraction and relaxation, and this was not reversed by mepyramine. SRS-A has not yet been identified chemically, but the properties of the partially purified preparation suggest that it is an acidic lipoid substance firmly bound to protein.[77] There is evidence that it is not present in the tissues as such but is formed as the result of the antigen-antibody reaction in the tissues.[78] Its release may also play a part in the symptomatology of human asthma as it is highly active in contracting the musculature of human bronchioles.

Another substance producing a slow type of contraction of guinea-pig ileum is *bradykinin*, a polypeptide formed by the action of proteolytic enzymes on plasma proteins. Elliott[79] described its formation in plasma by the action of a plasma enzyme distinct from plasmin. Using a trypsin digest of pseudo-globulin from ox-blood he succeeded in purifying it and characterised it as a nonapeptide. It has recently been synthesised.[80] The pure nonapeptide contracts unstriped muscle, but its most dramatic action is to cause dilatation of blood vessels with increased capillary permeability. Bradykinin has been demonstrated in the plasma of shocked dogs.[81] Although it may be detected within 2 minutes of shock it is slow in forming, and in dogs that do not succumb, its concentration does not reach a maximum until some 90 minutes later. By this time the dog has recovered and its blood pressure has returned to normal. It would seem, therefore, that it plays little part in the symptomatology of shock in the dog but may account for late shock sometimes found after apparent recovery.

The permeability globulin (PF/dil) discovered by Miles (see Chapter 2) exists in the serum of a number of species, including man, as an inactive profactor which can be activated by dilution in saline to give esterase actively demonstrable by its action on TAME. There was no evidence that the level of PF/dil changes in anaphylactic shock or that it is activated by an antigen-antibody reaction, and it probably plays no role in the manifestation of anaphylactic shock.[82]

5-*Hydroxytryptamine* (5HT) is present in the mammalian body, mainly in the gastro-intestinal mucosa and brain tissue. It is also present in the platelets of the rabbit, guinea-pig and dog, and in the mast cells of the rat and mouse, but not in those of other species. Humphrey and Jaques[83] showed that 5HT was released from rabbit platelets *in vitro* by an antigen-antibody interaction. It has been found *in vivo* during anaphylaxis in the rabbit.[84] Rabbit lung contains 5HT which, together with histamine, is increased in shock due to the accumulation of platelets and liberation of 5HT from them. However, since the specific inhibitor of 5HT, dibromolysergic acid diethylamide, has no protective action on anaphylaxis in the rabbit, and 5HT could not be detected in the lung of the guinea-pig, it is unlikely that it plays a part in anaphylaxis in these two species. In the rat and mouse, there is evidence that it may be more important. It is present together with histamine in the mast cells. Unstriped muscle of the rat and mouse, which fails to contract to histamine, is susceptible to the action of 5HT and the contraction can be inhibited by lysergic acid diethylamide.

Summary

Anaphylactic shock may be produced in animals of many species by an injection of an antigen after they have become sensitised by a previous injection given some days earlier. The sensitising dose may be given by any route and may be exceedingly small. A latent period must then elapse and the shocking dose be given directly into the circulation. Sensitisation may be effected by antigens or, in some cases, by simple chemical compounds able to unite with body protein to form antigens. The shocking agent, either the whole antigen, or the hapten part of the antigen if a large molecule, must be identical or have a close immunological relationship to the sensitising agent. Simple radicles of small molecular size fail to produce shock, but specifically inhibit shock if given before the shocking dose of antigen. The main manifestations of shock can be accounted for by contraction of smooth muscle and damage to capillary endothelium. The signs and symptoms, however, differ in different species of animals, depending on the organ in which these tissues are mainly affected. In the guinea-pig the muscle of the bronchioles, in the dog that of the hepatic venous tree, and in the rabbit the muscle of the arteries, particularly the pulmonary arteries, are mainly involved. In all animals there is a leucopenia and thrombocytopenia.

The anaphylactic state can be transferred passively in the serum of sensitised animals both systemically and to a local area of skin *in vivo* (passive cutaneous anaphylaxis, PCA), or by sensitisation of unstriped muscle with antibody globulin *in vitro* to contract on the addition of specific antigen (Schultz-Dale reaction, S-D). Labelled gamma globulin is readily adsorbed to strips of guinea-pig ileum, minced lung and mesentery. It cannot be removed by washing but may be eluted with unlabelled gamma globulin. Adsorption may or may not lead to sensitisation, depending on the nature of the gamma globulin and the species of animal from which it was obtained. Sensitisation of guinea-pig tissues by homologous gamma globulin is, both quantitatively more effective than, and qualitatively different from, sensitisation by heterologous gamma globulin, and depends on an electrophoretically faster immunoglobulin (IgG_1) which fails to fix complement with antigen. Sensitisation of guinea-pig tissues with rabbit antibody is due to the slower moving classical complement-fixing IgG (IgG_2). It may or may not precipitate with antigen. Guinea-pig *homologous* IgG_2 not only fails to sensitise but blocks sensitisation by homologous IgG_1. The macromolecular 19S (IgM) homologous or heterologous immunoglobulins will not sensitise guinea-pig tissues. Heterologous sheep, horse and chicken antibody adsorbs to guinea-pig tissues, but fails to sensitise.

A reversed S-D reaction can be obtained by "sensitising" the guinea-pig ileum with normal rabbit gamma globulin (antigen) and adding guinea-pig anti-rabbit gamma globulin to the sensitised tissue. The cells involved in fixation are probably the mast cells of the tissue and not the vascular endothelium or muscle fibres. In the rabbit, the main manifestations of anaphylaxis are due to union of antigen and antibody in the circulation. Clumps of platelets, leucocytes and perhaps immune precipitate may collect in the terminal branches of the pulmonary arteries. Preformed antigen-antibody complexes containing excess of antigen, and of small molecular size, may produce shock in non-sensitised mice and guinea-pigs after a latent period.

The antigen-antibody reaction *in vivo* liberates histamine which is free, or held in a loosely bound state, in the granules of mast cells and in other cells. Histamine may also be formed *de novo* by activation of a histidine decarboxylase present in vascular endothelium. Liberation of histamine from mast cells depends on the presence of Ca^{++} ions, is temperature-dependent, requires a thermolabile factor present in tissues, is dependent on SH groups and needs a glycolytic mechanism as energy source. There is evidence that it depends on the activation of an esterase perhaps from the mast cell itself. Complement is not involved. In anaphylaxis due to homologous sensitisation of guinea-pig, rat and man (Chapter 39) it is not fixed. However, complement is probably involved in the release of histamine from mast cells in reversed passive sensitisation and in the release of histamine from rabbit platelets.

Other substances may be liberated during shock, for example 5-hydroxytryptamine, bradykinin, and a slow reacting substance (SRS-A) of unknown nature. With the exception of SRS-A, it is unlikely that any of these substances plays a part in the manifestations of shock in guinea-pigs, or dogs, but 5-HT probably plays the major role in anaphylactic reactions in the mouse and rat and may be involved in anaphylaxis in the rabbit. SRS-A is liberated from the guinea-pig lung, and may be responsible for a slow type of contraction of unstriped muscle which is found (in addition to the rapid contraction due to histamine) in the Schultz-Dale reaction, and which is not inhibited by antihistamine drugs.

A local area of inflammation, hæmorrhage and necrosis, the Arthus phenomenon, may be produced by an injection of antigen into the skin or other organs of actively, or passively, sensitised rabbits, or passively sensitised guinea-pigs. The phenomenon depends on the amount of precipitating antibody in the serum and is due to an antigen-antibody reaction in the circulation at the local site of injection. There is some evidence that the formation of an immune precipitate plays a part in the phenomenon. The phenomenon is due to damage to the walls of blood vessels, probably caused by the action of the acid products of glycolysis and by the mechanical blockage to blood vessels, brought about by leucocytes attracted to the site by complement fixed to the immune complex. The cells collect in the local area and may form small emboli which block arterioles and hence bring about necrosis. The release of histamine probably plays little part, if any, in the phenomenon.

REFERENCES

1. RICHET, C. (1913). *Anaphylaxis* translated by J. M. Bligh, Liverpool University Press. London: Constable & Co.
2. OTTO, R. (1906). *von Leuthold Gedenkschrift*, **1**, 153.
3. LANDSTEINER, K. (1945). *The Specificity of Serological Reactions*, Chapter 5. Cambridge, Mass.: Harvard University Press.
4. TILLETT, W. S., AVERY, O. T., and GOEBEL, W. F. (1929). *J. exp. Med.*, **50**, 551.
5. FELDBERG, W., and MILES, A. A. (1953). *J. Physiol. (Lond.)*, **120**, 205.
6. BURRAGE, W. S., IRWIN, J. W., PETERSEN, I. G., and GORDON, P. (1953). *Ann. Allergy*, **11**, 137.
7. WEIL, R. (1917). *J. Immunol.*, **2**, 525.
8. DIXON, F. J., and WARREN, S. (1950). *Amer. J. med. Sci.*, **219**, 414.
9. SIMONDS, J. P. (1923). *Amer. J. Physiol.*, **65**, 512.
10. BAUER, W., DALE, H. H., POULSSON, L. T., and RICHARDS, D. W. (1932). *J. Physiol. (Lond.)*, **74**, 343.
11. SIMONDS, J. P., and BRANDES, W. W. (1927). *J. Immunol.*, **13**, 1.
12. MAEGRAITH, B. G., ANDREWS, W. H. H., and WENYON, C. E. M. (1949). *Lancet*, **2**, 56; *Ann. trop. Med.*, **43**, 225.
13. DEAN, H. R., and WEBB, R. A. (1924). *J. Path. Bact.*, **27**, 51, 65.
14. MANWARING, W. H. (1910). *Z. Immun.-Forsch.*, **8**, 1.
15. WATERS, E. T., and MARKOWITZ, J. (1940). *Amer. J. Physiol.*, **130**, 379.
16. MANWARING, W. H., BEATTIE, A. C., and MCBRIDE, R. W. (1923). *J. Amer. med. Ass.*, **80**, 1437.
17. WEBB, R. A. (1924). *J. Path. Bact.*, **27**, 79.
18. GROVE, E. F. (1932). *J. Immunol.*, **23**, 101.
19. VALLERY-RADOT, P. (1949). *Précis des Maladies allergiques*, p. 18. Paris: Flammarion et Cie.
20. ABELL, R. G., and SCHENCK, H. P. (1938). *J. Immunol.*, **34**, 195.
21. JAQUES, L. B., and WATERS, E. T. (1940). *Amer. J. Physiol.*, **129**, P389.
22. MONKHOUSE, F. C., FIDLER, E., and BARLOW, J. C. D. (1952). *Amer. J. Physiol.*, **169**, 712.
23. DOERR, R., and RUSS, V. K. (1909). *Z. Immun.-Forsch.*, **3**, 181.
24. KABAT, E. A. (1947). *Amer. J. Med.*, **3**, 535.
25. KABAT, E. A., and LANDOW, H. (1942). *J. Immunol.*, **44**, 69.
26. KABAT, E. A., and BENACERRAF, B. (1949). *J. Immunol.*, **62**, 97.
27. HEIDELBERGER, M., TREFFERS, H. P., and MAYER, M. (1940). *J. exp. Med.*, **71**, 271.
28. OVARY, Z., BLOCH, K. J., and BENACERRAF, B. (1964). *Proc. Soc. exp. Biol. (N.Y.)*, **116**, 840.
29. HUMPHREY, J. H., and MOTA, I. (1959). *Immunology*, **2**, 19, 31.
30. BLOCH, K. J. (1967). *Progr. Allergy.*, **10**, 84.
31. BENACERRAF, B., and KABAT, E. A. (1949). *J. Immunol.*, **62**, 517.
32. SCHULTZ, W. H. (1910). *J. Pharmacol. exp. Ther.*, **1**, 549.
33. DALE, H. H. (1913). *J. Pharmacol. exp. Ther.*, **4**, 167.
34. GROVE, E. F. (1932). *J. Immunol.*, **23**, 147.
35. KULKA, A. M. (1943). *J. Immunol.*, **46**, 235.
36. MONGAR, J. L., and SCHILD, H. O. (1962). *Physiol. Rev.*, **42**, 226.
37. AUSTEN, K. F., and HUMPHREY, J. H. (1963). *Advanc. Immunol.*, **3**, 1.
38. BROCKLEHURST, W. E., HUMPHREY, J. H., and PERRY, W. L. M. (1961). *Immunology*, **4**, 67.

39. Nielsen, C. B., Terres, G., and Feigen, G. A. (1959). *Science*, **130,** 41.
40. Feigen, G. A., Nielsen, C. B., and Terres, G. (1962). *J. Immunol.*, **89,** 717.
41. Biozzi, G., Halpern, B. N., and Binaghi, R. (1959). *J. Immunol.*, **82,** 215.
42. Ovary, Z., and Karush, F. (1961). *J. Immunol.*, **86,** 146.
43. Benacerraf, B. (1965). *Molecular and Cellular Basis of Antibody Production.* Symp. Czech. Acad. Sci., p. 223. Ed. Šterzl, J. Prague: Czech. Acad. Sci.
44. Ovary, Z., Benacerraf, B., and Bloch, K. J. (1963). *J. exp. Med.*, **117,** 951.
45. Baker, A. R., Bloch, K. J., and Austen, K. F. (1964). *J. Immunol.*, **93,** 525.
46. Humphrey, J. H. (1959). *Cellular and Humoral Aspects of the Hypersensitive States* (Symp. N.Y. Acad. Med. **9,** Chap. I, p. I.). Ed. Lawrence, H. S. New York: Hoeber-Harper.
47. White, R. G., Jenkin, G. C., and Wilkinson, P. C. (1963). *Int. Arch. Allergy*, **22,** 186.
48. Dixon, F. J. (1959). *Mechanisms of Hypersensitivity.* (Henry Ford. Hosp. Internat. Symp., **8,** p. 209). Eds. Shaffer, J. H., LoGrippo, G. A., and Chase, M. W. Boston, Mass.: Little, Brown & Co.
49. McKinnon, G. E. (1959). Ref. 48, Chap. 11, p. 163.
50. Walter, J. B., Frank, J. A., and Irwin, J. W. (1961). *Brit. J. exp. Path.*, **42,** 603.
51. Walter, J. B., and Frank, J. A. (1959). *Brit. J. exp. Path.*, **42,** 609
52. Arthus, M. (1903). *C.R. Soc. Biol. (Paris).* **55,** 817.
53. Seegal, B. C. (1949). *Ann. N.Y. Acad. Sci.*, **50,** 681.
54. Benacerraf, B., and Kabat, E. A. (1950). *J. Immunol.*, **64,** 1.
55. Ovary, Z., and Bier O. G. (1953). *J. Immunol.* **71,** 6.
56. Rich A. R. (1951). *The Pathogenesis of Tuberculosis*, p. 414, 2nd edit. Oxford: Blackwell Scientific Publications.
57. Stetson C. A. (1951). *J. exp. Med.*, **94,** 347.
58. Tokuda, S., and Weiser, R. S. (1958). *Science*, **127,** 1237.
59. Germuth, F. G., Jr., and McKinnon, G. E. (1957). *Bull. Johns Hopk. Hosp.*, **101,** 13.
60. Benacerraf, B., Sebestyen, M., and Cooper, N. S. (1959). *J. Immunol.*, **82,** 131.
61. Trapani, I. L., Garvey, J. S., and Campbell, D. H. (1958). *Science*, **127,** 700.
62. McCluskey, R. T., Benacerraf, B., Potter, J. L., and Miller, F. (1960). *J. exp. Med.*, **111,** 180.
63. Schayer, R. W. (1963). *Ann. N.Y. Acad. Sci.*, **103,** 164.
64. Bloom, G., Larsson, B., and Aberg, B. (1958). *Zbl. Vet.-Med.*, **5,** 443.
65. Rogers, G. E. (1956). *Exp. Cell Res.*, **11,** 393.
66. Mota, I., and Dias da Silva, W. (1960). *Nature (Lond.)*, **186,** 245.
67. Mota, I. (1963). *Ann. N.Y. Acad. Sci.*, **103,** 264.
68. Mota, I. (1962). *Immunology*, **4,** 11.
69. Benditt, E. P., Holcenberg, H., and Lagunoff, R. (1963). *Ann. N.Y. Acad. Sci.*, **103,** 179.
70. Austen, K. F., and Bloch, K. J. (1965). *Complement*, p. 281. Ciba Foundation Symp. Eds. Wolstenholme, G. E. W., and Knight, J. London: J. & A. Churchill.
71. Winn, H. J. (1965). Ref. 70, p. 133.
72. Gocke, D. J., and Osler, A. G. (1961). 4th Int. Congr. Allergol. Excerpta Med. Int. Congr. Ser., p. 432.
73. Schild, H. (1936). *J. Physiol. (Lond.)*, **86,** 51.
74. Kellaway, C. H. (1930). *Brit. J. exp. Path.*, **11,** 72.
75. Kellaway, C. H., and Trethewie, E. R. (1940). *Quart. J. exp. Physiol.*, **30,** 121.
76. Brocklehurst, W. E. (1953). *J. Physiol. (Lond.)*, **120,** 16.
77. Brocklehurst, W. E. (1962). *Progr. Allergy*, **3.**
78. Brocklehurst, W. E. (1960). *J. Physiol. (Lond.)*, **151,** 416.
79. Elliott, D. F. (1963). *Ann. N.Y. Acad. Sci.*, **104,** 35.

80. Boisonnes, R. A. (1963). *Ann. N.Y. Acad. Sci.*, **103**, 5.
81. Beraldo, W. T. (1950). *Amer. J. Physiol.*, **163**, 283.
82. Becker, E. L. (1961). *Int. Symp. Immunol. Path.*, **2**, 37.
83. Humphrey, J. H., and Jaques, R. (1955). *J. Physiol. (Lond.)*, **128**, 9.
84. Waalke, T. P., and Cobru, W. (1959). *J. Allergy*, **30**, 394.

Chapter 39

REACTIONS TO EXOGENOUS ALLERGENS: ATOPY AND DELAYED HYPERSENSITIVITY

By G. P. Gladstone

In the last chapter we considered experimental anaphylaxis, a condition brought about by an immunological reaction taking place within the body tissues to a foreign antigen introduced parenterally. In this chapter we shall consider certain other disorders brought about by immunological reactions to foreign allergens* *in vivo* which differ from experimental anaphylaxis in a number of ways.

Many pathological conditions resulting from immunological reactions *in vivo*, the so-called allergic diseases, have been described, occurring either as natural diseases, or as the result of certain artificial therapeutic measures such as administration of serum antitoxin or drugs. In many infectious diseases, also, the body tissues become specifically sensitive to products of the infecting organism. For instance, patients convalescent from pneumococcal pneumonia show two types of hypersensitivity. They will react to the intracutaneous injection of the type specific polysaccharide of their infecting pneumococci by an immediate inflammatory reaction with local œdema (weal) and surrounding flare. They will also react to an intracutaneous injection of the species specific protein of the pneumococcus by a more slowly developing local lesion with less œdema but more cellular induration. Neither the polysaccharide nor the protein gives any reaction in a normal individual. There is in fact little doubt that the manifestation of many infectious diseases, particularly those of long duration, are in part determined by allergic elements, but it is not always easy to establish that this is so. We shall confine our attention to those disorders where there is strong evidence that the predominant features are allergic, that is they are the result of an antigen-antibody reaction *in vivo*.

Allergic diseases are not confined to those in which the allergen is introduced from without. We may legitimately extend the term to include those conditions where the allergen is one of the constituents of the body. We may thus classify allergic disorders into two groups. In the first group, considered in this chapter, the disorders depend on an immunological response to an exogenous allergen; in the second, considered in Chapter 40, they depend, either on antibody introduced from without, or on an immune response by the individual to antigens of his own tissues (auto-immunisation). Sometimes the antigen is a complex consisting partly of exogenous material and partly of endogenous tissue protein or cells (e.g. drug allergy). The allergic response to tissue grafts (the homograft reaction) is considered in Chapter 41.

Disorders due to allergens of exogenous origin may be conveniently sub-

* The term "allergen" is used rather than antigen, since, as will be seen, not all agents inducing hypersensitive reactions are antigenic.

divided according to the rate of development of the hypersensitive reaction following contact with the allergen into:

1. **Allergy of the immediate type.**—This is typically shown by the immediate urticarial skin reactions when the allergen is injected intradermally; antibodies are present in the serum; the manifestations are due to damage to capillary endothelium and contraction of unstriped muscle, as they are in anaphylactic reactions in animals.

2. **Allergy of the delayed type.**—The allergic reaction of this type does not appear until 24 hours after contact with the allergen; it is more indurated and less œdematous than that of the immediate type; circulating antibodies may or may not be present but play no part in the reaction; the manifestations are not due to damage to capillaries or to contraction of unstriped muscle, but consist of a slowly developing local inflammatory reaction with infiltration of mononuclear cells with or without necrosis. The immediate cause of the reactions is not known, but probably stems from a direct action on certain mesenchymal cells.

3. **Allergy of the serum sickness type.**—Here the signs and symptoms only develop 7–10 days after the injection of large amounts of antigen, e.g. horse serum antitoxin; the lesions are essentially œdematous and are mediated by circulating antibodies. The manifestations are due to vascular damage rather than to contraction of unstriped muscle.

Allergy of the Immediate Type

General Anaphylaxis and Atopy in Man

With rare exceptions, such as that following the rupture of an hydatid cyst into the peritoneal cavity, anaphylactic shock is not found in the course of natural diseases in man, because the sudden entry of a large amount of antigen into the circulation of a sensitised subject is not likely to occur naturally. However, the therapeutic use of horse serum antitoxin which, although not introduced directly into the circulation, is injected in large doses into the tissues, might be expected to bring about anaphylactic shock in sensitised individuals. Fortunately, even when large doses of horse serum are administered, allergic reactions leading to general systemic anaphylaxis with fatal outcome are rare. When such reactions do take place, in apparent contrast to anaphylaxis in the guinea-pig, they usually bear no relation to the amount of antigen administered. In fact, exceedingly small amounts of protein introduced parenterally, or even by feeding or inhalation, may be sufficient to produce fatal shock. For instance, shock may develop a few minutes after as little as 0·05 ml. of horse serum is injected subcutaneously. Even more remarkable are the few but well-authenticated cases of anaphylaxis developing as a result of stings from bees and wasps.[1] These individuals are not hypersensitive to the pharmacological action of the venom. Successive stings may produce progressively more severe systemic reactions with a final fatal outcome, or sensitivity may suddenly develop. It is difficult to understand how, even in the most sensitive individual, sufficient antigen from the minute amount injected can be carried throughout the body to bring about these dramatic results. It has been suggested that the fatal cases of anaphylactic shock are the result of a chance injection of venom into a vein, but even if this were so, considerable dilution of the venom antigen would take place in the blood volume. It is possible that the affinity of antigen for antibody fixed to sensitised cells is so great that the antigen becomes concentrated on these cells.

The symptoms and signs of anaphylactic shock in man are those of acute respiratory distress with subsequent vascular collapse. Respiratory obstruction may be due to broncho-constriction or, in some cases, laryngeal œdema. There is profound fall in blood pressure with syncope and often convulsions. Death occurs in a few minutes to an hour. At autopsy, there is usually pulmonary congestion and œdema with emphysema and petechial hæmorrhages in skin, mucous and serous membranes. It is probable, but not certain, that mast cells in the respiratory tract are the target cells as in the guinea-pig, with liberation of histamine which contributes to the obstructing laryngeal œdema and broncho-constriction. There is evidence, discussed later, that SRS-A (Chapter 38) plays a major part in broncho-constriction.

Atopy.—Almost all anaphylactic reactions in man are confined to certain individuals who have a predisposition to develop immediate type hypersensitive reactions on contact with foreign allergens. These individuals are said to be suffering from the condition known as atopy. The term, literally meaning a strange disease, was coined by Coca to denote a group of allergic diseases of the immediate type which are subject to an hereditary influence. It is not always possible, however, to find an hereditary influence in conditions resembling atopy in all other ways, and the term has, therefore, been broadened to include such conditions.

It is well known that some individuals are unable to eat common articles of food without suffering from acute symptoms which vary in severity from urticarial rashes to acute gastro-intestinal upset and asthma. Others are particularly sensitive to the inhalation of dust from animal or vegetable sources, reacting with acute coryza or asthma. Hay fever, due to inhalation of grass pollens in the height of summer, is a particularly common form of such hypersensitivity.

The reactions of atopy usually start a few minutes after contact with the allergen and are often specifically related to a single type of allergen. The specificity may be of a very high degree. For example, persons may be sensitive to strawberries grown only in certain districts. On the other hand, persons liable to be sensitive to one type of allergen are often equally liable to become sensitive to others. This is particularly shown in hay fever, in which sufferers are usually sensitive to many types of pollen.

The particular "shock tissue" involved is determined in two ways. (1) The *route* through which the allergen makes contact with the body cells. Substances reaching the body by inhalation tend to produce nasal œdema or bronchiolar spasm. Articles of food usually produce acute gastric and intestinal symptoms, but eczematous and urticarial rashes are common. (2) *Individual peculiarities.* Thus one of twins sensitive to cow's milk reacted with generalised urticaria, the other with abdominal pain, vomiting and diarrhœa.[2] In some cases the reaction may vary in the same individual. The eczema of infancy and childhood may give way to asthma or hay fever in later life.

A characteristic of atopy is the local skin reaction that can be elicited by introducing the allergen into the skin by injection or via a scratch. The reaction occurs *within a minute or so of the introduction of the allergen* and consists of an urticarial weal surrounded by an area of erythema, and does not in fact differ from Lewis's non-specific "triple response". It may be obtained in cases where the skin is not normally involved, as in asthma, and may be considered as a local anaphylactic type of reaction, the primary vascular response being due to a contraction of the smooth muscle of the arterioles accompanied by changes in the permeability of the capillary walls.[3]

Blood and tissue *eosinophilia* frequently accompany atopy. In acute manifestations of allergy, however, as in anaphylactic shock, there is a fall in the number of circulating leucocytes, including the eosinophils. Subsequently, the eosinophils may increase to 6 per cent or more. Eosinophils may be present in the mucous secretion of the nose and bronchi in hay fever and asthma. A differential diagnosis can often be made between infective and allergic sinusitis by the nature of the cells in the secretion. The significance of eosinophils in allergic diseases is unknown.

In comparing atopic hypersensitivity with classical anaphylaxis, we have to consider: (1) the nature of the allergen; (2) the influence of heredity; (3) how sensitisation is brought about; and (4) passive transference.

(1) The Nature of the Sensitising Agent

Many allergens are proteins, their activity being destroyed by proteolytic enzymes or denaturation by cooking. Horse dander is of this type, and eggs and milk, the most common food allergens, depend on their proteins for their allergenic nature. In some cases, however, cooking may actually produce an allergen, as in the classical sensitivity of Küstner to a species of fish when the fish had been cooked but not when it was raw (see below). Occasionally it is not the food as partaken that is the allergen but certain metabolic products of the food. In these cases symptoms do not appear until some hours after ingestion owing to the necessity for metabolic breakdown.[4] The chemical nature of the allergens of plant pollens has been extensively studied (for review see ref. 5). Those of grass pollen[6] and house dust[7] contain carbohydrate. The allergens of ragweed appear to be polypeptides of small molecular weight (about 5,000) which resist proteolysis.[8] In considering the elicitation of the hypersensitive reaction, it need cause no surprise that an allergen is not necessarily an antigen. Anaphylactic shock can be brought about in a sensitised animal by injecting a hapten. If atopy is analogous, then a protein-free hapten might well be an adequate excitant.

(2) The Influence of Heredity

It is usually found that one or both parents of the individual are also sensitive, though it is not the sensitivity to a particular allergen but *the predisposition to become sensitive* that is inherited. However, there is some tendency for parent and offspring to react in the same way although to different allergens. Occasionally there may be an inherited sensitivity to the same allergen. The hereditary factor, however, would appear not to be absolutely essential, and in many otherwise typical cases of hay fever and asthma, no hereditary factor can be found. It is probable that all individuals have the capacity to react to particular antigens that reach the tissues in an unaltered form, provided the sensitising stimulus is sufficiently large or prolonged. Some allergens produce sensitivity in normal people even in small doses. It has been repeatedly observed that *Ascaris lumbricoides* antigen in small doses will sensitise normal individuals, but they may vary widely in the rate at which they can be sensitised. This has also been observed with diphtheria toxoid.[9] The sensitivity of normal people to these allergens does not differ noticeably from that of individuals in whom a definite family history of atopy can be obtained.

It has been suggested that the hereditary element distinguishes atopy from experimental anaphylaxis in the guinea-pig. Although it is true that all guinea-pigs can be sensitised, strains exist which show a tendency to become more readily sensitised than others. If due allowance is made for the greater sensitivity of guinea-pigs as a whole compared with man, the differences that exist are more of degree than of kind.

(3) **Acquirement of Sensitivity**

In patients where the sensitivity is specific for a single allergen, it is very likely that sensitisation has been brought about by a previous contact with the allergen, although it may not be possible to obtain a history of such contact. With allergens such as pollens, or dusts of animal origin, it is impossible to exclude a previous contact because of their ubiquitous nature, and with some allergens the history of previous contact may be quite evident.

Sensitisation may occur very early in life, but whether it occurs *in utero* is still a matter of controversy. If it does occur, it is not due to a passive transfer from the mother, but an active sensitisation brought about by contact with allergens, perhaps in the mother's diet. There is little doubt that the newborn child can be sensitised by the proteins in the mother's diet transmitted via the milk. It has been repeatedly shown that the absorption into the circulation of unaltered protein in the food is a physiological phenomenon occurring throughout life, but particularly in newborn infants, in sensitive and non-sensitive subjects alike. It would seem possible, therefore, that proteins in the mother's diet pass into her circulation unchanged, from there to her milk and then pass, still unchanged, through the child's intestinal wall. Since only minute quantities are probably required to sensitise, this route of sensitisation may not be so unlikely as it first appears. Infants fed only on human milk have been shown to be sensitised to cow's milk by five weeks of age,[10] and it can only be inferred that this was due to cow's milk in the mother's diet.

(4) **Passive Transfer of Sensitivity**

Human antibodies of the classical type (IgG) will effectively sensitise guinea-pigs for anaphylactic shock. In this they resemble rabbit antibodies, so much studied in anaphylaxis in the guinea-pig (Chapter 38). As with these, there is a direct relation between anaphylactic sensitisation and the content of antibody demonstrable by *in vitro* tests (complement fixation and precipitation). However, sera from atopic sensitive individuals fail to sensitise guinea-pigs or any other laboratory animal with the exception of the monkey. Nor can antibodies be demonstrated by *in vitro* tests. Transfer however, is possible in man. Atopic blood donors have been known to transmit their sensitivity passively to

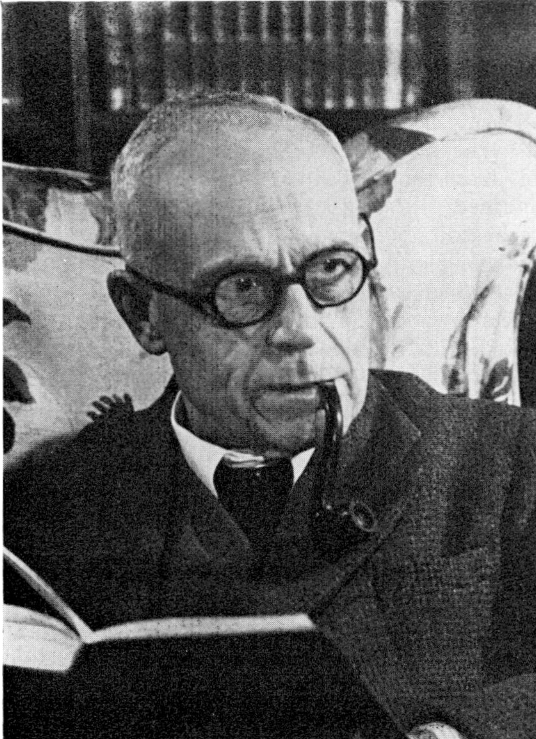

39/FIG. 1.—Carl Prausnitz (Giles) 1876–1963, from a portrait kindly supplied by himself.

recipients, and Prausnitz (FIG. 1) and Küstner in 1921 discovered that serum from atopic individuals injected into the skin of normal individuals would produce local sensitivity confined to the area of injection. An immediate weal and flare reaction developed when allergen was injected into the same site. The test has been used extensively as being the only definitive test available for the study of the sensitising antibodies in atopic sera.

Prausnitz-Küstner (P-K) Reaction.[11]—Küstner was sensitive to a certain species of cooked fish. If some of his serum was injected intracutaneously into the skin of a normal subject, followed by a small quantity of an extract of this fish into the same site twenty-four hours later, a local weal was produced within one and a half hours. In such a test the prepared site is extraordinarily sensitive to allergen. As little as 1/3200 ml. serum is required for sensitisation and as little as $1/10^{10}$ of egg albumin has been known to produce a reaction when the site has been prepared with serum from a person highly sensitive to egg albumin. The allergen need not be injected into the site, but will react even if it is taken by the mouth—further evidence of the absorption of unaltered protein. A latent period of twenty-four hours is usually necessary for fixation of the antibody to the skin before a reaction can be obtained, but in some cases this may be shortened to as little as forty-five minutes. The site remains sensitive for as long as 4–6 weeks. Following a positive Prausnitz-Küstner reaction, the site loses its sensitivity.

The P-K reaction has its counterpart in the passive cutaneous anaphylactic reaction (PCA) in laboratory animals (Chapter 38). It will be recalled that wealing does not occur in these animals, the reaction being demonstrated by injection of a vital dye intravenously which diffuses into a cutaneous site where antigen and antibody have previously been injected.

Just as *homologous* antibodies able to sensitise guinea-pig tissues to general anaphylaxis and PCA (IgG_1) differ in certain ways from antibodies of the classical type (IgG_2), even greater differences are found between sensitising antibodies and those of the classical type in man. For this reason, the sensitising antibodies have been called *reagins*.

We may summarise the properties of reagins as follows: 1. Reagins cannot be demonstrated by the usual *in vitro* techique of complement fixation or precipitation. In this they differ from the guinea-pig "anaphylactic" antibodies (IgG_1) which precipitate with antigen, although they fail to fix complement (Chapter 38). 2. As we have seen, they will not sensitise animals, except monkeys, to anaphylactic shock, or to a passive cutaneous anaphylactic reaction (PCA), but they will sensitise human skin to a P-K reaction. Guinea-pig anaphylactic antibodies are also selective, but have a wider range, being able to sensitise not only their own tissues but those of rats and mice (see ref. 12). 3. Reagins are destroyed at 56° C. for 1 hour, and the activity is not restored by adding fresh non-allergic serum. The thermolability, therefore, is not due to complement.[13] The guinea-pig IgG_1 is thermostable and is not destroyed at 56° for 4 hours. 4. Reagins will not pass from mother to fœtus *in utero*, so that passive sensitisation is never found. In this they resemble antibodies of the 19S type. The evidence suggests, however, that they are of smaller size resembling more closely the 7S antibodies (see below). Their failure to pass the placental barrier may be due either to their affinity with, and binding to, placental tissue or their ability to complex with other serum proteins particularly α_2 macroglobulins. Guinea-pig anaphylactic antibodies are readily transmitted *in utero*. 5. Reagins will not neutralise the allergen, i.e. will not prevent the allergen from producing a P-K reaction in a prepared site. Guinea-pig IgG_1 readily unites with antigen and prevents the union of antigen with fixed IgG_1.

Although in general reagins have the properties listed above, the so-called reagin antitoxin described by Kuhns and Pappenheimer[14] is an apparent exception. After repeated injections of diphtheria toxoid, the serum of both atopic and normal subjects, contained, in addition to antitoxin of the classical type, a skin sensitising type which however united with and neutralised toxin, fixed complement and sensitised guinea-pigs to anaphylactic shock. Although the toxoid used was of a high state of purity, the possibility that reagins had developed from a trace impurity as the result of a prolonged course of immunisation could not be excluded.[15] The existence of a reagin with antitoxic properties must therefore remain unproven.

Numerous attempts have been made to demonstrate reagins and measure their titre in the serum of sensitive subjects by reactions carried out *in vitro*. Agglutination tests with allergens linked to red blood cells have not proved satisfactory, because reagins are almost always accompanied by antibodies of the classical type (blocking antibodies) having the same specificity and equally active in hæmagglutination.

More success has been obtained by the measurement of histamine release from leucocytes when allergen is added to the blood of sensitive individuals. This observation, made 25 years ago by Katz and Cohen,[16] has been fully confirmed by Noah and his colleagues,[17] who have demonstrated a relation between the degree of sensitivity of the individual and the quantity of histamine released *in vitro*. Reagins are firmly bound to leucocytes and cannot be removed by washing, so that leucocyte suspensions from allergic individuals represent a stable system for gauging the degree of sensitivity and hence the quantity of reagin in a patient's serum. By this and other tests it has been estimated that sera of sensitive subjects may contain as little as 0·02 μg antibody N/ml.

Sensitisation of leucocytes could be transferred passively. When leucocytes from normal individuals were treated with serum from sensitive subjects, then thoroughly washed and exposed to allergen, histamine was released, the rate and quantity being determined by the concentration of the reagin in the serum.

The physico-chemical nature of reagins.—In spite of extensive investigations into the nature of reagins by the physico-chemical methods which have proved so fruitful with other antibodies, we are still largely ignorant of their nature. This is partly due to the very low concentrations present in serum, even from highly sensitive individuals, the loss of activity that occurs during quite mild purification processes[18] and the tendency for reagins to bind on to other serum proteins, particularly α_2 macroglobulin. It was at one time thought that at least some of the reagin antibodies were in the fast moving gamma globulin fraction designated IgA.[18, 19, 20] However, recently, considerable doubt has been cast on the possible relation between IgA and reagins by finding that reagins can be present in sera completely devoid of IgA (see 18); also, by the observation that a new type of rapidly migrating gamma globulin, designated IgE, antigenically different from IgA, IgG, or IgM and present in the serum of atopic subjects, has reaginic activity.[22] The further finding by Johansson and Bennich[23] of a patient with myelomatosis having abundant myeloma protein in the serum similar to IgE, may open the way to a study of this new type of immunoglobulin.

Binding of reagins to tissues.—The most characteristic property of reagins which distinguishes them from other types of antibody is the rapid and prolonged fixation to human tissues. Ragweed reacting reagin, transferred to a normal individual, fixes most readily to skin but also to conjunctiva, nasal mucous membranes, linings of the stomach and intestine and leucocytes. It also has an affinity for bronchiolar tissue, as shown by the production of a Schultz-Dale reaction (Chapter 38) with bronchiole rings from a pollen-sensitive asthmatic subject.[24] Passive sensitisation for a S-D reaction of human uterus, appendix and ileum and monkey ileum has also been claimed (for refs. see 12). In human skin removed by biopsy, the site of fixation of pollen reactive reagin appears to be the epithelial cells rather than the underlying mesenchymal tissue. No fixation takes place in skin heated to 60° for 30 minutes, so making it unlikely that adsorption is non-specific (for refs. see 13). The mechanism of fixation is unknown, but some ingenious suggestions have been made as to its nature.

In Chapter 38 we saw that the part of the gamma globulin molecule determining fixation in anaphylactic sensitisation was that part of the H chain designated Fc. In the guinea-pig, homologous sensitisation was determined by the Fc part of IgG_1, antigenically different from that of IgG_2 which failed to sensitise. In the rabbit and man, the Fc fragment of their respective IgG antibodies sensitise guinea-pig, but not homologous, tissues.[2]

With analogies such as these it might be thought that the Fc fragment of the immunoglobulin reagins was concerned in the fixation to human skin. However, the attachment of reagins to human tissues is much firmer and more permanent than the attachment of homologous IgG_1 to guinea-pig tissues, being still present in a passively prepared site after 28 days, whereas IgG_1 only persists for 2–4 days. This suggests that a more active and specific attachment is involved. It has, therefore, been suggested that it is not the Fc fragment of the molecule that is concerned in the fixation and sensitisation by reagin, but the Fab fragment containing the specific antibody (antigen combining) groups. This means that reagin in its fixation to human skin is acting like an antibody to some component of the epithelial cell; in fact an autoantibody. But reagin is an antibody specific for the allergen. To get over the difficulty of postulating a bispecific antibody, which has never been found in the natural state, Stanworth[25] makes use of the known ability of reagin to form complexes with other proteins, and suggests that a dimer is formed between reagin (postulated as an autoantibody to some antigen of the cell) and IgG (a classical type antibody with a specificity directed to the allergen). Two adjacent pairs of dimers fixed to the cell by the Fab areas on the reagin part of the dimer unite with allergen through the free Fab groups of the IgG half of the dimer. There is as yet no experimental data to support this ingenious suggestion.

Desensitisation

In certain types of atopy, particularly hay fever, it has been found that the injection of gradually increasing doses of allergen enables the patient to tolerate larger and larger doses, and gives rise to considerable amelioration of symptoms on exposure to natural contact. At first sight this would appear irrational. If a patient has a hereditary predisposition to produce the reagin type of antibody which does not block the allergen, an increased production of the reagin would, if anything, increase his sensitivity. An explanation was suggested by the work of Cooke and his colleagues,[26] and later of Loveless.[27] Although an actual increase in the amount of reagin may be found, the serum of a patient after treatment with pollen extracts contains a type of blocking antibody more nearly akin to the classical type in failing to fix to human skin, in being thermostable, in having a high affinity with the allergen and in passing the placental barrier. It was found to be of the IgG_2 type. By uniting with the allergen in the circulation, it prevents its union with cell bound reagin. However, the titre of blocking antibody is not directly correlated with the clinical improvement of the patient, suggesting that other factors also play a part.

The Evidence that Atopy depends on the Release of Histamine and SRS-A from Cells

The role of histamine in atopy is less certain than its role in classical anaphylaxis. Brocklehurst[28, 29] has shown that histamine and a slow reacting substance (SRS-A) similar to that found in anaphylaxis were both liberated from isolated preparations of the bronchioles of a boy who reacted to pollen by an attack of asthma. Human bronchioles appeared to be more susceptible to the action of SRS-A than those of other animals, and Brocklehurst suggested that SRS-A is of particular importance in the manifestations of atopy. He showed that SRS-A also lowered the threshold tolerance of the tissues to histamine, and this may explain the increased sensitivity to histamine observed in the atopic subject.[30]

We have already seen that histamine is released from blood leucocytes (basophils) when allergen is added to the blood of atopic subjects.[16, 17]

Further evidence that histamine plays a part in atopy is the relief afforded by the use of antihistamine drugs. These seem to be more effective in the manifestations of atopy due to increased vascular permeability than in those due to contraction of unstriped muscle. This observation supports Brocklehurst's view that factors other than histamine are important in atopic asthma.

Serotonin (5-hydroxytryptamine) appears to play no part in human allergy.[31]

The Delayed Type of Allergy (DTA)

We have now to consider a type of allergy whose manifestations, in contrast to those of the immediate type, appear some hours after contact with the allergen and cannot be directly related to the presence of circulating antibody. This delayed type of allergy is sometimes known as "infective allergy" or "tuberculin type allergy", because it is typically seen in tuberculosis. However, the term "infective allergy" is misleading, for, not only is it not confined to infective disease, but allergy of infective disease is not confined to the delayed type. We have already noted, for instance, that in patients with pneumococcal pneumonia, immediate type allergy can be demonstrated when the type specific polysaccharide of the infecting pneumococcus is injected intracutaneously. Although DTA may play an important part in the pathology of infective disease (e.g. tuberculosis see Chapter 42), it may also be important in the manifestation of such non-infective conditions as contact dermatitis and autoimmune disease (Chapter 40) and the homograft reaction (Chapter 41).

DTA is not confined to man, but can equally well be demonstrated in some, but not all, laboratory animals. The guinea-pig, particularly is a very suitable animal for its manifestation, and in fact DTA was first described in connection with experimental tuberculosis in this animal by Robert Koch (42/Fig. 3). Koch's observations, known as the *Koch phenomenon*, were concerned with the altered reactivity of the guinea-pig to superinfection with the tubercle bacillus compared with that to a primary infection. He described the march of events as follows:

> "If a normal guinea-pig is inoculated with a pure culture of tubercle bacilli, the wound, as a rule, closes and in the first few days seemingly heals. After 10 to 14 days, however, there appears a firm nodule which soon opens, forming an ulcer that persists until the animal dies. Quite different is the result if a tuberculous guinea-pig is inoculated with tubercle bacilli. For this purpose it is best to use animals that have been infected 4 to 6 weeks previously. In such an animal, also, the little inoculation wound closes at first, but in this case no nodule is formed. On the first or second day, however, a peculiar change occurs at the inoculation site. The area becomes indurated and assumes a dark colour, and these changes do not remain

limited to the inoculation point, but spread to involve an area 0·5 to 1·0 cm. in diameter. In the succeeding days it becomes evident that the altered skin is necrotic. It finally sloughs, leaving a shallow ulcer which usually heals quickly and permanently, and the regional lymph nodes do not become infected. The action of tubercle bacilli upon the skin of a normal guinea-pig is thus entirely different from their action upon the skin of a tuberculous one. This striking effect is produced not only by living tubercle bacilli, but also by dead bacilli, whether killed by prolonged low temperature, by boiling or by certain chemicals."

It was later found that if a smaller dose of bacilli than that used by Koch was given, the accelerated inflammation was not attended by sloughing.

Extracts of tubercle bacilli called by Koch "tuberculin" were highly potent in eliciting the reaction. Doses of 0·01 ml., which had no effect on normal guinea-pigs, killed tuberculous animals within a few hours, and as little as 0·00001 ml. injected intracutaneously produced as well-marked inflammatory reaction. The active agent has since been shown to be a protein, tuberculoprotein (PPD), of molecular weight about 10,000. The reaction can readily be obtained in man who is even more easily sensitised than the guinea-pig. The reaction is said to be "delayed" because it does not appear macroscopically for 12–18 hours after injection and reaches its maximum intensity in 24 hours. However, changes can be observed much earlier microscopically. The reaction is an important diagnostic test for tuberculous infections, inapparent or overt, in man and can be performed in a number of ways, the most satisfactory being by the intracutaneous injection of PPD (Mantoux). The response consists of a raised indurated erythematous nodule which may show papules. In severe reactions, necrosis to a variable degree occurs. The histology of the reaction is considered in a later section.

DTA differs in a number of ways from atopy:

(1) **Nature of the Allergen**

Whereas in atopy and anaphylactic sensitisation, the specific allergen can be either polysaccharide or protein, in DTA only proteins are effective.[32, 33] These proteins need not necessarily be derived from infective organisms; by certain procedures discussed below DTA may be produced to serum proteins or to egg albumin.

(2) **Inherited Predisposition**

There is no hereditary predisposition to sensitivity as there is in atopy. Differences in response between individuals, as for instance in the extent of a tuberculin reaction, are not due to some innate inherited difference in the individuals but to differences in the extent of their tuberculous lesions.

(3) **Acquirement of Sensitivity**

The first thing to note is that DTA cannot be produced by introducing the allergen alone into the tissues. For example, guinea-pigs injected with tuberculoprotein will not develop DTA, although they will develop anaphylactic shock on a second application as they would with any other protein. Likewise repeated injections of tuberculoprotein into a tuberculin negative human individual will not produce sensitivity though there is evidence that it will increase the sensitivity of a subject already tuberculin positive (for refs. see Uhr[34]). Sensitivity can, however, be produced by dead tubercle bacilli provided the dose is adequate.

A further advance in our understanding of the mechanism of this type of allergy was made when Dienes[35] found that small amounts of egg albumin or serum proteins, which in ordinary circumstances sensitised guinea-pigs only to anaphylactic shock, produced delayed type sensitisation when injected into a tuberculous focus in a guinea-pig. Subsequently it was found that sensitisation could also be brought about by injecting the protein together with killed tubercle bacilli. By this means sensitivity was acquired not only to the antigen, but to the tuberculoprotein as well.

Some factor in the tubercle bacillus must therefore act as an *adjuvant*. We have already seen that dead tubercle bacilli in Freund's adjuvant enhance the immune response of the classical type to antigens incorporated in it (Chapter 34). Freund's adjuvant has been found to be a highly effective agent also in producing DTA. In fact, as we shall see, sensitivity can be acquired to most proteins, even of homologous and autologous origin, by incorporating them in this adjuvant, which has thus become an important tool in the experimental investigation of the mechanism of DTA. The active agent in the tubercle bacillus appears to be the same as that enhancing the antibody response, namely Wax D, a lipopolysaccharide peptide complex of the wall of the bacillus[36] (see Chapter 34). Thus, antigens incorporated in Freund's adjuvant give rise to two types of immune response: DTA and production of antibody. The time relations of these two responses are different, DTA developing sometimes several days before antibody can be detected.

Attempts have been made to obtain DTA in the absence of an antibody response by using (1) minute doses of antigen injected intracutaneously,[37] (2) antigen complexed with antibody in great excess so blanketing the antigenic groups,[38] (3) protein of low immunogenicity conjugated with large amounts of a hapten (for refs. see 34), which stimulates the production of antibody to the hapten, but only DTA to the protein. These methods have in common the reduction in number of antigenic determinants for antibody production. The first two methods, however, in addition to DTA, stimulate the production of potential immunity (see Chapter 34) and eventually of antibody.[39] Moreover, it has been claimed that the DTA reaction obtained by these methods differs in certain ways from DTA of the tuberculin reaction, or of that produced by protein incorporated into Freund's complete adjuvant. It has been called the "Jones-Mote" type of hypersensitivity[40] from the original description by these authors in 1934.[41] How far the difference is qualitative or merely dependent on intensity of sensitisation is still controversial.

The relation between the production of DTA and antibody is discussed in a later section.

(4) Passive Transfer

No satisfactory evidence, either clinical or experimental has been produced to show that delayed hypersensitivity is dependent on circulating antibodies and can be passively transferred in serum. Indeed, as noted above, it may be found under conditions in which the formation of antibody is suppressed. Nevertheless, successful transfer has certainly been achieved with suspensions of cells. Chase[42] transferred a typical tuberculin-type sensitivity from a tuberculous guinea-pig by using peritoneal exudates produced by injection of paraffin oil, and cells from spleen and lymph gland. The cells were injected intraperitoneally and gave rise to a generalised tuberculin sensitivity of the whole skin, which developed within 1–3 days. This important observation has been repeated many times in animals, and transfer has also been successful in man using blood cells of the buffy layer from a sensitive donor. The factors involved have been studied in some detail by Lawrence[43] who has succeeded in transferring the delayed type of sensitivity to tuberculin, to various streptococcal antigens and to diphtheria toxoid from man to man with blood cells from the buffy coat.

The degree of sensitivity of the recipient depends on the number of cells transferred and the degree of sensitivity of the donor. If a small number of cells are taken from a moderately sensitive donor, the sensitivity produced in the recipient is confined to the site of injection as in the P-K reaction. To produce generalised sensitivity, at least 0·1 ml. of packed cells are necessary in man and considerably larger doses in animals. However, compared with the number of cells that become sensitised in the recipient, such doses are relatively very small.

Transfer in animals can only be achieved with living cells and presumably depends on their ability to survive and grow in the recipient animal. Thus the duration of sensitivity depends on whether the donor and recipient are from the same inbred strain or are cross bred. When donor and recipient are from different strains, tuberculin sensitivity is of maximal intensity immediately after transfer, but wanes over the next few days and disappears after a week. This is probably due to a homograft reaction against the transferred cells (Chapter 41). With inbred strains of guinea-pigs, it is possible to transfer enduring or even permanent tuberculin sensitivity (for refs. see 44). Passive transfer is not confined to tuberculin sensitivity but can be obtained in DTA to other proteins, to contact dermatitis (Chapter 40), to autoimmune diseases such as allergic encephalomyelitis (Chapter 40) and to transplantation immunity (Chapter 41).

It was natural to believe that the transferred cells took part in the hypersensitive reaction when the recipient was challenged with the allergen. However, transfer experiments undertaken with lymph node cells labelled with tritiated thymidine from sensitive donors have generally shown no accumulation of labelled cells in the vicinity of the challenge area, the majority of cells being unlabelled and hence of host origin. Moreover, when guinea-pigs were sensitised to two different allergens, one by active sensitisation and the other by passive sensitisation with cells labelled with tritiated thymidine, the labelled cells were equally distributed between hypersensitive lesions evoked with either allergen, showing that there was no specific attraction for the labelled cells to the deposit of allergen (for refs. see 34).

The major involvement of the host cells in passive transfer of delayed hypersensitivity suggests that there is a passage of information from the cells of the donor to those of the recipient. That some metabolic activity of the transferred cells is required is suggested by the observation that mitomycin C or actinomycin D, which inhibit RNA synthesis and, therefore, protein synthesis, prevented the cells from transferring hypersensitivity, although they remained viable and continued to synthesise about half the protein that would have been expected.[45] Moreover, unlike cells producing antibody, which continue to produce it when transferred to irradiated recipients, cells fail to transfer DTA to an irradiated recipient—further evidence that the host cell is involved.

Transfer in man.—Passive transfer of delayed hypersensitivity with cells from the buffy coat is particularly easy to achieve. The conditions for transfer differ in several features from those with laboratory animals and have been extensively investigated by Lawrence (for refs. see 34). Unlike transfer in guinea-pigs, dead cells disintegrated by freezing and thawing or by distilled water, and cell extracts treated with deoxyribonuclease until the Feulgen reaction became negative, or with ribonuclease, or even with trypsin were effective. The factor associated with the blood leucocytes on which transfer in man depends was obtained in a soluble form by allowing leucocytes from sensitive individuals to stand in fresh serum for $\frac{1}{2}$ to 1 hour at 37° C., when the factor passed from the cells to the serum. This so-called "transfer factor" could also be released specifically by addition of the specific antigen (allergen) to a suspension of the cells in serum. In spite of this specific release by antigen, transfer factor cannot be equated to antibody either of the classical or reagin type. It appears neither to combine with, or be neutralised by, antigen (e.g. diphtheria toxoid, tuberculin), nor to neutralise antigen itself (e.g. diphtheria toxin). Moreover, it is dialysable and has been estimated to have a molecular weight of less than 10,000.

Transfer factor has up till now eluded all attempts to discover its nature. Until more is known about its chemical structure, little profit is obtained by speculations concerning its mode of action.

Nature of the sensitised cell in DTA transference.—Although successful transfer has been achieved with various cell mixtures (blood leucocytes, peritoneal exudates, and cells from lymph nodes, spleen and bone marrow), there is strong evidence that the cell responsible both for active and passive sensitisation is the small lymphocyte: (1) Agents such as cortisone and X-rays suppress DTA in proportion to their effect in lowering the lymphocyte content of the blood; (2) As described in Chapter 5, removal of the thymus in early life results in low levels of circulating lymphocytes with virtual absence of small lymphocytes in lymph nodes and spleen. Such animals have a markedly lowered ability to become sensitised. The correlation between the depletion of small lymphocytes and the inhibition of sensitisation is very close. (3) Successful transfer of DTA is closely correlated with the number of small lymphocytes in the cell suspension. It has been shown that tuberculin sensitivity can be transferred with cells from the thoracic duct of which 95 per cent are small lymphocytes.[46]

It might be added that the above observations incriminating the small lymphocyte as the essential cell in DTA transfer might equally be applied to the production of antibodies, and merely implies that it is the key cell determining both immune responses. This subject is more fully discussed in Chapter 35.

Although the importance of the small lymphocyte in transfer of DTA is well established, the possibility of the macrophage also being concerned has not been entirely ruled out.[47] Certainly, as noted in the next section, it plays an important part in the manifestations of DTA.

Cellular Reactions in Delayed Hypersensitivity

In vivo.—The histology of the development of a delayed type allergic response such as the tuberculin reaction in the skin has been repeatedly studied, but there is still controversy about its nature (for refs. see 34, 48). Whereas some regard it as no different from a classic inflammatory reaction produced by non-specific toxic agents, others believe that the cellular infiltration is of a special kind. The careful observations of Spector and his colleagues[48] on the development of the tuberculin reaction in a large number of guinea-pigs suggest that the initial stages are no different from any other inflammatory reactions. They noted two waves of cell migration from the vessels. The first, occurring at 2–3 hours, consisted of leucocytes predominantly polymorphs, which came to lie in the perivascular zones. In 5–6 hours the polymorphs migrated from these zones leaving the mononuclears, which had migrated with them and had apparently become immobilised in the perivascular zones. In 8 hours, another and more intense migration of polymorphs and mononuclears took place with some fluid exudate, and the histological appearance at this time resembled any other acute inflammation. This was followed by migration of polymorphs into the tissues leaving the mononuclears surrounding the vessels as before. The infiltrate of mononuclear cells reaches its maximum in 24–48 hours and consists almost entirely of cells which have migrated from the blood, as shown by pre-treatment of the guinea-pig with tritiated thymidine.

The administration of tritiated thymidine during the development of the lesion shows that 5–10 per cent of the cells are dividing and frequent mitoses are seen. The infiltration may be so extensive as to produce ischæmia, and it has been suggested that the necrosis seen with intense tuberculin reactions may be due to this cause. Necrosis is not found with DTA to bland proteins.

The nature of the mononuclear cells is controversial, the small and large lymphocytes and monocytes all being considered as possible precursors. The evidence, however, is strongly suggestive that most, if not all, are derived from blood monocytes.[49] Whether the lymphocyte also participates in the reaction is still controversial.[50] Plasma cells are not present except sometimes late in the reaction with the possible development of a superimposed Arthus reaction due to circulating antibody.[51]

Apart from necrotic lesions, Gell and Hinde[52] describe fibrinoid degeneration in vessel walls in severe tuberculin reactions.

In summary.—The histological appearance of DTA reactions consists essentially of a biphasic inflammatory reaction of exaggerated intensity and delayed onset. Lymphocytes, although they are necessary for the development of sensitisation, probably take little or no part in the reaction, the cell predominantly involved being the blood monocyte, which becomes immobilised in the perivascular zone, changes its appearance and may undergo mitosis. These cells migrate from the vessels at the same time as the polymorphs but their numbers are not obvious until the polymorphs have migrated away from the perivascular zone. Necrosis may occur in intense tuberculin reactions probably due to ischæmia from the intense cellular infiltration.

In vitro.—Owing to the complexity of the conditions *in vivo*, attempts have been made to simplify the system by using a population of cells maintained *in vitro*. In 1932 Rich and Lewis[53] described inhibition of migration and cytotoxic changes in spleen and marrow cells in explants taken from highly sensitive tuberculin-positive guinea-pigs when the explants were exposed *in vitro* to PPD. This work has been repeated many times, not always with successful results. Sometimes, in fact, the reverse has occurred—actual stimulation of metabolic activity and proliferation of sensitive cells under the influence of the allergen. Waksman and Matoltsy,[54] for instance, describe the proliferation of "intermediate mononuclears" from the peritoneal cavity of tuberculin sensitive guinea-pigs and the development from them of mature macrophages under the influence of tuberculin, and Mackaness[55] observed increased synthesis of DNA and stimulation of mitosis in macrophages sensitised with bovine serum albumin on contact with the antigen.

In Chapter 37 we have already noted the observations of Mackaness that peritoneal macrophages previously sensitised under conditions leading to delayed hypersensitivity were stimulated to greater metabolic activity, destruction of facultative intracellular parasites and proliferation by contact with specific antigen (cellular immunity). On the other hand, Goldberg and his colleagues,[56] using electron micrographs of skin lesions produced by injection of ferritin into DTA sensitised guinea-pigs, noted degeneration and necrosis of histiocytes (macrophages) which had taken up the antigen.

The cytotoxic changes have been variously described as an inhibition of migration of cells from the explant, or a rounding up, granulation and vacuolation of cells with final death and disintegration. Unlike the cytotoxicity due to antibody and complement, the death of the cell is a slow process usually requiring several hours. Complement is not required.

There has been some controversy concerning the type of cell involved. Rich believed that most if not all cells of the body were sensitive, the inflammatory reaction of a tuberculin reaction being due to substances released from the damaged cell.

Current opinion confines the sensitive cell to certain mesenchymal cells particularly macrophages and fibroblasts. Macrophage migration from lymphoid explants can be inhibited with as little as 9 μg/ml. of antigen. Sensitivity in macrophages from explants of lung and focal lymph node first appears 5 days after sensitisation, when delayed skin reactions are first obtainable, and 2–4 weeks later spreads to macrophages from distal lymph nodes and spleen.[47]

A distinction must be made between cells from sensitised animals which are *sensitive* to the action of the allergen and those that are *sensitised*, that is capable of transferring sensitisation to other animals. We have already seen that the latter are represented by the small lymphocytes. The small lymphocyte, however, does not appear to be sensitive itself as shown by the failure of allergen to inhibit its migration from explants.[57]

Some recent observations of David and his co-workers throw light on this transference of sensitivity from one cell population to another (for refs. see 34, 47). They used an *in vitro* system consisting of cells from paraffin induced peritoneal exudates of guinea-pigs sensitised to tuberculin, diphtheria toxoid or ovalbumin. When these cells were placed in open ended fine capillary tubes and incubated in tissue culture chambers for 24 hours, extensive migration of the cells from the ends of the tubes occurred and spread out on the floor of the chamber. If the specific allergen in quite small doses was mixed with the cell suspension, however, migration was largely prevented (FIG. 2).[58] The reaction was highly specific and reflected the sensitivity of the animal from which the cells were obtained. Cells from guinea-pigs producing antibody, but immunised in ways that did not lead to DTA, were unaffected.

The effect was not shown with normal cells, or with normal cells in the presence of serum rich in antibody, or in the presence of serum from DTA sensitised donors. Normal cells allowed to stand in immune serum and washed were also unaffected, thus excluding "cytophilic antibody" found by Boyden[59, 60] to adsorb to macrophages and spleen cells. However, transfer of sensitivity to normal cells was achieved by mixing with them a proportion of sensitive cells.

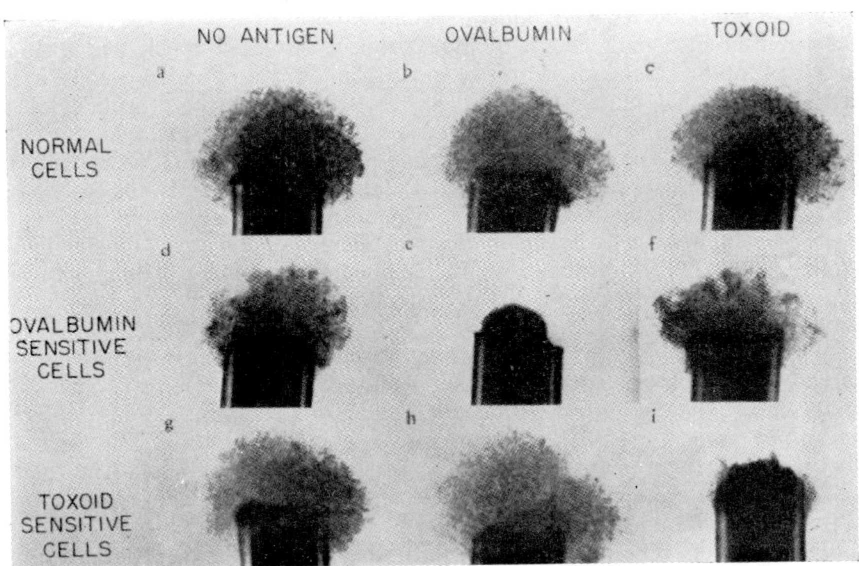

39/Fig. 2.—Effect of ovalbumin and diphtheria toxoid on the migration of peritoneal cells from guinea-pigs exhibiting delayed hypersensitivity to ovalbumin or diphtheria toxoid. Photographs were taken after 24 hr. of incubation. *a*, Normal cells without antigen; *b*, normal cells in presence of ovalbumin; *c*, normal cells in presence of toxoid; *d*, ovalbumin sensitive cells without antigen; *e*, ovalbumin sensitive cells in presence of ovalbumin, migration is inhibited; *f*, ovalbumin sensitive cells in presence of diphtheria toxoid; *g*, toxoid sensitive cells without antigen; *h*, toxoid sensitive cells in presence of ovalbumin; *i*, toxoid sensitive cells in presence of toxoid. Migration is inhibited. (From David, Al-askari, Lawrence and Thomas.[58])

When as little as 2·5 per cent of cells from the peritoneal exudate of a guinea-pig sensitised to a specific allergen was mixed with peritoneal cells from a normal animal, specific inhibition of migration of the whole population occurred on adding the allergen. Further work showed that transfer appeared to be an active property of the sensitive cell. Killed cells were inactive, and antibiotics such as actinomycin D and puromycin which inhibit protein synthesis, as shown by the failure of the cell suspension to incorporate C^{14} labelled leucine, also inhibited the effect of antigen on cell migration. There is thus a close parallel between transfer *in vitro* and *in vivo*, in which, as noted above, the same active synthetic ability was required for transfer from donor to recipient cells.

The paraffin induced peritoneal exudate consists mainly of mature macrophages with some "small round cells", some of which may be immature macrophages and others lymphocytes. While there is no doubt that it is the migration of sensitive macrophages which is inhibited by the allergen, it is likely, on the analogy of transfer *in vivo*, that it is the lymphocyte that transfers the sensitivity to it. Evidence supporting this possibility has been obtained by Bloom and Bennett.[61] They found that the migration of pure suspensions of macrophages from sensitised guinea-pigs containing less than 0·5 per cent lymphocytes was not inhibited by the specific allergen. If, however, 0·6 per cent or more pure suspension of lymphocytes were added, specific inhibition was obtained.

Extending this work, Bennett and Bloom[61a] obtained a cell free protein, capable of inhibiting the migration of macrophages *in vitro* and eliciting a DTA reaction in normal guinea-pig skin *in vivo*, from sensitised lymphocytes by incubating them in the presence of the specific allergen. This so-called *migratory inhibitory factor* (MIF) is produced by guinea-pigs exhibiting DTA sensitisation, but not from animals producing only circulating antibody. It is not to be confused with "transfer factor" which, it will be recalled, is also obtained from sensitised lymphoid cells by incubation with specific allergen. Transfer factor requires serum for its release, is only obtained from human cells and cannot itself elicite a DTA reaction, but transfers sensitivity from one lymphocyte population to another.

In summary.—Macrophages from sensitised animals show three types of changes in contact with specific allergen both *in vitro* and *in vivo*: (1) increased metabolic activity, migration from vessels and proliferation; (2) inhibition of migration; and (3) cytotoxic changes resulting in degeneration and necrosis. Whether these changes represent stages in a single process, or whether more than one factor operates in determining the fate of the macrophage is not understood. Quite small amounts of MIF, the active protein from sensitised lymphocytes, inhibit migration. The mechanism determining stimulation has yet to be discovered. The cytotoxic effect of degeneration and necrosis may be a secondary phenomenon, e.g. ischaemic necrosis due to blockage of vessels with cellular infiltrate. It has been suggested that liberation of lysosomal enzymes from damaged macrophages, and possibly from sensitised lymphocytes undergoing lymphoblastic changes (Chapter 35) also play a part in tissue damage.

DELAYED HYPERSENSITIVITY, IMMUNITY AND THE PRODUCTION OF ANTIBODIES

In spite of extensive research extending over more than half a century, the relation between DTA and immunity is still far from clear.

In the earlier chapters the term "immunity" has been used in two distinct senses: (1) to denote protection against infective disease and (2) in its more immunological sense, to denote induction and production of antibody to antigens which may be bland proteins quite unconnected with infective disease. DTA may be related to immunity used in both these senses.

Does DTA have a Protective Value in Infective Disease?

Its possible implication in cellular immunity to infections with intracellular parasitic bacteria and viruses has already been considered in Chapter 37.

What is the Relation between DTA and Antibody?

Is it an early stage in the formation of antibody, or a sensitisation of cells by preformed humoral antibody or an entirely different immune phenomenon?

These questions remain unresolved. Proponents of the view that DTA represents an early stage of antibody formation, perhaps the induction stage, have been impressed with the fact that the same type of cell, the lymphocyte, to which less than 20 years ago no function could be assigned, now appears to be the key cell determining antibody production (Chapter 35), delayed hypersensitivity, homograft reaction and transplantation immunity (Chapter 41) and some forms of autoimmunity (Chapter 40). Similarity in morphology of cell type, however, does not necessarily denote similarity of function; there is in fact evidence that the lymphocyte population is heterogeneous (Chapter 5).

We may briefly summarise some of the resemblances and differences between DTA and the early stages in antibody production. They are ably discussed in recent reviews.[32, 62]

(1) Phylogenetically, both DTA and antibody production appear at the same point in evolution, namely in the higher cyclostomes represented by the sea lamprey. As this is the most primitive animal to show evidence of lymphoid tissue, it is not surprising that the two appear together

(2) Ontogenetic development also runs parallel. With strong antigens such as phage øX in man, DTA and antibody can be produced *pari passu* by newborn infants, although the capacity of the infant is quantitatively deficient compared with adults.

(3) As we have seen, sensitisation to DTA with minute doses of allergen or antigen-antibody complexes intracutaneously, although not of itself producing antibody for several weeks, induces immunological memory quite early so that subsequent injections produce a secondary antibody response. However, there is doubt whether DTA sensitisation brought about by these procedures is typical.

(4) Both the development of immunological memory and DTA are markedly inhibited by X-irradiation. However, the dose required to depress the latter is 2–4 times greater than that required to suppress the former. The reverse is found with cortisone.

(5) Induction of immunological memory and production of antibody can be carried out without the appearance of DTA by immunising by routes not involving the skin and in the absence of Freund's adjuvant.

(6) We have already noted that DTA cannot be produced with polysaccharide antigen, or antigens whose specificity is determined by polysaccharide haptens, which are usually good stimulants of antibody production. Conversely, certain synthetic polypeptides will induce DTA but do not give rise to antibody.

(7) Passive transfer of immunogenesis and DTA by lymphocytes show certain differences. As already noted, DTA sensitised lymphocytes fail to transfer DTA to X-irradiated recipients, whereas lymphocytes from actively immunised animals produce antibody on transfer. Similarly, newborn infants and guinea-pigs cannot be passively sensitised to DTA by viable leucocytes from sensitive donors, although adoptive transfer of antibody forming cells is particularly effective in these immunologically immature neonates. These differences reflect

a difference in mechanism of transfer. Whereas in passive transfer of immunogenesis it is the transferred lymphocytes themselves which undergo changes to antibody producing cells (Chapter 35), in passive transfer of DTA further transfer of some factor from the donor to the cells (lymphocytes) of the recipient is necessary. If the host cells are deficient through X-irradiation or immaturity, DTA will not take place.

(8) Children suffering from the congenital form of hypogammaglobulinæmia (Chapter 34) who fail to produce antibody globulin, either as a primary or secondary response, can become tuberculin positive through natural infection or can be made so by immunisation with B.C.G. They may be sensitised also to contact dermatitis (Chapter 40).

(9) As noted in Chapter 40, when guinea-pigs are sensitised with certain antigens containing artifically introduced substituent haptens, the specificity to DTA, with a single exception mentioned below, is determined by the whole molecule including the carrier protein. On the other hand, antibody specificity, again with certain exceptions, is directed solely to the hapten group. The exceptions are: (*a*) *p*-azobenzene arsonate, which sensitises guinea-pigs to DTA specific for the hapten group and (*b*) the earliest formed IgM and IgG antibodies to a hapten-protein conjugate which have broad specificity directed to both hapten and carrier protein.[63]

(10) In the chicken, there is some evidence that DTA and antibody production are determined by two different populations of lymphocytes under the initial control of two different lymphoid organs, the bursa of Fabricius and the thymus. Surgical removal of the bursa in 8–9 week old chickens did not affect sensitisation to tuberculin[64] but produced marked suppression of immunological memory and antibody formation. On the other hand thymectomy at hatching had little effect on antibody formation in 6–9 week old chickens, but reduced the intensity of the tuberculin reaction and abolished certain autoimmune reactions determined by DTA (for refs. see 62, 65).

(11) The administration of antigen to newborn guinea-pigs some time before the sensitising dose is given in complete Freund's adjuvant, suppresses the later development of DTA and, temporarily, the formation of antibody (immune tolerance). However, when later the animal recovers its ability to produce antibody, it is still incapable of being sensitised to DTA.[62, 66]

From these considerations it would appear that the differences between DTA and the induction of the mechanism leading to the formation of antibody outweigh the similarities. However, until more is known about the nature of DTA and the mechanism of transfer, no conclusion is possible.

DTA and Cell Bound Antibodies

If DTA does not represent the initiation of antibody formation, is it the result of adsorption of preformed antibody to cells (cytophilic antibody)?

We have already seen that certain special types of antibody, e.g. IgG_1 in the guinea-pig and reagin type antibody in man, have a high affinity for certain cells of the body, e.g. mast cells and epithelial cells. Apart from these "anaphylactic" antibodies, Boyden and his colleagues[59] have described immune globulins, which they term "cytophilic" antibodies, that have an affinity for certain cells. These antibodies, which represent only a small fraction (0·1–1 per cent) of the humoral antibodies of the serum, are 7S in type and resemble the classical IgG antibodies of the serum. They appear to play no part in anaphylactic sensitisation. Certain of these antibodies have an affinity for macrophages and, in view of the importance of the macrophage in DTA, the possibility that DTA is related to adsorption of cytophilic antibodies on to macrophages must be considered.[67] However, we have already seen that such antibodies play no part in the inhibition of the migration of macrophages by allergen *in vitro* in David's experiments. Moreover, the inability to transfer DTA with serum, even when large quantities are used, is an insuperable difficulty to postulating any humoral mechanism for DTA, even if the antibody concerned is in trace amounts. The subject is discussed further by Nelson and Boyden[60] in a recent review.

Cytophilic antibodies are heterogeneous and probably include the cell-bound 19S antibodies to *Salm. typhi murium* of Rowley and his colleagues[68] which appear to be important in immunity to mouse typhoid (see Chapter 37), but there is no evidence that these are concerned in delayed hypersensitivity to antigens of this organism.

Allergy of the Serum Sickness Type

This term was first used by von Pirquet and Schick[69] to describe a multiplicity of signs and symptoms following the injection of therapeutic horse serum antitoxin in man. Unlike anaphylaxis, for which previous sensitisation is necessary, it develops after the first dose of serum, but only after a variable latent period of about a week. Relatively large doses of serum are required. For instance, von Pirquet and Schick found that 85 per cent of persons injected with 100–200 ml. of serum developed serum sickness, but with smaller doses the incidence fell off rapidly. With larger doses of 300–500 ml., the incidence also fell off.

The earliest sign is a localised urticarial rash appearing at the site of injection. This is followed by signs of a generalised reaction referable to increased permeability of the vascular endothelium, such as generalised urticaria, œdema and congestion of lymph glands draining the local site of injection, which may extend to other lymph glands, and œdema of the loose tissues of the eyelids and lips and dependent parts of the body. There is often pyrexia. As with anaphylaxis, a constant finding is a marked leucopenia affecting the polymorphonuclear leucocytes: cell counts may fall as low as 200/c.mm. The fall is rapid and coincident with the onset of symptoms. Evidence obtained from experimental serum sickness in rabbits, described below, suggests that the leucopenia is due to sequestration of leucocytes in the arterial walls particularly those of the heart, lung, mesentery, pancreas and spleen and beneath the endocardium of the valves of the heart. They have also been found in the œdematous lesions of the skin. Their possible role in the pathogenesis of the condition is discussed below.

The Mechanism of Serum Sickness

The occurrence of the disease is related to the presence of the antigens in horse serum, and bears no relation to the antitoxin content of the serum. The symptoms are due to an immune response taking place at a time when considerable amounts of the serum antigens are still present in the body. The incubation period of the disease (about 7–10 days) corresponds to the latent period which may precede an immune response to the primary injection of a soluble antigen. Dixon and his colleagues[70] extended their studies on the relation between the rate of elimination of labelled antigen and the development of the immune response in rabbits (see Chapter 34) to throw light on the mechanism of serum sickness. When they injected into rabbits a single large dose of bovine serum albumin labelled with I^{131}, a protein as effective as whole serum in producing experimental serum sickness but with a longer incubation period, they noted that the elimination of the foreign protein followed the usual three stage course they had observed with other labelled antigens (Chapter 34). A rapid fall lasting

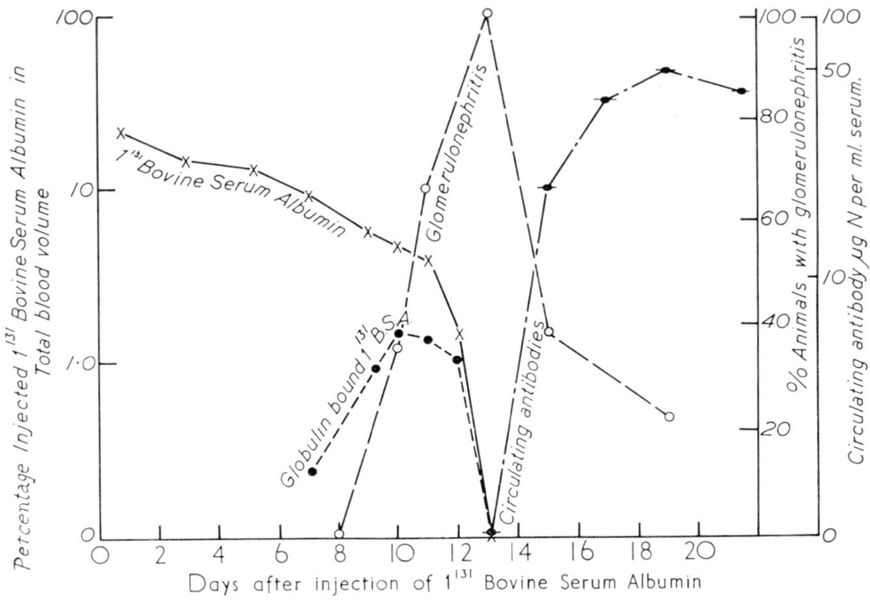

39/FIG.3—Time relations between fall of circulating antigen, formation of antigen-antibody complexes, lesions of serum sickness and rise of circulating antibody in rabbits injected with large doses of I^{131} labelled bovine serum albumin. (After Dixon *et al.*[70])

a few hours, due to equilibration between the blood and tissues, was followed by a slower fall due to metabolism of the foreign serum albumin at the same rate as that of the animal's own serum albumin. This lasted 10–11 days (rather longer than with bovine globulin (34/FIG. 2), which gives a more rapid immune response), and was followed by a greatly accelerated fall due to an increased rate of metabolism brought about by the development of an immune response to it (FIG. 3). This continued until about the 13th day when no circulating antigen was left. Towards the end of the second and beginning of the third phases, analysis showed that much of the labelled albumin remaining in the circulation was united to globulin and could be precipitated by half saturation with ammonium sulphate. There was evidence that these albumin-globulin complexes were soluble antigen-antibody complexes containing great excess of antigen. Free antibody was only detected after all the labelled antigen, either free or bound to antibody, had been removed both from the circulation and from the tissues.

There is no reason to believe that the type of antibody that forms these complexes with antigen is any different from the precipitating antibody of the classical type which eventually appears in the circulation. However, reagin type antibody is probably present as shown by the immediate weal and flare reaction when horse serum is injected intracutaneously, a reactivity which persists after the patient has become convalescent. Also the patient's serum will prepare a skin site for a P-K reaction. However, there are no other manifestations of atopy, e.g. those associated with muscular spasm, and indeed serum sickness must be clearly distinguished from serum atopy. Reagin, therefore, must play only a minor role in the serum sickness syndrome, being perhaps responsible for the urticarial rash.

It is of course well known that antibody-antigen complexes in the region of antigen excess are soluble, and it is probable that their rapid removal from the circulation and from the tissues coincident with the appearance of free antibody is brought about by the union of more antibody with the complex to make the proportion of antigen and antibody nearer the equivalence zone. Such antibody-antigen complexes at the equivalence zone, which are probably in too low a concentration to give a visible precipitate, are known to be taken up by the reticulo-endothelial system of the liver and spleen and are rapidly metabolised.[71] The soluble complexes formed initially, however, which contain great excess of antigen, and are consequently of smaller molecular size, are much less readily taken up by the recticulo-endothelial cells and continue to circulate with a half life of 2 days.[70]

In the few cases of serum sickness coming to autopsy characteristic inflammatory changes in the arteries of the internal organs, particularly the heart and kidneys, are found. Similar changes can be produced experimentally in rabbits injected intravenously with a large dose of serum,[72] and Dixon and his colleagues[70] also noticed these lesions in rabbits injected with a large dose of bovine serum albumin labelled with I^{131}.

Experimental Serum Sickness in Rabbits

A full account of the lesions following a single injection of a large dose of heterologous serum protein intravenously is given by McClusky.[73] The lesions consist of a glomerulonephritis with proliferation of the vascular endothelial cells, narrowing and obliteration of the capillary lumina with intracapillary deposition of fibrin. There is little polymorph infiltration. In contrast, the arterial lesions consist of focal segmental infiltration of the entire vessel walls with mononuclear cells and polymorphs with areas of necrosis in the media and proliferation of endothelial cells. The lesions are most marked in the smaller arteries of heart, lung, mesentery, pancreas and spleen but the aorta and larger pulmonary arteries are also affected. The inflammatory process may involve the aortic and mitral valve with subendocardial mononuclear and polymorph infiltration.

Dixon and his colleagues[70] using bovine serum albumin labelled with I^{131} showed that there was a definite time relation between the appearance and duration of glomerulonephritis and the appearance and duration of soluble antigen-antibody complexes in the circulation. The lesions commenced at the point of inflection of the curve of antigen elimination, where normal metabolic rate of antigen breakdown gave place to immune elimination (FIG. 3), and were approximately proportional in extent and severity to the amount of globulin-bound labelled antigen in the blood. With the increase in immune response, higher ratios of antibody to antigen in the complexes and more rapid removal from the blood by the reticulo-endothelial cells, the lesions abated.

That the lesions were the result of an antigen-antibody reaction with antigen excess and did not involve cellular factors (e.g. those of delayed hypersensitivity) was shown by Germuth and Pollack[74] who infused antibody into rabbits 24 hours after they had received a large intravenous dose of antigen. In this passively transferred serum sickness, lesions in arteries and glomeruli were observed within 25 hours, but little leucocytic infiltration was present.

The direct cause of the lesions of experimental serum sickness is still obscure. There is no doubt that both rabbit antibody and bovine antigen are present in the lesions as shown by immunofluorescent techniques. Heavy deposits were noted in the media of the arteries and glomeruli.[70] No deposition of antigen occurred before the immune response had developed, and no lesions were found if the response was inhibited by administration of nitrogen mustard or by X-irradiation. With the rise of antibody in the blood, the complexes segregated in the tissues disappeared.

It has been suggested that serum sickness is a generalised form of the Arthus phenomenon (Chapter 38), the lesions of which, it will be recalled, were attributed to a local collection of polymorphs attracted to components of complement fixed to the antigen-antibody complexes. As noted above, profound leucopenia may be associated with serum sickness and, in the experimental disease, many of these leucocytes have been found in the lesions. However, as we have seen, not all lesions contain polymorphs and in some the mononuclear infiltration is as marked as that of the polymorphs. It seems likely that polymorphs participate to some extent in the arterial and valvular lesions, but not in the glomerular lesions in which they are absent. Moreover, fibrinoid necrosis of arterial walls has been produced in experimental serum sickness in the virtual absence of polymorphs.[73] It would seem, therefore, that polymorphs do not play the major role in serum sickness that they do in the Arthus phenomenon.

Experimental Serum Sickness and the Production of Antibody

Not all rabbits develop serum sickness on intravenous injection with serum protein. Dixon and his colleagues[75] noted that rabbits repeatedly injected with bovine serum albumin responded in one of 3 ways according to the rapidity with which they made antibody. The first group, good antibody producers, suffered from only a transient glomerulonephritis which quickly abated as their reticulo-endothelial cells rapidly removed the antigen in immune complexes. The second, which failed to produce antibody sufficiently rapidly, developed chronic lesions of serum sickness with soluble complexes persisting in the circulation. The third group, poor producers of antibody, were devoid of lesions, and antigen in the uncombined state persisted in the circulation. These latter probably correspond to human subjects given excessively large doses of horse serum in which the immune response would be depressed (Chapter 41).

Immediate and Accelerated Serum Sickness in Man

Individuals given a second injection of serum antitoxin rarely develop anaphylactic symptoms unless they are atopic subjects, but do react with a greatly accelerated and sometimes immediate development of serum sickness. This is clearly due to accelerated antibody production brought about by a secondary response.

The Role of Histamine in Serum Sickness

That histamine may play a part in the œdematous lesion of serum sickness in man is suggested by the response to antihistamine drugs. It is possible that its release is a secondary result of damage to mast cells in the arterial lesions and, in the rabbit, to platelets, clumps of which have been shown in the vicinity of the lesion. Its release may be responsible for the œdematous lesions in skin and soft tissues.

Summary

Allergic disorders, determined by immunological reactions *in vivo*, may be the result of natural diseases, or may be brought about artificially by therapeutic agents or experimental procedures. The antigen concerned may be exogenous or endogenous. Disorders due to exogenous antigens are divided according to the rate of development of the hypersensitive reaction following contact with the exciting allergen into: (1) immediate. (2) delayed and (3) serum sickness type.

In the immediate type, the reaction begins within a few minutes and circulating antibody can usually be demonstrated in the serum. The lesions are those associated with increased permeability of capillary endothelium and contraction of unstriped muscle and are of short duration. They include experimental anaphylaxis in animals (Chapter 38) and atopy in man. Atopic subjects have an inherited tendency to develop acute reactions to foreign allergens, which may take the form of an anaphylactic shock, asthma, acute coryza, gastro-intestinal disorders and urticarial rashes. The skin and mucous membranes are usually sensitive to the allergen and respond to intracutaneous injection by an immediate weal and flare reaction. The serum of these subjects contains "anaphylactic" antibody of a special type called reagin. Reagins are probably a new kind of immunoglobulin (IgE). They differ from the classical IgG and IgM antibodies in a number of ways, particularly in having a high affinity for human epithelium and other human tissues. They cannot be demonstrated by the usual serological reactions *in vitro*, but will transfer sensitivity to other individuals but not to animals (Prausnitz-Küstner reaction). The addition of allergen to a suspension of leucocytes from a sensitive subject will liberate histamine from the cells, the amount liberated being determined by the concentration of reagin in the serum. Desensitisation by doses of allergen may be related to the formation of IgG antibody which unites with the allergen and blocks its union with fixed reagin. The symptoms and signs of atopic reactions are determined by the release of histamine and possibly also by the formation of SRS-A.

Delayed type allergy (DTA) occurs naturally in certain bacterial infections (e.g. tuberculosis) or it may be produced artificially by injecting the allergen with Freund's adjuvant. The reaction following contact of the tissues with allergen for a second time occurs after a delay of twenty-four hours and consists of a slowly developing indurated inflammatory reaction containing large numbers of mononuclear cells. The manifestations are not due to circulating antibody and are not the result of an action on vascular endothelium or on unstriped muscle. Passive transfer cannot be achieved with serum, but can be achieved with lymphoid cells from lymph nodes, spleen or buffy coat to recipients of the same species and preferably of the same strain. There is strong evidence that the cell concerned in transfer is the lymphocyte, but the donor cells are not concentrated in the lesions induced in the recipient by the allergen, which seem to contain mainly the recipient's own cells. In man, but not in animals, transfer has been achieved with a dialysable extract of sensitive cells. The nature and mode of action of this "transfer factor" is unknown. The origin of the inflammatory cells in the lesions of DTA is controversial. The evidence strongly suggests that they arise from the blood monocytes. Allergen specifically prevents migration of peritoneal macrophages from sensitised animals from a local site *in vitro*. The migration of normal macrophages is also inhibited if mixed with a small percentage of sensitised cells. There is evidence that the cell which transfers this property to normal macrophages is a sensitised lymphocyte. Sensitised lymphocytes incubated with the specific allergen release a protein which inhibits the migration of normal macrophages and produces a DTA reaction in normal guinea-pig skin.

DTA is probably not a step in the pathway to antibody synthesis.

Serum sickness is brought about by the injection of a relatively large amount of horse serum which is present in the tissues at the time when antibody is starting to be formed. It comes on six to ten days after the injection, and the manifestations are those due to increased capillary permeability due to histamine release. The lesions are probably due to localisation of soluble antigen-antibody complexes containing antigen in excess in the walls of the arteries of the internal organs. The symptoms and signs abate when free antibody appears in the circulation due to the rapid removal of these complexes. The antibody concerned is of the classical IgG and IgM types, although the reagin type may be responsible for the urticarial rash.

REFERENCES

1. Jensen, O. F. (1962). *Acta path. microbiol. scand.*, **54**, 9.
2. Ratner, B. (1945). *J. Amer. med. Ass.*, **127**, 696.
3. McMaster, P. D. (1959). *Cellular and Humoral Aspects of the Hypersensitive States*. (Symp. N.Y. Acad. Med., **9**, 319). Ed., Lawrence, H. S. New York: Hoeber-Harper.
4. Cooke, R. A. (1942). *Ann. intern. Med.*, **16**, 71.
5. Sherman, W. B. (1959). *Ann Rev. Med.*, **10**, 207.
6. Augustin, R. (1953). *Congr. int. Microbiol., VI. Riassunti di Commun.*, **1**, 432.
7. Rimington, C., and Maunsell, K. (1950). *Int. Arch. Allergy*, **1**, 115.
   Rimington, C. (1951) in Ref. 8, p. 252.
8. Abramson, H. A. (1951). *Treatment of Asthma*, p. 219. Baltimore: Williams & Wilkins.

9. Kuhns, W. J., and Pappenheimer, A. M., Jr. (1952). *J. exp. Med.*, **95,** 363, 375. Kuhns, W. J. (1953). *J. exp. Med.*, **97,** 903; (1954) **99,** 577; (1955) **101,** 109. Pappenheimer, A. M., Jr. (1955). *J. Immunol.*, **75,** 259.
10. Laroche, G., Richet, C. (Fils), and Saint-Girons, F. (1930). *Alimentary Anaphylaxis*, p. 74, trans. by M. P. Rowe and A. H. Rowe. Berkeley, California: University of California Press.
11. Prausnitz, C., and Küstner, H. (1921). *Zbl. Bakt.*, **86,** 160.
12. Bloch, K. J. (1967). *Progr. Allergy*, **10,** 84.
13. Stanworth, D. R. (1963). *Advanc. Immunol.*, **3,** 181.
14. Kuhns, W. J., and Pappenheimer, A. M., Jr. (1962). *J. Immunol.*, **89** 652.
15. Finger, J., and Kabat, E. A. (1958). *J. exp. Med.*, **108,** 453.
16. Katz, G., and Cohne, S. (1941). *Amer. J. Med.*, **3,** 545.
17. Noah, J. W., and Brand, A. (1961). *J. Allergy*, **32,** 236.
18. Sehon, A. H. (1965). *Molecular and Cellular Basis of Antibody Formation*, p. 227. Ed. Šterzl, J. New York: Academic Press.
19. Vaerman, J. P., Epstein, W., Fudenberg, H., and Ishizaka, K. (1964). *Nature* (*Lond.*), **203,** 1046.
20. Fudenberg, H. (1965). *Ann. Rev. Microbiol.*, **19,** 301.
21. Fireman, P., Vannier, W. E., and Goodman, H. C. (1963). *J. exp. Med.*, **117,** 603.
22. Ishizaka, K., Ishizaka, T., and Hornbrook, M. M. (1966). *J. Immunol.*, **97,** 75.
23. Johansson, S. G. O., and Bennich, H. (1967). *Immunology*, **13,** 381. Johansson, S. G. O., Bennich, H., and Wide, L. (1968). *Immunology*, **14,** 265.
24. Schild, H. O., Hawkins, D. F., Mongar, J. L., and Herxheimer, H. (1951). *Lancet*, **2,** 376.
25. Stanworth, D. R. (1965). *Int. Arch. Allergy*, **28,** 71.
26. Cooke, R. A., Barnard, J. H., Hebald, S., and Stull, A. (1935). *J. exp. Med.*, **62,** 733.
27. Loveless, M. H. (1940). *J. Immunol.*, **38,** 25; (1943) **47,** 165.
28. Brocklehurst, W. E. (1956). *Histamine*. CIBA Foundation Symp. edited by G. E. W. Wolstenholme and C. M. O'Connor, p. 175. London: J. & A. Churchill.
29. Brocklehurst, W. E. (1962). *Progr. Allergy*, **6,** 539.
30. Rose, B. (1947). *Amer. J. Med.*, **3,** 545.
31. Brocklehurst, W. E. (1956). *J. Physiol.* (*Lond.*), **120,** 16P.
32. Dienes, L. (1931). *J. Immunol.*, **20,** 333.
33. Freund, J., and Bonanto, M. (1944). *J. Immunol.*, **48,** 325.
34. Uhr, J. W. (1966). *Physiol. Rev.*, **46,** 359.
35. Dienes, L. (1929). *J. Immunol.*, **17,** 531.
36. White, R. G. (1967). *Brit. med. Bull.*, **23,** 39.
37. Salvin, S. R. (1958). *J. exp. Med.*, **107,** 109.
38. Uhr, J. W., Salvin, S. B., and Pappenheimer, A. M., Jr. (1957). *J. exp. Med.*, **105,** 11.
39. Coe, J. E., and Salvin, S. B. (1964). *J. Immunol.*, **93,** 495.
40. Martin, A. B., and Raffel, S. (1964). *J. Immunol.*, **93,** 937.
41. Jones, T. D., and Mote, J. R. (1934). *New Engl. J. Med.*, **210,** 120.
42. Chase, M. W. (1946). *J. Bact.*, **51,** 643.
43. Lawrence, H. S. Ed. (1959). *Cellular and Humoral Aspects of the Hypersensitive States*, p. 279, Chap. 7. (Symp. Sect. Microbiol., N.Y. Acad. Med.) New York: Hoeber-Harper.
44. Arnason, B. G., and Waksman, B. H. (1964). *Advanc. Tuberc. Res.*, **13,** 1.
45. Bloom, B. R., Hamilton, L. D., and Chase, M. W. (1964). *Nature* (*Lond.*), **201,** 689.
46. Wesslen, T. (1952). *Acta tuberc. scand.*, **26,** 38.
47. Dumonde, D. C. (1967). *Brit. med. Bull.*, **23,** 9.

48. SPECTOR, W. G. (1967). *Brit. med. Bull.*, **23,** 35.
49. VOLKMAN, A., and GOWANS, J. L. (1965). *Brit. J. exp. Path.*, **46,** 50, 62.
50. TURK, J. L. (1967). *Brit. med. Bull.*, **23,** 3.
51. GELL, P. G. H., and BENACERRAF, B. (1961). *Advanc. Immunol.*, **1,** 319.
52. GELL, P. G. H., and HINDE, I. T. (1951). *Brit. J. exp. Path.*, **32,** 516.
53. RICH, A. R., and LEWIS, M. R. (1932). *Bull. Johns Hopk. Hosp.*, **50,** 115.
54. WAKSMAN, B. H., and MATOLTSY, M. (1958). *J. Immunol.*, **81,** 220.
55. MACKANESS, G. B. (1967). *Progr. Allergy*, **11,** 89.
56. GOLDBERG, B., KANTOR, F. X., and BENACERRAF, B. (1962). *Brit. J. exp. Path.*, **43,** 621.
57. HEILMAN, D. H. (1963). *Tex. Rep. Biol., Med.*, **21,** 136.
58. DAVID, J. R., AL-ASKARI, S., LAWRENCE, H. S., and THOMAS, L. (1964). *J. Immunol.*, **93,** 264.
59. BOYDEN, S. V. (1963). *Cell Bound Antibodies*, p. 7. Eds. AMOS, B., and KOPROVSKI, H. Philadelphia: Wistar Institute Press.
60. NELSON, D. S., and BOYDEN, S. V. (1967). *Brit. med. Bull.*, **23,** 15.
61. BLOOM, B. R., and BENNETT, B. (1966). *Science*, **153,** 80.
61a. BENNETT, B., and BLOOM, B. R. (1968). *Proc. nat. Acad. Sci.* (*Wash.*), **59,** 756.
62. SZENBERG, A., and WARNER, N.L . (1967). *Brit. med. Bull.*, **23,** 30.
63. GELL, P. G. H., and WOLSTENCROFT, R. A. (1967). *Brit. med. Bull.*, **23,** 21.
64. JANOVIC, B. D., and ISVANESKI, M. (1963). *Int. Arch. Allergy*, **23,** 188.
65. WARNER, N. L., and SZENBERG, A. (1964). *Ann. Rev. Microbiol.*, **18,** 253.
66. TURK, J. F., and HUMPHREY, J. H. (1961). *Immunology*, **4,** 310.
67. KARUSH, F., and EISEN, H. M. (1963). *Science*, **136,** 1032.
68. ROWLEY, D., TURNER, K. J., and JENKIN, C. R. (1964). *Aust. J. exp. Biol. med. Sci.*, **42,** 237.
69. PIRQUET, C. VON, and SCHICK, B. (1905). *Die Serumkrankheit.* Leipzig; (1951). English transl. by B. SCHICK. Baltimore: Williams & Wilkins.
70. DIXON, F. J., VAZQUEZ, J. J., WEIGLE, W. O., and COCHRANE, C. G. (1959). See Ref. 43, Chapter 9, p. 354.
71. BENACERRAF, B., SEBESTYEN, M., and COOPER, N. S. (1959). *J. Immunol*, **82,** 131.
72. RICH, A. R. (1946–47). *Harvey Lect.*, **42,** 106.
73. MCCLUSKEY, R. T. (1965). *The Inflammatory Process*, p. 649, Chap. 20. Eds. ZWEIFACH, B. W., GRANT, L., and MCCLUSKEY, R. T. New York: Academic Press.
74. GERMUTH, F. G., and POLLACK, A. D. (1958). *Bull. Johns Hopk. Hosp.*, **102,** 245.
75. DIXON, F. J., FELDMAN, J. D., VAZQUEZ, J. J. (1961). *J. exp. Med.*, **113,** 899.

Chapter 40

REACTIONS TO ALLERGENS IN PART OR WHOLLY ENDOGENOUS: DRUG ALLERGY AND AUTOIMMUNITY

BY G. P. GLADSTONE

HAVING considered in the last chapter disorders due to allergens introduced from the external environment, we have to consider now disorders brought about by allergens derived in part or wholly from within the tissues of the sensitive individual. The reaction *in vivo*, which is the direct cause of these disorders, may be the result of an immune response of the sensitive individual to his tissues (autoimmunisation) or may be due to antibody introduced from without as in hæmolytic disease of the newborn. We shall begin by considering drug allergy, a type of allergy in which the allergen is partly introduced from without and partly derived from the body tissues.

DRUG ALLERGY

Drug allergy has been defined as hypersensitivity to chemical substances of a molecular weight less than 1000.[1]

It has frequently been observed that workers in chemical industries, chemists, pharmacists, doctors and patients treated with certain therapeutic drugs suffer from general or local reactions exhibiting many of the features of the hypersensitive states that we have considered in Chapter 39. The same signs and symptoms may be elicited by drugs of very different pharmacological action. The condition, therefore, must be clearly distinguished from drug intolerance which is a heightened susceptibility to the pharmacological action of the drug.

Although the agents responsible for drug allergy are many times smaller than proteins and clearly cannot be considered as antigens, there is strong evidence that the condition resembles other forms of allergy in being determined by an immunological reaction *in vivo*. There is usually a history of previous contact with the drug, or one closely related to it. When the drug is first used no reaction takes place. There may then be a latent period of some weeks, months or even years, after which subsequent contact with the drug brings about a reaction. This shows the same degree of specificity that one associates with an immune reaction, the more easily appreciated since the allergen is of known chemical composition, making it often possible to relate sensitivity to a particular easily recognised chemical group. Sensitivity to aspirin may thus be directed to its acetyl group or salicylic acid moiety or to the whole molecule. Sensitivity may be transferred passively either with serum or with cells of the sensitised donor. The transferred sensitivity shows the same specificity as that of the actively sensitised donor.

Linkage of Drugs with Tissue Proteins and Cells *in vivo*

How can these substances of low molecular weight induce immunological reactions which we normally associate with proteins? The clue to our understanding of this problem was first suggested by the classical work of Landsteiner and his colleagues,[2] to which reference has already been made (Chapter 38), who showed that guinea-pigs could be sensitised to anaphylactic shock by injecting simple compounds such as picryl chloride intracutaneously, or intraperitoneally in a water-in-oil emulsion with dead tubercle bacilli (Freund's adjuvant). They noted that these drugs readily united with serum protein and suggested that sensitivity in drug allergy is brought about by a spontaneous linkage of the drug with proteins of the body *in vivo*. Subsequent work by Eisen and his colleagues[3] has amply confirmed this view.

These authors compared eight 2,4-dinitrophenyl compounds, with a high degree of configurational uniformity, for their ability to elicit local reactions in the skin of sensitised persons. Only four of the compounds were effective, and these were shown to form covalent bonds with serum albumin *in vitro* and with skin proteins *in vivo*. The inactive compounds, on the other hand, formed no such linkages with protein. The conditions determining linkage of drugs to protein have been reviewed by Eisen.[1] The bond between drug and protein must be firm and covalent bonds, stable under physiological conditions, best satisfy these requirements. Co-ordinate bonds may also be sufficiently stable, but weaker bonds of van der Waals and ionic types, which are commonly concerned in binding many compounds of small molecular weight to serum albumin, and which are readily broken, are not effective. Union to protein takes place through such amino-acid residues as lysine, cysteine, tyrosine and histidine. Drugs capable of reacting with protein usually do so irrespective of the nature of the protein, but in at least one case a particular protein is required: 2,4-dinitrobenzene sulphonate reacts at neutral pH with the protein of epidermis and hair by splitting disulphide bonds to form 2,4-dinitrophenyl-cysteinyl residues but fails to form complexes with five other proteins including serum albumin and globulin. On the other hand it may happen that conjugation *in vivo* is different from that *in vitro*. For example, 2,4-dinitrochlorobenzene reacts *in vitro* equally readily with keratin and with collagen. In the skin of the guinea-pig, however, it will only react with keratin of the epidermis and not with collagen in the dermis, possibly because of interference in the latter site by mucopolysaccharides.

The protein may also have an importance in the manifestation of drug allergy. As will be seen later, drugs capable of sensitising the skin to contact dermatitis, a delayed type of drug allergy, although capable of uniting with many different proteins will only sensitise by union with a particular protein or proteins contained in the skin. The protein apparently contributes to the specificity of the drug-protein conjugate.

The ability of a compound to form firm bonds with protein is not the only factor that determines its ability to sensitise. Other factors are the rate of hydrolytic destruction of the complexes and the inherent antigenicity of the residual group determining specificity after it has united with protein.[4] A metabolic or degradation product of the drug, provided it retains the specificity of the drug, may be the inducer and this may account for the fact that most commonly used drugs, e.g. quinine, aspirin and sulphonamides, which are incapable of forming firm bonds with protein at physiological pH values, nevertheless induce hypersensitivity. Some drugs may sensitise by reacting with protein both in an unchanged state and after preliminary degradation *in vivo*. For instance, there is evidence (for refs. see 5) that sensitivity to penicillin may be brought about in either of these ways; pencillin may react directly with the ε-amino group of lysine in the protein or after rearrangement to its highly reactive isomer penicillenic acid. This isomer is formed spontaneously both *in vivo* and *in vitro*. Sensitisation is of the immediate (anaphylactic) type (see below). Penicillin may also react after hydrolysis *in vivo* through penicilloic acid to further degradation products which probably unite with cysteine residues in the protein. Reactivity through penicilloic acid leads to the delayed (contact dermatitis) type of sensitivity.*

Sometimes the antigen-antibody reaction involving the drug takes place on or in the vicinity of the platelets, red cells and leucocytes. This results in lysis of the cells by complement and brings about drug-induced thrombocytopenia, hæmolytic anæmia or agranulocytosis. Although the presence of the drug and antibody specifically determined by it are necessary, neither appears to be firmly bound to the blood cells. The mechanism involved in this form of drug allergy is discussed in a later section.

Classification of Drug Allergy

The manifestations of drug allergy may be any of the three types we have considered in Chapter 39.

(1) Allergy of the immediate type: anaphylaxis and drug atopy.

(2) Allergy of the delayed type: contact dermatitis.

(3) Allergy of the serum sickness type.

(4) A fourth type, mentioned above, due to union of drugs with the formed elements of the blood.

Not infrequently more than one of these types can co-exist in the same individual.

Anaphylactic Shock and Atopy due to Drugs

We have already seen (Chapter 38) that simple chemical substances of low molecular weight can be used to sensitise guinea-pigs, but anaphylactic shock cannot subsequently be induced unless the drug is conjugated artificially to protein. The protein here acts merely as a carrier and does not contribute to the specificity of the antigen. On the other hand, in man, anaphylactic shock may result from the injection of the unconjugated drug, although luckily such accidents are rare. However, there is one drug, penicillin, which has been used so universally that there can hardly be a person in civilised countries that has not received a dose at some time in his life. This has resulted in a sufficient number of fatal, or nearly fatal, accidents as to make the subject of some importance.[6] There is usually a history of repeated injection, inhalation, or oral administration of penicillin at some earlier period in the patient's life which, it must be presumed, has brought about sensitisation. In one case quoted by Feinberg[6] the patient, a sufferer from hay fever, had been shown to be sensitive to penicillium spores as well as to grass pollen and had been given repeated injections of

* The possibility has been raised recently[36, 37] that some cases of sensitivity to penicillin are due to a trace protein contaminant in commercial preparations of benzylpenicillin acting as a carrier. In other cases, high molecular weight polymers of penicillin which are formed on standing may be responsible.

extracts of these cells every summer for 17 years in an attempt to desensitise her. She was then given a single dose of penicillin intramuscularly and in a few minutes collapsed with acute symptoms of shock, but recovered. Subsequent scratch tests with crystalline penicillin O and G showed strong wealing within a few minutes. Although subjects sensitive to penicillin are often, as in this case, sensitive to other allergens, this is by no means invariable. There is usually a period of several weeks between the nonreacting (sensitising) and reacting dose. In some cases sensitisation may proceed from a "serum sickness" type of reaction (see later section) to accelerated "serum sickness" reaction and finally to immediate shock, a situation which is also seen in allergy due to other allergens (Chapter 39). The reacting dose is usually given by the intramuscular route but severe and even fatal reactions have been produced by intranasal instillation, insufflation or even oral administration.[7]

The less drastic signs and symptoms of drug atopy resemble those of atopy due to other allergens, that is urticarial rashes, coryza, asthma and gastro-intestinal disorders. However, it is only rarely possible to elicit a skin reaction in a sensitive subject with the unconjugated drug, unless the drug is highly reactive with the skin protein. Even then some time must elapse for efficient conjugation to take place. Sensitivity to penicillin is an exception. It is often possible to demonstrate sensitivity by a scratch test as in the patient quoted above. With less reactive drugs, such as aspirin, a positive immediate type reaction may be elicited when the drug is mixed with the patient's serum before injection or when a tablet of the drug is held against the mucous membrane of the mouth for some minutes. Reagins also can seldom be demonstrated by a Prausnitz-Küstner reaction, but with penicillin and sulphadiazine transfer of sensitivity to local areas of skin of normal individuals has been successfully achieved with serum from sensitive subjects, and a positive P-K reaction has been obtained by injecting these drugs, not as is usually done into the prepared skin site, but intramuscularly at a site distant from it. The reaction is of the usual rapidly developing weal and erythema type.

Drug Allergy of the Delayed Type: Contact Dermatitis

Contact dermatitis is by far the most common form of allergy due to chemical substances of low molecular weight. It occurs wherever persons are exposed to repeated skin contact with certain chemical substances and is found particularly in chemical industrial workers and among patients who have had repeated or prolonged local application of therapeutic agents. The clinical features are a superficial inflammation of the skin, generally with vesiculation more or less restricted to the area of contact of the exciting substance. The pathological process is essentially a superficial chronic inflammation of a local area of skin with swelling of the epithelial cells, vesicle formation and perivascular infiltration of the dermis with mononuclear cells. The lesion has many of the characters associated with that of other forms of delayed type hypersensitivity.

Individual Selection and Induction of Sensitivity

Although most human subjects may be made hypersensitive by repeated contact with many of the agents able to bring about this type of sensitivity, some individuals are more easily sensitised than others, and a few appear to be completely refractory. If a hereditary element exists, it is quite distinct from that determining atopy.

Contact dermatitis is not confined to man. Guinea-pigs may readily be sensitised to many of the drugs producing sensitivity in man. Much of the recent work on the specificity of drug allergy described in a later section has been carried out with this animal.

Acquirement of Sensitivity

Sensitisation can be brought about by the repeated local application of the agent to the surface of the skin. Experimentally this can be carried out by the "patch test", which is also used to test for sensitivity. This is performed in a variety of ways, ensuring intimate contact of the agent over a period of 24–48 hours with the skin surface, which may be previously scarified. Several such applications are usually required to induce sensitivity. It seems that, for sensitisation to occur, contact with the skin is essential, for it can be achieved by injection actually into the skin, but not by other parenteral routes or by feeding. Sensitisation develops in 8–21 days, as shown by a local reaction at the site of a patch test. This is typically a *delayed reaction*, occurring after 24 hours, like the tuberculin reaction, in contrast to the immediate weal and flare of the atopic skin test. With the lowest grade of sensitisation, it consists of an erythema; with high grades, papules, vesicles and confluent bullæ are found. The whole skin is sensitive and a positive patch test may be obtained anywhere on its surface. The reaction shows the same specificity as other immunological phenomena.

Nature of the Allergens

The sensitising agents are usually simple chemical compounds: formaldehyde, iodine, salicylates, substituted catechols from certain plants such as poison ivy, extracts of certain species of *Primula* and, less commonly, animal products such as wool and silk. Most of these are toxic when applied to the normal skin in concentrated form. However, a sensitive individual may react to amounts many hundred-fold lower than the minimal toxic dose.

Specificity of Allergens

We have already noted that specificity in drug hypersensitivity can readily be related to the chemical composition of the allergen in the same way that specificity of an antigen with artificially introduced chemical substituents is related to the nature of the chemical substituent (Chapter 32). Recent work on sensitisation to contact dermatitis, however, (reviewed in ref. 8) has shown that, unlike the specificity of the artificially conjugated antigens used for the production of antibody, specificity in contact dermatitis involves not only the drug but the protein as well. As the protein is normally that of the sensitised subject, contact dermatitis may be regarded as a form of autoimmunity. The relative parts played by drug and protein in the specificity of drug-protein complexes in experimental contact dermatitis in guinea-pigs have been investigated[8, 9] and compared with those determining the specificity of complexes used for the production of antibodies. In Salvin's experiments,[8] guinea-pigs were sensitised to dinitrofluorobenzene (DFB), (a drug reacting spontaneously with protein), by injecting it intracutaneously in Freund's incomplete adjuvant (i.e. water-in-oil emulsion without tubercle bacilli). This method of sensitisation is more reliable and rapid than repeated application to the skin surface. When he applied the drug to the skin 5 days after sensitisation, typical contact dermatitis was produced. After 9 days, antibody started to appear, detected by an Arthus reaction on injection of DFB conjugated to a heterologous protein (hen egg albumin (HEA)). The specificity of the antibody was determined entirely by the DFB, the carrier protein playing no part, as shown by the fact that HEA could be replaced by guinea-pig serum or other protein. However, when he used DFB coupled to HEA, or to a serum protein of the guinea-pig itself (GA), he failed to obtain contact dermatitis to DFB, although delayed type hypersensitivity could be elicited to the DFB–HEA or DFB–GA complexes and to the unconjugated proteins themselves. As before, the antibody that was subsequently formed was specific solely for the DFB hapten. Finally, he used DFB coupled to proteins from the guinea-pig's skin (GS). This time there was not only delayed hypersensitivity to the complex and to the unconjugated skin protein and subsequently antibody specific for DFB, but also contact dermatitis to DFB (Table1).

40/Table 1

The Relation Between Hapten and Carrier Protein in Contact Dermatitis in the Guinea-pig[8].

*Sensitising Agent**	*Test Agent*	*Contact Dermatitis to DFB*	*DTA† to Protein carrier*	*Antibody specific for DFB*
DFB	DFB	+		+
DFB-HEA	DFB	0	+	+
DFB-HEA	HEA	0	+	+
DFB-HEA	DFB-HEA	0	+	+
DFB-GA	DFB	0		+
DFB-GA	GA	0	+	+
DFB-GA	DFB-GA	0	+	+
DFB-GS	DFB	+	+	+
DFB-GS	GS		+	+
DFB-GS	DFB-GS		+	+

*Sensitising agent injected intracutaneously in Freund's incomplete adjuvant.

DFB Dinitrofluorobenzene.
HEA Hen egg albumin.
GA Guinea-pig serum albumin.
GS Guinea-pig skin extract

†Delayed type hypersensitivity

These results suggest that the specificity of contact dermatitis is determined, not only by the drug, but by certain protein or proteins present in the skin. These apparently cannot be replaced by heterologous protein or even by homologous serum proteins. On the other hand, when preformed conjugates of the drug are used, delayed type hypersensitivity may be produced to the conjugate or to the protein carrier of the conjugate, even when the protein is that of the guinea-pig itself. Contact dermatitis to the drug is not produced unless the particular homologous skin protein is the carrier. In all cases, antibodies that are eventually produced are specific only for the drug, the protein merely acting as a carrier to confer antigenicity on it.

Role of the Skin in Contact Dermatitis

From the observations noted in the last section, the skin appears to be essential for sensitisation to contact dermatitis. One of its probable functions is to provide the specific protein or proteins for conjugation. Eisen[1] showed that C^{14}-labelled 2,4-dinitrochlorobenzene applied to the surface of guinea-pig skin united with protein within 10–15 minutes, conjugation being maximal after 3 hours. Thereafter, it declined rapidly, but some persisted for very long periods of time. The conjugates appear to be localised in the epidermis and there is evidence that to be effective they must be in the inner malpighian layers. Another function of the skin may be to retain allergen long enough for its conjugation to protein. It is also possible that lipids of the skin may act as adjuvants in the same way that the wax D of the tubercle bacillus in Freund's adjuvant (Chapter 34) produces delayed type sensitivity to proteins injected with it.

Passive Transfer of Contact Dermatitis

As with delayed hypersensitivity of the tuberculin type, contact dermatitis is not dependent on the formation of circulating antibodies and no passive transfer has been achieved with serum. However, as with tuberculin sensitivity, successful generalised transfer has been achieved in animals and man with cells from the buffy coat and in animals with cells from lymph glands, spleen and peritoneal exudates.[10] Transfer can be achieved with whole cells, but not so far with certainty with killed or disrupted cells.[11]

Cells from sensitised agammaglobulinæmic subjects will transfer sensitivity to normal subjects, showing that contact dermatitis, like tuberculin type sensitivity, is not dependent on the capacity of the cells to make humoral antibody.

Drug Allergy of Serum Sickness Type

Certain drugs that are maintained at a constant level in the blood stream for a number of days, such as sulphonamides, arsphenamine and penicillin, may give rise in normal individuals to a condition resembling serum sickness, with the same latent period of from 7–10 days.[12] The common manifestations, as in serum sickness, are urticarial rashes, angio-neurotic œdema, arthropathies and arteritis affecting particularly the kidneys, and this sometimes leads to symptoms and signs of renal failure. The condition is rarely fatal and usually clears up rapidly. Patients who develop this type of hypersensitivity give no history of previous contact with the drug, are not necessarily hypersensitive to other allergens, and give no weal and erythema on scratch test even with drugs like penicillin which elicit a reaction in atopic subjects. No local or general passive transfer is possible, either when sickness develops or from convalescent donors. It thus differs from true serum sickness. The mechanism involved is still uncertain, but in the few cases that have come to post-mortem, glomerulitis and arteritis of the viscera, particularly involving the kidney and intestines are found. It is likely that the condition may have the same pathogenesis as experimental serum sickness in animals, the antigen being a conjugate of the drug with protein (Chapter 39).

Drug Allergy Involving Linkage of the Drug to Formed Elements of the Blood

Drug-induced Thrombocytopenic Purpura

This disease was first described by Loewy[13] more than 30 years ago in two patients following administration of the hypnotic drug "Sedormid". The condition has been extensively studied by Ackroyd (for refs. see 14, 15). The drugs most commonly involved are Sedormid, quinidine, quinine and sulphonamides. As with the other forms of drug allergy, there is a history of previous administration of the drugs, sometimes over weeks or even years without symptoms. Once sensitivity has developed, thrombocytopenia may commence within a few minutes to a few hours after taking the drug, with or without the development of purpura and hæmorrhage into mucous membranes. A purpuric reaction may often be obtained in these patients by applying to the skin a patch containing the drug in propylene glycol.

It is easy to demonstrate in the patients' serum *in vitro* an antibody which agglutinates, and in the presence of complement, lyses the patients' platelets and the platelets of normal individuals, but only when the specific drug is also present. This antibody may be IgG or IgM in type.

There are certain difficulties in accepting the obvious explanation of this condition, namely that the drug acts as a hapten uniting with the platelet as a carrier and stimulating the formation of antibody specific for the drug-platelet complex, and that antibody will then agglutinate and, in the presence of complement, lyse any platelet that has the drug on its surface.[15] Firstly, unlike the firm union between hapten and protein carrier required for antigenicity in other forms of allergy, the union of the drug with the platelet and the further union of antibody with the drug platelet complex are so loose that agglutination may be inhibited or reversed merely by removing the drug by dialysis. Secondly, it is generally found that the reaction between antibody, drug and platelet is not inhibited by excess of free drug. On the contrary, the reaction becomes more pronounced with increasing concentration of the drug. This is contrary to all reactions of conjugated antigens with their antibodies in which excess of hapten inhibits or reverses the reaction.

A second hypothesis suggests that a stable union between the drug and some soluble macromolecule takes place in the blood, and antibody is produced against the conjugate. The resulting antigen-antibody complex in the blood then becomes adsorbed to the platelets bringing about their non-specific agglutination. The platelet according to this hypothesis plays a purely passive role—an "innocent bystander".[16] This is similar to the part played by leucocytes and platelets in anaphylactic reactions in the blood of rabbits (Chapter 38) where the platelets and leucocytes become aggregated with the antigen-antibody complexes and are filtered off in the vascular pulmonary bed. However, in anaphylactic reactions there is no evidence that the platelets undergo lysis, although they liberate pharmacologically active substances, and if the animal survives, the platelet count returns rapidly to normal. In drug-induced thrombocytopenia, on the other hand, lysis of platelets occurs and the thrombocytopenia persists. Moreover, Cronin[17] made an artificial antigen by coupling to a protein a modified Sedormid molecule immunologically identical with Sedormid, but differing from it by being highly reactive with protein. Antibody added to this antigen in the presence of platelets *in vitro* united with the antigen, but the resulting complex had no effect on the platelet population. Also there was no evidence that antibody to this conjugate was present in the blood of Sedormid sensitive subjects. Further this "innocent bystander" hypothesis does not explain the failure of excess drug to inhibit the hypersensitive reaction.

Finally, it has been suggested (see ref. 15) that sensitisation is brought about not by the drug itself, but by some metabolic breakdown product of the drug which can form firm links with the platelet. When the whole drug is added to the platelets and patients' serum *in vitro* it "fits" the cell and the antibody not so well as the real hapten, so explaining the lability of the union with cell and antibody and failure of excess drug to inhibit the reaction. No evidence in support of this hypothesis, however, is yet available.

Drug-induced Hæmolytic Anæmia and Agranulocytosis

These diseases have a mechanism essentially similar to drug-induced thrombocytopenia, but are less frequently encountered. The drugs associated with hæmolytic anæmia are phenacetin, para-amino-salicylic acid, quinine, and quinidine. Agglutination of the patients' red cells and other compatible red cells with the patients' serum in the presence of the drug can usually be demonstrated *in vitro*, but it is not always possible to show hæmolysis. However, when hæmolysis does take place, it is complement determined.

Agranulocytosis due to drugs may or may not involve an immune mechanism, because certain drugs are toxic to leucocytes or to leucocyte precursors in the bone marrow in their own right. Antibodies to leucocytes, demonstrable by agglutination in the presence of the drug, however, can be shown in the serum of patients but are less easily demonstrated than platelet agglutinins in drug-induced thrombocytopenia.

Evidence that a specific anti-leucocytic agent is present in the blood of patients treated with amidopyrine was obtained by Moeschlin and his colleagues (for refs. see 18), who transfused normal subjects with the blood from a sensitive patient within 3 hours after taking the drug orally. An immediate fall in granulocytes occurred in the recipient reaching 800 per c.mm. in 40 mins. Similar observations were made when rabbits were transfused with the patients' serum. It would seem, therefore, that the source of leucocyte like the platelet is not important.

ALLERGIC DISORDERS DUE TO ANTIGENS WHOLLY OF ENDOGENOUS ORIGIN (BLOOD AND FIXED TISSUE CELLS)

The hypersensitive reactions considered so far involve an immunological response *in vivo* to exogenous antigens or allergens immunologically unrelated to those of the animal's tissues, except in so far as proteins or cells of the tissues are necessary to act as carriers of the allergen and in some cases to contribute to its specificity (contact dermatitis). We now have to consider disorders in the body brought about by reactions between antibody and the antigenic constituents of the individual's own tissues. The damage may be the result of clearly demonstrable circulating antibody introduced from without or by passage from the mother to the fœtus *in utero*. The reaction may also be induced by a graft of immunologically competent cells (spleen or lymph gland) from another animal and induced to "take" by the induction of immune tolerance (graft *v.* host reaction, see Chapter 41). Alternatively, it may be brought about by an immune response of the individual himself to his own tissue antigens (auto-immunisation).

Antibody introduced from without

When sera containing high titres of antibody to a particular cell type are introduced into an experimental animal, the cells of this type may be specifically destroyed. Thus hæmolytic anæmia, thrombocytopenia and leucopenia may be produced by antibodies to red cells, platelets and leucocytes respectively. The antibodies concerned are those of the classical type and are produced by injecting the tissue cells into animals of another species. They are specific for antigens on the cell surfaces, and there is no reason to believe that the damage to the cells is brought about by any other mechanism than lysis by complement after sensitisation by antibody.

Blood transfusion is the only comparable procedure in man which could bring about destruction of blood cells by antibody introduced from without. Since 1911, when group O individuals were first used as universal donors to transfuse individuals of all other groups, it was thought that the anti-A and anti-B isoantibodies in the blood of these donors would be so diluted in the recipient's blood as to be innocuous. This has, in general been borne out by experience. Many thousands of individuals have been transfused with group O blood without mishap. However, dangerous group O donors exist who appear to have a sufficiently high titre of anti-A antibodies to produce destruction of the red cells of a group A recipient. These donors often have, in addition to their anti-A isoantibodies (IgM) which are readily neutralised by group A substance in the recipient's blood and tissues, IgG antibodies, the result of unrecognised immunisation with substances cross reacting with blood group A substance, and these are not readily neutralised by soluble group A antigen. In two cases quoted by Mollison[19] the donors had high titres of anti-A IgG antibodies. There was a history of their having received pepsin refined anti-tetanus serum some months previously, which is known to stimulate the production of group A antibodies due to cross reacting antigen in the hog pepsin used in the refining process.

Hæmolytic Disease of the Newborn

This is a serious and often fatal hæmolytic disease of newborn infants due to antibodies to the fœtal red cell introduced by a more natural means than blood transfusion, namely through the placenta from mother to child. The child, if not stillborn, has severe anæmia and jaundice with enlargement of liver and spleen which are undergoing active erythropoiesis. The first child is usually born healthy, the disease becoming more severe with progressive pregnancies. The ætiology of the condition is well established and is determined by the absence of D antigen (one of the Rh antigens) in the blood cells of the mother and its presence in that of the father. As the presence of the antigen is genetically determined and dominant, it is also present in the red cells of the child. The immediate cause of the disease is the transplacental passage of fœtal red cells into the mother's circulation with consequent immunisation and passage of D antibodies back through the placenta into the fœtal circulation. The antibodies in the maternal circulation may be 19S as well as 7S in type but only the latter are transmitted. These are of the IgG type, but mostly differ from the classical antibodies in being incomplete and failing to agglutinate the infant's cells and to fix complement. They can be demonstrated on the surface of the infant's red cell by agglutination with anti-human gamma globulin serum (Coombs direct globulin test) and in the maternal circulation by treatment of any Rh positive red cells with her serum, washing and agglutinating the sensitised cells with anti-human gamma globulin serum (Coombs indirect globulin tests).

As these incomplete Rh antibodies fail to fix complement, immune lysis cannot be demonstrated *in vitro* and the profound destruction of the infant's red cells cannot be due to lysis by complement. The destruction is probably due to removal of the red cells by the reticulo-endothelial cells following opsonisation by Rh antibody.[19]

The ABO blood group system may also be concerned in the disease. The usual finding is that the mother is blood group O and her husband and child group A. The disease is much less severe than that involving the Rh system. This is probably due to (1) the presence in the maternal circulation of Group A isoantibodies which sensitise and rapidly remove chance entry of fœtal cells before they have a chance to produce an antigenic stimulus. (These isoantibodies being IgM in type fail to pass the placenta); (2) the presence of soluble group A substance in the plasma and body fluids of the group A child which unites with any maternal A antibodies which pass the placenta. However, in spite of these precautions immunisation of the mother may take place and IgG antibodies pass to the fœtus. As noted above, these are not readily neutralised by group A substance and may affect the cells of the fœtus.[20]

A few cases of neonatal thrombocytopenia having a similar origin have been described.[21]

Autoimmunity

In recent years it has become increasingly evident that antigens of the body tissues, normally recognised as "self" and as such tolerated by the animal, may for various reasons come to be regarded as "foreign" and induce an autoimmune response. This response to "self-antigens" may take the form of frank production of antibody or the development of delayed hypersensitivity, and often leads to secondary cytopathic effects which may be general, or may be confined to one organ or tissue. The mere finding of antibody in the circulation to some antigen of the body does not necessarily imply that an immunological response is the cause of a pathological condition; it could equally well be the result. A pathological process could change the tissues to such an extent that they become autoantigenic. The antibodies so formed could or could not then contribute to the pathological condition. Also, where delayed hypersensitivity and the presence of autoantibodies coexist, it is sometimes difficult to determine which, if either, is primarily concerned in the cytopathic effects.

Over the past few years numerous symposia, reviews and monographs have appeared on the subject of autoimmunity (e.g. refs. 22, 23, 24) and these should be consulted for a full account of the subject. It is not possible here to give more than a brief outline of the conditions that may contribute to autoimmune reactions.

Factors which may lead to the Development of an Immune Reaction by the Animal to its own Tissues

They have been ably summarised by Glynn.[25] The most important would appear to be the following:

1. *The formation of a complex between an exogenous hapten and host protein or cells in vivo* in such a way as to change the protein carrier or cells so that they become autoantigenic. We have already met examples in contact dermatitis. On the other hand, drug hypersensitivity of the immediate type (atopy) is not an example of autoimmunity because the immune response is directed to the drug, the body protein merely conferring antigenicity on it and taking no part itself in specificity.

It is possible that a hapten of an infecting organism may take the place of the drug and induce an immune response not only to itself but also to its autogenous carrier. There is some evidence that such a mechanism may operate in glomerulonephritis associated with a throat infection with certain types of *Streptococcus pyogenes* (types 5 and 12), a complex being formed between specific products of the streptococci and some protein in capillary basement membrane.

2. *The development of an immune reaction to antigens normally inaccessible to antibody forming cells.*—It is known that certain tissues and proteins of the body such as the lens and uvea of the eye, myelin and thyroglobulin, which do not normally come into contact with antibody forming cells, can be antigenic when injected into the same animal from which they have been removed. Conditions may arise, e.g. trauma or following virus infection, whereby these tissues get into the blood stream or are infiltrated with antibody forming cells. An example is sympathetic ophthalmia in which uveal pigment is released into the circulation from damage to one eye producing an immune response which affects the sound eye. Antibody to thyroglobulin following mumps thyroiditis may be another example.

3. *Alteration of host constitutive antigens by physical or chemical agents or by infection.*—It is not uncommon for patients to develop urticarial skin reactions on exposure to light. There is evidence that many if not all these reactions are brought about by an immediate type allergic sensitisation to an autologous antigen normally formed or released in the skin by exposure to light of a certain wave range. In one patient described by Baer and Harber,[26] extensive œdema in the skin developed on exposure to visible light of 4200–5000 Å range. The sensitivity could be passively transferred to normal skin with the patient's serum (Prausnitz-Küstner reaction).

Denaturation of proteins alter their immunological specificity and animals injected with denatured proteins from their own tissues will produce an immune response to them. In rheumatoid arthritis considered in a later section, an immune response occurs to partially denatured serum gamma globulin, but the cause of this change in the gamma globulin molecule is entirely unknown.

Infection may also bring about alterations in the antigenic structure of tissues and stimulate an immune response to new cellular antigens. It has been suggested that the cytopathic changes found in a number of diseases, e.g. mumps parotitis and orchitis, Hashimoto's thyroiditis and infective hepatitis, may be the result of an immune response to new antigens in or on the cells brought about by the presence of the virus. (For a discussion on the part played by myxoviruses in autoimmunity, see ref. 27.) The cytopathic action may be either the result of humoral antibody or more likely, particularly in the examples quoted in which lymphocytic infiltration is a marked feature, the result of delayed hypersensitivity. There is at present little evidence to support this suggestion in human diseases. However, recent observations on lymphocytic choriomeningitis of mice (LCM) (reviewed in ref. 28) strongly support a mechanism of this kind in this disease. Newborn mice infected intracerebrally with LCM virus, after a transient mild "runt" disease, remain healthy, in spite of the presence of large amounts of virus in almost all the organs of the body. They are immunologically tolerant to the virus, no immune response, either humoral or of the delayed type, being evident. Mice infected after immunological maturity, however, suffer from a fatal infection with lymphocytic infiltration of the organs containing the virus. Agents which depress the immune response such as X-rays, cortisone and amethopterin have a protective effect on such mice, but have no action on the extent of the viræmia or virus content of the organs. It would seem, therefore, that the cytopathic effect of LCM was entirely due to an immune reaction affecting the organs containing the virus but not the virus itself.

4. *Infection with organisms having antigens immunologically similar to those of the body tissues.*—Infection may also produce an autoimmune response when the determinant groups in the antigen of the infecting agent are similar to those of certain tissues of the body. The exogenous antigen is sufficiently dissimilar not to be regarded as "self" by the body tissues so that an immune response against the exogenous antigen is mounted which cross reacts with tissues of the body. There is little doubt that a mechanism of this kind operates in rheumatic fever. The well known association of the onset of rheumatic conditions with a preceding throat infection with β hæmolytic streptococci, has recently been clarified by Kaplan (for refs. see 23, Chapter 18). Using fluorescent antibody he demonstrated a cross reaction in rabbits between antigens in the sarcolemma of the heart myofibrils, the smooth muscle of blood vessels and endocardium and an antigen associated, but not identical, with the M protein of certain β hæmolytic streptococci. Similar cross reacting antibodies were demonstrated by precipitation in patients with rheumatic fever.[29] However, it must be stressed once again that the presence of such antibodies does not necessarily mean that they are the causal agents of the pathological effects of the disease.

5. *The development of a new tissue antigen subsequent to immunological maturation.*—On the assumption that tolerance to "self" antigens is established in the embryo and neonate by contact with potential antibody forming cells still in the immature state, self antigens that develop subsequent to maturation, might be expected to be regarded as foreign by the immune mechanism if they come into contact with antibody forming cells. Such antigens arise in connection with the sex cells. As with other antigens inaccessible to the antibody forming cells,

these do not normally stimulate an immune response. However, it is not uncommon to find antibodies to spermatozoa associated with sterility in men.

6. *Experimental breakdown of tolerance with Freund's adjuvant.*—We have already seen that Freund's complete adjuvant enhances the development of both types of immune response: delayed hypersensitivity and production of antibody (Chapters 34 and 39); and that in the former it enables certain proteins of the tissues of the animal to become immunologically reactive (e.g. the carrier protein in contact dermatitis). Autoimmunity on an even wider scale can be produced by emulsifying extracts of organs in the adjuvant before injection, a procedure which has been used extensively in the study of autoimmune reactions in animals and is considered in more detail below.

7. *Natural breakdown of homeostatic mechanism.*—According to Burnet's clonal selection theory of antibody formation, autoimmune disease associated with the formation of antibody to a single antigen, e.g. acquired hæmolytic anæmia or idiopathic thrombocytopenia, may be due to the mutation and development of an antibody forming clone of cells subsequent to maturation of the immune mechanisms, having resisted suppression (immunological paralysis) by excess of self antigen. Such homeostatic breakdown may be the result of pathological lesions in the thymus, the organ considered to be responsible for the regulation and primary production of lymphocytes, and hence of immunologically competent cells. While no lesions of the thymus can be related to the acquired hæmolytic anæmia of man (see below), there is a clear association between thymic hyperplasia and the appearance of germinal centres in the thymus and the natural hæmolytic anæmia affecting certain strains of mice which was discovered by Bielchowsky and his colleagues[30] (NZB/BL). These mice develop a spontaneous genetically determined hæmolytic anæmia associated with serum auto-antibodies to their red cells. Similar thymic changes have been observed in man with *myasthenia gravis*, a disease characterised by progressive weakness of the skeletal muscle and the appearance in the patient's serum of antibody reacting with the A-band of skeletal muscle, (demonstrated by fluorescent antibody techniques) and also with an antigen in the reticulo-endothelial cells of the thymus itself. Burnet considers that the thymus is normally concerned in the suppression of "forbidden clones" to self antigens. In myasthenia gravis, some antigenic stimulus arising in the thymus itself is not suppressed, but stimulates the formation of germinal centres and production of an antibody cross reacting with skeletal muscle.

In disseminated lupus erythematosus, also associated with thymic changes and considered in a later section, a more extensive breakdown of homeostasis involving many clones may be involved. The relation between the thymus and autoimmunity is discussed in refs. 22, 23 and 24.

8. *Variation in sensitivity of the immune mechanism of different individuals to antigenic differences.*—There is no doubt that considerable variation exists in the immune response of different individuals to a foreign antigen. In addition, individuals may vary in their ability to distinguish the degree of "foreignness" of an antigen. Tissue antigens which have undergone some change not sufficient to prevent their being still accepted as "self" by most individuals may be considered "foreign" by others. It has been suggested that such a mechanism may operate in producing the so-called "rheumatoid factor" in rheumatoid arthritis. This

factor is present in the serum not only of patients with rheumatoid arthritis but also in their near relatives and consists of antibody gamma globulin of the 19S type which reacts specifically with the individual's own gamma globulin of 7S type, if the latter has undergone some alteration from the native state, as produced for instance by treatment with mild heat or acid. Although the rheumatoid factor is present in trace amounts in the serum of normal individuals, its presence in relatively high concentration may reflect the ability of certain individuals to recognise slight alterations in the gamma globulin molecule which would be missed by normal individuals. As noted later, the rheumatoid factor appears to have nothing to do with the ætiology of the disease.

Before describing examples of natural autoimmune diseases of man, we may consider some examples of experimental autoimmune reactions in animals.

Experimental Induction of Autoimmunity in Animals

We have already noted that certain tissues in the body that do not normally come in contact with antibody forming cells, e.g. lens and uveal protein, thyroglobulin, myelin of the C.N.S., and spermatozoa may be antigenic when injected into the animal from which they have been removed, particularly if they are injected together with water-in-oil emulsion containing dead tubercle bacilli (Freund's adjuvant). With the exception of spermatozoa, these antigens appear to be organ specific, rather than species specific, that is heterologous, isologous or autologous antigens from a particular organ are immunologically equivalent. The appearance of antibodies in the circulation following experimental introduction of these tissues into animals is associated with lesions in the same organs as those from which the antigen is taken. Thus the injection of tissue from the C.N.S. not only produces antibodies which fix complement with the tissue but also produces an allergic encephalomyelitis characterised by focal areas of perivascular inflammation and demyelination within the brain and spinal cord. Similarly, the injection of thyroglobulin and uveal tissue not only gives rise to circulating antibodies to thyroglobulin and uveal tissue, but also produces thyroiditis and uveitis respectively. Delayed skin reactions to myelin, uveal pigment and thyroglobulin can be obtained in animals with experimental allergic encephalomyelitis, uveitis and thyroiditis respectively, and allergic encephalomyelitis can be transferred passively with lymphoid cells. None of these experimental diseases can be transferred passively with serum, suggesting that delayed type hypersensitivity plays the dominant role in their ætiology.

Some Examples of Autoimmune Diseases in Man

Diseases probably dependent on Delayed Hypersensitivity

The experimentally induced autoimmune reactions in animals considered above have their counterpart in *encephalomyelitis in man induced by the use of anti-rabies vaccine*. Since 1885, when Pasteur introduced his method of inoculation against rabies by injecting spinal cords of rabbits containing the fixed virus, a number of cases of encephalomyelitis closely resembling experimental allergic encephalomyelitis of animals has occurred. The condition, in fact, has the same ætiology, namely stimulations of an immune response to the brain tissue of the person immunised by rabbit spinal cord. Like the experimental disease, the immune response is thus organ- rather than species-specific.

Sympathetic ophthalmia is another condition in man resembling experimental allergic uveitis of animals, but here the immunological stimulus is brought about by trauma. In these patients it is possible to elicit a delayed type of hypersensitivity by intracutaneous injection of uveal tissue.

Hashimoto's thyroiditis is another example in which delayed type hypersensitivity probably plays the dominant role, although antibodies to antigens of the thyroid are present in the patient's serum. It is a natural disease of the thyroid having a close similarity to experimental thyroiditis produced by injecting thyroglobulin and other thyroid antigens with Freund's adjuvant into rabbits and guinea-pigs. It was first described by Hashimoto in 1912 as an extensive hyperplasia of lymphoid tissue in the thyroid with the formation of lymphoid follicles, enlargement of the gland and symptoms of hypothyroidism. However, its nature remained obscure until 1956 when Roitt, Doniach and their co-workers (see ref. 31) showed that the high level of serum gamma globulin observed in this disease was due, in part at least, to antibodies which precipitated with human thyroglobulin. These antibodies are 7S IgG in type and are specific for human thyroglobulin. They sensitise guinea-pigs to passive cutaneous anaphylaxis and aggultinate tanned red cells treated with thyroglobulin, but do not fix complement with thyroglobulin. In a smaller percentage of cases antibodies to a colloid antigen other than thyroglobulin or to a microsomal fraction in thyroid epithelial cells can be demonstrated by fluorescent anti-human globulin.

It is still not clear whether these antibodies play a part in the causation of the disease or are merely secondary, the result of an invasion of the thyroid tissue by immunologically competent cells. The titre of antibody in the patient's serum is not related to the clinical condition, but on the other hand some sera from patients with Hashimoto's disease have been shown to be cytotoxic to tissue cultures of human thyroid, the cytotoxicity being correlated with the content of anti-microsomal antibody in the serum.[32] Attempts have been made to demonstrate delayed type hypersensitivity in Hashimoto's disease, but owing to the high level of antibody, Arthus type reactions obscure the issue. However, the lesions in the thyroid are more closely correlated with delayed type hypersensitivity than with production of antibody. The causal factor which initiates the autoimmune response is quite unknown.

Other examples of autoimmune diseases in man in which delayed type hypersensitivity probably plays the dominant role are reviewed in ref. 22. The evidence that delayed hypersensitivity rather than humoral antibody is concerned in their pathology is summarised in ref. 33.

Autoimmune Disease due to Humoral Antibodies

There are certain natural autoimmune diseases of man in which humoral antibodies clearly play a part.

The idiopathic acquired hæmolytic anæmias were first described by Widal more than 50 years ago and have been extensively studied by Dacie.[34] There are two main forms of the disease associated with two different kinds of antibody in the patient's serum:

(1) *The Warm Antibody type* which is similar to hæmolytic disease of the newborn, affects all ages and varies in severity from a mild chronic anæmia to

severe hæmolytic disease with jaundice and splenomegaly. Gamma globulins reactive with red cells are present in the blood but cannot be detected by direct hæmagglutination or hæmolysis. However, addition of anti-human gamma globulin to red cells taken either from the patient himself or from normal individuals after prior treatment with the patient's serum, causes the cells to agglutinate (Coombs anti-globulin test), showing the presence of incomplete antibody globulin adsorbed to the cells. Although complement is not absorbed and apparently plays no part in the hæmolysis, the patient's own cells or normal cells from other individuals labelled with Cr^{51} and transfused have a life span considerably shorter than the normal.[19] Destruction *in vivo* is probably brought about by phagocytosis of the sensitised red cells by the reticulo-endothelial system. Maximum absorption of antibody occurs at 37°, hence the term warm antibodies. Like the Rh incomplete antibodies, they appear to be in the 7S IgG globulin range.

(2) *The Cold Antibody type of idiopathic hæmolytic anæmia* occurs mainly in elderly people and is characterised by hæmoglobinuria occuring in cold weather. Antibody globulin, reactive with the patient's own red cells or the red cells of normal people, can be demonstrated by direct hæmagglutination, but only if the test is carried out below 30–32° C. The agglutinin titre of the patient's serum appears to increase as the temperature is lowered to 4° C. Unlike the warm antibodies, the "cold antibodies" are found in the IgM (19S) serum fraction, fix complement and bring about hæmolysis *in vitro*, the optimal temperature for this reaction being cold enough to allow fixation of large amounts of antibody and warm enough for complement to cause lysis. Lysis does not occur at 37°, and therefore it is unlikely that the hæmolytic nature of the disease is due to lysis by complement *in vivo*. However, there is some evidence that complement is required for stabilising the fixation of the cold type antibody to the red cell. Normal red cells added to the patient's serum heated to 56° to destroy complement are agglutinated below 32°, but the "cold antibody" is dissociated and the cells dispersed when the temperature is raised to 37°. Although the addition of complement will not now allow the binding of antibody at 37°, dissociation (i.e. removal of antibody from the red cell) but not disaggregation (dispersal of the agglutinated cells) is prevented if complement is added at the lower temperature. That antibody and complement are still bound to the disaggregated cells is shown by adding anti-human globulin (Coombs direct anti-globulin test) which brings about agglutination. However, whereas the adsorption of the warm type of antibody was demonstrated by agglutination with *anti-gamma* globulin and was inhibited by free gamma globulin, adsorption of the cold type antibody and complement was shown by agglutination by antibody to a *non-gamma globulin fraction* and this was not inhibited by gamma globulin. Analysis showed that the non-gamma globulin adsorbed to the cell which reacted with anti-human globulin was probably the fourth component of complement which masked the much smaller amount of antibody gamma globulin required for fixation of the complement. The latter could be demonstrated, however, by weak agglutination with anti-gamma globulin serum after sensitisation with sera containing high titres of cold antibody.[34]

To summarise.—The warm type of idiopathic hæmolytic anæmia is due to fixation of non-agglutinating (incomplete) antibody IgG (7S) to an antigen in the patient's cells *in vivo*. This probably sensitises them to being removed and destroyed by the reticulo-endothelial system. Maximum adsorption is at 37°. Complement is not fixed and plays no part in the hæmolytic syndrome. The cold type of idiopathic hæmolytic anæmia is due to fixation of an agglutinating (complete) antibody IgM (19S) to the patient's cells. Fixation does not occur at body temperature *in vivo*. Exposure to cold, e.g. of an extremity, brings about fixation to chilled cells, and complement stabilises the fixed antibody when the cells are subsequently warmed to 37°. Although complement is adsorbed with the antibody it fails to bring about lysis at 37°, which probably takes place after removal by cells of the reticulo-endothelial system as with the warm type. *In vitro* at low temperatures both agglutination and hæmolysis with complement can be demonstrated but are not found *in vivo*.

The nature of the antigens in the red cell involved in these hæmolytic anæmias has received much attention. They seem to be fairly widely distributed in human cells but not in animal cells other than primates. There is evidence that one of the Rh antigens (e) present in the red cells of about 98 per cent of individuals is concerned in the warm type of anæmia. A new type of antigen (I) is probably concerned in most of the reactions of the cold type. This antigen is not present in fœtal red cells and develops slowly until at about 2 years of age it is present in all but 2 per cent of individuals. In the rare individuals lacking it, anti-I may be found in the serum, but has no pathological significance, behaving like other isoantibodies to blood group antigens.

Autoantibodies to platelets may be responsible for at least some cases of **idiopathic thrombocytopenic purpura**. Owing to the lack of platelets in these patients it is not easy to demonstrate sensitisation by antibody. However, thrombocytopenia has been produced in normal subjects by transfusion with the patients' blood, suggesting that an antibody to platelets is the cause of the thrombocytopenia. The development of purpura is not fully understood, but is probably accounted for by the early observation of Bedson that vascular endothelium and platelets possess a common antigen. Anti-platelet antibody and complement would produce a cytopathic action on the endothelium and allow leakage of red cells.

Diseases of Unknown Ætiology in which Autoimmunity may play a Dominant Role

Disseminated lupus erythematosus is a disease characterised by multiple lesions throughout the body particularly involving the connective tissue of the skin, mucous membranes, heart, kidneys, spleen and blood vessels. Thrombocytopenia and hæmolytic anæmia may also be present. A characteristic of the disease is the appearance in the connective tissue of irregular aggregations of hæmatoxylin staining material which absorb ultraviolet light at 2600 Å and are Feulgen positive. They represent collections of much altered nuclear material.

The serum of lupus patients contains a greatly increased concentration of gamma globulin. Much of this is found to be antibody reacting with a variety of tissues, particularly with the antigens of the nuclei. In smears of bone marrow or clotted blood taken from lupus patients, the so-called lupus erythematosus cell (LE cell) may be found. These are polymorphonuclear leucocytes containing chromatin inclusion bodies in their cytoplasm made up of whole or depolymerised nuclei of damaged cells. The formation of these LE cells can be observed *in vitro* when the serum from a lupus patient is added to a suspension of normal polymorphs. The nucleus of the leucocyte swells and is extruded into the surrounding medium, where it is taken up by another polymorph and comes to lie as an inclusion body within it.

Antinuclear antibodies which appear to react widely with nuclei, not only of different tissues, but of different individuals or even of different species of animal, may be demonstrated in lupus serum by fluorescent anti-globulin serum. When fresh tissue is exposed to lupus serum, washed and stained with fluorescent anti-globulin serum, all nuclei of mammalian cells from whatever source appear stained except mature spermatozoa. The nuclei of spermatozoa differ from those of immature sperm cells and of other cells in consisting of a DNA protamine not DNA histone. It would appear therefore that at least one kind of antibody present in lupus serum is to a DNA-histone complex[35] and this probably corresponds to the factors (antibody) associated with the formation of the LE cell. Other antinuclear globulins have been described reactive to parts of the complex and to other parts of the nucleus; nucleolus, DNA, histone and soluble protein in the nucleus. Antibodies to cytoplasmic constituents may also be found and are probably responsible for hæmolytic anæmia and thrombocytopenia, but except in these conditions the relations between the tissue lesions and the production of autoantibodies is obscure. Both 7S and 19S gamma globulin appear to be involved in the reaction of lupus serum, and the reaction may or may not fix complement.

The ætiology of the disease is still in doubt. The multiplicity of antibodies to a large number of tissue antigens suggests that a general breakdown in homeostasis has taken place, but these might equally well be secondary to the tissue changes. The thymus may or may not show hyperplastic changes.

Rheumatoid arthritis.—This condition is a generalised chronic inflammation of the joints with dense infiltration of plasma cells and lymphocytes, but other tissues are also involved such as the serous membranes, lymphoid tissue, heart and peripheral blood vessels. Subcutaneous granulomata developing at the points of pressure are characteristic features.

As we have seen, the serum of most, but not all, patients with this disease contains the so-called rheumatoid factor, (RF) a 19S gamma globulin containing 10 per cent polysaccharide and migrating as a fast component electrophoretically. This reacts specifically with partially denatured 7S gamma globulin not only of human origin but of other mammals also. The reaction may be demonstrated by precipitation, or by agglutination when the denatured globulin is adsorbed onto particulate cells or latex particles. The presence of bound RF on the plasma cells of synovial membrane, lymph nodes and subcutaneous nodules may be shown by heat aggregated 7S gamma globulin conjugated with fluorescein isothiocyanate. That the formation of RF is genetically determined is suggested by its presence in close relatives of patients, but attempts to implicate it in the pathogenesis of the disease have failed. It has been suggested that the lesions are the result of delayed hypersensitivity to certain products of inflammation brought about, for instance, by trauma in subjects genetically prone to detect and react to slight changes in structure of body proteins caused by inflammation. However, there is no evidence that a delayed hypersensitivity reaction can be elicited to inflammatory tissue such, for instance, as extracts of synovial membrane from an affected joint and the opinion is widely held that the immunological phenomena are secondary to a primary pathological process of as yet unknown ætiology. According to this view, rheumatoid arthritis should not be classified as an autoimmune disease proper as the immunological phenomena probably do not contribute to the lesions of the disease.

Summary

Drug-induced allergy is brought about by linkage of drugs or their degradation products to proteins in the tissues by covalent bonds and a subsequent immune response to the complex. The immune response may be of the immediate, delayed or serum sickness type. Linkage of drugs to the formed elements of the blood may also stimulate an immune response.

Anaphylactic shock and atopy occur as the result of previous sensitisation with the drug and may result in the same manifestations as those due to natural allergens. Weal and flare reactions to the cutaneous injection of the drug and positive Prausnitz-Küstner reactions can sometimes but not always be elicited with the unconjugated drug. Specificity is determined by the drug, the protein merely acting as a carrier. *Contact dermatitis*, a delayed type of drug allergy, is due to repeated contact of the drug with the skin. The specificity is determined not only by the drug but also by the skin protein. Sensitisation to preformed drug-protein complex in Freund's adjuvant brings about a delayed type hypersensitivity to both drug and protein carrier and later the production of antibodies whose specificity is determined by the drug but not the protein. Contact dermatitis can be passively transferred to animals and man with lymphoid cells but not with serum. In this it resembles other forms of delayed hypersensitivity. *Drug allergy of the serum sickness type* is found when drugs are maintained at a high level in the blood stream for several days during which an immune response to the drug develops. It has the same manifestations as serum sickness due to serum proteins and probably has the same pathogenesis, i.e. segregation of soluble complexes of antibody with excess antigen in the walls of the arteries with secondary glomerulonephritis and arteritis.

Drug-induced thrombocytopenia is due to the prolonged administration of certain drugs such as "Sedormid", quinidine, quinine and sulphonamide. Antibodies which agglutinate and lyse platelets, in the presence of complement, either of the patient or of other individuals when the drug is present can be demonstrated in the patient's serum. The drug appears to be loosely combined to platelets and to antibody because dissociation can be produced by dialysis. The reaction is not inhibited by excess drug. The mechanism of the reaction is not clear.

Drug-induced hæmolytic anæmia and agranulocytosis are similar to drug induced thrombocytopenia involving red cells and leucocytes respectively. A loose combination of drug, antibody and cell gives rise to agglutination or complement lysis.

Hæmolytic disease of the newborn.—Here the antigen is entirely endogenous (the fœtal red cell), the reaction being produced by transmission to the fœtus of anti-D (Rh) antibodies through the placenta from mother to child. The antibodies are for the most part incomplete IgG type which can be demonstrated on the red cell by agglutination with anti-human globulin serum, but not by direct agglutination or by complement fixation. Complement is not fixed and the hæmolysis is brought about by removal by the reticulo-endothelial cells and intracellular destruction.

Autoimmunity.—The conditions that could determine an immune response to an animal's own tissues are: (1) Formation of a complex between exogenous hapten and protein of the body in such a way that an immune response is formed not only to the hapten but also to the carrier protein. Drug contact dermatitis is an example. (2) Antigens normally inaccessible to the antibody forming mechanism becoming accessible either by trauma or by infection e.g. sympathetic ophthalmia. (3) Alteration and formation of new antigen in body tissues by physical, chemical or biological agents, e.g. allergic sensitisation of the skin by sunlight; lymphocytic chorio-meningitis of mice. (4) Cross reactivity between infecting bacteria and antigens of the tissues, e.g. rheumatic fever. (5) Development of new tissue antigens subsequent to immunological maturation and chance contact with the antibody forming mechanism, e.g. antibodies to spermatozoa leading to sterility in men. (6) The use of Freund's adjuvant to break down tolerance to the animal's own tissues. (7) Natural breakdown of the homeostatic mechanism from causes unknown, e.g. disseminated lupus erythematosus. (8) Ultra sensitivity of the immune mechanism to detect slight alterations in body antigens, e.g. rheumatoid factor in rheumatoid arthritis. Autoimmune disease may involve humoral antibodies or the development of delayed hypersensitivity or both.

Experimental allergic encephalomyelitis, uveitis and thyroiditis are examples of autoimmunity due to delayed type hypersensitivity induced experimentally in animals by injection with Freund's adjuvant of extracts of brain, uveal pigment and thyroglobulin respectively. Natural diseases in man of a like nature are encephalomyelitis due to rabies immunisation and sympathetic ophthalmia. Hashimoto's thyroiditis is probably also due to delayed hypersensitivity affecting the thyroid tissue, but antibodies to thyroglobulin and microsomal fraction of thyroid cells are also found. Autoimmune diseases in which antibody plays a part are the *immune hæmolytic anæmias, immune agranulocytosis* and *thrombocytopenia.* The hæmolytic anæmias are of two kinds, (1) warm type involving incomplete 7S immunoglobulin resembling that involved in hæmolytic disease of the newborn and (2) cold type characterised by attacks of hæmoglobinuria on exposure to cold due to a 19S autoantibody to the patient's own red cells which unites with the cells at temperatures below 32° C. Destruction of the sensitised red cells takes place in the liver and spleen after removal by reticulo-endothelial cells.

Disseminated lupus erythematosus, a disease of obscure ætiology is characterised by antibodies to antigens of the nucleus of the blood and parenchyma cells but whether this is the cause or result of the condition is not known.

Rheumatoid arthritis, also of obscure origin, is characterised by lymphocytic infiltration of the joints and other organs with the appearance of antibodies of the 19S type reacting with denatured gamma globulins of the 7S type (Rheumatoid Factor). It is generally thought that the immunological phenomena of the disease are secondary and play no part in its ætiology.

REFERENCES

1. EISEN, H. N. (1958). In *Cellular and Humoral Aspects of Hypersensitive States.* (Symp. N.Y. Acad. Med., **9,** Chap. 4, p. 89). Ed. LAWRENCE, H. S. New York: Hoeber-Harper.
2. LANDSTEINER, K. (1945). *The Specificity of Serological Reactions*, Chap. 5. Cambridge, Mass.: Harvard Univ. Press.
3. EISEN, H. N., ORRIS, L., and BELMAN, S. (1952). *J. exp. Med.*, **95,** 473.
4. GELL, P. G. H., HARRINGTON, C. R., and MICHEL, R. (1948). *Brit. J. exp. Path.*, **29,** 578.
5. LEVINE, B. B. (1965). *Fed. Proc.*, **24,** 45.
6. FEINBERG, S. M., FEINBERG, A. R., and MORAN, C. F. (1953). *J. Amer. med. Ass.*, **152,** 114.
7. TOMPSETT, R., SHULTZ, S., and MCDERMOTT, W. (1947). *J. Bact.*, **53,** 581.
8. SALVIN, S. B. (1965). *Fed. Proc.*, **24,** 40.
9. BENACERRAF, B., and GELL, P. G. H. (1959). *Immunology*, **2,** 219.
10. LAWRENCE, H. S. (1958). Ref. 1, Chap. 7, p. 279.
11. BLOOM, B. R., and CHASE, M. W. (1967). *Progr. Allergy*, **10,** 151.
12. DAMMIN, G. J. (1958). Ref. 1, Chap. 16, p. 581.
13. LOEWY, F. E. (1934). *Lancet*, **1,** 845.
14. ACKROYD, J. F. (1964). *Immunological Methods*, p. 453. Ed. ACKROYD, J. F. Oxford: Blackwell Scientific Publications.
15. ACKROYD, J. F. (1969). In preparation.
16. DAMESHEK, W. (1965). *Ann. N.Y. Acad. Sci.*, **124,** 6.
17. CRONIN, A. E. (1965). Ph.D Thesis, Camb. Univ. Quoted in Ref. 15.
18. MOESCHLIN, S. (1958). *Sensitivity Reactions to Drugs*, p. 77. Eds. ROSENHEIM, M. L., and MOULTON, R. Oxford: Blackwell Scientific Publications.
19. MOLLISON, P. L. (1967). *Blood Transfusion in Clinical Medicine*, Chap. 11, 4th edit. Oxford: Blackwell Scientific Publications.
20. KOCHWA, S., ROSENFIELD, R. E., TALLAL, L., and WASSERMAN, C. R. (1961). *J. clin. Invest.*, **40,** 874.
21. GARRETT, J. V., GILES, MCC., COOMBS, R. R. A., and GURNER, B. W. (1960). *Lancet*, **1,** 521.
22. *Annals of the New York Academy of Sciences* (1965). **124,** 1–411, 413–890.
23. GLYNN, L. E., and HOLBOROW, E. J. (1965). *Autoimmunity and Disease*. Oxford: Blackwell Scientific Publications.
24. MACKAY, I. R., and BURNET, F. M. (1963). *Autoimmune Diseases*. Springfield, Ill.: Charles C. Thomas.
25. GLYNN, L. E. (1963). *Modern Trends in Immunology*, **1,** Chap. 10, p. 206. Ed. CRUICKSHANK, R. London: Butterworth.
26. BAER, R. L., and HARBER, L. C. (1965). *Fed. Proc.*, **24,** S15.
27. ISACSON, P. (1967). *Progr. Allergy*, **10,** 256.
28. HOTCHIN, J. (1962). *Cold Spr. Harb. Symp. quant. Biol.*, **17,** 479.
29. KAPLAN, M. H. (1965). *Ann. N.Y. Acad. Sci.*, **124,** 904.
30. BIELSCHOWSKY, M., HELYER, B. J., and HOWIE, J. B. (1959). *Proc. Univ. Otago med. Sch.*, **34,** 9.
31. ROITT, I. M., and DONIACH, D. (1958). In *Mechanisms of Hypersensitivity* (Henry Ford Hosp. Symp., **8,** Chap. 21, p. 325). Eds. SHAFFER, J. H., LOGRIPPO, G. A. and CHASE, M. W. Boston, Mass.: Little Brown & Co.
32. PULVERTAFT, A. L. (1959). *Lancet*, **2,** 214.
33. TURK, J. L. (1967). *Delayed Hypersensitivity*, Chap. 11. Eds. NEUBERGER, A., and TATUM, E. L. Amsterdam: N. Holland Publ. Co.

34. Dacie J. V. (1962). *The Hæmolytic Anæmias*, Part II. The Autoimmune Hæmolytic Anæmias, 2nd edit. London: J. & A. Churchill.
35. Holborow, E. J., and Weir, D. M. (1959). *Lancet*, **1**, 809.
36. Batchelor, F. R., Dewdney, J. M., Feinberg, J. G., and Weston, R. D. (1967). *Lancet*, **1**, 1175.
37. Stewart, G. T. (1967). *Lancet*, **1**, 1177.

Chapter 41

THE IMMUNOLOGY OF TISSUE TRANSPLANTATION

By J. L. Gowans

In this chapter we shall be considering the reactions of animals to grafts of normal cells and tissues. The transplantation of tumours has already been discussed in Chapter 24 and we shall see how some of the principles which were established in these studies also apply to the behaviour of transplants of normal tissues.

There is one observation which will occupy a central place in our discussion. Many vertebrate tissues and organs can be excised and grafted to other positions on the same individual. Such *autografts* heal into place, re-establish their blood supply, and function normally for the life of the individual. Yet, if normal tissue from one animal is transplanted to another animal of the same species the graft will sooner or later be destroyed, although it may survive and function for a time. A graft which is transplanted from one member to another of the same species is called a *homograft* and the process which destroys it is the *homograft reaction*. Thus, the plastic surgeon uses autografts of skin to repair areas of the body surface which have been destroyed by severe burns or by disease; these survive for the life of the patient. A graft of skin from another individual—a homograft—would at first heal into place but would later die and slough away as a scab. Similarly, the scales of a goldfish can be transplanted to pockets prepared elsewhere on its surface and they will survive permanently; but the same scales transplanted to another goldfish would be destroyed by a homograft reaction.[1] In special circumstances homografts may survive permanently. This occurs, for example, when grafts are exchanged between identical twins. However, we shall see that these exceptions can all be explained in terms of the mechanism which destroys homografts: they are special examples of the way in which this mechanism is abolished or circumvented.

The homograft reaction appears to be a general feature of vertebrates for it has been observed in man and many other mammalian species, in birds, lizards, amphibia and goldfish. It is not clear in what way the homograft reaction is biologically "useful". In many ways it resembles the immunological response of animals to invading micro-organisms but the problem is to identify natural processes or hazards which are the equivalent of the experimental homograft.

The study of tissue transplantation is of great theoretical interest to immunologists and geneticists but it is also important for practical reasons. Although the immunosuppressive measures at present available will often allow the prolonged survival of organ transplants in man, they are far from ideal and the eventual fate of the graft always remains in doubt. The discovery of a safe method for permanently abolishing the homograft reaction in man would open the way for spectacular advances in the surgical use of tissue and organ transplants. We shall see that biologists have already shown that this problem is soluble in principle.

Grafts are classified according to the relationship of the donor to the recipient and to the anatomical position in which the graft is placed. We have already defined auto- and homografts; *heterografts* are transplants between members of different species; an *isograft* is one in which the donor and recipient are genetically identical. Transplants of these four kinds are described as autologous, homologous, heterologous and isologous. The terminology of tissue transplantation has recently been revised and, unfortunately, the old and new systems occur side by side in the literature. In the new system heterografts are called *xenografts*; grafts between members of the same species are described as *syngeneic* when the donor and recipient are genetically identical and *allogeneic* when they are genetically different. Homografts accordingly become *allografts*. An *orthotopic* graft is transplanted to an anatomically correct position in the recipient, e.g. skin to a bed prepared in skin. *Heterotopic* grafts are those which are placed in unnatural position, e.g. bone to subcutaneous tissue, thyroid to brain.

THE HOMOGRAFT REACTION

Skin Homografts

Our knowledge of the homograft reaction stems from the classical studies of Medawar[2–5] on the behaviour of orthotopic skin grafts in experimental mammals. Other tissues and organs, for example kidneys, submaxillary glands and nerves, are known to elicit a homograft reaction but skin possesses a number of particular advantages for experimental work. A skin graft is technically easy to apply; it causes no great inconvenience to either the donor or the recipient animal; and its survival time, which is a measure of the strength of the homograft reaction, can be accurately estimated by the day-to-day observation of its surface appearance, by making serial histological examinations, and by excising it and grafting it back on to its donor.

An autograft and a homograft of mammalian skin are indistinguishable for the first few days after transplantation. Both heal into place and rapidly acquire a new blood supply and both develop a lymphatic drainage. After about a week the homograft begins to differ both grossly and microscopically from the autograft. The homograft becomes darker in colour and thicker and harder to the touch and histological examination shows that the dermis and the graft bed have become invaded by mononuclear cells which include many lymphocytes together with plasma cells of varying maturity. The blood vessels of the graft become dilated, the flow of blood in them slows and eventually stops, and hæmorrhages develop as a result of rupture of the vessel walls. The final stage is reached in about two to three weeks when the epithelium is desquamated and the dermis, which is now necrotic, is shed as a scab. Meanwhile the autograft has healed firmly into place and survives for the life of the animal.

This sequence of events is typical of homografts of human as well as of animal skin, although in severely ill patients their survival may be somewhat prolonged. In man the process of healing which follows destruction of skin is attended by gross distortions as the edges of the wound are pulled by the contracting scar tissue. In many other mammals large defects will heal without any unsightly contractures since the skin is freely moveable on the body wall and not, as in man, firmly bound to the subcutaneous tissue. Skin grafting in man is thus a cosmetic necessity. In severely burned patients a skin graft serves the important immediate purpose of preventing fluid loss from the injured area and of guarding against the entrance of infection. Whenever possible the surgeon will apply grafts of the patient's own skin since these alone will survive, proliferate and repair the defect, but when very large areas of skin are destroyed, homografts of skin are sometimes employed to provide a temporary covering which may last a few weeks.

Genetics of Transplantation

An animal which receives a first homograft of skin will destroy it in a time which may vary from a few days to several months. In randomly bred laboratory animals and in man the breakdown of the graft is usually complete in two to three weeks. The most important factor which determines the survival-time of a homograft is the closeness of the genetic relationship between the donor and the host. When the donor and the host are genetically identical, as is the case with identical twins, skin grafts will never break down for they have the same constitution as autografts. The survival of grafts exchanged between identical twins is itself a demonstration that the factors which determine the acceptance or rejection of homografts are inherited. In fact, the survival of skin grafts exchanged between two individuals has been accepted as medico-legal proof that they are identical twins.

It is generally accepted that homografts are destroyed by an immunological reaction which is provoked by certain antigens present in the graft. These *histocompatibility antigens* are present in all the nucleated cells of the body and the particular set of antigens possessed by an individual is determined by his genetic constitution. The homograft reaction is therefore an expression of the genetic differences which exist between individuals belonging to the same species. Prolonged inbreeding, which progressively reduces genetic variance, can eventually eliminate these individual differences so that grafts exchanged between the members of a highly inbred strain will survive permanently, although grafts transplanted from one inbred strain to another are rapidly destroyed. The existence of highly inbred strains of mice has made possible the detailed analysis of the genes which control histocompatibility antigens. Such analyses have shown that each gene is dominant and that a graft will survive if the recipient possesses all the histocompatibility genes (and therefore all the antigens) which are present in the graft. It is of no consequence to the survival of the graft if the recipient possesses histocompatibility genes in addition to these.

Our understanding of the genetic basis of transplantation came originally from the study of transplantable tumours in mice and is associated particularly with the names of Little, Snell and Gorer. However, the methods devised by these workers have since been applied to the study of grafts of normal tissue and it will be instructive if we consider one such study in some detail. This will illustrate not only the genetic laws of transplantation but also one of their important practical consequences.

Barnes and Krohn[6] studied the fate of orthotopic skin grafts in two highly inbred strains of mice, the A-strain mouse (albino) and the CBA-strain mouse (agouti). It was found that grafts exchanged within either strain survived permanently while those exchanged between the two strains broke down in 10 to 13 days. When the two strains were crossed, the progeny (the F_1 generation) accepted grafts from either parent and from each other, but grafts from the F_1 to the parents were again destroyed in about two weeks. Skin which was grafted from the inbred parents to members of the F_2 generation ($F_1 \times F_1$) showed survival times which varied from 10 to 180 days; less than 2 per cent of the grafts were alive at 100 days and probably none of them survived permanently. The Mendelian interpretation of these results is as follows.

Highly inbred strains of mice are obtained by successive generations of brother-sister mating. Prolonged inbreeding results in a progressive increase in the number of homozygous loci, and when all grafts exchanged between the members of an inbred strain survive permanently then it can be assumed that the animals are homozygous at all their histocompatibility loci. If we assume that the two mouse strains differ by a pair of genes at a single histocompatibility locus then we can designate the genotypes of the two strains as AA and A′A′. The F_1 generation obtained by crossing these two strains will consist of individuals who all possess the genotype AA′. Since the members of the F_1 generation are all identical they will accept grafts from each other; they will also accept grafts from either parent for the F_1 will possess one representative of every gene present in the homozygous parents. If two F_1 individuals are mated then their genes will segregate in the progeny (the F_2 generation) in the proportions 1 AA, 2 AA′, 1 A′A′. It can be seen that grafts from either of the original inbred parents will be accepted by three-quarters of the individuals in the F_2 generation. If the inbred parent who is the skin donor differs from the other parent at *n* antigen-determining loci (and not at only one, as we have assumed so far), then its grafts will survive in $(\frac{3}{4})^n$ of the F_2 generation. In this way Barnes and Krohn calculated that the segregation of the genes by which their two inbred strains differed had occurred at about 15 loci. This was a minimum estimate since the analysis only revealed those genes which were not shared by the two strains. The great variability in the survival times in the F_2 showed that different loci were of very unequal strength, that is, some genes determine stronger antigens than others. In fact, one histocompatibility locus in the mouse, the H-2 locus, determines a series of antigens which are overridingly stronger than any others. An interesting weak transplantation antigen is that controlled by the Y chromosome; this results in the slow destruction of grafts transplanted from males to females, even within inbred strains of mice.[7]

The existence of so many histocompatibility loci means that the number of possible skin genotypes in the progeny of a cross between the two strains of mice which we have been considering must be extremely large. The number of possible skin genotypes in the whole species must be astronomical for we would have to take into account all the alternative allelic forms which can occupy each locus. For example, the H-2 locus can be occupied by at least 18 alleles.

The type of analysis we have just considered cannot, of course, be carried out in man but if the situation is comparable to that in mice then the number of different "tissue types" in the population is so large that the chance of finding a completely compatible donor for a patient who requires a homograft is for practical purposes non-existent, unless he has an identical twin. However, we saw that, in mice, the alleles at the H-2 locus control a particularly strong series of transplantation antigens. There is now also some evidence in man for the existence of a single strong locus (called HL-A) and the hope is that if human donors and recipients can be matched for the strong HL-A antigens then the reaction due to the very large number of weak antigenic differences may be easily controlled by immunosuppressive measures.

Tissue typing for human organ transplantation[8] is at present carried out with antisera which are thought to identify histocompatibility antigens on blood leucocytes. By applying a battery of such antisera to leucocytes from the recipient and the prospective donors and then observing the patterns of agglutination or cytolysis, the donor which matches best with the recipient is chosen. The sera come from individuals immunized against leucocytes either by repeated blood transfusions or, in multiparous women, by the repeated passage of fœtal leucocytes into the maternal circulation. Another possible method of tissue typing in man—the mixed lymphocyte reaction—will be explained in the section on graft-against-host reactions.

Mechanism of Homograft Reaction

An animal which has rejected a homograft acquires a prolonged state of sensitivity during which a second graft from the same donor will be destroyed more quickly. For example, an A-strain mouse will destroy a skin graft from a CBA-strain mouse in about 10 days, but a second CBA skin graft transplanted three weeks after the first will be destroyed in less than 6 days. The histological changes in such *"second-set" homografts* differ from those which accompany the destruction of the first graft. Whereas the cellular infiltration extends throughout the substance of a "first-set" graft, in the second-set reaction it is confined to the junction of the graft and the graft-bed and is inconspicuous in comparison. A second-set graft never acquires an efficient blood supply and its death is probably due to ischæmia. First-set grafts, on the other hand, enjoy a latent period during which a normal blood supply and a lymphatic drainage are established; only later does a reaction against the graft develop.

It has been shown in both man and experimental animals that the state of sensitivity which follows a first homograft is *specific* in that it is only directed against grafts from the original donor (or from individuals antigenically related to the donor); it is also *systemic*, for grafts transplanted to any position on the body are destroyed more quickly. The sensitivity induced by homografts has the characters of an actively acquired immunity and there is now general agreement that homografts are destroyed by an immunological mechanism. The problem is to decide the nature of this immunological mechanism.

The antigenic stimulus.—The state of sensitivity induced by a first homograft of skin causes a second skin graft to break down more quickly. It has been shown that spleen, bone marrow and ovary, among other tissues, will also sensitize an animal against a subsequent graft of skin provided, of course, that all the tissues come from the same donor or from animals belonging to the same inbred strain. Experiments of this kind have led to the belief that transplantation antigens are present in all the nucleated cells of the body. The phenomenon of immunological tolerance, which we will consider in a later section, makes it almost certain that the different tissues of an individual possess precisely the same transplantation antigens. Thus, a newborn mouse which is injected intravenously with a suspension of spleen cells will, in adult life, accept a homograft of adrenal tissue from the donor of the spleen cells.[9] This means that adrenal tissue can contain no antigen which is not also present in spleen cells, because if the adrenal homograft survives, immunological tolerance to every single one of its antigens must have been induced in the host. Transplantation antigens, then, are "individual specific" and not "tissue specific" and, as we explained earlier, they are under strict genetic control.

Transplantation antigens can be obtained in high concentration from the lipoproteins of cell surfaces, but their exact chemical nature is uncertain and it is not clear whether the cells of different tissues all contain the same amount.

The form in which antigens are released from homografts of living tissue is also unknown. The orthodox view is that antigenic material is released from the graft either in a soluble form or as the debris of wear and tear and that it passes by way of the afferent lymphatics to the regional lymph nodes. In favour of this view is the observation that grafts placed in peculiar sites which lack lymphatics, for example the hamster cheek pouch,[10] enjoy a prolonged survival; and that, as we shall see, the seat of the reaction which eventually destroys a homograft is the regional lymph node. On the other hand organ grafts, in which the blood vessels of the donor and recipient are joined surgically and in which a large blood flow is immediately re-established may sensitize their hosts by a different mechanism. Thus kidney grafts are destroyed even if they are prevented from making lymphatic connections with their host and sensitization must occur by way of the blood. There are two possibilities: either antigen is shed into the blood and carried to the spleen and lymph nodes; or circulating lymphocytes interact with antigens in the kidney itself and then migrate from the blood into lymphoid tissue from which the reaction against the graft is launched.[11] Small lymphocytes in the blood could well mediate this process of "peripheral sensitization" since, as we shall explain later, they have been identified as cells which can initiate transplantation reactions after stimulation with histocompatibility antigens.

Effector mechanisms.—Once a homograft has established an effective lymphatic connection with its host important changes occur in the draining lymph nodes. Large dividing cells with prominent nucleoli and a cytoplasm which stains strongly with pyronin arise in the cortical areas of the nodes. These cells, which are scattered in distribution and unrelated to germinal centres, have been variously termed large pyroninophilic cells, large lymphoid cells and immunoblasts. They are the morphological hallmark of a homograft reaction.

The importance of the changes in the draining nodes was first demonstrated by Mitchison[12] for tumour homografts in mice and his findings were later confirmed by Medawar and his colleagues[13] for orthotopic homografts of skin. The key observation was that homograft sensitivity, that is the ability to destroy a homograft more quickly, could be transferred to a normal animal by injecting it with cells prepared from the regional lymph nodes of previously sensitized animals. This is an example of "adoptive" immunization, a procedure that has already been discussed in Chapter 35. An actual experiment will illustrate the point. A normal CBA mouse was injected intraperitoneally with cells from the regional lymph nodes of other CBA mice which had been grafted 11 days before with skin from A-strain mice. The injected mouse was then found to destroy an

A-strain graft skin more rapidly than control CBA mice which had not received an inoculation of cells. Similarly, cells from the thoracic duct or the blood of sensitized animals will confer an adoptive immunity to homografts.[14] From experiments such as this it has been inferred that the agents which destroy an orthotopic skin homograft are lymphocytes which are formed in the regional lymph nodes in response to antigen, enter the efferent lymph, circulate in the blood and then migrate from the blood into the graft.[15, 16]

Recent experiments *in vitro* support the idea that direct contact between sensitized lymphocytes and the target tissue is important in the destruction of homografts. Wilson sensitized rats with homografts of skin and nine days later added their thoracic duct lymphocytes to a culture of cells derived from the skin donor. The target cells became surrounded by lymphocytes and were destroyed after incubation for 48 hours in the absence of any added complement or immune serum .[17] Little is known about the properties of lymphocytes from sensitized animals which enable them to destroy foreign cells. The current notion is that the effector cells synthesize a specific antibody which is bound to their surface and that this "cell bound" antibody interacts with graft cells (antigen) to initiate the destructive events. It is also possible that the interaction of lymphocytes with graft antigens *in vivo* may mobilize other cells from the blood, particularly macrophages, and that these also play a part in the destruction of the foreign tissue. Thus it has been shown that when sensitized lymphocytes are exposed to specific antigen *in vitro* they will liberate substances which have the property of immobilizing macrophages.[18] It will be clear that much remains to be learnt about the mechanism by which homografts are destroyed.

We have so far ignored the possibility that circulating antibodies play a part in the destruction of homografts. There is no doubt that homografts provoke the formation of serum antibodies and that in some circumstances these can exert a strong cytotoxic effect *in vivo*. They will certainly destroy first-set homografts which are inoculated as suspensions of dissociated cells, for example cell suspensions prepared from normal or malignant lymphoid tissue, and from normal bone marrow. On the other hand, first-set homografts of normal solid tissues which have a fibrous stroma and a blood supply can be, and probably are, destroyed by a cellular mechanism alone. Striking evidence for this conclusion is the observation that fœtal sheep, which are naturally agammaglobulinæmic, can destroy skin homografts *in utero*.[19] In this experiment the precaution was taken to neutralize *in vivo* any new antibody which may have been induced by the homograft. Similarly, sensitivity to skin homografts can be readily transferred in mice by means of lymphoid cells from sensitized donors but not by serum.

Circulating antibody can influence the survival of solid homografts but the effects are complex and unpredictable. If prior immunization has led to high concentrations of antibody in the circulating blood, skin or kidney grafts may die rapidly from vascular damage and failure of their blood supplies. The eventual failure of long-standing organ homografts in individuals receiving immunosuppressive drugs has also been attributed to a chronic attack on their vasculature by antibody. On the other hand, circulating antibody may actually protect some homografts from immunological attack.[20] Such "enhancing" antibody may act by shielding tissue antigens from the attention of immunological effector cells but the factors which determine whether antibody favours or prejudices the survival of a homograft are not clear.

There is thus some evidence for the view that the homograft reaction is mediated by lymphocytes which are released into the efferent lymphatics by the regional lymph nodes and pass by way of the blood to the graft. Experiments on graft-versus-host reactions, which we will consider later, suggest that these effector lymphocytes may be the progeny of the large pyroninophilic cells which arise and divide in the regional nodes, and that the large pyroninophilic cells arise in turn from small lymphocytes which initiate the immunological reaction, either centrally in the nodes or peripherally in the graft, following their stimulation by antigen.[21]

You will remember that in Chapter 39 the bacterial allergies were also described as immunological reactions which are mediated by lymphoid cells and not by circulating antibodies: the tuberculin reaction was a typical example. The analogy between the state of sensitivity which is revealed by a second-set skin homograft and that revealed by an intradermal injection of tuberculin into an individual who has already encountered the tubercle bacillus is a close one. Tuberculin sensitivity and homograft sensitivity can both be transferred to other animals by cells, but not by serum; and the analogy has been strengthened by the demonstration that guinea-pigs which have been sensitized with skin grafts react to the intradermal injection of antigenic material from the skin donor with a typical tuberculin-like skin reaction.[22] We may therefore regard the skin homograft reaction as one of the "cellular" immunities and the second-set reaction as a manifestation of delayed-type hypersensitivity.

Anatomical and Physiological Anomalies

Grafts of living tissue will survive if the recipient possesses all the antigens which are present in the graft. Thus, grafts will survive permanently if the donor and recipient are identical twins; if they are members of the same highly inbred strain; or if the recipient is a member of the F_1 progeny of a cross between two inbred strains and the donor is one of the inbred parents. These survivals have simple genetic explanations. Some grafts which are transplanted between genetically unrelated individuals will survive for other reasons.

Homografts of the cornea probably survive because they can neither provoke nor respond to a state of immunity: the cornea possesses neither lymphatics nor blood vessels. The evidence that orthotopic homografts of corneal tissue cannot respond to a state of immunity comes from experiments in which skin homografts were transplanted to the normal cornea of a highly immunised animal. Such grafts survived as long as they remained avascular.

Homografts of blood vessels are used clinically. They do not survive but provide a framework along which the host's own cells can grow. Cartilage homografts are also used clinically but these do survive, possibly because they possess no blood vessels and even an existing state of immunity cannot take effect.

There are many reports that grafts of endocrine tissue will survive when genetic considerations dictate that they should fail. Krohn has pointed out that most of these results become less convincing when the evidence is carefully examined, a view which is reinforced by his own finding that ovarian homografts in ovariectomized mice were readily destroyed and that the resulting sensitization was sufficient to cause a skin homograft to break down with the tempo of a second-set reaction.[23]

An interesting anomaly is the prolonged survival of homografts placed in the hamster cheek pouch. Such grafts become vascularized but they do not sensitize their hosts, probably due to the curious properties of the subcutaneous tissue of the pouch which lacks lymphatics.[10] Similarly, homografts placed on lymphatic-free pedicles of skin raised artificially on the backs of guinea-pigs enjoy a prolonged survival.[24] Both these examples can be taken as evidence against the importance of "peripheral sensitization" for small, slowly vascularized homografts.

Non-Specific Modification of the Homograft Reaction

The homograft reaction can be depressed by agents which impair the general immunological responses of an animal. For example, whole body X-irradiation, cortisone and certain antimetabolites, alkylating agents and antibiotics will all prolong the survival of homografts. When given alone these agents will only cause a significant prolongation of graft survival at dangerously high doses and they carry with them the hazard of rendering the recipient more susceptible to infections. In human organ transplantation the antimetabolite azathioprine, a derivative of 6-mercaptopurine, is often used together with corticosteroids as an immunosuppressive régime. The mode of action of these various agents is uncertain but in general they appear to act by depressing cell proliferation in lymphoid tissue.

Anti-lymphocyte serum (ALS).—The administration of antisera raised in one species against the lymphocytes of another species (for example rabbit-anti-mouse) may lead to a remarkable prolongation in the survival of homografts and even xenografts in the species providing the lymphocytes, with little general ill effect to the recipient.[25] For example, injections of rabbit-anti-mouse ALS allow the indefinite survival of skin homografts in healthy mice even when the donor and recipient differ at the strong H2 locus.[26] ALS also has the remarkable property of erasing the memory of prior immunization to homografts and of returning the animal to its virgin immunological state. The action is completely non-specific in that it will depress the response of the treated animals to homografts of widely different antigenic constitution and its efficacy is little affected by the antigenic disparity between donor and recipient. ALS appears to affect particularly the cell mediated immunities and leaves the ability to form circulating antibodies relatively unimpaired. The effective material in ALS is contained in the 7S gamma-globulin but its mode of action is not yet clear. Repeated injections eventually lead to a considerable destruction of lymphocytes in lymphoid tissue, particularly the long-lived small lymphocytes composing the recirculating pool. ALS has not yet been fully evaluated as an immunosuppressive agent for use in human transplantation.

Thymectomy.—It has been shown in mice and in several other species that the presence of the thymus during early life is essential for the normal development of lymphoid tissue.[27] Mice thymectomized at birth or early in the neonatal period show in adult life a depletion of small lymphocytes in the blood and lymphoid tissue and a severe impairment of their capacity to develop delayed hypersensitivity and to reject homografts and even xenografts. The ability of thymectomized mice to produce circulating antibodies varies with the antigen employed for immunization; for example, the response to sheep erythrocytes is severely depressed while that to hæmocyanin is little affected. During the first few months after neonatal thymectomy many animals develop a wasting disease which is eventually fatal and which is characterized by loss of weight, a ruffled, hunched appearance and diarrhœa. Germ-free mice do not develop this wasting syndrome after thymectomy suggesting that the immunological impairment in conventional mice leads to a fatal infection by some as yet unidentified agent.

The profound immunological deficiency which develops in neonatally thymectomized mice can be prevented by implanting a graft of intact thymic tissue from a young donor. The graft soon becomes colonized by the host's own cells and all the new lymphocytes in the restored lymph nodes are also finally of host origin. Experiments in which animals have been injected with cells carrying distinct chromosome markers have suggested that these host cells originate from stem cells in the bone marrow and that the migration from marrow → thymus → peripheral lymphoid tissue is the pathway by which functionally mature lymphoid tissue is normally built up. The influence which the thymus exerts on the marrow migrants may be hormonal since the deficiencies of neonatally thymectomized mice can also be made good by thymic tissue enclosed within small chambers which are impermeable to cells but not to large molecules.

Although thymectomy in adults has little obvious effect on immunological performance it is likely that the thymus continues to replenish peripheral lymphoid tissue with cells of marrow origin throughout life. Thus, heavily irradiated animals which are protected with bone marrow do not recover immunologically if they are also thymectomized; and thymectomy prevents the spontaneous return of reactivity which usually occurs in immunologically tolerant animals as the concentration of specific antigen in them wanes,[28] a point which will become clear later. That the intact thymus continues to export cells to the lymph nodes and spleen in adult animals has been demonstrated in experiments in which thymic cells were labelled *in situ* with tritiated thymidine.[29]

We mentioned earlier that as homografts are not normally encountered by animals in their environment the activity of lymphocytes in these reactions does not illuminate their normal function. One possibility, first suggested by Lewis Thomas, is that the homograft reaction is a mechanism for recognizing and eliminating neoplastic cells. This theory implies that the neo-plastic cells which are eliminated develop additional antigens which enable them to be recognized and attacked immunologically. Evidence for the existence of such a surveillance mechanism comes from the observation that tumours arise or can be more readily induced in certain animals with lymphoid aplasia, namely following neonatal thymectomy, in some chronic graft-against-host reactions, and, possibly, following prolonged treatment with antilymphocyte serum. The idea of surveillance by lymphocytes has aroused considerable interest but it must still be regarded as speculative.

Immunological Tolerance

The measures we have just considered lead to an indiscriminate depletion or destruction of lymphoid tissue and, consequently, to a non-specific depression of the homograft reaction. In contrast, the phenomenon of acquired immunological tolerance is a highly specific inhibition of immune responsiveness induced by the administration of antigen. It is best explained by an example. The example is based on the fact, which we have already discussed, that a normal A-strain mouse will destroy a skin homograft from a CBA mouse in about 10 days.

An A-strain embryo is injected on the 17th day of fœtal life with a suspension of living nucleated cells, for example blood leucocytes or bone marrow cells, from a CBA mouse of any age. Two months after birth the injected A-strain mouse receives a skin homograft from the donor of the CBA cells, or, if it is more convenient, from another mouse of the same highly inbred CBA strain. This homograft, far from being destroyed in 10 days, heals into place, grows a healthy pelt of agouti hair and survives for a prolonged period; it may even survive for the life of its A-strain host. Whereas the injection of allogeneic nucleated cells will immunize an adult mammal or bird against a skin graft from the cell donor, a similar injection into an embryo does just the opposite; it renders the individual tolerant of the graft. This remarkable phenomenon was first demonstrated experimentally by Billingham, Brent and Medawar[30] and illustrations of it are shown in Plate G.

The events leading to this experimental demonstration are of particular interest. Owen[31] reported in 1945 that the blood of dizygotic cattle twins sometimes contained a permanent mixture of two serologically distinct red cell types, one derived from each twin. Twin cattle are synchorial and apparently the precursors of red blood cells are freely exchanged *in utero* across the blood vessels of the fused fœtal membranes. Burnet and Fenner[32] in 1949 proposed a theory of antibody formation which was considerably influenced by Owen's observations. Central to this theory was an attempt to explain why an animal does not form antibodies against components of its own tissues. Burnet and Fenner suggested that during embryonic development the animal "learns" to recognize its own body constituents and to dispose of its worn-out cells without forming antibodies against them; they predicted that if an animal were injected with foreign antigenic material while still an embryo, it would be incapable of responding immunologically to this material in adult life. In 1951 Medawar and his colleagues complemented Owen's work by showing that the majority of twin calves would accept homografts of each other's skin and followed this in 1953 with the announcement that immunological tolerance to skin homografts could be produced by injecting fœtal animals with allogeneic living cells. We shall see later that the ability to induce tolerance is not restricted to antigens which are injected in the form of living cells and that tolerance can also be induced in adult animals.

Properties of Tolerance

Long lasting immunological tolerance is most readily induced if the genetic and therefore the antigenic relationship beween the donor and recipient is close; and it becomes progressively more difficult to induce as the animal develops its capacity to reject homografts. Thus, tolerance across a weak transplantation barrier can be readily induced in embryo or newborn mice by a small inoculum of the appropriate foreign cells, while tolerance to strong antigens in adults may require very large intravenous doses of foreign cells combined with a preliminary depression of the recipient's homograft response by means of drugs or whole body X-irradiation.

The point in development at which the capacity to reject homografts can be first demonstrated varies from species to species. In mice, tolerance can be easily induced as late as the first day after birth although even at this time the homograft reaction is sufficiently developed to destroy extremely small inocula of foreign cells. On the other hand, fœtal sheep can destroy skin homografts more than 50 days before birth. The time at which homograft reactivity develops in man is not known but there is no doubt that tolerance can be induced. Human twins have been reported in which the blood of each member contains erythrocytes of the other's type in addition to its own.[33] This must have arisen by an exchange of hæmopoietic cells in fœtal life and is the exact counterpart of the condition in dizygotic cattle twins. A human being or an animal in which cells from another individual coexist with its own is called a chimera. The condition we have just described is erythrocyte chimerism.

Immunological tolerance to homografts, like actively acquired immunity to homografts, is immunologically *specific*. Thus, the twin cattle which accepted grafts from each other rejected grafts from other donors; and mice of one inbred strain that are made tolerant of tissue from a second strain, retain unimpaired their ability to react against grafts from a third, unrelated strain. It also resembles homograft immunity in being individual specific and not tissue specific. The neonatal injection of allogeneic spleen cells in mice will induce tolerance, for example, to homografts of the donor's skin and adrenal glands.

Immunological tolerance is said to be a "central" failure of the immune response. The evidence for this view comes from the dramatic way in which tolerance can be abolished by injecting syngeneic lymphoid cells from a non-tolerant animal.[30] For example, if lymph node cells from a normal A-strain mouse are injected into a tolerant A-strain mouse bearing a long-standing graft of CBA skin, the graft will rapidly break down. This experiment shows that the graft retains its antigencity in the tolerant animal and that there is no block which prevents the effectors of graft destruction from reaching it. It is the lymphoid tissue of the tolerant animal which fails to respond: this failure is "central" not "peripheral". It is of some interest that the immunological apparatus of the tolerant animal can also be re-equipped by an injection of normal syngeneic lymphocytes from the thoracic duct.[21] This is further support for the idea that lymphocytes which normally circulate in the blood can initiate the reaction which destroys a homograft. FIGURE 1 illustrates an experiment of this kind in a tolerant rat.

Tolerance is not a phenomenon restricted to grafts of living tissue. There is ample evidence that tolerance of conventional "non-living" antigens can also occur, and such tolerance reveals itself by the failure of the animal to form dntibodies in response to antigenic challenge at an age when it would normally eo so.[34] A number of workers have injected soluble protein antigens, for cxample bovine or horse serum albumin, into newborn rabbits and have conaluded that the duration of tolerance depends on the amount of antigen originally injected and that repeated injections of antigen will prolong the period of

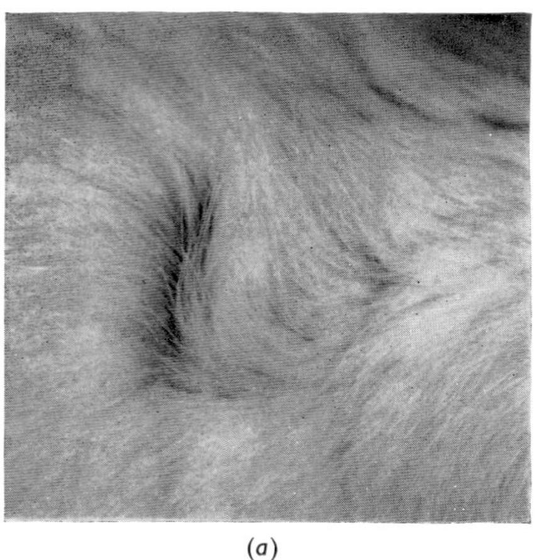

(a)

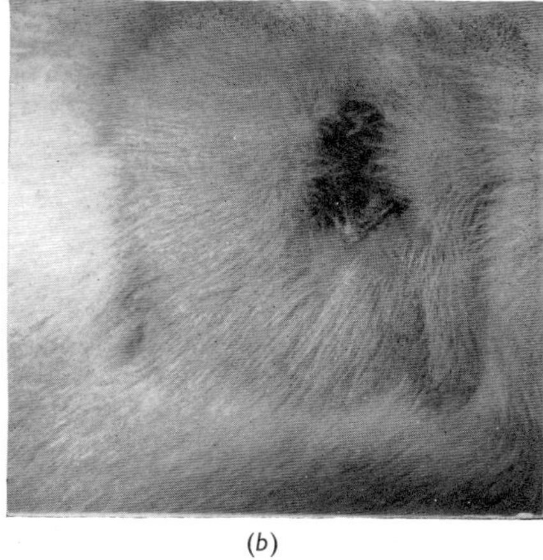

(b)

41/Fig. 1.—Destruction of homograft on a tolerant rat by the injection of normal isologous cells from the thoracic duct.

(*a*) Tolerant rat (T) of one inbred strain bearing a homograft of skin from rat (D) of another strain. The graft can be recognised by the direction of its hair growth. On the day of birth T had been injected intravenously with spleen cells from D to induce tolerance. At two months of age T was grafted with D's skin and the picture shows the graft 93 days later. A non-tolerant rat would have destroyed such a graft in about two weeks.

(*b*) The appearance of the same graft 18 days after the intravenous injection of 700 million lymphocytes from the thoracic duct of a normal rat of the same inbred strain as T. The hair has been clipped and the graft, now completely destroyed, appears as a dark contracted scab.

tolerance. A similar conclusion came from a study of the tolerance of chickens to foreign red cells: repeated transfusions of red cells starting at the birth would maintain the state of tolerance for many weeks, but tolerance disappeared if the transfusions were discontinued. A subsequent injection of red cells then resulting in an immune response.

The work on conventional antigens has established the important point that the maintenance of the tolerant state depends on the continued presence of antigen. The life-long tolerance of skin homografts which follows a single fœtal or neonatal injection of living cells also depends on on a persisting source of antigen. This is provided by the descendants of the originally injected cells for it has been shown that tolerant mice remain cellular chimeras.

Immunological tolerance to conventional antigens can also be produced in adult animals, but as with histocompatibility antigens, less readily than in very young animals. Adult rabbits can be made tolerant by means of large repeated doses of soluble protein antigens, the elimination of antigen from the blood proceeding at a non-immune rate for long periods. Similarly, tolerance to a soluble protein, bovine serum albumin, can be induced in mice by repeated large doses of antigen ("high zone" tolerance) but here the entry into the tolerant state is preceded by a period during which circulating antibody is formed. Surprisingly, repeated very small doses of bovine serum albumin will also induce tolerance ("low zone" tolerance) and the onset is more rapid than with the

(a)

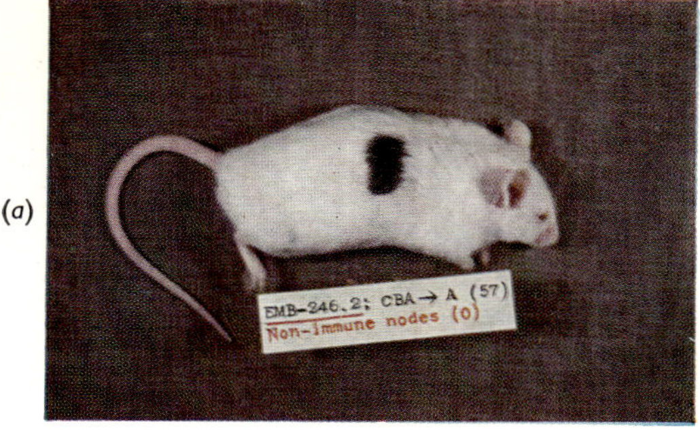

(b)

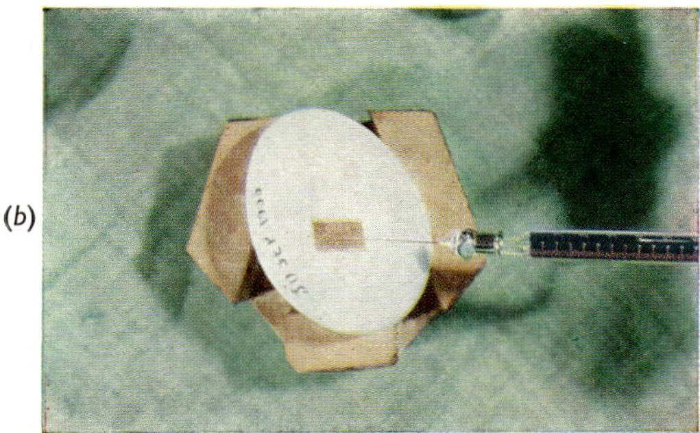

(c)

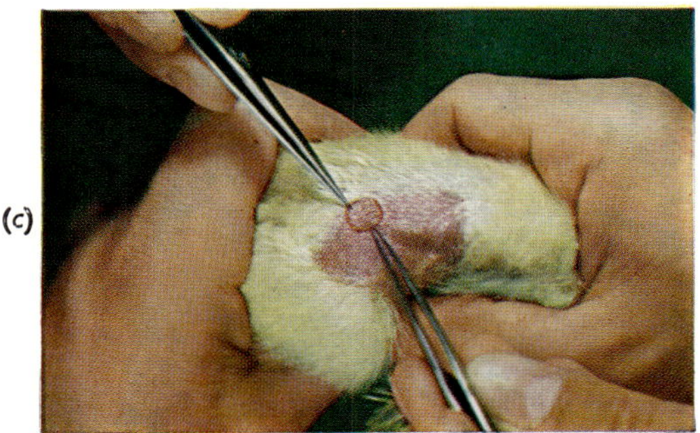

(d)

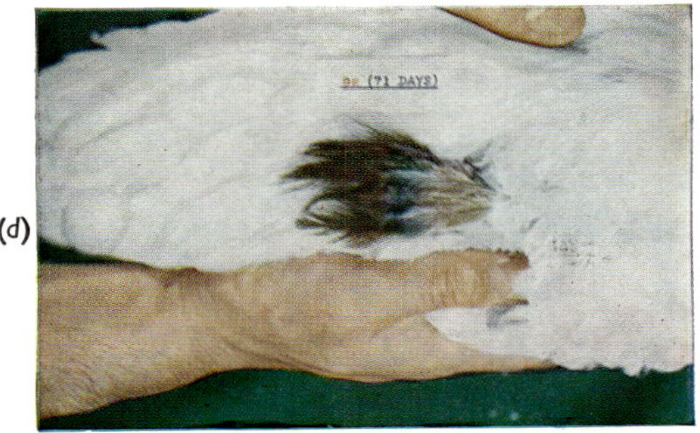

PLATE G

IMMUNOLOGICAL TOLERANCE

(*a*) A healthy CBA skin homograft 57 days after transplantation to a tolerant A-strain mouse which had been injected during uterine life with adult CBA tissue. A non-tolerant mouse would have destroyed such a graft in 10 days.

(*b–d*) Induction of tolerance in chickens.

(*b*) White Leghorn chick embryo being injected through chorio-allantoic vein with cells from a Rhode Island Red.

(*c*) White Leghorn chick, two weeks after hatching, being grafted with skin from the Rhode Island Red cell-donor.

(*d*) Rhode Island Red skin homograft 71 days after transplantation to tolerent White Leghorn chick. (From Billingham, Brent and Medawar.[30])

high zone régime and occurs without preceding antibody formation. In these experiments with mice,[35] tolerance was demonstrated by their failure to make antibody following a challenging dose of antigen in adjuvant.

Two other types of specific non-reactivity in adults deserve mention. Both were discovered before the demonstration of immunological tolerance by Medawar and it is necessary to consider their relationship to it. The first was called "immunological paralysis" by Felton[36] who showed that whereas mice can be protected against pneumococcal infection by immunization with small doses of specific pneumococcal polysaccharide, such immunization was ineffective if a very large dose of the specific polysaccharide had been given previously: no antibodies were formed and no protection against infection resulted. The immunological paralysis was specific since the mice responded normally to other antigens. It is still not clear whether antibody is produced in the paralysed mice and is continually neutralised by the vast excess of antigen which is known to persist for considerable periods in the tissues; or whether this is a true central failure of the immune response.

The second form of specific non-responsiveness in adults concerns the inhibition of sensitization to certain simple chemicals. In Chapter 40 we mentioned the delayed-type hypersensitivity which can be induced in adult guinea-pigs by the intradermal injection of certain simple chemical compounds. Chase showed that the ability of guinea-pigs to become sensitized in this way could be abolished if the compound in question was previously fed to the animal by mouth.[37] For example, if picryl chloride is injected intradermally the guinea-pig will later react to the application of picryl chloride to its skin with a delayed hypersensitivity reaction. But if picryl chloride had been previously fed to the animal the subsequent injection would fail to sensitize it. This inhibition of the immune response is long lasting, specific for the compound fed and can be regarded as a specific central failure of responsiveness.

Mechanism and significance of tolerance.—Acquired immunological tolerance was first thought to be a phenomenon which could only be induced in animals before they had developed the capacity to respond to the specific antigen in question. It is now clear that the same phenomenon can be induced in adults but that it requires large and often repeated dosage with antigen. At all ages tolerance will "break" unless antigen persists in the animal. The only comment to make is that it is obviously more difficult to maintain a suitable concentration of antigen in animals which have already developed the capacity to eliminate it. The effectiveness of "low zone" dosage in inducing tolerance to certain antigens in adults may simply reflect its failure to induce antibody formation. Similarly, if certain antigens are freed of aggregated or denatured components which are highly immunogenic (that is, efficient at inducing antibody formation) the remaining fraction may readily induce tolerance.

Although it is clear that the specific deficiency of a tolerant animal lies in its lymphoid tissue nothing is known at a cellular level about the mechanism by which antigen induces and maintains tolerance. It was at first suggested that all the specifically reactive cells in the animal were eliminated by the antigen, but as tolerance "breaks" when antigen disappears it is clear that potentially reactive cells are still present. The latter may be derived from the thymus because tolerance will not break spontaneously in thymectomized animals.[28] In other words, the return to normal reactivity is probably not due to the recovery of "tolerant cells" but to the provision of a new population of cells.

The possible biological function of tolerance has been discussed by Brent and Medawar.[38] It is argued that immunological tolerance is a device for preventing the occurrence of autoimmune reactions. Those body components which are potentially antigenic and which normally have access to the sites of antibody formation cannot provoke antibodies against themselves in adult life because, in the embryo, they had already induced immunological tolerance. Autoimmune diseases have been considered in detail in Chapter 40. The existence of erythrocyte chimerism in man and in cattle shows that immunological tolerance is a naturally occurring phenomenon and it is legitimate to think that it may play an important role in the developing organism.

GRAFT-AGAINST-HOST REACTIONS

In the kind of experiment we have been discussing the only activity we have assigned to the graft is that of providing an antigenic stimulus to the lymphoid tissue of the host. We will now consider the consequences for the host if the graft itself consists of lymphoid tissue. If such a graft survives it can theoretically react against the antigens of the host. This has now been shown to happen in several experimental situations, all of which can be fatal for the host. These situations amount to a list of the special circumstances under which homografts are accepted, namely, in very young animals, in F_1 hyrids given parental strain tissue and in immunosuppressed adults.

Allogeneic Lymphoid Grafts to Embryo or Newborn Hosts

Immunological tolerance to homografts of skin can be induced in mice by the intravenous injection of living cells into the newborn animal. As a matter of convenience the cells used to produce the state of tolerance are usually obtained from lymph nodes or spleen since a suspension suitable for intravenous injection can be readily prepared from them. Using this procedure Billingham and Brent[39] found that tolerance could be regularly produced between certain mouse strains and that the injected mice grew and developed normally. But if certain other strains were used the mice died a week of two after the injection. They grew normally at first but then growth ceased and the weight loss which followed was always associated with severe diarrhœa. The retarded, wasted appearance of these animals led to the condition being called "runt disease". Milder forms of the disease can occur, from chronic runting with a survival time of several months to a transient weight loss with complete recovery.

We have already described how the regional lymph nodes of the host are the seat of the immunological reaction which destroys a homograft. In runt disease the situation is reversed and the tissues of the host provide an antigenic stimulus for the lymphoid cells of the graft. The graft proceeds to mount an immunological attack against the host which damages its tissues and causes slight or severe illness or death. At the same time the host—the newborn mouse—is immunologically immature and cannot reject the graft which is so damaging to it.

The demonstration that runt disease is due to an immunological attack by the graft against the host comes from the following kind of evidence: (1) runt disease only occurs if the graft of lymphoid tissue survives. If the host is old enough to destroy it by a homograft reaction then no disease results. (2) Tissues which contain few or no lymphoid elements, for example, bone marrow, do not cause runt disease. (3) The incidence and severity of runt disease increase as the genetic disparity between donor and host becomes greater. Thus, runting never occurs when the mouse strains are closely related (e.g. CBA→C3H) but if there are wide antigenic differences between them then all the injected mice may die (e.g. C57→A). (4) Fœtal cells, which are incapable of an immune response, will not induce runt disease.

A condition in birds similar to runt disease was described quite independently by Simonsen.[40] The injection of allogeneic spleen cells or buffy coat blood leucocytes into chick embryos caused the death of the chick about two weeks after hatching with signs of wasting, an enlarged spleen and a hæmolytic anæmia. This condition was shown to be a graft-against-host reaction by experiments similar to those we have just described. Further evidence for this interpretation was the finding that in experiments with inbred chickens parental-line blood leucocytes caused gross splenic enlargement when they were injected into F_1 hybrid chicks, but that the injection of F_1 cells led to only minor changes in parental-line chicks. In other words, splenic enlargement only occurred when the host possessed antigens not present in the graft. This situation will be explained further in the next section.

Parental-strain Lymphoid Grafts to F_1 Hybrid Hosts

We explained that runt disease occurred because the newborn mouse: (1) had no power to reject the lymphoid graft; and (2) possessed antigens which were absent from the graft. A similar situation arises when an F_1 hybrid animal of any age is injected with lymphoid cells from one of its inbred parents. The injected cells will survive since they possess no antigen which is foreign to their F_1 host. But the host also contains the antigens of the other parent and these are "foreign" to the injected cells; consequently the injected cells will

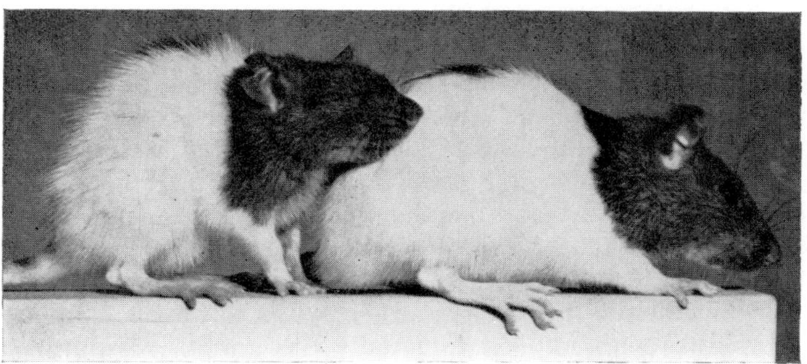

41/FIG. 2.—GRAFT-AGAINST-HOST REACTION.

Two F_1 hybrid littermates. The rat on the right is normal, that on the left had been injected 14 days previously with a suspension of small lymphocytes from a normal parental strain donor. The injected rat shows the typical signs of a graft-against-host reaction, namely profound weight loss, a ruffled, hunched appearance and skin lesions on the paws.

react immunologically against them. Lethal wasting disease has been produced in this way in adult mice[41] and rats.[42] The fatal disease in adult F_1 rats (FIG. 2) is characterised by skin lesions, extreme loss of body weight, enlargement of the spleen and lymph nodes, atrophy of the thymus, and atrophy and ulceration of the small intestine.

Mechanism of Graft-against-Host-Reaction

The earliest lesions in the host occur in its lymphoid tissue. The spleen and lymph nodes may enlarge considerably and later atrophy; in all cases the normal architecture becomes grossly disorganised. These changes are associated with the colonization of the host's lymphoid tissue by the injected lymphoid cells and it is thought that a proliferation of both donor and host cells contributes to the initial hypertrophy. It is likely that the host lymphoid tissue bears the main brunt of the immunological attack and that many of the pathological and clinical features of the disease are secondary to its destruction.[43] The nature of this immunological attack and the way in which it produces tissue destruction are unknown but it may be fundamentally similar to the mechanism of homograft destruction. In other words, the injected lymphoid cells mount a "cellular" type of immunological reaction against the tissues of the host. The idea that the host lymphoid tissue is the target for the attack is consistent with the greater sensitivity to the disease of lightly X-irradiated hosts. In such animals the lymphoid tissue has already been considerably damaged by the X-rays.

The immunological reaction which eventually kills the host is initiated by the interaction of the antigens of the host with certain cells in the graft. The identity of these cells became clear after the demonstration that pure suspensions of small lymphocytes prepared from either the blood or thoracic duct lymph will cause fatal graft-against-host reactions in newborn mice and adult F_1 hybrid rats respectively.[21] It has also been shown that some of the parental strain small lymphocytes which colonize and attack the lymphoid tissue of F_1 hybrids enlarge rapidly and start dividing; their progeny consist of more lymphocytes of progressively decreasing size.[44] These large dividing cells are identical morphologically with the large pyroninophilic cells which, as we have already mentioned, appear in the regional lymph nodes of animals rejecting homografts. There is no doubt that the antigens against which small lymphocytes react to initiate graft-against-host reactions and which also induce the transformation to large pyroninophilic cells are the foreign histocompatibility antigens of the host, because if the lymphocytes come from a specifically tolerant donor then they neither cause a graft-against-host reaction nor do they transform. The importance of these observations is that they have provided the first clue to the immunological function of small lymphocytes and also a plausible scheme for the cellular changes which underlie the homograft reaction.[45] Small lymphocytes can apparently interact with antigen to initiate the immune response, and it is possible, though not yet proven, that the new lymphocytes derived from them may be the effectors of graft destruction. Further evidence that small lymphocytes can initiate the homograft reaction comes from the rapidity with which homografts of skin break down in immunologically tolerant animals after an injection of small lymphocytes from a normal (non-tolerant) donor.[21]

When small lymphocytes from two genetically dissimilar individuals are incubated together *in vitro* each responds to the foreign histocompatibility antigens of the other and starts enlarging and dividing.[46] This "mixed lymphocyte reaction" is analogous to the transformation observed during graft-against-host reactions *in vivo* which we have just described. Attempts have been made to assess the antigenic disparity between pairs of human lymphocyte donors by measuring the degree of transformation and division which occurs, but the method is not yet regarded as giving a reliable guide for the selection of donors in human transplantation.

Another example of the stimulation of small lymphocytes by histocompatibility antigens is the "normal lymphocyte transfer reaction" and it again emphasizes the relation between graft-against-host and homograft reactions.[47] This transfer reaction shows itself as a delayed inflammatory response in the skin of normal guinea-pigs following the intradermal injection of allogeneic lymphocytes. If lymphocytes from one donor are injected into the skin of a group of outbred guinea-pigs then the intensity of these local graft-against-host reactions correlates with the order in which skin homografts from each member of the group are destroyed by the lymphocyte donor.

There have been speculations about the importance of graft-against-host reactions in human disease. It has been suggested that the extreme wasting and hæmoyltic anæmia which occur at a terminal stage in certain malignant conditions of lymphoid tissue may be due to an immunological reaction by the lymphoid tumour against the host. This postulates a change in the tumour which leads it to regard one or more antigens of the host as foreign.[48] Less speculative is the warning that if maternal blood lymphocytes leaked across the placenta they would be likely to attack the fœtus in precisely the same way as allogeneic lymphocytes will attack a fœtal mouse and cause runt disease.[39] This emphasizes the importance of the particularly effective barrier which normally separates the fœtal from the maternal circulation.

A further example of an experimental graft-against-host reaction and of its possible human counterpart will be described in the next section.

Repair of Radiation Injury

The bone marrow is one of the tissues that are highly sensitive to X-irradiation (see Chapter 26). In 1950 Jacobson showed that the mortality of mice from exposure to high doses of X-rays could be greatly reduced by shielding the spleen during irradiation. The hæmopoietic tissue which is normally present in the spleen of adult mice underwent a considerable hypertrophy in the protected animals and this was followed by recovery of the bone marrow.[49] It was then found that mice could be protected if living cells from the bone marrow or the spleen were injected immediately after irradiation. Early in this work it was realised that the beneficial effect of treatment with spleen or marrow was due to the rapid re-equipment of the irradiated animal with hæmopoietic tissue, but it was not clear how this came about. We shall see that an investigation of this problem is, in effect, a study in tissue transplantation. It need hardly be added that the possibility of treating radiation injury in man by injections of hæmopoietic cells has given the investigations in animals a particular interest.

Treatment with Hæmopoietic Tissue

High doses of X-irradiation cause extensive damage to the gut as well as to the bone marrow. The clinical picture at death depends upon which of these organs is the more severely affected and this, in turn, depends on the dose of radiation and the species of animal. Rats that receive a lethal dose of X-rays usually succumb from the effects of damage to the intestinal tract. In other species, of which the mouse is one, a large dose of radiation will destroy the intestinal epithelium and kill the animal in a few days, but with smaller doses which kill the mice between one and two weeks, damage to hæmopoietic tissue predominates. The treatment of radiation injury by injection of blood-forming cells has been studied mainly in mice using doses of radiation which will just kill all the animals. The "intestinal syndrome" caused by higher doses of radiation is not influenced by treatment of this kind.

Two rival theories were put forward to explain the recovery of lethally irradiated animals given injections of living hæmopoietic cells. Some argued that the injected cells proliferated in the host and provided it with a new functioning marrow. Jacobson, on the other hand, originally favoured the idea that a humoral factor derived from the injected cells stimulated the regeneration of the irradiated animal's own marrow. In support of this it was pointed out that rat marrow was effective in the treatment of irradiated mice and that rat marrow could not be expected to survive in the mouse: it would be destroyed by a homograft reaction.

The decision between these two theories clearly required methods which would distinguish the cells of the donor from those of the irradiated host. Several groups of workers were able to show beyond doubt that the resuscitation of lethally irradiated animals is due to the proliferation of the injected cells: the animal survives because it acquires a functional graft of bone marrow. The most elegant proof is due to Ford and his colleagues at Harwell.[50] They distinguished donor from host cells by examining chromosomes in squash preparations of the tissues. For example, when an irradiated mouse was treated with rat hæmopoietic cells it was found that all the mitoses in its "regenerated" marrow had chromosomes whose number and appearance were typical of those of the rat. Similarly, when syngeneic mouse marrow was used there was repopulation of the host by the donor's cells. In this case the marrow cells were identified by a chromosome translocation which was peculiar to the cells of the donor mice.

It has been shown by several other workers that treatment with allogeneic and xenogeneic marrow is followed by the appearance in the circulating blood of erythrocytes and granulocytes of donor origin. Lindsley[51] identified circulating donor-type erythrocytes in allogeneic rats by an agglutination reaction. Others have shown the presence of rat granulocytes in the blood of irradiated mice by applying a histochemical test for alkaline phosphatase: rat granulocytes give a positive reaction while those of the mouse do not.[52] Experiments of this kind have shown that the replacement of the host's circulating erythrocytes and granulocytes by those of the donor may, in some cases, be complete.

Cells from the donor's marrow also contribute to the regeneration of lymph nodes in irradiated animals, but lymphoid cells will not repopulate bone marrow and no protection can be obtained by transplanting them. This is an important observation since it militates strongly against the view that small lymphocytes can transform into marrow stem cells. This conclusion was emphasised by a study in which large numbers of syngeneic mouse thoracic duct cells, 95 per cent of which are small lymphocytes, were found to give no protection against a lethal dose of irradiation.[53] Before the animals died a considerable repopulation of their lymphoid tissue had occurred but there was no sign of regeneration in the bone marrow. The stem cell in marrow which is capable of restoring the hæmopoietic tissue in irradiated animals has not yet been identified morphologically. Although it is apparently not a lymphocyte it is certainly present in normal blood because irradiated animals can be protected with concentrates of blood leucocytes.

The early workers underestimated the degree to which the immunological responses of an animal are impaired by high doses of radiation. It is now clear that homografts and xenografts of marrow will survive in lethally irradiated hosts because no immune reaction is mounted against them. Such chimeras will subsequently accept skin grafts from the animal which provided the marrow cells. For example, a lethally irradiated mouse will accept a skin graft from the rat which provided it with the life-saving injection of marrow cells, although it will reject a skin graft from an unrelated donor. If the lymphoid tissue of the irradiated animal had been completely replaced by that of the donor the survival of the skin graft from the donor would not be surprising. But in cases where the host's lymphoid tissue recovers the survival of the foreign skin graft (and the marrow graft) requires an explanation. It has been suggested that the regenerating lymphoid tissue of the lethally X-irradiated host is in a condition comparable to developing lymphoid tissue in the fœtus, and is able to acquire immunological tolerance of the foreign donor cells.

Complications of Treatment

Although lethally irradiated animals can be rescued by injecting syngeneic, allogeneic or xenogeneic marrow, more cells are needed as the genetic disparity between the donor and the host increases. Thus about twenty times as many allogeneic as syngeneic marrow cells are required to give protection in mice, and successful xenogeneic treatment needs more still. The reason for this is not clear but there may be physiological or nutritional reasons why, for example, rat cells cannot establish themselves in a mouse environment as readily as can mouse cells.

The most serious complication of the treatment of radiation injury with foreign hæmopoietic cells is the development of the condition known in animals as "secondary disease".[54] This disease is another example of a graft-against-host reaction and it is thought to be due to lymphoid elements in the original inoculum of marrow cells which slowly proliferate and react against the tissues of the host. Secondary disease came to be noticed in the following way.

It is a convention in experimental work to regard "successful" treatment of radiation injury as that which permits the animal to survive for 30 days. However, it was pointed out by workers at Harwell that if the treated animals were observed for more than 30 days an important difference emerged between the allogeneic- and syngeneic-treated groups. Mice given allogeneic cells became sick soon after 30 days and by about 100 days they were all dead. This did not occur after treatment with syngeneic cells. The main signs of secondary disease are extreme wasting, skin lesions and diarrhœa and the condition is usually, though not invariably, fatal.

Several lines of evidence point to secondary disease as a graft-against-host reaction.[54] Animals with this condition can retain an intact donor-type bone marrow and also a healthy skin graft from the bone marrow donor. Death cannot therefore be due to the rejection of the transplanted marrow by the recovering lymphoid tissue of the host. Attempts to circumvent the development of secondary disease have added weight to the idea that it is a graft-against-host reaction. The transplantation of marrow from an F_1 hybrid to an irradiated parental-strain animal cannot result in a graft-against-host reaction, since the host will not possess antigens which are foreign to the graft. Several workers have reported that no secondary disease does, in fact, occur in such a combination. Further, there are claims that no secondary mortality occurs if embryonic rather than adult hæmopoietic tissue is transplanted.

Apparently against the idea that secondary disease is a graft-against-host reaction is the observation that an identical wasting disease occurs in lethally irradiated mice restored with small inocula of syngeneic bone marrow.[55] However, it is probable that the wasting syndrome in both cases is a consequence of lymphoid aplasia, in the first due to an immunological attack and in the second due to an inadequate number of lymphoid precursors in the syngeneic marrow inocula. We have already considered the similar wasting syndrome associated with lymphoid aplasia which occurs in neonatally thymectomized animals.

In man the occurrence of secondary disease remains a serious potential risk to any heavily irradiated patient who is given allogeneic marrow, and the therapeutic value of fœtal hæmopoietic tissue in radiation injury has not yet been firmly established. Allogeneic marrow grafts have been used in clinical practice in the treatment of accidental radiation injury and of marrow aplasia due to drugs. Attempts have also been made to eradicate malignant disease with high doses of radiation, the damage to the patient's hæmopoietic tissue being made good by a subsequent transplantation of marrow cells. In this last example it is likely that at least one patient has died from secondary disease, the new lymphoid cells from the graft of foreign marrow having mounted a lethal graft-against-host reaction. The benefit to patients who have been treated with marrow grafts is difficult to assess, but their potential therapeutic value is a strong incentive to work in this field.

REFERENCES

1. Hildemann, W. H. (1957). *Ann. N.Y. Acad. Sci.*, **64,** 775.
2. Medawar, P. B. (1944). *J. Anat. (Lond.)*, **78,** 176.
3. Medawar, P. B. (1945). *J. Anat. (Lond.)*, **79,** 157.
4. Medawar, P. B. (1946). *Brit. J. exp. Path.*, **27,** 9.
5. Medawar, P. B. (1946). *Brit. J. exp. Path.*, **27,** 15.
6. Barnes, A. D., and Krohn, P. L. (1957). *Proc. roy. Soc. B*, **146,** 505.
7. Eichwald, E. J., and Silmser, C. R. (1955). *Transplant. Bull.*, **2,** 148.
8. Bach, F. H. (1968). *Science*, **159,** 1196.
9. Medawar, P. B., and Russell, P. S. (1958). *Immunology*, **1,** 1.

10. Billingham, R. E., and Silvers, W. K. (1964). *Plast. reconstr. Surg.*, **34,** 329.
11. Strober, S., and Gowans, J. L. (1965). *J. exp. Med.*, **122,** 347.
12. Mitchison, N. A. (1954). *Proc. roy. Soc. B.*, **142,** 72.
13. Billingham, R. E., Brent, L., and Medawar, P. B. (1954). *Proc. roy. Soc. B*, **143,** 58.
14. Billingham, R. E., Silvers, W. K., and Wilson, D. B. (1963). *J. exp. Med.*, **118,** 397.
15. Gowans, J. L. (1965). *Brit. med. Bull.*, **21,** 106.
16. Wilson, D. B., and Billingham, R. E. (1967). *Advanc. Immunol.*, **7,** 189.
17. Wilson, D. B. (1965). *J. exp. Med.*, **122,** 143.
18. David, J. R. (1968). *Fed. Proc.*, **27,** 6.
19. Silverstein, A. M., and Kraner, K. L. (1965). *Transplantation*, **3,** 535.
20. Brent, L., and Medawar, P. B. (1961). *Proc. roy. Soc. B*, **155,** 392.
21. Gowans, J. L., and McGregor, D. D. (1965). *Progr. Allergy*, **9,** 1.
22. Brent, L., Brown, J., and Medawar, P. B. (1962). *Proc. roy. Soc. B*, **156,** 187.
23. Krohn, P. L. (1959). In *Biological Problems of Grafting*, p. 146. Eds., Albert F. and Medawar P. B. Oxford: Blackwell Scientific Publications.
24. Barker, C. F., and Billingham, R. E. (1968). *J. exp. Med.*, **128,** 197.
25. Wolstenholme, G. E. W., and O'Connor, M., Eds. (1967). Ciba Foundation Study Group No. 29, *Antilymphocyte Serum.* London: J. & A. Churchill.
26. Levey, R. H., and Medawar, P. B. (1966). *Proc. nat. Acad. Sci.* (*Wash.*), **56,** 1130.
27. Miller, J. F. A. P., and Osoba, D. (1967). *Physiol. Rev.*, **47,** 437.
28. Claman, H. N., and Talmage, D. W. (1963). *Science*, **141,** 1193.
29. Weissman, I. L. (1967). *J. exp. Med.*, **126,** 291.
30. Billingham, R. E., Brent, L., and Medawar, P. B. (1956). *Phil. Trans. B*, **239,** 357.
31. Owen, R. D. (1945). *Science*, **102,** 400.
32. Burnet, F. M., and Fenner, F. (1949). *The Production of Antibodies*, 2nd edit. Melbourne: Macmillan & Co.
33. Dunsford, I., Bowley, C. C., Hutchison, A. M., Thompson, J. S., Sanger, R., and Race, R. R. (1953). *Brit. med. J.*, **2,** 81.
34. Dresser, D. W., and Mitchison, N. A. (1968). *Advanc. Immunol.*, **8,** 129.
35. Mitchison, N. A. (1964). *Proc. roy. Soc. B*, **161,** 275.
36. Felton, L. D. (1949). *J. Immunol.*, **61,** 107.
37. Chase, M. W. (1946). *Proc. Soc. exp. Biol.* (*N.Y.*), **61,** 257.
38. Brent, L., and Medawar, P. B. (1959). In *Recent Progress in Microbiology*, p. 181. (Symposium of VIIth Int. Congr. Microbiol.) Ed. Tunevall G. Stockholm: Almqvist and Wiksell.
39. Billingham, R. E., and Brent, L. (1959). *Phil. Trans. B*, **242,** 439.
40. Simonsen, M. (1957). *Acta path. microbiol. Scand.*, **40,** 480.
41. Cole, L. J., and Ellis, M. E. (1958). *Science*, **128,** 32.
42. Gowans, J. L. (1962). *Ann. N.Y. Acad. Sci.*, **99,** 432.
43. Billingham, R. E., Defendi, V., Silvers, W. K., and Steinmuller, D. (1962). *J. nat. Cancer Inst.*, **28,** 365.
44. Ford, W. L., Gowans, J. L., and McCullagh, P. J. (1966). In *The Thymus: Experimental and Clinical Studies*, p. 58. Eds. Wolstenholme, G. E. W., and Porter, R. London: J. & A. Churchill.
45. Gowans, J. L., McGregor, D. D., Cowan, D. M., and Ford, C. E. (1962). *Nature* (*Lond.*), **196,** 651.
46. Bain, B., Vas, M. R., and Lowenstein, L. (1964). *Blood*, **23,** 108.
47. Brent, L., and Medawar, P. (1966). *Proc. roy. Soc. B*, **165,** 281.
48. Kaplan, H. S., and Smithers, D. W. (1959). *Lancet*, **2,** 1.
49. Jacobson, L. O., Simmons, E. L., Bethard, W. F., Marks, E. K., and Robson, M. J. (1950). *Proc. Soc. exp. Biol.* (*N.Y.*), **73,** 455.

50. Ford, C. E., Hamerton, J. L., Barnes, D. W. H., and Loutit, J. F. (1956). *Nature* (*Lond.*), **177,** 452.
51. Lindsley, D. L., Odell, T. T., and Tausche, F. G. (1955). *Proc. Soc. exp. Biol.* (*N.Y.*), **90,** 512.
52. Nowell, P. C., Cole, L. J., Habermeyer, J. G., and Roan, P. L. (1956). *Cancer Res.*, **16,** 258.
53. Gesner, B. M., and Gowans, J. L. (1962). *Brit. J. exp. Path.*, **43,** 431.
54. Barnes, D. W. H., Ford, C. E., Ilbery, P. L. T., and Loutit, J. F. (1958). *Transplant. Bull.*, **5,** 101.
55. Barnes, D. W. H., Loutit, J. L., and Micklem, H. S. (1962). *Ann. N.Y. Acad. Sci.*, **99,** 374.

The following reviews not already listed in the references may be consulted:

Billingham, R. E., and Silvers, W. K. (1963). *Ann. Rev. Microbiol.*, **17,** 531. Sensitivity to homografts of normal tissues and cells.

Brent, L., Ed. (1965). *Brit. med. Bull.*, **21,** 97–180. Transplantation of tissues and organs.

Medawar, P. B. (1958). *Harvey Lect.*, **52,** 144. The immunology of transplantation.

Medawar, P. B. (1958). *Proc. roy. Soc. B*, **148,** 145. The homograft reaction.

Micklem, H. S., and Loutit, J. F. (1966). *Tissue Grafting and Radiation.* New York: Academic Press.

Simonsen, M. (1962). *Progr. Allergy*, **6,** 349. Graft versus host reactions. Their natural history, and applicability as tools of research.

Chapter 42

CHRONIC INFLAMMATION AND TUBERCULOSIS

By J. C. F. Poole and H. W. Florey

We have so far considered the local cellular reactions that occur in response to an acute insult to the tissues and those occurring when damaged tissues are healing. There are, however, a number of conditions in which inflammation is not of the acute type, i.e. characterised by the exudation of fluid and the accumulation of polymorphs, but is marked by the presence of cells particularly of the mononuclear type, i.e. macrophages and lymphocytes. This latter type of lesion is that associated with chronic inflammation. It may be caused by the presence of irritating material such as silica or asbestos; it may occur when there is a near balance between the resistance of the body and the inroads of an infecting agent such as the organism of tuberculosis or syphilis; or it may occur following long-continued mechanical irritation, such as that caused by a jagged tooth; or as a result of impaired nutritional conditions such as are present in a viscus whose blood supply is reduced or in the ulcers of the leg that result from venous stasis due to varicose veins.

Tissue subject to chronic inflammation may contain cells of many kinds. There may be a mobilisation of macrophages and lymphocytes and at the same time attempts at healing are shown by much fibroblastic activity. In addition giant cells, probably formed by the fusion of macrophages, may accumulate especially around insoluble foreign bodies—hence the name they frequently receive of "foreign body giant cells". Plasma cells and sometimes eosinophils may also be a prominent feature.

A number of serious diseases caused by micro-organisms are of a chronic inflammatory nature almost from the beginning. In such diseases, the cellular responses to infection vary according to the organism concerned. For example, in tuberculosis, as we shall see, macrophages, cells derived from macrophages and smaller numbers of lymphocytes are found. On the other hand in the early lesions of syphilis, lymphocytes and plasma cells predominate. In actinomycosis—rather surprisingly—there is a polymorph response.

Tuberculosis is of such widespread occurrence and has so many interesting pathological facets that we will devote the rest of this chapter to its consideration.

TUBERCULOSIS

Tuberculosis is an extremely common bacterial infection. Even in advanced countries with good health services the proportion of people who become infected may be of the order of 50 per cent, but because of great variations from one part of a country to another, precise figures have little meaning. Happily, for most people it is an exceedingly trivial condition which passes unnoticed and has no long term results apart from the desirable one of conferring increased resistance to subsequent infection.

Almost every organ or tissue can on occasion be involved in the disease. However, much the commonest organs to become infected are the lungs. Pulmonary tuberculosis is also known as consumption of the lungs and as phthisis but both terms are obsolescent. Parts of the alimentary tract are fairly often infected; so are bones and joints—hunchbacks are usually people who have had tuberculosis of the spine. In some parts of the world tuberculous infection of the skin is common and leads to the distressing and disfiguring condition known as lupus vulgaris.

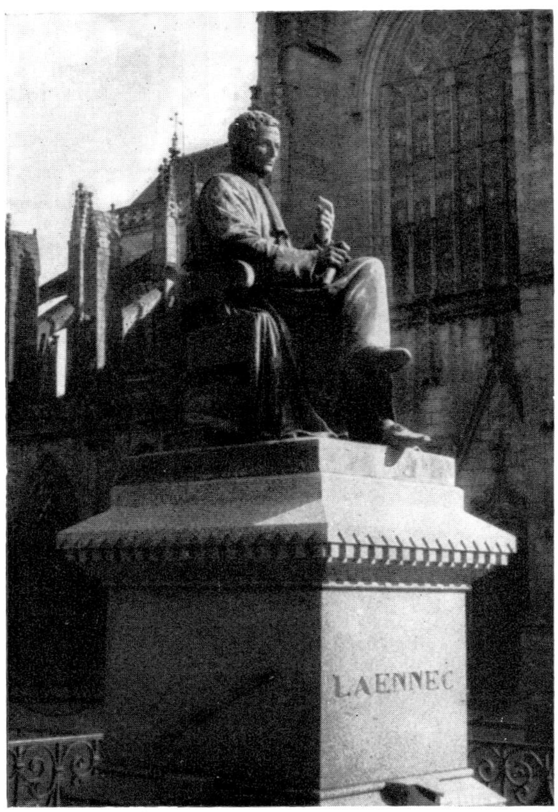

42/FIG. 1.—René-Théophile-Hyacinthe Laennec (1781–1826). Statue erected in the Place Saint-Corentin, Quimper, his birthplace in Brittany.

Historical

Tuberculosis was known in antiquity, for its ravages can be recognised in lesions of bones that have survived. Probably the first known example of disease of the vertebral column dates to the Neolithic period (about 5000 B.C.). There is evidence of bony lesions in Egyptian mummies and the disease may have been common in the predynastic period of Egypt. A clay statuette dating from about 4000 B.C. shows the distortion of the spine often associated with tuberculosis (illustrated in Sigerist[1]). It does not seem that tuberculosis of the lungs was common in Egypt, for no description of this form of the disease exists, but phthisis was recognised by the Greeks, and described by their physicians, e.g. in the Hippocratic writings (*ca.* 400 B.C.).* Tuberculous disease of the lungs is also mentioned in the Indian Rig-Veda (about 1500 B.C.), and there are a number of representations of the disease among the primitive statuettes of the New World. The idea of tuberculosis as a separate disease did not emerge until 1671 when Francis Sylvius (De le Boë) used the term *tubercula minora vel majora* to describe the appearances of lesions of the lungs of consumptives. Very accurate descriptions of the macroscopic appearances of tuberculous lesions were given by William Stark (1740–70), whose work appeared in 1788, and by Matthew Baillie (1761–1823), who published his observations in 1793. This work influenced the French school, the most distinguished members of which were perhaps Louis (1787–1872) and Laennec (1781–1826) (FIG. 1). The latter, who was himself a consumptive, introduced the stethoscope into medicine. At this time certain pathologists, for instance Bayle (1774–1816) of France, held the view that miliary tuberculosis was a different disease from what was called caseous phthisis, a view supported and expanded by Virchow (1821–1905). Laennec propounded the modern doctrine that tuberculosis is a morbid process that may occur in various parts of the body and that consumption is tuberculosis of the lungs.

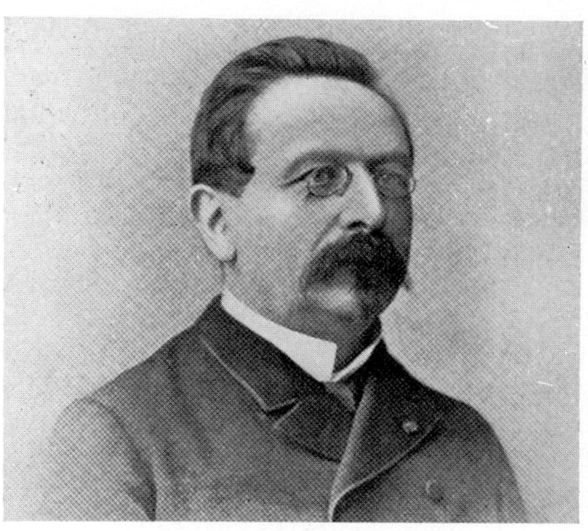

42/FIG. 2.—Jean-Antoine Villemin (1827–1892).

The ancients such as Galen (*ca.* A.D. 130–200) expressed a popular view in stating that the exhalation of a phthisical patient is dangerous, and a number of observers in the sixteenth and eighteenth centuries thought of phthisis as contagious, but by the early nineteenth century these views were submerged and the disease was thought to be associated with "constitution" and to be of an hereditary nature. Thus by the middle of the nineteenth century pathologists and physicians, with a few exceptions, considered that tuberculosis was not communicable.

That tuberculosis is indeed an infective disease was shown by J.-A. Villemin (1827–92) (FIG. 2), who was a French army surgeon. Amongst other things, he caused tuberculosis in guinea-pigs by the inoculation of human tuberculous material, and infected rabbits with material from tuberculous lesions of cattle. Villemin's work was eventually completely confirmed, though not all were at first successful in repeating it. The final proof of the infective and bacterial

* A continuous tradition links phthisis of the early Greek medical writers with pulmonary tuberculosis as we understand it now. Many of these early descriptions are rather vague and may have referred to other conditions. The disease described in the Hippocratic writings in Epidemics, III, xiii, could well have been pulmonary tuberculosis.

nature of tuberculosis was provided by Robert Koch (1843–1910) (FIG. 3), who announced his discovery in 1882.[2] The essential features of Koch's demonstration lay in his proof that the tubercle bacillus was constantly present in lesions, that it could be isolated from them in pure culture, and that the injection of these pure cultures produced tubercles in healthy animals.

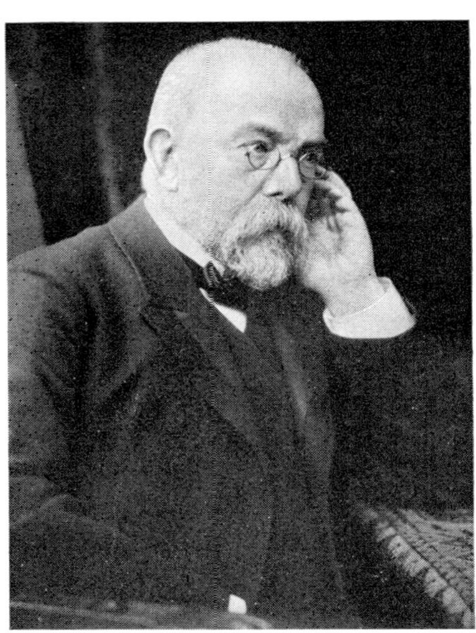

42/FIG. 3.—Robert Koch (1843–1910).

Mycobacterium tuberculosis

The disease in man and animals is caused by a number of types of the one species of micro-organism, *Mycobacterium tuberculosis*. The mycobacteria are characterised by certain distinguishing features. They do not stain readily, but when treated with a suitable mordant the stained bacilli resist decolorisation by acids. The bacterial cell has a high content of lipoid material. Although one lipoid component, mycolic acid, has been reported to show acid-resistant staining, it is by no means settled that this physical property of mycolic acid is the cause of acid-fastness in the intact bacterial cell. A third characteristic of pathogenic strains of mycobacteria is that they multiply slowly.

There are several types of the tubercle bacillus. Both the *human type* and the *bovine type* commonly cause disease in man and in certain other animals. The distinction between the two types was not at first appreciated, but it is now clear that the strains which Koch isolated and studied in his early experiments[3] included examples of both. The fact that two distinguishable types of the tubercle bacillus could cause disease in man began to become clear in the early years of this century, and it was found that they differed not only in cultural characteristics but also in their range of host specificity (see below). An attenuated strain of the bovine type of tubercle bacillus was prepared by Calmette and Guérin in 1924[4] and has been extensively used for active immunisation in man. It is known as "Bacille Calmette-Guérin", or BCG for short, and will be considered further in a later section. The *avian type* can infect birds and some mammals but not man. The *cold-blooded type* causes disease in many fish, amphibia and reptiles but cannot infect any warm-blooded animal. A fifth type of tubercle bacillus, the *vole bacillus*, was discovered by Wells in 1937[5] as a natural parasite of wild voles captured in certain areas of England, Scotland and Wales. This organism produces only localised disease when injected into the skin of man, and, like BCG, has been used for active immunisation in experimental animals and in man. The *dassie bacillus* is an organism very similar to the vole bacillus which was discovered in 1958[6] in South Africa in the lungs of the dassie or Cape Hyrax (*Procavia capensis*): it has not so far been tried in man for active immunisation, but promising results have been obtained in animal experiments.[7, 8]

Sources of Infection for Man

As far as human infection is concerned, the greatest natural source of tubercle bacilli is provided by persons with open tuberculous lesions of the lung. Bacilli, often in millions, are expectorated in the sputum or sprayed as droplets into the air during talking, coughing or sneezing. When sputum has dried, the bacilli can remain alive for a long time in the dust which it yields. Either droplets or dust containing tubercle bacilli may be inhaled by healthy persons, especially those in close contact with the infected individual, who often does not know that he is a danger to those around him. It is perhaps a comfort, when contemplating the pavements, to believe that sunlight may quickly kill the tubercle bacillus, at least when it is moist.

The experiments of Koch,[3] which were confirmed by many others, suggested that infection in animals could be initiated by the inhalation of droplets or fine particles of dust containing tubercle bacilli. There was, however, considerable controversy over this matter, for many pathologists at the beginning of the present century maintained that tubercle bacilli gained entrance to the lungs after absorption from the alimentary tract. This may be so in a very small number of cases. Cobbett[9] discussed the evidence at some length and supported the view that tubercle bacilli could be inhaled into the lung, by showing that the organism *B. prodigiosus* (now known as *Chromobacterium prodigiosum* or *Serratia marcescens*) penetrated to the margins of the lungs of animals a few minutes after they had been exposed to a culture sprayed into the air.

Estimates vary, but the number of inhaled bacilli necessary to cause infection in a susceptible animal may be quite small. Improved techniques have been devised whereby bacilli can be introduced into the air in known numbers and, since the bacilli tend to clump together into "bacillary units", in known degrees of dispersion. Rabbits and other animals can be made to inhale the infected air for a given time. Experiments using this technique indicate that about three very fine bacillary units composed of virulent bovine bacilli were required to produce one tuberculous focus in the lung of a rabbit possessed of some genetic resistance to the disease. It was much more difficult to infect with larger aggregates of bacilli, since these probably do not reach the alveoli so readily as the smaller units, but fall on ciliated mucosa and are swept upwards to the pharynx and are swallowed. The deduction made from these experiments was that the inhalation of a few tubercle bacilli in fine droplets expelled from the mouth or nose is more likely to lead to infection of the lung than the inhalation of a much larger number of organisms in relatively coarse particles of dust or large droplets.[10, 11] It is possible that some of the larger aggregates may be arrested in the upper respiratory tract and may gain entrance to the body via the tonsil or mucous membrane of the nasal cavities. But swallowed organisms are often rendered harmless. Thus it was found that 10,000 bacilli, from a culture of which a very few bacilli would produce tubercles in the lung, could be ingested by the rabbit without producing an observable effect. This observation confirmed earlier studies which have been summarised by Cobbett.[9]

Another source of infection is milk from cows with infected udders. Bacilli swallowed in milk gain entrance into the body through the tonsils or the wall of the intestine. This form of infection can be controlled by doing away with the source of bacilli. Thus in the United Kingdom, the United States of America and in several other countries, where tuberculous cattle have been almost completely eliminated by slaughter, and where pasteurisation of milk is well-nigh universal, infection due to the bovine bacillus is very rare indeed.

Occasionally infection occurs at the site of injury in butchers who cut themselves with knives contaminated with bovine bacilli, or in surgeons and nurses who prick or cut themselves when operating on or dressing infected tissues, or in pathologists who injure themselves while making post-mortem examinations. Tubercle bacilli may also gain entry to the skin through abrasions and cracks, causing the tuberculous disease of the skin known as lupus vulgaris. It is doubtful whether they can penetrate intact skin. Perhaps they can enter the lymphatics or nasopharynx from the conjunctival sac, which is exposed to air-borne droplets. *Mycobacterium balnei*, a closely related acid-fast bacillus, has been shown to be responsible for infection of the skin with the production of tubercles in bathers using infected swimming-pools.[12]

Widespread Nature of Disease

As recently as 1950 it was stated that 5,000,000 people die of tuberculosis every year, and that there are 50,000,000 people in the world afflicted with the disease.[13] Although these figures have no accurate statistical basis they are not an unreasonable guess and will give some idea why it is considered that tuberculosis is still the most important bacterial disease affecting man.

It is sometimes supposed that tuberculosis is more widespread in cold countries than in hot, but there are no grounds for believing that this is so. Tuberculosis occurs in all the countries of the world.

Decrease in Mortality and Incidence of Disease

In many places where hygiene is not so highly developed as in Western countries the death-rate from tuberculosis is still high. In certain countries there has been a striking and continuous fall in the death-rate during the last century. The decline in mortality in England and Wales is indicated in the following table:

Standardised Mortality Ratios for England and Wales, 1851–1965. (Base years 1950–1952 taken as 100)

1851–1860	1438	1931–1939	245
1861–1870	1346	1940–1944	221
1871–1880	1190	1945–1949	174
1881–1890	1004	1950–1954	85
1891–1900	815	1955–1959	36
1901–1910	649	1960–1964	22
1911–1920	541	1965	16
1921–1930	362	1966	16
		1967	14

In terms of actual numbers of deaths, for the years 1851–1860 the average number of people who died of tuberculosis each year was 65,887, while in 1965 the number was 2,282. It will be noticed that the standardised mortality ratio has shown a ten-fold reduction in the last twenty years, as big a proportional decrease as in the previous century. It would be unreasonable not to attribute this accelerated fall in numbers of deaths from tuberculosis in part to the advances in methods of treatment, prevention and early diagnosis which have been a feature of the post-war period. This great reduction in numbers of people dying of tuberculosis has been accompanied by some remarkable alterations in the age and sex distribution of fatal cases. In the latter part of the nineteenth century, there was a very high infant mortality, a relatively low incidence among older children and a second peak in the curve in early middle age. Both peaks have now disappeared and tuberculosis has become largely a disease of old age: about three-quarters of those who died of the disease in 1965 were aged 55 or more. There has been a surprising change in the sex ratio of fatal cases. A hundred years ago the numbers dying each year were very similar for the two sexes and it may have appeared that sex had no bearing on tuberculosis mortality. Gradually, however, a large sex difference has emerged, and at present about three times as many deaths occur among males as among females. For some reason this sex difference only applies to the older age groups: below the age of 35 the numbers of deaths, though small, are very similar for both males and females.[14]

Until recent years up to 90 per cent of adult members of "civilised", or shall we say highly organised, communities were believed to have contracted the disease at some time, though the vast majority were never aware of having it, as they recovered without manifesting sufficient illness to draw attention to their infection. Modern methods for detecting early or past infection, such as X-ray examination and tuberculin testing, make it fairly clear that at the present time, in such countries as Great Britain and the United States of America, a substantial proportion of the young adult population has not contracted the disease. There are now enough young people who have never been infected, and therefore give a negative reaction to tuberculin, to make the tuberculin test a useful aid to diagnosis in some cases of obscure illness. This is a reflection of the decrease in the reservoir of infection which is provided by the infected persons from whom the disease is mostly spread.

Disease in Animals

Tuberculosis often occurs in animals other than man. Many domestic animals are susceptible, notably cattle, pigs and fowls and also cats and dogs. Wild animals in captivity are often infected but seldom if ever acquire the disease in their natural environment. Mention has already been made of the naturally occurring infections of the vole and of the dassie with special types of tubercle bacillus which appear to be nonvirulent for other mammalian species. It is of course very possible that other such diseases await discovery.

The bovine type of tubercle bacillus is probably capable of infecting all mammals but the human type is much more restricted in its host range. Monkeys are very susceptible to the human type and perhaps acquire the disease from tuberculous human beings chattering at them through the bars of their cages. Dogs are more often infected by the human than by the bovine type. The guinea-pig is highly susceptible to both the human and the bovine strain and has therefore been widely used both in experimental and in diagnostic work. In contrast the rabbit develops a rapidly fatal disease when injected with bovine tubercle bacilli but only a small local lesion if the human type is used, a difference which, incidentally, provides a reliable method for distinguishing the two types.

In considering the susceptibility of various animals to infection by *Myco. tuberculosis* it is necessary to distinguish between infection by natural routes (e.g. inhalation) and experimental infections in which bacilli are injected. Thus the rabbit, although highly susceptible to the bovine type of bacillus when given by injection, seldom contracts tuberculosis spontaneously, even in captivity. It should also be noted that differences in susceptibility to the two types may be of a quantitative rather than an all-or-nothing nature. For example, the vole can be infected both by the human and by the bovine types, but about 10,000 times as many human type organisms are needed to produce effects comparable to those obtained with a minimal infective dose of bovine bacilli.[15]

Events following Infection

Lungs

What happens after the inhalation of tubercle bacilli? Knowledge of the first stages of the tissue reaction that occurs in man after infection is negligible, but there are good reasons for supposing that the earliest changes seen in animals such as rabbits and guinea-pigs are essentially the same as those in man.

There is a striking difference between the reaction produced in an animal that has never been infected with tubercle bacilli and that occurring in an animal which is already suffering from tuberculosis, or which has been vaccinated with dead tubercle bacilli or with a bacillus of low virulence such as BCG or the vole bacillus.

When a guinea-pig inhales a few bacilli in very fine droplets the organisms reach the lung alveoli, where they are taken up by the mononuclear phagocytic cells in the alveolar walls. During the first few days after infection a vaccinated animal has a very active cell reaction around the bacilli, but in an unvaccinated animal bacilli may remain in the lung without any surrounding cell reaction even up to 6 days after infection. In the vaccinated animal the bacilli appear to remain unchanged in the large mononuclear cells, while in the unvaccinated the bacilli multiply intracellularly, so that by the 6th day 20 to 40 bacilli may be found in one cell. About the 8th day or after, by which time hypersensitivity to the bacillus has begun to develop, many tubercle bacilli are present and a cell reaction begins in the unvaccinated animal and takes place rapidly, leading on to the formation of a central necrotic area. At a comparable time after infection necrosis is less in vaccinated animals in which, although the number of cells is great, the number of bacilli remains small. This may be because the intensity of the reaction is determined by the number of organisms present at the site of the lesion.

Other portals of entry.—The reactions occurring soon after the inhalation of tubercle bacilli have been considered, but what happens when the bacilli are swallowed? It has been established in animals that considerably larger doses of bacilli are needed to produce infection through the alimentary tract than through the lungs. Perhaps the most dramatic demonstration of the fact that ingested bacilli cause infection was given by the Lübeck disaster in which 251 newly-born infants swallowed 3 doses of human tubercle bacilli given to them by mistake mixed with the immunising organism BCG. Probably almost all the infants became infected. Of 174 who survived 127 were later shown by radiography to have calcified, that is healed, tuberculous lesions in the mesenteric lymph nodes. In those who died the bacilli had in most cases reached the lungs and caused pulmonary tuberculosis.

Exactly how the bacilli penetrate the intestinal mucosa has not been elucidated, though it has been known for a long time that they can pass into the lymph flowing in the regional lymphatics, and cause lesions in the lymph nodes, without apparently infecting the gut wall itself. No lesions either microscopic or macroscopic were detected even after keeping a concentrated suspension of tubercle bacilli in a loop of guinea-pig intestine for many hours, though whether they had penetrated the mucosa in that time was not determined.

If, as seems probable, bacilli can gain entry to the body through the tonsil, they pass into the regional lymphatics and reach the cervical lymph nodes. Tuberculosis of the cervical nodes is, or was, quite a common disease, but often there is no apparent tuberculous lesion in the tonsil.

When tubercle bacilli are accidentally implanted in the human skin they usually give rise to a tumour-like lesion composed of cells typical of tuberculous infection. The lesion is in consequence sometimes called a tuberculoma—a term, however, which is customarily applied to solitary tuberculous lesions in the brain. Natural tuberculous infection of the skin—lupus vulgaris—usually gives rise to a more diffuse reaction in the cutis.

Intravenous injection of bacilli.—Though experimental infection by the lungs no doubt corresponds most nearly with natural pulmonary infection in man, information of interest concerning the earliest stages of the development of a tubercle has been gained by injecting suspensions of bacilli intravenously into rabbits. Some tubercle bacilli lodge in the capillaries of the lungs, and it seems that, unlike those reaching the lungs by the airways, they are surrounded at first by polymorphonuclear leucocytes which phagocytose the bacilli. This is the normal response to the intravenous injection of any form of particulate matter. By about 14 hours after the injection mononuclear cells appear and ingest some of the polymorphs, which are then digested, and so the bacilli are freed in the protoplasm of the mononuclear cells.[16] With the passage of time the latter become the most marked constituent of the developing tubercle. Eventually they form the great bulk of all cells present. This is true of all tuberculous lesions, wherever they develop.

Productive and Exudative Lesions

As is the case with all inflammation, the reaction to the tubercle bacillus has two components—cells and fluid exudate. The commonest tuberculous lesion is mainly cellular, and its development is sometimes called a "productive" or "proliferative" process. When the proportion of exudate is larger the lesion is said to be "exudative", and as this type of process has some distinctive characters it will be considered separately later.

Structure of the Young Proliferative Lesion

Thus, though it is not certain that the first reaction following inhalation is precisely the same as that following intravenous injection, there is no doubt that a young experimental tubercle is in the main a collection of cells around the implanted bacilli. In man the process of formation is essentially the same as that in animals, though by the time lesions are recognised there is no sign of a preliminary polymorph reaction, if indeed it was ever present. An early microscopic tubercle in the liver of man is shown in FIG. 4.

It will be seen from the figure that a young tubercle, the reaction to the presence of one or a few tubercle bacilli, consists of a substantial mass of cells. So far we have referred to mononuclear cells, but in the tubercle some of these cells come to have a distinctive appearance, and are usually still known by

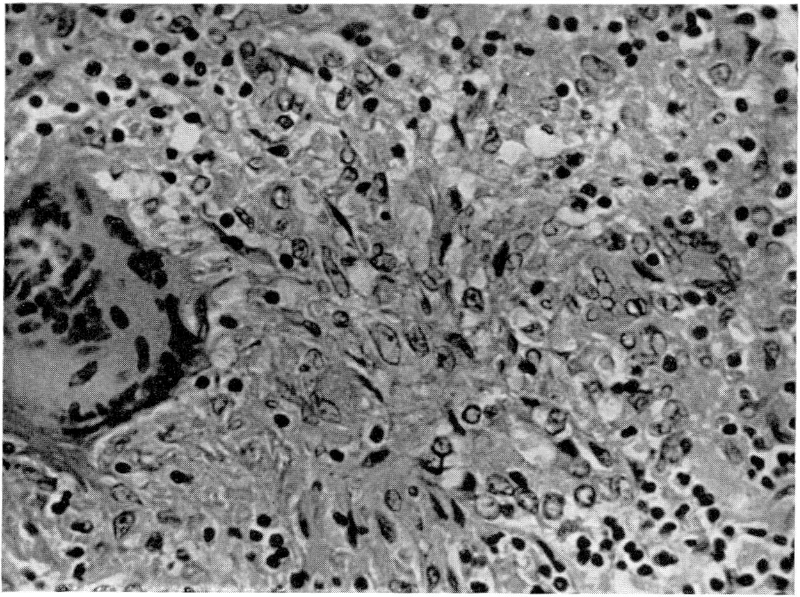

42/FIG. 4.—The centre of a young tubercle in the liver of man, showing a well-marked epithelioid cell reaction, a giant cell and a peripheral zone of lymphocytes. The vesicular nuclei of the epithelioid cells and the cytoplasmic extensions of the giant cell are well shown.

their old name of epithelioid cells, though they do not arise from epithelium and look only vaguely like epithelial cells. These cells, which form a palely staining tissue, have elongated vesicular nuclei and a faintly outlined cell boundary which is irregular, forming branches that apparently connect with neighbouring cells. In relationship with these cells there are frequently to be seen large multinucleate giant cells, known as Langhans giant cells, which contain several nuclei—occasionally up to a hundred or more—usually arranged at the periphery of the cell or towards one side. The giant cells also send out protoplasmic processes among the surrounding epithelioid cells.

At the periphery of the epithelioid cells is a zone of small round cells that are usually considered to be lymphocytes, and with them unaltered exudative mononuclear cells are often to be seen. The collection of epithelioid cells and lympho-

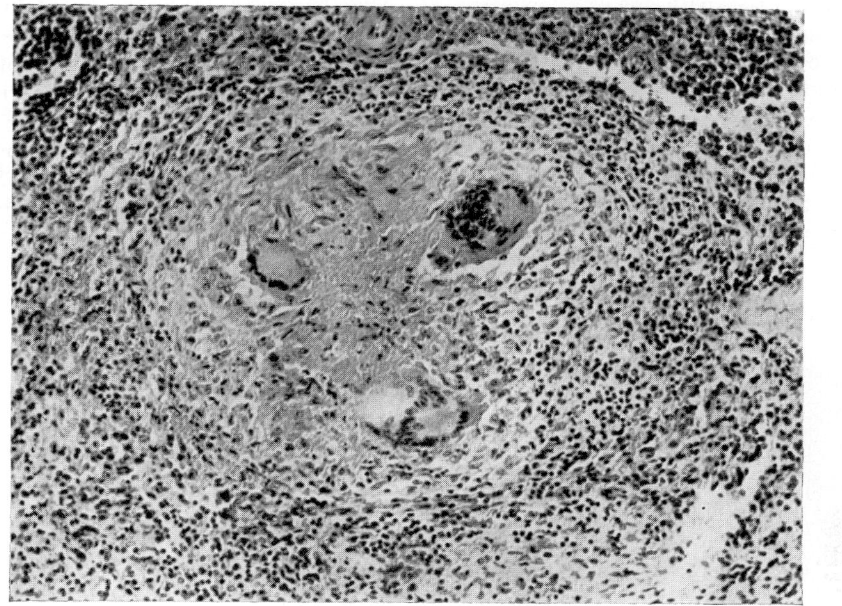

42/Fig. 5.—Microscopical tubercle in the spleen of man. At the centre of the palely staining mass of epithelioid cells the earliest signs of necrosis can be seen.

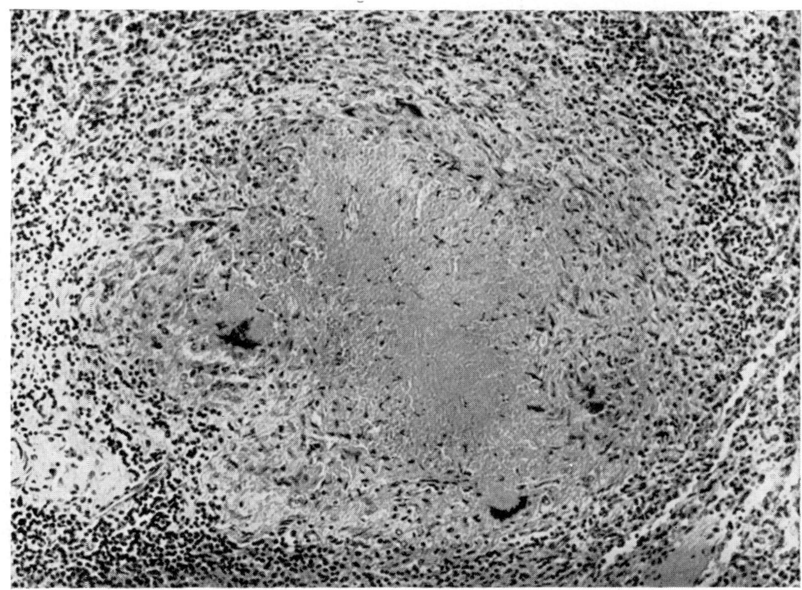

42/Fig. 6.—Microscopic tubercle in the spleen of man, showing well-marked central caseation. There is probably also some early fibroblastic reaction at the periphery.

cytes, often with one or a few giant cells near the centre, is known as a giant cell system or microscopic tubercle. With increasing age the cell mass grows in size and may necrose at its centre. Because of its cheese-like appearance the necrosed tissue is referred to as caseous material; and the process is known as caseation. These later stages in the development of the tubercle are illustrated in FIGS. 5 and 6.

Concurrently with the process described above fibroblasts at the periphery of the lesion begin to form collagen in those individuals or species, of which man is usually one, who have relatively great resistance to the growth of the bacilli. In very susceptible species such as the guinea-pig, such fibrous tissue is not formed, but nevertheless reticulin fibres are greatly increased in number (FIG. 7).

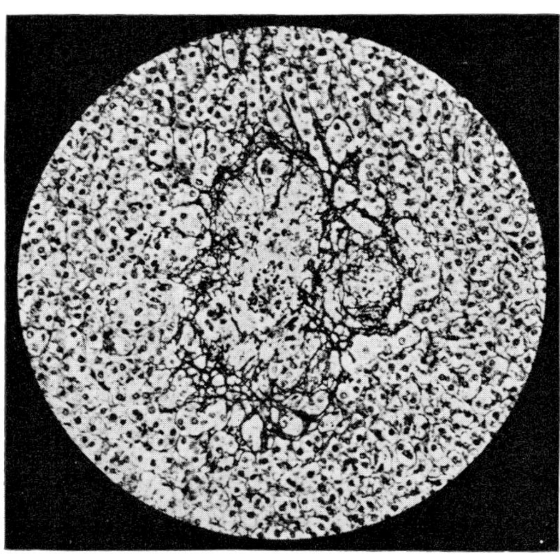

42/FIG. 7.—An increase in the number of reticulin fibres (stained black by silver) can be seen around this microscopic tubercle in the liver of a guinea-pig. In this species fibrous tissue is not formed around tubercles.

Growth of the Tubercle

Unless healing, which we will consider later, takes place, the mass consisting of epithelioid cells, giant cells and lymphocytes with a central area of caseation increases in size by the centrifugal growth of the original tubercle, or by the formation of satellite tubercles. The latter arise near the original lesion, and may be caused by the migration of mononuclear leucocytes carrying tubercle bacilli or by the transmission of bacilli along lymphatics or in the tissue fluids. As the new tubercles enlarge they coalesce with the original lesion and with one another. This process may go on until large lesions are produced.

As you will have realised, the original lesion caused by the lodgement of tubercle bacilli is microscopic but, with growth, the tubercles eventually become visible as minute bodies, at first less than a millimetre in diameter. They are seen as firm, rounded, sharply demarcated grey structures. These small tubercles are frequently referred to as miliary tubercles, as they are supposed to be about the size of millet seed—better known as canary seed. With increase in size and the occurrence of central caseation they change to a yellow colour. When such tubercles extend by the formation and coalescence of satellites, the term conglomerate tubercle is applied. Such lesions may be largely composed of caseous material with a rim of tissue consisting of cells such as occur in young tubercles.

Though it is convenient to describe the "centre" and the "periphery" of a tubercle, it must not be assumed that such an arrangement can always be made out in human material. It is found in young lesions, such as those of miliary tuberculosis, and foci with the same general arrangement can sometimes be found in older and more complex lesions, but often it is not possible to divide up the lesion in any particular way and many of the cells appear to be mixed up with no special orientation. This type of tissue response is often referred to as tuberculous granulation tissue.

Histogenesis

From what cells do the epithelioid and giant cells arise, and what is the cause of the central caseation? The view most commonly accepted to-day of the origin of epithelioid cells is that they are formed from monocytes—or macrophages—which for the most part arrive at the point of infection by the blood stream, i.e. as blood monocytes, though some maintain that the connective tissue macrophages play an important part. It seems unlikely that the cells are formed by local cell division, as mitoses are rarely seen in a tubercle. The mononuclear cells, as we have seen, ingest the growing tubercle bacilli, whose presence in the cells, it is believed, alters the macrophages in such a way that they have the appearance characterised by the name epithelioid cell. When, however, one inspects certain lesions one is struck by the large development of epithelioid cells in the apparently almost total absence of bacilli demonstrable by staining. Possibly monocytes are transformed into epithelioid cells if they are only near cells containing bacilli. While tubercle bacilli or some of their constituents may produce epithelioid cells, this cell transformation is not specific; it is seen, for instance, in the lesions of brucellosis and tularæmia, and insoluble foreign bodies such as paraffin sometimes produce a similar reaction. In the disease known as sarcoidosis, large numbers of cells with all the characteristics of epithelioid cells are developed, though no acid-fast or, for that matter, any other organisms can be demonstrated in the lesions.

There is no question that the mononuclear cells from which the epithelioid cells arise can phagocytose tubercle bacilli, but it is by no means clear that epithelioid cells can do so. It is true that tubercle bacilli are sometimes found inside epithelioid cells, but they could have entered while the cells were still of the phagocytic mononuclear type.

From animal experiments, in which tubercle bacilli and an inert particulate substance such as carbon have both been injected intravenously, it has been learnt that the epithelioid cells of a tubercle may contain carbon which has reached them from the blood stream (FIG. 8). But it seems most probable that such carbon was abstracted from the blood stream by ordinary mononuclear cells that have subsequently been turned into epithelioid cells by the presence of tubercle bacilli. At present the consensus of opinion is that epithelioid cells are not phagocytic.

The typical cellular structure of a tubercle, in particular the epithelioid and giant cells, can be formed in animals not only by the injection of live bacteria

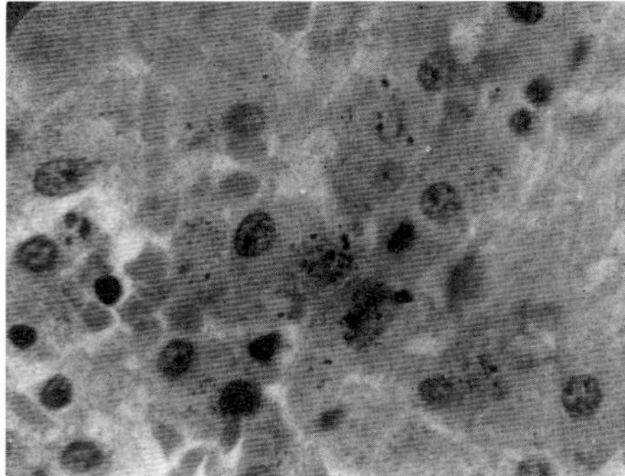

42/FIG. 8.—The edge of a tuberculous lesion in the lung of a rabbit which had been injected intravenously with india ink. Ten daily injections, which began 18 days after infection, were given. Note the fine dusting of carbon particles present in the epithelioid cells. (From Markham and Florey.[17])

that multiply in the tissues but by heat-killed bacilli or even by saprophytic acid-fast organisms such as the timothy grass bacillus (FIG. 9).

The main ways in which the response of the tissues to dead bacilli differs from that to living bacilli may be summarised as follows:

1. Much larger numbers of dead bacilli are needed to produce quantitatively comparable results.

2. Dead bacilli produce lesions that are almost entirely cellular unless a massive inoculation is used, when caseation may follow.

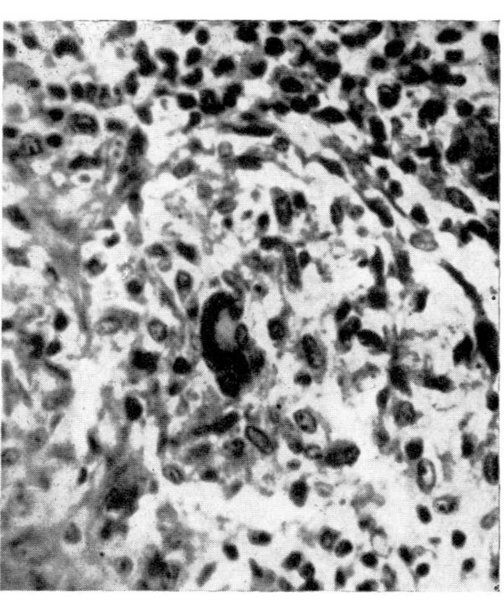

42/FIG. 9.—A lesion showing epithelioid and Langhans-type giant cells produced by the injection of dead bacilli into the testis of a rat, an animal in which "typical tubercles" are not produced by live bacilli.

3. Lesions due to dead bacilli develop only at the site of inoculation, with the exception of occasional slight spread through the transport of bacilli along the lymphatics.

But the cell reaction in the two cases is essentially the same. It is perhaps significant that the mononuclear phagocyte responds chemotactically to the tubercle bacillus, and it might be reasonable to suggest that the bacilli contain certain substances that can change phagocytic cells into those types that are characteristically seen in the tubercle.

Anderson and his colleagues obtained a number of fractions from tubercle bacilli. They were proteins, carbohydrates, fatty acids and waxes. This work has been extended by Lederer and his colleagues and it is now certain that a large number of compounds of novel type can be extracted. Attempts have been made to find out which fractions are responsible for the formation of epithelioid cells. The waxes and branch-chain fatty acids induced epithelioid cell formation when injected into animals, but at present there are certain difficulties in accepting that these are the actual substances responsible for the tissue changes in the disease. In the first place the extracted compounds are not necessarily the same as those in the living bacilli, and secondly much more of them is needed to produce the reaction than is likely to be formed by bacilli in the tissues.

Giant Cells

There are two possible ways in which the giant cells could be formed. They might be due to the coalescence of monocytes or to the division of nuclei without cytoplasmic fission. As mitosis is never seen in these cells, the former hypothesis seems much more likely.

It has been suggested that the distribution of the nuclei at the periphery of the cell is due to the presence in its centre of ingested granular material into which the nuclei cannot penetrate. The same reason possibly accounts for the finding that organisms, or other particulate matter, are usually distributed in the periphery of epithelioid cells.

There is much evidence to show that giant cells arise from mononuclear phagocytes, such as those lining the liver sinusoids and those occurring in the tissues, but there is little if any certain knowledge of the reasons why most macrophages or monocytes turn into epithelioid cells while only a few turn into giant cells.

The "small round cells" at the periphery of a microscopic tubercle are usually considered to be lymphocytes. Their function is unknown. The mononuclear phagocytic cells and fibroblasts are of the ordinary types.

Fate of Lesions

In man, lesions such as we have been discussing may be arrested at an early stage, with subsequent regression of the cellular changes and the formation of fibrous tissue at the site of the lesion. Sometimes there is extension of the process with necrosis of the centre of the lesion, but even then the balance may be turned at some stage in favour of the defensive mechanisms of the body and the area of cellular change and necrosis may be encapsulated by fibrous tissue. In course of time the fibrous tissue may gradually replace the whole lesion. Very commonly healing processes may be going on in one part of an affected organ while extension is taking place in another.

We will now consider these processes in greater detail.

Caseous Necrosis

Sooner or later the centre of the microscopic tubercle, or agglomeration of tubercles, composed of newly accumulated cells, undergoes necrosis. This necrosis of tuberculous tissue is known as caseation because the dead material has the appearance of cheese. In experimental tuberculosis of animals it is sometimes slight, varying with the species and the state of immunity of the animal, but in human tuberculosis it nearly always occurs early and is an important feature.

At first sight it would appear to be easy to explain caseation. It might be supposed that the necrosis occurring in the developing tubercle was directly due to some poisonous substance produced by the tubercle bacillus, just as pyogenic organisms such as the staphylococcus produce toxins which directly kill tissue cells in the neighbourhood of the growing bacteria. But it is difficult to show that anything of the sort occurs with the tubercle bacillus. Large quantities of dead tubercle bacilli, and some of their lipid components, are toxic for normal animals, but there is no undoubted evidence that this toxicity is responsible for the necrosis which can be caused by even small numbers of live bacilli.

The effect of tubercle bacilli on cells has been studied in tissue cultures. A number of observers have described how tubercle bacilli can grow and live in cells that have phagocytosed them. Macrophages containing enormous numbers of certain strains of bacilli have been seen to wander about for days in culture medium.

It has been suggested that virulent mammalian strains of the tubercle bacillus can interfere with the motor activities of granulocytes that have taken them up, and that when ingested in sufficient numbers they can kill them; whereas avirulent strains do not do this. Macrophages also are damaged after the ingestion of virulent tubercle bacilli. Small numbers of bacilli grow freely within the cytoplasm of unsensitised mononuclear phagocytes until, with an increase in their number, they kill the host cell. If this intracellular growth of bacilli is prevented by including small quantities of streptomycin in the suspending medium, the macrophages survive as well as uninfected cells.

The killing of macrophages by intracellular organisms may be the result of a direct toxic action of the bacillus or may result from the metabolic activity of a large number of intracellular bacilli acting to deprive the host cell of some essential requirement such as oxygen.

Although a cytolytic effect can be demonstrated in tissue culture, the study of the earliest histological changes in the intact animal does not indicate that the cells that accumulate in the neighbourhood of the invading bacteria are killed at first in significant numbers, even though they may contain numerous bacteria.

The tubercle bacillus seems not to secrete any exotoxin in the usual sense of the term, but a substance called "cord factor", which is produced in cultures of certain mycobacteria, must be mentioned briefly. Middlebrook, Dubos and Pierce[18] claimed that virulence among strains of *Myco. tuberculosis* was associated with growth of the bacilli in cord-like structures in liquid media. Bloch[19] isolated a substance from such strains which he called "cord factor" which was toxic for isolated leucocytes and for mice injected intraperitoneally. It was not suggested that this substance was responsible for growth in cords but it seemed for a time that it might have something to do with the pathogenic action of tubercle bacilli. Noll, Bloch, Asselineau and Lederer[20] identified cord factor as trehalose-6,6′-dimycolate. However, Hart and Rees[21] showed that the original claim that cord-formation and virulence were associated might not be correct, as they found that a non-virulent strain of the tubercle bacillus known as

H37Ra was able to form cords. Furthermore, "cord factor" has been isolated from cultures of BCG, of the smegma bacillus (which does not grow in cords) and of a strain of human origin which was shown to be non-virulent for mice.[22] "Cord factor" is a substance not without interest, but it is at present difficult to see how it can be concerned in caseous necrosis, or, indeed, in any other manifestation of the disease.

As we shall see later, the vessels round a tubercle may go into stasis and become thrombosed, but it is difficult to determine whether this follows or precedes necrosis.

The main cause of necrosis or caseation appears to lie in the severe reaction of an allergic nature that occurs in an animal sensitised to a protein component of the tubercle bacillus. The sensitisation can result from a previous vaccination or infection, but it can also develop during the course of the primary disease.

Our understanding of this altered response of the tissues to the tubercle bacillus is based on an important experiment described by Koch in 1891[23] and usually known as the "Koch phenomenon". This experiment and the conclusions which can be drawn from it in the light of subsequent investigations have been considered in detail in Chapter 39. It will be convenient to summarise the main points here.

Koch found that if he inoculated a normal guinea-pig subcutaneously with tubercle bacilli nothing obvious happened for about 10–14 days. Then a nodule formed at the site of inoculation, enlarged and broke down to form an ulcer which gradually enlarged until the animal died. At the same time the regional lymph nodes became severely infected. If while this process was going on a *second* subcutaneous inoculation of tubercle bacilli was given to the animal at a different site, the consequences were very different indeed. (Koch found that the effect was best demonstrated if the second inoculation was given 4–6 weeks after the first). Instead of a delay of 10–14 days before anything striking could be seen, marked changes were noted after 1–2 days. The skin round the site of inoculation became thickened and dark and a few days later became necrotic and sloughed off. But this second lesion healed quickly and permanently and there was no significant lymph node involvement. Moreover the sloughing of the skin round the site of inoculation did not appear to be due to any action of live bacilli because dead bacilli produced the same effect.

Why does the animal respond in such a strikingly different way to the second inoculation of tubercle bacilli? The reason, as we now know, is that it has *both* become allergic to certain protein constituents of the bacillus *and* developed a degree of immunity to tuberculosis. The rapid sloughing of the skin round the site of inoculation is a typical allergic response to the delayed type; the lesion heals promptly and the lymph nodes do not become infected because of the immunity. If the immunity is sufficient to demolish the bacilli in the second inoculation why can the animal not cope with the consequences of the original infection? The answer is probably that by the time immunity develops many of the bacilli descended from those in the original inoculum remain in areas of caseous necrosis where they are not accessible to the animal's immune defences. We shall return to the problems of immunity and allergy in tuberculosis in a later section.

When tissue is killed by the staphylococcus it is liquefied by the liberation

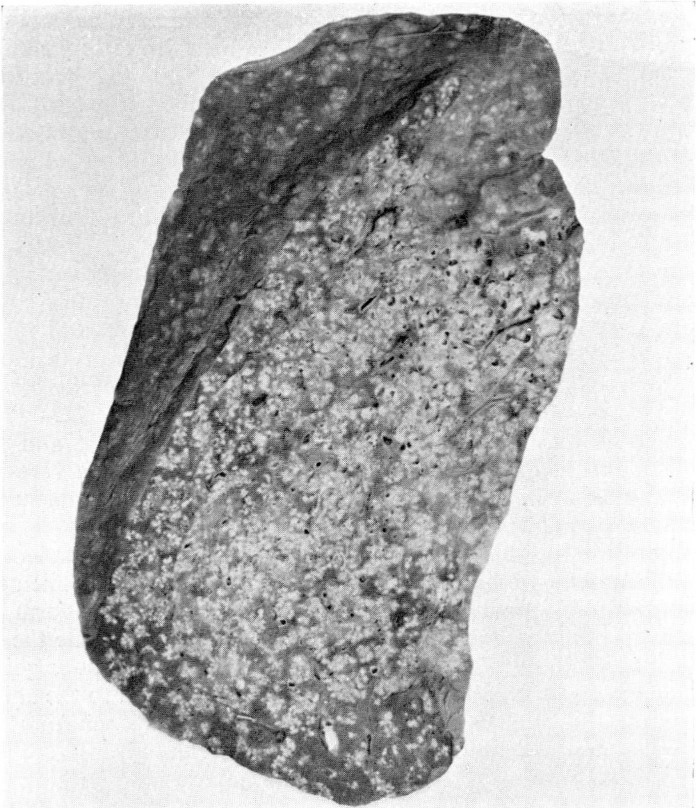

42/FIG. 10.—Acute tuberculous broncho-pneumonia. Spread of infected material took place by the bronchial tree, and the lesions can be seen in little clusters, corresponding with the distribution of the smaller bronchi and bronchioles. In some places small "acute cavities" can be seen, where softened caseous material has been discharged through the bronchi.

of enzymes from the dead cells, especially the polymorphonuclear leucocytes, and turned into pus. In the necrotic material produced by the presence of the tubercle bacillus enough autolysis occurs for the cells to lose their structure, and in the caseous mass no cell structure can generally be recognised. Only in exceptional circumstances does the necrotic material become liquefied in the early stages (FIG. 10); instead, it becomes coagulated to form an inspissated cheesy mass. This is probably because enzymes from the granules of polymorphs are much more active in producing autolysis than are those from the lysosomes of monocytes.

Softening

Eventually the cheesy caseous material may soften and become liquid. Probably polymorphs enter the lesion and by virtue of their content of enzymes carry on autolysis to liquefaction. It is generally held that polymorphs are present in areas where softening takes place. They can sometimes be seen in large numbers, but in other cases they appear to be scanty, or again it may be that enzymes enter from the blood plasma and the tissue may become more acid and so allow autolytic enzymes to act. Whatever the cause, the necrosed material becomes fluid, sometimes only in one part of a lesion, and usually only in some of a number of lesions. At the same time as the lesion liquefies tubercle bacilli increase greatly in number. In caseous material they are usually present, but often only in very small numbers. Softened material may be teeming with them. Again it cannot be said whether the tubercle bacilli divide because the liquefied material provides them with better conditions for growth or whether the increase in the number of bacilli precedes softening and plays a part in it.

It is sometimes stated that softening occurs only when the lesion is secondarily infected with pyogenic organisms. It can be stated with assurance that secondary infection is not necessary for softening, though it may sometimes be its cause.

A result of the liquefaction is the formation of a tuberculous abscess, which may approach a surface. As there is none of the vascular dilatation, redness and increased temperature of the skin that are associated with a pyogenic abscess, the fluctuant swelling containing the liquefied caseous material is called a cold abscess. The pus of a cold abscess may track for long distances before reaching a surface. One of the most striking examples is the passage of tuberculous pus from tuberculous vertebræ into the sheath of the psoas muscle and thence beneath the inguinal ligament. It may come to the surface there or even farther down the thigh. The cavity and the track through which the discharge reaches the surface becomes lined with tuberculous granulation tissue which has the cellular characters of non-tuberculous granulation tissue but contains giant cells and epithelioid cells sometimes arranged in quite well-defined tubercles.

The more or less lengthy track, known as a sinus, is very liable to become infected with pyogenic organisms and it may persist for months or years without healing. The tuberculous pus that is discharged is a structureless granular mass in which degenerating cells can sometimes still be recognised.

If the softened area should be in the lung, the material may be discharged through the bronchi leaving a cavity that may heal with great difficulty, if at all.

Calcification.—Caseated areas may, instead of softening, become calcified. Again, exactly what happens is not clear, but over the course of months in man, and more rapidly in the rabbit, calcium carbonate and phosphate are deposited in fine dust-like particles or in extensive solid masses. Although calcified, these lesions may still harbour viable bacilli. This process of calcification occurs particularly in lymphatic nodes, and it makes old tuberculous lesions clearly visible by X-ray.

Healing.—If the tubercle bacilli are in some way prevented from dividing or are killed, i.e. where resistance to the tubercle bacilli is sufficiently great, as it usually is in man, fibrous tissue forms around and in lesions, or, if they are large, encapsulates them, so that the progress of the disease is arrested. The resulting nodules of fibrous tissue may become hyalinised. Frequently, however, the lesion becomes chronic, that is, healing, or at least fibrosis, may be occurring at one point, while at another progressive destruction may be taking place, so that in this way extensive fibrotic lesions are produced.

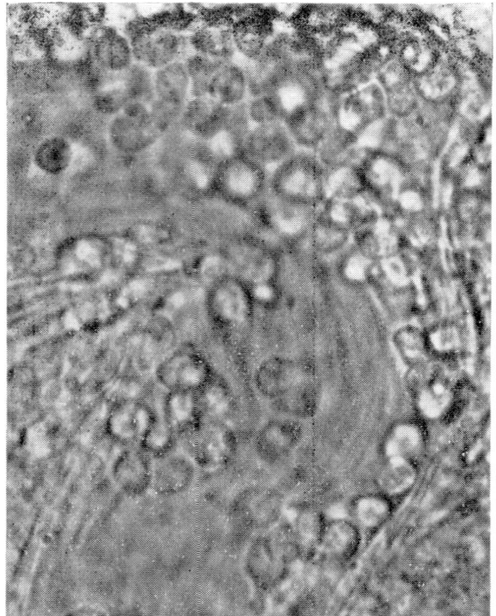

42/FIG. 11.—Leucocytes sticking to the walls of vessels near a growing tubercle.

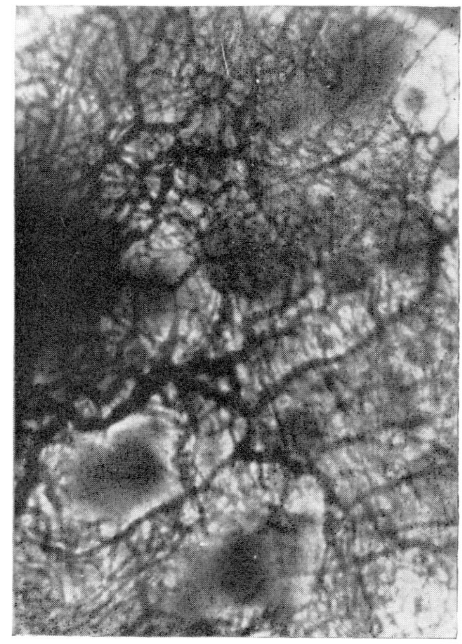

42/FIG. 12.—Tubercles developing in a chamber in which the tissue was much thicker than that shown in FIGS. 13 to 16. Note the isolated avascular areas (tubercles) surrounded by a rich vascular network of dilated blood vessels.

Avascularity of a Tubercle

Observations *in vivo*.—A tubercle is usually described as an avascular structure, though some maintain that new capillaries can be found in it and that its avascular nature is exaggerated. Nevertheless the blood supply is poor, as it is difficult to inject any vessels even at the periphery of a growing tubercle. It is, however, adequate to maintain the nutrition of the cells at least at the periphery of the lesion.

Does the diminution of blood supply in the neighbourhood of the growing tubercle contribute to caseation? Some light has been thrown on this question by observations on tubercles developing in transparent chambers in rabbits' ears.[24] The thin layer of tissue in the chamber was inoculated with bovine tubercle bacilli through a hole in the back of the chamber. The manipulations caused some damage to the tissue and it was impossible to determine, during the few days required for this to clear up, whether the changes seen were due purely to trauma or partly to the presence of tubercle bacilli. However, some time between the 10th and 24th days a rapid change occurred, characterised at first by vascular dilatation and the sticking of leucocytes to the vessel walls (FIG. 11). The changes were progressive and led to hæmoconcentration, stasis and thrombosis. The end result of these changes was the formation of small avascular tubercles with necrotic centres similar to those seen in FIG. 12.

We have made similar observations using chambers with a thinner and more rigidly confined layer of tissue. It was possible to observe that opacities developed 10 days or so after infection. They were probably composed of dead cells and were to be seen in the neighbourhood of vessels carrying a good blood supply. FIGURES 13 and 14 show such an early tubercle traversed by a vessel which has been compressed by a cellular accumulation of which the centre appears necrotic. As the tuberculous processes extended, vessels at the periphery of the growing tubercle passed into stasis and were seen to disintegrate in the spreading necrosis (FIGS. 13, 14, 15 and 16). It seemed that the vessels were severely damaged by the tuberculous process which was already causing necrosis, rather than that the primary damage was to the vessels.

It may be concluded that the destruction of the blood supply near an expanding tubercle cuts down the supply of nutriment to the cells but is itself not the primary cause of necrosis.

Exudative Lesions

Attention so far has been concentrated on the development and properties of the most usual manifestation of tuberculosis—the tubercle—but in some situations and in some circumstances this so-called productive lesion may not develop. Instead, the tissue reaction is characterised by a large amount of inflammatory exudation—the exudative lesion.

Whereas the focal tuberculous lesion that we have been describing develops slowly, and is usually classed as a chronic inflammation, the exudative inflammations are generally much more acute. They often occur when tubercle bacilli reach serous membranes such as the pleura, pericardium, peritoneum or meninges. On these membranes the exudate may form a fibrin clot, and polymorphonuclear cells may be present as well as lymphocytes and mononuclear

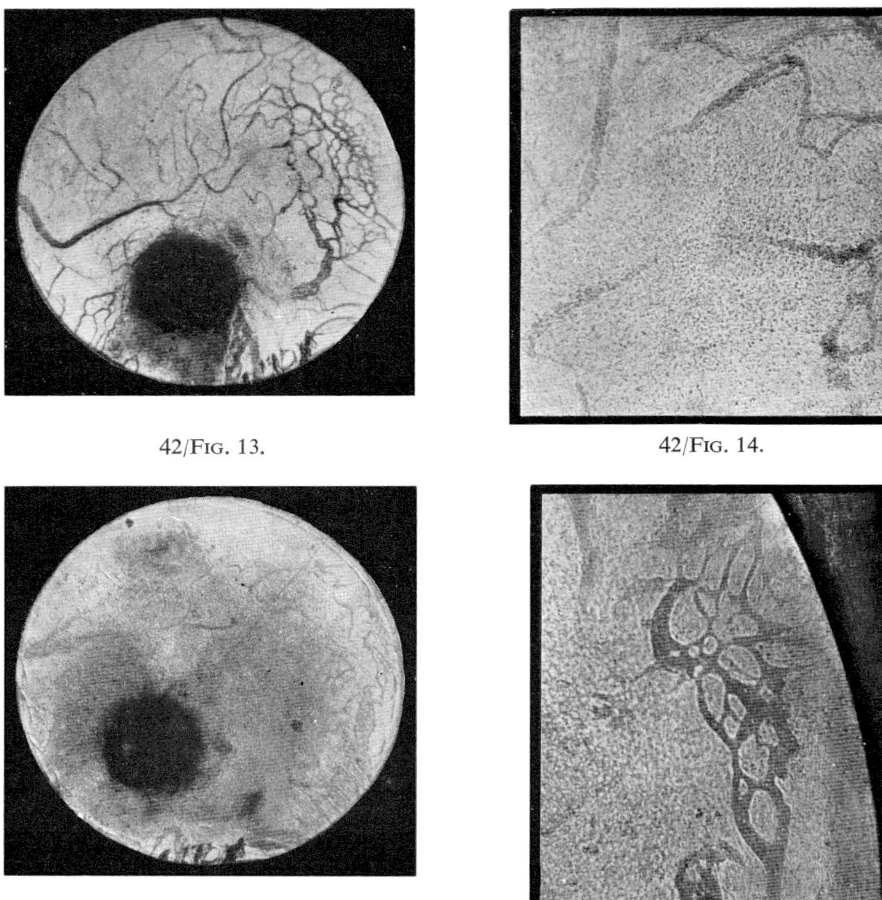

42/FIG. 13.

42/FIG. 14.

42/FIG. 15.

42/FIG. 16.

42/FIG. 13.—A chamber in which tuberculous changes are occurring. The black circle at the lower left-hand side of the chamber is a silver pin closing a hole through which tubercle bacilli were introduced 10 days before this photograph was taken. The beginning of necrosis is to be noted to the right of the centre of the field. This is seen more highly magnified in FIG. 14. (×3 approx.)

42/FIG. 14.—A portion of the chamber shown in FIG. 13. An area of increased opacity, probably due to the necrosis of accumulated cells, can be seen. A compressed vessel is passing through the area. At the time the photograph was taken, this vessel still carried a vigorous flow of blood. 16 mm. objective.

42/FIG. 15.—The same chamber as shown in FIG. 13. This photograph was taken 6 days after FIG. 13. The tuberculous process to the right of the pin has extended considerably and a focus in the upper portion of the field is apparent. The dark area is free from blood vessels some of which at the periphery are in stasis.

42/FIG. 16.—Vessels in complete stasis at the edge of an advancing tuberculous process. The same chamber as shown in FIGS. 13, 14 and 15. Photograph taken 16 days after inoculation. (From Sanders, Florey and Wells.[26])

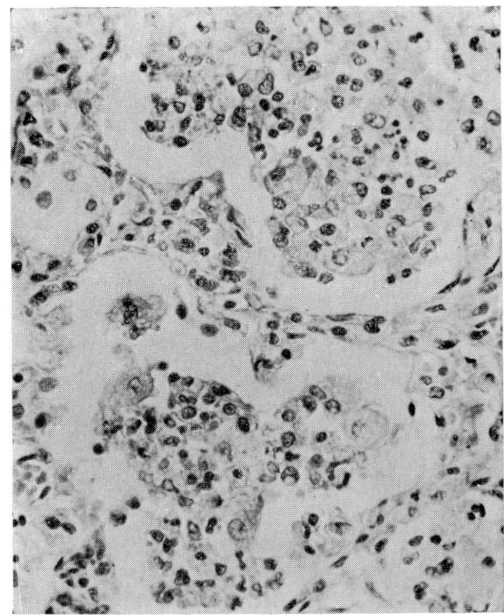

42/FIG. 17.—An area of tuberculous broncho-pneumonia, showing an early cellular exudate in which mononuclear cells predominate. Such lesions frequently contain vast numbers of bacilli and are likely to undergo massive necrosis.

leucocytes. If the exudative reaction occurs in the lungs, tuberculous pneumonia results (FIG. 17). The exudate with its content of cells is similar to that seen on the serous surfaces, and varies greatly in extent, sometimes involving a whole lobe or more.

No one factor can be held to be responsible for producing an exudative rather than a productive lesion, but the factors tending to produce the one or the other have been summarised by Pinner, whose modified scheme is shown below. It should be emphasised that each of the points noted indicates a general trend, and is in no way absolute.

Productive reaction	**Exudative reaction**
A. Factors in the bacillus	
Small dose	Large dose
Low virulence	High virulence
B. Factors in the host	
Inherited and constitutional resistance	Inherited and constitutional susceptibility
Compact tissue structure (e.g. liver)	Loose tissue structure (e.g. lung, meninges)
Possibility hypersensitivity relatively small	Hypersensitivity relatively great
C. Factors in the process of infection	
Many small deposits of bacilli	Few large deposits of bacilli

Though the situation of the bacilli in the looser tissues and their presence in large numbers are important factors in the production of exudative tuberculosis, it seems to be fairly certain that the inflammation is the result of previous sensitisation of the body and has a large allergic component. Nevertheless, experimentally, the primary implantation of large numbers of bacilli in the lung of rabbits with inherited low resistance can give rise to a tuberculous pneumonia.

Just as the centre of a cellular tubercle may caseate, so the acute tuberculous exudate may necrose and caseate. The necrosis is probably due to the same causes as those operating in a productive tubercle, but it may be particularly associated with the presence of enormous numbers of bacilli. Although necrosis occurs in most cases, there is good evidence that the exudate can sometimes resolve completely, leaving only microscopical residues.

The Dissemination of Tubercle Bacilli in the Body

We have seen how tubercle bacilli can gain entry into the body and have followed the development of the lesion at the portal of entry under various conditions. How do the bacilli spread about the body from the local lesion?

Lymphatic Spread

In an unsensitised animal the bacilli are very soon disseminated from the point of lodgement into lymphatics along which they are carried to the regional lymphatic nodes. Perhaps they travel as free bacilli, but it is equally likely that they are transported inside phagocytic cells. In any case, when they reach the nodes they lodge in the sinusoids where they initiate the tuberculous changes that we have already discussed. Thus when the primary infection is in the lung the nodes at the hilum are almost invariably found to be infected and to have

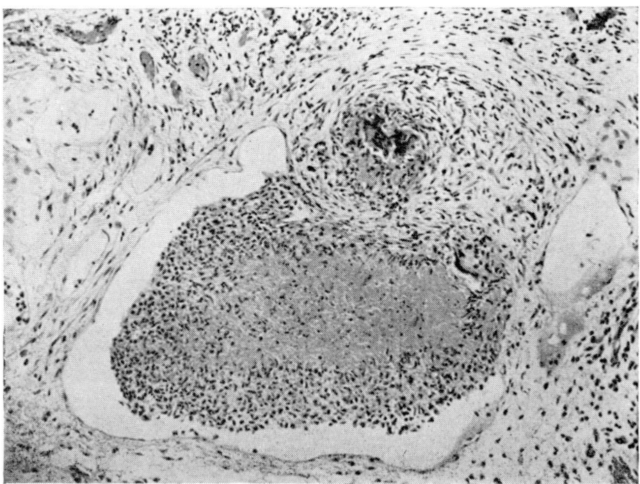

42/Fig. 18.—Lymphatic spread of tuberculosis. A tubercle in a subserous lymphatic of the small intestine. The lesion consists of an older giant cell system with peripheral fibrosis in the wall of the lymphatic, and a more recent accumulation of mononuclear cells within the lumen. The latter also contains a giant cell that has undergone central necrosis.

undergone tuberculous change. When the bacilli enter the body through the intestine the mesenteric nodes are affected, when through the tonsil the corresponding cervical nodes.

Usually a healthy lymph node acts as an efficient filter, but as lesions develop infection may pass from one to another along a chain of nodes; later, bacilli may enter the thoracic duct from a caseating lymph node and thus reach the blood stream, by which they can be widely disseminated. Sometimes bacilli lodge in the walls of lymphatic vessels, where tubercles then develop. This is often seen well in tuberculosis of the intestine, where chains of small tubercles may show the course of the sub-peritoneal lymphatics (FIG. 18). While this lymphatic spread is almost universal in first infections the same is not true of subsequent infections. Here, because the local reaction is rapid and intense, the bacilli are not readily dispersed. Therefore gross tuberculosis of the lymph nodes is much commoner in children than in adults.

Spread by the Blood Stream

Dissemination by way of the blood stream most frequently occurs when a vein is eroded by an extending tubercle, and caseous material, rich in bacilli, is discharged into the blood (FIG. 19). In this way many tubercles may be seeded in a number of organs at about the same time. If the infection is massive it usually kills the patient in a short time, but chemotherapy may influence this type of tuberculosis very favourably. As little time elapses in untreated cases between spread by the blood stream and death, the tubercles seen post-mortem scattered in the various organs are still small—"miliary"—and the condition is known as miliary tuberculosis (FIG. 20).

Though miliary tuberculosis is the form of blood-borne tuberculosis most often described, the hæmatogenous spread is not always of such massive proportions as to lead rapidly to the death of the patient. Instead, a few bacilli may be lodged and then multiply in tissues such as the kidney, spleen, liver, bone, testes or ovaries, giving rise to large, sometimes solitary, tuberculous lesions with the morphological and other characteristics we have already discussed.

Some organs seem to have a resistance to the tubercle bacilli spread by the blood stream, thus it is rare to find either miliary or other tubercles in the thyroid gland, the pancreas, the heart or the voluntary muscles.

Spread through Tubes

Another way in which tubercle bacilli are spread is by passage along tubes such as the bronchial tree and the ureters. In the case of pulmonary tuberculosis bronchial spread is of very great importance and is one of the chief hazards to those suffering from tuberculosis of the lung. Growing tubercles may impinge on and then destroy the wall of a bronchiole or bronchus (FIG. 21). It is easy to understand how, if the lesion is caseous, and particularly if the caseous material is fluid, infected material may be aspirated along neighbouring bronchi during coughing, reaching hitherto unaffected lung tissue, and setting up the growth of new tubercles. In this way very extensive lesions of the lungs may be established in a short time, and sometimes rapidly fatal tuberculous broncho-pneumonia may result (FIGS. 10 and 27).

Tubercle bacilli from the lungs pass up the main bronchi when necrotic

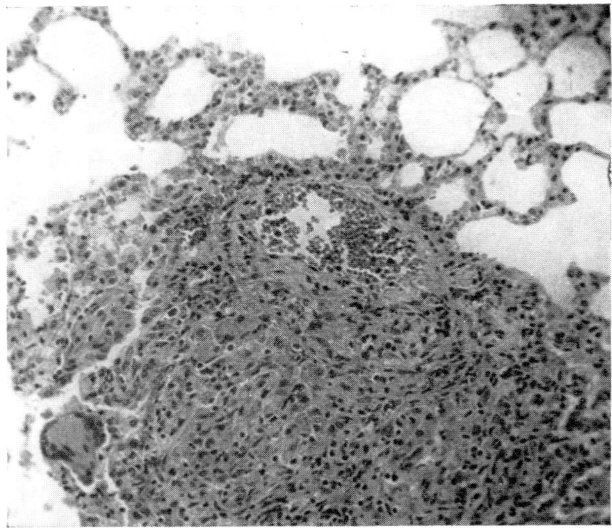

42/FIG. 19.—A tuberculous lesion in the lung of a rabbit. The tuberculous tissue has invaded the vein and has obliterated half the lumen. Some fibroblasts are growing in and over the projection. (From Markham.[27])

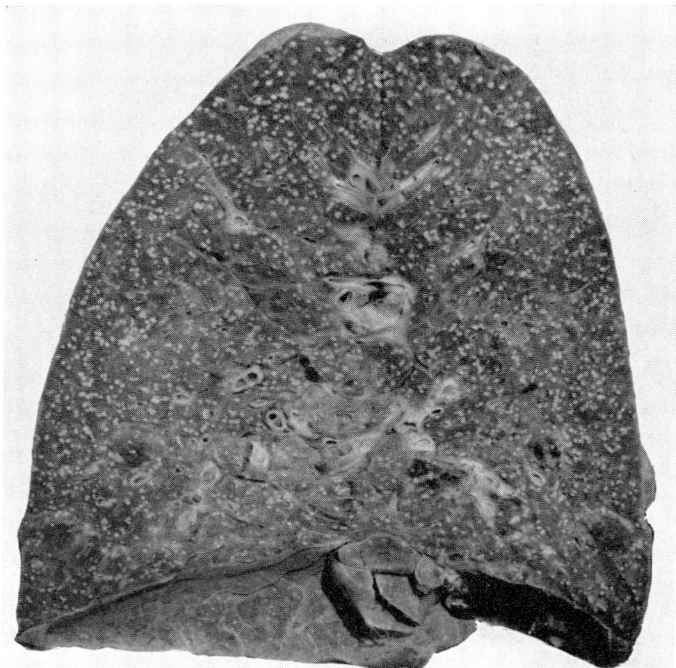

42/FIG. 20.—Lung showing well-developed miliary tubercles distributed uniformly throughout the lung and visible through the pleura over the base.

material is expectorated, and may lodge in and infect the larynx. They may be swallowed and, if in sufficient numbers, give rise to tuberculous lesions in the intestine.

Another example of spread through tubes is furnished by the course of tuberculosis of the kidney which, originating from a hæmatogenous infection, often extends into the ureter and urinary bladder.

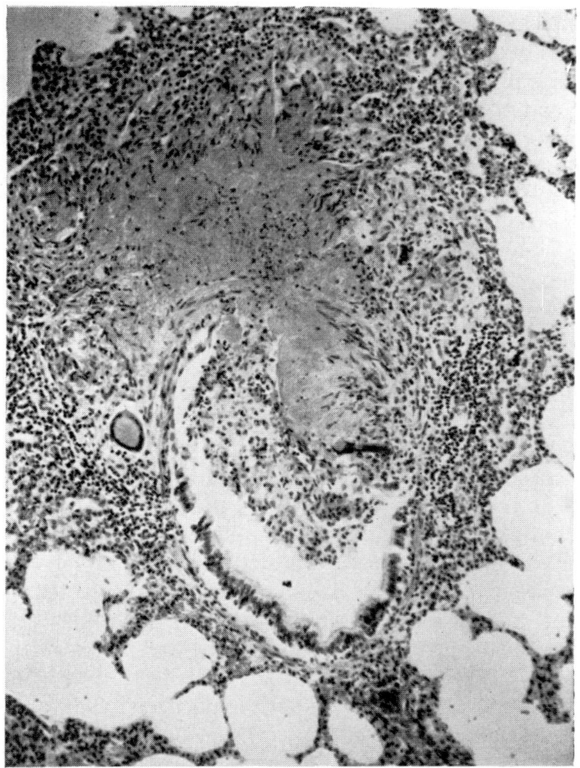

42/FIG. 21.—Spread of tubercle bacilli by the airways. Part of the wall of a bronchiole has been destroyed in a caseous focus. In this way necrotic material, containing tubercle bacilli, becomes free in the airway.

Dissemination in Cavities

Dissemination of bacilli may also occur after a tuberculous focus has invaded the wall of a serous cavity. Thus there may be widespread dissemination in the pleural cavity from a sub-pleural focus or in the peritoneal cavity from tuberculous mesenteric glands, resulting in a tuberculous pleurisy or tuberculous peritonitis. Sometimes a tuberculous process spreading from the lung or mediastinal lymph glands may invade the pericardium and be disseminated through the serous sac.

Tuberculous meningitis is a special and important example of invasion of a membrane. The organisms may reach the meninges from the blood, and the meningitis is sometimes part of a generalised miliary tuberculosis. In other cases the meninges seem to be infected from a focus in the brain. There is often considerable exudate, which may clot, and the bacilli may spread widely through the cerebrospinal spaces.

The Behaviour of Tubercle Bacilli in Lesions

It has already been noted that bacilli are found in the epithelioid cells and macrophages of the tubercle and that they often occur in particularly large numbers in caseous material. Nevertheless their growth in the caseous centre of a closed tubercle is probably slow, for the bacillus needs a good supply of oxygen for maximum growth and the oxygen tension in the caseous material is thought to be low. It has also been pointed out[17] that growth of the tubercle bacillus is inhibited *in vitro* by the fatty acids that are known to be present in considerable amounts in caseous material. Acids such as lactic and capric acids powerfully inhibit the growth of the tubercle bacillus and may kill it if the pH of, and the oxygen tension in, the lesion are low.

If a tuberculous lesion of the lung discharges caseous material into a bronchus, a cavity is formed which is connected with the air passages and is therefore well aerated. This improves the conditions for growth of the organisms in the walls of the cavity, by improving oxygenation and removing inhibitory substances, and millions of organisms may begin to appear in the sputum of the patient. The growth of bacilli may also be stimulated by the entry of blood constituents into a caseating tubercle, for it has been shown *in vitro* that serum albumin, for instance, neutralises the effects of fatty acids.

What happens to the tubercle bacilli contained in cells? As we have previously learnt, pyogenic organisms are frequently both killed and dissolved by polymorphonuclear cells that have ingested them. Can the mononuclear leucocytes do the same to tubercle bacilli? There is no doubt that sometimes, especially in man and in animals that have been previously infected, tubercle bacilli can disappear from tissues in which they are placed without giving rise to any lesion. It is commonly assumed that this is due to "digestion" of the organisms by mononuclear cells whose action has been in some way strengthened during the development of immunity.

Many attempts have been made to observe the fate of intracellular tubercle bacilli, especially by the use of tissue cultures. It seems reasonably certain that in circumstances that have not been accurately determined intracellular bacilli can be killed and broken up, the statement frequently being made that they are reduced to a brownish pigment. Estimates of the speed at which this can be accomplished vary from a few hours to many days—the latter time seems to be the more likely. How the bacteria are killed and by what enzymes they are digested remains a problem to be solved. It is interesting that ignorance on this point should be so profound, since many investigators, as will be seen later, place the most important defence of the body against the tubercle bacillus in the mononuclear cell.

Childhood and Adult Tuberculosis

In children.—It has long been noted that the manifestations of disease in infants and children are different from those in adults. In spite of the fact that

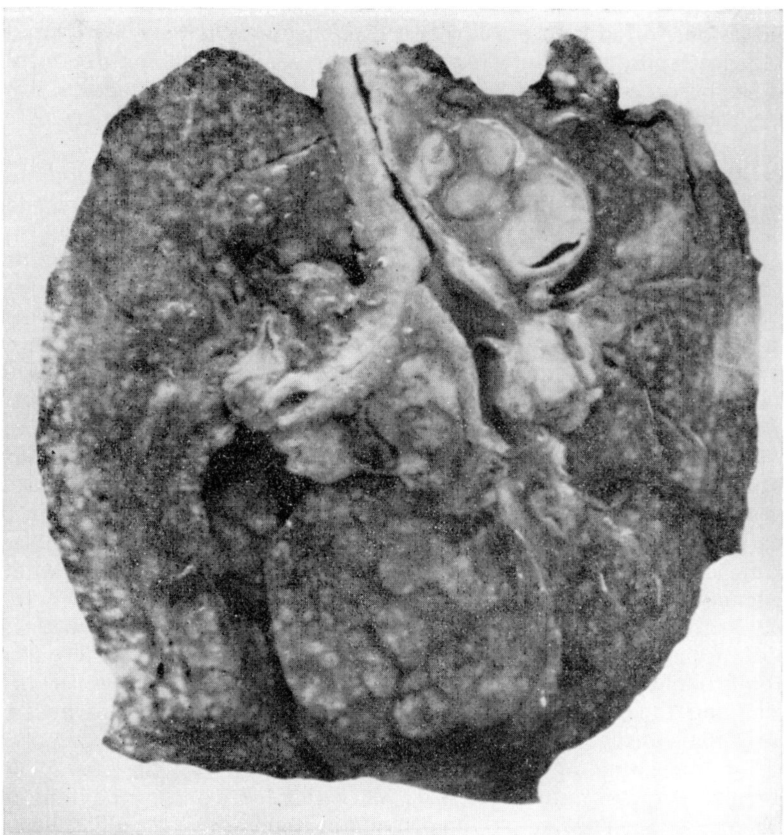

42/FIG. 22.—Fatal primary tuberculosis in infancy. The primary lesion is situated just beneath the pleura towards the base of the upper lobe (right of picture). From this the tracheo-bronchial lymph nodes were infected. At some point the enlarged caseating nodes invaded the blood stream, producing a terminal miliary tuberculosis, clearly seen in the lungs. This infant, who died at the age of 9 weeks, was infected by the father who had pulmonary tuberculosis. Two other children in the family died of tuberculous meningitis.

bovine infection was at one time relatively common in children, leading to some primary lesions of the tonsil or intestine, or their associated lymph glands, there is little doubt that the lung is the commonest portal of entry of the tubercle bacillus, even in the young, or that tuberculosis of the lung is the most important manifestation of the disease at this age. In the child the first infection in the lung usually takes the form of a solitary lesion with the usual histological structure near the pleural surface of the lower part of the upper lobe or in the lower lobe. This may grow to a centimetre or so in diameter and caseate (FIG. 22).

What is more important than the local lesion is that bacilli pass from it to the lymph glands at the hilum of the lung where large caseating masses are usually produced. In most instances this primary infection heals leaving a small scar in the lung and sometimes calcified hilar glands. Or there may be extension of the lesions, often with erosion of a bronchus near the involved glands, with subsequent aspiration of infected material further into the lung. By this time the child has become allergic to the tubercle bacillus and its products, and with the entrance of large numbers of bacilli into the lung lobular areas of caseous pneumonia are produced.

In some cases infected material may find its way into the blood stream as previously described, initiating widespread tuberculosis or sometimes localised solitary lesions, which are particularly common in the bones.

In adults.—Infection occurring in adults is due either to activation of an infection that started in childhood, or, probably more commonly, to a new infection. In the adult the lesion is nearly always close to the apex of one lung, more often the right, for reasons that have never been fully explained. Some workers hold that the apical localisation of re-infection tuberculosis is due to the fact that the stream of blood which enters the superior vena cava passes into the pulmonary artery and thence to the upper right lobe, with little mixing of blood entering the heart from the inferior vena cava. This stream can be contaminated by infected material from the diseased lung and regional lymph nodes that arrives in the venous system via the thoracic duct.[29, 30] The lesion in this region, which histologically consists of macrophages, epithelioid cells, fibroblasts and multinucleated cells is a localised broncho-pneumonia with very slight evidence of œdema. After a certain amount of growth and caseation have taken place it may heal, leaving a scar over which the pleura is usually thickened. In those who do not so satisfactorily overcome their infection a great variety of morbid anatomical changes can be produced, depending on the number of bacilli present and the resistance of the host. In a partially resistant host chronic phthisis may ensue, with gradual extension of the process accompanied by caseation and softening; and if the lesions connect with the airways, cavities are formed sometimes of great size. When there is extensive cavitation blood vessels may be seen crossing them or lying prominent in the walls. Their lumina have for the most part been obliterated by thrombosis or by obliterative endarteritis (FIG. 23), though occasionally vessels are eroded, causing serious or even fatal hæmorrhage. Fibrous tissue is formed in the neighbourhood of the active process in large amounts, and may replace or encapsulate lesions, but it may itself undergo necrosis. The name "chronic fibro-caseous tuberculosis" is sometimes given to this type of disease (FIG. 24). Cavities may also be associated with much more acute areas of inflammation and necrosis produced by the aspiration of bacilli to hitherto unaffected parts of the lungs. The tissues of the host are by this time highly sensitive, and if a substantial number of bacilli or much of their degradation products passes by the bronchi to unaffected parts, tuberculous broncho-pneumonia may be initiated. An abundant exudate consisting of fluid, fibrin, polymorphonuclear and mononuclear leucocytes, and lymphocytes may fill the alveoli. Extensive necrosis rapidly occurs and in exceptional cases caseation of a whole lobe may occur. FIGURES 24 and 25 illustrate some of the end results of such processes. This kind of rapid spread through the lung is often the last and fatal result of long-standing fibro-caseous disease.

One characteristic of all forms of adult tuberculosis is that the regional lymph nodes are not generally affected by caseating tuberculosis, though occa-

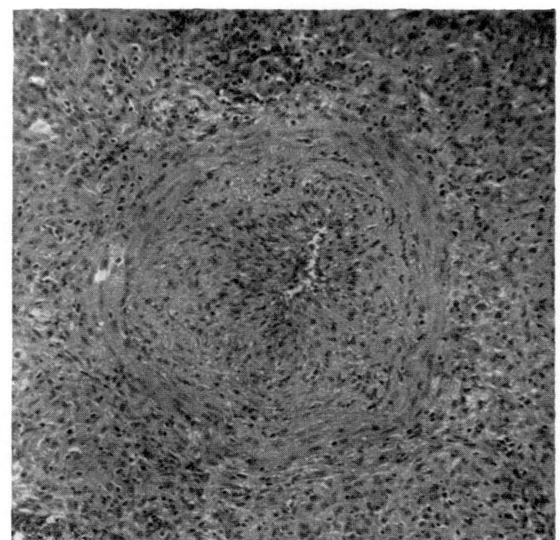

42/FIG. 23.—An artery showing well-marked endarteritis obliterans. This vessel passed through a tuberculous lesion in the lung of a rabbit.

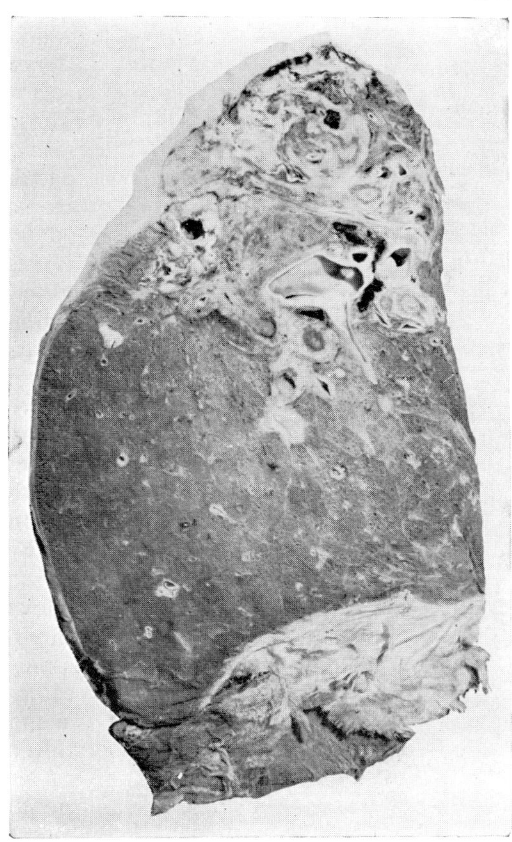

42/FIG. 24.—Chronic fibro-caseous tuberculosis. The whole of the upper lobe has been destroyed by tuberculous infection. The pleura over most of the lung surface has become greatly thickened.

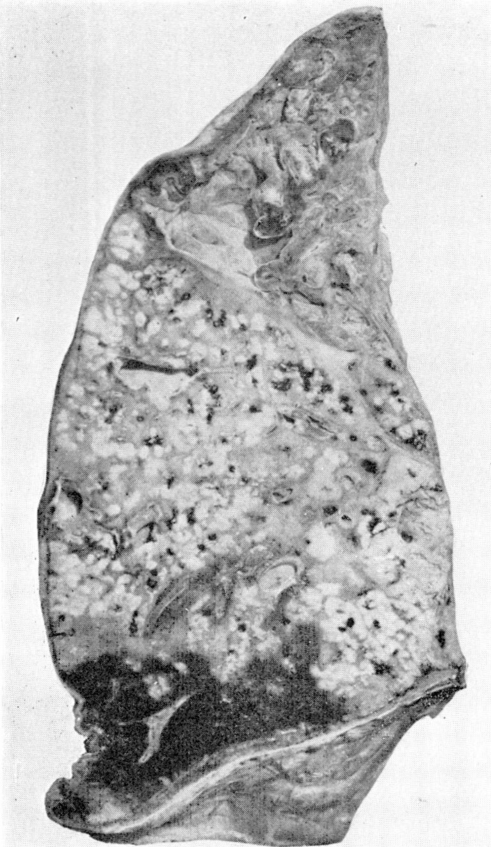

42/FIG. 25.—The upper lobe is the seat of an old cavitated fibro-caseous lesion and has been largely destroyed. The remainder of the lung is involved in a more recent caseous broncho-pneumonia. In some areas the lobular distribution of the process is clearly seen.

sionally small tubercles may be present in them. In other words, there is not nearly as much lymphatic spread as in children.

The differences between the disease in children and adults used to be attributed to the fact that adults had generally had a previous infection, and that the allergic and immune state can greatly influence the picture. Though no doubt there is something in this view, the position is now thought not to be so clear cut. Children rapidly become allergic and probably immune during the course of their first infection, but still they very rarely show adult types of lesion. And it appears that many adults now reach maturity without having had a tuberculous infection, but nevertheless the "childhood" type of infection is seldom found in them (though it has been described as occurring in American negroes).

There is now a tendency to associate the difference between childhood and adult tuberculosis with intrinsic changes in the reaction of the body associated with age.

RESISTANCE TO TUBERCULOSIS

Natural Resistance

It is known that factors such as the species of animal contribute to natural resistance to tuberculosis. For example, tubercle bacilli will grow in the mononuclear phagocytic cells of the hamster, and appear to do no damage to them. The rat does not become sensitive to tuberculin and, though it reacts to the presence of the bacillus by mobilising large numbers of mononuclear cells, caseation and softening do not occur in the lesions. If the animal dies from the infection, death

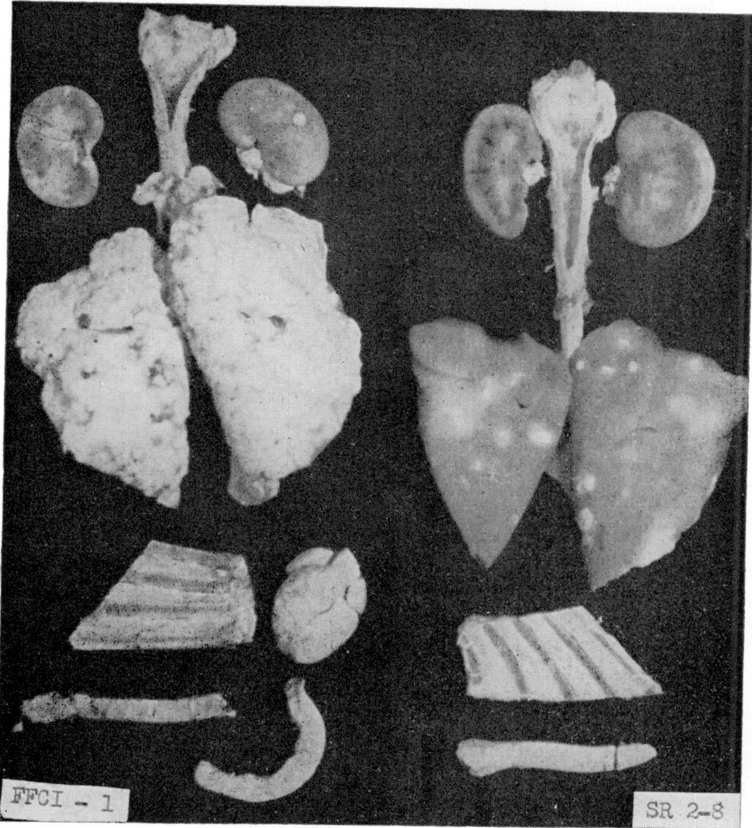

42/Fig. 26.—The organs of the genetically susceptible rabbit, FFCI–1, and of the genetically resistant rabbit, SR2–8, four months after the simultaneous inhalation of an estimated number of 30 isolated bovine tubercle bacilli of the Ravenel strain. Rabbit FFCI–1 died of massive caseous pneumonia with enlargement and caseation of the draining tracheo-bronchial lymph nodes, pleural tuberculosis, hæmatogenous tuberculosis of both kidneys, tuberculosis of the bone marrow and of the appendix. Rabbit SR2–8 was killed on the day rabbit FFCI–1 died. There were a few slowly progressive tubercles in both lungs; one of these, in the middle of the left lung, near its mesial border, has undergone central liquefaction. The disease is strictly localised to the portal of entry in the lung; there is no lymphogenous or hæmatogenous dissemination. (From Lurie, Heppleston, Abramson and Swartz.[11])

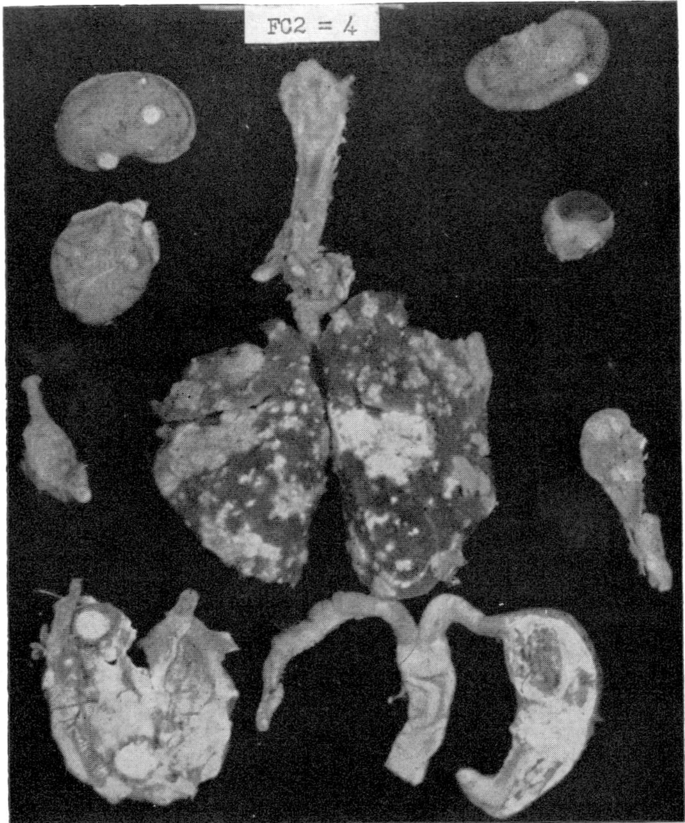

42/Fig. 27.—The organs of the genetically susceptible rabbit, FC2–4, and of the genetically resistant rabbit, SRI–6 (*opposite*), after the simultaneous inhalation of an estimated number of 30 isolated bovine tubercle bacilli of the Ravenel strain. Rabbit FC2–4 died 179 days after exposure, with large caseous pneumonic lesions in both lungs and caseation of draining tracheo-bronchial lymph nodes. Diaphragmatic and pericardial tuberculosis are seen in the lower left corner and below the left kidneys, respectively. Hæmatogenous tuberculosis in the lungs, kidneys, and ileocæcal junction, the latter between the heart and the diaphragm, is evident. Tuberculosis of the sclera of the left eye is depicted on the right. Below it may be seen the disease in the head of the left femur and of the bone marrow. Tuberculosis in the intra-uterine inspissated fœtus is depicted in the lower right corner. Rabbit SRI–6 died of asphyxia from tuberculous laryngitis 212 days after infection. Every lesion in the lung is excavated and encapsulated. There is no lymphogenous or hæmatogenous dissemination. (From Lurie *et al.*[11])

appears to be the result of mechanical blocking of the lung by large collections of cells.

The rabbit is resistant to the human type of bacillus—that is, infection either produces no lesions or, if a sufficiently large dose of the organism is given, a lesion that heals. But even small numbers of the bovine bacillus cause progressive tuberculosis, and invariably kill. It has been shown that human bacilli do, in fact, multiply in the rabbit but that at the same time they stimulate the development of enough resistance to enable the rabbit to free itself of them. It is suggested that man's usual reaction is like that of the rabbit to the human bacillus, for the majority of infected mankind recover completely from their first infection.

Genetic factors in susceptibility to tuberculosis are known to operate in guinea-pigs, rabbits and mice and also in man. We will consider the evidence from animal experiments first. Lurie[31] succeeded in breeding highly susceptible and highly resistant strains of rabbits as well as some with intermediate qualities. He was able to show that under conditions of respiratory infection the genetic constitution determined whether rapidly progressive generalised tuberculosis, localised chronic pulmonary disease or something between the two was initiated. Examples of the lesions produced by Lurie in animals of differing susceptibility are shown in FIGS. 26 and 27. He considered that the responses to infection of the resistant race of rabbits were more rapid than those of susceptible animals. He found that the accumulation of bacilli both within and without cells was less, while the cellular reactions, caseation and liquefaction took place more rapidly in resistant than in susceptible animals.[32] Tuberculin sensitivity developed more rapidly in resistant animals. The difference in behaviour between the two strains was due essentially to the fact that resistant animals destroyed the bacilli in the lungs more effectively than did the poorly resistant animals.

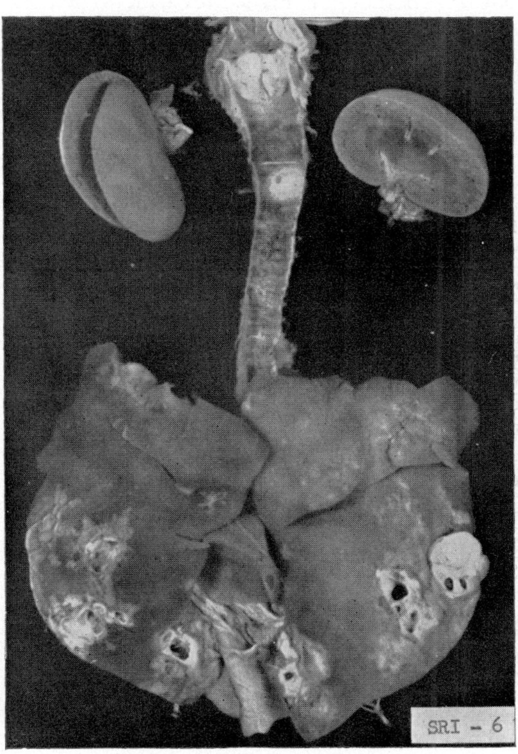

42/FIG. 27 (*opposite*).

From a similar point of view Gray and his colleagues[33] have concluded that not only strain, but species differences in susceptibility may be dependent on the rate at which immunity develops during the course of the infection.

Dubos and his co-workers[34] have also produced evidence that the local biochemical environment of the inflammatory reaction may influence the fate of invading micro-organisms. They have shown that a number of metabolites, notably lactic acid, which are thought to accumulate in areas of inflammation and necrosis, are toxic to tubercle bacilli at a low pH and a low oxygen tension. The biochemical reactions may be related to genetical constitution.

Besides genetical constitution there is evidence that the size of the infecting dose of organisms has a great influence on the lesion produced; thus if rabbits of high natural resistance receive a large enough dose, the type of disease may be the same as that caused by small doses in animals with low resistance.

It has long been suspected that there might be genetic variations in the susceptibility of man to tuberculosis. Tuberculosis tends to run in families, but this tendency might not be due to heredity, because a tuberculous patient is particularly likely to infect close relations. Since the time of Hippocrates it has been widely held that thin people are especially likely to contract the disease. If this is true, the physical type might well be genetically determined. The idea that underweight subjects have a relatively high tuberculosis morbidity has been confirmed comparatively recently in a study of American naval personnel.[35] More convincing evidence for genetic factors in human tuberculosis in man has come from twin studies. The idea was to collect pairs of twins one of whom was known to be tuberculous and look for evidence of the disease in the other twin. As environmental influences affecting monozygotic twins are unlikely to be appreciably different from those affecting dizygotic twins, if the disease occurs in both twins more often with monozygotic than with dizygotic twins this would provide evidence for a genetic predisposition. Four studies have been extensive enough to provide statistically significant evidence that such is indeed the case. The results are summarized in the following table:

Authors, date, country	*Percentage of twin-pairs of whom both were tuberculous*		*Total number of twin-pairs studied*
	Monozygotic	*Dizygotic*	
Diehl & von Versucher, 1936, Germany[36]	65	25	205
Kallmann & Reisner, 1943, U.S.A.[37, 38]	62	18	308
Harvald & Hauge, 1956, Denmark[39]	38	19	143
Simonds, 1963, U.K.[40]	32	14	205

The question arises as to whether the decline in mortality from tuberculosis referred to above could be attributable to natural selection with genetically susceptible strains of the human race being gradually eliminated from the population. No doubt this has been a contributory factor but it may not have been a very important one.

Other factors affecting the incidence of tuberculosis in man.—The influence of *age* and of *sex* on tuberculosis mortality have already been considered. *Race* has an effect, but it is particularly difficult to be certain to what extent racial differences are due to heredity rather than to environment. There is, however, general agreement that the American negro, American Indian and Eskimo, quite apart from their usually lower economic status, suffer more acutely from tuberculosis than the white man; for example caseous necrosis is much greater and extensive hæmatogenous generalization more common.

There is no question that tuberculosis is a disease greatly influenced by *environment*. It is a disease of poverty and dirt, so much so that it has been stated that "statistically, the incidence of clinical tuberculosis is inversely proportional to the amount of the family income". Clearly the remedying of overcrowding and poor hygiene will do much to reduce reservoirs of infection and hence prevalence of the disease. *Nutrition* may be an economic factor of importance. The tuberculous person may be very thin, and one of the features of active tuberculosis is the progressive loss of weight of the patient, but it is probable that malnutrition in itself, especially lack of proteins and probably of vitamins, impairs resistance to tuberculosis. During a war the tuberculosis rate may increase very considerably, and an important factor in this is probably deprivation of food in whole populations.

Both environment and malnutrition are closely related to *occupation*, and occupations in which tuberculous persons work in relatively confined spaces may result in the ready passing of the disease to those previously unaffected. Occupations associated with dust containing silica are also particularly associated with tuberculosis. The presence of silica, and possibly of other dusts, in the parenchyma of the lungs excites a massive fibrous-tissue reaction with which tuberculous infection is very frequently associated. Although the reason for the association is not yet known, it has been shown in experimental animals that attenuated strains of the tubercle bacillus will cause progressive disease in silicotic lungs though not in normal ones. Workers in gold mines where there is much quartz, in coal mines such as those in South Wales and in such occupations as knife grinding, if proper precautions are not taken, are particularly liable to this form of tuberculosis. Another form of occupational risk is that of nurses, medical practitioners, students and social workers, all of whom have frequent contact with tuberculous patients.

Acquired Resistance

The mechanism of acquired resistance to tuberculosis and complications introduced into the problem by the co-existence in the infected animal of delayed-type hypersensitivity, have been considered in detail in Chapters 37 and 39. The main points will be recapitulated briefly.

An individual who has had tuberculosis and recovered is much less likely to contract the disease again than is one who has never been infected. So far, however, it has proved impossible to achieve a degree of immunity against tuberculosis anything like as complete as can exist against such diseases as diphtheria, poliomyelitis, smallpox or tetanus. Consequently, when considering tuberculosis, we often talk about "acquired resistance" or "increased resistance to subsequent infection" to indicate that the immunity is relatively inefficient. As in previous chapters the terms "allergy" and "hypersensitivity" will be used interchangeably in the following discussion.

When an animal is infected with *Myco. tuberculosis* three responses of an immunological nature are known to take place:

(1) Soluble antibodies appear in the serum.

(2) Delayed-type hypersensitivity develops to certain protein constituents of the tubercle bacillus (these are known collectively as "tuberculo-proteins").

(3) There is increased resistance to subsequent infection.

We will consider each of these responses in turn.

Soluble antibodies.—These can be dismissed rapidly. Such antibodies cannot passively transfer either acquired resistance or delayed-type hypersensitivity to a normal animal. So far as can be ascertained their presence is neither beneficial nor harmful: they do not appear to influence the course of the disease in any way.

Delayed-type hypersensitivity.—In considering the Koch phenomenon it was pointed out that an infected guinea-pig responds to an inoculation of living or dead tubercle bacilli by a sloughing of the surrounding skin which begins in 1–2 days. Koch showed further that it was unnecessary to use intact bacilli to obtain this effect: tuberculo-proteins produced the same result. These he obtained from the filtrate of a liquid culture of tubercle bacilli and the rather crude material prepared by his original method is called Koch's Old Tuberculin (O.T.). Nowadays it is customary to use a purified protein derivative (P.P.D.). Either substance may be referred to simply as tuberculin. If small quantities of tuberculin are injected into the skin of an infected animal or human being there is no sloughing but a transient reddening of the skin occurs: this is known as the tuberculin reaction.

In characterising this immunological response as an allergic or hypersensitive reaction we have made the concealed assumption that it is a harmful consequence of infection with the tubercle bacillus. But is this right? Could this be a protective reaction enabling the animal to get rid of the bacilli by sacrificing the tissue in their immediate neighbourhood? Apparently not, because in experimental animals it is possible to produce delayed-type hypersensitivity without any increased resistance to subsequent infection and *vice versa*. Raffel[41] showed that injection of a wax extracted from the bacilli produced delayed-type hypersensitivity* but no increased resistance. Wells and Wylie[42] found that if guinea-pigs were actively immunised with the vole bacillus both increased resistance and a positive tuberculin reaction were produced; after about eleven months the tuberculin reaction became negative; six months later still the animals' resistance to injection was unimpaired. Bocquet and Nègre[43] demonstrated that methanol extracts of tubercle bacilli could be used to produce a fair degree of immunity which was not accompanied by a positive tuberculin reaction. Thus, as far as their practical consequences are concerned, acquired resistance and delayed-type hypersensitivity seem to be independant immunological responses to infection with tubercle bacilli. It would, however, be too sweeping to say that there is no connexion whatever between immunity and allergy in tuberculosis. We will return to this point later but it will be convenient to consider next the principal immune mechanism in tuberculosis.

Increased resistance to subsequent infection.—If acquired resistance to infection with the tubercle bacillus is not due to soluble antibodies and is not due to the delayed-type hypersensitivity reaction, how does it function? There is now no doubt that the main difference between a normal animal and one with

* Note that the injection of tuberculin does not produce delayed-type hypersensitivity. It may however sensitise an animal to anaphylaxis as might the injection of any foreign protein.

acquired resistance lies in altered properties of the resistant animal's macrophages. That this might be the case was indicated nearly thirty years ago in an experiment by Lurie, who took macrophages from normal and resistant animals, allowed them to ingest bovine tubercle bacilli and placed them in the anterior chambers of rabbits' eyes, where they would be inaccessible to soluble antibody. The macrophages from resistant animals inhibited the multiplication of the bacilli to a much greater extent than did macrophages from normal animals.[44] These and other early observations have been confirmed and greatly extended in recent years and it has become clear that in tuberculosis we have a cellular as opposed to a humoral type of immunity. This is an immune mechanism profoundly different from that operating in most bacterial infections, but it is not absolutely unique. Something very similar seems to occur in infections with certain species of *Listeria*, *Brucella*, and *Salmonella*. Interestingly enough, there seems to be cross immunity between infections by bacteria of these four genera, which are quite unrelated in respect of antigens which can give rise to classical antibodies. There is now evidence that immune macrophages differ from normal macrophages in the following ways: they are mobilised more rapidly and are stimulated to divide following infection; they possess greater powers of phagocytosis; and they destroy engulfed organisms more efficiently.[45]

Possible relationships between acquired resistance and delayed-type hypersensitivity.—(1) Although soluble *antibodies* seem to have no protective effect in tuberculosis, the body fluids and tissues of tuberculous animals contain soluble substances which have a non-specific toxic action on tubercle bacilli. These soluble substances seem to be tissue breakdown products and metabolites among which lactic acid may be particularly important. Perhaps, therefore, delayed-type hypersensitivity can assist the main cellular immune mechanism in overcoming infection, but at the heavy price of destroying tissue. This finding in no way upsets the conclusion that delayed-type hypersensitivity *alone* has no protective action.

(2) A hint of a much more fundamental connection between delayed-type hypersensitivity and cellular immunity comes from experiments on the interaction of antigen, immunologically active lymphocytes and macrophages which have been considered in Chapters 37 and 39. It appears that under certain experimental conditions large doses of antigen cause death of macrophages while smaller amounts will stimulate them to divide. Thus delayed-type hypersensitivity and cellular immunity may be divergent pathways from a common initial route in the animal's immunological response to infection. If this is so, it would not necessarily affect the conclusion that one pathway leads to killing bacteria and the other to destroying the host's tissue.

Active immunisation against tuberculosis.—Before the end of the nineteenth century attempts had been made to produce active immunity against tuberculosis with tuberculin. The results were disappointing as would now be expected in view of what has since been learnt about the immunological properties of tuberculin. Dead tubercle bacilli have been used on many occasions and good results have often been claimed but the method seems to have fallen into disuse, perhaps unjustifiably.[46]

BCG, the attenuated bovine strain introduced by Calmette and Guérin in 1924, has been extensively used for active immunisation in man: it has already been given to 250,000,000 people, according to a recent estimate.[47] Unfortunately the early studies tended to be unsatisfactory for one reason or another and as late as 1947 Wilson[48] could not but conclude that there was no absolutely convincing evidence that BCG had any protective value. Since then, however, several investigations have been reported which have established its efficacy. During the same period it has been shown that the vole bacillus gives at least as good a degree of protection.

As an example, we will consider a trial conducted by a Medical Research Council Committee on 56,700 schoolchildren, aged 14–15½ when they were examined in 1950–52. Of those who were tuberculin-negative, some were given BCG, some the vole bacillus and a third group served as controls. Over 90 per cent were followed up until at least 1957. The results as reported in 1959[49] were as follows:

	Total number	*Number of cases of Tuberculosis*	*Annual incidence per* 10,000
Controls	13,300	153	2·30
BCG	14,100	27	0·38
Vole bacillus	6,700	11	0·33

It was calculated that BCG had produced an 83 per cent reduction in tuberculosis morbidity and the vole bacillus an 87 per cent reduction: the difference in results between the two methods was not statistically significant but the value of both was clearly established. A further report in 1963[50] gave substantially similar results but the follow-up since the 1959 report was less thorough.

In this trial the vole bacilli used were fully virulent for voles. Sula[51] in Czechoslovakia compared BCG with an attenuated strain of the vole bacillus and found over a period of five years that 13 out of 76,631 children given BCG developed tuberculosis as against 3 out of 32,772 who received the vole bacillus. Again there is a suggestion that the vole bacillus may be more effective but again the difference is not statistically significant. If there is little to choose between BCG and the vole bacillus on the grounds of efficacy, is there any reason to prefer the one to the other in respect of undesirable side-effects? In some trials of the vole bacillus unpleasant skin reactions reminiscent of lupus vulgaris were reported[49, 52] but it has been pointed out that this only happened when the number of immunising organisms used was (as can be seen in retrospect) unnecessarily large.[53] Generalised tuberculosis following BCG inoculation has been reported by some investigators and four cases have been described in which fatal tuberculosis is said to have been caused by BCG (for references see Andersen *et al.*, 1959[54]); an attempt has been made to discredit the reports of fatal cases[55] but it is not completely convincing. No case of fatal tuberculosis has so far been ascribed to the vole bacillus but it must be realised that BCG has been used on a far greater scale.

All in all, there seem to be no powerful reasons at present for preferring BCG to the vole bacillus or *vice versa.*

Not all studies of the effectiveness of BCG as an immunising agent have given such good results as the English investigation described above. For example, Palmer, Shaw and Comstock[58] in a large and well-controlled trial in certain areas of the southern United States found that BCG reduced the annual tuberculosis morbidity rate from 0·22 per 1,000 only to 0·14 per 1,000. It has been suggested that in these areas there exists a widespread inapparent infection with atypical mycobacteria which confer increased resistance to tuberculosis and that therefore BCG can add little to the fairly high level of immunity which the population has already acquired.[53, 57]

There is probably a good case for immunising people such as nurses and medical students who are exposed to an exceptionally high risk of contracting tuberculosis. The case for immunising all tuberculin-negative individuals in a population is much less convincing. Perhaps it may be advisable in countries where the incidence of tuberculosis is high and the level of resistance is low.

REFERENCES

1. SIGERIST, H. E. (1951). *A History of Medicine*, Vol. 1, Plate IV, FIG. 10. London: Oxford Univ. Press.
2. KOCH, R. (1882). *Berl. klin. Wschr.*, **19,** 221.
3. KOCH, R. (1884). *Mittheilungen aus dem Kaiserlichen Gesundheitsamte*, 2, 1. An English translation by S. Boyd is available in: *Recent Essays by Various Authors on Bacteria in Relation to Disease*. Ed. WATSON CHEYNE, W., London: New Sydenham Society, **115,** 67, 1886.
4. CALMETTE, A., and GUÉRIN, C. (1924). *Ann. Inst. Pasteur*, **38,** 371.
5. WELLS, A. Q. (1937). *Lancet*, **1,** 1221.
6. WAGNER, J. C., BUCHANAN, G., BOKKENHEUSER, V., and LEVISEUR, S. (1958). *Nature (Lond.)*, **181,** 284.
7. SMITH, N. (1960). *Tubercle (Edinb.)*, **41,** 203.
8. SMITH, N. (1965). *Tubercle (Edinb.)*, **46,** 58.
9. COBBETT, L. (1917). *The Causes of Tuberculosis*, pp. 136–185. Cambridge Public Health Series. London: Cambridge Univ. Press.
10. WELLS, W. F., RATCLIFFE, H. L., and CRUMB, C. (1948). *Amer. J. Hyg.*, **47,** 11.
11. LURIE, M. B., HEPPLESTON, A. G., ABRAMSON, S., and SWARTZ, I. B. (1950). *Amer. Rev. Tuberc.*, **61,** 765.
12. LINELL, F., and NORDÉN, Å. (1954). *Acta tuberc. scand.*, Suppl. No. 33.
13. AMBERSON, J. B. (1950). *Amer. J. Med.*, **9,** 571.
14. *Annual Report of the Chief Medical Officer of the Ministry of Health* (1967). London: H.M.S.O.
15. WELLS, A. Q. (1938). *Brit. J. exp. Path.*, **19,** 324.
16. VORWALD, A. J. (1932). *Amer. Rev. Tuberc.*, **25,** 74.
17. MARKHAM, N. P., and FLOREY, H. W. (1951). *Brit. J. exp. Path.*, **32,** 25.
18. MIDDLEBROOK, G., DUBOS, R. J., and PIERCE, C. (1947). *J. exp. Med.*, **86,** 175.
19. BLOCH, H. (1950). *J. exp. Med.*, **91,** 197.
20. NOLL, H., BLOCH, H., ASSELINEAU, J., and LEDERER, E. (1956). *Biochem. biophys. Acta (Amst.)*, **20,** 299.
21. HART, P. D'A., and REES, R. J. W. (1954). *J. gen. Microbiol.*, **10,** 150.
22. NAGASUGA, T., TERAI, T., and YAMAMURA, Y. (1961). *Amer. Rev. resp. Dis.*, **83,** 248.
23. KOCH, R. (1891). *Dtsch. med. Wschr.*, **17,** 101.
24. EBERT, R. H., AHERN, J. J., and BLOCH, R. G. (1948). *Proc. Soc. exp. Biol. (N.Y.)*, **68,** 625.
25. PINNER, M. (1945). *Pulmonary Tuberculosis in the Adult*. Springfield, Ill.: Charles C. Thomas.

26. SANDERS, A. G., FLOREY, H. W., and WELLS, A. Q. (1951). *Brit. J. exp. Path.*, **32,** 352.
27. MARKHAM, N. P. (1950). Thesis presented for the Degree of Doctor of Philosophy, Oxford. The effect of the injection of colloidal dyes and particles on the cells of tubercles caused by *Mycobacterium tuberculosis.*
28. DUBOS, R. J. (1950). *Amer. J. Med.*, **9,** 573.
29. SMITH, D. T., ABERNATHY, R. S., SMITH, G. B., Jr., and BONDURANT, S. (1954). *Amer. Rev. Tuberc.*, **70,** 547.
30. ABERNATHY, R. S., SMITH, G. B., Jr., and SMITH, D. T. (1954). *Amer. Rev. Tuberc.*, **70,** 557.
31. LURIE, M. B. (1950). *Amer. J. Med.*, **9,** 591.
32. LURIE, M. B., ZAPPASODI, P., and TICKNER, C. (1955). *Amer. Rev. Tuberc.*, **72,** 297.
33. GRAY, D. F., GRAHAM-SMITH, H., and NOBLE, J. L. (1960). *J. Hyg. (Lond.)*, **58,** 215.
34. DUBOS, R. J. (1954). *Biochemical Determinants of Microbial Diseases.* Cambridge, Mass.: Harvard Univ. Press.
35. PALMER, C. E., JABLON, S., and EDWARDS, P. Q. (1957). *Amer. Rev. Tuberc.*, **76,** 517.
36. DIEHL, K., and VON VERSUCHER, O. (1936). *Der Erbeinfluss bei der Tuberkulose.* Jena: Gustav Fischer.
37. KALLMANN, F. J., and REISNER, D. (1943*a*). *Amer. Rev. Tuberc.*, **47,** 549.
38. KALLMANN, F. J., and REISNER, D. (1943*b*). *J. Hered.*, **34,** 269, 293.
39. HARVALD, B., and HAUGE, M. (1956). *Dan. med. Bull.*, **3,** 150.
40. SIMONDS, B. (1963). *Tuberculosis in Twins.* London: Pitman.
41. RAFFEL, S. (1946). *Amer. Rev. Tuberc.*, **54,** 564.
42. WELLS, A. Q., and WYLIE, J. A. H. (1952). *Brit. J. exp. Path.*, **33,** 405.
43. BOCQUET, A., and NÈGRE, L. (1923). *Ann. Inst. Pasteur*, **37,** 787.
44. LURIE, M. B. (1942). *J. exp. Med.*, **75,** 247.
45. MACKANESS, G. B., and BLANDEN, R. V. (1967). *Progr. Allergy*, **11,** 89.
46. WEISS, D. W. (1959). *Amer. Rev. resp. Dis.*, **80,** 340, 495, 676.
47. HART, P. D'A. (1967). *Brit. med. J.*, **1,** 587.
48. WILSON, G. S. (1947). *Brit. med. J.*, **2,** 855.
49. Medical Research Council Tuberculosis Vaccines Clinical Trials Committee (1959). *Brit. med. J.*, **2,** 379.
50. Medical Research Council Tuberculosis Vaccines Clinical Trials Committee (1963). *Brit. med. J.*, **1,** 973.
51. SULA, L. (1958). *Tubercle (Edinb.)*, **38,** 10.
52. FREW, H. W. O., DAVIDSON, J. R., and REID, J. T. W. (1955). *Brit. med. J.*, **1,** 133.
53. HART, P. D'A. (1967). *Amer. Rev. resp. Dis.*, **96,** 1.
54. ANDERSON, A. S., *et al.* (1959). *Brit. med. J.*, **1,** 1423.
55. VAN DEINSE, F. (1956). *Rev. Tuberc. (Paris)*, **20,** 44.
56. PALMER, C. E., SHAW, L. W., and COMSTOCK, G. W. (1958). *Amer. Rev. Tuberc.*, **77,** 877.
57. COMSTOCK, G. W., and PALMER, C. E. (1966). *Amer. Rev. resp. Dis.*, **93,** 171.

The following comprehensive works may be consulted with profit:

RICH, A. R. (1951). *The Pathogenesis of Tuberculosis*, 2nd edit. Springfield, Ill.: Charles C. Thomas.

DUBOS, R., and DUBOS, J. (1953). *The White Plague—Tuberculosis, Man and Society.* London: Victor Gollancz.
This book is strongly recommended not only for the clear presentation of problems associated with tuberculosis, but for its historical background to present-day thinking on the disease.

LURIE, M. B. (1964). *Resistance to Tuberculosis: Experimental Studies in Native and Acquired Defensive Mechanisms.* Cambridge, Mass.: Harvard Univ. Press.

INDEX

INDEX

[NOTES]

[NOTES]

[NOTES]

[NOTES]

[NOTES]